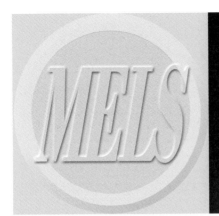

Mastery of Endoscopic and Laparoscopic Surgery

Mastery of Endoscopic and Laparoscopic Surgery

THIRD EDITION

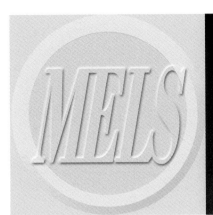

Edited by

Nathaniel J. Soper, MD

Loyal and Edith Davis Professor and Chair
Department of Surgery
Northwestern University Feinberg School of Medicine
Chicago, Illinois

Lee L. Swanström, MD

Clinical Professor of Surgery
Oregon Health Sciences University
Director, Division of Minimally Invasive Surgery
Legacy Health System
Portland, Oregon

W. Stephen Eubanks, MD

Professor and Chairman
Hugh E. Stephenson Jr. Department of Surgery
University of Missouri School of Medicine
Columbia, Missouri

in conjunction with

Michael E. Leonard

Medical Illustrator
Clement, California

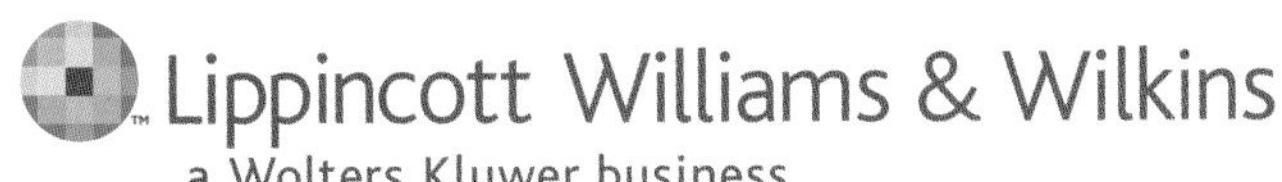

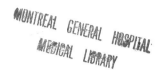

Lippincott Williams & Wilkins
a Wolters Kluwer business
Philadelphia • Baltimore • New York • London
Buenos Aires • Hong Kong • Sydney • Tokyo

Acquisition Editor: Brian Brown
Managing Editor: Julia Seto
Project Manager: Nicole Walz
Marketing Manager: Lisa Parry
Cover Designer: Karen Quigley
Production Services: GGS Book Services PMG

530 Walnut Street
Philadelphia, PA 19106
LWW.com

Printed in China

Library of Congress Cataloging-in-Publication Data

Mastery of endoscopic and laparoscopic surgery/edited by Nathaniel J. Soper, Lee L. Swanström, W. Stephen Eubanks; in conjunction with Michael E. Leonard, medical illustrator.—3rd ed.
p.; cm.
Includes bibliographical references and index.
ISBN-13: 978-0-7817-7198-6
ISBN-10: 0-7817-7198-6
1. Endoscopic surgery. 2. Laparoscopic surgery. I. Soper, Nathaniel J. II. Swanström, Lee L. III. Eubanks, Steve, 1959-
[DNLM: 1. Endoscopy. 2. Laparoscopy. WO 505 M423 2009]
RD33.53.M38 2009
617′.05—dc22 2008027028

10 9 8 7 6 5 4 3 2 1

To my wife, Cindy, who has supported me unwaveringly in this and all other career endeavors. And to my three sons, who give me much-needed perspective and grounding in my life.

NJS

I would like to dedicate this book to those who motivate me to explore new frontiers in surgery: especially Dr. Ron Passi, who instilled in me a love of flexible endoscopy and a fearlessness in its application. To my Comrades in Arms and great friends, Nat Soper, John Hunter, and Jeff Peters. And to my always supportive partners: Christy, Mark, and Paul, who put up with my projects and help care for my patients. Thanks to you all.

LLS

To the fellows, residents, and students who have submitted to my teaching and mentorship. Your eagerness and willingness to learn from me has made my life as a surgical educator truly rich. Your accomplishments and successes have given me my greatest professional joy.

WSE

Contents

Contributing Authors

SAJIDA AHAD, MD
University of Washington Medical Center,
Seattle,
Washington

LEAQUE AHMED III, MD
Chief, Section of Endocrine Surgery,
Associate Professor of Clinical Surgery,
College of Physicians and Surgeons of Columbia University,
New York,
New York

TRACEY D. ARNELL, MD
Assistant Professor of Surgery,
Columbia University College of Physicians and Surgeons,
Department of Surgery;
Vice-Chair Medical Education,
Program Director,
Residency Training Program,
New York,
New York

MAURICE E. ARREGUI, MD, FACS
Chairman, Department of General Surgery,
St. Vincent Hospital,
Indianapolis,
Indiana

SHARON L. BACHMAN, MD
Minimally Invasive Surgery Fellow,
Department of General Surgery,
University of Missouri,
Columbia,
Missouri

DONALD BLAIR, MD
Program Director,
Cancer Cell Biology Branch,
National Cancer Institute,
Frederick,
Maryland

MATTHEW BLUM, MD
Section Head of General Thoracic Surgery,
Northwestern Memorial Hospital,
Chicago,
Illinois

FRED BRODY, MD, FACS, MBA
Associate Professor of Surgery,
Department of Surgery,
The George Washington University Medical Center,
Washington,
District of Columbia

BORIS BRONFINE, MD
St. Vincent Hospital,
Indianapolis,
Indiana

CHRISTOPHER J. BRUCE, MD
Clinical Assistant,
Professor of Surgery,
New York Medical College,
White Plains,
New York

L. MICHAEL BRUNT, MD
Department of Surgery,
Washington University School of Medicine,
St. Louis,
Missouri

GORDON BUDUHAN, MD, MSC, FRCSC
Fellow,
Thoracic Surgery,
Division of Thoracic Surgery,
University of British Columbia;
Fellow,
Division of Thoracic Surgery,
Vancouver General Hospital,
Vancouver,
British Columbia,
Canada

RACQUEL S. BUENO, MD
Clinical Fellow,
Minimally Invasive and Robotic Surgery,
Department of Surgery,
University of Illinois at Chicago,
Chicago,
Illinois

CATHERINE CAGIANNOS, MD
Assistant Professor,
Division of Vascular Surgery,
The Michael E. DeBakey,
Department of Surgery,
Houston,
Texas

ROBERT A. CATANIA, MD
Fellow and Visiting Instructor,
Minimally Invasive Surgery,
University of Maryland Medical Center,
Baltimore,
Maryland

JOHN A. COLLER, MD
General Surgery,
Colon and Rectal Surgery,
Lahey Clinic,
Burlington,
Massachusetts;
Assistant Clinical Professor of Surgery,
Tufts University School of Medicine,
Boston,
Massachusetts

KEVIN C. CONLON, MD
Department of Surgery,
Memorial Sloan-Kettering Cancer
Center,
New York,
New York

BRIAN R. DAVIS, MD
Research Fellow,
Department of Surgery,
University of Louisville,
Louisville,
Kentucky

ALBERTO DE HOYOS, MD
Assistant Professor,
Department of Surgery,
Northwestern University;
Department of Surgery,
Northwestern Memorial Hospital,
Chicago,
Illinois

AUREO LUDOVICO DE PAULA, MD
Director,
Department of Surgery,
Hospital de Especialidades,
Goiania,
Brazil

ANTONIO LUIZ DE VASCONCELLOS MACEDO, MD
General Surgeon,
Department of Surgery,
Albert Einstein Hospital,
São Paulo,
Brazil

ASOK DORAISWAMY, MD
Clinical Fellow,
Department of Surgery,
Cedars-Sinai Medical Center,
Los Angeles,
California

BRIAN J. DUNKIN, MD
Associate Professor of Surgery,
Chief of the Division of
Laparoendoscopic Surgery,
University of Miami, Miller School of
Medicine,
Miami,
Florida

AMR M. EL SHERIF, MD
Research Fellow,
Department of Surgery,
Creighton University School of
Medicine,
Omaha,
Nebraska

W. STEPHEN EUBANKS, MD
Professor and Chairman,
Hugh E. Stephenson Jr. Department
of Surgery,
University of Missouri School
of Medicine,
Columbia,
Missouri

EDWARD L. FELIX, MD, FACS
Director of California Institute of
Minimally Invasive Surgery,
Clinical Assistant Professor of Surgery
(UCSF Fresno),
Fresno,
California

LORENZO E. FERRI, MD
Department of Surgery,
Faculty of Medicine,
McGill University Health Centre,
Montreal,
Quebec,
Canada

CHARLES J FILIPI, MD, FACS
Professor of Surgery,
Creighton University Medical Center,
Department of Surgery,
Creighton University School of
Medicine,
Omaha,
Nebraska

RICHARD J. FINLEY, MD, FRCSC, FACS
Professor of Surgery,
Division of Thorasic Surgery,
University of British Columbia;
Surgeon,
Division of Thorasic Surgery,
Vancouver General Hospital,
Vancouver,
British Columbia,
Canada

PIERO M. FISCHELLA, MD
Assistant Professor of Surgery,
Stritch School of Medicine,
Loyola University;
Director,
Esophageal Motility Center,
Loyola University Medical Center,
Maywood,
Illinois

JAMES F. FITZGERALD, MD
Washington Hospital Center,
Section of Colon and Rectal Surgery,
Washington,
District of Columbia

JAMES W. FLESHMAN, MD
Chief, Section of Colon and Rectal
Surgery,
Department of Surgery,
Division of General Surgery,
Washington University School of
Medicine,
St. Louis,
Missouri

DENNIS L. FOWLER, MD
Surgical Professor of Clinical Surgery,
Department of Surgery,
Columbia University of Physicians and Surgeons;
Vice President and Medical Director,
Perioperative Services,
New York Presbyterian Hospital,
New York,
New York

GERALD M. FRIED, MD, FRCS(C), FACS
Adair Family Chair of Surgical Education,
Department of Surgery,
McGill University;
Steinberg-Bernstein Chair of Minimally Invasive Surgery and Innovation,
Department of Surgery,
McGill University Health Centre,
Montreal,
Quebec,
Canada

BRICE GAYET, MD, PHD
Professor of Surgery
Department of Digestive Diseases
Institut Mutualiste Montsouris
University Paris V
Jourdan,
Paris,
France

MOUZA T. GOOVA, MD
University of Texas Southwestern Medical Center,
Dallas,
Texas

JON C. GOULD, MD
Associate Professor,
Department of Surgery,
University of Wisconsin School of Medicine and Public Health;
Co-Medical Director,
Bariatric Surgery Program,
Department of Surgery
University of Wisconsin School of Medicine and Public Health,
Madison,
Wisconsin

IGOR S. GOUSSEV, MD
Fellow in Surgical Endoscopy and Hepatobiliary and Pancreatic Surgery,
Department of Surgery,
University of Louisville,
Louisville,
Kentucky

TAGORE M. GRANDHI MD, FRCS
Bariatric Fellow,
Legacy Health System,
Portland,
Oregon

FREDERICK L. GREENE, MD
Clinical Professor,
Department of Surgery,
University of North Carolina;
Chairman,
Department of Surgery,
Carolinas Medical Center,
Charlotte,
North Carolina

ANDREW A. GUMBS, MD
General Surgery,
New York Presbyterian Hospital,
Columbia University Medical Center,
New York,
New York

PAUL D. HANSEN, MD
The Oregon Clinic,
Portland,
Oregon

KARIN HARDIMAN, MD
Research Fellow,
Department of Surgery,
Oregon Health and Science University,
Portland,
Oregon

B. TODD HENIFORD, MD
Chief,
Division of Gastrointestinal and Minimally Invasive Surgery,
Department of Surgery,
Carolinas Medical Center,
Charlotte,
North Carolina

FERNANDO A.M. HERBELLA, MD
Professor,
Surgery and Oncology,
Department of Surgery,
University of Rochester;
Chairman,
Department of Surgery,
Strong Memorial Hospital,
Rochester,
New York

JAMES R. HINES, MD
Professor and Interim Chair,
Department of Surgery,
Northwestern University,
Feinberg School of Medicine,
Chicago,
Illinois

WILLIAM W. HOPE, MD
Laparoscopic Fellow,
Department of Surgery,
Carolinas Medical Center,
Charlotte,
North Carolina

KATHERINE E. HSU, MD
Department of Surgery,
Faculty of Medicine,
McGill University,
McGill University Health Centre,
Montreal,
Quebec,
Canada

ERIC S. HUNGNESS, MD
Assistant Professor of Surgery,
Department of Surgery,
Northeastern University;
Staff Surgeon,
General Surgery Department,
Northwestern Memorial Hospital,
Chicago,
Illinois

JOHN HUNTER, MD
Professor and Chairman,
Department of Surgery,
Oregon Health and Science University,
Portland,
Oregon

SAYEED IKRAMUDDIN, MD
Department of Surgery,
University of Minnesota,
Minneapolis,
Minnesota

WILLIAM B. INABNET III, MD
Associate Professor of Clinical Surgery,
Department of Surgery,

Columbia University;
New York Presbyterian Hospital,
New York,
New York

MOHAMMAD JAMAL, MD

Assistant Professor,
Department of Surgery,
University of Iowa Carver College of Medicine,
Iowa City,
Iowa

GLYN G. JAMIESON, MD

Professor of Surgery,
University of Adelaide Department of Surgery,
Royal Adelaide Hospital,
Adelaide,
South Australia

DANIEL B. JONES, MD

Associate Professor,
Department of Surgery,
Harvard Medical School;
Chief,
Section Minimally Invasive Surgery,
Department of Surgery,
Beth Israel Deaconess Medical Center,
Boston,
Massachusetts

NAMIR KATKHOUDA, MD, FACS

Professor of Surgery,
Chief,
Minimally Invasive Surgery,
Department of Surgery,
Keck School of Medicine,
University of Southern California.
Los Angeles,
California

TODD A. KELLOGG, MD

Assistant Professor of Surgery,
Center for Minimally Invasive Surgery,
Department of Surgery,
University of Minnesota,
Minneapolis,
Minnesota

KENT W. KERCHER, MD

Chief,
Minimal Access Surgery,
Carolinas Medical Center,
Charlotte,
North Carolina

LEENA KHAITAN, MD, MPH, FACS

Associate Professor,
Department of Surgery,
Case Western Reserve University,
Cleveland Ohio;
Director,
Minimally Invasive and Bariatric Surgery,
Geauga Medical Center,
Chardon,
Ohio

RALF KOLVENBACH, MD, PHD

Department of Vascular Surgery and Endovascular Therapy,
Augusta Hospital and Catholic Clinics,
Duesseldorf,
Germany

PETER F. LALOR, MD

Clinical Fellow,
Bariatric Institute and Division of Minimally Invasive Surgery,
Cleveland Clinic Florida,
Weston,
Florida

RODNEY LANDRENEAU, MD

Director,
Comprehensive Lung Center,
University of Pittsburgh Medical Center Shadyside,
Pittsburgh,
Pennsylvania

BRIAN D. LAYTON, DO

Chief Resident,
Department of Surgery,
Carolinas Medical Center,
Charlotte,
North Carolina

DANIEL A. LAWES, MD

Assistant Professor of Surgery,
College of Medicine;
Fellow in Laparoscopic Colorectal Surgery,
Department of Colorectal Surgery,
Mayo Clinic—Arizona,
Scottsdale,
Arizona

DANIEL B. LESLIE, MD

Assistant Professor,
Division of Gastrointestinal Surgery,
Department of Surgery,
University of Minnesota,
Minneapolis,
Minnesota

EDWARD LIN, DO, FACS

Assistant Professor of Surgery,
Department of Surgery,
Emory University School of Medicine;
Director,
Emory Bariatrics,
Chief,
Emory GI Surgery,
Department of General Surgery,
Emory Crawford Long Hospital,
Atlanta,
Georgia

CEDRIC S. F. LORENZO, MD

Fellow,
Minimally Invasive Surgery,
Northwestern University Feinberg School of Medicine,
Olson Pavilion,
Chicago,
Illinois

BRUCE MACFADYEN, MD

Chairperson of Surgery,
Moretz/Mansberger,
Distinguished Chair of Surgery,
Section Chief of General Surgery,
Professor of Surgery,
MCG Health System,
Augusta,
Georgia

JEFFREY M. MARKS, MD

Associate Professor,
Department of Surgery,
Case Medical Center;
Faculty,
Department of Surgery,
University Hospitals,
Cleveland,
Ohio

BRENT D. MATTHEWS, MD, FACS

Associate Professor,
Department of Surgery,
Washington University;
Chief,
Section of Minimally Invasive Surgery,
Department of Surgery,

Barnes-Jewish Hospital,
St. Louis,
Missouri

JOHN MELLINGER, MD, FACS

Professor of Surgery,
Program Director,
General Surgery Residency Program;
Chief,
Section of Gastrointestinal Surgery,
Medical College of Georgia,
Augusta,
Georgia

W. SCOTT MELVIN, MD

Professor of Surgery,
Chief,
Division of General and Gastrointestinal Surgery,
Director,
Center for Minimally Invasive Surgery,
The Ohio State University,
The Ohio State University Hospitals
Columbus,
Ohio

KENRIC M. MURAYAMA, MD

Professor of Surgery and Association,
Chair,
Robotics and Emerging Technologies,
Department of Surgery,
John A. Burns School of Medicine,
University of Hawaii,
Honolulu,
Hawaii

NINH T. NGUYEN, MD

Associate Professor,
Department of Surgery;
Chief,
Division of GI Surgery,
University of California,
Irvine Medical Center,
Orange,
California

BRANT K. OELSCHLAGER, MD

Associate Professor,
Department of Surgery,
University of Washington;
Director,
Center for Videoendoscopic Surgery,
Swallowing Center, and Bariatric Surgery,
University of Washington Medical Center,
Seattle,
Washington

RAYMOND P. ONDERS, MD, FACS

Associate Professor of Surgery,
Department of Surgery,
Case Western Reserve University School of Medicine;
Director of Minimally Invasive Surgery,
University Hospitals Case Medical Center,
Cleveland,
Ohio

ADRIAN PARK, MD, FRCSC, FACS

Campbell and Jeannette Plugge Professor of Surgery,
Chief,
Division of General Surgery,
University of Maryland Medical Center,
Baltimore,
Maryland

EMMA J. PATTERSON, MD, FACS, FRCSC

Medical Director,
Legacy Good Samaritan Obesity Institute;
Clinical Assistant Professor,
Department of Surgery,
Oregon Health and Science University,
Portland,
Oregon

MARCO G. PATTI, MD

Professor of Surgery,
Director,
UCSF,
Center for Esophageal Disorders,
Fellow,
Laparoscopic Surgery,
University of California—San Francisco,
San Francisco,
California

JONATHAN P. PEARL, MD

LCDR,
MC,
USN,
Department of Surgery,
National Naval Medical Center,
Bethesda,
Maryland

KYLE PERRY, MD

Laparascopic Fellow,
Department of Surgery,
Oregon Health and Science University,
Portland,
Oregon

JEFFREY H. PETERS, MD

Professor,
Surgery and Oncology,
Department of Surgery,
University of Rochester;
Chairman,
Department of Surgery,
Strong Memorial Hospital,
Rochester,
New York

EDWARD H. PHILLIPS, MD

Associate Professor,
Department of Surgery,
University of Southern California;
Vice-Chair,
Department of Surgery,
Cedars-Sinai Medical Center,
Los Angeles,
California

JEFFREY L. PONSKY, MD

Oliver H. Payne Professor and Chairman,
Department of Surgery,
Case Western Reserve School of Medicine,
Cleveland,
Ohio

ERIC C. POULIN, MD, MSC, FRCSC, FACS

Wilbert J Keon Professor and Chair of Surgery,
University of Ottawa,
Ontario,
Canada;
Surgeon-in-Chief,
The Ottawa Hospital,
Ottawa,
Canada

KINGA POWERS, MD, PhD

General Surgery,
Minimally Invasive Surgery,
Cambridge Health Alliance, Whidden Campus,
Everett,
Massachusetts;
Cambridge Health Alliance, Cambridge Campus,
Cambridge,
Massachusetts

VIVEK N. PRACHAND, MD
Assistant Professor of Surgery,
Department of Surgery,
University of Chicago Medical Center,
Chicago,
Illinois

BRUCE J. RAMSHAW, MD
Chief of Surgery and Associate Professor,
Department of General Surgery,
University of Missouri,
Columbia,
Missouri

SCOTT T. REHRIG, MD, LTC MC
General Surgeon,
Department of Surgery,
Walter Reed Army Medical Center,
Washington,
District of Columbia

WILLIAM RICHARDS, MD, FACS
Ingram Professor of Surgical Sciences,
Director of Laparoscopic Surgery,
Medical Director of the Center for Surgical Weight Loss,
Department of Surgery,
Vanderbilt University Medical Center,
Nashville,
Tennessee

STEVEN S. ROTHENBERG, MD
Clinical Professor of Surgery,
Department of Surgery,
Columbia University,
The Morgan Stanley Children's Hospital,
New York,
New York;
Chief of Pediatric Surgery,
Chairman,
Department of Pediatrics,
The Rocky Mountain Hospital for Children,
Denver,
Colorado

BASHAR SAFAR, MD
Clinical Resident,
Department of Colorectal Surgery,
Cleveland Clinic Florida,
Weston,
Florida

BARRY SALKY, MD
Chief,
Division of Laparoscopic Surgery,
Mount Sinai School of Medicine,
New York,
New York

VLADIMIR SCHRAIBMAN, MD
Associate Physican,
Gastrointestinal Surgery,
Federal University of São Paulo;
General and Gastric Surgeon,
Department of Surgery,
Albert Einstein Hospital,
São Paulo,
Brazil

STEVEN D. SCHWAITZBERG, MD
Visiting Associate Professor of Surgery,
Harvard Medical School,
Boston,
Massachusetts;
Chief of Surgery,
Department of Surgery,
Cambridge Health Alliance,
Cambridge,
Massachusetts

DANIEL J. SCOTT, MD, FACS
Associate Professor of Surgery,
Director,
Southwestern Center for Minimally Invasive Surgery,
University of Texas Southwestern Medical Center,
Dallas,
Texas

CAROL EH SCOTT-CONNER, MD, PHD
Professor,
Surgeon,
Department of Surgery,
University of Iowa Carver College of Medicine,
Iowa City,
Iowa

KENT R. VAN SICKLE, MD
Assistant Professor of Surgery,
Division of General and Laparoendoscopic Surgery,
University of Texas Health Science Center,
San Antonio,
Texas

C. DANIEL SMITH, MD
Professor and Chairman,
Department of Surgery,
Mayo Clinic—Florida,
Jacksonville,
Florida

LEE E. SMITH, MD, FACS
Director,
Section of Colon and Rectal Surgery,
Washington Hospital Center,
Washington,
District of Columbia

NATHANIEL J. SOPER, MD
Loyal and Edith Davis Professor and Chair,
Department of Surgery,
Northwestern University Feinberg School of Medicine,
Chicago,
Illinois

STEVEN M. STRASBERG, MD, FRCS(C), FACS, FRCS(ED)
Pruett Professor of Surgery,
Section of HPB Surgery,
Washington University in Saint Louis;
Pruett Professor of Surgery,
Section of HPB Surgery,
Barnes-Jewish Hospital,
St. Louis,
Missouri

LEE L. SWANSTRÖM, MD
Clinical Professor of Surgery,
Oregon Health Sciences University,
Director,
Division of Minimally Invasive Surgery,
Legacy Health System,
Portland,
Oregon

SAMUEL SZOMSTEIN, MD
Clinical Assistant Professor,
Department of Surgery,
NOVA Southeastern University,
Fort Lauderdale,
Florida;
Associate Director,
Bariatric and Metabolic Institute and Division of Minimally Invasive Surgery,
Cleveland Clinic Florida,
Weston,
Florida

DERON J. TESSIER, MD
Instructor,
Department of Surgery,

Washington University;
Minimally Invasive Surgery Fellow,
Department of Surgery,
Barnes-Jewish Hospital,
St. Louis,
Missouri

SARAH K. THOMPSON, MD

Assistant Professor of Clinical Medicine,
Penn Medicine at Radnor,
Radnor,
Pennsylvania

DESMOND P. TOOMEY, MD

Professional Surgical Unit,
The University of Dublin,
Trinity College,
Adelaide and Meath Hospitals
Incorporating the National Children's Hospital,
Tallaght,
Dublin,
Republic of Ireland

ALFONSO TORQUATI, MD, MSCI

Associate Professor of Surgery,
Department of Surgery,
Duke University;
Director of Obesity Research,
Department of Surgery,
Duke University Medical Center,
Durham,
North Carolina

ALFRED TRANG, MD

Division of Laparoscopic Surgery,
Mount Sinai School of Medicine,
New York,
New York

COREY E. VAN HOVE, MD

Oregon Health and Sciences University,
Portland,
Oregon

KHASHAYAR VAZIRI, MD

Assistant Professor,
Department of Surgery,
George Washington University,
Washington,
District of Columbia

GARY C. VITALE, MD

Professor of Surgery,
Department of Surgery,
University of Louisville,
Louisville,
Kentucky

JOSH WALKER, CCP

Perfusionist,
Department of Surgery,
Division of Cardiothoracic Surgery,
University of Texas Health Science Center at San Antonio,
San Antonio,
Texas

STEVEN D. WEXNER, MD

Department of Colorectal Surgery,
Cleveland Clinic Florida,
Weston,
Florida

BRENT C. WHITE, MD

Fellow of Minimally Invasive Surgery,
Department of Surgery,
Emory University School of Medicine,
Atlanta,
Georgia;
Staff Surgeon,
Department of Surgery,
Bassett Hospital,
Cooperstown,
New York

MARK WHITEFORD, MD

Clinical Assistant Professor of Surgery,
Oregon Health and Science University;
Gastrointestinal and Minimally Invasive Surgery Division,
Legacy Portland Hospitals,
Portland,
Oregon

SAMUEL ERIC WILSON, MD

Professor of Surgery,
Department of Surgery,
University of California—Irvine,
Orange,
California;
Chief,
Surgical Healthcare Group,
Department of Surgery,
Veterans Affairs Medical Center,
Long Beach,
California

TONIA M. YOUNG-FADOK, MD

Chair,
Division of Colon and Rectal Surgery,
Professor of Surgery,
Mayo Clinic College of Medicine,
Phoenix,
Arizona

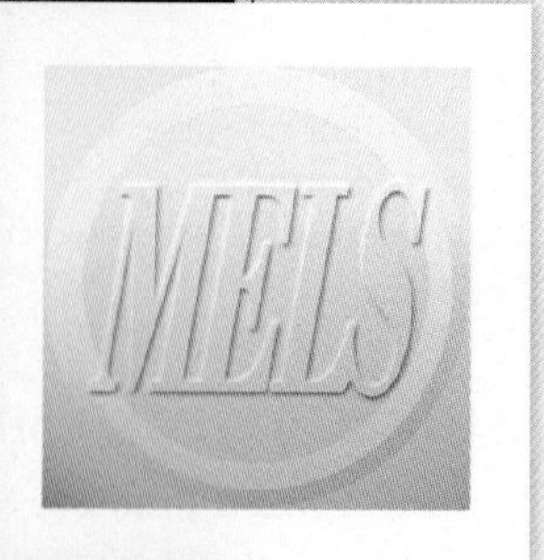

Preface

It has now been two decades since the "laparoscopic revolution" swept through the surgical world. This revolution, fueled by surgical innovators and patient demand, left many traditional surgeons and surgical approaches in its wake. Huge strides have been made in the ensuing decades, and the benefits of minimally invasive (or minimal access) surgery have now become universally acknowledged and confirmed by well-designed studies. Numerous advances have occurred over the eight years since the first edition of this textbook was published. There are many operations described in this book that were thought to be investigational or experimental at the time of inception of the first edition. This field of surgery has matured to the point where most of these same procedures are now the gold standard by which other operations are measured.

Over the last few years there has been a major increase in interest in the possibility of performing surgery with no external incisions whatsoever: so-called Natural Orifice Transluminal Endoscopic Surgery (NOTES). At the same time as this new approach to procedures has emerged, there has been a resurgence in commitment to flexible endoscopy by surgeons. We have included early descriptions of this new and exciting field of surgery in this textbook. We have also stressed the importance of flexible endoscopy as a valuable surgical tool for most of the body systems we work with. Many surgeons, especially those who were not early adopters of laparoscopy, are eagerly awaiting clinical trials of NOTES to assess whether this is a field with real potential.

The textbook has been reorganized to be more organ-based, with a common approach to diseases and disorders of each major organ system. All of the chapters have been updated, and most have been completely rewritten to give our readership access to the most up-to-date knowledge. Readers will also find the text richly illustrated with the outstanding artwork of Michael Leonard and appreciate the inclusion of color photography throughout. As is traditional with a Mastery of Surgery series, the editors have attempted to put each chapter in perspective with an accompanying commentary section.

Whether the scope is flexible or rigid and whether it is inserted through an incision or through a natural orifice, endoscopic techniques will continue to exert a tremendous influence on surgery of the major body cavities. The editors believe it is crucial for surgeons to maintain a mastery of flexible endoscopic techniques as we anticipate further development of endoluminal and transluminal techniques and technologies. Whether or not NOTES surgery assumes a major role in clinical treatment algorithms, an ability to perform flexible endoscopic manipulations will be necessary for the "complete" surgeon of tomorrow. Even if NOTES does not take off, the instruments developed in the effort will likely be used for other purposes, such as endoluminal or single-incision procedures. The surgical profession must continue to push the limits of the envelope while insisting on technical competence and evidence-based processes.

The editors have managed to persuade many of the world's experts to share their wisdom in this textbook. We are indebted to these masters for their time and effort and willingness to adhere to tight timelines to ensure the readership has access to the latest information. It is because of the authors and other surgical luminaries that the field of surgery has been able to offer "kinder and gentler" therapies to our patients.

Putting together a textbook and ensuring that it adheres to the highest standards is a major undertaking. The editors wish to thank Julia Seto and Brian Brown for their shepherding of the process.

General Topics

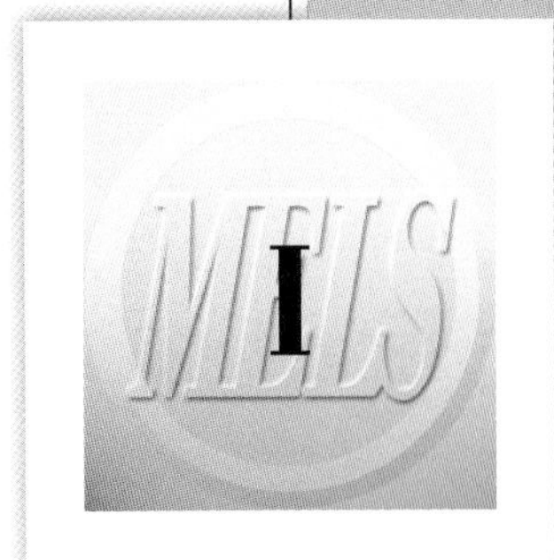

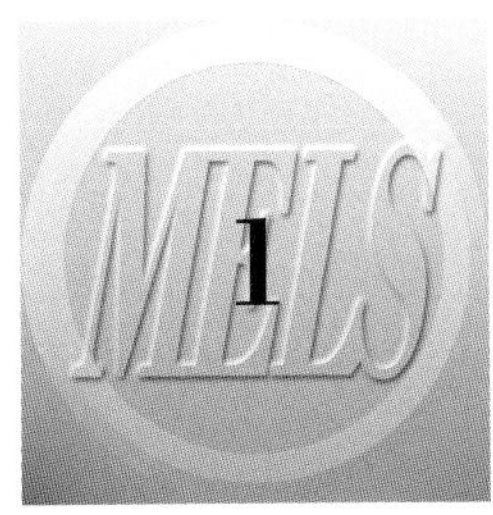

The Dominant Role of Endoscopy in Gastrointestinal Surgery

JONATHAN P. PEARL AND JEFFREY L. PONSKY

INTRODUCTION

Nearly all interventions in the field of gastrointestinal surgery can be performed using minimally invasive techniques, whether by laparoscopy or endoscopy. At its inception, endoscopy was used strictly for diagnosis, but today's expanding field of interventional endoscopy is broadening the applications in the gastrointestinal tract. As we move forward, novel endoscopic techniques are being developed for management of gastrointestinal diseases, and the field of gastrointestinal surgery will likely be dominated by endoscopic surgery.

Surgical endoscopy has a rich tradition, as many of the pioneers in interventional endoscopy were surgeons. In 1968 McCune et al. reported the first cannulation of the ampulla of Vater, in a precursor to endoscopic retrograde cholangiopancreatography. Shinya and Wolff introduced colonoscopic polypectomy in 1975, leading to the delineation of the adenoma-to-carcinoma sequence in colon polyps and highlighting the utility of the screening colonoscopy. The first percutaneous endoscopic gastrostomy, which extended endoscopy outside of the gastrointestinal tract, was peformed by Ponsky and Gauderer in 1979. Shortly thereafter, Stiegman applied the concept of band ligation of hemorrhoids to esophageal varices.

Endoscopic Procedures

Many conventional gastrointestinal operations have been supplanted by surgical endoscopic procedures. From esophagus to rectum, endoscopic approaches to diagnosis, hemostasis, foreign body removal, resection, tissue ablation, treatment of strictures, and palliation are widely available. These approaches have been embraced for their favorable results and are seen to offer the beneficial cosmetic and side effect profile of other minimally invasive techniques.

Today's interventional endoscopic procedures borrow from steadfast surgical principles. Hemostasis, tension-free apposition of tissues, and adequate margins of resection are familiar themes to gastrointestinal surgeons. To preserve favorable patient outcomes in the minimally invasive era, these principles should be devoutly observed regardless of the means of access to the gastrointestinal tract.

Esophagus

Creative methods of ablation and resection for Barrett disease have arisen. For example, the standard protocol for surveillance of Barrett esophagus without dysplasia or with low-grade dysplasia has been periodic surveillance with endoscopic biopsy, and resection is considered when biopsy suggests high-grade dysplasia. Today,

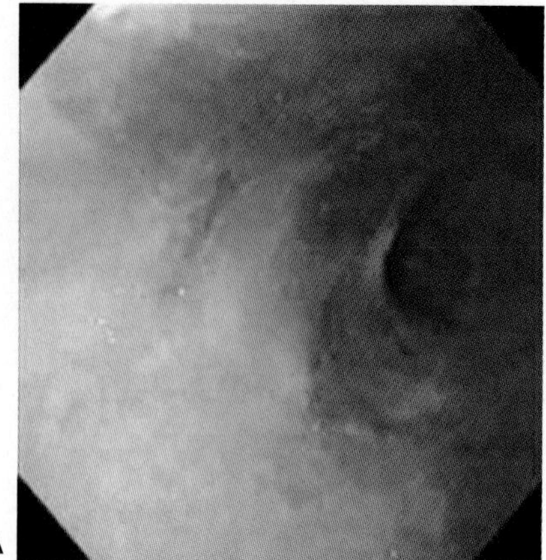

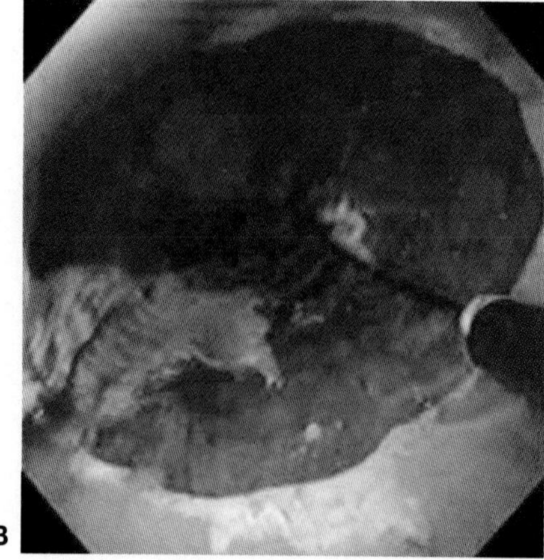

Fig. 1-1. A. Endoscopic view of Barrett esophagus. B. Endoscopic view after circumferential bipolar ablation of Barrett esophagus.

new techniques of endoscopic ablation of Barrett esophagus are gaining prominence. Both cryotherapy and bipolar coagulation have been shown to be effective in ablating intestinal metaplasia with a low rate of complications (Fig. 1-1). Whether ablation of Barrett disease without dysplasia provides benefit is as yet unclear.

Some groups are using endoscopic application of bipolar coagulation to ablate Barrett esophagus with high-grade dysplasia. This technique is currently viewed as an alternative to esophagogastrectomy in those patients unfit for a major thoracoabdominal operation. More experience will determine the efficacy of ablating high-grade dysplasia.

Endoscopic mucosal resection (EMR) has been used by some endoscopists to extirpate Barrett esophagus. The technique of EMR typically involves a saline (or other liquid) injection in the submucosa, which serves to lift the lesion. Then, using a cautery device, the specimen is removed at the junction of the mucosa and submucosa. Accomplished endoscopists are capable of resecting lesions of several centimeters in diameter.

Another EMR technique is the "suck-and-cut" technique, often used for polypoid lesions in the esophagus and other areas of the gastrointestinal tract. In this technique, a specialized cap is placed on the tip of the endoscope. Suction is applied to the lesion, which is delivered into the cap. A band is then placed at the base of the lesion, and the lesion is amputated.

Endoscopic hemostasis has been adopted as first-line therapy for bleeding esophageal varices. Initial reports advocated injection of vasoconstricting or sclerosing agents, but band ligation and injection of epinephrine are now most commonly employed. The results have been salutary, with endoscopic hemostasis and other minimally invasive techniques (such as transjugular intrahepatic portacaval shunts) displacing most emergency and elective surgical portacaval shunts.

Chemotherapy, radiotherapy, and surgery are standard methods for treating both adenocarcinoma and squamous cell carcinoma of the esophagus. In some instances, esophageal stenting may be appropriate for palliation, whether for unresectable disease without response to chemotherapy or as a short-term means to facilitate oral nutrition.

Both metal and plastic stents are available for endoscopic deployment (Fig. 1-2). The lesion is identified endoscopically, and the stents are commonly placed under fluoroscopic guidance. Metal stents are typically constructed of nitinol (a nickel-titanium alloy) and may be bare or covered with a material such as polyurethane.

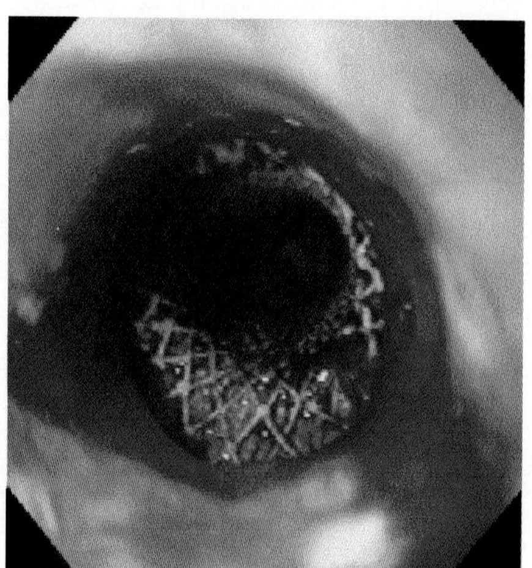

Fig. 1-2. Endoscopic view of metal esophageal stent placed for palliation of malignancy.

These stents are considered permanent and serve to maintain luminal patency in the face of malignancy. Plastic stents, in contrast, are used to bridge either benign or malignant esophageal strictures and are typically removed after 30 to 60 days. Plastic stents may be coated with silicone (i.e., covered), which inhibits passage of fluid into the stent's interstices, making them potentially useful for treating anastomotic dehiscences, tracheoesophageal fistulae, or esophageal perforations.

Stomach

Endoscopy is the primary means of diagnosis and treatment of upper gastrointestinal (GI) bleeding. Ulcers, vascular ectasia, and Mallory-Weiss tears are all amenable to endoscopic treatment. Available modes of hemostasis include cautery, argon coagulation, injection, banding, and clips. These techniques have significantly reduced the morbidity and mortality of upper GI hemorrhage and are efficacious in high-risk cases, such as visible vessels and recurrent bleeds, although operative hemostasis is still necessary on occasion.

One of the most commonly performed endoscopic interventions is percutaneous endoscopic gastrostomy for enteral nutritional support. Standard methods of placement include the pull and push methods. In cases of head and neck cancer there have been reports of seeding of the gastrostomy tract using both the push and pull techniques; therefore, alternative endoscopic means of enteral feeding tube placement have been devised. The SLiC technique involves endoscopic insufflation of the stomach followed by a modified percutaneous technique. Following endoscopic insufflation the gastrostomy tube is introduced percutaneously, without traversing the oropharygeal region, using a dilating laparoscopic trocar and a replacement-type gastrostomy tube.

For patients with contraindications to percutaneous endoscopic gastrostomy such as ascites, carcinomatosis, or trismus, an alternate percutaneous gastrostomy method has been developed. Championed in Japan, percutaneous transesophageal gastrostomy accesses the gastrointestinal tract through the cervical esophagus. No endoscopy is used, but ultrasound guidance permits needle access to the esophagus. After a guidewire is placed, a dilator and peel-away sheath facilitate placement of an indwelling balloon catheter into the stomach. This method has been shown to be safe and effective.

Numerous endoscopic methods have been developed for the management of gastroesophageal reflux disease. Submucosal injection of bioprosthetics has been mired with complications, but full thickness suturing devices and radiofrequency energy have yielded favorable outcomes with limited side effects. Currently, pharmacotherapy or fundoplication may be the preferred treatment of reflux, but as technology advances these modalities might be replaced by endoscopic therapy.

Endoscopic dilation can be used in the management of strictures or gastric outlet obstruction. Balloon dilation under direct visualization may be used for dilating anastomotic strictures after bariatric operations or gastric resection. In fundoplication patients who complain of dysphagia, intraluminal dilation of the wrap may provide relief. Patients with gastric outlet obstruction or impaired gastric emptying may benefit from dilation of the pylorus, occasionally combined with injection of Botulinum toxin for further relaxation of the pyloric musculature.

The placement of temporary plastic stents may be a solution to postoperative anastomotic leaks. Reports have described stenting of gastrojejunostomy leaks after gastric bypass and esophagogastrostomy leaks after esophageal resection. Reoperation or other drainage procedures should be considered standard, especially in early leaks after gastric bypass, but advances in endoscopic stent technology may result in a less invasive solution to anastomotic leaks.

Foreign body retrieval is often best accomplished endoscopically. A variety of devices is available to aid in retrieval. Specialized forceps, nets, and bags can be advanced through the scope to capture the foreign body. Overtubes or hoods placed on the tip of the scope are employed when retrieving sharp objects in order to protect the esophagus during withdrawal.

An underappreciated application of endoscopy is intraoperative endoscopy during gastrointestinal procedures. Foregut operations are especially conducive to endoscopy. When performing a Heller myotomy for achalasia, for example, endoscopic examination can ensure an adequate length of myotomy and can be used to search for violation of the mucosa. Endoscopy can also be used to locate the esophagogastric junction during paraesophageal hernia repair and again search for any injuries to the stomach or esophagus. Similarly, endoscopy can be used in fundoplications to ensure no injury has occurred and to examine the configuration of the wrap, thereby providing a reference point should future endoscopy be indicated.

A useful technique in intraoperative endoscopy is the leak test, in which the operative site is filled with saline, and the lumen of the esophagus or stomach insufflated. A leak manifests itself as bubbles in the operative field and is subsequently repaired, thereby averting the morbidity of a postoperative leak.

Yet another application of endoscopy is in combination with laparosocopy for resection of gastric masses. Large case series have reported success with intragastric resection of GI stromal tumors. An endoscope is used to insufflate the stomach, followed by percutaneous access using laparoscopic trocars and instruments. The resection is then carried out with endoscopic visualization using the laparoscopic instruments.

Endoscopy can also aid in assessing the margins of laparoscopic resection of GI stromal tumors. A laparoscopic dissection is initially performed. Before resecting the lesion, commonly with a linear stapler, the proposed margin of resection is inspected endoscopically. The endoscope can be also be used to ensure no encroachment on the esophagogastric junction occurs and to test for leaks for the staple line.

Duodenum

As with the esophagus and stomach, endoscopic hemostasis is first-line management for bleeding duodenal ulcers. A broad armamentarium is available to achieve hemostasis, with endoscopically applied clips showing utility for actively bleeding and visible vessels in the base of duodenal ulcers.

Endoscopic resections of periampullary adenomas (Fig. 1-3), localized adenocarcinomas, and small duodenal carcinoid tumors have been described with favorable outcomes. Adequate margins and hemostasis can be obtained using a needleknife or snare for dissection. Side-viewing duodenoscopes, as are used for endoscopic retrograde cholangiopancreatography (ERCP), are ideal for endoscopic interventions in the periampullary region.

Endoscopic stenting has shown utility for the palliation of unresectable periampullary tumors or in cases of external compression causing duodenal obstruction. When combined with biliary stenting, a double bypass of the gastrointestinal and biliary systems may be achieved without the morbidity of a conventional operation.

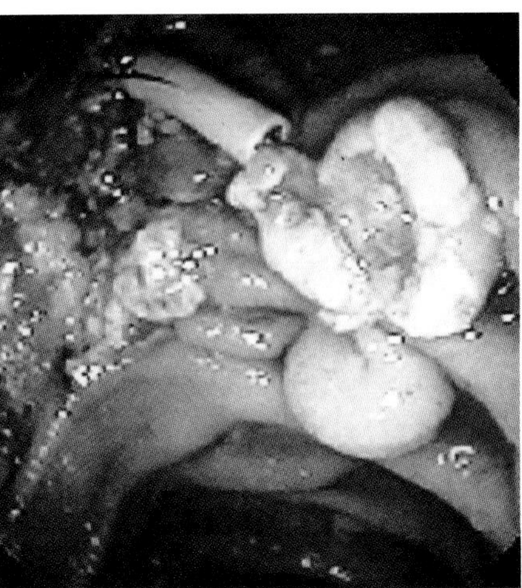

Fig. 1-3. A periampullary lesion undergoing endoscopic resection. A transpapillary plastic stent has been placed.

Biliary Tree

In most instances, ERCP is reserved for therapeutic interventions of the biliary tree and pancreatic ducts. Radiographic tests, such as standard ultrasonography, endoscopic ultrasound, CT scans, and magnetic resonance cholangiopancreatograms, have replaced ERCP as a diagnostic tool. ERCP, however, remains the procedure of choice for most biliary and pancreatic interventions.

Choledocholithiasis, a clear indication for laparotomy and conventional common duct exploration just a few short decades ago, is now routinely managed with stone extraction and sphincterotomy via ERCP. Bile duct leaks, as might occur after cholecystectomy, hepatic resections, or trauma are commonly stented in order to hasten their resolution. Both benign and malignant strictures of the bile duct are amenable to stenting for the relief of obstructive jaundice. Plastic stents, as are employed for benign strictures, remain patent for 3 to 6 months, and expandable metal stents provide a long-term egress of bile in the case of malignant strictures.

Obscure syndromes, such as sphincter of Oddi syndrome and papillary stenosis, are suitable for endoscopic treatment rather than duodenotomy and sphincteroplasty. Endoscopic manometry of the sphincter of Oddi is employed in the diagnosis of sphincter of Oddi syndrome. If confirmed by history and objective findings, an endoscopic sphincterotomy might provide relief. Similarly, a patient with obstructive jaundice without a clear etiology could receive relief from sphincterotomy of a stenotic papilla.

Pancreas

As with the biliary tree, pancreatic duct abnormalities are suitable for treatment by ERCP. As a primary means of diagnosing pancreatic adenocarcinoma, ERCP has been supplanted by radiologic tests, including endoscopic ultrasound. However, ERCP still has a role in relief of jaundice in periampullary lesions, with plastic stents inserted for temporary relief in preoperative patients and expandable metal stents used in patients deemed unresectable.

Pancreatic fistulae can be a vexing problem for gastrointestinal surgeons. Endoscopic stenting of the pancreatic duct has been reported to provide a low-pressure outlet for pancreatic secretions, leading to earlier closure of the pancreatic fistula. Sphincterotomy and stenting of the pancreatic duct can also provide relief in patients with chronic pancreatitis or, rarely, pancreas divisum.

The management of symptomatic pancreatic pseudocysts usually consists of internal drainage of the cyst into the stomach, duodenum, or jejunum. This can be accomplished conventionally, laparoscopically, or endoscopically. Pseudocysts bulging into the posterior stomach are especially suitable for endoscopic cystogastrostomy (Fig. 1-4). The location of the pseudocyst is typically assessed using endoscopic ultrasound through the gastric wall. The stomach is then punctured and the cyst cavity entered. The channel is subsequently dilated, commonly with a balloon, and stents are placed across the cystogastrostomy to maintain patency.

Symptomatic pseudocysts in communication with the main pancreatic duct may be relieved by transpapillary drainage. An ERCP is performed, and a pancreatic stent is placed across the papilla. This provides a low-pressure outlet for pancreatic secretions and may result in the diminution of the pseudocyst's size.

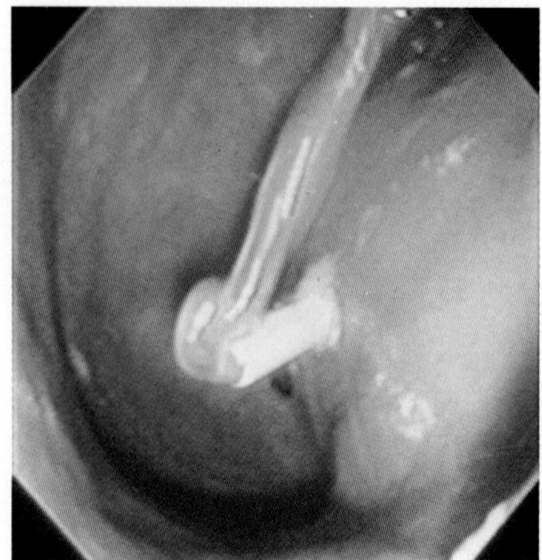

Fig. 1-4. Endoscopic cystogastrostomy with stent placement for a symptomatic pancreatic pseudocyst.

There are case series of transgastric endoscopic debridement of pancreatic necrosis. Much like pseudocyst drainage, the area of necrotic pancreas is localized through the posterior gastric wall using endoscopic ultrasound. A gastrotomy is made, and the necrotic debris is removed using endoscopic instruments such as Dormia baskets. These reports, which come from investigators with a special interest in the field, point to the expanding influence of endoscopy in gastrointestinal disease.

Small Bowel

Until recently, the diagnosis of small bowel pathology has eluded conventional radiographic and endoscopic methods. Commonly, laparotomy or laparoscopy was necessary to assess the jejunum and ileum. Two endoscopic innovations have made the small bowel accessible: capsule endoscopy and double-balloon enteroscopy. In capsule endoscopy, a wireless miniaturized camera is swallowed by the patient. A series of images are stored while the camera passes by peristalis through the GI tract. Capsule endoscopy has been shown to be useful in the diagnosis of occult bleeding in the small bowel, benign and malignant neoplasms, and inflammatory bowel disease.

While capsule endoscopy provides for diagnosis of small bowel pathology, double-balloon enteroscopy allows for both diagnosis and treatment. In double-balloon enteroscopy a long enteroscope is combined with an overtube, both of which have balloons capable of fixing their position. Through a sequence of advances and reductions, much of the small bowel is accessible. The enteroscope has working channels that permit biopsy, hemostasis, dilation, and resection of small bowel lesions.

Direct enteral access for feeding into the jejunum is occasionally desirable. A percutaneous endoscopic jejunostomy technique, similar to that used for a pull-type gastrostomy, has been developed. In an endoscopy suite with fluoroscopic capability an enteroscope is passed into the proximal jejunum. The position is confirmed fluoroscopically, and the safe tract technique is used to enter the desired loop of bowel. A standard catheter and wire are then used to perform a pull-type percutaneous endoscopic jejunostomy.

Colon and Rectum

Colonoscopy has long been used for screening and polypectomy. Today's endoscopists are pursuing more aggressive resections using endoscopic mucosal resection techniques. Large villous polyps are amenable to resection using the saline lift and cautery technique. Instruments currently under development may allow full thickness resections of polyps with endoscopic serosa-to-serosa closure of the colotomy.

Colonic conditions that might have warranted urgent operations in the past are now temporized using endoscopic means. Sigmoid volvulus is now routinely untwisted using either a flexible or rigid sigmoidoscope in a prepared bowel on an elective basis. Refractory colonic pseudo-abstruction is also commonly managed with colonoscopic decompression.

Intraoperative colonoscopy has utility during colonic resections. Prior to a laparoscopic colon resection, a lesion can be identified and tattooed by the surgeon, ensuring accurate localization for the minimally invasive operation. A bubble test can also be performed to locate an anastomosis, as with upper GI operations.

Stenting is useful for circumferential colon lesions, especially in the descending and sigmoid colons. Expandable metal stents are available for palliation in unresectable lesions, and temporary plastic stents are capable of traversing a narrowed lumen and allowing preoperative preparation of the colon. Covered plastic stents may be used to treat anastomotic dehiscences, but the length and stiffness of the delivery system limits the application to distal anastomoses. In many circumstances stenting may spare the patient a temporary diverting colostomy and allow a better quality of life.

Tomorrow's Surgical Endoscopy

As is evident, endoscopy plays a major role in gastrointestinal surgery. Every organ in the gastrointestinal tract can be approached with the endoscope, and interventional endoscopy is flourishing. Tomorrow's surgical endoscopy will continue its expansion in gastrointestinal surgery, possibly making today's conventional and laparoscopic operations obsolete.

Bariatric surgery has blossomed in the era of laparoscopy. A future endoscopic procedure might offer the benefits of a restrictive operation without the need for incisions or general anesthesia. An endoscopically placed reservoir could serve as the gastric pouch, as could a pouch created with a plicating device. A long, narrow stent could function similar to a vertical banded gastroplasty. Endoscopic gastrojejunostomy has been reported in laboratory animals, with anastomoses created using magnets and endoscopic sewing devices.

A new generation of interventional capsule endoscopes is in the developmental stages. These devices might be capable of traversing the entire GI tract, including the colon, and localizing pathologic lesions. Thereafter, interventions such as radiofrequency ablation of polyps or elution of topical hemostatic agents will automatically occur when the findings indicate.

Endoscopic full thickness resections will likely be possible in the near future. Instruments initially conceived for gastroplication for reflux will likely be adapted for use in other organs. A suturing device will be capable of delivering full thickness sutures to close a defect after transmural resection of a large colon polyp, and an endoscopic stapler could be used to close a gastrotomy for peritoneal access.

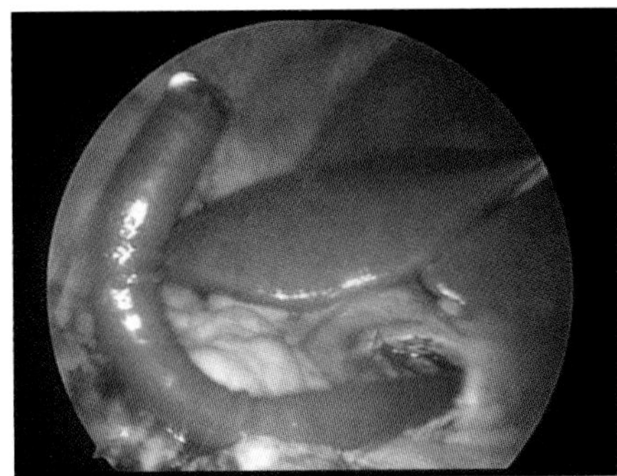

Fig. 1-5. Laparoscopic view of transgastric endoscopic peritoneoscopy.

Beyond conventional intraluminal endoscopy and its multitude of applications, transluminal endoscopic surgery is on the horizon (Fig. 1-5). Using the mouth and rectum to access the peritoneal cavity is a natural extension of conventional endoscopy. Many technical advances are needed to create a stable operative field capable of bimanual manipulation of tissues with adequate optics, but routine scarless transgastric appendectomy or cholecystectomy is not beyond the imagination.

We may be entering the new golden age of endoscopy with an explosion of endoscopic advances. Combining surgical principles with endoscopic techniques could generate a host of new endoscopic applications in the gastrointestinal tract, with endoscopy fortifying its dominant role in gastrointestinal surgery.

SUGGESTED READING

Gauderer MW, Ponsky JL, Izant RJ Jr. Gastrostomy without laparotomy: a percutaneous endoscopic technique. *J Pediatr Surg* 1980;Dec;15(6):872–875.

Mackey R, Chand B, Oishi H, et al. Percutaneous transesophageal gastrostomy tube for decompression of malignant obstruction: report of the first case and our series in the US. *J Am Coll Surg* 2005;Nov;201(5):695–700.

Ono H, Kondo H, Gotoda T, et al. Endoscopic mucosal resection for treatment of early gastric cancer. *Gut* 2001;Feb;48(2):225–229.

Sabnis A, Liu R, Chand B, et al. SLiC technique: a novel approach to percutaneous gastrostomy. *Surg Endosc* 2006;Feb;20(2):256–262.

Yamamoto H, Sugano K. A new method of enteroscopy: the double-balloon method. *Can J Gastroenterol* 2003;Apr;17(4):273–274.

COMMENTARY

Drs. Pearl and Ponsky have highlighted the importance of flexible endoscopy in diagnosing and treating diseases of the gastrointestinal tract. They point out that surgeons were among the early innovators in endoscopy. As we are painfully aware, gastroenterologists have assumed the dominant role for performing elective flexible endoscopy in most medical centers. Most surgeons abdicated their role in flexible endoscopy to concentrate on more traditional surgical pursuits in the operating room. Over the last 20 years, great advances have been made in endoscopic techniques. Many of these procedures have assumed the primary treatment modality for diseases and disorders previously treated surgically. Technologies have been developed that allow injection, resection, ablation, and apposition of tissues using the flexible endoscopic platform.

What was once a bright line separating the field of gastroenterology and surgery has become increasingly blurred. With the advent of endoluminal treatments and the possibility of transluminal interventions, it is clear that surgeons must step back into the fray of flexible endoscopy. The surgical establishment has responded to these developments by increasing the required number of flexible endoscopic procedures that must be performed during the course of a general surgery residency.

This chapter sets the scene for the remainder of the text. Subsequent chapters will go into more details of the performance of flexible and rigid endoscopic procedures. Suffice it to say that endoscopy, and more specifically endoscopic intervention, will be an integral component of the comprehensive management of patients with diseases of the gastrointestinal tract. Surgical gastroenterologists must learn how to perform and apply flexible endoscopy for the total care of their patients.

NJS

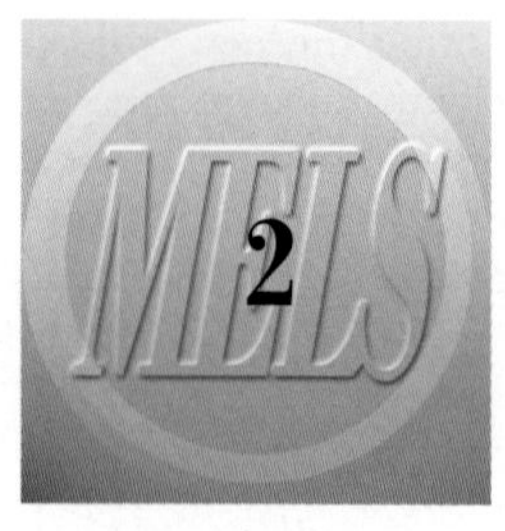

Patient Selection and Practical Considerations in Surgical Endoscopy

MOHAMMAD K. JAMAL AND CAROL E. H. SCOTT-CONNER

INTRODUCTION

Minimal access surgery is like other forms of surgery in that patient selection involves weighing a series of factors and risks. This chapter will discuss these, as well as the manners in which risk may be mitigated. Practical considerations common to most minimal access procedures will also be discussed. Subsequent chapters deal with specific procedures.

Patient Selection

Several questions need to be considered when a patient is evaluated for minimal access surgery. First, does the patient need surgery? What are the alternatives? What is the patient's individual risk for surgery? Is a minimal access approach feasible? Does the option of a minimal access approach alter indications for surgery? Are there special factors that might render such an approach infeasible? Will the patient tolerate the equivalent open procedure if conversion is required? Finally, will the patient tolerate any potential complications of the procedure?

Every operation described in this text has a set of accepted indications for which surgery is considered the best treatment. In the context of laparoscopic appendectomy (LA), acute appendicitis is an example of such an indication. Currently, appendectomy is the recommended treatment, and the only question is whether to perform this laparoscopically or by an open approach. There is considerable variability in practice. Some surgeons use LA almost exclusively, whereas others rarely use it, insisting that they can perform an appendectomy through a small muscle-splitting incision with excellent outcomes. Meta-analysis of published series has shown surprisingly little difference between LA and open appendectomy. The open procedure has a higher incidence of wound infection, and LA has a slightly higher incidence of postoperative intraabdominal abscess formation. Unanswered questions, such as the optimum duration of antibiotic therapy when LA is performed for acute appendicitis, cloud these issues. Many use LA preferentially for women of childbearing age who require surgery for right lower quadrant pain, reasoning that enhanced visualization of the pelvic organs during LA assists in accurate diagnosis and treatment. Conversely, the patient with neglected retrocecal appendicitis might be better served by open appendectomy. Interval appendectomy after percutaneous drainage of appendiceal abscess and appendectomy for tumors of the appendix represent indications for elective surgery. LA might be used in the former case. In the latter, concern over spillage of tumor cells and adequacy of excision would argue in favor of open surgery.

Although it is generally accepted that the indications for surgery should not change simply because a minimal access approach is feasible, there is no question that the number of cholecystectomies increased dramatically after the introduction of the laparoscopic cholecystectomy (LC). This has been interpreted to mean that patients formerly unwilling to undergo surgery are now consenting and that physicians may be making earlier referrals. A similar phenomenon seems to be occurring with bariatric surgery.

Assessment of the patient's fitness for surgery is part of preoperative planning. A patient's medical history and a physical examination provide much of the information needed to make an initial assessment of risk. The astute clinician will recognize that a common recurring theme in the following discussion is to control any treatable disease. For example, hypertension and diabetes should be controlled, and any correctable cardiac condition should be addressed before surgery. Surgery that involves entering a body cavity increases the patient's risk over that associated with surgery that does not involve entering a cavity; thus laparoscopic or thoracoscopic surgery by its nature entails an additional component of risk. It is important to reiterate that these "minimal access" surgical procedures are not truly minimally invasive in terms of potential physiologic alterations and the risk of surgery and anesthesia.

ASSESSMENT AND QUANTITATION OF RISK

During the past half century, the general risk of death associated with anesthesia has declined from 1 in 10,000 cases to 1 in 100,000. The American Society of Anesthesiologists (ASA), with its Physical Status Classification (also commonly referred to as ASA classification), provides a standardized ranking system used in operating rooms around the country (Table 2-1). Preoperative evaluation by an anesthesia care provider includes not only assessment of physical status but also assessment of the airway, any individual or family history of difficulties during surgery or anesthesia, idiosyncratic drug reactions or allergies, and a detailed medication history. Characterizing

TABLE 2-1. AMERICAN SOCIETY OF ANESTHESIOLOGISTS PHYSICAL STATUS CLASSIFICATION DESCRIPTION

PS-1	A normal, healthy patient
PS-2	A patient with mild systemic disease that results in no functional limitation
PS-3	A patient with severe systemic disease that results in functional limitation
PS-4	A patient with severe systemic disease that is a constant threat to life
PS-5	A moribund patient who is not expected to survive without the operation
PS-6	A declared brain-dead patient whose organs are being removed for donor purposes
Modifier: E	Emergency operation

the surgical risk of a patient for a specific form of anesthesia involves a detailed and concerted preoperative assessment among the anesthesiologist, surgeon, and the primary care physician. This should entail a thorough but a cost-effective effort to define the patient's risk of morbidity specific to individual organ systems as well as the overall risk of death from the procedure. Hence, the decision to proceed with surgery should be made within the context of anesthetic and surgical risk.

Preoperative assessment begins with a thorough history and physical examination of the patient and serves to elucidate information that will impact the choice of anesthetic technique, the type of anesthesia, monitoring, and specific postoperative recovery requirements. This should be complemented with selective laboratory and diagnostic testing based on the findings of the history and physical examination.

Conditions that elevate the overall risk of surgery and anesthesia include recent myocardial infarction, uncontrolled congestive heart failure, uncontrolled hypertension, and diabetes (Table 2-2). This risk elevation is independent of the modality of anesthesia used. It is unclear whether a minimal access (as opposed to an open) approach changes the risk in any way. Laparoscopy may be fundamentally different from thoracoscopy in this respect. Whereas the intraoperative physiologic alterations caused by pneumoperitoneum tremendously affect anesthetic management, thorascopic surgery is performed under single-lung ventilation in a manner similar to that of thoracotomy. During the postoperative phase, both offer more rapid healing with decreased pain compared with the analogous open approach.

TABLE 2-2. FACTORS THAT MAY INCREASE THE GENERAL RISK OF ANESTHESIA AND INTRAABDOMINAL OR INTRATHORACIC SURGERY

- Active coronary artery disease
- Congestive heart failure
- Dysrhythmias
- Chronic obstructive pulmonary disease
- Cirrhosis
- Asthma
- Diabetes
- Hemodynamically significant aortic stenosis
- Age >70 yrs
- Emergency operation
- Renal failure

Physiologic Consequences of Laparoscopic Surgery

Laparoscopic surgery is most commonly performed with carbon dioxide pneumoperitoneum, because it is cheap, does not support combustion, and is rapidly eliminated from the body, decreasing the risk of gaseous embolism. Although alternatives exist, including abdominal wall lift devices, these have not found widespread application. Essentially all the systems of the body, from cardiopulmonary and renal effects through intracranial pressure and mesenteric blood flow, are affected by laparoscopy (Table 2-3, page 8). Most of these are consequences of elevated intraabdominal pressure and the use of carbon dioxide as the insufflating agent. Because these effects should be considered in patients undergoing laparoscopy, before, during, and after the completion of the procedure, and should guide patient selection and further clinical management, they will be briefly summarized here.

Systemic Effects of the Pneumoperitoneum

Carbon dioxide pneumoperitoneum produces well-known effects upon the cardiopulmonary system, including a reduction in venous return, causing a reduction in the preload and a consequent reduction in stroke volumes and cardiac output. This results in a compensatory increase in heart rate and elevated systemic and pulmonary vascular resistance. The degree of alteration of these parameters is dependant on several factors including the type of anesthetic agent, the cardiopulmonary status of the patient, and metabolic and acid-base factors. The degree of hypercarbia also plays an important role in determining the degree of acidosis that may result and thus, alter the acid-base balance. The degree of hypercarbia depends in turn on the duration of procedure, the pressures used, and any preexisting pulmonary disease.

The reduction in stroke volume and subsequent cardiac output are the direct result of myocardial depression from carbon dioxide pneumoperitoneum, as well as elevated transdiaphragmatic and transmediastinal pressures. Elevated systemic vascular resistance results from a combination of compensatory mechanisms in response to the elevated intraabdominal pressure. The increased peritoneal pressure compresses the aorta, the vena cava, and the splanchnic vasculature, decreasing preload. The release of renin and vasopressin tend to increase the afterload. The final result of these chemical and mechanical responses is an overall reduction in cardiac output and peripheral blood flow, as well as increased systemic vascular resistance.

Most patients tolerate these changes quite well, particularly with good anesthesiology support. Patients in ASA class I or II generally do well. Patients in class III or IV must be approached with caution, as they may have significant underlying cardiopulmonary disease and may not be able to compensate for the physiologic changes during laparoscopic surgery. If a patient develops cardiopulmonary decompensation during laparoscopic surgery and is not actively hemorrhaging, decreasing the amount of pneumoperitoneum or completely desufflating the abdomen is generally an appropriate first response.

In contrast to the indirect cardiac effects, almost all respiratory effects of the carbon dioxide pneumoperitoneum are secondary to the mechanical effects exerted by an increase in intraabdominal pressures. This in turn causes an increase in diaphragmatic excursion increasing peak airway pressures and reducing vital capacity, functional residual capacity, and compliance. Diaphragmatic displacement can further increase intrathoracic pressures and increase dead space and ventilation-perfusion mismatch. The combination of these factors may require an increase in the minute ventilation during laparoscopic procedures by nearly 15%, even in healthy subjects, to compensate for the respiratory effects of the pneumoperitoneum.

Thoracoscopic surgery is generally performed with single-lung ventilation. The tracheobronchial tree is intubated with a special endotracheal tube that allows selective ventilation of a single bronchus. Absorption atelectasis rapidly produces collapse of the nonventilated lung with corresponding cardiopulmonary alterations. Hypoxic pulmonary vasoconstriction in the collapsed lung is a normal physiologic response that minimizes shunting. Occasionally, low-pressure CO_2 insufflation is used to increase exposure. When this is done, the possibility for mediastinal shift and hemodynamic compromise must be kept in mind. The *Suggested Reading* section at the end of this chapter gives detailed information about these alterations.

Renal

General anesthesia can pose several challenges in the patient with chronic renal failure undergoing laparoscopic surgery.

TABLE 2-3. COMPLICATIONS AND ADVERSE EFFECTS OF THE CARBON DIOXIDE PNEUMOPERITONEUM

Complication/adverse effect	Possible mechanism
CARDIOPULMONARY	
Adverse effects:	
Tachycardia	Sympathetic response to impaired venous return and hypercarbia
Hypertension	Sympathetic response to impaired venous return and hypercarbia
Increased vascular resistance	Sympathetic response to impaired venous return and hypercarbia
Increased myocardial oxygen demand	Sympathetic response to impaired venous return and hypercarbia, tachycardia, increased afterload
Decreased cardiac output	Reduced venous return, increased afterload, impaired contractility from hypercarbia
Bradycardia	Vasovagal response to peritoneal stretching and irritation
Cardiac arrhythmias	Hypercarbia, hypoxia, catecholamine response
Hypotension	Vena caval compression, decreased venous return
Pneumomediastinum	Diaphragmatic perforation
Reduced lung compliance	Reduced lung volumes, elevated diaphragm
Increased airway resistance	Increased intrathoracic pressure from transmitted increased intraabdominal pressure
Ventilation-perfusion mismatch	Reduced lung volumes from elevated intrathoracic pressures
Hypercarbia/acidosis	Carbon dioxide retention
Atelectasis	Collapse of lung bases secondary to high diaphragmatic pressures
Complications:	
Tension pneumothorax	Barotrauma, diaphragmatic perforation, or hiatal dissection
Myocardial infarction	Reduced myocardial blood flow in the presence of increased oxygen demand
Metabolic acidosis	Inadequate metabolic perfusion due to reduced cardiac output, increased peripheral resistance, and hypercarbia
Hypoxia	Atelectasis and reduced lung volumes
Hypercarbia	Increased carbon dioxide retention
Respiratory acidosis	Increased carbon dioxide retention
Aspiration	Increased risk of regurgitation of gastric contents
Air embolus	Entry of carbon dioxide through injured blood vessels
Subcutaneous emphysema	Insufflation of carbon dioxide into the subcutaneous tissues
Shoulder pain	Irritation of diaphragm
NEUROLOGIC	
Increased intracranial pressure	Increased intracranial blood flow from hypercarbia
Potential cerebral edema	Increased intracranial blood flow from hypercarbia
Brain stem herniations	Increased intracranial pressure
RENAL	
Oliguria	Decreased renal blood flow from elevated intraabdominal pressure and low cardiac output
Renal failure	Decreased renal blood flow from elevated intraabdominal pressure and low cardiac output

The carbon dioxide pneumoperitoneum can induce oliguria and a severe respiratory acidosis that can further exacerbate already existent acid-base and electrolyte abnormalities in these patients. Ideally, all patients with chronic renal failure should be considered for preoperative dialysis to correct any preexisting electrolyte abnormalities. This is especially true for patients with hyperkalemia, as the coronary effects of this are all too common and are usually exhibited as severe arrhythmias in the perioperative period. The choice of anesthetic agents is determined by the presence of renal failure as most nondepolarizing muscle relaxants are at least partially excreted in the urine. Cisatracurium remains the agent of choice as it is degraded by nonspecific esterases and Hoffman degradation. All prophylactic antibiotics should be administered in renal doses and the use of subcutaneous low-molecular weight heparin for deep venous thrombosis prophylaxis should be used with caution.

There appears to be sufficient evidence to conclude that both renal function and renal blood flow (RBF) are decreased during pneumoperitoneum. The magnitude of the decrease is dependent on factors such as preoperative renal function, level of hydration, level of pneumoperitoneum, patient positioning, and duration of pneumoperitoneum. The increased intraabdominal pressures during laparoscopy cause vena caval and aortic compression and a subsequent reduction in renal perfusion.

Data from several large reviews demonstrate compelling evidence that RBF decreases during pneumoperitoneum. This decrease is pressure dependent (with 12 to 15 mmHg being the most common values used), worsened with some positions (head up), improved with fluid hydration, and not dependent on the gas used. The magnitude of the decrease is also likely to vary with each specific animal model, the method of RBF measurement, and the experimental design chosen. Although this decrease in RBF is well documented, it is unclear whether this is of any clinical significance. It is likely that these changes in RBF are not significant in healthy patients under most normal conditions, but may be important in cases wherein RBF is already compromised.

Five studies (one human and four animal studies) demonstrated no decrease in renal function during pneumoperitoneum in normal subjects. The magnitude of the decrease in renal function likely varies with the numerous factors described previously for RBF. Furthermore, the decrease appears to be temporary, with function returning to normal a variable time after pneumoperitoneum is released. In conclusion, although the data demonstrate that renal function is decreased during pneumoperitoneum, the clinical significance of this phenomenon is not certain because it appears that renal function returns to normal after pneumoperitoneum is released. However, every effort should be made to achieve an adequate renal perfusion by maintaining fluid balance during laparoscopic procedures.

Cardiovascular

Cardiovascular risk factors need to be extensively assessed prior to proceeding with general anesthesia for a laparoscopic procedure. This is especially important in patients with known cardiac disease or risk factors for heart disease. Patients with diabetes, hypertension, and hypercholesterolemia form a higher risk group of patients and should be investigated for existing heart disease with preoperative cardiac testing, which might reveal the presence of silent heart disease that could be the deciding factor between medical and surgical treatment options. The physiologic impact of the carbon dioxide pneumoperitoneum and positional changes previously described could potentially cause increased stress on the cardiovascular system, especially in a patient with existing cardiac disease.

An electrocardiogram as the sole preoperative assessment tool may be generally enough in the vast majority of asymptomatic males above the age of 40 years and females beyond 50 years of age. The American College of Cardiology and the American Heart Association Guidelines for Perioperative Cardiovascular Evaluation for Noncardiac Surgery places intraperitoneal and intrathoracic procedures at an intermediate cardiac risk. A thorough cardiac evaluation is mandatory in patients with preexisting cardiac risk factors with limited functional reserve and the presence of major or intermediate clinical predictors. These include recent acute myocardial infarction, unstable angina, large previous irreversible myocardial ischemic changes, uncompensated congestive heart failure, arrhythmias, and severe valvular heart disease. Patients with these coronary syndromes should undergo noninvasive cardiac testing with stress echocardiogram and a Cardiolite scan along with a specialty cardiology evaluation.

Hypertension should be adequately controlled prior to any elective surgical procedure requiring a general anesthetic. Beta-blockers have received special consideration in recent years and all patients with hypertension are generally started on perioperative beta blockade that is continued into the postoperative period. The objective should be to titrate the dose to a heart rate of 50 to 60 beats per minute, which appears to decrease the perioperative risk of a major coronary event in high-risk patients.

Diabetics undergoing general anesthesia pose another relatively high risk group of patients. Serum glucose levels should be tightly controlled in the perioperative period as elevated levels have been associated with poor wound healing, higher infection rates, and dehydration. An optimal blood glucose level of 150 to 200 mg/dL should be maintained, ideally with intravenous rather than subcutaneous insulin. Cautious monitoring of serum glucose levels is essential, and significant hypoglycemia should also be avoided as hypoglycemic somnolence in a sedated patient may be wrongly attributed to the effects of drugs and anesthetic agents.

Pulmonary

A thorough pulmonary evaluation is essential in patients undergoing a general anesthetic for laparoscopic procedures who have preexisting severe chronic obstructive or restrictive pulmonary disease and asthma. All efforts should be made to optimize these medical conditions prior to an elective procedure. In select patients at higher risk of pulmonary complications, pulmonary function testing and a specialty pulmonary consultation should be obtained. Patients who smoke should be advised to quit smoking for at least a period of 8 weeks, although some evidence suggests a higher incidence of perioperative pulmonary complications (bronchospasm, pneumonia, and a need for respiratory therapy) in those patients who have recently ceased smoking.

The management of a patient recovering from a recent upper respiratory tract infection (URI) has been the topic of discussion for several decades. There is evidence to suggest that the impact of a URI on pulmonary risk may be present for as long as 6 weeks following the reduction of symptoms. Therefore, the decision to proceed with surgery should be made on an individual basis and guided by the urgency of the procedure, the existence of other medical conditions that may substantially increase the overall risk, and presence of other alternatives to a general anesthetic.

A potentially fatal complication of anesthesia, especially in patients with preexisting pulmonary disease (asthma and chronic obstructive pulmonary disease) could arise from severe laryngospasm. This can be recognized by the presence of severe inspiratory stridor and in extremes of cases, total absence of breath sounds. The immediate administration of 100% oxygen and in some cases, a small dose of succinylcholine (0.1 mg/kg), will relax the vocal cords and usually provide an effective treatment for this condition.

Practical Considerations

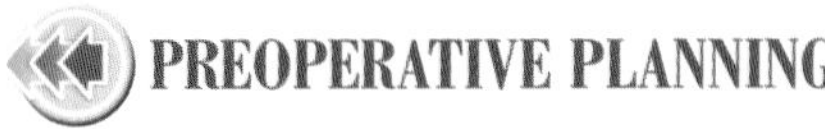

PREOPERATIVE PLANNING

Laboratory testing should be selective and guided by the patient's history and the physical examination. Most literature suggests that the medicolegal implications of missing an abnormal test are usually greater than if the test was never performed. According to a report by Kaplan et al., only 60% of the 2800 tests performed in their patient population were actually indicated and only 0.22% yielded significant results. Other studies have found similar low yield of routine preoperative testing prior to a surgical procedure. In addition, testing performed in the preceding 6 to 8 months may be adequate unless significant changes in the patient's medical history have occurred that mandate new or further testing of the involved systems.

Patients undergoing routine low risk laparoscopic procedures including laparoscopic cholecystectomy, appendectomy, and tubal ligation should ideally have a complete blood count, a basic metabolic panel, and a coagulation profile drawn prior to surgery. Males older than 40 and females older than 50 years of age should undergo an EKG to rule out any existing heart disease. Further testing should be guided by the suspicion or presence of associated comorbidities. Pulmonary function testing in the presence of severe pulmonary disease, thyroid function testing in the presence of a known thyroid abnormality, and pregnancy testing in women of childbearing age are some examples. A chest radiograph is useful in patients with known cardiac or pulmonary disease. These recommendations should be used as general guidelines, and all diagnostic testing should be cost-effective and individualized to suite a patient's particular needs.

Monitoring during Surgery

Standard monitoring for all procedures performed under general anesthesia as defined by the American Society of Anesthesiologists include continuous EKG, pulse oximetry, noninvasive blood pressure measurements at least every 5 minutes, capnography, and inspired oxygen and tidal volume measurements. Monitoring of the end-tidal carbon dioxide (CO_2) is essential in all laparoscopic procedures, as diffusion of the pneumoperitoneum can potentially raise the arterial CO_2 concentration. This may require adjusting the minute ventilation to compensate for the increased CO_2

load. As the relationship between end-tidal and arterial CO_2 may change considerably with increasing dead space and ventilation perfusion mismatch during general anesthesia, close monitoring of these values is essential to prevent severe acid-base abnormalities. This is especially true for patients with serious pulmonary or cardiac disease who may not withstand long durations of rising acidemia. In such instances, invasive arterial monitoring, either with an arterial line and frequent arterial blood gases, may be essential.

Capnography may also indicate the presence of complications of a pneumoperitoneum such as a pneumothorax. The sudden elevation of peak inspiratory pressures combined with an absence of breath sounds on clinical examination may indicate the presence of this entity, whereas a rapid rise in end-tidal CO_2 with a reduction in cardiac output usually indicates a venous air embolism. Invasive arterial monitoring for patients with severe coronary artery disease is generally fraught with complications. Frequent positional changes as well as the increased intrathoracic pressure secondary to the pneumoperitoneum generally falsely raise the central venous, pulmonary arterial, and wedge pressures, making it difficult to interpret the results. A more useful entity for intraoperative cardiac monitoring is the use of a transesophageal echo (TEE) in high-risk cardiac patients. This would provide detailed information on the atrial and ventricular function and the presence of any segmental myocardial wall hypokinesis associated with an intraoperative cardiac event. A TEE is also useful to determine functional cardiac output when combined with Doppler technology.

In the ambulatory surgery arena, the use of EEG monitoring devices is becoming more common. These devices, such as the bispectral index (BIS) monitor (Aspect Medical Systems, Newton, MA), uses a proprietary algorithm to calculate a BIS value to indicate the level of hypnosis. This BIS value can be used to titrate the level of inhalational agents, typically at lower doses than with standard monitoring devices alone. This can be of potential benefit in speedy emergence and early hospital discharge.

POSTOPERATIVE MANAGEMENT

Nausea and Vomiting

Laparoscopic surgery in itself has been known to be an independent risk factor for postoperative nausea and vomiting (PONV). This was reported to occur in as high as 70% of patients after minor laparoscopic procedures such as gynecologic laparoscopy and Nissen fundoplication. The outcomes can be minor and include patient dissatisfaction and late discharge from the recovery room or catastrophic, including aspiration pneumonitis, Nissen wrap disruption, and herniations.

Several steps can be taken to prevent PONV. Inhalational agents such as nitrous oxide (N_2O) should be avoided as their use has been associated with perioperative ileus, small bowel distention, and the resultant PONV. The use of a totally intravenous agent such as propofol, although relatively more expensive than other inhalational agents, may be preferred in patients with a history of severe PONV despite antiemetic prophylaxis. Increased oxygen inhalation peri- and postoperatively, as well as adequate hydration with intravenous fluids intraoperatively, has been shown to reduce the incidence of PONV. The use of nonnarcotic analgesics such as nonsteroidal antiinflammatory drugs (NSAIDs) and local anesthetics may also be of some benefit in reducing PONV.

Pharmacologic prophylaxis remains the mainstay of preventing postoperative emesis. Most patients undergoing laparoscopy should receive at least one prophylactic agent, if not combination therapy. The judicious use of agents including intravenous steroids (dexamethasone), anticholinergics (scopolamine), serotonin receptor antagonists (ondansetron), butyrophenones (droperidol), phenothiazines (promethazine), and histamine-1 receptor antagonists (dimenhydrinate) has been shown to be useful in preventing PONV in patients undergoing laparoscopic procedures.

Pain Control

Although minimally invasive procedures are generally associated with significantly less pain than their open counterparts, they are far from being pain free. Patients should be adequately counseled regarding the presence and treatment of postoperative pain following laparoscopic procedures. Pain associated with laparoscopic procedures is multifactorial and may include pain emanating from visceral organs, diaphragmatic irritation from the pneumoperitoneum, and musculoskeletal pain from laparoscopic port placement.

Preemptive pain control in the form of local anesthetic infiltration at port sites has been shown to be effective in controlling pain and reducing narcotic analgesic requirements following laparoscopy. Another alternative is the use of intravenous analgesics such as ketorolac and postoperative Patient Controlled Anesthetic (PCA) devices utilizing either morphine or hydromorphone. More recently, patient controlled narcotic transdermal patches and long acting bupivacaine pumps inserted into the subcutaneous tissue have been introduced and become more widely available for common use after procedures that employ a higher number or location of laparoscopic incisions, such as the laparoscopic Roux-en-Y gastric bypass and colon resections.

Laparoscopic Surgery in Special Conditions

In the early days of LC, conditions such as obesity, pregnancy, previous surgery, and cirrhosis were considered contraindications. Gradually techniques have evolved for dealing with most of these. While they are no longer considered contraindications, they are complicating factors. These are listed in Table 2-4 and will be considered briefly here.

Obesity

In the United States, nearly 61% of adult are classified as overweight and another 27% obese. Obesity causes and exacerbates a multitude of problems including hypertension, diabetes, sleep apnea, venous stasis disease, coronary artery disease, and hyperlipidemias. These obesity-related comorbidities account for nearly 300,000 to 325,000 deaths in the United States each year. Consequently these patients signify a group of higher risk individuals for general anesthesia. Hence, special consideration to planning for any laparoscopic procedure in this patient group becomes more essential.

Before surgery, all patients should undergo a thorough preoperative anesthesia evaluation. Special attention should be

TABLE 2-4. FACTORS THAT MAY COMPLICATE OR INCREASE THE DIFFICULTY OF LAPAROSCOPIC SURGERY

Morbid obesity
Cirrhosis
Pregnancy
Previous surgery in the region

given to the presence of a difficult airway that may require advanced maneuvers like awake intubation and nasotracheal or fiberoptic intubation. The presence of sleep apnea as well as certain anatomic findings such as a short muscular neck should alert the anesthesiologist of a possible difficult airway.

Furthermore, these patients should undergo thorough laboratory testing including a complete blood count, basic metabolic panel, coagulation profile, and liver function testing. Thyroid function tests and an electrocardiogram should also be obtained if there is any evidence to suggest preexisting thyroid function abnormality or coronary artery disease. A chest X-ray should also be obtained if there is any evidence of preexisting pulmonary disease including obstructive sleep apnea, obesity hypoventilation syndrome, and asthma. Specialty medical consultations should be obtained in the event of any existing serious medical condition. As a rule, all morbidly obese patients should receive preoperative placement of compression devices and low-molecular weight heparin to prevent deep venous thrombosis. Preoperative antibiotics should also be administered to prevent postoperative wound complications.

Adequate patient positioning is the key to a successful laparoscopic procedure in the obese. All pressure points including the elbows, knees, and ankles should be adequately padded and strapped in place using tape or Velcro to avoid nerve compression injuries. A foot board facilitates placing the patient in extreme positions including the reverse Trendelenburg and side tilting of the bed. These maneuvers are crucial to provide adequate exposure in certain anatomic regions in the abdomen. For example, placing the patient in steep reverse Trendelenburg provides an excellent exposure to the right upper quadrant for the performance of a laparoscopic cholecystectomy when a generous omentum might obscure the view. Similarly, this position also provides an excellent view of the esophageal hiatus after adequate left liver lobe retraction, for the performance of hiatal dissection for an antireflux or bariatric surgical procedure.

Trocar placement follows the similar principle of the "rule of triangulation." In addition, when operating on a morbidly obese patient, extra-long trocars should be available in case the patient's body habitus and the thickness of the abdominal wall prevents adequate placement of a normal length trocar. The use of non-bladed trocars in this patient group is suggested to avoid development of a trocar site hernia in the future. As a general rule, these trocar sites do not require closure unless they are 10 mm or larger in diameter and when placed in the midline. Closure of port sites in a morbidly obese patient could be challenging and require the use of special fascial closure devices. In addition, most of these non-bladed or dilating trocars are ribbed to prevent dislodgement during introduction of endomechanical devices, which could be a source of surgeon frustration and extra time spent in the operating room.

Angled laparoscopes are the key to a successful laparoscopic procedure. These include the 30- and 45-degree scopes that are the armamentarium of an advanced laparoscopic surgeon and provide excellent visualization, especially around blind corners. Extra long laparoscopes may be required when dealing with an obese patient with a deep chest cavity. This is sometimes essential for performing supra-mesocolic procedures, such as esophageal or gastric resection and bariatric surgical procedures. Creation of a pneumoperitoneum can be efficiently achieved using the Veress needle in the upper abdominal quadrants, although this approach should be used cautiously in a previously operated abdomen. The chances of an iatrogenic injury can be minimized with the use of optical trocars that allow placement under direct laparoscopic vision.

Obese patients already have elevated intraabdominal pressures and will commonly require higher insufflation pressures to achieve a pneumoperitoneum. Generally, a pneumoperitoneum to a pressure of 18 mmHg can be safely created to provide adequate visualization of the peritoneal cavity.

Pregnancy

Laparoscopy was first used for the evaluation of acute abdominal pain in pregnancy in 1980 by gynecologists. There was much controversy then as there is now, due to the high rate of complications and mortality. In the next decade, newer equipment and a better understanding of the physiology of the mother and fetus during the procedure made it safer for laparoscopy in pregnancy.

The major advantages of minimally invasive surgery can also be utilized in the treatment of surgical disorders of the pregnant patient. With advancements in laparoscopic surgery, its use in pregnant patients is now becoming widely accepted. Any surgeon treating the pregnant patient must have a thorough understanding of the physiology of the pregnant patient and risks and benefits of laparoscopic surgery. The most commonly reported laparoscopic procedures performed during pregnancy include laparoscopic cholecystectomy, appendectomy, diagnostic laparoscopy for bowel obstruction, and the treatment of associated gynecological pathologies including adnexal mass, ovarian torsion, ovarian cystectomy, and the management of an ectopic pregnancy.

Lachman et al. analyzed 518 pregnant patients undergoing surgery and found that laparoscopic cholecystectomy was the commonest (45%), followed by adnexal surgery (34%) and appendectomy (15%). The possible drawbacks of a laparoscopic exploration are possible injury to the uterus during Veress needle insertion, potential reduction of uterine blood flow secondary to increased intraabdominal pressure, risk of CO_2 absorption to the mother and child, and the technical difficulty of laparoscopic surgery. Physiologic and anatomic changes occurring during pregnancy introduce certain risks unique to the gravid patient. The potential risks include poor visualization due to the gravid uterus, uterine injury during trocar placement, decreased uterine blood flow or premature labor from the increased intraabdominal pressure, and increased fetal acidosis or other unknown effects due to CO_2 from pneumoperitoneum.

Decreased uterine blood flow from pneumoperitoneum remains hypothetical. It is postulated that this is unlikely to be a major concern given the frequent pressure alternations induced during maternal Valsalva, coughing, and straining. Furthermore, it is maintained that a pneumoperitoneum may well be safer and better tolerated than manual uterine retraction during open appendectomy or cholecystectomy. Fetal hemodynamic abnormalities (tachycardia and hypertension) that can potentially occur are generally attributed to fetal hypercarbia. The latter can be easily reversed by maintaining mild maternal respiratory alkalosis. Monitoring maternal arterial blood gases has proven superior to maternal capnography in this regard.

Patient positioning in a pregnant patient by far remains one of the most important factors in determining an adequate fetal circulation. In the supine position, compression of the inferior vena cava may cause decreased venous return and reduced cardiac output. The ideal position is the lateral recumbent position, as it tends to increase the maternal cardiac output by nearly 20% and the increased venous return from the lower limbs reduces the risk of deep vein thrombosis. Nonetheless, hypovolemia can easily occur and will cause decreased cardiac output with decreased placental perfusion. Strict replacement of intravascular volume is also essential during the course of the procedure.

Pregnancy also affects the maternal pulmonary function. For example, as pregnancy progresses, functional residual capacity and residual volume decreases due to an elevated diaphragm. The blood has an increased oxygen-carrying capacity and increased oxygen consumption that can lead to hypoxemia. Hence, there tends to be a chronic state of mild respiratory alkalosis that has to be maintained during surgery.

Another important change relevant to fetal well-being is the maternal acid-base status. Carbon dioxide rapidly diffuses between maternal-fetal circulations and during laparoscopy, and CO_2 in the maternal circulation may increase, partly due to CO_2 insufflation. Thus, there is all the more need to keep pneumoperitoneal pressures as low as possible in all laparoscopic procedures. If partial pressure of carbon dioxide (pCO_2) increases to more than 40 mmHg, decreased removal of fetal CO_2 occurs, leading to severe fetal acidosis. This can be overcome by hyperventilating the lungs during surgery, therefore maintaining a slight respiratory alkalosis. Capnography is adequate to monitor CO_2 levels in routine cases. However, for prolonged and difficult cases, serial maternal arterial blood gas determinations are necessary.

The motility of the gastrointestinal tract is also affected by hormonal changes during pregnancy. Gastroesophageal reflux is common in pregnancy due to decreased lower esophageal sphincter tone, delayed gastric emptying, and mechanical compression by the enlarging uterus. Nasogastric tube suction and strict airway management is mandatory for all pregnant patients undergoing laparoscopic surgery to prevent aspiration pneumonitis. Pro-phylactic antibiotics are used in all cases because pregnant women are mildly immunocompromised.

Gaining access to the intraabdominal cavity remains a controversial issue in pregnant patients undergoing laparoscopic exploration. The safest technique appears to be an open Hasson port placement. However, in the early part of the first trimester, creation of the pneumoperitoneum via a Veress needle access in the upper abdominal quadrants has been reported and may be deemed feasible. The consideration to gain access using these different maneuvers also largely depends on the expertise of the laparoscopist along with duration of pregnancy.

Despite concerns, good outcomes using laparoscopy in pregnancy have increasingly been reported. In one review, the rates of fetal loss and other complications, as well as the length of the procedure, were similar for laparoscopic surgery and open appendectomy. Another source demonstrated the feasibility of laparoscopic surgery during all trimesters; others have described it as safe during the first two trimesters and generally contraindicated during the third. The second trimester has been reported the safest for performing laparoscopy.

Previously Operated Abdomen

Laparoscopy has become the mainstay of surgical treatment of common surgical disorders including acute appendicitis and acute cholecystitis. However, previous abdominal surgery has been considered to be a contraindication for laparoscopic surgery. Although this may be true in certain instances, several reports have discussed the impact and safety of laparoscopic procedures in a previously operated abdomen. In fact, laparoscopic management may become the standard of care for all morbidly obese patients needing surgical exploration and patients with recurrent ventral and inguinal hernias, as these groups of patients benefit most from a minimally invasive approach.

With advances in laparoscopic skills and instruments, previous abdominal surgery has become a relative, but not an absolute, contraindication to laparoscopic surgery. Laparoscopic cholecystectomy is one of the most commonly performed laparoscopic procedures in the United States. Several studies reporting patients undergoing LC after previous abdominal surgery have demonstrated that this procedure is feasible and without an increased risk of complications. In other reports, however, previous abdominal surgery, especially upper abdominal surgery, has been associated with increased conversion to open surgery and increased postoperative complication rates for LC. It is important to classify previous abdominal surgery as upper and lower explorations as patients requiring a laparoscopic exploration of a previously unexplored compartment appear to be at similar risk for iatrogenic injury. This is especially true for patients who have undergone a previous lower abdominal surgery. These patients are often women, because of the percentage of lower abdominal surgeries that are cesarean sections and gynecologic operations.

One major concern about laparoscopic exploration after previous abdominal surgery is the risk of bowel or vessel injury during the insertion of the Veress needle or placement of the first trocar. Because adhesion formation due to previous abdominal surgery is difficult to predict preoperatively, it may be advisable to use an open Hasson technique for insertion of the first trocar in patients with previous abdominal surgery. Another concern in laparoscopic exploration following a previous abdominal surgery is the need for adhesiolysis. Laparoscopic adhesiolysis in itself may be associated with an increased risk of conversion, intraoperative complications, and longer operative time. The expertise and the experience of the operating surgeon plays a crucial role in determining whether laparoscopic exploration after a previous open exploration is feasible in this group of patients. In conclusion, several reports show that previous abdominal surgery, whether upper or lower, generally has no significant impact on laparoscopic exploration with respect to conversion rates, intraoperative and postoperative complication rates, operative time, and overall hospital stay.

Cirrhosis

Cirrhosis significantly increases the risk of any abdominal surgery because of coagulopathy, decreased hepatic reserve, and increased periportal collaterals. Cirrhotics have an increased incidence of gallstones, and most reports in this patient population concern LC. Although biliary surgery is particularly fraught with hazard in cirrhotics because of collateral vessels, LC seems to be neither more nor less safe than open cholecystectomy in patients with Childs-Pugh class A or B cirrhosis. Surgery in patients with Childs-Pugh class C cirrhosis carries a significant risk of death, and there are very little data on the use of laparoscopy in this patient population.

In conclusion, with careful patient selection and preoperative preparation, it has been possible to offer an endoscopic alternative for most patients in whom surgery is indicated. The chapters that follow detail specifics relative to each particular procedure.

General Considerations in Laparoscopic and Thoracoscopic Surgery

Ergonomics

Room layout and trocar placement can facilitate minimal access surgery or render it miserable at best, impossible at worst. Specific positioning tips for each surgical procedure are given in the chapters that follow, but some general advice will be given here. Usually, the surgeon stands directly across from the anticipated pathology; directly facing the primary monitor, which is arranged to provide an unobstructed and glare-free view. The laparoscope or thoracoscope should face in the same direction, and operating ports are positioned on both sides to allow access. Whenever possible, think of the port with the scope as your head and the two primary ports through which you will operate as your left and right hand. This will help you place these ports in a triangulated fashion on both sides of the scope. Allow sufficient distance between ports to avoid dueling instruments. Secure the patient to the table and thoroughly pad all pressure points, so that you can tilt the table as needed to use gravity to advantage. Some procedures (for example, laparoscopic splenectomy) are best performed in a lateral decubitus position; others, such as Nissen fundoplication, may be performed with the patient's legs spread to allow the surgeon to stand between the legs and face the hiatus directly. Regardless of patient position, the surgeon should be able to stand in a comfortable, relaxed stance and manipulate instruments freely. Repetitive stress injuries can occur, particularly if your position requires unnatural flexion or extension of your wrists as you operate. Instruments have generally been optimized for a certain size and physical build; surgeons who have much smaller or larger hands may have difficulties. If you find you are having problems, try different instruments and strive to adopt a body position that allows you to keep your wrists in a neutral position as you work.

Choice of Laparoscope

Excellent visibility is crucial. Laparoscopes are classified as straight or angled. Straight scopes look directly ahead, and are therefore simple to aim and use. Angled scopes are available in a series of preselected options: 30 degrees and 45 degrees are particularly popular. An angled scope allows you to effectively look around corners, a bit like a periscope, but requires some facility in use. If used incorrectly, the angle of the scope can actually hinder your visualization of a structure. For some procedures, it is essential. All minimal access surgeons should gain facility with the use of a variety of straight and angled scopes.

The ability to troubleshoot your equipment is essential, particularly if you perform laparoscopic procedures, such as LA, at night or with inexperienced teams. Flexible scopes and scopes with binocular vision are available but have not come into common use. Most surgeons compensate for the lack of depth perception by moving the tissue in question, palpating it with the tip of an instrument, examining it from several perspectives with an angled scope, or opting for a trial dissection.

Suturing and Knot-Tying

Facility with suturing and knot-tying are essential. Special needles have been developed for laparoscopic suturing, but many surgeons find that, with practice, a normal needle can be used. Figure 2-1 shows how a standard needle can be introduced into the abdomen. Excellent laparoscopic needle holders, capable of securely gripping the needle, are critical. These are available with gentle curves to facilitate needle passage (Fig. 2-2). Most surgeons perform intracorporeal instrument ties in a manner very similar to that used during open surgery (Fig. 2-3). The Aberdeen knot (Fig. 2-4) is an alternative that some use instead. Some surgeons place a clip over the knot of a tied suture for extra security. This also serves as a radiopaque marker.

Hand-Assisted Laparoscopy

Laparoscopic procedures can be performed completely via a laparoscopic approach (such as LC or LA), as laparoscopic-assisted procedures in which a small incision is made for specimen removal and/or anastomosis (such as laparoscopic right colon resection), or as hand-assisted procedures. In hand-assisted laparoscopy (HALS), a small incision is made during initial trocar placement. A special sealing device allows the surgeon

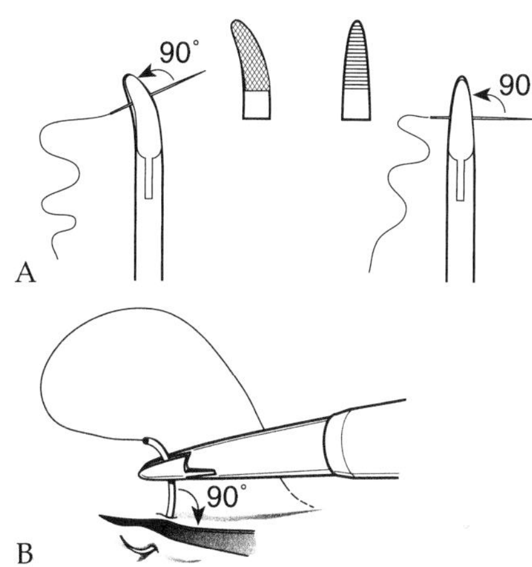

Fig. 2-2. A. Curved, tipped needle drivers give added flexibility to needle position. **B.** This allows the needle to always be at a right angle to the suture line.

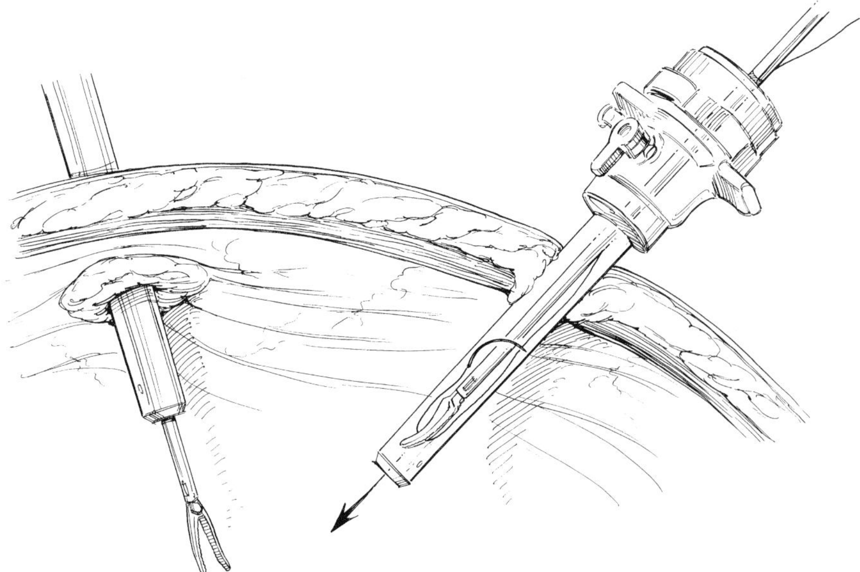

Fig. 2-1. A needle is inserted into the abdomen by grasping it 2 cm from the needle and placing it through an adequate-sized port. The assisting needle holder or grasper can then grasp the suture to prepare the needle for loading onto the suturing needle holder (right).

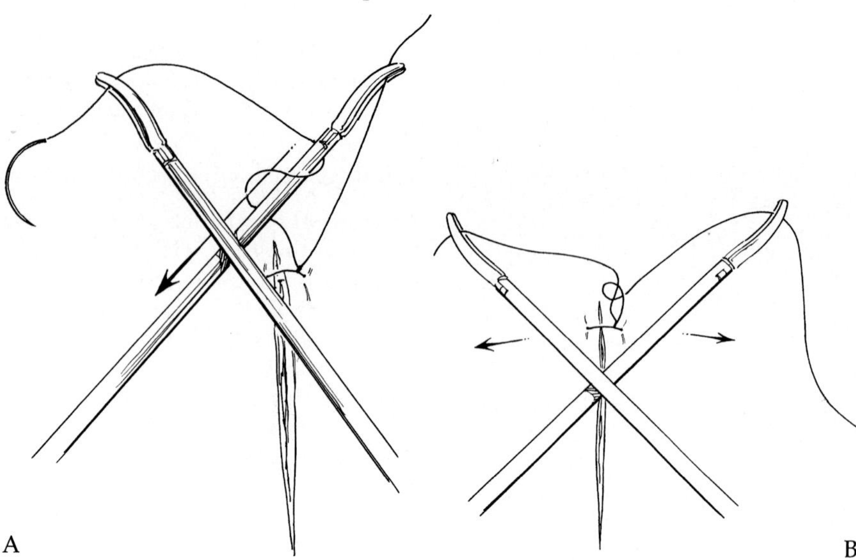

Fig. 2-3. Intracorporeal knot-tying with crossed needle drivers. **A.** The tail of the suture is placed away and to the right for subsequent easy grasping. With this technique, the right hand never has to release the suture. The tail is grasped with the left-hand grasper and pulled through the loop. **B.** The instruments are crossed right over left to place a second flat tie and complete the square knot. Subsequent throws can be similarly placed for reinforcement.

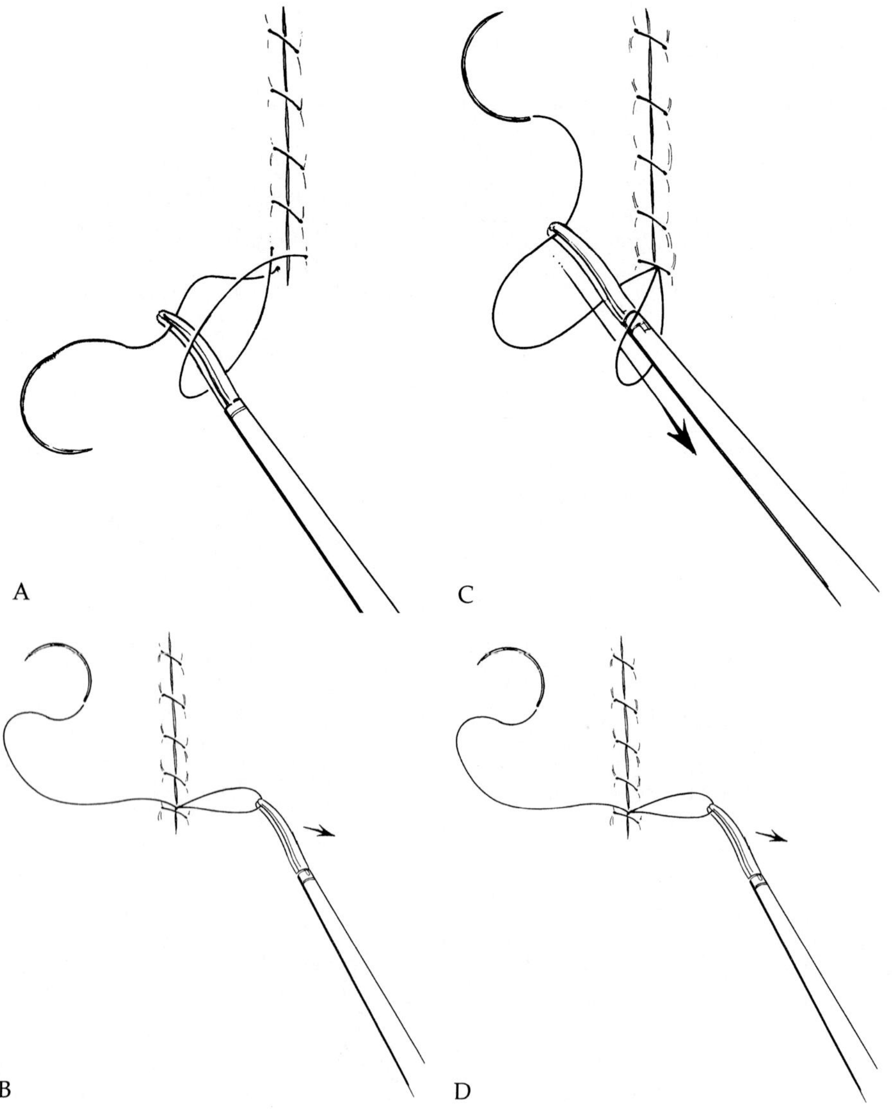

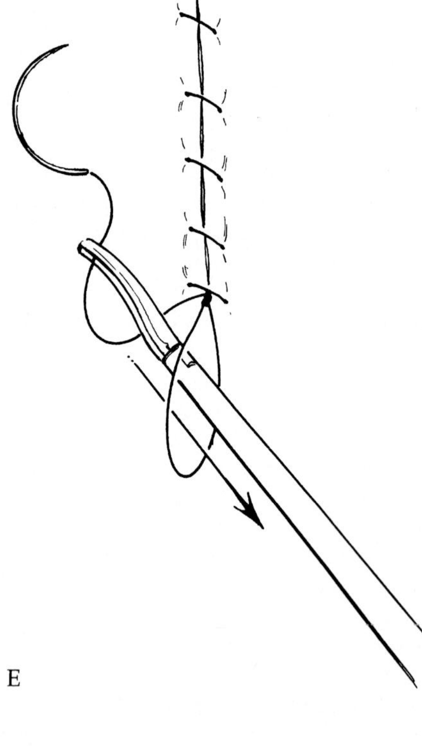

Fig. 2-4. An Aberdeen knot used to complete a running stitch. The needle end is grasped close to the tissue and pulled part way through the loop to create a knot. The Aberdeen knot is completed by pulling a loop of the needle side of the suture through to create a new loop every time. The needle side is then brought completely through the last loop to cinch the knot. (Adapted from Laws HL. Suturing Techniques. In: Arregui ME, Fitzgibbons RJ, Katkouda N, et al., eds. *Principles of laparoscopic surgery*. New York, Springer-Verlag 1995; 35–45.)

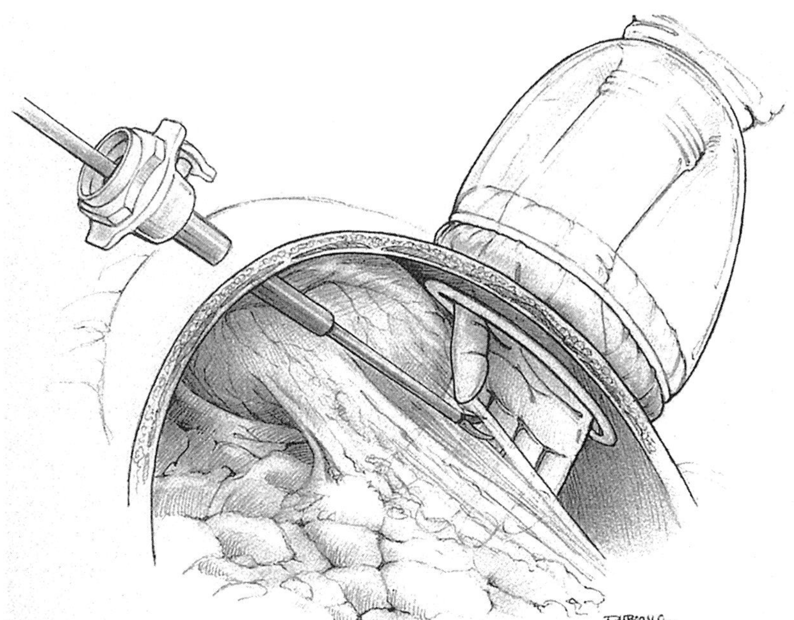

Fig. 2-5. Hand-assisted laparoscopic surgery (HALS) device in use. (From Czerniach DR, Novitsky YW, Litwin DEM. Hand-Assisted Approach to Splenectomy. In: Katkhouda N, ed. *Problems in general surgery: surgical diseases of the spleen.* Philadelphia: Lippincott Williams & Wilkins, 2002;19:36–47. Reprinted with permission.)

to insert a hand into the abdomen. This provides tactile feedback and the most effective retraction possible (Fig. 2-5).

CONSIDERATIONS IN FLEXIBLE ENDOSCOPIC PROCEDURES

In contrast to laparoscopy and thoracoscopy, flexible endoscopic procedures are commonly performed under a combination of topical anesthesia and conscious sedation. In conscious sedation, the patient retains protective mechanisms and is drowsy but arousable. This actually represents a kind of general anesthesia, such that careful preoperative assessment, procedural and postprocedure monitoring, and sufficient recovery are essential for safety.

SUGGESTED READING

Eypasch E, Sauerland S, Lefering R, et al. Laparoscopic versus open appendectomy: between evidence and common sense. *Dig Surg* 2002;19:518–522.

Fleisher LA. Risk indices: what is their value to the clinician and patient? *Anesthesiology* 2001;94:194–204.

Gilbert K, Larocque BJ, Patrick LT. Prospective evaluation of cardiac risk indices for patients undergoing non-cardiac surgery. *Ann Intern Med* 2000;133:356–359.

Naitoh T, Ganger M, Garcia-Ruiz A, et al. Hand-assisted laparoscopic digestive surgery provides safety and tactile sensation for malignancy or obesity. *Surg Endosc* 1999;13:157–160.

O'Malley C, Cunningham AJ. Physiologic changes during laparoscopy. *Anesthesiol Clin North Am* 2001;19:1–19.

Poggio JL, Rowland CM, Gores CJ, et al. A comparison of laparoscopic and open cholecystectomy in patients with compensated cirrhosis and symptomatic gallstone disease. *Surgery* 2000;127:405–411.

Practice Advisory for Preanesthesia Evaluation. A report by the American Society of Anesthesiologists Task-Force on Preanesthesia Evaluation. *Anesthesiology* 2002;96:485–496.

Shah JS, Bready LL. Anesthesia for thoracoscopy. *Anesthesiol Clin North Am* 2001;19:153–171.

Szegedi LL. Thoracic anesthesia: pathophysiology of one-lung ventilation. *Anesthesiol Clin North Am* 2001;19:435–453.

Physiologic Changes

Buunen M, Gholghesaei M, Veldkamp R. Stress response to laparoscopic surgery: a review. *Surg Endosc* 2004;18:1022–1028.

Demyttenaere S, Feldman LS, Fried GM. Effect of pneumoperitoneum on renal perfusion and function: A systematic review. *Surg Endosc* 2007;21:152–160.

Neuhaus SJ, Watson DI. Pneumoperitoneum and peritoneal surface changes: a review. *Surg Endosc* 2004;18:1316–1322.

Nguyen NT, Wolfe BM. The Physiologic Effects of Pneumoperitoneum in the Morbidly Obese. *Ann Surg* 2005;241(2):219–226.

Strickland AK, Martindale RG. The increased incidence of intraabdominal infections in laparoscopic procedures. Potential causes, postoperative management, and prospective innovations. *Surg Endosc* 2005;19:874–881.

Anesthesia

Alessandri F, Lijoi D, Mistrangelo E. Effect of presurgical local infiltration of levobupivacaine in the surgical field on postsurgical wound pain in laparoscopic gynecological surgery. *Acta Obstet Gynecol Scand* 2006;85(7):844–849.

American Society of Anesthesiologists Task Force on Sedation and Analgesia by Non-Anesthesiologists. Practice guidelines for sedation and analgesia by non-anesthesiologists. *Anesthesiology* 2002;96(4):1004–1017.

Eagle KA, Berger PB, Calkins H, et al. ACC/AHA guideline update for perioperative cardiovascular evaluation for noncardiac surgery: executive summary a report of the American College of Cardiology/American Heart Association Task Force on Practice Guidelines (Committee to Update the 1996 Guidelines on Perioperative Cardiovascular Evaluation for Noncardiac Surgery). *Circulation* 2002;105(10):1257–1267.

Gerges FJ, Kanazi GE, Jabbour-Khoury SI. Anesthesia for laparoscopy: a review. *J Clin Anesth* 2006;18(1):67–78.

Hanly EJ, Fuentes JM, Aurora AR. Carbon dioxide pneumoperitoneum prevents mortality from sepsis. *Surg Endosc* 2006;20(9):1482–1487. Epub 2006 Jul 24.

Lawrence VA, Cornell JE, Smetana GW. Strategies to reduce postoperative pulmonary complications after noncardiothoracic surgery: systematic review for the American College of Physicians. *Ann Intern Med* 2006;144(8):596–608.

Nesek-Adam V, Grizelj-Stojcic E, Rasic Z. A comparison of dexamethasone, metoclopramide, and their combination in the prevention of postoperative nausea and vomiting after laparoscopic cholecystectomy. *Surg Endosc* 2007;21(4):607–612. Epub 2007 Feb 7.

Obesity

Frezza EE, Shebani KO, Robertson J. Morbid obesity causes chronic increase of intraabdominal pressure. *Dig Dis Sci* 2007;52(4):1038–1041. Epub 2007 Mar 7.

Kurzer E, Leveille R, Bird V. Obesity as a risk factor for complications during laparoscopic surgery for renal cancer: multivariate analysis. *J Endourol* 2006;20(10):794–799.

Simopoulos C, Botaitis S, et al. The contribution of acute cholecystitis, obesity, and previous abdominal surgery on the outcome of laparoscopic cholecystectomy. *Am Surg* 2007;73(4):371–376.

Pregnancy

Al-Fozan H, Tulandi T. Safety and risks of laparoscopy in pregnancy. *Curr Opin Obstet Gynecol* 2002;14:375–379.

Amos JD, Schorr SJ, Norman PF, et al. Laparoscopic surgery during pregnancy. *Am J Surg* 1996;171:435–437.

Bisharah M, Tulandi T. Laparoscopic surgery in pregnancy. *Clin Obstet Gynecol* 2003;46:92–97.

Chawla S, Vardhan S, Jog SS. Appendicitis during pregnancy. *MJAFI* 2003;59:212–215.

Conron RW Jr, Abbruzzi K, Cochrane SO, et al. Laparoscopic procedures in pregnancy. *Am Surg* 1999;65:259–263.

Lachman E, Schienfeld A, Voss E, et al. Pregnancy and laparoscopic surgery. *J Am Assoc Gynecol Laparosc* 1999;6:347–351.

Manmoodian S. Appendicitis complicating pregnancy. *South Med J* 1992;85:19–24.

Palanivelu C, Rangarajan M, Parthasarathi R. Laparoscopic appendectomy in pregnancy: a case series of seven patients. *JSLS* 2006; 10:321–325.

Previously Operated Abdomen

Akyurek N, Salman B, Irkorucu O. Laparoscopic cholecystectomy in patients with previous abdominal surgery. *J Soc Laparoendosc Surg* 2005;9:178–183.

Curet MJ. Special problems in laparoscopic surgery: previous abdominal surgery, obesity, and pregnancy. *Surg Clin North Am* 2000; 80:1093–1100.

Diez J, Delbene R, Ferreres A. The feasibility of laparoscopic cholecystectomy in patients with previous abdominal surgery. *HPB Surg* 1998;10:353–356.

Karayiannakis AJ, Polychronidis A, Perente S. Laparoscopic cholecystectomy in patients with previous upper or lower abdominal surgery. *Surg Endosc* 2004;18:97–101.

Liu SI, Siewert B, Raptopoulos V, et al. Factors associated with conversion to laparotomy in patients undergoing laparoscopic appendectomy. *J Am Coll Surg* 2002;194:298–305.

Schirmer BD, Dix J, Schmieg RE Jr, et al. The impact of previous abdominal surgery on outcome following laparoscopic cholecystectomy. *Surg Endosc* 1995;9:1085–1089.

Wu JM, Lin HF, Chen KH, et al. Impact of previous abdominal surgery on laparoscopic appendectomy for acute appendicitis. *Surg Endosc* 2007;21(4):570–573. Epub 2006 Nov 14.

COMMENTARY

It is the hope of the editors that the number of pages dedicated to patient selection and preoperative preparation is not a relative indication of the importance of the topic. Rather, it is our hope that the importance of excellent surgical judgment and patient preparation permeates the entire book. The authors selected to prepare this chapter have condensed a broad and difficult topic into a concise and helpful overview.

The times during which a surgeon, internist, and anesthesiologist work independently without communication to prepare a patient for surgery should be long past. This antiquated silo mentality does not lead to proper patient care or the safest possible operation or perioperative experience. Whether the topic is postoperative nausea and vomiting (PONV) and the need to address two of the three main nausea centers pharmacologically or the appropriate level of blood pressure control through alpha-blockade in the patient presenting with a pheochromocytoma, communication between specialties is needed in order to optimize patient care and outcomes.

The importance of a thorough history and physical exam as the patient is prepared for surgery is emphasized from the earliest days of medical school. Additionally, documentation of these findings in the proper verbiage has recently taken on increased importance. The accurate description of our patients and all of their comorbidities has become an important part of the evaluation of our surgical outcomes, potentially impacting reimbursement or, the case of credentials, the ability to perform specific procedures. Opportunities are emerging for small increases in reimbursement for counseling patients regarding smoking cessation or screening patients for drug and alcohol addiction.

The myriad of tests and procedures available in the preoperative evaluation and preparation of the surgical patient must be applied in a logical manner with an eye towards available evidence that these test results and procedures will lead to better patient care. Inappropriate tests and procedures are expensive, time-consuming, and inconvenient for patients and they can be dangerous. When combined with technical skills and expertise, the proper preparation of surgical patients provides the greatest opportunity for excellent surgical care.

WSE

Tools of the Trade

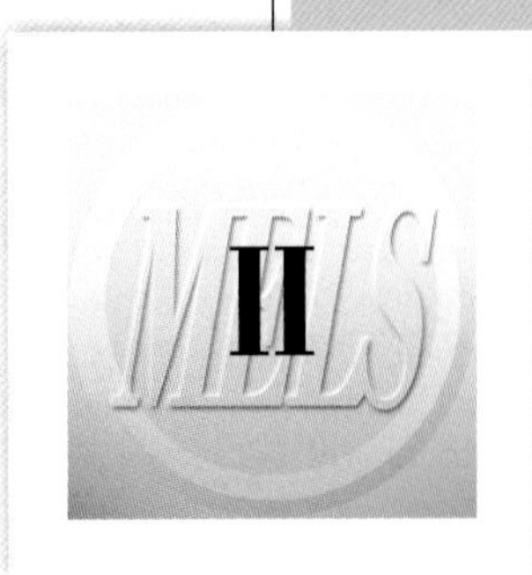

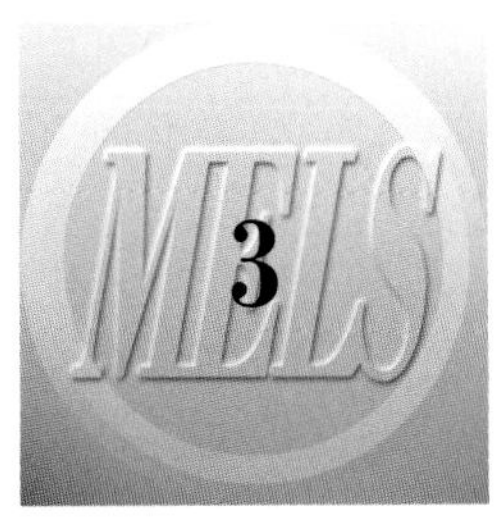

New Technology in Endoscopy

JONATHAN P. PEARL AND JEFFREY M. MARKS

INTRODUCTION

Although the basic platform of flexible endoscopes is similar to that devised 50 years ago, numerous recent technological advances are becoming available to the endoscopist. Novel self-propelled endoscopes and shape-conforming overtubes may permit simpler colonoscopic exams. An abundance of new imaging modalities may facilitate early detection of dysplasia and other pathologic entities. While many of these techniques remain investigational and are currently in clinical trials to determine patient benefit, it is clear that as endoscopic technology and its indications progress in tandem, the endoscopist's armamentarium will continue to expand.

Standard Endoscope Technology

The flexible fiber-optic endoscope was first introduced in 1957. Videoendoscopy has replaced fiber optics (although light sources remain fiber-optic), but the central design of the endoscope has remained largely unchanged. A plastic sheath surrounds the optical, directional, irrigation, and insufflation mechanisms. Four-way tip deflection using dual controls, first available in 1970, permits up to 210 degrees upward deflection, 100 degrees downward deflection, and 90 degrees left and right deflection. Outer diameters range from 4.3 to 11.3 mm, and instrument channels range from 2.8 to 4.2 mm in diameter. Some of the larger diameter therapeutic endoscopes have dual working chambers for instrumentation.

Videoendoscopy permits electronic transmission of real-time images via a charge-coupled device (CCD). The CCD is composed of multiple solid-state image sensors made of silicon semiconductor material. The image sensors are divided into numerous discrete photosites, known as picture elements (pixels), with a higher density of pixels producing sharper images. The image is transmitted to a video processor and subsequently to a television screen for viewing, in contrast to viewing through the scope with fiber-optic technology. The progression to video technology has permitted education of trainees and allowed for advanced therapeutics, as assistants can fully participate by viewing the television monitor.

Newer generation endoscopes produce high-resolution images by combining white light with high-resolution CCDs. With some CCDs composed of up to one million pixels, the quality of the displayed image in high-resolution endoscopy allows for precise examination of fine mucosal details. The role of high-resolution technology for early detection of dysplastic lesions is currently being investigated.

LOOP-RESISTING MECHANISMS

One of the impediments of modern endoscopy, especially in the colonoscopy, is the formation of undesired loops in the shaft of a flexible scope. Loop formation may prohibit expeditious and safe passage to the cecum by transmitting the force of insertion to the colon wall or mesentery rather than to forward progression. Common adjunct maneuvers used to combat loop formation are the application of external abdominal pressure and alteration of patient positioning. Although oftentimes successful, these maneuvers are labor-intensive and may hinder the efficiency of the endoscopy unit. Two technical advances aim to prevent loop formation: variable stiffness endoscopes and shape-locking overtubes.

Variable Stiffness Endoscopes

Conventional colonoscopes have a static level of column strength throughout the length of the insertion tube. The column strength determines the amount of buckling of the instrument that occurs during insertion and the level of elasticity that remains during reduction of loops. Variable stiffness endoscopes permit alteration of the column strength through an adjustable tensioning coil. The aim is to produce a colonoscope with a flexible tip for negotiating tight angulations and a stiffer proximal portion to resist loop formation. Variable stiffness endoscopes are equipped with a stiffness control ring located just distal to the control mechanisms. The stiffness control ring regulates a tensioning wire that runs the length of the insertion tube and allows for variable degrees of stiffness.

During routine use of the variable stiffness mechanism, the colonoscope remains at maximum flexibility for traversing the sigmoid colon. At that point, any loops are reduced using torque and withdrawal maneuvers and then the stiffness is increased to prevent further loop formation. If a loop again forms, the stiffness is zeroed and the loop reduced. Again, the stiffness is augmented for passage to the cecum. Finally, the stiffness is returned to the default setting for withdrawal.

The data from studies comparing variable stiffness colonoscopes to conventional scopes are inconclusive. Some studies report faster cecal intubation using variable stiffness endoscopes with less need for adjunct maneuvers, while other similar studies report no significant differences. The technique appears safe, with few reports of complications directly attributable to the variable stiffness mechanism. Despite the inconclusiveness of the clinical studies, there may be some advantage to using pediatric variable stiffness colonoscopes in patients with difficult anatomy.

Shape-Locking Devices

Overtubes have long been employed in attempts to reduce sigmoid looping during colonoscopy, but these earlier devices are considered cumbersome by most users and may cause perforation. To overcome some of these shortcomings, a new generation overtube that converts from a flexible to a rigid state on demand has been developed. The ShapeLock Endoscopic Guide (USGI Medical, Inc.; San Clemente, CA) consists of a reusable skeleton of multiple titanium links, a disposable inner plastic lining, an atraumatic foam tip, and a disposable smooth external skin. A squeeze handle at the base of the device converts it from a flexible mode to a rigid mode. The shape-locking device is made in 40 and 60 cm lengths with an inner diameter of 20 mm.

In proposed usage, the device is back-loaded over the insertion tube of a colonoscope. The scope is passed through the sigmoid colon, and any existing loops are reduced. The shape locking overtube is then advanced while in flexible mode and subsequently converted to rigid mode. The aim is to transmit the force of insertion to forward propulsion of the colonoscope, protecting the wall of the large bowel.

A small clinical study has been reported using the shape-locking device. No device-related complications were noted, but the optimal strategy for employing the device was uncertain. Additionally, a separate report extolled the ability to rapidly redeploy the colonoscope when using the shape-locking device should specimen retrieval and reinvestigation of the colon be necessary.

New Scope Technology

While the construction of standard endoscopes remained largely unchanged over many decades, today novel scope designs are being developed to either simplify colonoscopic examinations or enhance mucosal visualization. Other than double-balloon enteroscopy, these technologies are chiefly limited to small clinical trials, but their application could gain momentum in the coming years.

Self-Propelled Colonoscopes

In an effort to simplify the process of colonoscopic screening, self-propelled endoscopes are in development. The Aer-O-Scope (GI View, Ltd; Ramat Gan Israel) is a user-independent, self-propelled, self-navigating colonoscope (Fig. 3-1). The device consists of a disposable rectal introducer, supply cable, and a scope embedded within a scanning balloon. The introducer is inserted, and

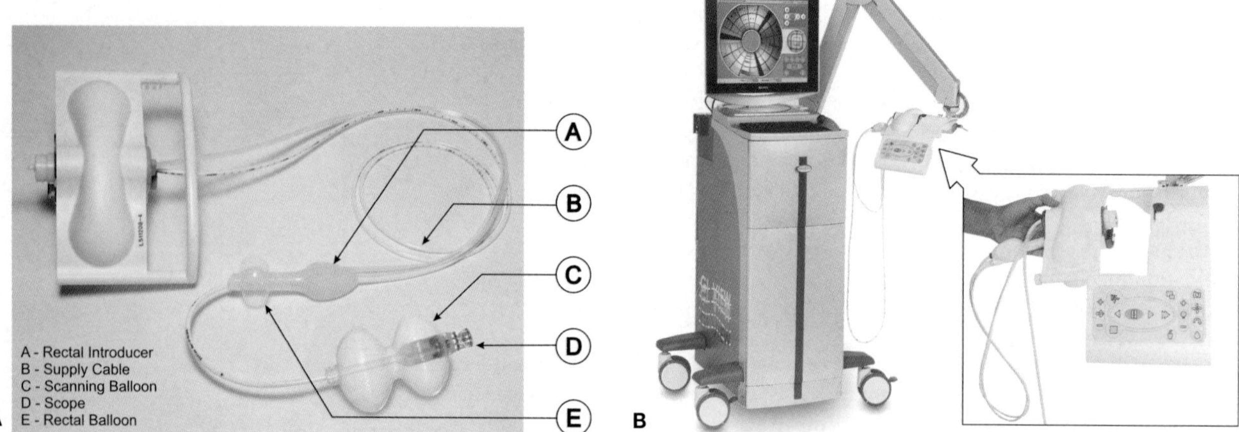

Fig. 3-1. A. The disposable Aer-O-Scope self-propelled colonoscope. **B.** The multipurpose Aer-O-Scope personal computer system. (Photographs used with permission from GI View, Ltd.)

the scope with its scanning balloon is passed through the hollow tube of the introducer. The silicone balloon at the introducer is inflated at the anus, forming a seal to prevent leakage of insufflated CO_2. The soft scanning balloon is inflated, and gas is insufflated between the balloons, thereby generating adequate pressure to propel the device. For safety, pressures within, in front of, and behind the balloon are continuously monitored and adjusted through a computer algorithm. Once the cecum is reached, the pressure in and behind the balloon is reduced while the area in front of the balloon is infused with CO_2, thereby creating the pressure gradient to reverse the scope and examine the colon. The captured images are transmitted through the supply cable, displayed in real time on the monitor, and recorded on a compact disk.

A small pilot study examined the proof of concept of the Aer-O-Scope. In a cohort of young volunteers (ages 18 to 43 years), the device successfully reached the cecum in 83% of cases. There were no device-related complications. The device contains no working channel for therapeutic interventions; therefore it is intended for screening purposes only.

Another self-propelled colonoscope, the ColonoSight (Stryker Corporation; Kalamazoo, MI) employs air-assisted propulsion in a disposable system. A pneumatic mechanism generates the pressure to create the forward force while an operator directs the scope using handles. The system uses light-emitting diode optics, rather than video or fiber optics, and has disposable working channels. A pilot study for the ColonoSight reported intubation of the cecum in 88% of cases at a mean time of 12 minutes without any device-related complications.

Computer-Controlled Partially Automated Colonoscope

The NeoGuide Endoscopy System (NeoGuide Systems; San Jose, CA) is designed to avoid loop formation by adjusting an endoscope's insertion tube to match the configuration of the colon. The distal tip is guided similarly to conventional colonoscopy, and the insertion tube is composed of multiple steerable segments connected to an actuation control unit. Using a sophisticated computer program, data from physician-determined tip orientation and insertion depth is used to create a three-dimensional map of the colon. This, in turn, permits computer control of the shape and orientation of the insertion tube, using motors embedded within the system's console.

Use of this guidance system is reportedly transparent to the endoscopist. The distal tip is controlled by the physician, while the system automatically constructs the three-dimensional map and configures the insertion tube. The scope includes a working channel that permits instrument exchange, and the guidance system can be disabled for colonoscopy in the passive mode. The system has yet to be tested in a clinical trial.

Miniature Auxiliary Imaging Device

To detect mucosal lesions situated behind haustral folds, an auxiliary imaging device has been developed. The Third Eye Retroscope (Avantis Medical Systems, Inc.; Sunnyvale, CA) is passed through the working channel of a standard colonoscope. The 3.4-mm device then provides a retroflexed image of haustral folds, a perspective that might be absent when using a forward-viewing colonoscope. In an *in vitro* study, the auxiliary imaging device was shown to enhance the detection of polyps located on the proximal aspect of haustral folds.

Double-Balloon Enteroscopy

The most frequent methods of small bowel endoscopic examination are push enteroscopy and capsule endoscopy. The technical demands of push enteroscopy often result in forceful pressure exerted on the small bowel. Capsule endoscopy allows examination of much of the small bowel mucosa, but interventions are not possible. To remedy these shortcomings, double-balloon enteroscopy was developed. The double-balloon system consists of a dedicated 200-cm endoscope with a balloon, mounted distally, combined with a 145-cm overtube with a balloon. The purpose of the overtube is to prevent stretching of the small bowel through which the enteroscope has already traversed. The balloons, whose pressure measures 45 mmHg when inflated, serve to maintain the position of the scope and overtube.

During insertion for upper enteroscopy, the scope and overtube are concurrently advanced into the proximal small intestine. A series of balloon inflations, deflations, and system advancements permits progression through the small bowel. After advancing, the system is gently withdrawn to pleat the small bowel onto the overtube. Balloon fixation and shortening maneuvers continue for up to half the length of the small bowel.

Double-balloon enteroscopy has many distinct advantages. The system can be inserted orally or per anus in order to examine the jejunum and ileum. Working channels are available that permit biopsy, polypectomy, and hemostasis. The distal tip is very maneuverable, and a specific segment of small bowel can be repeatedly inspected by inflating the balloon on the overtube and sequentially advancing and withdrawing the endoscope.

Endoscopists dedicated to the practice of double-balloon enteroscopy report favorable results. Clinical studies have documented an 88% success rate in the complete examination of the small bowel in total enteroscopy (upper and lower) cases. The technique has been used in the diagnosis and treatment of small bowel strictures, tumors, and hemorrhage. There are few reported complications, with a single case of perforation noted among 178 cases in one large series. Thus, when mastered, the technique of small bowel enteroscopy can be useful in the detection and treatment of suspected small bowel mucosal lesions.

Imaging Advances

There have been many recent advances in endoscopic imaging techniques. The purpose of most of these techniques is the early detection of dysplasia, which might elude standard endoscopic visualization. Clinical use of new imaging is limited principally to specialized centers, but future widespread application of an imaging method for early dysplasia detection is a certainty.

Chromoendoscopy

The technique of chromoendoscopy is used extensively in Asian countries, but has lagged behind in Europe and the United States. In chromoendoscopy, conventional videoendoscopes are used to examine gut mucosa after application of a vital dye. Little specialized equipment is necessary, except for a catheter to evenly spray the staining solution.

The aim of chromoendoscopy is to detect subtle mucosal abnormalities. Commonly used agents include Lugol's solution, methylene blue, indigo carmine, Congo red, and phenol red. Both Lugol's solution and methylene blue are absorbed by the secretory cells of the gastrointestinal tract. Indigo carmine is not absorbed by cells, but accumulates in pits and valleys,

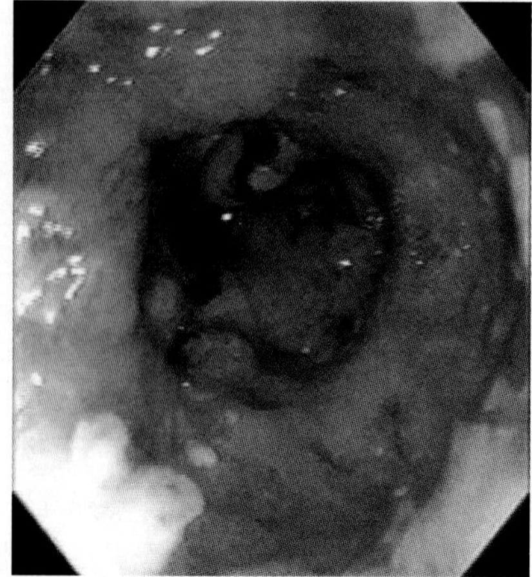

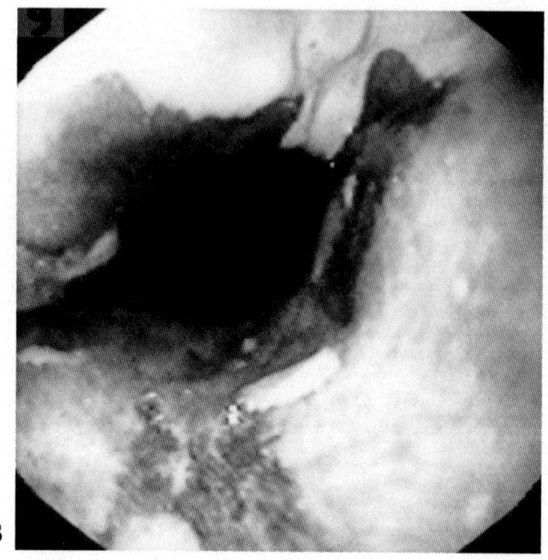

Fig. 3-2. A. Endoscopic view of esophagogastric junction with findings suspicious for Barrett esophagus. **B.** Endoscopic view after application of methylene blue. The cells harboring intestinal metaplasia take up the dye more readily than the surrounding mucosa. (Photographs courtesy of Amitabh Chak, MD.)

thereby highlighting mucosal architecture. Both Congo red and phenol red react to changes in acid secretion, although Congo red is no longer approved by the Food and Drug Administration.

A 2% to 3% solution of potassium iodide (Lugol's solution) reacts with glycogen in keratinized squamous epithelium. Normal squamous epithelium stains a deep brown, but inflammation, dysplasia, and carcinoma do not stain because of a lack of glycogen. Lugol's solution has been shown to be effective in detecting Barrett esophagus as well as screening for squamous cell carcinoma of the esophagus.

One of the most common uses of chromoendoscopy is the application of methylene blue for detection of Barrett esophagus (Fig. 3-2). Before using methylene blue, intestinal surface mucus is removed using N-acetylcysteine. Next, methylene blue is applied, and the area is vigorously irrigated with saline. Cells with intestinal metaplasia take up methylene blue readily, but normal gastric mucosa and esophageal squamous epithelium do not. Chromoendoscopy with methylene blue has been shown to enhance the detection of Barrett esophagus, even in patients whose esophagogastric junction appeared normal on conventional endoscopy.

Another significant use of chromoendoscopy is the detection of nonpolypoid colonic lesions. Flat adenomas and depressed colonic mucosal lesions may be difficult to detect due to their subtle findings, yet depressed lesions may harbor up to a 30% chance of malignancy. Chromoendoscopy, typically with a 0.5% solution of methylene blue and a conventional endoscope, aids in the detection of the subtle depressions, disruption in vasculature, and color changes associated with nonpolypoid colonic lesions.

Magnification Endoscopy

In magnification endoscopy, a cap with a magnifying lens is fitted to the tip of an endoscope. The mucosa in contact with the lens is thus magnified without impairing the maneuverability of the scope. Degrees of magnification range from 1.5 to 115× and can be changed on the scope by turning a dial at the hand controls. Some specialized scopes are equipped with a motor-driven lens that is controlled by foot pedals. This feature changes the focal distance of the mucosa, thereby providing for magnification.

The technique of magnification endoscopy is frequently used in conjunction with chromoendoscopy (Fig. 3-3). Chromoendoscopy is used for the broad surveillance of the mucosa followed by a focused examination of suspicious lesions in magnification mode. This combined examination has been reported in case series to enhance the detection of Barrett esophagus, chronic gastritis, Helicobacter pylori infection, gastric dysplasia, and early gastric cancer. Despite the favorable reports, the data are inconclusive regarding improvement in patient outcomes.

Confocal Fluorescence Microendoscopy

Standard endoscopy uses white light to visualize a large surface area with relatively low resolution. In contrast, confocal endoscopy aims to visualize the mucosa and submucosa with subcellular resolution, a technique deemed optical biopsy. The process of confocal magnification reduces out-of-focus light from above and below the focal plane at a magnification of 1000×. The system is designed to measure tissue fluorescence; therefore an exogenous fluorophore (a molecule that causes another molecule to be fluorescent) is usually administered. Varying depths of tissue are examined by altering the focal plane, and images from different depths are stacked together to create an optical slice of tissue; thus, the term optical biopsy.

Confocal microendoscopy may serve to complement conventional endoscopy. In current practice, a confocal probe is either passed through a working channel or

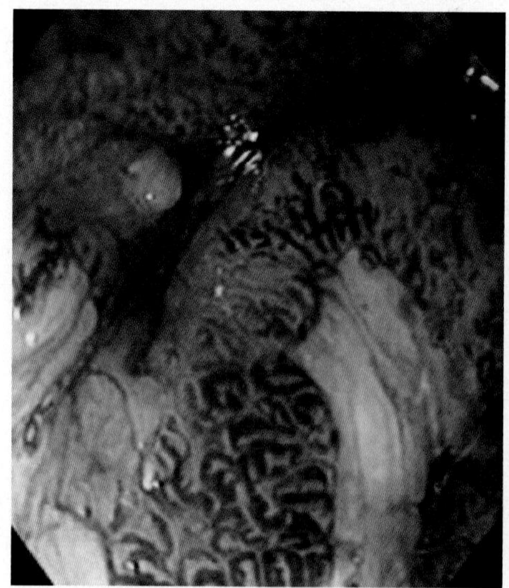

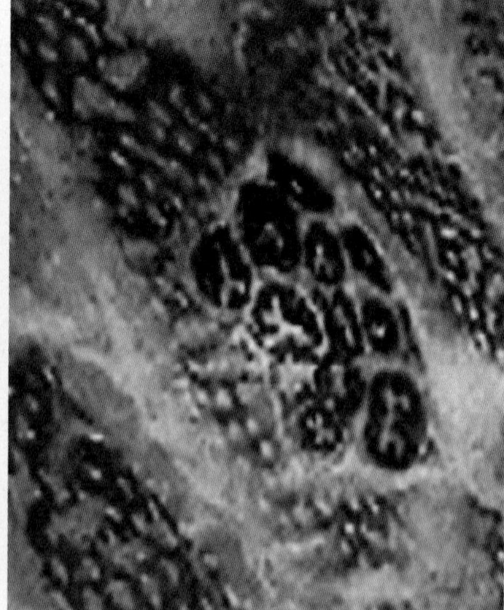

Fig. 3-3. Magnification endoscopy combined with chromoscopy. Both the standard magnification (35×) and high-magnification (115×) views of the esophagogastric junction depict islands of intestinal metaplasia. (Photographs courtesy of Amitabh Chak, MD.)

attached to the end of an endoscope. Intravenous fluorescein and topical acriflavine are administered to create the fluorescence contrast necessary, similar to hematoxylin and eosin in light microscopy. Tissue depths from 100 to 300 μm are interrogated at a 488-nm excitation wavelength.

Confocal fluorescence microendoscopy is an emerging technology not yet studied in large-scale trials. There are reports of a high correlation between optical biopsy and tissue biopsy for early colonic dysplasia, Barrett esophagus, and Helicobacter pylori infiltration of antral mucosa. The technique might be used after chromoendoscopy reveals a suspicious region of gastrointestinal mucosa. The proposed benefits of confocal fluorescence microendoscopy are many: detection and grading of premalignant lesions, reducing health care costs by avoiding physical biopsy, and minimizing the risks associated with physical biopsy.

Narrow Band Imaging

Detailed examination of the intestinal mucosa has been shown to facilitate the detection of dysplastic lesions. In addition to chromoendoscopy, narrow band imaging permits such an examination, but without the administration of dyes. In narrow band endoscopy, filtered light is used to preferentially enhance the mucosal surface, especially the network of superficial capillaries (Fig. 3-4). Ordinary white light is passed sequentially through red, green, and blue light filters whose wavelength ranges are narrower than conventional filters. The mucosa is illuminated predominantly with intensified blue-green light, with light filters narrowed to bandwidths centered on 415 and 540 nm. Blue light, with a longer wavelength than red light, penetrates only superficially and therefore is ideal for examining intestinal mucosa.

Narrow band imaging is often combined with magnification endoscopy. Both adenomas and carcinomas have a rich network of underlying capillaries and are enhanced in narrow band imaging, thereby appearing dark brown against a blue-green mucosal background.

Endoscopes with specialized light filters are necessary to perform narrow band imaging. These scopes can be used in white light mode and subsequently switched to narrow band imaging by turning a dial. Narrow band imaging might offer many advantages over chromoendoscopy; there is no need for spraying vital dyes and using specialized catheters, and alternating between conventional and narrow band imaging is simple.

Because narrow band imaging is in its nascent stages, the findings are still being interpreted. Detection of intrapapillary capillary loops by narrow band imaging might correlate with the depth of invasion of esophageal cancer. Narrow band imaging has shown utility in the early detection of dysplastic lesions in patients with chronic ulcerative colitis and Barrett esophagus.

Autofluorescence

All tissues produce fluorescence when illuminated with short wavelength light. The fluorescence is emitted from constituent biomolecules termed fluorophores, such as collagen, elastin, aromatic amino acids, NADH, and porphyrins. Hemoglobin is the principal chromophore, absorbing light but not emitting fluorescence. When illuminated with ultraviolet light, the submucosa normally emits a bright green autofluorescence. Thickened mucosa, however, such as might be seen in dysplasia, attenuates the strong signal from the submucosa.

Autofluorescence endoscopy relies on several principles: tissue architecture changes such as mucosal thickening dampen submucosal autofluorescence; neovascularization alters the light emitting and scattering properties of surrounding tissue; the biochemical microenvironment, such as high oxidation-reduction activity, alters autofluorescence; and different tissue types have unique distribution of fluorophores.

First-generation autofluorescence endoscopes used a probe inserted through an accessory channel that emitted ultraviolet light. Point autofluorescence using the small probe was useful in examining visually apparent lesions, but was limited to a sampling area of only 1 to 3 mm^3. Prototype second-generation autofluorescence endoscopes capable of scanning a large surface area have been developed. These models use blue light excitation with detection of autofluorescence by highly sensitive CCDs. The reflected blue light is filtered out, and the low-intensity autofluorescent light is registered through CCDs. The image sensors then create a real-time pseudocolor image with dysplastic tissue displayed as dark red and normal tissue as light blue.

Autofluorescence endoscopy has been shown in pilot studies to improve the detection of dysplasia in Barrett esophagus and chronic ulcerative colitis. There is no need for administration of exogenous fluorophores, and detection of dysplastic lesions has been reported with a high degree of fidelity with histological specimens. Technological advances might broaden its future applications.

Optical Coherence Tomography

Endoscopic optical coherence tomography is an emerging technology analogous to endoscopic ultrasound (Fig. 3-5). The technique uses reflection of near-infrared light to produce real-time two-dimensional cross-sectional images of the gastrointestinal tract. These true anatomic images correspond to the histologic layers (mucosa, submucosa, and muscularis propria). The images obtained have a resolution that is ten times greater than endoscopic ultrasound.

The optical coherence image is produced by emitting near-infrared light into tissue and measuring the back scatter. A low-coherence light source is emitted and divided by an optical fiber splitter. After being split, one light is directed to the tissue via an optical fiber, and one light is directed to a mirror at a precisely controlled distance. Back-scattered light from

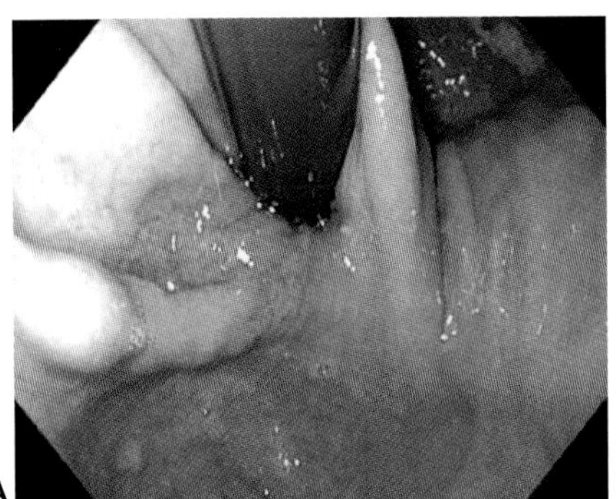

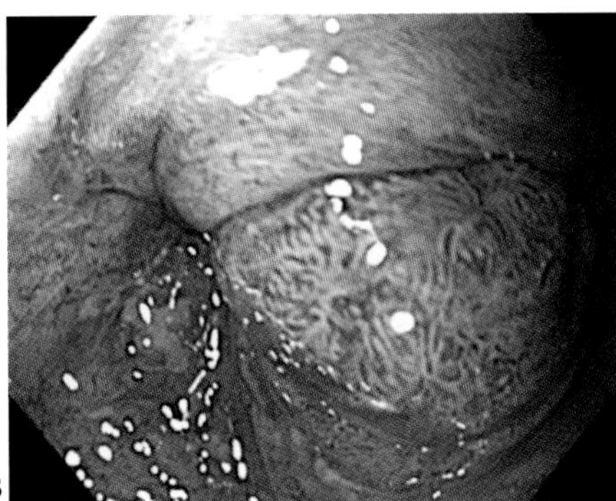

Fig. 3-4. A. Retroflexed view of the esophagogastric junction. **B.** Antegrade view of the esophagogastric junction with narrow band imaging. The superficial network of capillaries is enhanced with this imaging technique. (Photographs courtesy of Amitabh Chak, MD.)

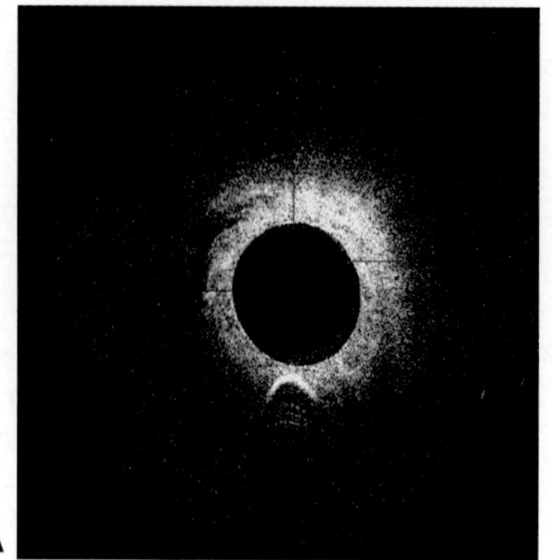

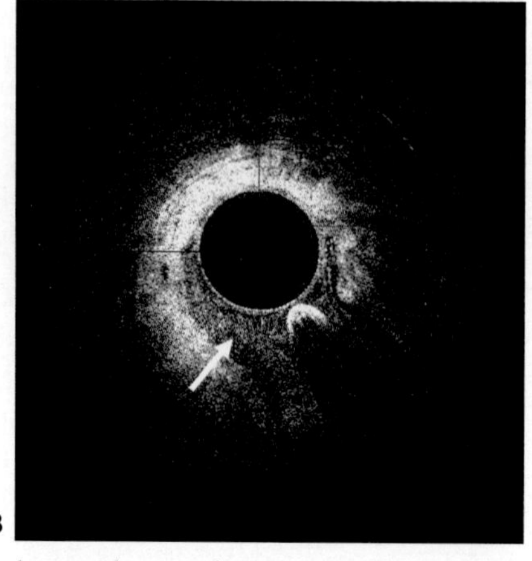

Fig. 3-5. A. View of a normal common bile duct with optical coherence tomography. **B.** A common bile duct optical coherence tomogram. The white arrow indicates the location of a cholangiocarcinoma. (Photographs courtesy of Gerard Isenberg, MD.)

the tissue combines with reflected light from the mirror to produce interference. The interference produces reflection, which is detected to create an image. In order to visualize various depths, the mirror is adjusted to produce a different degree of interference and back scatter.

In practice, specialized optical coherence catheters are passed through the working channel of standard endoscopes. The image can be obtained without apposing the catheter to the tissue. Standard optical coherence resolution of 20 μm allows identification of glands, crypts, and villi, thereby mandating a familiarity of histopathology by the endoscopist. Using second- and third-generation catheters and software, a high-resolution image can be obtained in 0.25 seconds.

Endoscopic optical coherence tomography is not yet in widespread use. At its current resolution, optical coherence optical biopsy cannot replace standard histology, but initial clinical studies have reported favorable results. A high sensitivity and specificity has been reported for staging of esophageal cancer and detection of dysplasia in Barrett esophagus. Other potential applications include the surveillance of high-grade dysplasia and distinguishing hyperplastic from adenomatous polyps.

Light Scattering Spectroscopy

Light scattering spectroscopy mathematically analyzes the intensity and wavelength of reflected light to estimate the size and degree of crowding of surface epithelial nuclei. The technique relies on the absorption and scattering of white light. Absorption depends on the concentration of specific compounds, such as hemoglobin, that absorb some wavelengths of light but reflect all others. Scatter varies as the size and density of space-occupying structures, such as collagen and organelles, changes. Scatter occurs as light interacts with and passes through the space-occupying structures.

Results from the epithelial light absorption and scatter are entered into a mathematical model. The biochemical nature of the examined area can be determined from absorption, and scatter provides information on the size and density of the organelles within a given tissue.

Small clinical trials using light scattering spectroscopy have shown efficacy in detecting Barrett esophagus and early colonic dysplasia. The technique relies on graphing mathematical computations rather than an optical biopsy, as in other emerging imaging techniques. Light scattering spectroscopy might be used in combination with optical biopsy for detection of early dysplasia.

Other Investigational Imaging Modalities

Raman spectroscopy relies on changes induced by light in the vibrational and rotational states of molecular bonds. Each molecular species has its own set of molecular vibrations that, when stimulated with light, results in unique Raman spectra of peaks or bands. Alterations in relative contributions of certain molecules in tissues influence the Raman spectra. Raman spectroscopy could potentially detect differences in nucleotide, amino acid, and lipid distribution, thereby detecting dysplastic lesions before they are grossly visible.

Stereoendoscopy projects a three-dimensional (3-D) image of the gastrointestinal mucosa. A prototype device has been developed based on the makeup of insect eyes. An array of prisms, each facing different directions, is constructed with overlapping fields of view. The input from each prism is computed to convert the 2-D input into a 3-D image. Thus, depth perception during endoscopy would be enhanced, potentially facilitating detection and treatment of neoplastic lesions.

Another technology at an investigational stage is immunophotodiagnostic endoscopy. The technique takes advantage of the ability to specifically target a tumor-related antigen with a fluorescent-labeled monoclonal antibody. The aim is to target dysplasia-associated biomarkers for early dysplasia detection; however, finding unique dysplasia-associated markers is difficult. As the understanding of tumor biology advances, unique targets may be discovered, and this technique may find clinical utility.

The Future

There is a broadening armamentarium available in gastrointestinal endoscopy, especially imaging techniques for the early detection of dysplasia. These techniques are certain to continue their brisk evolution, and those that offer the greatest clinical benefit will likely achieve widespread clinical application.

While the basic platform of the endoscope has remained largely unchanged over the past 50 years, endoscopists may someday be freed from the confines of the standard endoscope. Certainly, wireless digital technology and advances in light sources will eliminate the omnipresent cords and wires. Derivations from robotic technology will likely provide enhanced maneuverability of the endoscope tip and manipulable instruments providing fine dexterity.

In the near future, there will likely be a multifunctional endoscope with a combination of imaging technologies available. Standard white light will be used for screening and surveillance, and then the scope might be switched to autofluorescence mode for guidance to a neoplastic lesion. With the same scope, confocal microscopy might then be used to perform an optical biopsy, and optical coherence could be used to grade the depth of the lesion. If necessary, the same scope might have several working channels for interventions.

New endoscopic technology stirs the imagination as the application of endoscopes expands from intraluminal to transluminal therapy. Shape-locking devices or guided endoscopes could be used for stabilization of the transluminal operative field. High resolution and magnifying scopes could enhance the optics of an operative field, and other advanced imaging technology could be applied to solid organs for detecting neoplastic lesions. Scopes specifically designed for transluminal endoscopic surgery are likely to be developed. Thus, as the technology expands, so too will the applications of advanced endoscopic therapy.

SUGGESTED READING

Chiu HM, Chang CY, Chen CC, et al. A prospective comparative study of narrow-band imaging, chromoendoscopy, and conventional colonoscopy in the diagnosis of colorectal neoplasia. *Gut* 2007;56(3):373–379.

Isenberg G, Sivak MV Jr, Chak A, et al. Accuracy of endoscopic optical coherence tomography in the detection of dysplasia in Barrett's esophagus: a prospective, double-blinded study. *Gastrointest Endosc* 2005;62(6):825–831.

Monkemuller K, Weigt J, Treiber G, et al. Diagnostic and therapeutic impact of double-balloon enteroscopy. *Endoscopy* 2006;38(1):67–72.

Ponsky JL. Endoluminal surgery: past, present and future. *Surg Endosc* 2006;20 Suppl 2:S500–S502.

Sivak MV Jr. Gastrointestinal endoscopy: past and future. *Gut* 2006;55(8):1061–1064.

COMMENTARY

Drs. Pearl and Marks have provided an overview of current and future advances in endoscopy. Endoscopes in use today are little different from those used 50 years ago, albeit with the images now viewed on a video screen. However, efforts are underway at numerous sites to revolutionize the way endoscopy is performed and the format by which images are obtained. It is likely that screening endoscopy will ultimately be able to be performed using a self-propelled scope controlled by a nonphysician, becoming a true disruptive technology. It is also likely that cumbersome and time-consuming biopsy methods will be replaced by real-time "optical biopsy" technology. Certainly, new ways of imaging the gastrointestinal mucosa will become mainstream in the near future. Those involved in diagnostic endoscopy will need to retool their skill sets in order to keep abreast of these advances.

NJS

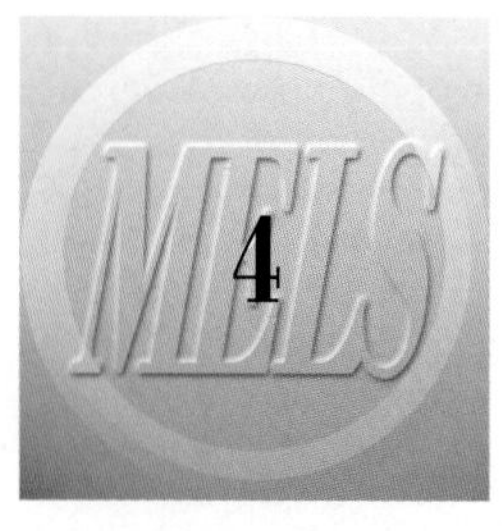

New and Evolving Laparoscopic Instrumentation

DANIEL J. SCOTT AND MOUZA T. GOOVA

INTRODUCTION

"What mankind can dream, research and technology can achieve."

C. Walton Lillehei (1918–1999), the "father of open heart surgery"

Despite its widespread acceptance, the field of laparoscopy and minimally invasive surgery is still in its infancy. The modern era of laparoscopic surgery arguably has occurred only over the past 20 years, while the roots of the field date back over 200 years. The idea of using an imaging system and a light source to visualize internal organs can be traced back to 1806, when German physician Philipp Bozzini reported an invention called the "Lichtleiter." This prototype endoscope used a tube, candlelight, and a system of mirrors. Although a revolutionary concept, it was not well accepted and not used in humans until 1853 by French surgeon Antoine Jean Desormeaux. With the invention of the lightbulb by Thomas Edison in 1880, subsequent pioneering work was made possible by Georg Kelling, Hans Jacobaeus, and others. Throughout the early 20th century, laparoscopy remained an experimental endeavor with limited clinical utility.

Major technological breakthroughs included the "cold light source" introduction by Max Fourestier in 1952, the Hopkins rod-lens system in 1953, and CCD (charged-coupled device) video imaging in 1985. As significant advancements in instrumentation were made, laparoscopy evolved from a predominantly diagnostic modality used almost exclusively by gynecologists in the 1970s to a burgeoning therapeutic modality embraced by general surgeons in the 1980s. Indeed, the first laparoscopic appendectomy was performed in 1980 by Kurt Semm, a German gynecologist. By 1985, the first cholecystectomy had been performed by Erich Mühe, a German surgeon, with well-known accounts of similar successes reported in 1987 by Phillipe Mouret in France and in 1988 by J. Barry McKernan and William Saye in the United States. After an initial period of considerable skepticism, the use of minimally invasive techniques exploded, with the successful application of laparoscopy to numerous operations and the benefit to patients clearly established.

At the core of this evolution is technology. For example, in the 1980s, Mühe was only able to perform a laparoscopic cholecystectomy after commissioning an instrument maker to create a prototype operating laparoscope and trocar system, which he called the "galloscope." At this time, instruments were crude at best, with only rudimentary grapsers and hand-held gynecologic instruments available. McKernan and Saye ligated the cystic duct using suture material, as no clip appliers were yet available. Similarly, until the computer chip television camera was introduced, the surgeon used one hand to hold the laparoscope and had only one hand available to operate. Thus, much of the work throughout the 1990s was aimed at relatively fundamental improvements in instrumentation, such as creating robust graspers, multifire clip appliers, staplers, energy sources, access ports, and imaging systems. With the establishment of these platforms, routine performance of complex procedures became possible.

Now, much of the focus on innovation lies in several novel areas, including robotics, high-definition imaging, and natural orifice approaches, which will be covered in separate chapters. But what about laparoscopic instrumentation? There are a number of central themes that continue to guide instrument innovation, in an effort to overcome clinical problems that remain limitations to the laparoscopic approach. First, as we know from psychomotor learning theory, surgical simulation, and real-life practice of laparoscopy, these techniques are difficult, with constraints such as decreased range of motion, a fulcrum effect, and diminished tactile feedback. Thus, many advancements in instrumentation are designed to make surgery easier by increasing range of motion (articulating instruments), automating functions (suturing, stapling, clipping, and tacking devices), or restoring tactile feedback (hand access ports). A second strategy involves making surgery safer and minimizing morbidity. For example, nonbladed trocars decrease the risk of injury or port site hernias, absorbable tack materials decrease the risk of adhesions, and computer-assisted devices (staplers, energy sources) may decrease the risk of mechanical failures. Finally, there is a clear evolution towards less invasion, as postoperative pain, recovery, and inflammatory response have been directly correlated with incision length. Intracorporeal instruments that can be deployed through a single access point, either transabdominally or via a natural orifice, will foster this less invasive shift by obviating the need for trocars. Hence, some of this technology may be truly disruptive, by dramatically changing the way surgery is performed.

The goal of this chapter is to highlight examples of instrumentation that illustrate these concepts. In no way is this chapter designed to be comprehensive, as including all of the devices that we would like to mention is not possible given our space limitations.

Articulating Handheld Instruments

Because laparoscopy uses trocars fixed to the abdominal wall, range of motion is inherently limited. One of the advantages of the da Vinci robotic system (Intuitive Surgical, Inc.; Sunnyvale, CA) is that the instruments articulate at the "wrist," near the end of the effector tip. This intracorporeal articulation has proven useful by improving range of motion and facilitating intricate maneuvers within confined spaces and at difficult angles. For example, articulating robotic instruments have dramatically increased the number of prostatectomies performed laparoscopically, as the urethral anastomosis may be constructed more easily. This anastomosis is difficult to perform, as the retropubic space is small and requires suturing at challenging angles. Articulation also facilitates knot-tying as looping the suture over a needle driver during instrument tying is easily achieved. Perhaps to a lesser extent, articulating instruments may afford superior retraction in some circumstances; certainly, "off angles" may be achieved even with parallel instrument approaches, facilitating tissue triangulation in confined spaces, such as during the mediastinal dissection for transhiatal esophagectomy. It should also be emphasized that the utility of instrument articulation using robotic systems is enhanced by the fluidity of the control system, because a surgeon's hand manipulating a joystick-type control allows movements in all directions without interruption. The obvious limitation of this technology is the very high, as seen with the da Vinci system.

As a lower-cost alternative, companies have devised ways of increasing the range of motion using traditional handheld instruments. One of the first platforms that introduced articulation is the Roticulator (Covidien; Norwalk, CT); it requires rotating a collar located just beyond the handle to advance the tip of the instrument in a forward curving fashion, until the tip articulates to 90 degrees. While the articulation may make some tasks easier (such as passing a Penrose drain through the retroesophageal space during a Nissen fundoplication), this and similar instruments made by other manufacturers have not been widely used. Many surgeons feel that such instrumentation is not necessary if appropriate techniques are used with conventional instrumentation (similar to the arguments heard concerning robotic systems) and that the instruments can be cumbersome to operate. For example, the Autosuture grasper platform requires two hands to perform the articulation maneuver and the ergonomics are poor; fluidity of movement, as achieved by robotic joysticks, is not possible.

In contrast, newer articulating instruments attempt to offer similar control afforded by robotic systems but in a handheld configuration through relatively creative handpiece and system designs. The Radius Surgical System (Tuebingen Scientific Medical GmbH; Tübingen, Germany) closely mimics the functionality achieved by da Vinci instruments, with wrist articulation very close to the effector tip (Fig. 4-1). The Radius Surgical System consists of two 10-mm instruments, one for the right hand and one for the left, with each instrument providing 6 degrees of freedom. The effector tips can be deflected up to 70 degrees by bending the palm-held handle and rotated 360 degrees by rotating a knob between the thumb and index finger. Compressing and releasing the handle closes and opens the jaws of various interchangeable, disposable tips, including graspers, scissors, and needle holders. The movement transmission is effected through the interaction of a gear rod, a push rod, and several gear wheels; the 10-mm shaft size is currently needed to accommodate these mechanisms and is a limitation of this system.

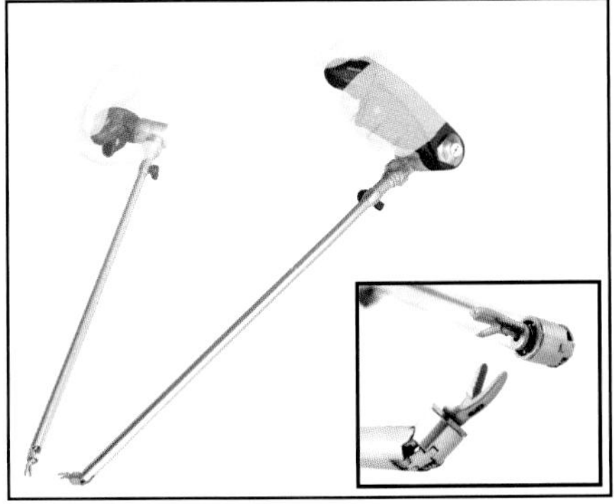

Fig. 4-1. The Radius System for articulating instruments uses 10-mm left- and right-handed instruments with gears that allow tip deflection and rotation.

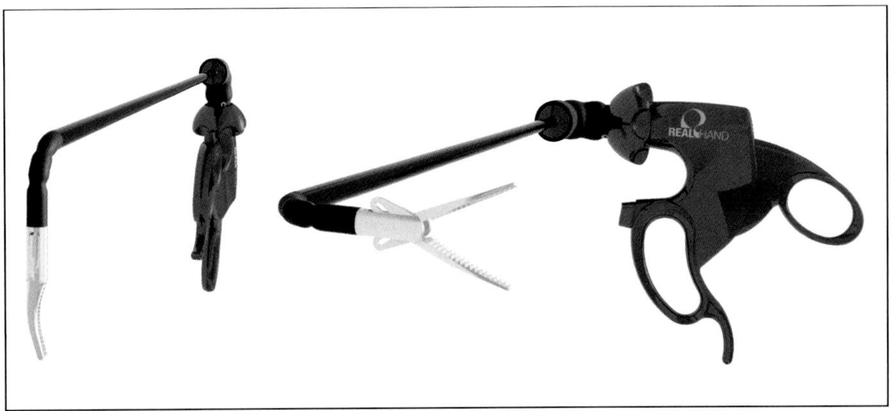

Fig. 4-2. RealHand instruments are 5-mm "high dexterity" instruments that allow the effector end to be deflected in any direction as the handle is manipulated in a pivoting fashion.

RealHand instruments developed by Novare Surgical Systems, Inc. (Cupertino, CA) allow broad sweeping motions with a substantial portion of the distal instrument deflecting in a fashion that mimics the movement of the surgeon's hand (Fig. 4-2). The manufacturer describes these as "high dexterity" instruments. When the surgeon's hand moves the instrument handle in any direction, the instrument tip follows exactly, offering 7 degrees of freedom, with real-time movement translation. The instrument handle appears similar to traditional handheld instruments, but pivots freely at the shaft-handle junction to activate a matrix of wire scaffolding that translates the handle motions to the effector tip. This technology affords 5-mm instrument shafts with numerous tip configurations. Future iterations are expected to incorporate a locking sleeve, which will allow the instrument to be locked in a straight or articulated form, aiding in stability.

Cambridge Endo (Framingham, MA) offers an articulating handheld platform approved by the Food and Drug Administration in 2006 called Autonomy Laparo-Angle Instrumentation (Fig. 4-3). The instruments offer 7 degrees of freedom and use a 5-mm shaft. The unique ergonomic handle is designed for single-handed (left- or right-handed) control; needle holders are currently available, with scissors, dissectors, and hook cautery instruments expected soon.

While these handheld articulating instruments seem innovative and may solve problems related to isolated circumstances involving hard-to-reach areas, their utility in performing routine tasks is less clear. Some of the early versions of the newer equipment suffer from stability problems, in that the instruments are so maneuverable that they become somewhat flaccid and hard to control. No data are available suggesting that these instruments will outperform conventional laparoscopic instruments. However, as we see an evolution towards less invasion, such articulating technology may be *enabling*. Specifically, if a single access port is used, multiple articulating instruments, inserted in a parallel configuration, may then diverge intracorporeally and offer true tissue triangulation.

Suturing Technology

It is well known that laparoscopic suturing is a difficult skill to master and requires significant training before proficiency is reached. For some time now, various suturing devices have been available that

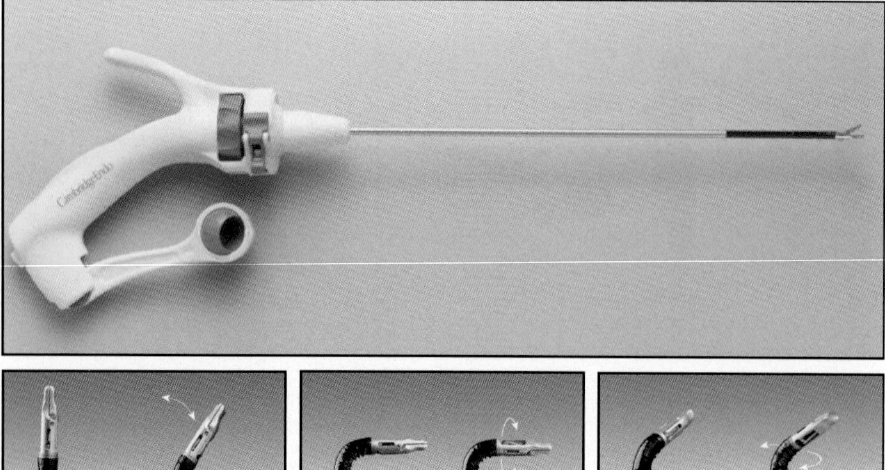

Fig. 4-3. The Cambridge Endo Autonomy Laparo-Angle Needle Holder allows 7 degrees of freedom with full control via a unique hand piece design.

make suturing easier by alleviating various steps of the task. For example, the ENDO STITCH device (Covidien; Norwalk, CT) automates needle positioning and the Suture Assist device (Ethicon Endo-Surgery, Inc.; Cincinnati, OH) automates knot-tying. Studies have shown that such devices can decrease procedural time, potentially offsetting the increased device cost compared to using conventional suture materials.

Suture Materials

Recently, a different approach has been pursued by innovations in the suture material configuration rather than the suturing instruments. One solution is the U-Clip Anastomotic Device (Medtronic, Inc.; Minneapolis, MN), which consists of a nitinol wire attached to a pop-off suture and needle (Fig. 4-4). For laparoscopic applications, a conventional needle driver is used to pass the suture through the tissue until the end of the nitinol segment is reached; the needle and pop-off suture are then disengaged from the nitinol segment, which closes into a ring-like configuration based on the shape-memory properties of the metal, thereby approximating the two pieces of tissue without the need for knot-tying. A wealth of experience has been reported with creating hand-sewn coronary artery bypass grafts using this technology with good results. The technology can also be used in conjunction with an automated device for proximal (vein graft to aorta) anastomosis creation with deployment of six U-Clip sutures simultaneously. Much less experience has been gathered with this technology for laparoscopic operations, but preliminary results are promising for applications such as Nissen fundoplication and other gastrointestinal procedures.

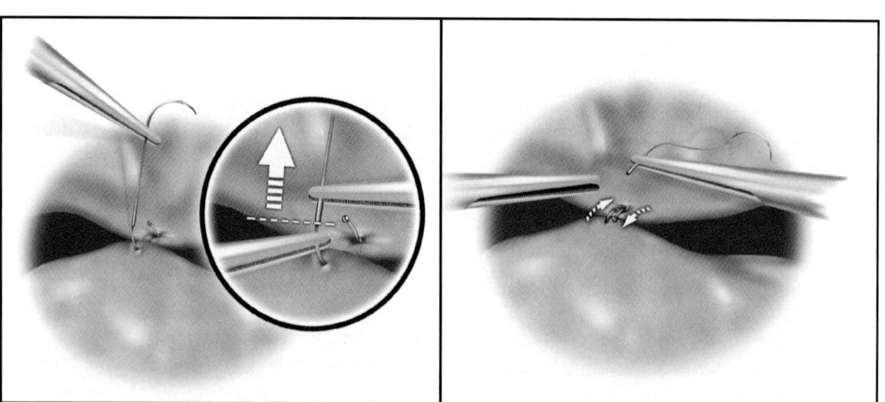

Fig. 4-4. The U-Clip Approximation device uses a nitinol wire attached to a pop-off suture and needle to approximate tissue without knot-tying.

A slightly different approach based on suture material modifications may also increase the efficiency of laparoscopic suturing. In January 2007, Angiotech Pharmaceuticals, Inc. (Vancouver, Canada) launched the Quill SRS (self-retaining system), which uses a patented barb design that eliminates the need for knots (Fig. 4-5). Tiny opposing barbs are cut into the surface of a monofilament suture in a bidirectional fashion, such that the midpoint of the suture is placed in the midpoint of the wound and the two suture strands are run in opposite directions. As the suture is pulled through the tissue, the barbs (cut in a spiral array) hold the suture tension in a constant fashion, without having to maintain tension manually. Placed in a running configuration, sufficient retentional forces are created to obviate the need for tying knots. One rationale, championed by plastic surgeons, is that cosmetic closures using this suture technology may result in less tissue inflammation because less foreign body material (suture knots) is used. For laparoscopic or endoscopic suturing, the potential benefits could be significant in terms of the relative simplicity of the "suture that doesn't need knots" concept. Experimental data on wound closure and, to a lesser extent, gastrointestinal suturing for anastomoses, suggest that adequate closures may be achieved simply by running the barbed suture and cutting off the excess, with no knot-tying.

Absorbable Tacks

Mesh fixation remains controversial for laparoscopic inguinal hernia repair, but is a routine part of almost all described techniques for laparoscopic incisional hernia repair. While seemingly essential for appropriate mesh fixation, traditional permanent tacks can cause significant adhesions, even if nonadhesiogenic mesh is used. Recently, instruments that use absorbable tack materials have been introduced. The I-Clip Tissue Fixation System (Covidien; Norwalk, CT) is a 10-mm single-use device with 20 polylactic acid constructs (Fig. 4-6). The I-shaped constructs have a height of 7.5 mm, which provides penetration almost twice as deep as other tacking devices, possibly aiding in fixation strength. The clips are designed to completely resorb within 12 months. The EasyTac Anchor Device (MedChannel LLC: Milton Village, MA) is a 5-mm single-use device with either 5 or 12 PLA (polylactide) constructs (Fig. 4-7, page 28). The conical,

A

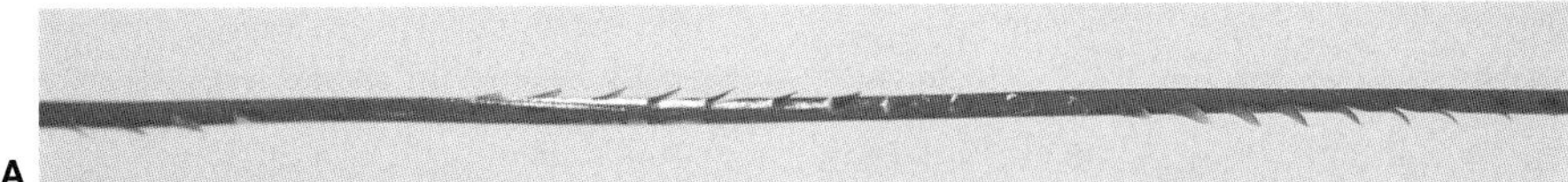

B

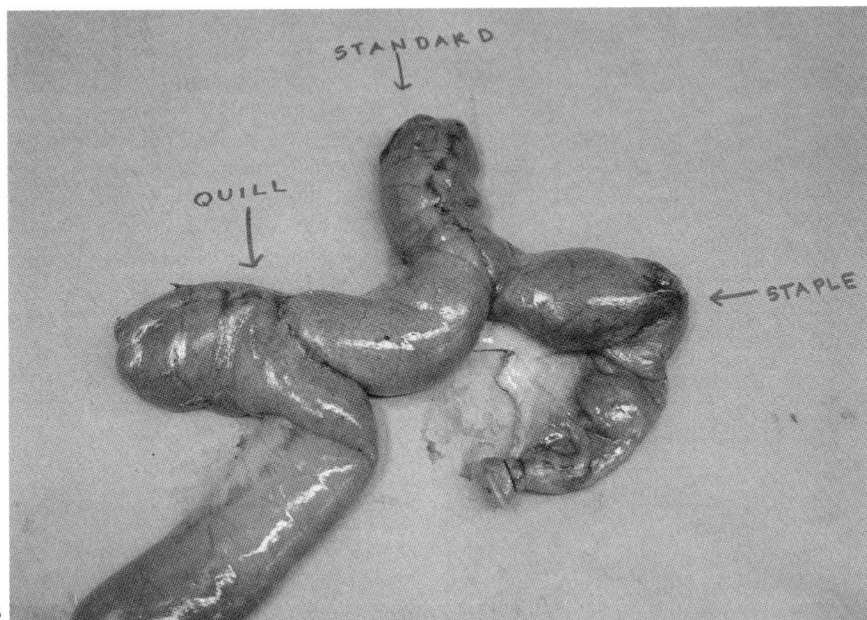

Fig. 4-5. The Quill Self-Retaining System uses barbed suture material placed in a bidirectional running pattern that holds the suture securely in the tissue without placing knots. **A.** A magnified view of the barbed configuration. **B.** Porcine side-to-side small bowel anastomoses using the Quill barbed suture, conventional suture, and staples with equivalent test results but significantly shorter operative times for the Quill group.

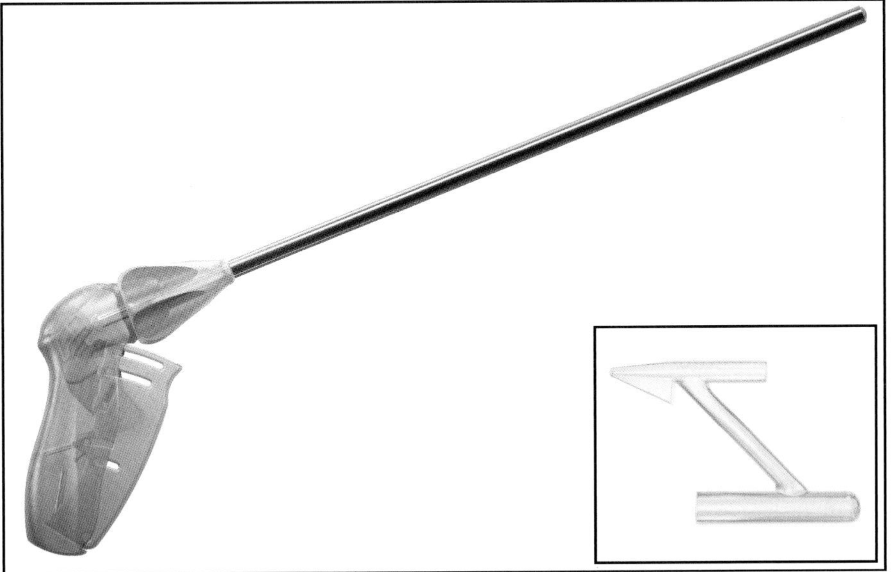

Fig. 4-6. The I-Clip Tissue Fixation System uses absorbable polylactic acid tacks for mesh fixation during hernia repair.

barbed constructs have a relatively generous height of 6.4 mm; they are designed to have 90% stability at 3 months post implantation and total degradation within 2 years.

Data are limited to support these new platforms, but studies are underway aimed at documenting benefit in terms of decreased adhesion formation.

Computer-Assisted Staplers

Laparoscopic stapling equipment rapidly evolved during the 1990s as complex gastrointestinal procedures such as the colectomy and gastric bypass became established. In recent years, though, few significant advances have been made. However, Power Medical Interventions (Langhorne, PA) has introduced a potentially significant paradigm shift by combining stapling and computer technologies, as well as developing a flexible shaft platform for potential endoluminal or transluminal deployment (Fig. 4-8). Approved by the Food and Drug Administration in 2000, the SurgASSIST platform provides a unique level of precision and monitoring during the application and firing of circular and linear staples. The system uses a computer-assisted power console connected to a loading unit via a 2.13-m long flexible shaft. The computer monitors tissue compression during stapler closure and appropriately matches compression to staple height. Programming eliminates overcompression with resultant tissue injury or ischemia and prevents the firing of the stapler if adequate compression cannot be achieved, as might be the case with thickened or inflamed tissues and a staple height mismatch. Since the power source for compression and firing is cable-driven and located well away from the stapling unit, there is no torque on the tissue during the firing sequence. This level of precision is touted to increase the reliability and safety of the system beyond that of conventional handheld staplers. Limited comparative data in animal models have not yet shown any difference, and no controlled clinical trials are available. Nonetheless, one large case series of open gastric bypass operations (403 cases) documented no anastomotic leaks and a very low stricture rate (1.7%), supporting the system's potentially high level of efficacy.

Only one flexible shaft system from Power Medical has an ability to be steered; the circular shaft stapler head can be tilted in four directions using the remote keypad. Limited reports of using this technology for endoluminal resections are available. As the technology continues to evolve, undoubtedly maneuverability similar to that achieved with flexible endoscopy would be desirable and hopefully pursued, as well as onboard imaging capabilities. Such a versatile instrument platform would likely have significant utility for single-access laparoscopy as well as

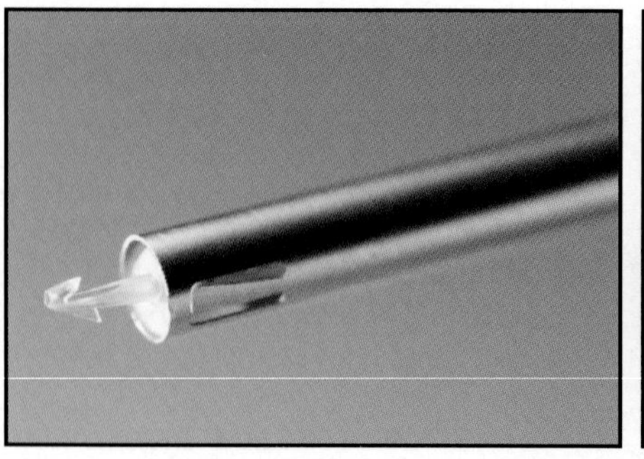

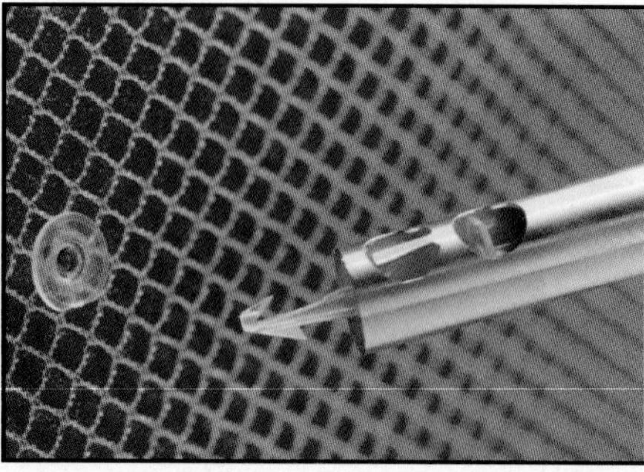

Fig. 4-7. The EasyTac Anchor is a 5-mm single device that deploys absorbable PLA (polylactide) constructs.

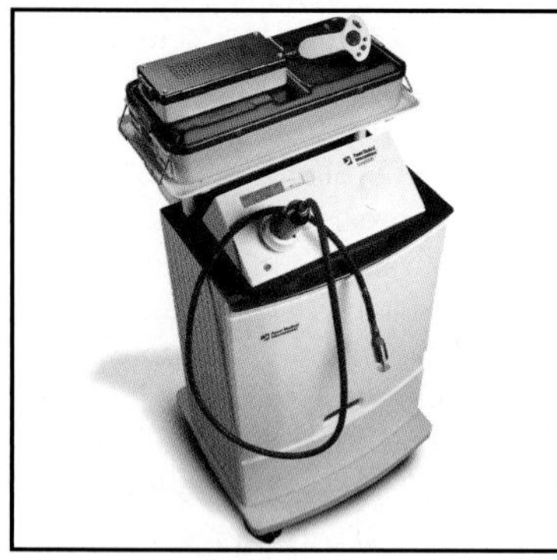

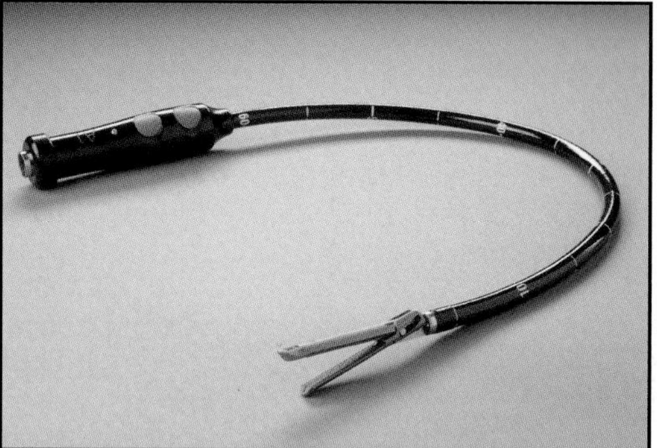

Fig. 4-8. The SurgASSIST Stapler platform uses computer-assisted stapling in an effort to increase precision and safety and allows novel endoluminal and transluminal applications via its flexible shaft.

Natural Orifice Transluminal Endoscopic Surgery (NOTES).

Deployable Intracorporeal Instruments

With the advent of NOTES, there is a clear focus on technologies that will foster a less-invasive approach than traditional laparoscopy can afford. One paradigm may be single-port-access, transabdominal laparoscopy with a solitary umbilical trocar and numerous small instruments that can be deployed intracorporeally; such a strategy would minimize the violation of the abdominal wall and also obviate the potential risk of complications that could accompany a NOTES approach (e.g., peritonitis from a gastrointestinal leak). Alternatively, many of these intracorporeal devices might be ideal for deployment via natural orifices, should methods for these approaches prove safe and reliable. In either case, the working premise is that a single access port can be used as an entry point for multiple instruments, and several devices are now under development for this purpose.

One of the most obvious targets for designing instrumentation of this type would be a video imaging system. Such a deployable camera would mean that a traditional laparoscope would not be needed and that a view of the operative field could be maintained even as the access port was used for other instrumentation. Investigators from Columbia University in New York, led by Dennis Fowler, MD, have designed a novel stereoscopic three-dimensional (3-D) imaging device that can be inserted and attached in the body cavity using a peritoneal clip (Figs. 4-9 and 4-10). The device is contained within an 11/16-inch diameter stainless steel tube and includes two motorized, miniature, remotely controlled cameras with 5 degrees of freedom each. The cameras collapse within the shell for insertion and are exposed once inside the abdomen. Moved in concert, the cameras can provide 3-D imaging; alternatively, the cameras can be moved separately, providing simultaneous 2-D views of two different areas. Preliminary inanimate and animate testing of this device has been promising.

A group from the University of Nebraska, led by Dmitry Oleynikov, MD, has developed a deployable video imaging platform termed "in vivo camera robots." This platform includes two systems, one that is mobile and one that is stationary. The mobile system (Fig. 4-11) originally was introduced as a 15-mm diameter, 75-mm long, 25-gm robot but was enlarged to a 20-mm diameter, 100-mm long, 50-gm robot to accommodate mechanisms for variable focus; this iteration is

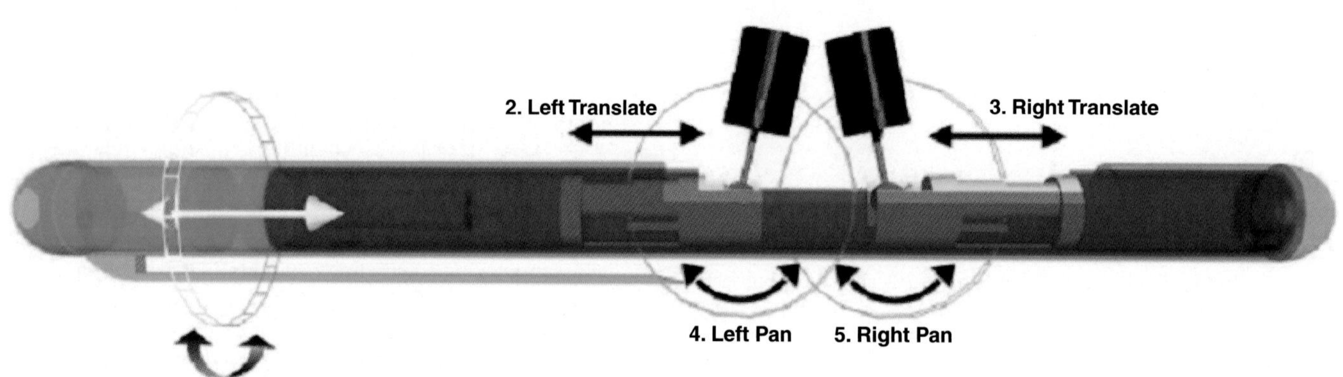

Fig. 4-9. Schematic diagram of a 3-D Stereoscopic Camera (Columbia University, New York) that can be deployed intracorporeally. (Reproduced with permission from Miller A, Allen P, Fowler D. In Vivo stereoscopic imaging system with 5 degrees of freedom for minimal access surgery. In: *Medicine meets virtual reality 12.* Westwood JD, et al., eds. Amsterdam: IOS Press; 2004:234–240.)

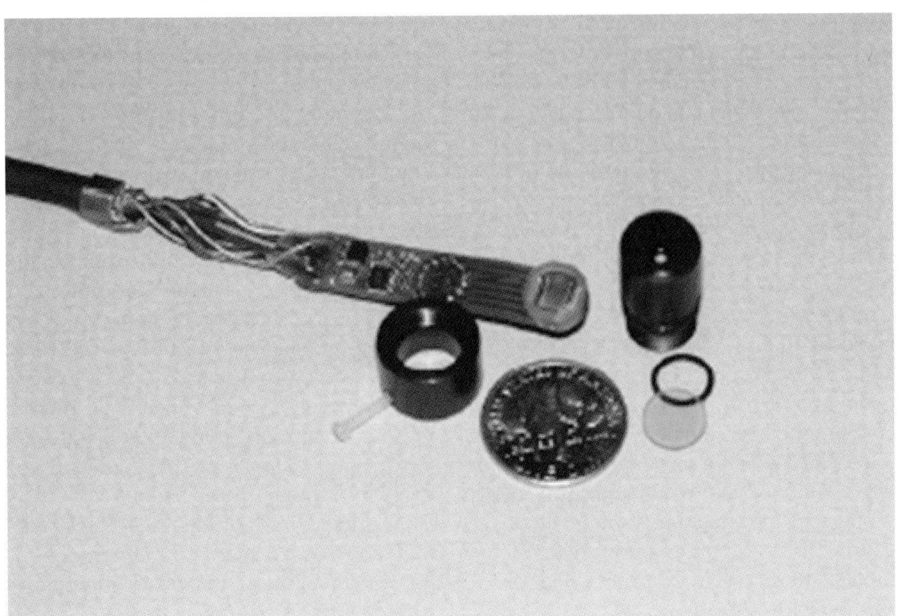

Fig. 4-10. The 8-mm CCD package with a 2.4-mm lens, lens mount, and color filter for in vivo stereoscopic imaging (Columbia University, NY). (Reproduced with permission from Miller A, Allen P, Fowler D. In Vivo stereoscopic imaging system with 5 degrees of freedom for minimal access surgery. In: *Medicine meets virtual reality 12*. Westwood JD, et al., eds. Amsterdam: IOS Press; 2004:234–240.)

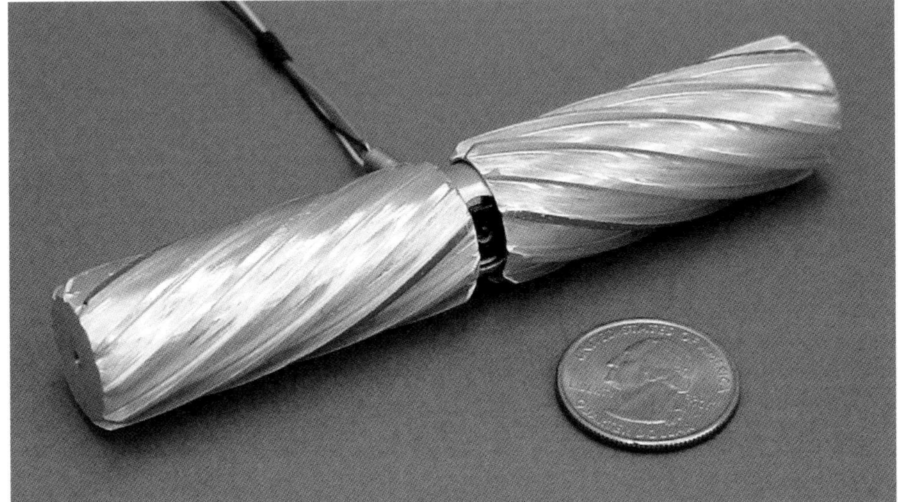

Fig. 4-11. The Mobile Adjustable-focus Robotic Camera (MARC) device has been developed by University of Nebraska investigators as a wheeled in vivo imaging system and has been successfully used during laparoscopic cholecystectomy experiments in pigs. (Reproduced with permission from Rentschler ME, Dumpert J, Platt SR, et al. Mobile in-vivo camera robots provide sole visual feedback for abdominal exploration and cholecystectomy. *Surg Endosc* 2006;20:135–138.)

termed "mobile adjustable-focus robotic camera" or MARC. The concept is that this robot may be deployed through an access port and maneuvered throughout the abdominal cavity to provide visualization. Incorporated into the housing of the device (on either side of the lens apparatus) are two helical wheels that are independently driven by direct current (DC) motors. The wheels allow the robot to propel itself over abdominal organs with capabilities of going forward, reversing, or turning. Although future devices are expected to use wireless technology, current iterations use wires connected to digital processors externally for imaging signal transmission. These wires exit the device in a "tail" that provides stability. As the device reverses its direction, the tail flips over the device's body; before the device flips in this fashion, sufficient torque is generated to allow 15 degrees of tilt. The MARC instrument can "roam" around the abdomen and provide real-time video imaging from any location. Current prototypes do not include onboard lighting; light from a laparoscope has been used for imaging. This system has been used as the sole source of visual imaging during laparoscopic cholecystectomy in a porcine model with good results. Insertion into the abdomen requires a 20-mm incision but future iterations are expected to be compatible with a 15-mm port size. In experimental models, injuries to abdominal organs from the device's wheels have not been noted. One limitation, however, is that since the device rests on the abdominal viscera, the view from the camera is directed either towards tissue very close to the camera in a downward direction or towards nonadjacent tissue in an upward viewing fashion. The traditional panoramic downward view used during most laparoscopic procedures is not possible. Investigations are underway to couple a grasping tool with the MARC system that would allow tissue biopsy.

As an alternative to the MARC system, the Nebraska group has also developed a stationary platform (Fig. 4-12). This system is designed to rest on top of the abdominal viscera using a set of three legs; because the device is 3 inches tall, a downward-looking view is possible. Similar to the MARC device, the current instrument is tethered (external wires) and

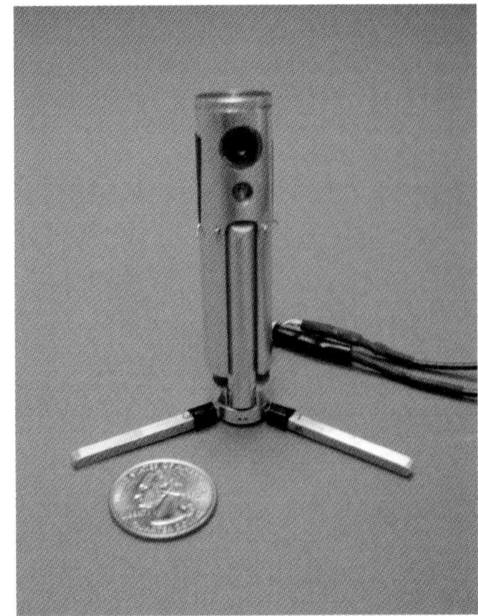

Fig. 4-12. The Pan and Tilt Camera Robot (University of Nebraska) is a 3-inch tall stationary platform that allows a downward-looking view.

uses the laparoscope as a light source. Onboard motors allow pan and tilt, and the device has a 15-mm outer diameter.

Investigators at the University of Texas (UT Southwestern Medical Center and UT Arlington) have also developed instruments for intracorporeal deployment, including video imaging, retraction, and dissection instrumentation (Figs. 4-13 to 4-17). In 2001, minimally invasive urologist Jeffrey Cadeddu developed the idea of using a Magnetic Anchoring and Guidance System (MAGS) to facilitate single-port-access laparoscopy. This technology involves the use of two components: (1) an internal component consisting of a surgical instrument attached to a baseplate containing permanent magnets and (2) an external component consisting of a handheld permanent magnet. The two components are held together via magnetic coupling such that the internal component may be directly manipulated (guided) by moving the external component. Once the internal component is positioned in a desired location (almost anywhere within the peritoneal cavity), the external component can be optionally exchanged for an 18-gauge percutaneous, threaded needle anchor, which provides secure, rigid, hands-free fixation.

Early work was aimed towards magnetic platform optimization with shielding and focusing permanent magnets made from neodymium iron boron (NdFeB) to yield coupling forces sufficient to control the 25- to 45-gm instruments. Proof-of-concept was established and the system proved advantageous in facilitating a minimally invasive nephrectomy in a nonsurvival porcine model, using a MAGS camera (Fig. 4-13) and retractor instruments (Fig. 4-14) while reducing the number of laparoscopic trocars to two. With the addition of a MAGS robotic cautery dissector (Fig. 4-15), the number of laparoscopic trocars was reduced to one (single-port nephrectomy) in a subsequent study. The initial design parameters were an outer diameter of 15 mm to allow instrument passage through a large laparoscopic trocar. For the laparoscopic approach, electrical (camera and cauterizer) and pneumatic (cauterizer) tethers are fed externally for signal transmission, electrical energy, and robotic control. The cautery dissector (Fig. 4-15) uses pneumatic pistons, remotely controlled using a joystick, to offer 8 degrees of freedom (three onboard and five via magnetic manipulation).

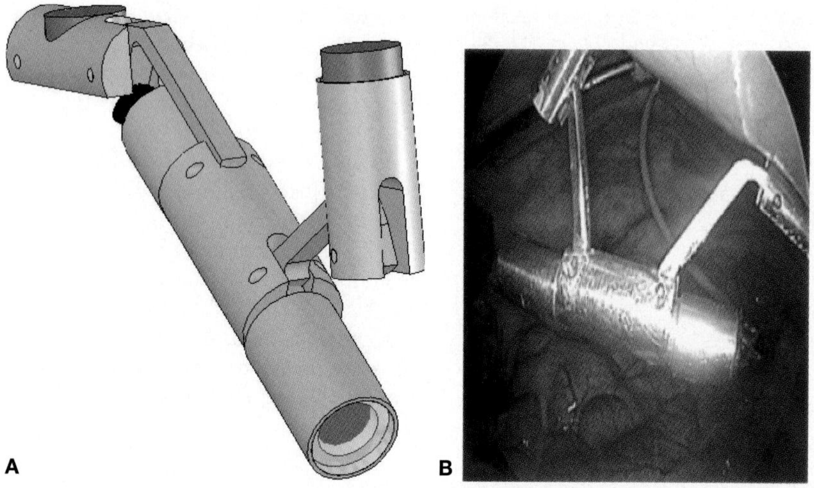

Work led by Daniel Scott, MD, has furthered research using the MAGS tool suite for general surgical and NOTES applications. Various generations of MAGS cameras, gallbladder tissue retractors, and cauterizer instruments have been successfully deployed via transabdominal and NOTES (transgastric, transcolonic, and transvaginal) approaches for use in cholecystectomies (porcine model). In all cases, the gallbladder has been completely dissected free from the liver attachments using only the MAGS cauterizer. Because of instrument limitations, laparoscopic assistance was required during initial experiments. Limitations included fogging of the camera and a lack of sufficient lighting (despite an onboard LED), requiring laparoscope and flexible endoscope assistance for visualization, and retractor dislodgement and inadvertent magnetic coupling between instruments, requiring laparoscopic rescue. Through successive investigations using rapid prototyping, subsequent MAGS platforms proved more robust and obviated the need for laparoscopic assistance.

The University of Texas investigators currently prefer a transvaginal route for cholecystectomy, as a large (25-mm outer diameter), rigid prototype access port (Fig. 4-17) may be used for instrument passage and pneumoperitoneum maintenance. Additionally, the transvaginal approach allows acceptable sterility via standard skin and vaginal preparation (using povidone-iodine) and secure closure (using conventional, open surgical instruments) without risk of peritonitis from a gastrointestinal leak. The tissue retractor (Fig. 4-16) includes a magnetic cradle (18-mm diameter) that is maneuvered to the right-upper quadrant using the external magnet and then exchanged for the 18-gauge needle anchor. Suspended from the cradle are two flexible graspers that allow tissue retraction

Fig. 4-13. Schematic **(A)** and intraabdominally **(B)** deployed views (porcine model) of intracorporeal MAGS camera (University of Texas), held externally using magnetic coupling. (Reproduced with permission from Park S, Bergs R, Eberhart R, et al. Trocar-less laparoscopy: magnetic positioning of intraabdominal camera and retractor. *Ann Surg* 2007;245:379–384.)

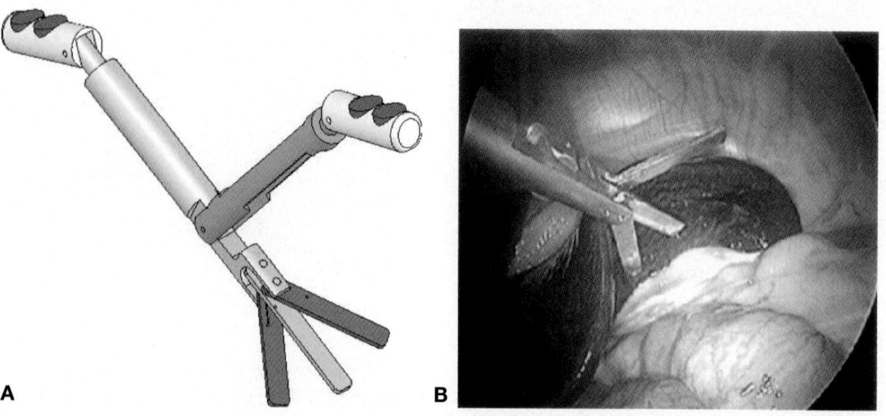

Fig. 4-14. Schematic **(A)** and intraabdominally **(B)** deployed view of intracorporeal MAGS retractor (University of Texas), shown elevating a porcine spleen. (Reproduced with permission from Park S, Bergs R, Eberhart R, et al. Trocar-less laparoscopy: magnetic positioning of intraabdominal camera and retractor. *Ann Surg* 2007;245:379–384.)

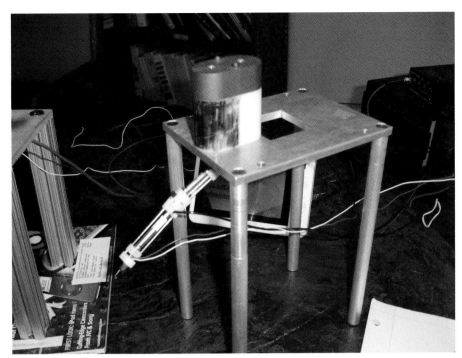

Fig. 4-15. Ex vivo view of external handheld permanent magnet (black and white oval cylinder) holding the MAGS robotic cautery dissector (University of Texas) in place; this device uses onboard pneumatic activation, is remotely controlled via a joystick, and offers 8 degrees of freedom.

via pushing and pulling the graspers' cables externally. The cauterizer (16-mm diameter) has a pneumatically activated arm that allows deployment in a collapsed fashion and extension of the instrument arm to a 45-degree angle once inside the abdomen (Fig. 4-17). Using the MAGS retractor and cauterizer, along with a standard single-channel flexible endoscope (for visualization, suction-irrigation, clips, grasper, and snare), these investigators have successfully performed completely NOTES transvaginal cholecystectomy on both nonsurvival and survival (14-day) porcine models with no complications or infections. Additional work is needed to improve the rigidity and versatility (such as use in thick tissue) of the retractor, and a robust MAGS camera system is still needed.

CONCLUSION

Ultimately, wireless and robotic technology may allow the full realization of the concept of intracorporeal deployment of

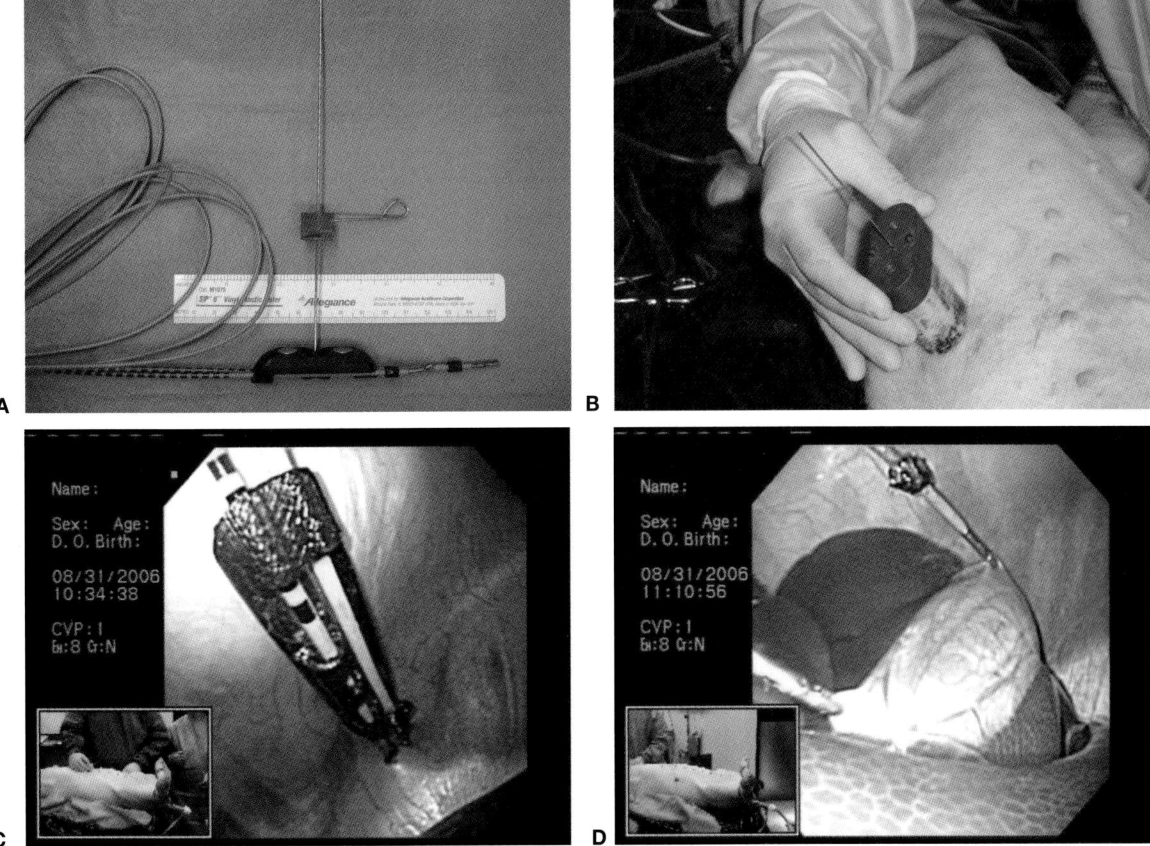

Fig. 4-16. MAGS tissue retractor (University of Texas) during a porcine transvaginal NOTES cholecystectomy experiment. **A.** Ex vivo view showing the 18-gauge needle anchor threaded into the internal cradle component, which holds the cable-driven graspers. **B.** The external magnet is used to maneuver the internal component into place and can then be exchanged for the needle anchor. **C.** The internal component is held rigidly in place on the peritoneal surface using the needle anchor, which allows for hands-free retraction (inset). **D.** While additional rigidity would be desirable, the flexible graspers allow sufficient retraction of the gallbladder to facilitate triangulation and a relatively broad exposure.

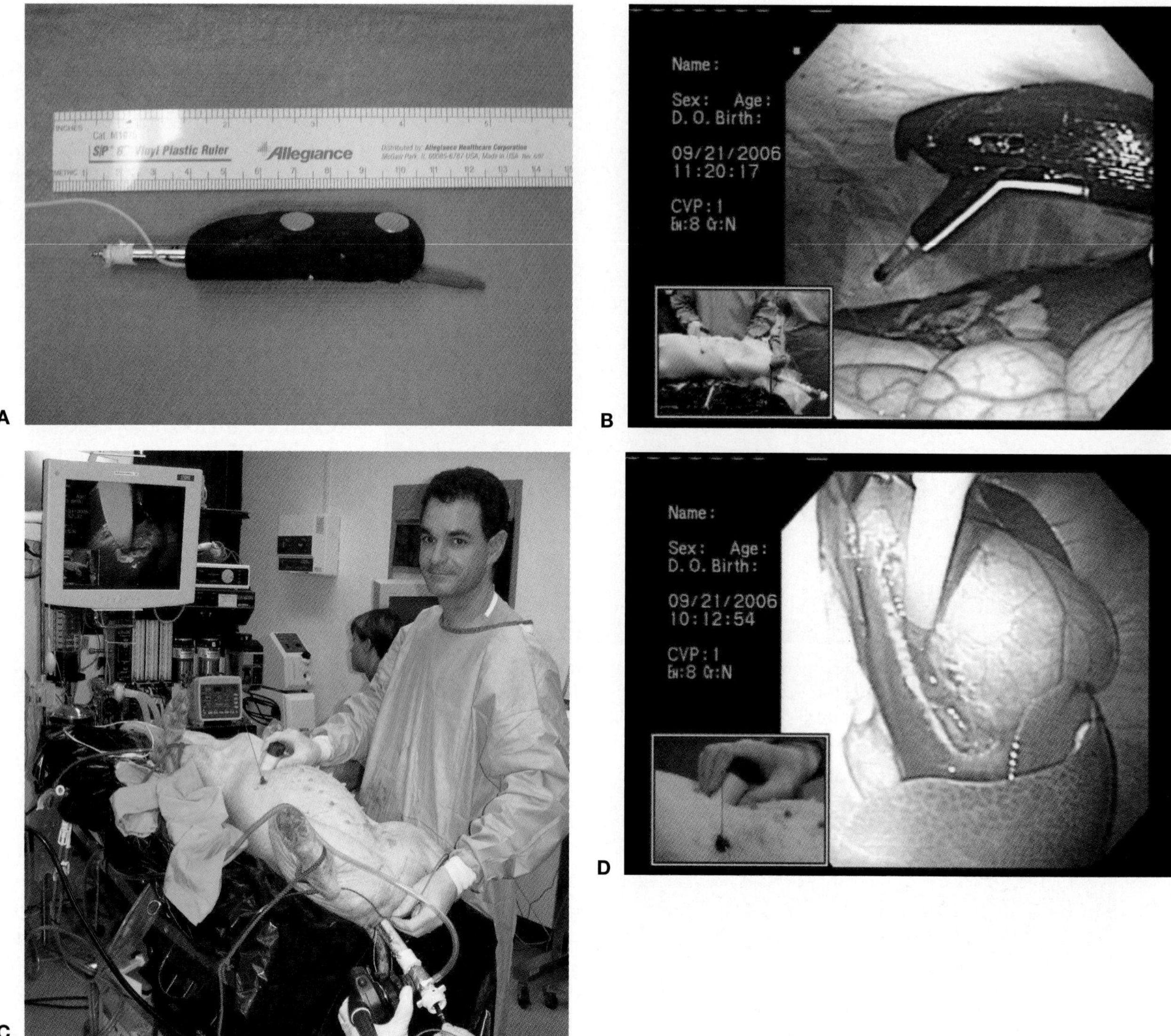

Fig. 4-17. MAGS cautery dissector (University of Texas). **A.** Ex vivo view of the pneumatically powered robotic cautery instrument. **B.** Once placed inside the abdomen, the arm is deployed to a 45-degree operating position. **C.** Daniel Scott, MD performing a transvaginal cholecystectomy (porcine model), manipulating the external magnet for cautery dissection in one hand and the grasper cables in the other. **D.** The cautery dissector is manipulated by positioning the external magnet (inset) and deforming the abdominal wall to provide blunt and sharp dissection.

a wide array of highly effective surgical instruments. As technologies from other industries, such as cellular telephones, computer games, military weapons, space navigation, aviation, and industrial automation, are applied to the field of surgery, such realizations may occur. With miniaturized equipment and powerful onboard or transmitted (radiofrequency, perhaps) energy sources, complex intracorporeal surgery may be possible without the use of abdominal incisions. While futuristic in concept, this "holy grail" for minimally invasive surgery may not be too far off.

SUGGESTED READING

Kaehler G, Grobholz R, Langner C, et al. A new technique of endoscopic full-thickness resection using a flexible stapler. *Endoscopy* 2006;38:86–89.

Liem RK, Niloff PH. Clinical experience using the computerized digital stapling system in open gastric bypass for morbid obesity. *Obes Surg* 2003;13:837–841.

Miller A, Allen P, Fowler D. In-Vivo stereoscopic imaging system with 5 degrees of freedom for minimal access surgery. In: Westwood JD, et al., eds. *Medicine meets virtual reality 12.* Amsterdam: IOS Press; 2004:234–240.

Park S, Bergs R, Eberhart R, et al. Trocarless laparoscopy: magnetic positioning of intra-abdominal camera and retractor. *Ann Surg* 2007;245:379–384.

Rentschler ME, Dumpert J, Platt SR, et al. Mobile in-vivo camera robots provide sole visual feedback for abdominal exploration and cholecystectomy. *Surg Endosc* 2006;20: 135–138.

Scott DJ, Tang SJ, Fernandez R, et al. Completely transvaginal NOTES cholecystectomy using magnetically anchored instruments. *Surg Endosc* 2007;21(12):2308–2316.

Tirabassi MV, Banever GT, Moriarty KP, et al. Feasibility of thoracoscopic U-Clip esophageal anastomosis: an alternative for esophageal atresia. *Reconstr J Ped Surg* 2004;39:851–854.

COMMENTARY

Drs. Scott and Goova have provided a snapshot of some of the newer instruments available for use in laparoscopic surgery, as well as several that are under development. Although for today's young surgeons laparoscopy seems to have been practiced forever, only 2 decades have passed since laparoscopic surgery was first used for general surgery applications. The early days were spent developing and improving basic rigid instruments, access ports, and safe devices for delivering pneumoperitoneum gas and transmitting light and images to the operator's eyes. There has also been much energy devoted to developing tools for hemostasis, suturing, and anastomosis. Laparoscopy continues to be hindered by several technical shortcomings, each of which is being addressed. These limitations include: the need for multiple access ports, rigid handheld instruments with reduced degrees of freedom of motion, the fulcrum effect of the ports, 2-D imaging, optics directed by an assistant, and a relative lack of haptic sensation. The evolution of surgical practice is clearly toward less and less "invasion" of the patient's body to carry out diagnostic or therapeutic procedures. Will this lead to the continued evolution of "traditional" laparoscopic instruments? Will this lead to the development of devices that will allow single-port access? Will this lead to the the development of natural orifice transluminal endoscopic surgery? Will this lead to the deployment of miniaturized robots to carry out the procedures themselves? Investigators around the world are looking at each of these areas as fertile ground for research and development, and both start-up companies and multinational corporations continue this quest toward maximal patient benefit with minimal invasion. This is certainly an interesting era in which to be practicing surgery, and we surgeons must help to drive the technological developments that will shape our future.

NJS

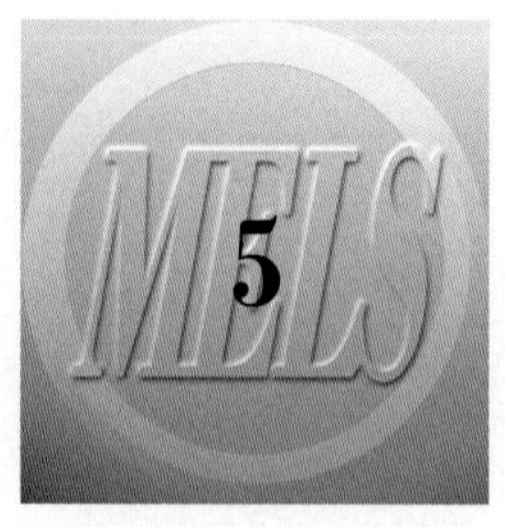

Imaging Systems in Minimally Invasive Surgery

STEVEN D. SCHWAITZBERG

INTRODUCTION

Laparoscopic and endoscopic procedures are so ubiquitous today that the technology that makes it possible is generally taken for granted. We as operating surgeons and assistants have an obligation to understand all of the central technologies of our craft in order to optimize the safety, cost-effectiveness, and efficiency of these procedures. The presentation of the visual information that we interpret in order to perform laparoscopic surgery has been in continuous evolution for more than a century. Georg Kelling, a pioneer at the dawn of the 20th century, was among those who developed the esophagoscope and early "coelioscopy" techniques. He was confronted with a complex task, demanding a means of access, lighting, and viewing capabilities to see inside of the abdominal cavity in order to make gynecologic or hepatic diagnoses. Those of his day had to rely upon drawn artwork rather than photography for documentation. Over the intervening years, the technology slowly developed and procedures advanced from purely diagnostic to include therapeutic techniques. Still, laparoscopy was pretty much a one-person show, with a single operating surgeon peering down the telescope. Fortunately, video technology would be developed that would find its way into the surgical arena and revolutionize minimally invasive surgery (MIS).

In the late 1980s, the laparoscopic cholecystectomy was the first minimally invasive procedure to gain widespread acceptance in the general surgery community. This procedure was the first of a juggernaut that overtook many open procedures by storm, replacing them with less invasive versions. However, a careful analysis will reveal that is was not the development of any one procedure such as laparoscopic cholecystectomy that serve as a catalyst, rather it was the development of *video-directed* laparoscopy, allowing a team approach to these procedures, that really was responsible for the growth of MIS. Assistants could now help the surgeon by retracting and providing tension in ways similar to open procedures, paving the way to accomplishing complex procedures previously deemed impossible.

Berci developed the first miniature camera for endoscopy in 1962. Later, William Chang would invent the first 1-Chip, solid-state camera using the Metal-Oxide-Semiconductor pick-up device in 1982, which further facilitated the development of the medical video camera system (personal communication). Since then, innumerable changes and improvements have resulted in the high-quality camera systems used today. Remarkably, the seemingly revolutionary camera systems available around 1987 or so would be considered unfit for clinical duty by today's standards due to the improvements all along the *imaging chain* since then.

The Imaging Chain

The philosopher and psychologist William James (1842–1910) is credited as saying, "A chain is no stronger than its weakest link, and life is after all a chain." Thus, the production of an excellent laparoscopic image requires that *all* of the links be in place and functioning else our wonderful (and expensive) systems will be rendered impotent by a worn-out light cable or magnetized monitor in need of degaussing. The classic imaging chain starts with the telescope, continues through the camera, and ends in the monitor, requiring seven pieces of equipment, known as the Magnificent Seven: light source, fiber-optic light cable, laparoscope, camera head, video signal processor, video cable, and monitor (Fig. 5-1). This results in eight places where the picture can be compromised, as the telescope has both a visual channel and fiber-optic light channel. The surgeon and the operating room team must work together to ensure optimal equipment function through careful handling of the equipment in the operating room and during the sterilization process. Accepting a poor video image is unacceptable and potentially dangerous. Yet, when the image is poor, many operating teams become paralyzed, unable to function without the aid of a medical engineer. "Understanding can overcome any situation, however mysterious or insurmountable it may appear to be." Accordingly, understanding the video system will allow the operating surgeon to do the basic troubleshooting for his or her system and not be totally dependent on nursing or technical staff, especially at night when experienced personnel may not be available. The advent of integrated operating suites has not changed the principles of this basic idea.

Today, we rarely see the imaging chain in its purest form. The Magnificent Seven are often supported by a cast of VCRs, photo printers, or digital capture devices. The cleanest images, that is, those with the least distortion, will be those whose video passes through the least number of devices. This is especially true of analog formats. Each time the signal passes through a device, the signal is degraded a bit. In "chain" configurations, peripheral devices such as printers and VCRs are placed in the imaging chain as well, to poor effect. Even the light source in some systems inputs the video signal so that automatic light adjustments can be made before that signal is sent to the monitor (Fig. 5-2). This type of arrangement is to be avoided as the operating image delivered to the surgeon is unquestionably suboptimal. Moreover, the recordings and prints will be degraded as well. The "distributed" configuration, in contrast, takes advantage of the fact that the video signal processor has multiple outputs of the identical video image, which can be disseminated to the various destinations. This allows each recipient device to obtain the cleanest image possible without cross interference (Fig. 5-3).

The modern imaging chain can be complex indeed, but the direction of the signal flow can always be followed with a little patience. While some institutions may purchase complete and well-integrated systems from telescope to monitor, a majority of laparoscopic system in use is the result of initial acquisition and subsequent upgrade of individual components.

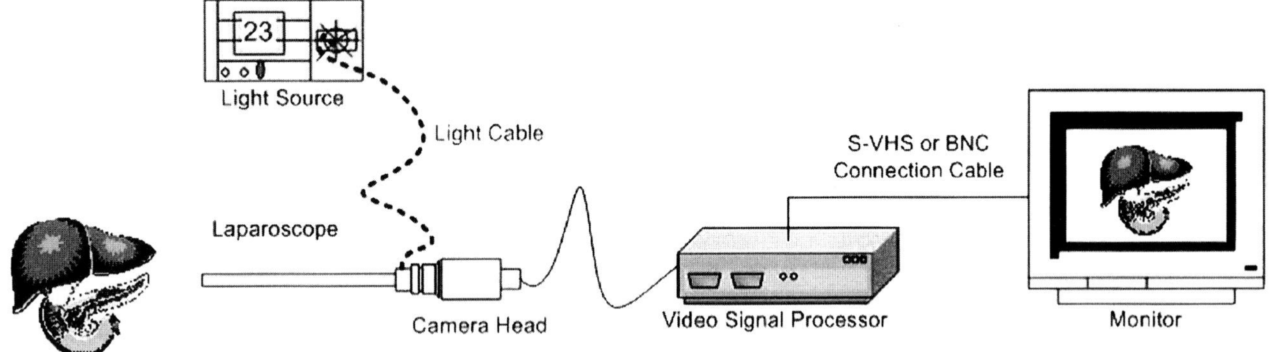

Fig. 5-1. The "Magnificent Seven" of the basic imaging chain.

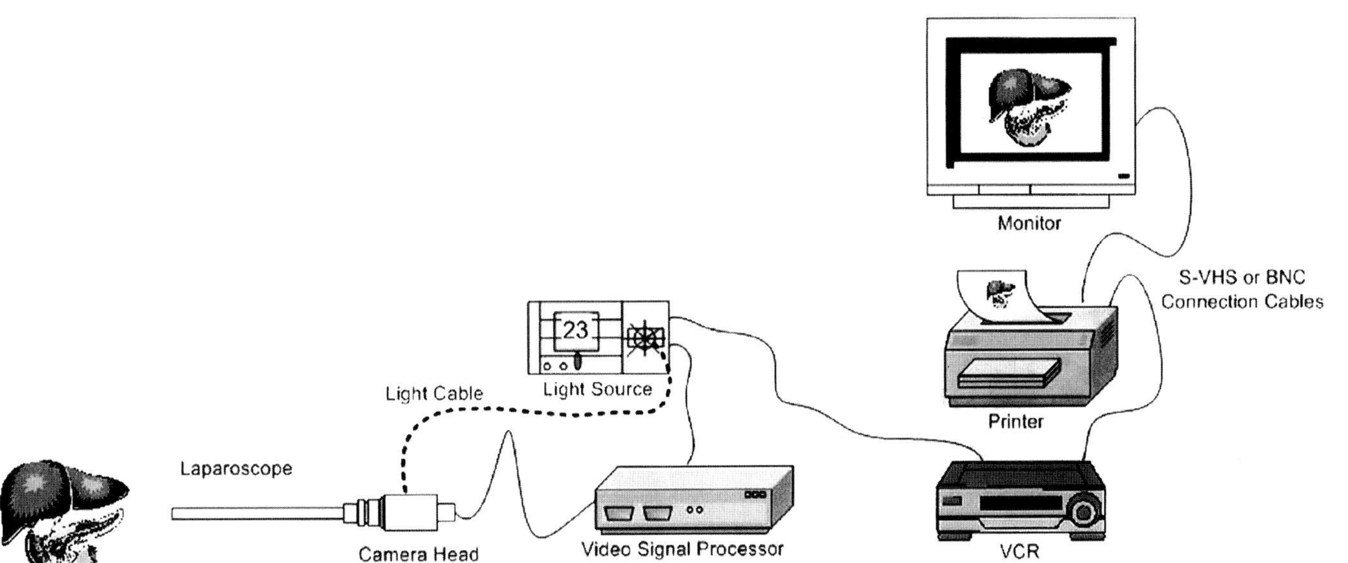

Fig. 5-2. Standard video setup with sequential pass-though of the video signal through each of the video components. This arrangement degrades the signal at each step of the chain.

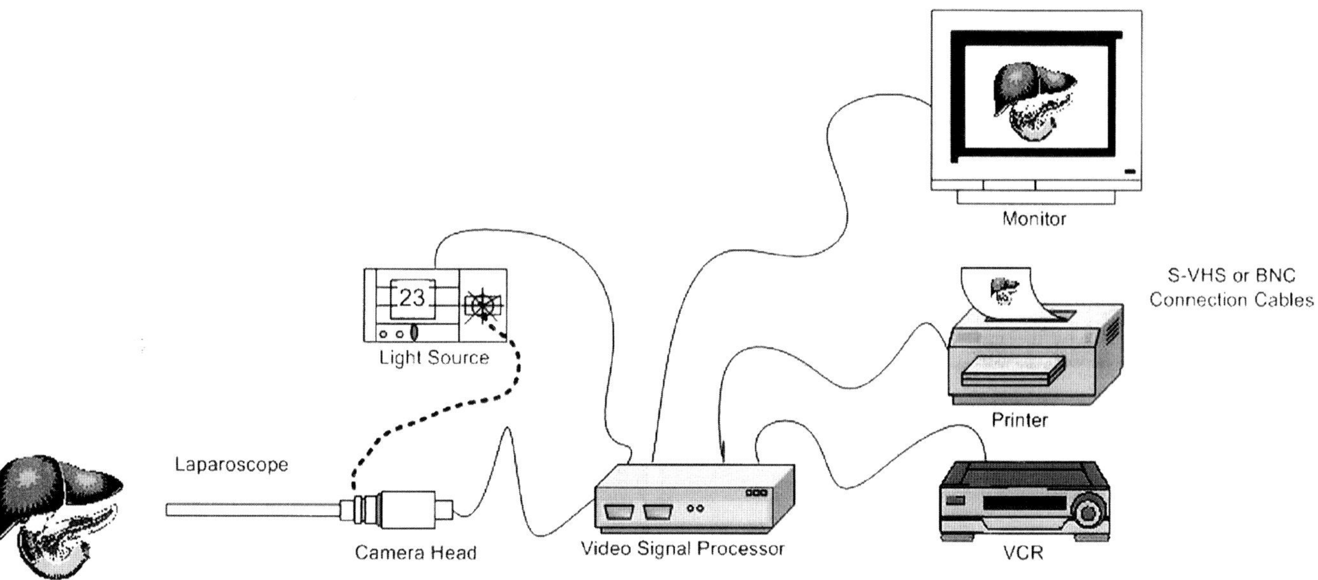

Fig. 5-3. Standard video setup utilizing a distributed approach to the video signal array.

As a result, the components of the new system may not be well matched in terms of signal impedance and visual resolution. Ultimately, the resolution will be limited to that of the lowest resolution component in the imaging chain rendering a potential high-resolution (and often expensive) device less than effective.

Light Source, Light Cable, and the Telescope Fiber Bundle

It is simple: no light, no laparoscopy. The light source is the often-overlooked soldier of the video laparoscopic system. Most of the light sources today utilize a halogen (150-watt), metal halide (250-watt), or xenon (300-watt) bulb, producing a very bright picture when used in an optimal imaging chain. While very powerful, these bulbs are also the Achilles' heel of the entire laparoscopic system. When the bulb fails, the entire system is out of commission until either the bulb is replaced or a new light is brought to bear. Many light sources record and display the hours of service and alert the biomedical medical engineer (or the well-informed surgeon) when it is time to make a change. When the lifetime rating of the bulb has been exceeded, the subsequent performance of the light source becomes unpredictable, often slowly dwindling until the surgeon just can't produce a well-lit scene despite the fact that a bright light seems to emanate from the laparoscope (Fig. 5-4). Typically, a metal halide bulb will be good for about 250 hours, while a Xenon will last for approximately 500 hours. The performance of xenon bulbs in the latter stages of life tends to be better than metal halide bulbs.

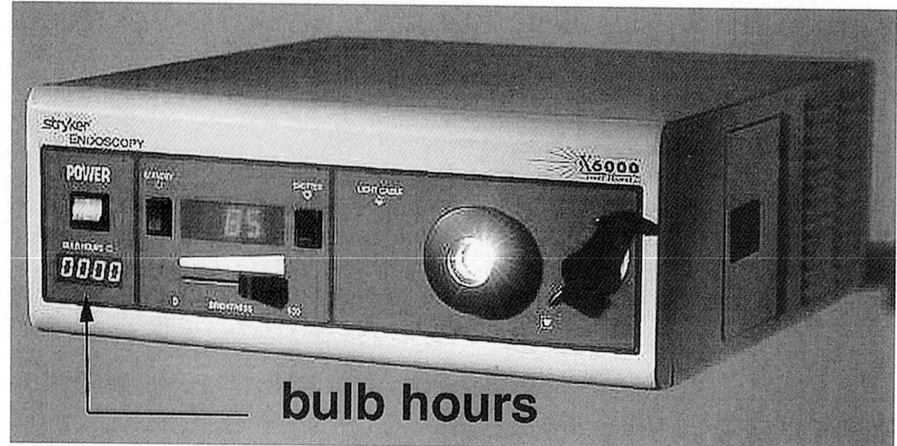

Fig. 5-4. Xenon light source: bulb-life display is shown. (Courtesy of Stryker Endoscopy; Santa Clara, CA.)

Finally, while it is remarkable how little heat is delivered to the tip of the laparoscope, the effects are cumulative. A lighted laparoscope or fiber-optic bundle in direct contact with paper drapes or the patient's skin will cause a burn after 20 or 30 seconds and must be avoided.

The fiber-optic cable and the fiber bundle in the laparoscope must be in excellent working order so as to achieve an optimal well-lighted picture. Some fiber-optic cables have a clear casing so the user can see the number of broken bundles in the light cord. Once the picture degrades and the number of visible breaks in the cable becomes extreme, it is time to replace this piece of equipment. If a broken light cable is suspected, a new cable should be placed without changing any setting on the system until the new image is evaluated. If the image is rectified, then the light cable that was replaced should be sent out for repair or discarded. Returning a bad light cable to general use is poor etiquette.

Identifying a laparoscope with a broken light bundle is a little trickier. In this instance, the surgeon sees a dark picture that does not improve with changing the light cable or the light source (assuming that they were functioning well to begin with). When the telescope is changed, the picture improves. If the biomedical technician *looks* down the laparoscope, the view is perfect and bright, thus implying the problem is caused by a broken fiber bundle inside of the telescope (Fig. 5-5). Table 5-1 illustrates the entire troubleshooting scheme for the "low light" scenario.

Too often, surgeons are tempted to find and adjust the "gain" control on the video signal processing box or the brightness knob on the monitor to brighten the picture when confronted with suboptimal lighting. This is occasionally necessary when excess blood in the field absorbs the light, but there are two good reasons why it should not be done at the beginning of a routine procedure just to get started. First, inadequate light at the beginning of the procedure is an indication that a piece of equipment is malfunctioning, a situation that should be rectified before getting too involved with the procedure. Second, the use of "gain" comes at the expense of picture resolution, resulting in a somewhat grainy image on the monitor, while turning the brightness knob to maximum produces a very washed-out picture. A good general rule of thumb to follow is to look in the right upper quadrant and visualize the space over the liver. The entire dome of the liver and right lateral diaphragm should be well lit and easily seen. If not, then the lighting system should be evaluated and optimized prior to beginning the dissection (Fig. 5-6, page 38).

Laparoscopes

The laparoscope is eye of the minimally invasive surgeon. In the beginning of the laparoscopic cholecystectomy era, the most commonly used telescope was the 10-mm straight lens, based on the Hopkins rod-lens design. Designs such as the thin lens system, which uses a series of objective lenses to transport the image down the laparoscope, are used less commonly (Fig. 5-7, page 38). Although smaller telescopes were available at that time, they had been designed to work in smaller spaces and, when used in the abdominal cavity, insufficient light and field of view precluded routine use. Since then, laparoscopes as small as 1 mm have been produced for diagnostic use. The field of view and picture brightness are dramatic improvements over early designs. "Mini" or "micro" 2-mm laparoscopy is reported for diagnostic and even advanced procedures. Rosser, Alimeda, and others has shown that these tiny laparoscopes can even be placed in patients who are awake.

One of the problems with working with these smaller laparoscopes (particularly those less than 3.4 mm OD, or outside diameter) is that they tend to bend easily, leading to potential damage during surgery. Full screen 5-mm laparoscopes with images comparable to many 10-mm systems are now available. When used with autoclavable camera systems, telescope changes

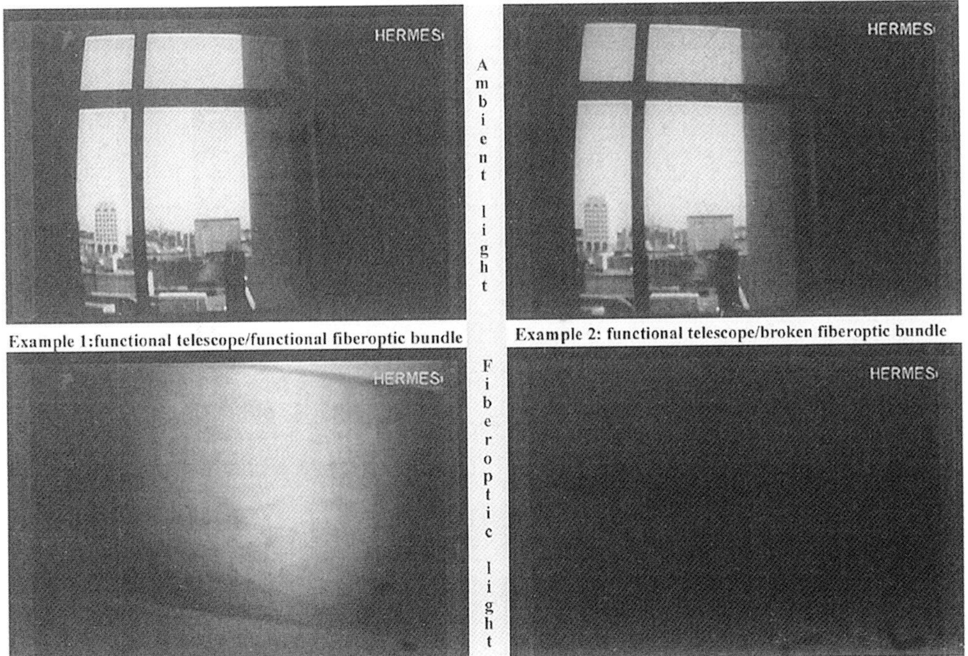

Fig. 5-5. Approach to the diagnosis of a broken fiber bundle within a lens-based laparoscope. The left-side images represent a functional telescope. On the right-side images, the fiber bundle is broken. The right upper photo utilizes the lens system only. The right lower photo is darkened because the fiber bundle is broken.

TABLE 5-1. MANEUVERS FOR TREATING THE "LOW LIGHT" SCENARIO

Step	Maneuver	Comments
1	Increase light source intensity.	Gain should be off—not needed in routine situations.
2	Reset monitor to default values.	Improvement indicates previous user adjustment.
3	Set light source shutter to manual.	Improvement indicates auto-shutter malfunction.
4	Set camera shutter to manual.	Improvement indicates auto-shutter malfunction.
5	Change laparoscope.	Improvement indicates broken fiber bundle in telescope—needs repair.
6	Change light cable.	Improvement indicates broken fiber bundles—needs replacement.
7	Change light source or bulb.	Bulbs should be replaced at the end of stated lifetime.

are accomplished rapidly, and cannula sizes can be kept to a minimum to allow for a view from a variety of port sites. However, 10-mm laparoscopes will remain the workhorse of MIS instrumentation until the durability of the smaller telescopes is improved.

The advanced laparoscopist works with an assortment of angled laparoscopes in order to achieve an optimal view. The advantages derived can be applied to just about any laparoscopic procedure. During laparoscopic cholecystectomy, when the transverse colon is prominent or a view behind the cystic duct facilitates dissection, the 30-degree or even 45-degree laparoscope is tremendously useful. Every operating center should have a full array of angled laparoscopes if for no other reason than safety. *If you can't see, you can't operate (safely).*

Digital laparoscopes, in which the laparoscope and camera head are a single unit with the imaging sensor at the end of the laparoscope, have been available since the early 1990s (Fig. 5-8, page 39). This "chip on a stick" was interesting, but suffered from the inability to focus clearly at close distances to the tissue and simply never really caught on. Recent improvements in the distal chip design have revitalized these systems. Today, high-definition unified video systems are available that provide excellent quality imaging (Fig. 5-9, page 39). The major characteristic of these systems is the integration of the laparoscope, light cable, and interface to the digital signal processor. The advantage of this approach is a well-tuned system capable of providing an optimal video display. The disadvantage is the lack of compatibility with legacy video systems that employ a separate rod–lens-like the scope. Using the same integrated proprietary technology, this has allowed the introduction of flexible video laparoscopes, thus bringing to laparoscopy advances originally developed for flexible endoscopy (LTF-V2; Olympus America, Inc; Center Valley, PA). These laparoscopes have four-way deflection for great versatility of viewing angles (Fig. 5-10, page 39). Despite the fact that flexible viewing options require a sophisticated camera operator and that its role during MIS is unclear, its use will likely increase in the future. Other innovations in laparoscope design include

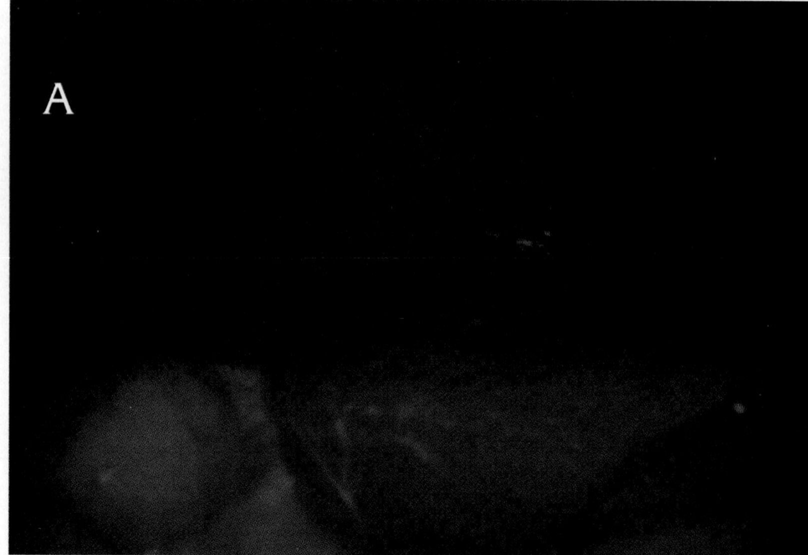

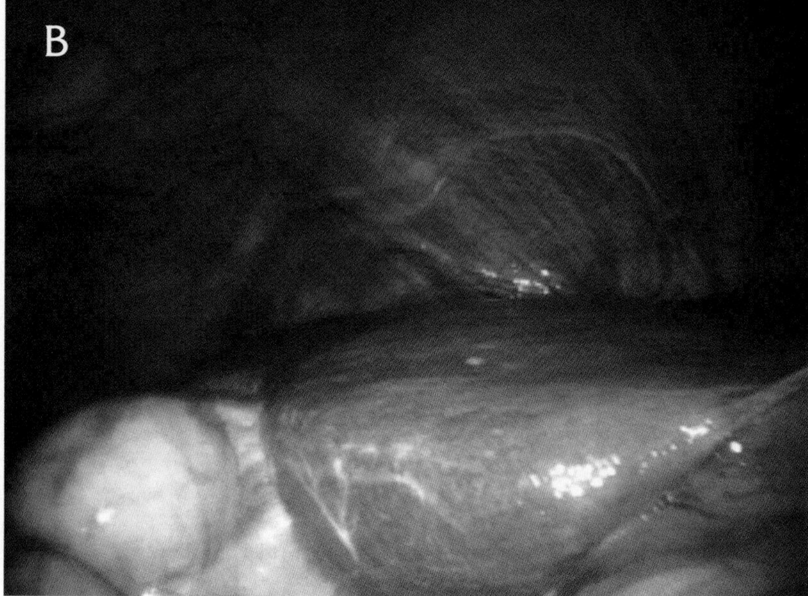

Fig. 5-6. Gallbladder lighting scene. **A.** Poorly lit right upper quadrant. The diaphragm is barely visible. **B.** Same patient after faulty light cable is replaced.

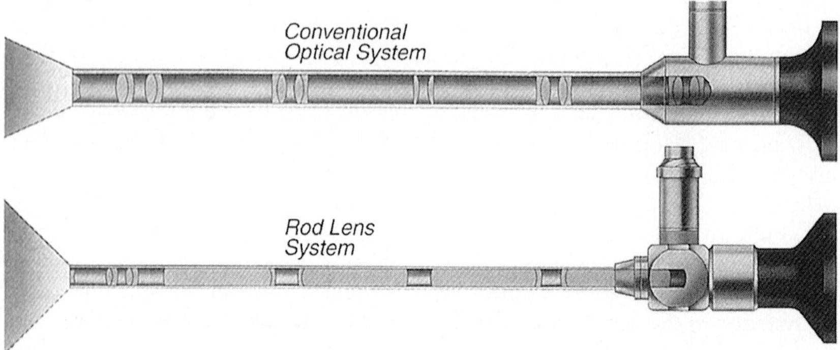

Fig. 5-7. Thin lens (conventional) and rod-lens designs used in laparoscopes today. (Courtesy of Karl Storz America Inc; Culver City, CA.)

auto-stabilizing imaging that uses two dual-axis accelerometers (DCI, KARL STORZ; Endoscopy-America, Inc.; Culver City, CA) so that the picture on the monitor is always upright.

Three-dimensional (3-D) laparoscopes are of two basic designs: single channel or dual channel. Dual channel laparoscopes provide a more striking 3-D picture than single channel telescopes. The wider the distance between the two optical channels, the more effective the 3-D effect is in simulating binocular vision. On the other hand, single channel 3-D laparoscopes can be angled, which is a big benefit inherent in this design.

Laparoscopes are sealed complex systems exposed to tremendous wear stress over their years of service. If the seal fails during surgery or sterilization, the image will become cloudy due the accumulation of moisture under the lens system. The impact of repeated sterilization cannot be overemphasized in terms of the wear and tear on the telescopes. Poor handling techniques will decrease the life span of these delicate instruments. Furthermore, the cost of repair of a broken laparoscope is invariably in excess of $1500, in our experience.

Camera Systems

The heart and soul of any laparoscopic image is the camera system. In general, this refers to the camera head that attaches to the laparoscope via a coupler and the signal-processing or camera control box that the camera head plugs into (Fig. 5-11, page 40). Similarly, it could also refer to the pure digital systems that include charge-coupled device (CCD) chips at the end of the laparoscope that plug directly into signal-processing boxes. Although discussed separately (see below), the monitor cannot be left out of this equation as optimal performance can only be achieved when camera resolution and display capabilities are similar. Camera heads come as either "one-chip" or "three-chip" devices. In a single-chip device, the CCD silicon wafer is made up of a grid of tiny image sensors, referred to as "pixels." Pixel density directly correlates with image resolution. In this example, multiple color sensors are deployed on the one chip, providing a colored image. The three-chip camera system is the one most commonly used today. Some three-chip cameras are capable of more than 950 lines of resolution, compared to about 550 lines for one-chip cameras (see below). A prism in the camera head is used to split the

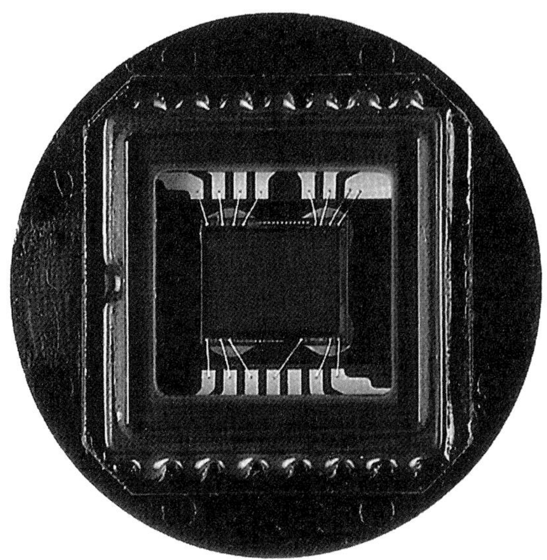

Fig. 5-8. Imaging acquiring CDD chip (enlarged).

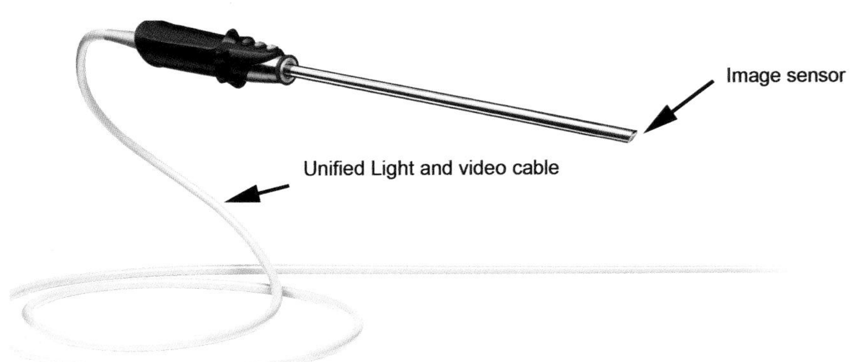

Fig. 5-9. In the unified digital design, the image sensor is moved to the tip of the laparoscope and the lens optics are eliminated. The video cable and light cable can be bundled together, somewhat simplifying their use. These are dedicate systems and cannot be interchanged. (Courtesy of Olympus Surgical.)

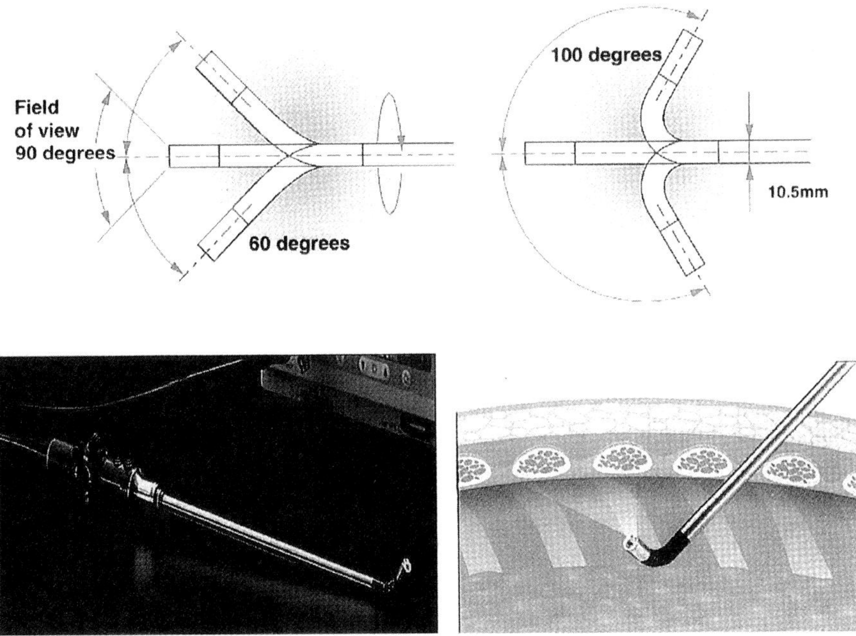

Fig. 5-10. Flexible digital video laparoscopes. This system provides unique viewing angle opportunities. (Courtesy of Olympus America Inc; Melville, NY.)

incoming lighted image into its three primary color (red, blue, and green) components, each falling on to its own CCD chip (Fig. 5-12, page 40). In each CCD, there are a number of sensor cells that convert the light that strikes it into an electrical charge. The charge is typically collected for 1/60 of a second, producing a field when the information from all of the cells is integrated. A high-resolution camera may contain more than 450,000 pixels. Each two fields make up a frame. Standard National Television Standards Committee (NTSC) format consists of 60 fields/30 frames per second outputted to a television monitor or VCR, rendering a natural smooth motion effect. This three-chip design provides the highest resolution and truest color rendition in cameras of this type. Three-chip camera systems today can provide more than 900 lines of horizontal resolution, producing extraordinary images on those systems capable of displaying such high-quality pictures.

Inherent in the modern camera is the ability to work in darker (low lux) settings than when these devices were first employed in the operating room. An interesting innovation in selected camera systems is the ability to view infrared light emission, such as with the InfraVison Imaging System (Stryker Endoscopy; San Jose, CA). Infrared-emitting nasogastric tubes to facilitate esophagus identification (Fig. 5-13, page 41) and ureteral stents to aid in ureter localization are available. These tools may be particularly useful in reoperative procedures or other instances where the tissue planes are distorted from inflammation or tumor.

Three-dimensional camera systems introduced in the early 1990s generated substantial interest but ultimately little following. Monitor-based systems usually required the viewers to wear special glasses that allowed the integration of the two image channels into a single image with apparent depth. Three-dimensional heads-up display systems routing the visual image through two separate computer video boards and onto separate liquid crystal displays provided a more binocular approach to the problem, such as the device shown in Figure 5-14, page 41 (Vista HMD; Vista Medical Technologies; Carlsbad, CA). The fact that the image is routed through a computer leads to possible future information integrations applications directed to the wearer's display. Computer video processing cards are now capable of outputs with resolutions as high as 2048 (horizontal) × 1536 (vertical) dpi. Although a number of surgeons have advocated for the

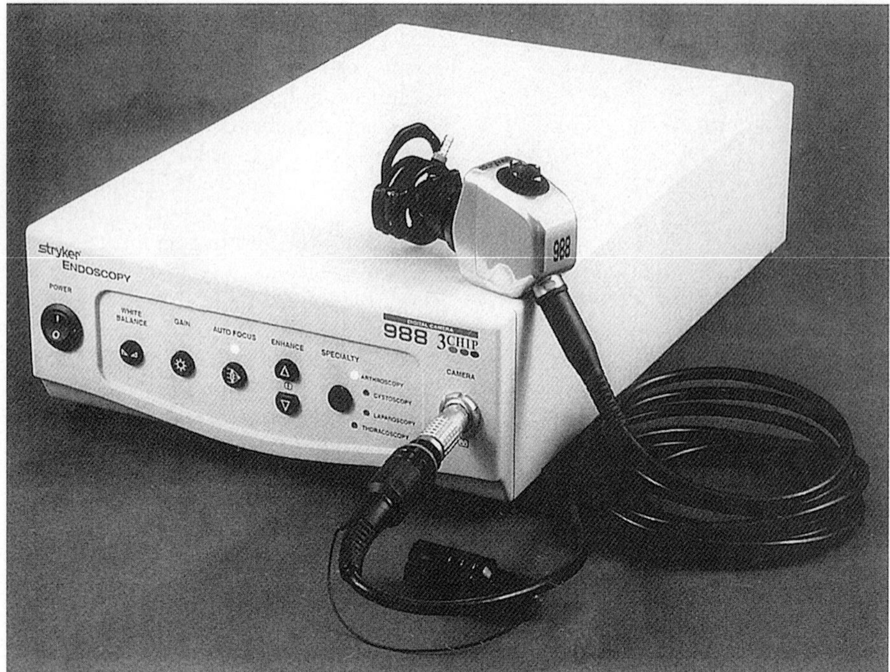

Fig. 5-11. A typical three-chip camera in use today. (Courtesy of Stryker Endoscopy; San Jose, CA.)

use of 3-D camera systems in certain procedures such as laparoscopic spinal surgery, bariatric surgery, and minimally invasive cardiac surgery, this technology has experienced limited diffusion into operating rooms perhaps due to limited data demonstrating added value to offset the added cost, causing a number of corporate enterprises to fail. Recent advancements in this area may stimulate a resurgence of this concept, including the development of software-driven image processing in order to provide a more natural stereoscopic image with improved depth perception.

Various authors have tried to quantify a benefit by operating in a 3-D environment, with inconsistent results. The recent appearance of computer-aided surgical operating systems for cardiac, urologic, and general surgical procedures (da Vinci; Intuitive Surgical Inc.; Sunnyvale, CA) has renewed interest in 3-D camera systems (Fig. 5-15, page 42). Relatively primitive haptic feedback exists for the operator using these remotely controlled "arms." The use of 3-D imaging display provides depth information used by the operator as a surrogate for haptics to the extent it is possible. Thus, at least for now, 3-D camera systems are a useful adjunct in the emerging "robotic" surgical arena.

Video Signal Processor (Camera Control Unit) and Video Output Format

Most manufacturers allow for multiple outputs from the video signal processing box, all of which carry the same picture so that the monitor, still printer and analog VCR, digital tape recorder, or digital capture device can each receive a clean image (Fig. 5-16, page 42). This can be a bit confusing as many of the signal boxes put out more than one type of video signal. Furthermore, these outputs can be analog or digital in nature. The three most common analog formats are composite, super video (Y/C), and RGB (red, blue, green). Composite signals carry the light and color information in a single channel that can be plugged directly into televisions, monitors, or VCRs using a variety

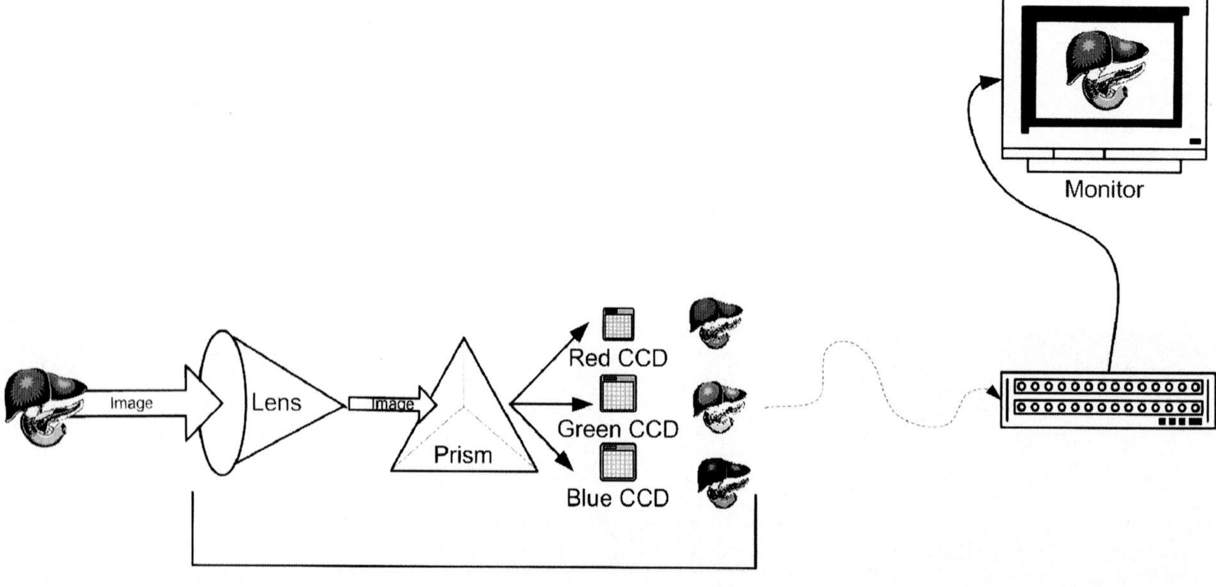

Fig. 5-12. A three-chip camera. Light enters the lens and is split into red, blue, and green components by a prism, allowing each color band to fall on its specified CCD.

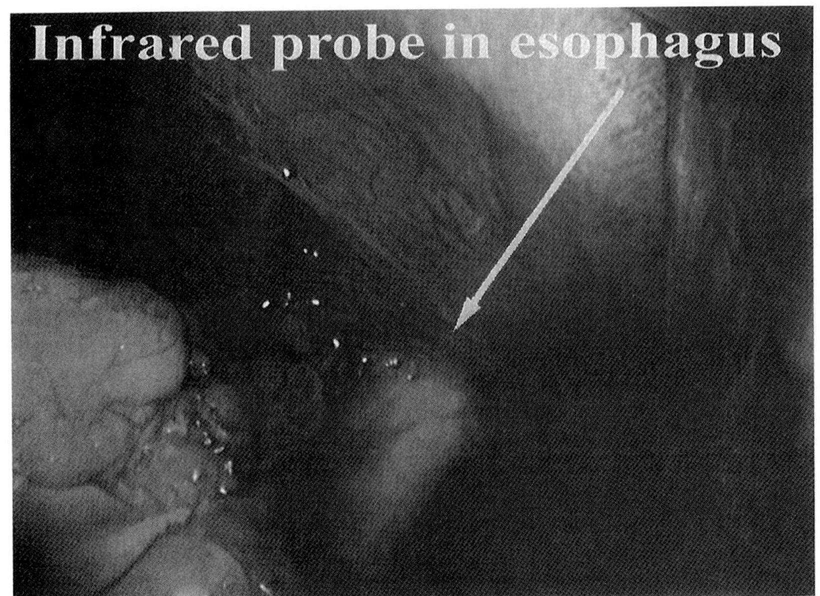

Fig. 5-13. An infrared-emitting probe built into nasogastric tube placed in the esophagus is observed using the InfraVision Imaging System. (Courtesy of Stryker Endoscopy; San Jose, CA.)

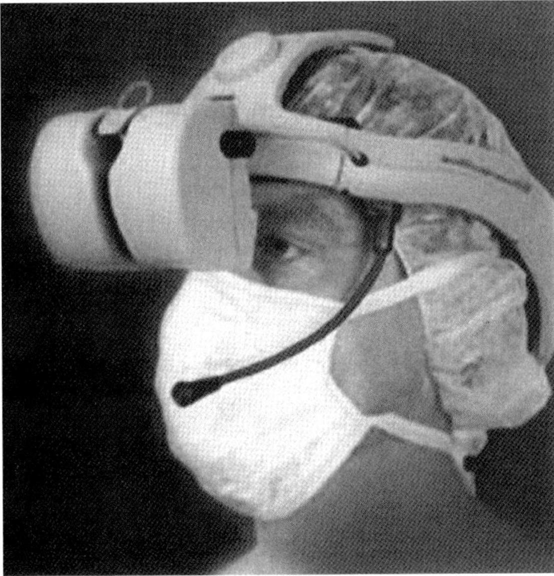

Fig. 5-14. A 3-D heads-up display provides stereoscopic images on liquid crystal displays. The headset is connected via cable into a computer, where the image is processed through dual video cards. (Courtesy of Vista Medical Technologies; Carlsbad, CA.)

of connectors such as RCA or BNC. Super video (S-VHS) or Y/C signals carry the light and color information on separate channels. This improves the resolution and minimizes distortion as the signal passes though devices or is videotaped, but requires devices with special inputs to receive or record the signal. S-VHS video recorders require special tape to record in the S-VHS format. These tapes will fit into but not play properly in standard VHS recorders. On the other hand, S-VHS tape decks will play VHS tapes without distortion and even record on them in a VHS format because the S-VHS decks will detect which type of tape it is and adjust accordingly. RGB signals are divided amongst four wires, each terminating with its own BNC connector. The first three wires carry a unique color signal, and the fourth channel is for synchronization of the image. Consumer DVD players offer this choice as well providing an optimal signal to higher-end televisions that can accept this signal. The image produced in this way offers somewhat more resolution than composite or even Y/C choices when tested on the same monitor. If available, this option this should be routinely selected by the operating surgeon.

There are a variety of digital outputs as well. The most well known is the DV output commonly carried via IEEE 1394 interface, also known as FireWire or i-LINK. Generally, these are for recording devices only, as currently there a limit to how long the cable from the source can be. Moreover, the DV output is a compressed format that must be "uncompressed" for viewing on a monitor. This adds about a 1/10-second delay and thus is *not* recommended for live surgical procedures. Digital recorders utilizing digital tape formats such as MiniDV, DVCAM, and DVCPRO all have bidirectional FireWire ports, meaning there are no input and output distinctions. Later, the digital recorders can be utilized to feed the recorded video into computers with an IEEE 1394 port for digital editing with no generational loss in the transfer. That is to say, perfect copies are made. When edited, the final digital segments are identical to the original or master source. The final video can be exported in a variety of ways such as to videotape, CD, or web-based material. In order to edit analog tapes (VHS or S-VHS) digitally on the computer, the analog signal must be digitized. This can be accomplished in a variety of ways, such as computer-based analog capture boards, rerecording the video to digital tape, or passing the analog video through a digitizing bridge device and channeling this output to an IEEE 1394 computer port. The digital visual interface (DVI) and the serial digital interface (SDI) are digital outputs that can be routed effectively to monitors without the the distance limitations that beset the IEEE 1394. The most recent video signal processors will output to a variety of analog and digital output devices that effectively meet the wide variety of operating room recording needs.

Video Capture and Export

An interesting and often forgotten aspect of these camera systems is that the images are all digital before being converted to the analog output displayed on most monitors. In this era of digital still and video photography, this feature can be particularly useful. The first generation of digital capture units stored bitmap images on floppies, Zip compatible media, or minidisks. The newer generation devices are more useful

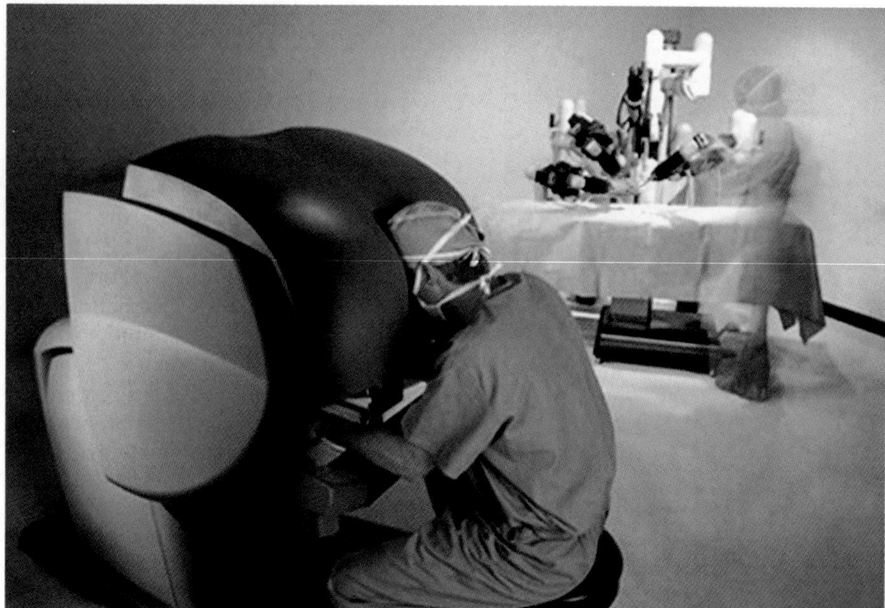

Fig. 5-15. A da Vinci surgical system. The 3-D video image is displayed to the surgeon at an image and telemanipulation console. (Courtesy of Intuitive Surgical, Inc; Sunnyvale, CA.)

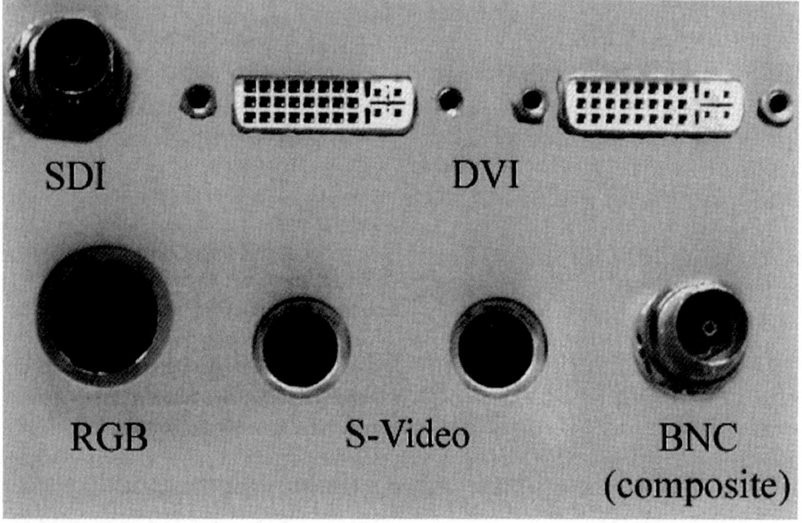

Fig. 5-16. A variety of analog and digital outputs available from the video signal processor (camera controller unit).

in a variety of ways. One system allows images to be captured on a SmartMedia card (OTV-S7V Visera Video System Center; Olympus America, Inc.; Center Valley, PA). This same memory card can also be placed in consumer or professional digital cameras, expanding the photographer's flexibility (Fig. 5-17). Images on SmartMedia (or CompactFlash or SD) cards can be imported easily into personal computers. Most systems today have both image and video capture capability, allowing these files to be written to a CD or DVD. Writing video files to large storage DVD will simplify digital video editing of these procedures because the expensive and often complicated digitization of videotape becomes unnecessary. Current DVD recording systems capture the video as MPEG 1 (352 × 240 pixels) or MPEG 2 (640/720 × 480 pixels) video allowing for several hours of video to be captured on a single DVD. In addition, systems that export the captured still or video images through file transfer protocol (FTP) to a hospital's computer network provide the opportunity for remote image storage, storage in electronic medical records, or hospital-wide (or beyond) observation. Examples include the SDC Pro video recorder and Stryker Switchpoint Infinity 2 video router (Stryker Endoscopy; San Jose, CA) and the Condor Control System (Smith and Nephew, Inc; Andover, MA). One of the more flexible features to emerge on some systems is the appearance of the Universal Serial Bus (USB) ports on the capture system. This innovative addition merges medical and consumer platforms. The surgeon can now download images to flash memory cards or portable hard drives, eliminating the need to print paper records (unless required for the medical record) or to collect CDs to store images (Fig. 5-18).

Monitors

The image on the monitor is similar to the old adage "all that the patient sees is the incision." It does not matter how technologically sophisticated the imaging system is if the picture on the monitor looks bad. Medical grade monitors can handle three types of input: composite video via a BNC connector, Y/C (super video via a 4-pin mini DIN) connector, and component RGB via the multi head BNC cable connector. Laparoscopic camera systems generally output to the first two choices, with Y/C pictures being slightly sharper with the newer systems possessing a RGB output as well. Given a choice, the surgeon should select the RGB option since this is consistently the most superior image.

The monitor is not subjected to as much wear and tear as most of the other components of the imaging chain, but the image can be degraded at this point in a few common ways. The most obvious is the manipulation of the monitor controls by a previous user to overcome some other defect in the video pathway. In general, this does not work well. Identifying the actual problem is, untimately, the superior solution. Second, monitors are subject to magnetic distortion, which often appears as a purplish fringe around the periphery of the image. This can be corrected by activating the "degauss" function present on many monitors. Third, unterminated video signals can feed back into the monitor and distort the image. This happens when a video cable is left attached to the primary monitor's output but free on the other end. The video signal has nowhere to go but back up the cable, degrading the image and often appearing as solarization on the monitor. Disconnecting the unneeded slave cable or, in some instances, activating the 75-ohm termination switch present at the output terminal on some monitors will correct this problem.

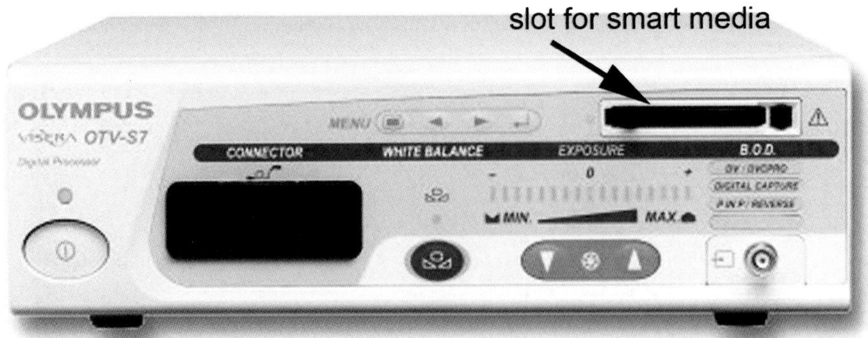

Fig. 5-17. Digital capture system utilizing SmartMedia cards. These cards can also be used in commercially available digital cameras. (Courtesy of Olympus America Inc; Melville, NY.)

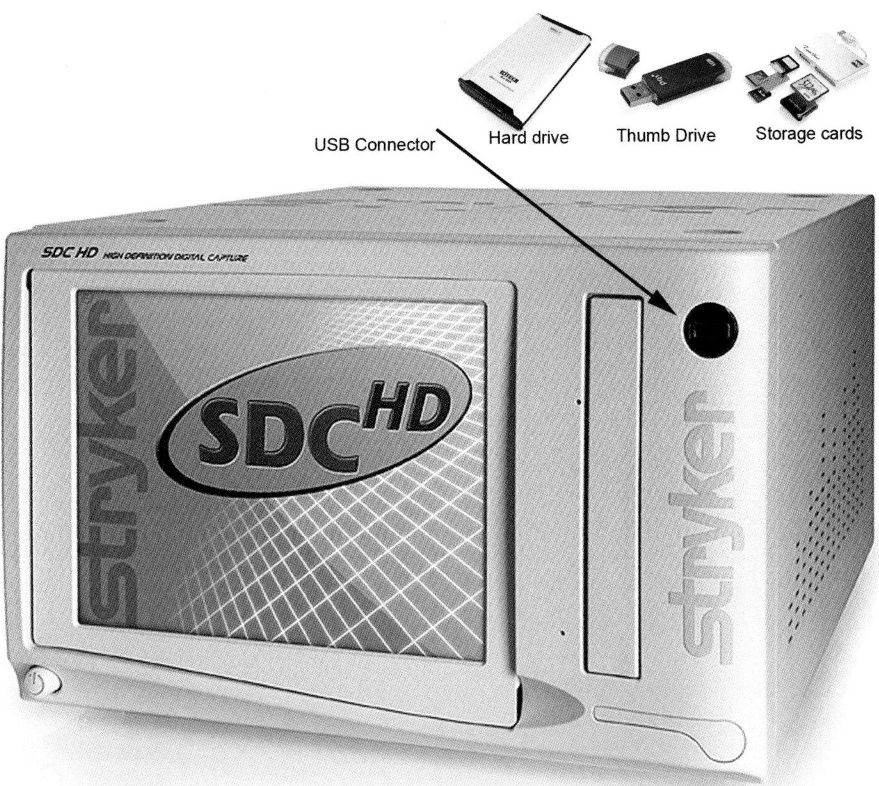

Fig. 5-18. The presence of a USB connector on the capture system allows for great flexibility in image storage to devices such as hard drives, thumb drives, or storage cards. (Courtesy of Stryker Endoscopy; San Jose, CA.)

The standard monitor in most operating rooms has a horizontal resolution of up to 600 lines. The obvious implication from this is that very high-resolution camera systems will require high performance monitors to achieve optimal image presentation. Solutions for this situation include high-end analog monitors, but the greatest potential for the future exists for digital monitors. For instance, digital flat panel displays that connect to computer systems using the DVI interface are commercially available. This is essentially the digital equivalent to the analog RGB standard in image quality. This standard specifies a single connector that allows for both the new digital and legacy VGA interfaces. This creates a common digital connectivity specification for digital displays and high-performance PCs while allowing for existing analog support. DVI handles bandwidths in excess of 160 MHz, and thus supports UXGA and HDTV (both high-definition video formats). This provides remarkable opportunities in the operating room for high-resolution camera systems. DVI should accelerate the trend to routine support of digital displays by PC-based controllers, thus reducing the cost of digital liquid-crystal monitors used in flat panel and laptop displays. Such systems are currently available (Stryker Endoscopy; San Jose, CA). One downside is that the cabling is limited to about 5 meters.

Another digital option is the Serial Digital Interface (SDI). This uses the SMPTE (Standards Committee of the Society of Motion Picture) 259M protocol, which is a serial digital video data stream consisting of video plus four audio channels, making up a 270 Mbps transmission, or 360 Mbps for wide-screen (16:9 aspect ratio). This is a very high quality broadcast signal and, unlike the other digital transmissions standards mentioned above, there is no limitation on cable length. These are exciting developments that are beginning to make their way into our operating rooms.

Flat panel displays lend themselves nicely to ceiling mounted operation. The substantial reduction in weight from about 50 pounds for CRT monitors to about 13 pounds for an LCD monitor allows for a much lower cost for boom installation. Analog/digital flat panel displays with resolutions of 1280 × 1024 pixels with S-VHS, Composite, XS-VGA, and DVI-D inputs are currently available (Fig. 5-19, page 44). The downside of these monitors is the need to be squarely in front of the image; otherwise, it will appear to be washed out and suboptimal. Large (42 inches and higher) high-resolution plasma displays are recently finding their way into operating rooms, now that the once prohibitive price points have fallen dramatically. Often wall mounted, these displays are useful in dedicated "endosuites" for teleconferences, telepresence, or mentoring activities.

Ergonomic Considerations

Ergonomic evaluations of optimal monitor placement suggest rethinking the standard tower placement and bringing the display down in the general direction of the operative field. Certainly, monitors placed above eye level are in suboptimal alignment with the surgeon's positioning. Recent reports show that laparoscopic surgeons complain of a variety of head, neck, and shoulder ailments, some of which may relate to monitor placement. In addition to ceiling-mounted flat panel designs, a few other options are available. One such is a sterile disposable screen in the surgical field that receives a boom-mounted

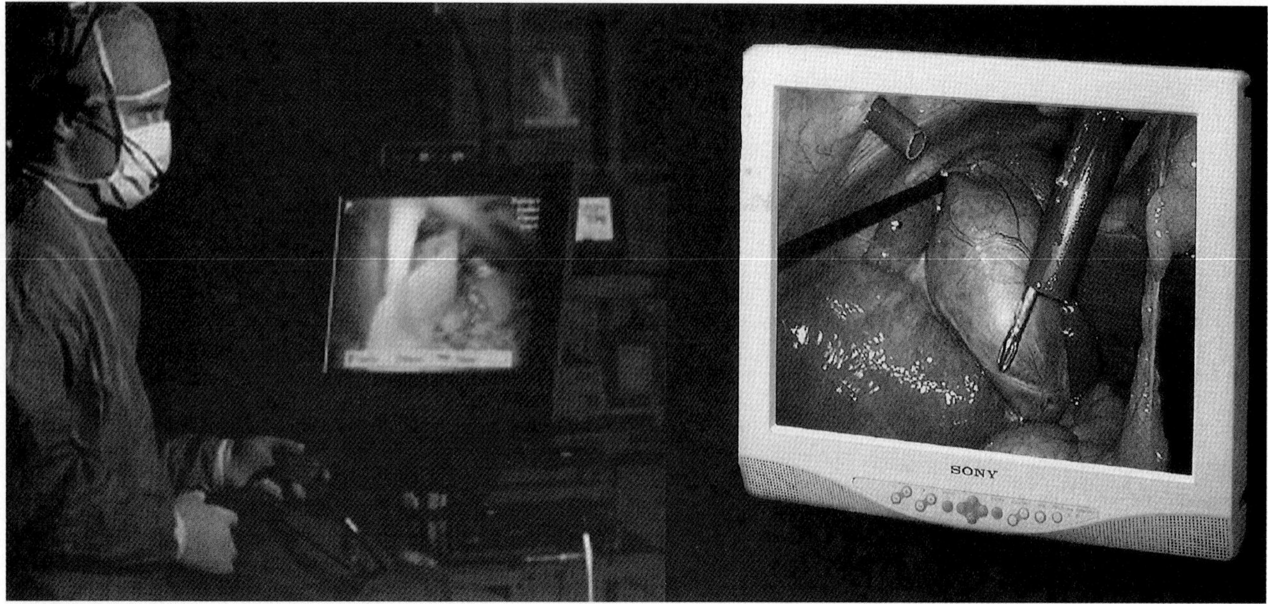

Fig. 5-19. Flat panel displays used in the operating room. These displays can be brought into ergonomically preferable locations, reducing operator stress. (Courtesy of Stryker Endoscopy; San Jose, CA and Sony Medical; Park Ridge, New Jersey.)

projection. This can be placed in optimal ergonomic position, and the surgeon can direct assistants or trainees by pointing to relevant structures directly on the screen. One example is InsideView (LSI Solutions; Victor, NY) (Fig. 5-20). Heads-up displays offer another ergonomic approach to this problem. In addition to the system mentioned earlier, which connects the wearer to the camera system by a cable, high-resolution cable-free "glasses" are becoming available. The video signal is passed to the headset via an infrared transmission, allowing substantial freedom for the surgeon (Fig. 5-21).

Resolving the Image

Image differences between inputs or systems can be subjective. For many years, the television industry has used test patterns for measuring monitor resolution. The classic RCA black-and-white Indian Head test card first appeared in the late 1930s and was used to evaluate the system (Fig. 5-22). The detailed patterns let people fine-tune the focus and resolution on their TVs. For national television system committee (NTSC) monitors, the vertical resolution is fixed at 525 lines of resolution. That means 525 horizontal scan lines are painted on the monitor to construct the image. Horizontal resolution is changeable and measurable using test patterns. Video system sharpness is determined by measuring "lines of resolution,"

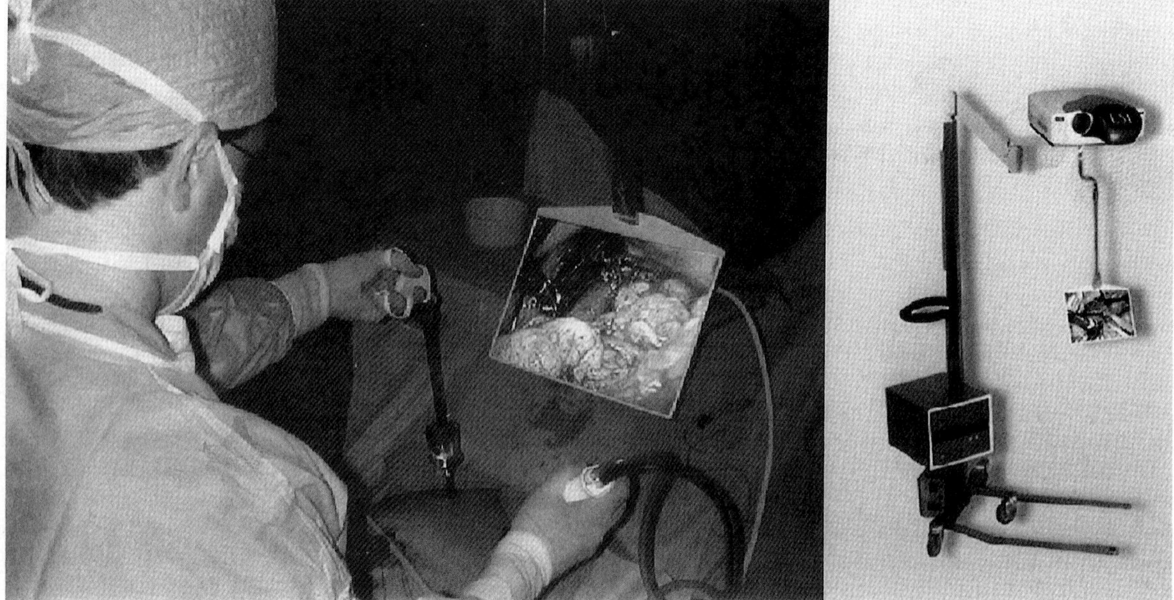

Fig. 5-20. Sterile "on the field" monitor. This monitor can be placed in just about any position imaginable. The surgeon can direct his or her team by pointing out important anatomy directly on the screen. (Courtesy of LSI Solutions; Rochester, NY.)

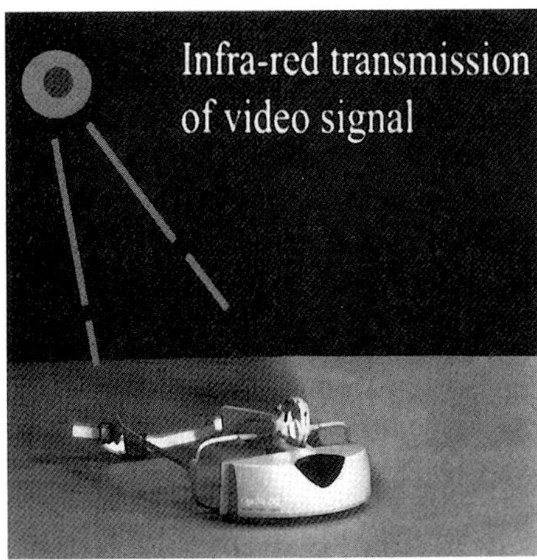

Fig. 5-21. Image display "glasses" without cables. An overhead infrared transmitter mounted on the ceiling or on a boom transmits the video information to this device. (Courtesy of Stryker Endoscopy; San Jose, CA.)

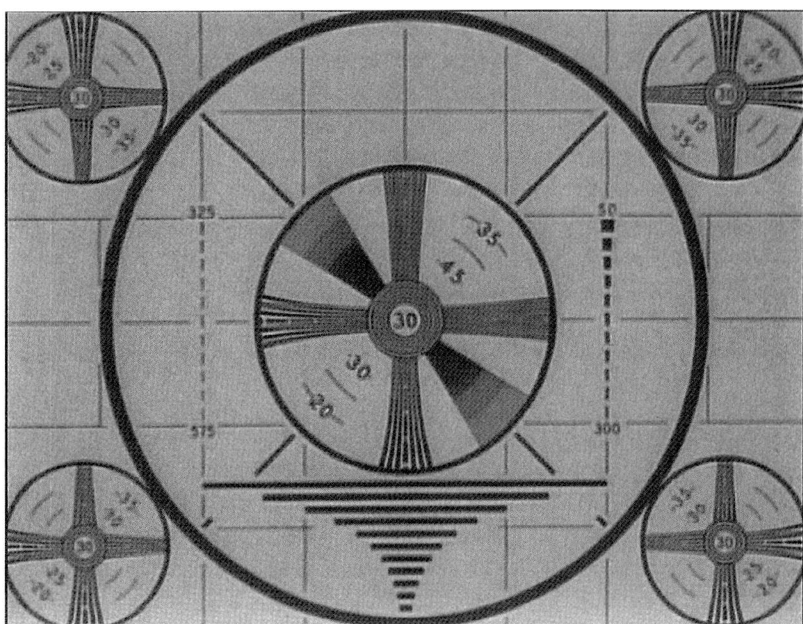

Fig. 5-22. Classic "Indian Head" test card developed by the RCA Corporation in 1939.

that is, the number of alternating black and white lines that a system is able to discriminate on a test pattern. Berber et al. described a simple method for evaluating the horizontal resolution of the laparoscopic video system. The one-chip cameras tested demonstrated a horizontal resolution of 640 lines with Y/C or RGB connections, whereas the-three chip cameras were able to resolve up to 800 lines with a RGB connection to the monitor from the camera (Fig. 5-23). Standard NTSC television broadcasting is maximized at only 330 lines regardless of television capability. DVD players display about 500 to 565 lines when connected optimally. For the surgeon, this math is relevant when using or purchasing a high-end camera system with 800 lines of horizontal resolution but displaying on a monitor capable of displaying only 500 lines. The benefits will not be realized, once again demonstrating that the imaging chain will only be as strong as its weakest link! Similarly, displaying an image from a camera capable of emitting a signal with only 500 lines of resolution on a monitor with much greater capability will not improve the image. The number of pixels that can be displayed vertically or horizontally such as those mentioned above is the rating scheme for digital monitors. Despite extensive monitor capability, the standard video signal is composed of 640 pixels horizontally by 480 pixels vertically, or 720 × 480 pixels (such as with MiniDV signals). The latter translates into about 540 lines of horizontal resolution. Once all of those pixels are accommodated, the image will not improve with more capable displays.

High-Definition Camera Systems

Recently, high-definition video cameras were introduced into minimally invasive surgery. There are two major formats for high-definition video: 720p and 1080i. They share in common a 16:9 display format, sometimes referred to as the *letterbox format*. This differs from standard definition television, which has been traditionally displayed in the 4:3 format. The 720p refers to the 720 scan lines from top to bottom in a *progressive* display and the 1080i refers to the 1080 scan lines from top to bottom in an *interlaced* display. Either of these formats produces twice the vertical and horizontal resolution of a standard definition television picture. The interlacing technique is used to produce a higher resolution than the monitor actually delivers. This is achieved by displaying every other horizontal scan line at each screen refresh. For example, that may mean that the image actually changes every 60th of a second, requiring two of these screen passes to produce a complete image. Interlaced images are associated with flickering artifact. Progressive scan means that the image is built by displaying the screen lines from top to bottom. Obviously, these events happen very quickly and are generally unnoticeable to the naked eye.

A high-definition video camera requires a display capable of taking advantage of the increased resolution. The classic cathode ray tube (CRT) television set can display only 550 scan lines. Thus, it is obvious that an upgrade to high definition is truly

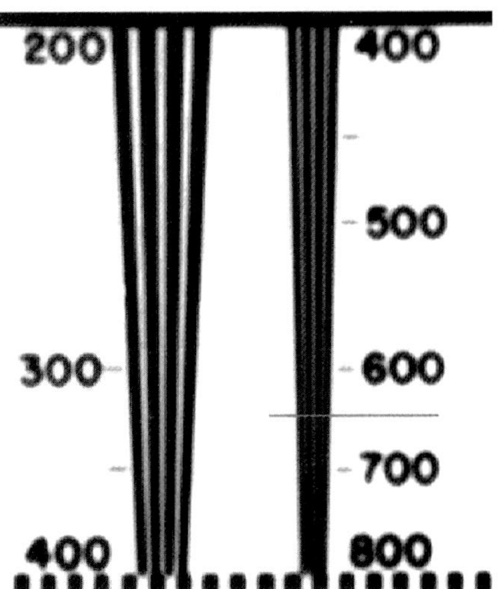

Fig. 5-23. Vertical wedge test pattern used to assess horizontal resolution. The photograph may not reflect the original image. In this case, the resolution was determined to be 650 lines of resolution.

a system upgrade. The related problem is how to record in these formats. Super video, VHS, or standard definition formats and thus are insufficient for recording high-definition images. The MiniDV recording format is 720 × 480 and, thus, is a high-definition format. But remembering that the chain is only as strong as the weakest link, one has to be certain that the signal being delivered to such a recording deck is actually a high-definition signal. Thus, recording a video onto a miniDV deck through the super video cable is only a standard definition recording. Similarly, connecting the high-definition monitor to the high-definition camera box via the standard definition cable is suboptimal.

High-definition DVD formats are also being developed. The two major formats are HD DVD and Blu-ray DVD. Both of these formats are capable of delivering a true HD image. This format war will rage on for some years to come. The major distinguishing factor at this time is that the Blu-ray DVDs are more expensive and have a theoretical capacity (200 GB, or gigabytes) that is over three times that of HD DVD. Most operating recording will continue on standard DVD, standard VHS, or miniDV recording systems for some time to come.

High-definition video signals should be transmitted from a camera box to the flat-panel display using Digital Visual Interface (DVI) cables. A single-link DVI cable is capable of transmitting a picture up to 1980 × 1080 pixels. Dual-link DVI cables are capable of even greater resolution. One of the limitations of the DVI cable is that the maximum effective length is rated at 16 feet. This means that the camera box needs to be reasonably close to the display monitors to use this format. There is an upcoming trend in the commercial home theater high-definition video market to use High-Definition Multimedia Interface (HDMI). This interface is capable of transmitting extraordinary bandwidth of over 10 Gpbs, more than five times what is needed to transmit HDTV. In addition to this extraordinary amount of video data, this single cable will also be capable of carrying eight channels of audio within the same plug and cable arrangement.

The real question that the operating team faces is whether or not the upgrade to HDTV is worth the investment. Recognizing that the past decade and a half has been notable for constant iterative upgrades in video quality, we can finally look forward to a stable platform for at least a while. These systems are available in both camera systems connected to classic rod-lens laparoscopes as well as the integrated all-digital systems. There is little data to indicate that surgical outcomes will be directly affected by a transition from standard definition video image to high-definition video image. That said, early users of HD systems find a clear improvement in the visual quality of the image displayed; reports of a 3-D–like effect are common. Furthermore, to truly take advantage of the high-definition image, the 16:9 letterbox format ideally would be displayed. The impact (value) of switching from a 4:3 format to a 16:9 format requires further study.

The Last Mile

In the near term, the "Holy Grail" for the world of digital video imaging in the operating room is a system that would allow the surgeon to select images and video at the end of the case to append to the medical record. The magnitude of this undertaking should not be taken lightly. Given the wide disparity of electronic medical record (EMR) systems available today and the numerous manufacturing concerns, a commodity solution (equivalent to plugging in a printer or recorder) is not readily available. Problems such as storage format, storage size, and route to specific

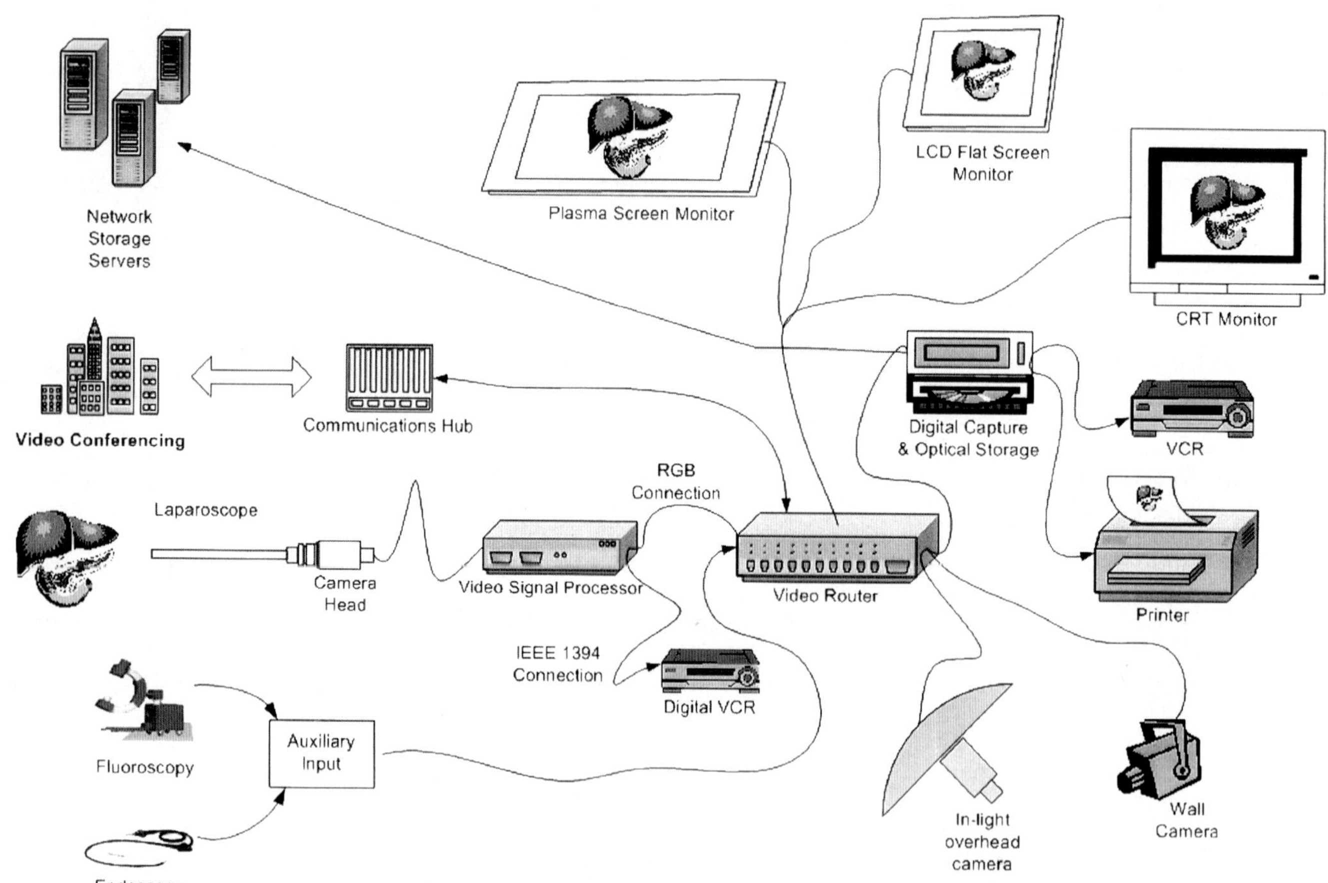

Fig. 5-24. The "totally integrated" operating theatre. The video image is capable of being directed into and out from the operating room by a central video router. This also allows for the integration of a variety of peripheral devices into the system.

EMR destination will require the creation of application standards that simply do not exist today. A custom solution, vendor by vendor and hospital by hospital, is required until that day comes.

CONCLUSION

The future of the imaging chain is bright. Careful attention to each aspect of the process will produce an excellent environment in which to operate. There are now a seemingly infinite number of ways the surgical video system can be configured. The simple laparoscopic tower on a rolling cart has morphed in the last decade into the dedicated endoscopic operating endosuite deploying the full array of video technologies in an integrated fashion. It has become just as easy to transmit the laparoscopic image to a location 1000 miles away as it is to print the captured input of a fluoroscopic cholangiogram for the chart. Figure 5-24 depicts a number of the possibilities available when utilizing a fully integrated operating endosuite. These environments will allow for the future developments in teaching, documentation, and image manipulation that we can expect to continue in our immediate futures.

SUGGESTED READING

Almeida OD, Val-Gallas JM. Office microlaparoscopy under local anesthesia in the diagnosis and treatment of chronic pelvic pain. *J Am Assoc Gynecol Laparosc* 1998;5: 407–410.

Berber E, Pearl JM, Siperstein AE. A simple device for measuring the resolution of videoscopic cameras and laparoscopes in the operating room. *Surg Endosc* 2002;16: 1111–1113; discussion 1114.

Berci G. Endoscopy and Television. *Br Med J* 1962;11610.

Berci G, Schwaitzberg SD. The importance of understanding the basics of imaging in the era of high-tech endoscopy: part I. Logic, reality, and Utopia. *Surg Endosc* 2002;4:377–380.

Berci G, Schwaitzberg SD. The importance of understanding the basics of imaging in the era of high-tech endoscopy: part II. Logic, reality, and Utopia. *Surg Endosc* 2002;16: 1518–1522.

Herron DM, Lantis JC, Maykel J, et al. The 3-D monitor and head-mounted display. A quantitative evaluation of advanced laparoscopic viewing technologies. *Surg Endosc* 1999;13:751–755.

James W. The Varieties of Religious Experience, Lectures 6-7, "The Sick Soul," 1902.

Litynski GS. *Highlights in the History of Laparoscopy: The Development of Laparoscopic Techniques—A Cumulative Effort of Internists, Gynecologists, and Surgeons*. Frankfurt/Main: Barbara Bernert Verlag;1996:xiv, 367.

Mueller MD, Camartin C, Dreher E, et al. Three-dimensional laparoscopy. Gadget or progress? A randomized trial on the efficacy of three-dimensional laparoscopy. *Surg Endosc* 1999;13:469–472.

Peale N. *Positive Thinking Every Day*. New York: Fireside; 1993.

Rosser JC, Palter SF, Rodas EB, et al. Minilaparoscopy without general anesthesia for the diagnosis of acute appendicitis. *J Soc Laparoendosc Surg* 1998;2:79–82.

Schauer PR, Ikramuddin S, Luketich JD. Minilaparoscopy. *Semin Laparosc Surg* 1999; 6:21–31.

Schwaitzberg SD. Use of microlaparoscopy in diagnostic procedures: a case report. *Surg Laparosc Endosc* 1995;5:407–409.

Vara-Thorbeck C, Toscano R, Felices M. Preperitoneal hernioplasty performed with needlescopic instruments (microlaparoscopy). *Surg Laparosc Endosc Percutan Tech* 1999;9: 190–193.

COMMENTARY

The author, a practicing surgeon who understands the frustrations and problems encountered on a day-to-day basis by the laparoscopic surgeon, has taken the complex topic of imaging systems that are utilized in minimally invasive surgery and broken them down into easy-to-read, understandable information. He has provided excellent help in understanding approaches to troubleshooting and the rudimentary knowledge that the surgeon should possess in order to effectively work with imaging systems.

The surgeon is frequently called upon to provide information to the hospital regarding the necessity for upgrades in imaging systems. Many times, this may be as simple as selecting the vendor for an integrated operating room. More frequently, the surgeon is put in the position of complaining about outdated or malfunctioning equipment and must badger those in charge of hospital budgets to provide adequate equipment, in order to perform safe laparoscopic surgery.

The information provided in this chapter is extremely useful to the surgeon regarding an appropriate assessment of available technology. The surgeon should take from this chapter a clearer understanding that an upgrade, small or large, of some component of the system might not result in the desired effect. The "weakest link of the chain" theory is emphasized in this chapter, meaning that if a surgeon upgrades multiple components of their system yet leaves in place one weak link the image will not be optimal.

The author also provides information that will help the surgeon to sort through the many claims made by various salespeople regarding image capabilities, and helps the surgeon to understand that a high-resolution camera system paired with an antiquated monitor will not provide the desired image.

It is certain that by the time this book has reached its useful lifespan, technology will have moved forward very rapidly and many of the descriptions of leading edge technology will appear old and even obsolete. This field of biomedical and optics engineering is advancing rapidly, and it is extremely difficult for the surgeon and hospital to maintain current or leading edge technology. Furthermore, it is very costly to take advantage of every advance. It is hoped that this chapter will provide guidance for the surgeon and hospital personnel who must make these difficult decisions in determining where expenditures will lead to true benefit.

WSE

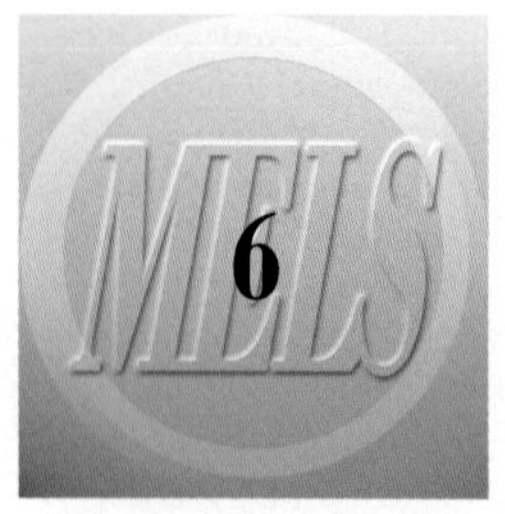

Surgical Robotics

JON C. GOULD AND W. SCOTT MELVIN

INTRODUCTION

Laparoscopy has come a long way since its introduction to general surgery in 1988. Since the early days of laparoscopic cholecystectomy, numerous advances have been made in the areas of imaging, instrumentation, and skills training. A new generation of surgeons has been trained in the era of laparoscopy. Numerous procedures have been adapted for a minimally invasive approach, and many patients have benefited as a result. In fact, the refinement of certain laparoscopic procedures such as cholecystectomy, fundoplication, and gastric bypass has led to a dramatic increase in the number of procedures performed per year. The impetus for this has been multifactorial and driven by industry, physicians, and patients alike. Minimally invasive surgery has become very much a part of the surgical culture.

Not all procedures lend themselves well to a laparoscopic approach, however. There are certain technical limitations that have limited the dissemination of laparoscopy to all areas of surgery:

- Standard laparoscopic instruments are rigid and provide finite freedom of movement.
- Natural tremor tends to be amplified at the tip of these instruments.
- Visualization during the procedure is typically flat and in two dimensions.
- During complex procedures, the surgeon is forced to stand in ergonomically awkward positions for sometimes extended periods of time.
- Camera holders are subject to fatigue, abrupt movements, and distractions during lengthy laparoscopic procedures, providing an unstable image.
- The "fulcrum effect" of the laparoscopic ports causes the instrument tips to move in the direction opposite to that of the surgeon's hands.

Recently, new technical devices have been introduced to address some of these limitations. The da Vinci Surgical System (Intuitive Surgical Inc; Sunnyvale, CA) is the only telerobotic system approved by the Food and Drug Administration (FDA) for clinical use that is commercially available at the time of this writing.

DEFINITIONS

These devices are commonly referred to as "robots," but this is not an entirely accurate label. A more precise description is computer-assisted telemanipulator. A robotic device is technically a "powered, computer-controlled manipulator with artificial sensing that can be preprogrammed to move and position tools to carry out a wide range of surgical tasks." This describes devices such as the orthopedic surgery tool Robodoc (Integrated Surgical Systems; Sacramento, CA). The Robodoc device is positioned and programmed to create a precise defect within the femoral shaft for placement of a prosthetic. The surgeon does not actually drill the hole; the robot moves according to a specific set of instructions and variables.

Computer-assisted devices are not true robots because they lack independent motions or preprogrammed actions. The term *telemanipulator*, or telesurgery, implies that there is a distance interposed between the surgeon and the patient. The surgeon sits at a console remote from the patient and manipulates controls for the surgical instruments. The surgeon's position is more comfortable and ergonomic at the console than at the bedside. The computer enhances the interaction between the surgeon and the bedside robotic device by eliminating tremor and scaling all motions to a selected degree. This makes very fine and precise movements of the surgical instruments possible. In addition, the robotic instruments are multi-articulated and capable of a full range of motion. This allows complex maneuvers not possible with standard laparoscopy. High-definition, three-dimensional visualization provides image detail and depth superior to that of a standard laparoscopic system. A robotic arm manipulates the camera, providing a steady view that is directed by the operating surgeon. The hand and instrument tip movements are synchronous. These features translate into numerous advantages for the operating surgeon and patient.

History and Evolution of Surgical Robotics

AESOP

Yulun Wang, Ph.D., developed the AESOP system with research funding from the Pentagon's Defense Advanced Research Projects Agency (DARPA) program in advanced medical biotechnologies. The acronym AESOP stands for Automated Endoscopic System for Optimal Positioning. AESOP was the first robotic device to receive approval from the FDA for clinical use in 1994. The first generation of AESOP was manipulated manually, either with a foot switch or hand control. Later, AESOP was directed with voice commands. AESOP attaches to the side of a standard operating table and will accept any rigid laparoscope (Fig. 6-1). When used for camera positioning and navigation in laparoscopy, the AESOP system may be helpful in facilitating solo-surgeon procedures. Several surgeons have reported the successful performance of solo-surgeon laparoscopic inguinal hernias, cholecystectomies, and Nissen fundoplications using this system. The robot holds the camera steady and maneuvers without abrupt or jerky movements. In addition, the robot will not become fatigued or distracted, which human camera operators are prone to do. However, the AESOP moves much more slowly than a skilled, attentive assistant. Repeated voice commands are required for every movement. These limitations and a few others prevented the universal dissemination of AESOP among laparoscopic surgeons.

Zeus Surgical System

The Zeus Surgical System (Computer Motion Inc; no longer in operation) was designed specifically for cardiac procedures. The FDA granted the Zeus system approval for use in abdominal operations in October 2001. The Zeus Surgical System was composed of a remote surgeon workstation, AESOP, and two AESOP-like robotic

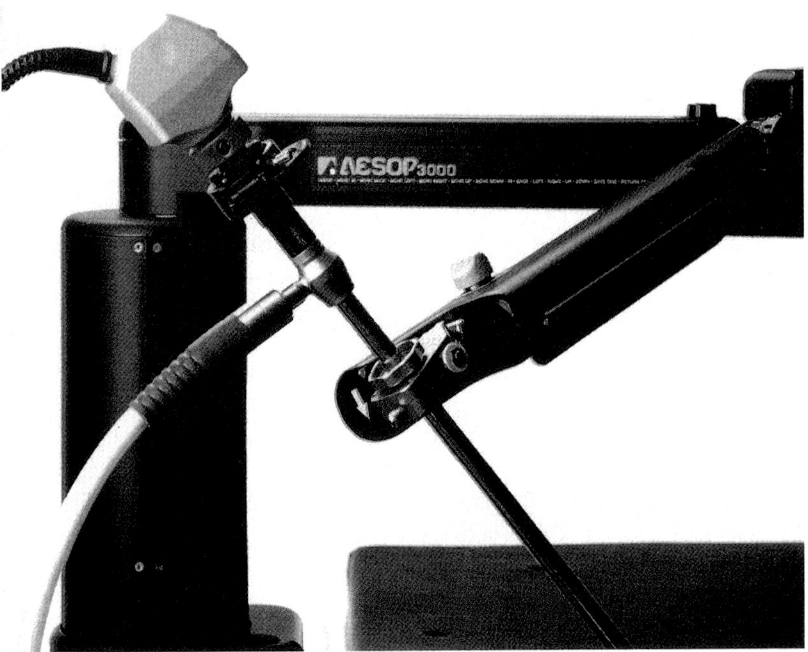

Fig. 6-1. AESOP robotic camera manipulator.

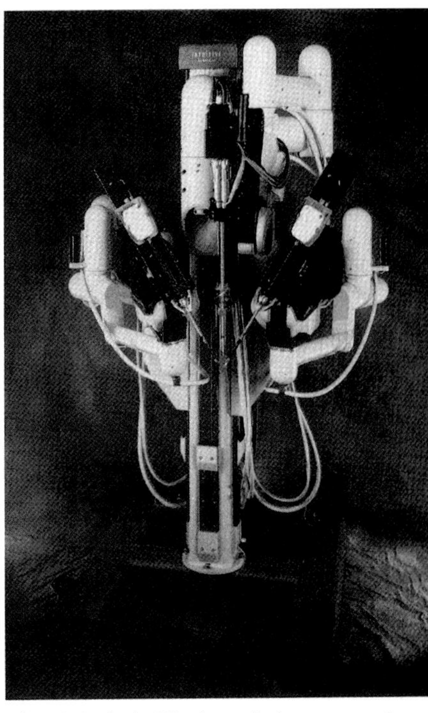

Fig. 6-3. A da Vinci surgical system patient-side cart.

arms for surgical instruments. In March 2003, Computer Motion (Zeus) and Intuitive Surgical (da Vinci Surgical System) merged. Zeus is no longer a supported or commercially available product.

da Vinci Surgical System

As mentioned, da Vinci is the only robotic surgical system commercially available with FDA approval for use in clinical surgery. Frederick Moll, MD, formed Intuitive Surgical in 1995 and developed the da Vinci surgical system by using robotic surgical technology from SRI International (Menlo Park, CA), formerly known as Stanford Research Institute. The original da Vinci system was designed specifically to enable the performance of closed chest coronary artery bypass grafting. The first FDA approval for clinical use was for abdominal laparoscopy in July 2000. The da Vinci system is now approved and used for a wide variety of minimally invasive robotic procedures.

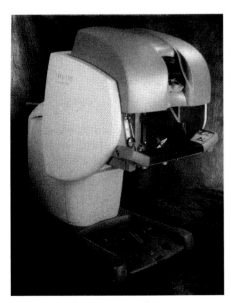

Fig. 6-2. A da Vinci Surgical System surgeon console.

The da Vinci Surgical System consists of the control console (Fig. 6-2), a tower for the insufflator and video electronics, and the patient-side cart. The surgeon sits at the control console, remote from the operative table but typically in the same room. This console is designed to provide the surgeon with an ergonomically comfortable position in which he or she can manipulate the "masters," or controls. Surgeon movement of the masters is translated into precise, real-time movements of the robotic instruments. The masters manipulate the camera when a foot switch is depressed. The surgeon's head rests on the console itself, and a stereoscopic image is displayed below his or her hands. This gives the impression that the patient is directly in front of the surgeon. Visualization is high definition and three dimensional, made possible with dual-lens, three-chip digital cameras.

The patient-side cart provides two or three robotic arms and one endoscopic arm that execute the surgeon's commands (Fig. 6-3). In the original model, operations were largely completed by the two-arm device. In addition to the third working arm, instruments have become available with a diameter of 5 mm, reducing abdominal wall trauma. Only two working arms can be used at a time; the device allows the arms not in use to be kept in a static configuration while control is toggled to another arm. This allows many general surgical procedures to be performed without the need for an additional skilled assistant. The robotic arms pivot at the 1-cm operating port. This eliminates excessive torque or tension on the patient's abdominal wall during movements. The da Vinci robotic surgical instruments are designed to provide a full 7 degrees of freedom to mimic the dexterity of the human wrist.

There are several limitations to the da Vinci system at the current level of technology. The patient-side cart is quite large and obtrusive. At times, this device limits the anesthesiologist's access to the patient. Using the da Vinci surgical system in smaller operating rooms is impractical, and the system often requires its own room for storage. The robotic arms are not attached to the operating table. Intraoperative table position changes (e.g., increased Trendelenberg) require removal of the robotic arms from the patient and replacement after repositioning.

There is currently no haptic feedback from the da Vinci surgical system to the surgeon. The system is capable of generating a tremendous amount of force with the robotic arms. Surgeons must rely on visual cues and need to be wary of movements made outside the field of view. Similarly, the surgeon cannot judge how tightly the robotic instruments are grasping tissue. This situation may lead to suture fraying and crushed tissue.

The da Vinci surgical system is cable-driven. Surgeons must be careful not to continuously rotate instruments in the same direction, because the device will become incapable of certain maneuvers until the cable is unwound. This is easily accomplished by rotating the instrument in the opposite direction, but this usually requires releasing the tissue or needle that the robotic arm was holding at the time the cable became locked.

The newer da Vinci S system was made available in 2006 and has some time-saving features such as quick-connect docking ports. Newer features also include an updated visualization system and an optional scope with a separate wide-angle image. However, the actual footprint and size of the device is very similar to the original design.

Robotic Endoscopic and Laparoscopic Procedures (Early Results)

GENERAL SURGERY

Robotic surgical systems have been utilized in a wide variety of minimally invasive abdominal surgical procedures. Cadiere et al. published a description of their experience using the da Vinci Surgical System, with 146 robotic laparoscopic cases: 48 cholecystectomies, 39 antireflux procedures, 28 tubal reanastomoses, ten gastroplasties for obesity, three inguinal hernias, three intrarectal procedures, two hysterectomies, two cardiac procedures, two prostatectomies, two arteriovenous fistulas, one lumbar sympathectomy, one appendectomy, one laryngeal exploration, one varicocele ligation, one endometriosis cure, one neosalpingostomy, and one deferent canal. The Academic Robotics Group, a group composed of surgeons from Johns Hopkins University School of Medicine, East Carolina University, University of Illinois School of Medicine, and Ohio State University, presented its combined experience with 211 robotic-assisted surgical procedures using the da Vinci system. In this multi-institutional study, 69 antireflux surgeries, 36 cholecystectomies, 26 Heller myotomies, 17 bowel resections, 15 donor nephrectomies, 14 left internal mammary artery mobilizations, seven gastric bypasses, seven splenectomies, six adrenalectomies, three exploratory laparoscopies, four pyloroplasties, two gastrojejunostomies, one distal pancreatectomy, one duodenal polypectomy, one esophagectomy, one gastric mass resection, and one lysis of adhesions were conducted. There were no adverse outcomes that could be attributed to the robotic system in either of these reports, which involve more than 350 cases. There is clearly a wide variety of potential applications for these technical devices.

Robotic Fundoplication

There are currently several prospective trials that compare standard laparoscopic and computer-enhanced robotic fundoplication. At Ohio State University, 20 consecutive robotic Nissen fundoplications were compared with 20 consecutive laparoscopic Nissen fundoplications. The robotic fundoplications took an average of 45 minutes longer but were associated with similar clinical outcomes. Clinical outcomes were assessed with a symptom survey administered on follow-up.

Cadiere's group conducted a prospective randomized trial of robotic versus laparoscopic Nissen fundoplication in 21 patients. Of these patients, eleven were treated with conventional laparoscopic surgery and ten were treated with computer-assisted surgery. The rate of blood loss, length of stay, and perioperative morbidity were similar in each group. The only significant difference was the mean operative time.

At the University of Turin, Morino et al. conducted a prospective randomized trial of robot-assisted vs. laparoscopic Nissen fundoplication in 50 consecutive patients. Twenty-five patients underwent robot-assisted surgery using the da Vinci surgical system and 25 patients had a standard laparoscopic fundoplication. Total operating time and skin-to-skin time were significantly shorter for conventional laparoscopy. The cost of a robot-assisted procedure was significantly higher than that for standard laparoscopic fundoplication (3157 euros vs.1527 euros; $P < 0.001$). There were no significant differences in clinical, endoscopic, or functional outcomes between groups.

Nakadi et al. conducted a prospective randomized study to compare the benefits and the costs associated with laparoscopic and robot-assisted Nissen fundoplication in 20 patients. Robot-assisted Nissen fundoplication was associated with longer operative times and higher costs compared to the laparoscopic approach. Increased cost for the robot-assisted cases was related to many causes, including the initial investment and maintenance for the technology, additional nursing costs, and the added cost of a specialized robotic instrumentation with a limited number of uses.

At Ohio State University, a study examined the feasibility of using the fourth robotic arm in computer-assisted fundoplication. Five Nissen fundoplications were completed in a mean operating room time of 134 minutes (80 minute robot time) with no intraoperative complications. When the fourth robotic arm is actively used in robotic fundoplication, the bedside surgeon has less of a role in operative exposure. The operating surgeon in these cases needs to be very aware that the fourth arm can represent a fixed retractor against which tissue could be damaged during manipulation with the other robotic arms. With the lack of tactile feedback provided, care must be taken to pay attention to visual clues of tissue tension as well as position, tension, and grip strength of the robotic instruments.

The relevant literature appears to demonstrate that robotic antireflux surgery is feasible and safe, but there seems to be no major difference in clinical outcomes when compared to standard laparoscopic antireflux surgery. Operating time and costs are increased for computer-assisted antireflux surgery compared to the conventional laparoscopic approach. At the current level of technology, computer-assisted antireflux surgery does not appear to offer major clinical advantages to patients with access to skilled and experienced laparoscopic surgeons.

Robotic Heller Myotomy

In robotic-assisted laparoscopic Heller myotomy, the high-definition, three-dimensional visualization helps a great deal. Experience shows that it is subjectively easier to see individual muscle fibers and to be certain that the myotomy is complete. This is significant because incomplete myotomy is the most common reason for the failure of a Heller myotomy. The use of a robotic surgical system in laparoscopic Heller myotomy may also help decrease the incidence of esophageal mucosal perforation. This event occurs in approximately 4% to 5% of laparoscopic Heller myotomies and requires advanced laparoscopic suturing skills to correct.

A recently published multi-institutional study investigated the outcomes following computer-assisted Heller myotomy and partial fundoplication for achalasia in 104 patients. The average overall operative time was 140.5 minutes for the entire series. This time decreased from 162.6 minutes for cases performed in the years 2000 to 2002 to 113.5 minutes for procedures performed during the latter part of the study, in 2003 to 2004 (P = 0.0001). There were no esophageal perforations in any of these 104 patients during surgery. Symptoms improved to a significant degree in all patients following myotomy, and no patient required reoperation for recurrent symptoms during the time period for the study.

Horgan et al. performed a prospective non-randomized trial of robotic-assisted vs. laparoscopic Heller myotomy in 121 patients. In this study, 62 patients were treated with conventional laparoscopic surgery, and 59 with robotically-assisted surgery. Operative time was significantly longer in the da Vinci group (141 ±49 vs. 122 ±44 minutes; P <0.05). In the last 30 cases, there was no difference in operative time between the groups (108 vs. 104 minutes; p = not significant). Intraoperative esophageal perforation was more frequent in the laparoscopic group (16% vs. 0%; P <0.01).

In 2006, Iqbal et al. reported their experience with minimally invasive Heller myotomy using both the da Vinci robotic system and conventional laparoscopy. In 19 robotic myotomies, there were no intraoperative esophageal perforations. Iqbal's group reported a 7.8% mucosal perforation rate for standard laparoscopic Heller myotomy in this series (four of 51 cases).

Although experience with robotic Heller myotomy is limited to specialized centers to date, it does appear as if there are certain clinical advantages to a computer-assisted approach when compared to the conventional laparoscopic approach. The primary advantage may lie in the capacity to minimize the occurrence of a mucosal perforation during myotomy in computer-assisted surgery. Presumably, this difference is attributed to superior visualization and improved range of motion during robotic myotomy.

Robotic Bariatric Surgery

Procedures that require extensive intracorporeal suturing and knot tying are ideally suited to a robotic approach. Sutured gastrojejunostomy in gastric bypass surgery for obesity is a technique perfected by several surgeons, but this technique has not been disseminated widely throughout the bariatric surgical community because of its complexity. The use of the robotic device with its multi-articulated instruments and increased freedom of movement may help to make a hand-sewn gastrojejunostomy in gastric bypass a more plausible approach for many surgeons. In a robotic-assisted gastric bypass, the robotic device is used for suturing the gastrojejunostomy. The rest of the procedure is typically conducted with standard laparoscopic techniques.

Ali et al. reported their experience with 50 robot-assisted laparoscopic Roux-en-Y gastric bypass (RYGB) procedures. Robot setup time, robot operative time, total operative time, and operative outcomes were tracked prospectively. Robot setup time and total operative time decreased as their series matured. There were few complications, with one intraoperative leak repaired during the original procedure and one stenosis reported on limited follow-up.

Mohr et al. recently reported their experience with totally robotic RYGB procedures. In the manuscript, the authors compare the operative times and perioperative complications of their first ten totally robotic RYGB cases with a retrospective matched sample of ten patients who underwent RYGB using conventional laparoscopic techniques. The median surgical time (169 vs. 208 minutes; P = 0.03) and median operative time divided by body mass index (BMI) (3.8 vs. 5.0; P = 0.04) were significantly lower for the totally robotic procedures. This same group also recently reported a retrospective review of the operative times and complications for their first 75 totally robotic RYGB procedures. Results were compared between three minimally invasive surgery fellows to examine learning curves for totally robotic RYGB. Each laparoscopic fellow reached a five-case running average metric of 3.5 min/BMI by 6th, 7th, and 9th cases, with a learning curve of 10 to 15 cases. This was significantly faster than that of laparoscopic RYGB, where the authors averaged 3.7 min/BMI for their first 100 cases and 2.9 min/BMI for their second 200 cases. The authors of this study concluded that totally robotic RYGB was superior to laparoscopic RYGB and that it is associated with a shorter learning curve.

Robotic surgical systems have also been successfully used in adjustable gastric band placement. Horgan et al. reported operative outcomes for 32 robot-assisted adjustable gastric band placements. Robotic gastric band placement was associated with a low complication rate and a similar length of stay as gastric bands placed with conventional laparoscopy. While operative times were greater for robotic-assisted band placements, the surgeons comment in their manuscript that the computer-assisted telemanipulator does facilitate gastric band placement in super-obese patients in particular. Experience with robotic gastric banding is quite limited to date.

The relevant literature suggests that computer-assisted robotic bariatric surgery is feasible and safe. While some surgical groups found that operative times were increased in robotic cases, other groups found that the robotic technology actually led to decreased operative times in bariatric surgical procedures. It is possible that robotic surgical systems may shorten the learning curve for complex bariatric cases like RYGB when compared to the conventional laparoscopic approach. Minimally invasive bariatric surgery may also be subjectively easier using a robotic device in a patient with an elevated BMI. Further research is necessary to answer these questions.

Other Robotic General and Vascular Surgical Procedures

Procedures that require complex laparoscopic skills such as suturing or knot-tying and are limited to single quadrants of the abdomen are the ones best suited for robotic assistance. In contrast, procedures that are simple, require navigation to multiple quadrants of the abdomen, or call for frequent table position changes are not as well suited to a da Vinci robotic approach as some of the procedures described above. In 1997, the first robotic telesurgical procedure was performed on a patient in Brussels, Belgium. Jaques Himpens, MD, and Guy Cadiere, MD, performed this robotic cholecystectomy with the da Vinci surgical system. Kornprat et al. in Austria prospectively compared robot-assisted da Vinci cholecystectomy to standard laparoscopic cholecystectomy in 46 patients. In the robotic cases, time for pre-procedure equipment set-up, cut-to-close times, and camera and trocar insertion times were significantly longer. Net dissection time for cystic artery, cystic duct, and gallbladder did not vary with technique. These authors felt that while robot-assisted cholecystectomy was feasible without system-related morbidity, it offered no appreciable clinical benefit and led to longer operative times.

Robotic solid organ surgery has been described for splenectomy, pancreatic resections, and adrenalectomies. For most of these procedures, individual series are small. In general, most authors find that the various robotic solid organ procedures are technically feasible and safe. In series where the robotic approaches to solid organ procedures are compared to a conventional laparoscopic approach, most investigators find that the robotic procedure is associated with an increased operative time and cost. Morino et al. in Turin, Italy, conducted a prospective randomized trial comparing laparoscopic to robotic adrenalectomy in 20 patients. The conversion rate, operative time, morbidity, and cost were greater in robotic cases.

Robotic surgical systems have been used successfully in colorectal surgery. D'Annibale et al. in Padova, Italy, compared the outcomes for 53 consecutive robotic colorectal cases to those of 53 standard laparoscopic colorectal cases performed in the same time interval. Complications, specimen length, number of lymph nodes, total time of surgery, length of stay, and return of bowel function did not differ between the two groups. The authors felt that the robotic system was particularly helpful at specific stages, including takedown of the splenic flexure, dissection of a narrow pelvis, identification of nervous plexus, and hand-sewn anastomosis. Other authors with experience in robotic colorectal surgery have commented that colorectal procedures spanning multiple quadrants of the abdomen and requiring table repositioning are difficult with the robotic surgical system.

SURGICAL SUBSPECIALTIES

Urologic Surgery

Robotic prostatectomy is the fastest growing treatment of prostate cancer worldwide. The FDA approved the da Vinci system for robotic radical prostatectomy in 2001. That year, less than 1% of all prostatectomies were performed with the aid of a robot. In 2005, an estimated 20% of all prostatectomies were performed robotically, and it is expected that this rate will continue to have a rapid growth rate. Prostatectomy is a case ideally suited to a computer-assisted robotic approach: the operative site is in the narrow confines of the male pelvis, and the multi-articulated instruments are well suited for the difficult urethral to bladder anastomosis. The standard laparoscopic radical prostatectomy was not embraced as readily by urologists as robotic prostatectomy has been, due mostly to the fact that the laparoscopic approach was quite difficult with an extensive learning curve.

There are now multiple large series of robotic prostatectomies published in the literature. Compared to open prostatectomy, the robotic technique seems to be associated with a similar oncologic outcome. Demonstrated benefits of robotic prostatectomy include a shorter hospital stay, less pain, less blood loss and fewer transfusions, and even better erectile function outcomes than conventional open nerve-sparing prostatectomy. Many urologists now consider robotic radical prostatectomy to be the gold standard.

Cardiac Surgery

Although originally designed for use in closed chest cardiac surgery, most of the clinical work using the da Vinci system to date has been in other areas. The da Vinci system has been given FDA clearance for internal thoracic artery mobilization, cardiac tissue ablation, mitral valve repair, endoscopic atrial septal defect closure, and mammary to left anterior descending coronary artery anastomosis for cardiac revascularization with adjunctive mediastinoscopy.

Robotic surgical systems have been used successfully in minimally invasive mitral valve repair and replacement with good results, including a shorter length of stay and fewer blood transfusions than in open mitral valve surgery. A multi-institutional study of robotically assisted totally endoscopic coronary artery bypass grafting was recently published. Ninety-eight patients requiring single-vessel left anterior descending coronary artery revascularization were enrolled. In 85 patients, the procedures were completed totally endoscopically with no mortality and low morbidity, angiographic patency, and reintervention rates comparable with published data from more traditional approaches. In the future, it is likely that multi-vessel or off-pump totally endoscopic robotic coronary artery bypass will be possible.

Thoracic Surgery

The da Vinci Surgical System has been used successfully for thymectomy, lobectomy, esophagectomy, and resection of mediastinal tumors. Robotic devices have proven to be particularly beneficial in minimally invasive thymectomy as a treatment for myasthenia gravis. The thymus is located in the anterior mediastinum in an anatomic area difficult to access with traditional thoracoscopy. Robotic instrumentation with a full 7 degrees of articulation can maneuver around corners, vital vessels, and nerves (phrenic) encountered in the tight confines of the anterior mediastinum. Rea et al. in Italy have utilized the da Vinci system in 33 thymectomies with good results and minimal morbidity. These authors feel that the robotic devices, when compared to traditional rigid thoracoscopic instruments, allow easier and safer access to the thymus in the neck region and the contralateral hemithorax.

Gynecologic Surgery

Robotic surgical systems may also have utility for gynecologists. Minimally invasive tubal reanastomosis with a robotic surgical system has been reported in small numbers of patients. The scaled motion and lack of tremor allow for precise suturing with interrupted 8-0 sutures, similar to that used in open microsurgical tubal reanastomoses. Several series of robotically assisted laparoscopic surgical hysterectomies have been reported, with generally good results. Several case reports and practices have discussed the advantages of robotic assistance for radical hysterectomy with associated lymph node dissection. Current studies are underway to evaluate the efficacy of robotic versus laparoscopic surgical procedures.

Pediatric Surgery

Experience in robotic pediatric surgery is currently limited. Robotic surgical systems may soon enable minimally invasive surgical procedures never before possible in children and infants. Motion scaling, tremor filtration, and high-definition visualization will prove to be essential advantages in minimally invasive procedures for these smaller patients.

Currently, the smallest available instruments for the da Vinci system are 5-mm. The imaging system still requires a 12-mm scope.

Several small case series and case reports of robotic pediatric pyeloplasty, robotic Heller myotomy, and robotic antireflux surgery have been published, mostly in adolescents.

Emerging Applications

Robotic interventions can be applied throughout the body, anywhere the advantages of remote control and motion scaling may be of benefit. With the advent of some emerging devices, the amount of motion scaling may be significant, allowing, for example, retinal surgery via ultra microdissection techniques with image-guided intervention and movement timed to pulsations of the retina.

Flexible platforms with inline vision systems and articulated working arms have been demonstrated with the endoVia surgical workstation. These types of devices may hold promise for a family of new procedures performed via a single access port or via natural orifices. The advantage of robotics is that multiple end effectors may be controlled from a single workstation with optimal platforms.

Emerging applications will also include procedures performed via the mouth and performed in the pharynx or hypopharynx. Neurosurgical applications are being evaluated and developed as well, perhaps utilizing image enhancement and motion scaling for minimally invasive approaches to the spine, brain, and skull base.

TRAINING AND EDUCATION

Robotic surgical systems, at the current level of technology, offer relatively few advantages in procedures such as cholecystectomy and Nissen fundoplication for the experienced laparoscopist. These procedures do not require fine movements in a confined space or extensive suturing and knot-tying. The improved ergonomics and visualization are nice features, but not critical. Inexperienced laparoscopists may find the computer-assisted approach to be easier early in their training. It has been shown that novice surgeons are able to complete a laparoscopic skills exercise more rapidly with a robotic system than with standard laparoscopic instruments. Robotic systems also allow novice surgeons to perform complex tasks with more consistency and precision than is possible with standard laparoscopic instruments. Robotic surgical systems may allow inexperienced laparoscopic surgeons to quickly and easily become comfortable with advanced laparoscopic procedures.

TELEPRESENCE SURGERY

Casualty data from the Vietnam War revealed that although improvements had been made in the overall mortality rate, survival of soldiers on the front lines with life-threatening injuries was no better than it had been in the Civil War. Robotic telesurgery was conceived as a technology designed to bring the surgeon to the wounded soldier without nearing the combat area. SRI International has developed an experimental advanced telepresence surgery system that enables a surgeon located in a Mobile Army Surgical Hospital (MASH) unit to perform emergency surgical procedures on soldiers in an armored surgical vehicle located in the combat zone. The robotic manipulator arms are mounted on an operating table in this vehicle, known as a Medical Forward Advanced Surgical Treatment vehicle. A microwave telecommunications link allows surgery to be performed up to a distance of 5 km. This system is designed to provide wounded soldiers who would otherwise exsanguinate with just enough surgery to control the hemorrhage until they can be transported to the MASH unit. The system has yet to be used in an actual combat situation.

Latency in telerobotic surgery is the time from when the handle of the instrument at the workstation is moved until the robotic surgical instrument itself moves. This is related to the time required to transfer the electronic signal from the workstation to the robotic arm. Humans can compensate for a latency of up to 200 msec, after which the delay is too great for accuracy. Until recently, issues of latency limited remote robotic surgery to short distances. In September 2001, however, surgeons in New York removed the gallbladder of a woman in France with the Zeus system. This was accomplished with a latency of approximately 150 msec using a high-bandwidth fiber-optic transatlantic cable connection.

In Canada, surgeons at McMaster University in Hamilton, Ontario, and at North Bay General Hospital, located 400 km north of Hamilton, established a telerobotic surgical service. Twenty-one telerobotic procedures, including 13 fundoplications, three sigmoid resections, two right hemicolectomies, one anterior resection, and two inguinal hernia repairs, were completed over a commercially available network with 15 Mbps bandwidth. There were no complications and mean hospital stays were equivalent to those in the tertiary institution for standard laparoscopy.

FUTURE DIRECTIONS

Future robotic surgical systems will incorporate precise haptic feedback and a sense of touch. The surgeon may someday be able to feel texture, temperature, and tension on tissues from the workstation. The bedside robotic device will become smaller and easier to set up and maintain. Additional robotic arms will be added to these systems, allowing complex procedures to be performed by a single surgeon with minimal assistance at the bedside. The cost of robotic surgical systems will decrease, making this technology more accessible to all surgeons.

Robotic devices may one day become so small and flexible that they may be placed in natural body orifices to perform endoluminal procedures. At the University of Nebraska, surgeons and engineers have been working to develop in vivo miniature robots. In a porcine model, these devices have been successfully deployed transgastrically into the peritoneal cavity to navigate, visualize, and even to grasp and manipulate tissue.

Signal transfer from the surgeon's console to the bedside robotic device will become possible over great distances with minimal latency, even wirelessly. Surgeons may someday be able to practice and plan complex procedures using virtual reality and patient-specific digital radiographs. Such a system may also serve to train residents and surgeons in robotic surgical procedures. Digitized images may ultimately help surgeons to operate on structures not visible in the operative field. As robotic surgical systems become more sophisticated, they may someday independently perform procedures after programming by a surgeon, much like the Robodoc system used in orthopedic surgery. Alternatively, robots may become capable of using artificial intelligence and sensing technology to operate with minimal human interaction. The future of robotic surgery is promising. These systems hold great potential to extend the capabilities of surgical performance beyond human limitations.

ACKNOWLEDGMENTS

Funded in part by a grant from the Covidien Corporation.

SUGGESTED READING

Ali MR, Bhaskerrao B, Wolfe BM. Robot-assisted laparoscopic Roux-en-Y gastric bypass. *Surg Endosc* 2005;19:468–472.

Anvari M, McKinley C, Stein H. Establishment of the world's first telerobotic remote surgical service: for provision of advanced laparoscopic surgery in a rural community. *Ann Surg* 2005;241(3):460–464.

Argenziano M, Katz M, Bonatti J, et al. Results of the prospective multicenter trial of robotically assisted totally endoscopic coronary artery bypass grafting. *Ann Thorac Surg* 2006; 81(5):1666–1674.

Cadiere GB, Himpens J, Germay O, et al. Feasibility of robotic laparoscopic surgery: 146 cases. *World J Surg* 2001;25:1467–1477.

D'Annibale A, Morpurgo E, Fiscon V, et al. Robotic and laparoscopic surgery for treatment of colorectal diseases. *Dis Colon Rectum* 2004;47(12):2162–2168.

Kaul S, Bhandari A, Hemal A, et al. Robotic radical prostatectomy with preservation of the prostatic fascia: a feasibility study. *Urology* 2005;66(6):1261–1265.

Lehman AC, Rentschler ME, Farritor SM, et al. Endoluminal minirobots for transgastric peritoneoscopy. *Minim Invasive Ther Allied Technol* 2006;15(6):384–388.

Marescaux J, Leroy J, Gagner M, et al. Transatlantic robot-assisted telesurgery. *Nature* 2001; 413:379–380.

Melvin WS, Dundon JM, Talamini M, et al. Computer-enhanced robotic telesurgery minimizes esophageal perforation during Heller myotomy. *Surgery* 2005;138:553–558.

Melvin WS, Krause KR, Needleman BJ, et al. A prospective trial of laparoscopic vs. computer assisted robotic Nissen fundoplication. *J Gastrointest Surg* 2002;6:11–16.

Morino M, Pellegrino L, Giaccone C, et al. Randomized clinical trial of robot-assisted versus laparoscopic Nissen fundoplication. *Br J Surg* 2006;93:553–558.

Rea F, Marulli G, Bortolotti L, et al. Experience with the "daVinci" robotic system for thymectomy in patients with myasthenia gravis: report of 33 cases. *Ann Thorac Surg* 2006;81(2):455–459.

Talamini MA, Chapman W, Melvin WS, et al. A prospective analysis of 211 robotic assisted surgical procedures. *Surg Endosc* 2002;16:205.

COMMENTARY

Drs. Gould and Melvin describe the history and current status of "robotic surgery." More properly entitled computer-assisted telemanipulation, robotic systems are designed to address many of the limitations of traditional laparoscopic surgery. These include improving dexterity by eliminating tremor, providing motion scaling, allowing true motion of instruments and wrist-like articulation, offering better visualization by allowing the surgeon to direct the optics with a very stable platform using high-definition three-dimensional imaging; improving ergonomics for the surgeon, and potentially allowing telesurgery applications. However, the robots also come at both a true and figurative price: there is an absence of haptic feedback, the equipment is bulky and technologically complex, the initial equipment is expensive, and the per-case disposable and personnel costs are significant. At the current time, there are relatively few operations that have been proven to be improved by the use of robotics. Probably the biggest "winner" to date is the robotic prostatectomy, which in many centers, has become the new standard of care. There are suggestions, but an absence of randomized data, that robotic Heller myotomy leads to fewer intraoperative mucosal perforations than standard laparoscopic myotomy. There is no doubt, however, that aficionados of robotic surgery will ultimately be able to convince even skeptics like this editor that certain operations *should* be performed using a computer-assisted telemanipulator.

Robotic surgery is clearly in its infancy. It is likely that the evolution of robotics will include much smaller systems that can be brought into the operative field for specific portions of operations best suited to their use. The addition of haptic feedback will also likely occur. Ultimately, a lower sticker price will be important to allow more widespread dissemination of the technology. It is important that surgeons such as Drs. Gould and Melvin are involved in the developmental phase of robotic surgery to help guide this evolutionary sequence.

NJS

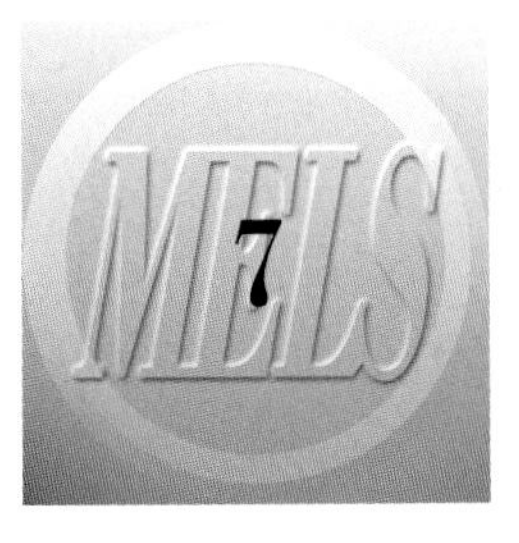

Simulators and Simulation

SCOTT T. REHRIG, KINGA POWERS,
AND DANIEL B. JONES

INTRODUCTION

"I will impart knowledge of the Art by precept, by lecture, and by every mode of teaching. . . ."

The Oath of Hippocrates

In the past decade, the place of medical simulation in surgical training and education has moved from a fringe movement to the mainstream. It has expanded from parts task training on physical box trainers to whole task training in virtual reality (VR) simulators. Additionally, it has evolved to include comprehensive surgical team training in mock operating room environments using crew resource management techniques.

Dr. Richard Satava stated in his paper *Disruptive Visions* that "traditional models of surgical education are struggling to keep abreast of the radical changes occurring throughout the healthcare profession. From the financial constraints of decreased funding due to the realignment of reimbursement policies to the demand for more oversight for patient safety and resident work hours, the burden upon providing quality surgical education has never been greater. Combine these challenges with the decreasing clinical opportunities and increasing complexity of the practice of surgery, and it is obvious that incremental changes to the system will not suffice."

Other individuals and groups have also called for changes in surgical residency training. Recently, the American Surgical Association's Blue Ribbon Panel on surgical education recommended medical simulators be broadly introduced into surgical education both for teaching as well as for the verification of competence of practicing surgeons. This panel further recommended that the ultimate goal should be to define a curriculum of surgical skills that trainees must acquire outside the operating room on simulators prior to performing surgical procedures on actual patients.

Building on the recommendations of the Blue Ribbon Panel, Dr. Carlos A. Pellegrini, in his Presidential Address to the American Surgical Association, called for the greater implementation of medical simulation in the education of surgical trainees. He defined simulation technology as a vital component to the future of surgical education. Pelligrini further stated that simulation provides an ideal learning environment in which the learner has permission to fail, and to do so repeatedly and without consequences. Simulation was not only seen as a means to train but also to accurately measure performance.

Additionally, in a recent editorial on surgical simulation and surgical crisis management training, Dr. Richard Reznick stated that there is an urgent need to augment our efforts in surgical simulation. He noted the "days of a slow ascent to competence, through trial and error on real patients, will not be part of our educational heuristics." He furthered that simulated environments needed development and validation.

The United States government is also committed to the advancement of medical simulation as a means of reducing medical error and improving patient outcomes. For example, Congressman J. Randy Forbes, the founder and chair of the Congressional Modeling & Simulation Caucus, is a strong supporter of simulation research. He and the members of his caucus are dedicated to improving patient safety, reducing medical errors, ensuring medical provider competency, and reducing health care costs.

These key leaders, visionaries, and politicians share a common goal: the integration of medical simulation into the training of surgical residents.

Reasons for Simulation to be Incorporated into Surgical Training

The Pretrained Novice

In an article in the *Annals of Surgery* in 2005, Dr. Richard M. Satava et al. called for the immediate implementation of surgical simulation in surgical education and training. Specifically, the authors described the educational and psychological factors key to successfully implementing simulation in surgical education. One of the most important factors identified was the idea of attentional resources. The authors explained that human beings are limited in the number of stimuli that they can interpret simultaneously; in other words, that humans have finite attentional resources.

Anyone who has experienced laparoscopic surgery understands that it requires a very different set of skills compared to open surgery. As Satava et al. explain, laparoscopic surgery requires the operator to devote attentional resources to the areas of psychomotor performance, depth/spatial judgments, operative judgment/decision making, and finally to the comprehension of instructions. If expert surgeons were compared to novice surgeons, expert surgeons would utilize fewer attentional resources in performing a case than novice surgeons. Therefore, novice surgeons are focusing their limited attentional resources on basic performance parameters, such as knowing where their instruments are at all times, instead of focusing their resources on learning the steps of the procedure, interpreting instrument feedback, and avoiding surgical errors.

The difference in attentional resources between expert and novice surgeons is what Satava calls an "attentional resource buffer." Essentially, this buffer allows the expert surgeon to devote more attentional resources to reducing surgical errors, thus, ensuring patient safety. As Satava et al. describe, if implemented properly, simulation can potentially create the "pretrained novice."

By training using simulation technology, the novice can develop psychomotor and spatial judgment skills to the point where they become "automated." The pretrained novice can devote more cognitive resources to mastering the steps of the procedure, learning how to handle or avoid intraoperative errors, and ultimately assisting the expert surgeon to perform safer surgery.

Evidence from Randomized Controlled Trials

In a recent meta-analysis published in the *Annals of Surgery* in March 2006, Sutherland et al. reported on 30 randomized controlled trials (RCTs) with 760 subjects. The authors' goals were to evaluate the effectiveness of surgical simulation and to assess the validity of current simulators for technical skills training. A summary of the results is shown in Table 7-1.

These authors found that surgical simulation was not superior to standard Halstedian training methods. However, the authors cited several systematic problems as potential reasons for the failure of the studies to show significant advantages of simulation technology over standard training methods. First, all of the studies suffered from small sample sizes. In addition, the studies posed multiple and confounding comparisons, leading to low statistical power. Compounding this was a lack of widely accepted validated metrics of performance for surgical simulation studies. Furthermore, the majority of the studies used nonblinded assessors, introducing bias because of the use of subjective global rating scales. It was felt that meaningful comparisons of one system or simulator could not take place between studies.

Despite these criticisms, the authors concluded, "surgical simulation may be just as good as other forms of surgical training." They found that most RCTs studied were able to show that both simulator and control groups improved significantly from the baseline. Surgical simulation in its current state can, therefore, provide an adjunct to standard surgical training.

Medical Simulation in Context

In a 2006 editorial on the topic of medical simulation in surgery, Sanjeev Dutta et al. placed the issue of the validation of simulation technology into broader context by asking whether a comprehensive strategy of competency-based training, using multiple modalities including simulation and supervised clinical care, yields better outcomes for patients, fewer errors, or more efficient patient care and education than does the current system of mostly apprenticeship-based training. The importance is not whether simulators are a superior means of training but rather if simulation as part of a competency-based curriculum is an effective pedagogical (teaching) strategy as compared to the current apprenticeship-based system.

In defense of the poor showing of the RCTs reported by Sutherland et al., Dutta noted that the findings of the meta-analysis were not surprising. Dutta explains the RCTs in medical simulation to date have been poorly funded because "[surgical] education and training . . . is at the bottom of the ladder and is no one's cash cow." He cites a lack of research funding as the major inhibitor to large multi-institutional, long-term studies that would address many of deficiencies in the studies noted by others.

Rather than being rejected by the surgical profession, simulation technology should serve as an adjunct to current surgical training practices. Other high-stakes professions like aviation, nuclear power, and the military have adopted simulation as a way of life. Dutta et al. note that no hazardous industry has anything remotely approaching level 1A evidence to support simulation practices. Medical simulation in its current form can have an immediate impact in surgical education and training in select circumstances. The ultimate success will depend on major policy changes in education, training, and performance assessment in health care.

TABLE 7-1. SUMMARY OF RESULTS FROM 30 RANDOMIZED CONTROLLED TRIALS

Comparison	Results
Computer vs. no training	• Six-ninths (66%) computer training performed better than no training.
Computer vs. standard training	• Five studies involving MIST-VR and URO mentor system • Three-fifths studies showed the computer training to be superior to standard training. • Many confounding variables • Overall effect was less pronounced than no training studies.
Computer simulation vs. video simulation	• Overall computer simulation showed mixed results better in some studies and not in others. • Four-sevenths showed superiority to video box trainers.
Computer simulation vs. physical box trainers	• One study compared computer simulation to physical box trainer and found it superior.
Video simulation vs. no training	• Six studies failed to show consistent benefit vs. no training.
Video simulation vs. other	• No difference in five studies.
Physical model vs. other including no training	• Mixed results in four studies.
Cadaver vs. standard training	• No statistical difference between groups in one study.

From Sutherland LM, Middleton PF, Anthony A, et al. Surgical stimulation: a systematic review. *Ann Surg* 2006;243(3):291–300.

Advances in Task Trainers

A recent review of surgical simulation in the *New England Journal of Medicine* described the range of simulators available, including bench, animal, cadaver, human patient simulators (HPS), and virtual reality (VR). Until very recently, animal and cadaver simulations have been the gold standard in surgical training and education. Bench models based on the Fundamentals of Laparoscopic Surgery (FLS) program, which is in turn based on the McGill Inanimate System for Training and Evaluation of Laparoscopic Skills (MISTELS) (see Fig. 7-1), and Rosser Top Gun Laparoscopic Skills and Suturing Program are widely used in surgical education for parts task training. In 2006, a multi-institution study demonstrated that the FLS examination was valid and reliable in its ability to discriminate between different levels of surgeon experience and training.

Several studies using bench models to train basic laparoscopic skills such as suturing have demonstrated that the skills are

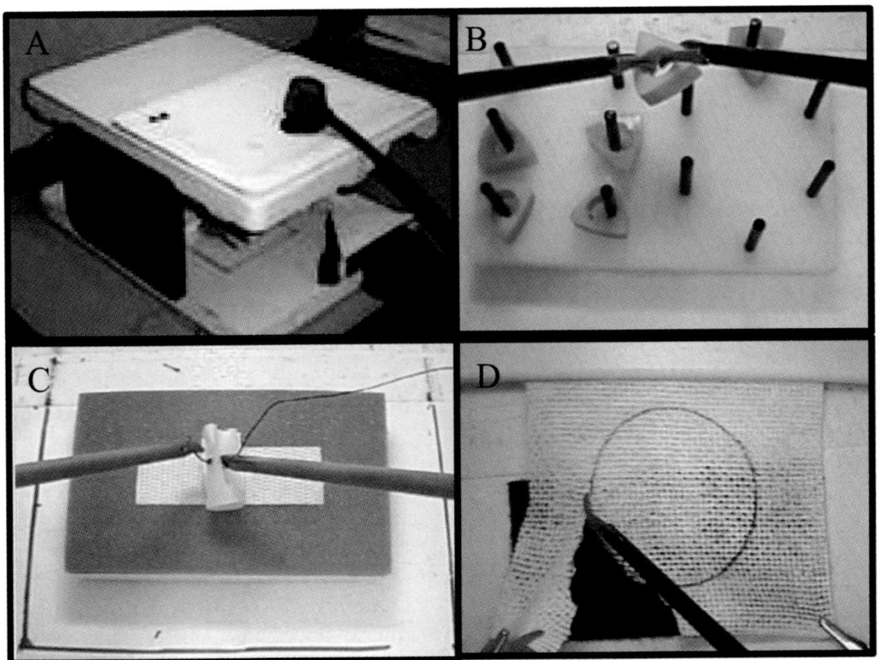

Fig. 7-1. A. FLS box trainer system with examples of tasks: **(B)** transfer task, **(C),** intracorporeal suture task, and **(D)** precision cutting task.

transferable from the training environment to the live operating room. For example, training on bench trainers using a set of five tasks—the checker board, bean drop, triangle move, rope drill, and endostitch (Fig. 7-2)—improved performance compared to standard training on bench trainers and translated into improved operative performance. Additionally these skills will deteriorate and require ongoing training in order to maintain proficiency.

While demonstrating that the practice of specific skills improved specific task performance in the operating room, this study did not necessarily prove that trainees learned the overall content of an operation. Dr. Elizabeth Hamilton et al. developed the laparoscopic total extraperitoneal (TEP) hernia simulator and curriculum. The model was a replica of a pelvis that allowed laparoscopic hernia repairs to be performed (Fig. 7-3, page 58). The multimodality curriculum included the TEP simulator, a TEP operative video, and an interactive CD-ROM. In this study, 21 PGY3 and PGY4 surgical residents (n = 21) were evaluated while assisting on a laparoscopic hernia repair. Half the group underwent formal training 30 minutes daily for 10 days, including the use of the model, watching an edited video of a laparoscopic hernia repair, and using an interactive CD-ROM. The other half of the residents received no additional formal training during their general surgery rotation. Afterwards, all residents performed a laparoscopic hernia repair as a posttest. Not only did the trained residents show significant improvement in time and motion, operation flow, use of assistants, and overall performance, for the first time Hamilton was able to demonstrate increased knowledge of the specific procedure in the operating room. In short, training in a simulated environment not only improved task performance, but also knowledge.

Virtual Reality Simulation Efforts by Surgical Specialties

All specialties within the broad profession of surgery are facing similar challenges to provide education and training to residents and practicing surgeons. Nearly all of the surgical specialties are turning to simulation as a way to meet these new training challenges. While the surgical specialties are embracing simulation technology, they also realize that their use of this technology must be research-based.

Currently, there are wide varieties of simulators available, and new systems are continually under development. To be effective educational tools, simulators must be reliable and valid. The validation process for surgical simulation is obviously complex and multifaceted. Validating a simulator generally requires numerous studies so that sufficient data can be accrued over time. It is, thus, appropriate that much of the research in simulation focuses on establishing the reliability and validity of various devices (Table 7-2, page 58). On a practical level, simulators must also be cost-effective and easily integrated into surgical education curricula. The surgical community realizes that it is essential to scrutinize this new simulator technology with the same rigor applied to other domains of surgery.

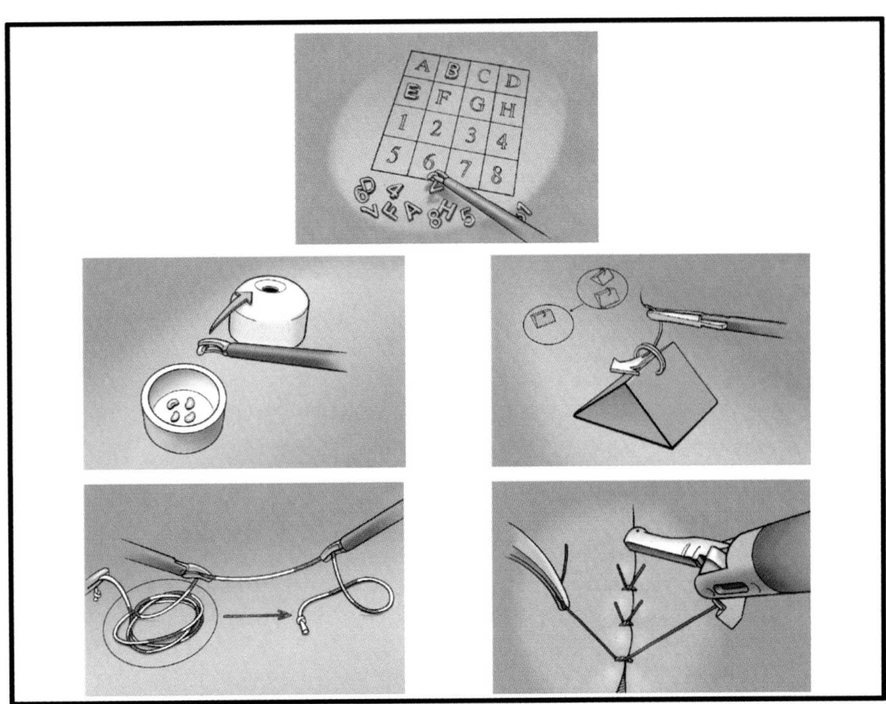

Fig. 7-2. Five tasks: the checker board, bean drop, triangle move, run rope, and endostitch.

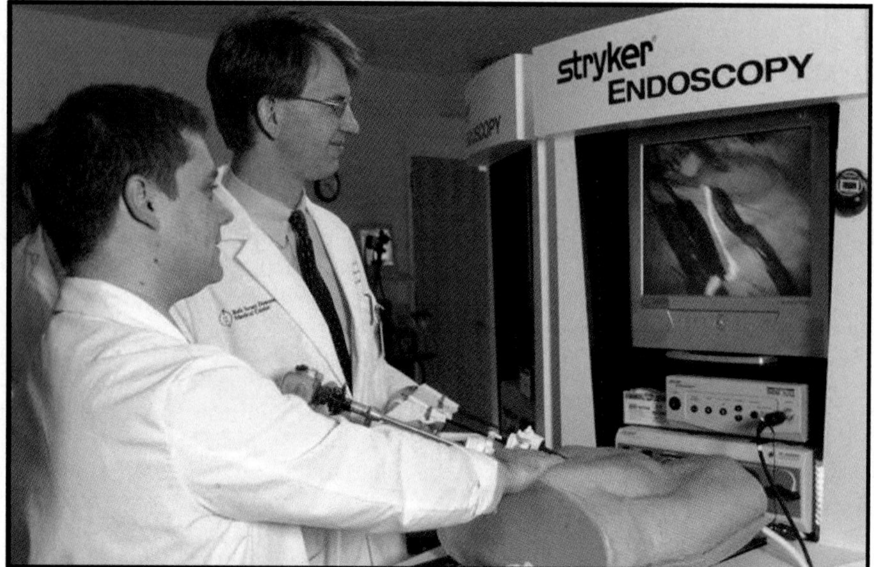

Fig. 7-3. A laparoscopic hernia simulator.

TABLE 7-2. DEFINITIONS OF RELIABILITY AND VALIDITY USED IN STUDIES OF SURGICAL SIMULATION

Reliability	
• The precision of a device • Robust and durable to afford consistent practice so that results are reproducible • Statistically scored from 0 to 1.0, between R = 0.5 to 0.8 is moderate, >0.8 is high	
Validity—the simulator's ability to measure what it was designed to measure	
Content validity	• The extent to which all relevant dimensions within a given domain are measured
Construct validity	• The ability to detect differences between groups with different levels of competence, supporting the notion that the test is measuring what it claims to measure
Concurrent validity	• Results of the test correlate with the criterion standard known to measure the same domain
Predictive validity	• Capacity to predict future performance
Face validity	• Extent that the simulation resembles the real task

Adapted from Soper NJ, Swanström LL, Eubanks WS, eds. *Mastery of endoscopic and laparoscopic surgery*. 2nd ed. Philadelphia: Lippincott Williams & Wilkins; 2005.

Vascular Surgery

In 2002, a Residency Review Committee of the Accreditation Council for Graduate Medical Education (ACGME) mandated that graduating fellows in vascular surgery have experience as the primary surgeon on 50 angiograms and 25 catheter-based endovascular cases. Because of this, and the fact that in major academic centers up to 70% of vascular cases are partially catheter-based, simulators that allow training in interventional procedures have been developed. One such system is the Procedicus Vascular Interventional System Trainer (VIST), developed by Mentice AB, Gothenburg, Sweden (Fig. 7-4). This is a multimedia device designed to simulate endovascular procedures for the treatment of carotid, renal, and iliofemoral occlusive disease. Additional modules allow for training in pacemaker lead placement, vena caval filter placement, cardiac catherization, and electrophysiology lead placement. It consists of a standard desktop PC with software that contains a representation of the human arterial system. The system uses a haptic interface that accurately recreates the vascular-catheter physical interaction. The simulation replicates hemodynamics, blood flow, and dye contrast media such that the operator can use standard angiographic catheters and guidewires, inject contrast dye, perform angioplasty, deploy stents, and perform digital subtraction angiography.

The VIST was validated in a randomized prospective study involving 20 general surgery residents at Columbia University. The residents, who had no prior endovascular experience, were randomized to train on the VIST or receive no training at all. Within 2 weeks of randomization, the residents completed two catheter-based endovascular cases. Staff vascular surgeons blinded to resident training status conducted evaluations using a Likert scale checklist and a global rating scale. Results demonstrated that VIST training improved resident performance in the operating room. Specifically, there was noted improvement during the procedural steps of an endovascular procedure as well as in the global rating scores of performance. This study is important in that it marks the first work that demonstrates transferability of endovascular simulation skills from the laboratory to the operating room.

In addition to providing fundamental endovascular skills training for resident training, the VIST has also been studied as a means for high-stakes assessment in interventional carotid angiography and stenting. Patel et al. studied whether VR training could be used to train 20 highly experienced interventional cardiologists without prior experience in carotid interventional techniques. Results demonstrated significant improvements in technical performance measured as procedure time, fluoroscopy time, contrast volume, and catheter handling errors comparing the subjects' first and last trials ($P < 0.05$). Additionally the internal consistency of the VIST simulator was very high (coefficient $\alpha > 0.8$) in all metrics except fluoroscopy time.

Urologic Surgery

A major focus of virtual reality surgical simulation efforts in urology has been on the fielding and validation of systems that allow for training of endourology skills. The most widely used VR simulator for dedicated endourologic training is the URO Mentor (Simbionix USA Corp.; Cleveland, OH). The University of Washington partnered with private industry to produce a VR-based simulator for the transurethral resection of the prostate (TURP). Matsumoto et al. of McMaster University, Ontario, Canada, performed a

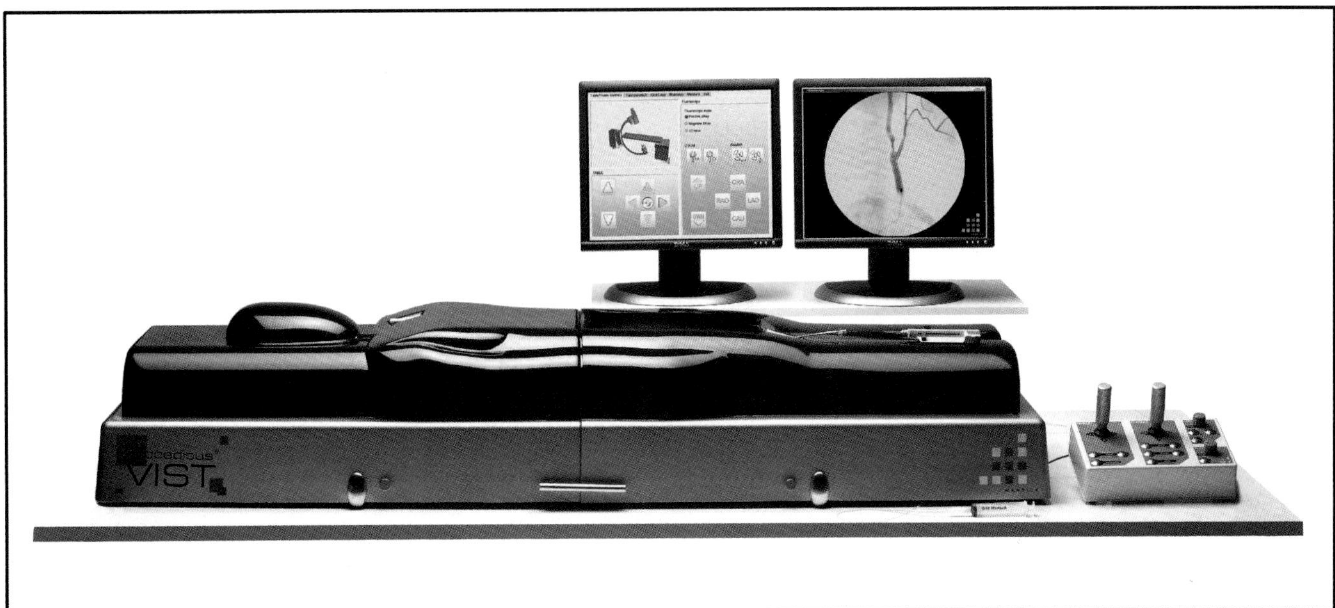

Fig. 7-4. Procedicus Vascular Interventional System Trainer (VIST) system.

validation study of this system. The authors compared senior and junior trainees' performance in endourologic technical skills such cystoscopy, guidewire insertion, and ureteric stone extraction using wire baskets. The VR performance was compared to a standardized high fidelity bench model. Results demonstrated significantly higher performance for senior vs. junior trainees. The authors concluded that the VR system was "a useful tool" for resident assessment. They also stated that the VR system was "comparable" to the validated bench model for endourologic skills training.

In a study from the University of California, medical students were randomized into two groups. The first group was given basic endourologic skills training on a VR simulator, while the other group was trained on a physical bench model. Eight weeks later, the endourologic skills performance of both groups was assessed using a live tissue kidney/ureter model. Results demonstrated no significant difference in technical performance between the VR and bench model trained groups. The conclusion was that the VR system was equivalent to the bench model and that the incorporation of simulation training may be useful for preliminary urologic resident training.

Sweet et al. performed the preliminary work on the University of Washington Virtual TURP Surgical Simulator. In a study of 72 staff urologists and 19 residents, this system's face, content, and construct validity were established. Experts performed predictably better with fewer errors compared to residents, demonstrating a significant difference in basic endourologic skills.

Obstetrics and Gynecologic Surgery

Current simulation efforts in obstetrics and gynecology have focused on the development of software modules to complement existing technologies for general laparoscopy skills training. Currently, two major commercial VR simulation technologies have dedicated obstetrical and gynecologic applications: the LAP Mentor (Simbionix USA Corp.; Cleveland, OH) and the LapSim Gyn (Surgical Science Sweden AB; Gothenburg, Sweden). VR modules exist that allow for training in hysteroscopy (such as Immersion Medical's Hysteroscopy AccuTouch system) and tubal ligation.

A recent study from the Imperial College of London assessed the validity of the LapSim Gyn (Fig. 7-5). Gynecologists were stratified into three groups based on levels of experience and performed a laparoscopic salpingectomy for ectopic pregnancy. Their results demonstrated significant differences between groups for overall time to complete the procedure, blood loss, and instrument path length (smoothness). The study established construct validity for the module. They concluded that

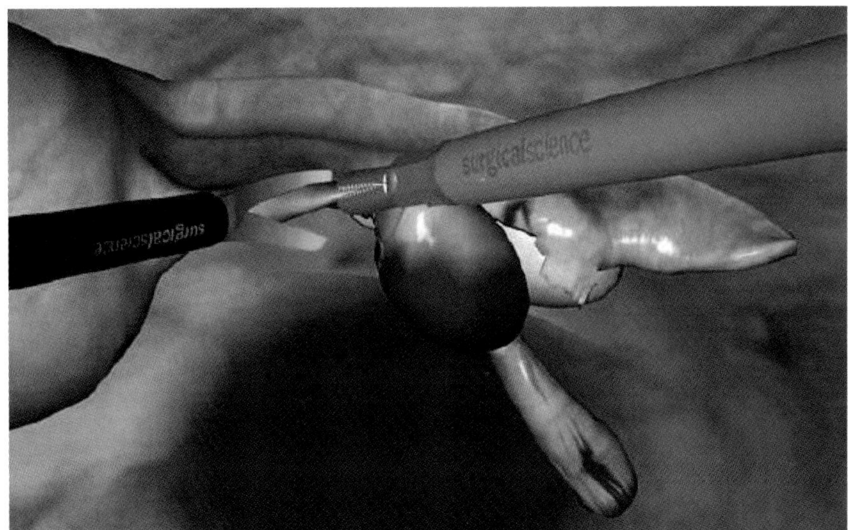

Fig. 7-5. A salpingectomy module for the LapSim Gyn. (Courtesy of Surgical Science Ltd., Gothenberg, Sweden.)

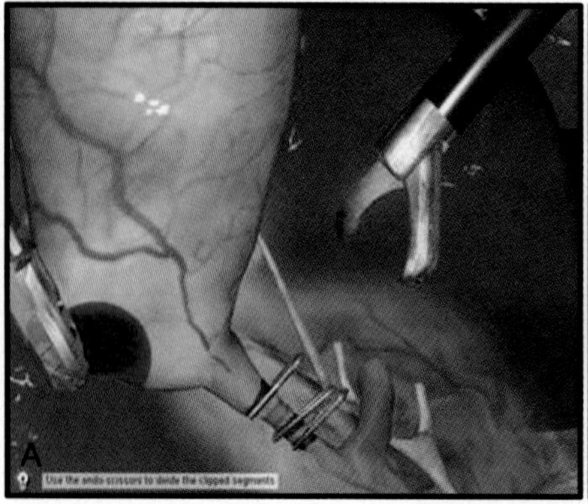

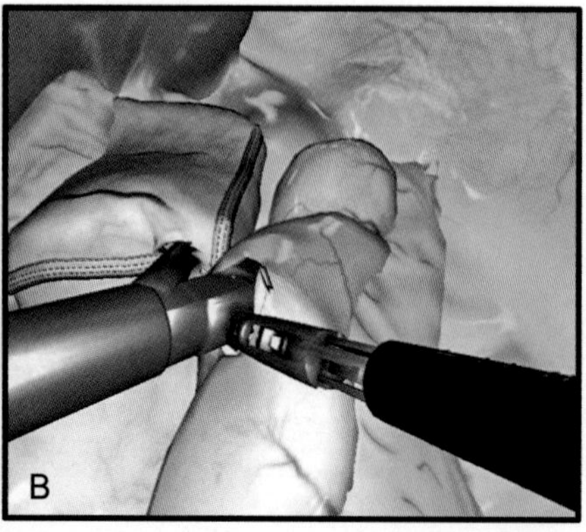

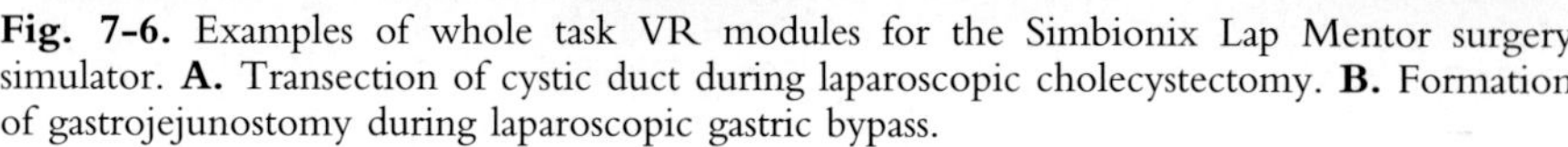
Fig. 7-6. Examples of whole task VR modules for the Simbionix Lap Mentor surgery simulator. **A.** Transection of cystic duct during laparoscopic cholecystectomy. **B.** Formation of gastrojejunostomy during laparoscopic gastric bypass.

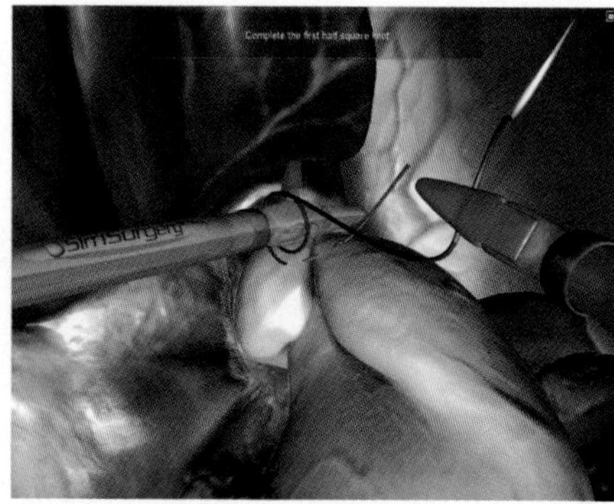
Fig. 7-7. A suturing module for laparoscopic fundoplication. (SimSurgery Surgical Education Platform (SEP) trainer.)

for inexperienced gynecologists, VR simulation might have a benefit, but for experienced operators the learning curves would likely not dramatically improve.

General Surgery

To date, the majority of efforts in VR simulation have focused on technologies that involve general surgery skills training. The medical literature is replete with studies that describe all aspects of medical simulation as it relates to general surgery. In 2002, two studies demonstrated the successful transfer of laparoscopic skills gained on the MIST-VR trainer to the operating room environment during the performance of a live laparoscopic cholecystectomy.

Several VR simulator companies have developed software modules that allow for the practice of whole procedures. The Simbionix LAP Mentor surgical trainer has a variety of procedural modules, including laparoscopic cholecystectomy, ventral hernia repair, and Roux-en-Y gastric bypass (Fig. 7-6). Surgical Science's LapSim surgical trainer, in addition to its basic skills module, has a software module for laparoscopic cholecystectomy called the LapSim Dissection. Additionally, other systems like the SurgicalSim Education Platform (SimSurgery AS; Oslo, Norway) allow for suture practice during laparoscopic fundoplication procedures (Fig. 7-7).

Recently, the European Association of Endoscopic Surgeons (EAES) completed a review of available simulator systems for laparoscopic and endoscopic surgery training and published consensus guidelines of their findings. Using widely accepted criteria for levels of evidence and levels of consensus recommendation, the EAES evaluated eight simulator systems. Tables 7-3 and 7-4 illustrate their findings. The EAES concluded that the available

TABLE 7-3. EUROPEAN ASSOCIATION OF ENDOSCOPIC SURGEONS CONSENSUS STATEMENT ON SURGICAL SIMULATORS: SUMMARY OF RESULTS

Flexible endoscopy simulators	**Overall consensus findings**
[1]Accutouch Lower GI	Diagnostic module—Level 2 recommendation Therapeutic module—0 consensus
[1]Accutouch Upper GI	EGD/Gastroscopy—0 consensus ERCP—0 consensus
[2]GI Mentor Colonoscopy	Level 3 recommendation
[2]GI Mentor Cyberscopy/Gastroscopy	Level 2 recommendation
Laparoscopic procedural simulators	**Overall consensus findings**
[3]Procedicus MIST	Level 2 recommendation
[4]LapSim Basic	Level 4 recommendation
[5]ProMIS	Level 3 and 4 recommendation
[2]Lap Mentor Basic	0 Consensus

[1]Immersion Medical, San Jose, CA
[2]Simbionix, Cleveland, OH, USA (www.simbionix.com/Media_validation_LAP.html)
[3]Mentice, Gothenburg, Sweden (www.mentice.com)
[4]Surgical Science, Göteborg, Sweden (www.surgicalscience.com/main/default/default.cfm)
[5]Haptica, Dublin, Ireland (www.haptica.com/id11.htm)
From Carter FJ, Schijven MP, Aggarwal R, et al. Consensus guidelines for validation of virtual reality surgical simulators. *Surg Endosc* 2005;19:1523–1532.

TABLE 7-4. EUROPEAN ASSOCIATION OF ENDOSCOPIC SURGEONS CONSENSUS STATEMENT ON SURGICAL SIMULATORS: LEVEL OF RECOMMENDATION CRITERIA

1. Based on one systematic review (1a) or at least two independently conducted research projects classified as 1b
2. Based on at least two independently conducted research projects classified as level 2a or 2b, within concordance
3. Based on one independently conducted research project level 2b, or at least two trials of level 3, within concordance
4. Based on one trial at level 3 or multiple expert opinions, including the opinion of Work Group members (e.g., level 4)

From Carter FJ, Schijven MP, Aggarwal R, et al. Consensus guidelines for validation of virtual reality surgical simulators. *Surg Endosc* 2005;19:1523–1532.

literature concerning VR task trainers for general surgery lacks uniformity in design, execution, and metrics of assessment.

Despite the lack of consensus as to the validity of the various commercial simulation technologies, it is clear that as the forces of educational change mentioned above continue to evolve and, as computer technology improves, ever-increasing examples of valid and reliable medical simulation will be possible. Ultimately, this will only be realized if government, industry, and academia continue to partner in ways that make the research and development cost-effective.

TABLE 7-5. TYPES OF EDUCATIONAL MODELS AND SIMULATORS THE AMERICAN COLLEGE OF SURGEONS WILL INVENTORY IN EDUCATION INSTITUTES

Airway model	ProMIS
Anesthesia simulator	Prostate model
Bench models	Pelvic model
Breast model	Trauma Man
Devices used to do open procedures	Simulators
Inguinal hernia model	Ultrasound simulator
Lap Chole simulator	Upper endoscopy simulator
Lower endoscopy simulator	Urology simulator
Mirror trainers	Ventral hernia model
Mist VR	Video trainers
Operating microscope	

Efforts to Improve Simulation-Based Education

At the national level, several groups, including the American College of Graduate Medical Education (ACGME) and the American College of Surgeons (ACS), have recently initiated efforts to standardize simulation-based education. The ACGME Residency Review Committee recently stated that all general surgery residencies should have access to a basic skills lab by 2008. Moreover, the ACS has established specific criteria for learners, curriculum, personnel, and resources for centers seeking ACS Accreditation as a Comprehensive Education Institute (CEI) or a Basic Education Institute (BEI). For example, the CEIs must provide education to at least three different learner groups (physicians, residents, medical students, nurses, allied health professionals) in addition to surgeons. Activities would include: collaboration with other centers, curriculum development, expansion of practice, interdisciplinary training, introduction of new skills, long-term follow-up of the learner, maintenance of skills, team training, and remediation of practice. The curriculum should incorporate psychomotor and cognitive skills, and the facility should accommodate at least 20 trainees in no less than 1200 contiguous square feet. An additional 4000 square feet would accommodate conference rooms, storage, vivarium, teleconferencing, and offices. The BEIs would require less space and resource commitment and fewer personnel, but would have explicit educational goals, appropriate models and simulators to meet learning objectives, and a formal assessment of educational programs. A variety of different models and simulators exist, and the ACS will inventory resources to facilitate collaboration between institutes (Table 7-5). In 2006, the ACS and the Association of Program Directors in Surgery initiated a working committee to establish a skills-based 5-year curriculum for all surgery trainees that includes modules for basic and advanced laparoscopy.

Simulation, Crisis Management, and Surgical Team Training

Single task training represents only one aspect of simulation in surgical education. Recently, the simulation movement in surgery has broken out from the realm of technical task trainers to the pursuit of completely simulated operating room environments for the training of surgical teams in both technical and nontechnical performance. A major technology that allows these simulated operating room environments to function is the human patient simulator.

History of Mannequin Simulators

The specialty of anesthesia has been at the forefront of medical simulation training since its inception. Dr. Jeffrey Cooper of the Center for Medical Simulation (Cambridge, MA) traces the origin of human patient simulators (HPS) to Norway in the 1960s, when Asmund Laerdal created a mannequin for training mouth-to-mouth resuscitation. Laerdal collaborated with Norwegian anesthesiologist Dr. Bjorn Lind to develop the model that later evolved into the well-known Resusci Anne simulator used for cardiopulmonary resuscitation training. The first computer-based HPS was developed at the University of Southern California in the mid-1960s as a collaboration between Dr. Judson Denson and military defense contractors. The "Sim One" HPS marked the first true anesthesia simulator that allowed basic algorithm training.

Current HPS are the evolution of these original technologies. Both Medical Education Technologies, Inc. (METI; Sarasota, FL) and Laerdal, Corp. (Fig. 7-8, page 62) produce simulators that are in extensive use worldwide. For example, both the METI HPS and the Laerdal SimMan consist of a mannequin and control rack of computer software. The mannequin is a lifelike adult or pediatric body that includes cardiovascular, pulmonary, and other systems that respond automatically to a user's interventions and to the environment.

HPS mannequins allow users to perform a variety of technical and nontechnical performance measures. Examples of technical procedures include physical exams, cardiopulmonary resuscitation (CPR), and advanced trauma life support (ATLS) procedures. HPS systems provide subjects with nontechnical feedback such as heart and lung sounds, pulses, and a variety of physiologic parameters including EKGs, blood pressures, and oxygen saturation.

The mannequins were primarily developed for anesthesia training, and are, thus, programmed with pharmacologic parameters for over 60 intravenous and gaseous drugs. When a drug is administered, the simulator takes into account "patient" weight and physical condition to obtain onset and offset times and dose-dependent systemic effects. Drug interactions are also calculated and reflected in the vital signs.

Lessons Learned from Anesthesia

Surgical residency programs have only recently begun implementing the use of HPS as part of their education and training

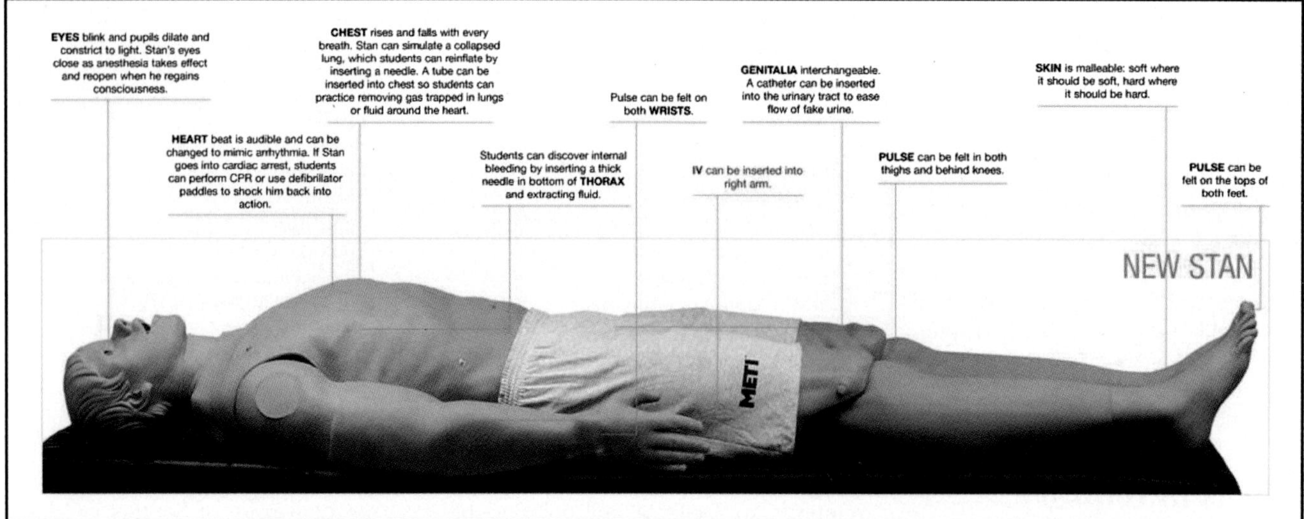
EYES blink and pupils dilate and constrict to light. Stan's eyes close as anesthesia takes effect and reopen when he regains consciousness.
CHEST rises and falls with every breath. Stan can simulate a collapsed lung, which students can reinflate by inserting a needle. A tube can be inserted into chest so students can practice removing gas trapped in lungs or fluid around the heart.
Pulse can be felt on both **WRISTS**.
GENITALIA interchangeable. A catheter can be inserted into the urinary tract to ease flow of fake urine.
SKIN is malleable: soft where it should be soft, hard where it should be hard.
HEART beat is audible and can be changed to mimic arrhythmia. If Stan goes into cardiac arrest, students can perform CPR or use defibrillator paddles to shock him back into action.
Students can discover internal bleeding by inserting a thick needle in bottom of **THORAX** and extracting fluid.
IV can be inserted into right arm.
PULSE can be felt in both thighs and behind knees.
PULSE can be felt on the tops of both feet.
NEW STAN
METI

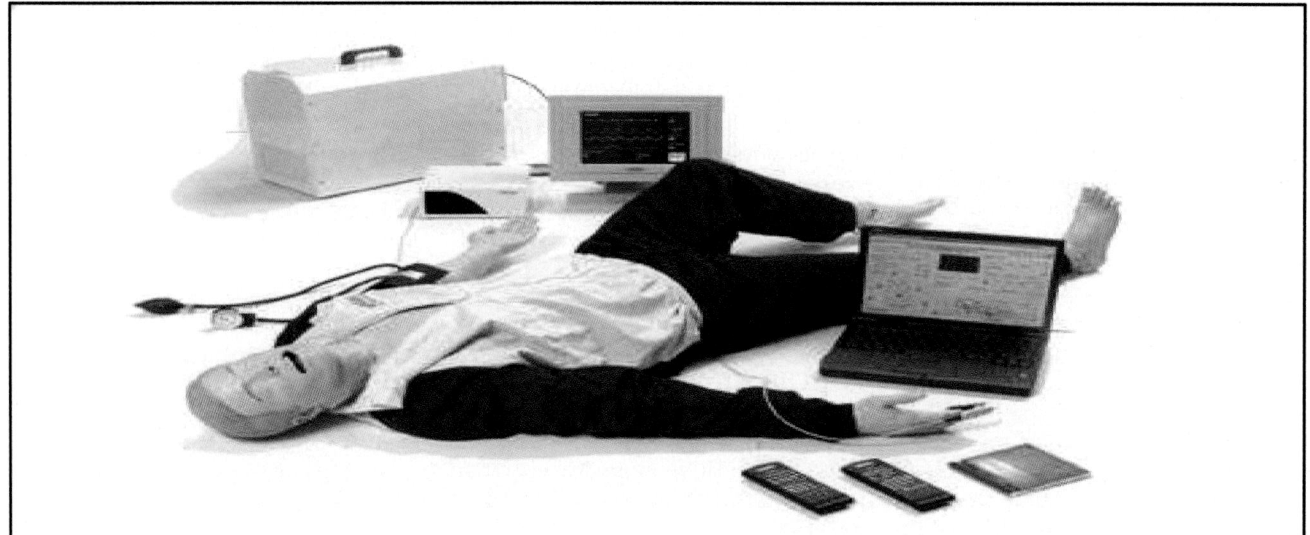

Fig. 7-8. METI HPS (top) and Laerdal SimMan (bottom).

programs. Thus, there is extensive research in the area of skills training relating specifically to surgical residency training, but there are few examples of surgical research involving human patient simulators. However, anesthesia residencies have been using simulators in their training programs for several decades, and there are numerous studies examining their use. The two examples that follow describe the use of HPSs for training and performance assessment to be used in high-stakes testing situations such as board certifications.

In 1998, Gaba et al. published one of the first comprehensive simulation studies evaluating both the technical and nontechnical performance of anesthesiologists in crisis situations. Teams were videotaped and assessed using the Line/LOS Checklist measurement instrument, which was adapted from the aviation industry. The researchers measured the performance of subjects during a malignant hyperthermia (MH) and cardiac arrest scenario. Results demonstrated high scores on technical performance (0.78 ±0.08 for MH; 0.83 ±0.06 for cardiac arrest) but poor scores for nontechnical performance (28% for MH; 14% for cardiac arrest). This study is important in that it demonstrated the feasibility of using simulation as a means to measure the technical and nontechnical performance of anesthesia teams during operating room crisis events.

In 2005, Savoldelli et al. reported a prospective study in which HPS systems were used to assess senior anesthesia trainees and compared this to standard assessment tools such as an oral examination modeled on a board certification examination. Twenty senior residents were tested on resuscitation and trauma scenarios, using a mock oral board examination and then the two simulator scenarios. The results showed good interrater reliability across scenarios and modalities. Concurrent validity—a measure of how well the simulation-based examination correlated to the validated oral examination—was moderate for the resuscitation (r = 0.52) and trauma (r = 0.53) scenarios. The authors concluded that the simulation-based examination was a good tool in terms of ability to discriminate levels of trainees. Additionally they concluded that simulation might be a useful adjunct to the oral examination in medical certification testing. While conclusive studies of the effectiveness of the HPS in surgical training programs have yet to be completed, the anesthesia studies suggest that the HPS could become a useful adjunct to traditional surgical training and performance assessment.

Crisis Management Training

The HPS has allowed the surgical simulation field to expand to include the comprehensive training of surgical crisis management (SCR) and crew resource management (CRM) in mock operating rooms. These are simulated environments only in the sense that the patient is a simulated mannequin; the equipment and participating personnel follow scripted operating room scenarios.

The aviation industry was the first to embrace the concept of CRM training. Healy et al. reviewed the history of CMR in the aviation industry and described the elements of the training in relation to performance in the operating room environment. The authors detailed research that demonstrated aviation accidents occur not because of equipment failure but rather because of crew member failure to work together efficiently during crises. In the 1970s, psychologists studied flight crew performance and determined that often crew members recognized problems early on but were reticent to bring them to their superiors' attention for fear of retribution. Based on these findings, the aviation community began a reducing their emphasis on team hierarchy, encouraging subordinate team members to raise concerns immediately related to safety; and training senior team members to listen to subordinate team members and to view these concerns as honest concerns rather than defiance.

In 2000, the Institute of Medicine report *To Error Is Human: Building a Safer Health System* called for a reduction in medical error via formal training in teamwork analogous to SCR and CRM. As a response to this, the American College of Surgeons presented general sessions and postgraduate courses on SCR/CRM at the 2004 and 2005 Clinical Congresses in an effort to educate it membership, based on the concept that the same techniques that are used in the aviation industry can be implemented in the operating room. Examples include preprocedure briefs (OR final timeout), routine use of standard operating procedures (clinical care pathway), checklists, and the promotion of open team communication.

Surgical Research Involving Surgical Crisis Management/Crew Resource Management

Sir Ara Darzi et al. at the Imperial College of London, United Kingdom, performed a validation experiment using a bleeding crisis in a simulated operating theater in 2006. The study assessed surgical residents' technical abilities and nontechnical team/human factors skills during crises. The crisis scenario involved the use of a synthetic model of a 5-mm femoral vein laceration mounted to an HPS. Also present were a standardized operating room team comprising an anesthetist, a scrub nurse, and a circulating nurse. Researchers used global rating scales to assess the technical and nontechnical performances of junior and senior surgical residents. Variables measured included time to diagnosis, time to inform team members of crisis, time to achieve control, and time to close laceration. The study demonstrated high levels of face validity (95% agreement) and usefulness as a training and assessment tool for technical and SCR/CRM teaching. The evaluation of technical skills such as the ability to control femoral vein bleeding showed significant differences between the performance of senior and junior trainees (median ± interquartile range, 68 ±13 vs. 51.8 ±14.9, $P = 0.001$). Interestingly, there was not a major difference in nontechnical performance between the groups. Leadership skills' scoring showed a trend favoring senior trainees, but was not significant. Metrics of time revealed several significant differences between groups, including time to diagnosis of bleeding ($P = 0.01$), time to control bleeding ($P = 0.001$), and time to close laceration ($P = 0.001$).

This sentinel study represents the first published results describing the application of SCR/CRM techniques in a model of open surgery. The Imperial College simulation group built a synthetic model with high face validity. They developed and validated the metrics necessary to measure technical and nontechnical performance. Finally, they proved that surgery must be a "team sport."

Others centers are also developing and validating SCR/CRM techniques in mock operating environments. The Beth Israel Deaconess Medical Center has recently established a mock laparoscopic endosuite operating room in their Carl J. Shapiro Simulation and Skills Center (SASC) in Boston, MA. Face, content, and construct validity was established for simulated laparoscopic crisis scenarios in a mock laparoscopic endosuite, which replicates a real operating theater. All standard laparoscopic surgical equipments, as well as an anesthetic simulator, are present. The novel synthetic body used allows for placement of a Veress needle, abdominal CO_2 insufflation, trocar insertion, and simulation of intraperitoneal hemorrhage. The operative model deserves recognition as the first published example of a true operable abdomen. It consists of a series of commercially available off-the-shelf synthetic abdominal organs that are accurate in dimension and appearance (Fig. 7-9, page 64). This model, draped in surgical drapes, is used in conjunction with a METI HPS to provide realism and, more importantly, physiologic feedback to the subjects on the anesthesia monitors after each operative intervention, with the manipulation of the mannequin's hemodynamic parameters performed through a software program in an adjacent control room.

The study validates the mock endosuite system as a potential teaching tool for surgical team training specifically for crisis management during minimally invasive surgical cases (Fig. 7-10, page 64). Results demonstrate high face validity for the laparoscopic model. As depicted, (Fig. 7-11, page 65) novice and expert surgeons gave median scores of 4.29 and 4.43 respectively for face validity, compared to the scrub nurses, who deemed face validity to be higher (4.71) although not significantly different. The internal consistency of face validity questions was high, indicating good scale reliability among the questions. The majority of experts (80%) considered the simulation suitable for initial training in general surgery, thus establishing its content validity. To establish construct validity, the study evaluated the technical and nontechnical performances of novice and expert laparoscopic surgeons throughout a simulated intraabdominal hemorrhage during a laparoscopic cholecystectomy. In assessing nontechnical skills, experts scored significantly higher (90% ±6) than novices (51% ±15; $P < 0.001$). For technical skills measurement, no difference was observed in Veress safety and laparoscopic equipment setup between groups. However, there was a significant overall difference between the two groups in their ability to identify bleeding (63% ±19 vs. 94% ±6) and hemodynamic instability (52% ±21 vs. 93% ±5), their decision to convert to an open laparotomy (54% ±24 vs. 90% ±11), and in their control of intraabdominal hemorrhaging (48% ±24 vs. 93% ±15). Interestingly, experts took a shorter time to control the bleeding, but ultimately persisted longer laparoscopically attempting to salvage the case. The protocol significantly discriminated between the technical and nontechnical performance of novices and experts (Fig. 7-12, page 65).

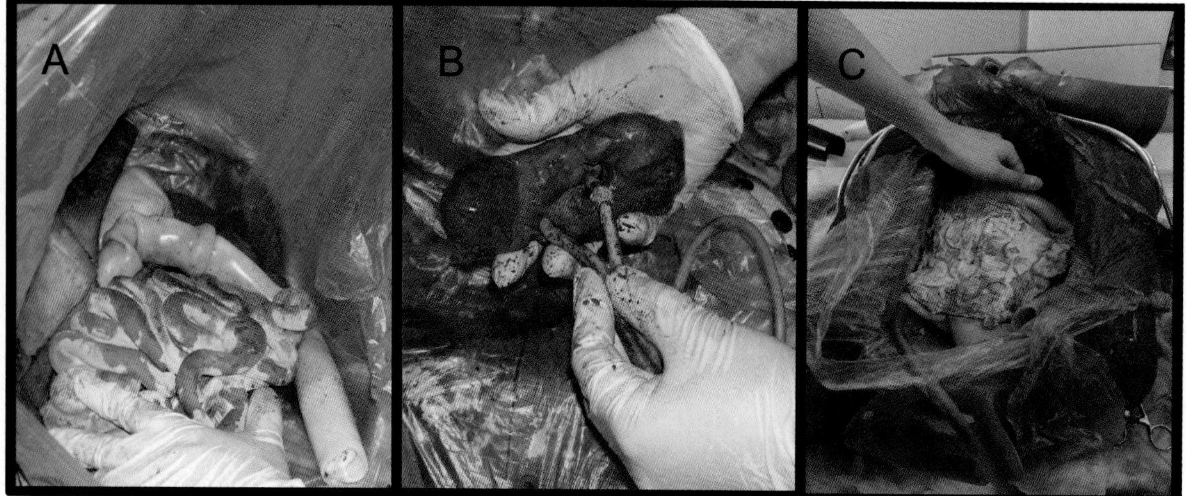

Fig. 7-9. A. Denotes simulated bowel. **B.** Denotes spleen with vasculature. **C.** Completed model ready for simulation. (Developed by Noel Irias, SASC, 2006.)

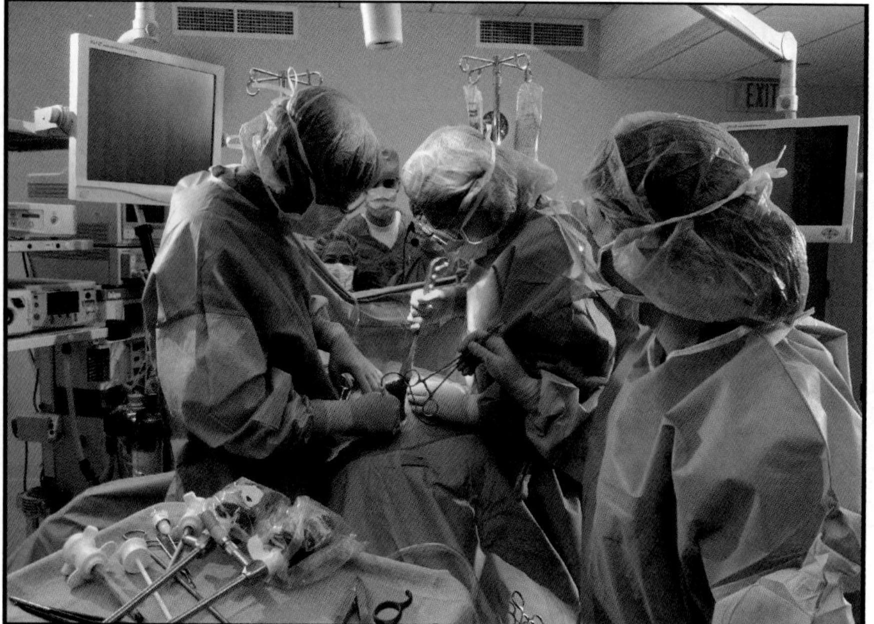

Fig. 7-10. Conversion to open surgery after a simulated laparoscopic surgical crisis. (Courtesy of Shapiro Simulation and Skills Center; Beth Israel Deaconess Medical Center; Boston MA; www.bidmc.harvard.edu/sasc.)

Medical Simulation and the United States Military

Funding Innovation in Medical Simulation

Currently, the Department of Defense (DOD) funds innovative programs developing all aspects of simulation technology through the Telemedicine and Advanced Technology Research Center (TATRC), a subordinate element of the United States Army Medical Research and Materiel Command (USAMRMC). TATRC manages core Research, Development, Test, and Evaluation (RDT&E) efforts and congressionally mandated projects in telemedicine and advanced medical technologies. To support its RDT&E efforts, TATRC maintains a productive mix of partnerships with federal, academic, and commercial organizations. TATRC also provides short-term technical support (as directed) to federal and defense agencies; it develops, evaluates, and demonstrates new technologies and concepts; and it conducts market surveillance with a focus on leveraging emerging technologies in health care and health care support. Since 1997, TATRC, which is largely funded by the U.S. Army, has funded 44 projects totaling $12,555,000 and is expected to have funded 174 projects totaling $74,811,000 in 2007.

Simulation Training for Combat Medics and Forward Surgical Teams

At the U.S. Army Medical Department (AMEDD) Center and School, the Department of Combat Medic Training (DCMT) is one of the largest users of HPS systems worldwide. They currently have 139 METI "trauma man" human patient simulators.

DCMT provides combat medics with instruction on the basic skills necessary to be successful in accomplishing their military duties. Training up to 7200 soldiers a year, students receive 17 hours of HPS-based instruction in the following areas: vital signs, airway practical exercise, medical assessment practical exercise, trauma assessment practical exercise, cardiac/respiratory practical exercise, OB/GYN practical exercise, and emergency cricothyroidotomy/needle chest decompression. This culminates in a field training exercise involving HPS causalities in a mock desert village with 13 casualties (both military and civilian) suffering injuries from an improvised explosive device as well as embassy bombing mass casualty exercise with 13 casualties suffering blast injuries (Fig. 7-13, page 66).

The use of HPS, although it accounts for less than 5% of total training time, is critical in learning specific tasks. These

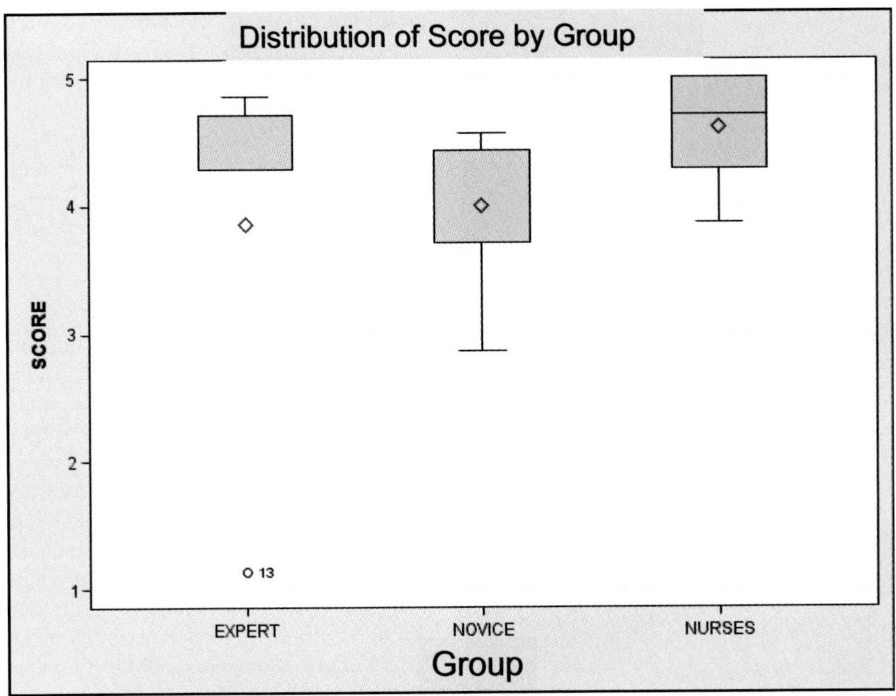

Fig. 7-11. Face validity scored on 5-point Likert scale.

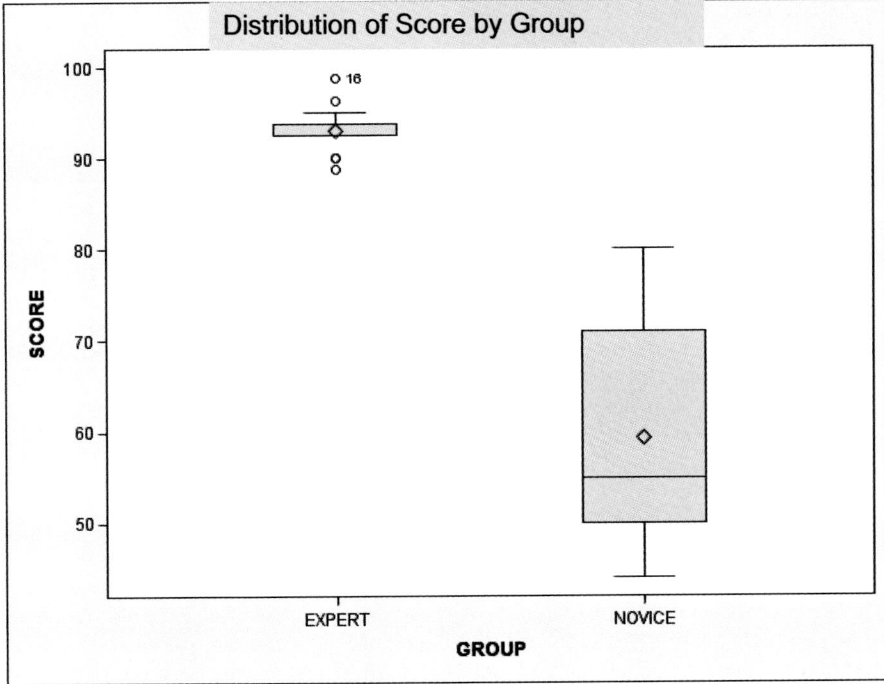

Fig. 7-12. Total Technical Skills Assessment Scores.

simulators are excellent tools for our soldiers to learn heart and breath sounds on the battlefield and for practicing procedures not possible on live patients such as needle chest decompression and surgical cricothyroidotomy. Soldiers can practice hemorrhage control using various tourniquets to stop the simulator from "bleeding."

The primary mission of the surgical assets of the U.S. military's tri-service medical system is to provide far forward acute trauma care to wounded DOD personnel in times of conflict. Prior to the global war on terrorism, which began in September, 2001, most military trauma providers did not provide daily care to acutely injured trauma patients. In response to this problem, one initiative to help maintain trauma skills has been to rotate military forward surgical teams through month-long rotations at civilian level-one trauma centers prior to combat deployments.

Holcomb described a study that evaluated U.S. military trauma providers at the beginning of a 28-day trauma rotation using standardized trauma scenarios. Performance was measured using scored and timed tasks involving evaluation and treatment of trauma patients. At the end of the rotation, the teams were reevaluated. Results demonstrated significant improvement in four out of the five scored tasks and six of the eight timed tasks. The authors concluded that HPS systems were a valid teaching and evaluation tool in the complex field of trauma resuscitation.

Additionally, the DOD has funded many innovative projects involving novel simulators for trauma training. One example is a combined HPS and VR simulator from the Center for Integration of Medicine & Innovative Technology (CIMIT) in Boston, MA. The VIRGIL system, developed by CIMIT's Simulation program, fuses an HPS with a computer interface that tracks the internal position of tube thoracostomy during placement. VIRGIL provides realistic force feedback during the skin incision, dissection through intercostal muscle and pleura, and subsequent placement of a 36-Fr chest tube (Fig. 7-14, page 66).

Guidelines for Team Training Using Surgical Simulators

Investment in simulation technology alone will not produce improved surgeons or highly effective interdisciplinary medical teams. In a recent review article on team training, Burke et al. explained that while the surgical community has focused on teaching technical skills, as the use of interdisciplinary health care teams continues to evolve, technical task training will no longer be adequate. In addition to skills training, the surgical community must develop teamwork skills that are cognitive, behavioral, and attitudinal to allow surgeons to work efficiently as part of interdisciplinary teams. Burke et al. provided guidelines for team training that have been adapted from over 20 years of military and aviation team training. The guidelines cover three areas: pre-team training factors, implementation, and post-team training factors.

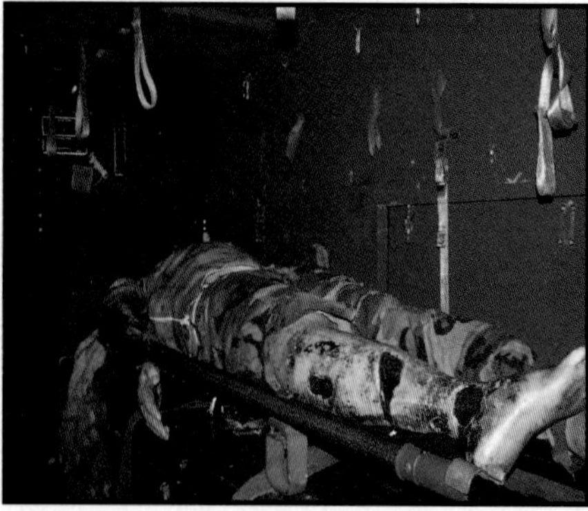

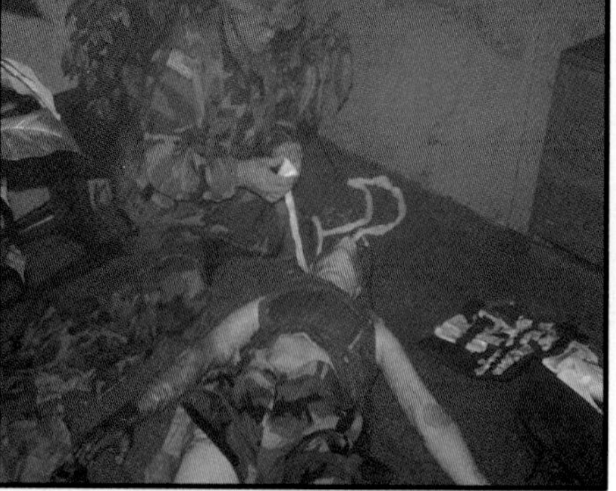

Fig. 7-13. Combat medic field training exercise using HPS at the U.S. Army's AMEDD Center and School, Fort Sam Houston, TX. (Used with permission from LTC David Hernandez, U.S. Army.)

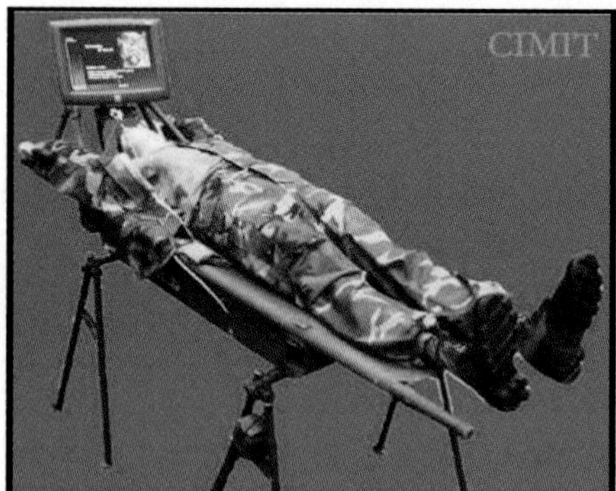

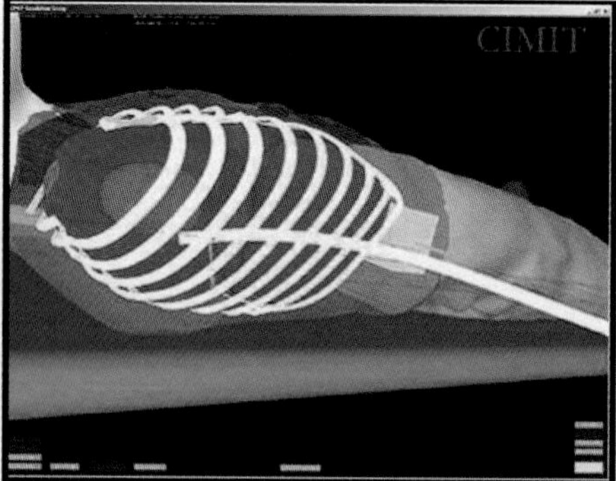

Fig. 7-14. A VIRGIL combined HPS and VR simulator from the Center for Integration of Medicine & Innovative Technology (CIMIT).

Pre-Team Training Phase

The pre-team phase set ups the training environment. It includes the introduction and analysis of the task. This may call for the identification of the teaching of specific skills and the assignment of these skills to team members. Introduced at this point are tasks that require more than one team member; team members must then plan how they will cooperate to complete them. The use of pre-training tools (such as written materials given to the participants in advance of the training) will maximize the benefit of the training. Finally, leaders must emphasize the positive aspects of the training and demonstrate its usefulness in the participants' work situation.

Implementation Phase

The study's implementation phase includes six key guidelines. The first and perhaps most important is the emphasis on teaching the five core teamwork components. Research identifies the five components of teamwork: (1) team leadership, (2) mutual performance monitoring, (3) backup behavior (or the ability to anticipate team members' needs and to come to their assistance when necessary), (4) adaptability, and (5) team orientation (or placing the team goals above any individual goals). Health care professionals are often leaders within their specialties, but this specialty area leadership does not necessarily translate into the ability to anticipate the needs of other team members, the willingness to place team goals over individual goals, or the ability to lead an interdisciplinary team. Teaching what Burke calls the "big five of teamwork" will help orient individuals to place more emphasis on the success of the team rather than individual success.

Several of the other guidelines identified by Burke et al. in the implementation phase reinforce the core teamwork competencies. These include teaching team members to be flexible and to adapt, especially as it relates to providing backup assistance to others. Team training must also teach team members to be sensitive and understanding of other members and to promote a learning environment where junior team members feel confident to identify problems and senior team members respond respectfully to junior members' concerns. Additionally, training should include the use of closed loop communication so that all verbal interactions are clearly understood.

The final guideline identified in the implementation phase is guided practice. Guided practice is a strategy that is widely used by the military and aviation communities as well as by professional educators. Task exposure by itself does not assume learning; participants must practice working as a team and receive intermittent feedback during this practice. This feedback reinforces positive behaviors and allows corrective action to be taken during the exercise.

Post-Training Phase

The success of the implementation phase must be measured. During the post-training phase, the leader evaluates all aspects of the training, including the participants' abilities to meet the stated goals as well as their reactions to the trainers and the training environment. A team of experts does not make an expert team. For example, team members might focus on their particular aspect of the operation to the point where they do not notice potential problems. Some members might see potential problems but are hesitant to identify them for fear of retribution. Teaching the five core components of teamwork, as well as the other guidelines identified by Burke et al., can help teams focus on their ultimate goal, patient safety.

CONCLUSION

The military, aviation, and other high-risk industries first embraced simulation technology several decades ago. In these fields, the companies building complex systems (weapons systems, aircraft, nuclear power plants, etc.) provide simulators to their end users for training and performance assessment. As relative newcomers to the field of simulation, surgeons have embraced the benefits of simulation as an adjunct to surgical education and as a means to improve patient safety.

The business model that medical simulation companies currently pursue is to project what type of simulators will be most marketable to the surgical community for training and performance assessment. This model has led to major advances in technology, but, as we have noted, many of the systems developed lack validation for a variety of reasons.

Due to the low profitability of medical simulation as a business model, U.S. government agencies like the Agency for Healthcare Research and Quality (AHRQ), the medical safety proponent of the U.S. Department of Health and Human Services, and the U.S. Army's TATRC will continue to represent a major source of funding for research and development in medical simulation. Despite these sources, current funding is inadequate. Ultimately, surgeons will have to find innovative ways to partner with hospitals, foundations, and philanthropy to fund education research.

Simulation technology alone will not improve surgical residency training or produce highly skilled surgeons. Simulation technology must be paired with a curriculum that is based upon sound educational principles. For instance, the American College of Surgeons' initiatives to develop basic and advanced laparoscopic module as well as the college's Accredited Education Institutes are prime examples of efforts to develop curricula for surgical education. Without steps like these, simulation technology is not likely to reach its potential.

A classic case study from the aviation industry illustrates what can happen in the face of inadequate team training. In January 1982, the pilot and copilot of Air Florida Flight 90, sitting on the tarmac of the Washington National Airport, began a series of events that became a tragic example of what can go wrong when teams fail to communicate effectively. On the afternoon of the crash, freezing temperatures and snow paralyzed the nation's capital. Despite these conditions, the pilot did not follow the aircraft's guidelines for deicing. While the copilot noticed instrument anomalies, he did not forcefully insist that the takeoff be aborted. The crash that followed, in which 78 people were killed, became the catalyst for the mandated implementation of crew resource management training in the aviation industry.

In the 1970s, much was written about crew resource management, but few pilots willingly embraced this new approach to safety. Many parallels exist between the aviation industry of the 1970s and the surgical profession today. Although much has been written about crew resource management as a means to ensure patient safety, not all surgeons are fully invested in this new paradigm. The aviation industry forced pilots to change their leadership styles to assure airline safety and simulation. In order for surgeons to fully meet their obligations to patient safety, the medical simulation community must strive to provide surgeons with the same realistic simulated environments that the aviation industry provided pilots over 2 decades ago.

SUGGESTED READING

Burke CS, Salas E, Wilson-Donnelly K, et al. How to turn a team of experts into an expert medical team: guidance from the aviation and military communities. *Qual Saf Health Care* 2004;13:96–104.

Cao CGL, Zhou M, Jones DB, et al. Can surgeons think and operate with haptics at the same time? *J Gastrointestinal Surg* 2007; 11:1564–1569.

Carter FJ, Schijven MP, Aggarwal R, et al. Consensus guidelines for validation of virtual reality surgical simulators. *Surg Endosc* 2005;19:1523–1532.

Debas HT, Bass BL, Brennan MF, et al. American Surgical Association Blue Ribbon Committee Report on Surgical Education: 2004. *Ann Surg* 2005;241:1–8.

Dutta S, Gaba D, Krummel TM. To simulate or not to simulate: what is the question? *Ann Surg* 2006;243:301–303.

Healy GB, Barker J, Madonna G. Error Reduction Through Team Leadership: Applying Aviation's CRM Model in the OR. *Bulletin American College Surgeons* 91[2]. 2006.

Hoover SJ, Berry MP, Rossick L, et al. Ultrasound-guided breast biopsy curriculum for surgical residents. *Surg Innov* 2008;15(1): 52–58.

McIntyre T, Monahan T, Villegas L, et al. Teleconferencing surgery enhances effective communication and enriches medical education. *Surg Laparosc Endosc Percutan Tech* 2008;18(1):45–48.

Moorthy K, Munz Y, Forrest D, et al. Surgical crisis management skills training and assessment: a simulation[corrected]-based approach to enhancing operating room performance. *Ann Surg* 2006;244:139–147.

Powers KA, Rehrig ST, Irias N, et al. Simulated laparoscopic operating room crisis: approach to enhance the surgical team performance. *Surg Endosc* 2008;22(4):885–900.

Reznick RK, MacRae H. Teaching surgical skills—changes in the wind. *N Engl J Med* 2006;355:2664–2669.

Reznick RK. Surgical simulation: a vital part of our future. *Ann Surg* 2005;242: 640–641.

Satava RM. Disruptive visions: surgical education. *Surg Endosc* 2004;18:779–781.

Seymour NE, Gallagher AG, Roman SA, et al. Virtual reality training improves operating room performance: results of a randomized, double-blinded study. *Ann Surg* 2002; 236: 458–463.

Sutherland LM, Middleton PF, Anthony A, et al. Surgical simulation: a systematic review. *Ann Surg* 2006;243:291–300.

Swanstrom LL, Fried GM, Hoffman KI, et al. Beta test results of a new system assessing competence in laparoscopic surgery. *J Am Coll Surg* 2006;202:62–69.

COMMENTARY

These authors have detailed the current status of virtual reality tools and simulators for teaching minimally invasive surgery. This is an area of intense investigation and is in a constant state of evolution; by the time this text is published, there will likely be several new simulators available in the laboratory or marketplace. Nevertheless, this chapter discusses the background supporting the current efforts and puts it in the context of the aviation industry, which set the standard for simulation training decades ago. The living, breathing human patient is very different from the easily modeled airspace surrounding an aircraft. Only in recent years has computing power achieved a level sufficient to allow early attempts at realistic, interactive simulation of clinically relevant tasks and portions of operations. Most current virtual reality simulators remain "cartoonish," with graphics of lower fidelity than most video games. Realistic appearing interfaces between human and machine are just being developed. The ability to model tissue characteristics, particularly deformability, and the addition of haptics are improving the "reality" aspect of the virtual space. Great strides have been made in all of these areas just within the past few years.

Clearly, the "see one, do one, teach one" era in surgical education is a relic of the past. Effective means of teaching surgical skills outside of the increasingly expensive operating room environment, allowing trainees to enter the operating theatre with background knowledge and skills sets, are fundamentally important to surgical education. Many first- and second-generation simulators are currently available and have been covered in this chapter. Limited applications and high price tags hamper these devices, each with their advantages and disadvantages. For the field to evolve and develop, surgical educators must be involved in the development and application of these technologies. The authors, who have been involved in these efforts, give the reader a unique vantage point on this rapidly evolving field.

Finally, team training is discussed, and its importance emphasized, along with the use of simulated operating room environments. Individuals' reactions and team interactions in both routine and crisis management modes can be assessed and improved. In the complex milieu of surgery, simulated environments will take on a larger role in the training and evaluation of competency among surgical providers.

NJS

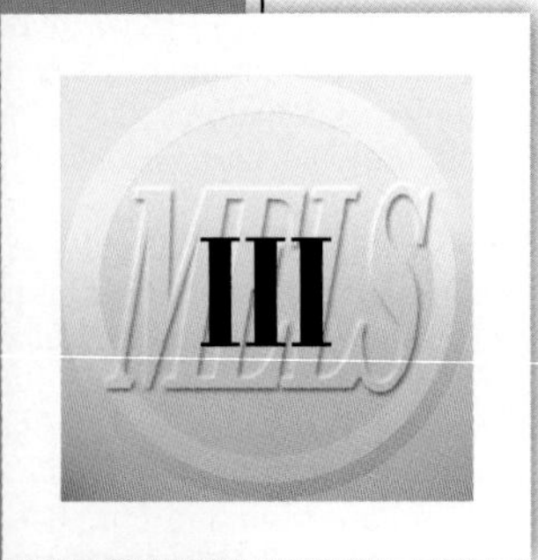

III Diseases of the Esophagus

A. Benign Disorders

Gastroesophageal Reflux

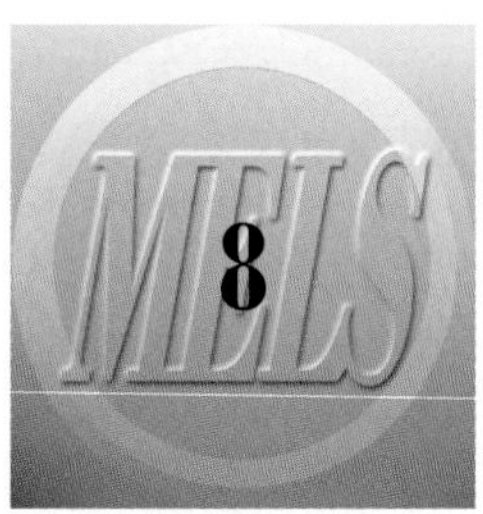

8 Anatomic and Physiologic Tests of Esophageal Function

FERNANDO A. M. HERBELLA
AND JEFFREY H. PETERS

INTRODUCTION

The goals of preoperative evaluation of esophageal function include the following:

1. Elucidation of symptoms that might be attributable to esophageal diseases, as well as symptoms potentially attributable to other foregut abnormalities.
2. Identification of associated anatomic abnormalities, such as Barrett esophagus, shortened esophagus, esophageal stricture, and large sliding or paraesophageal hiatal hernia.
3. Assessment of functional disorders of the foregut.
4. Estimation of the probability of a successful symptomatic response to surgical therapy.
5. Planning the type of the operative approach, including laparoscopic and open transabdominal or transthoracic, and the likelihood of needing to perform an additional procedures such as a Collis gastroplasty.
6. Assessment of comorbidities that might impact candidacy for surgery, the surgical approach, and perioperative complications.

The most common preoperative diagnostic studies include:

1. X-ray esophagram.
2. Upper gastrointestinal endoscopy.
3. Esophageal manometry.
4. Ambulatory esophageal pH monitoring.

Further investigations, in particular gastric emptying studies and radionuclide biliary imaging, are added depending on the findings of standard testing and the presence of symptoms that warrant further study.

Symptoms

A careful, structured assessment of the patient's symptoms is critical. Despite the fact that symptomatic improvement is usually used as the determinant of success, symptom assessment is often among the most superficial of all evaluations. Esophageal symptoms can be grouped as typical (heartburn, regurgitation, dysphagia) or atypical (for example, extraesophageal symptoms such as chest pain, cough, laryngitis, etc.). Symptoms of delayed gastric empting (e.g., nausea, vomiting, early satiety) should also be documented, as they may be part of the physiopathology of the disease. The patient's perception of each symptom should be explored in an effort to avoid misinterpretation. Of equal importance is to classify symptoms as primary or secondary to allow an estimate of the probabilty of relief. Symptomatic response to medications is of importance as it can predict outcomes following surgery. Although symptoms are used to screen patients for tests and to measure satisfaction with and the success of treatment, they are in fact an unreliable method to diagnose actual esophageal pathology.

Tests

Video Contrast Esophagram

Radiographic assessment of the anatomy and function of the esophagus and stomach is an important part of the preoperative evaluation. A carefully performed video esophagram provides anatomic as well as functional information. It is best done using a standardized protocol allowing quantification of findings and video-recorded so that the operating surgeon can view the dynamic study. For assessment of esophageal body function, the protocol includes five separate 10-cc swallows of barium, 15 seconds apart, in the prone oblique position. Solid bolus transport can be evaluated with a contrast-coated hamburger swallowed in the erect position. Esophageal diameter is measured after rapid swallow of several gulps in the prone oblique position to maximally distend the esophagus (Fig. 8-1). Specific protocols include:

- Evaluation of the relationship of the esophagogastric junction to the diaphragmatic hiatus: [2 to 3 individual swallows in the supine position focused on the distal esophagus and esophagogastric junction (EGJ)].
- Evaluation of cricopharyngeal function: [lateral and anteroposterior (AP) views of the oropharynx and upper esophagus in the erect position].
- Specific imaging for mucosal detail: [spot films of the collapsed esophagus].
- Evaluation of the reducibility of hiatal hernias: [1 to 2 swallows with gas distention, in the upright position].
- Evaluation of esophageal emptying, especially in patients with achalasia: [timed barium swallow with the patient placed upright. The height of the barium column is measured and recorded 1 and 5 minutes after ingesting a fixed volume of barium].

The benefit of videotaping these studies cannot be overemphasized. Doing so provides the surgeon with a real-time assessment of esophageal peristaltic function, bolus transport, and the size and reducibility of hiatal hernias. More information can be gained from such a dynamic assessment than from intermittent spot films.

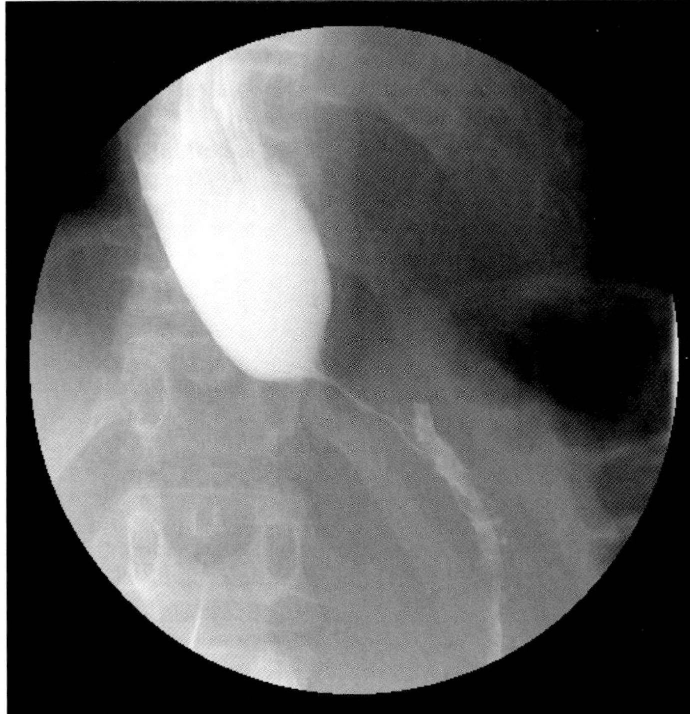

Fig. 8-1. Barium esophagram of a patient with achalasia. There is a narrowing of the esophagogastric junction (bird's beak sign) and dilatation of the esophagus.

Obstructive lesions (rings, strictures, tumors, etc.) and the presence and characteristics of hiatal hernias (size, type, and reducibility) are anatomic variables of interest particularly to surgeons. Although hiatal hernias can be detected with other methods (e.g., computerized tomography, manometry, and endoscopy) a well-performed esophagram is an accurate and easy method (Fig. 8-2, page 70).

Functional information provided by X-ray studies includes an assessment of esophageal motility patterns and the effectiveness of bolus transport. The video esophagram adds to and/or complements the information obtained by esophageal manometry (Table 8-1, page 70). For example a patient with poor esophageal motility on manometry studies but normal bolus transport on video esophagram and no dysphagia may be treated differently than the typical dysmotility patient.

As a method to detect gastroesophageal reflux disease (GERD), barium esophagography has a low sensitivity, meaning that a negative study does not preclude the presence of GERD. Only 40% of patients with classic symptoms of GERD will have spontaneous reflux observed by the radiologist at the time of contrast evaluation. Provocative maneuvers, such as the Trendelenburg position and abdominal compression, can enhance the sensitivity of the test, at the expense of specificity. Specificity is also compromised in patients with motility disorders that cause retrograde peristalsis, which in turn causes retrograde barium transit to be mistaken for reflux.

Endoscopy

Upper endoscopy serves as the "physical examination" of the esophagus. It should be performed in all patients undergoing esophageal surgery, ideally by the operating surgeon. There is no substitute for the firsthand visualization of pharyngeal, laryngeal, esophageal, and gastric mucosal as well as anatomic pathology in the decision for and selection of the appropriate operative procedure. Endoscopy allows assessment of anatomic correlates such as the presence of a large hernia, intrathoracic stomach, esophageal dilation, or a twisted previous fundoplication, which may influence treatment decisions.

Endoscopy provides objective evidence of the presence or absence of reflux-induced complications such as esophagitis, stricture, or columnar lined (Barrett) esophagus (Fig. 8-3, page 71). The severity grade of esophagitis, from A

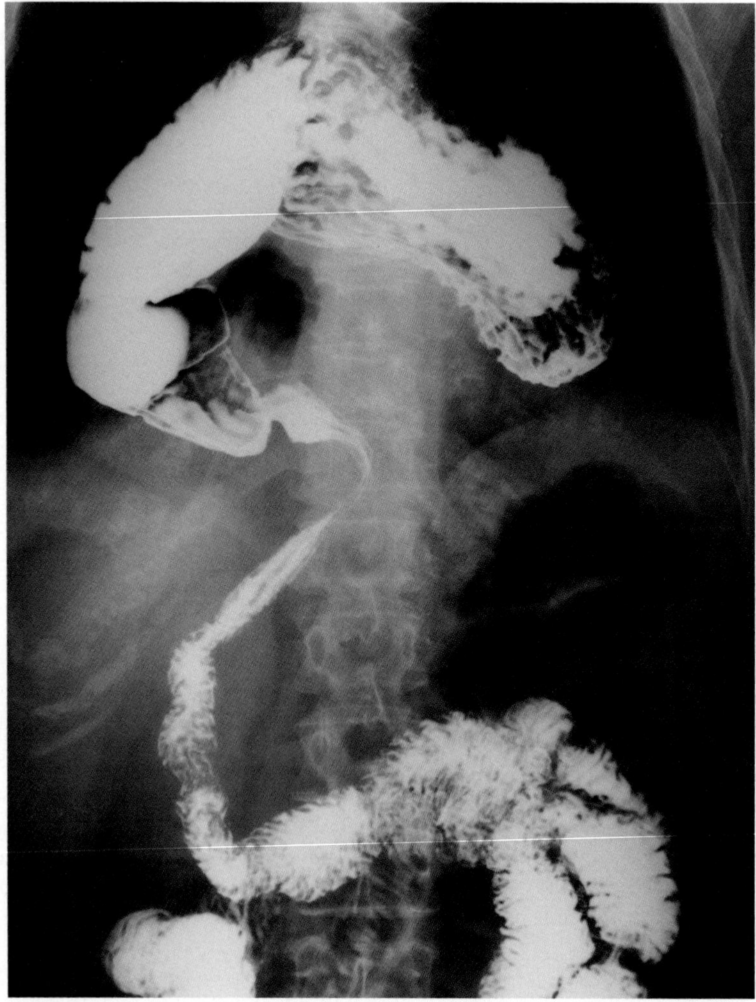

Fig. 8-2. Barium esophagram demonstrates a large hiatal hernia with an intrathoracic stomach and gastric volvulus.

TABLE 8-1. PROTOCOL FOR VIDEO ESOPHAGRAM STUDIES

Patient position	Purpose	Technique
Prone, right anterior oblique (RAO) position	Esophageal body function	Five separate 10-cc swallows, 15 seconds between each; follow bolus on videotape
		Video swallow over thoracic inlet and another over distal 1/3 of esophagus without panning
	Esophageal diameter	Rapid swallow of several gulps to maximally distend esophagus
	Gastric function	Videorecord activity of stomach and duodenum for 30 seconds in prone position
Supine	Relationship of GE junction to hiatus	Two to three individual swallows, focused on distal esophagus and GE junction
Erect	Cricopharyngeal function	Lateral and anteroposterior (AP) views of oropharynx and upper esophagus
	Mucosal injury	Spot of collapsed esophagus for mucosal detail
	Reducibility of hernia	Video images of one to two swallows focused on distal esophagus and GE junction
		Gas distention of distal esophagus
Erect	Solid bolus transport	Record video images of passage of two contrast-coated hamburger boluses from oropharynx to stomach

to D, is known to correlate with the severity of the disease. Biopsy results are also important. Biopsies of the gastric antrum, cardia just distal to the squamocolumnar junction (SCJ), and the esophageal body 2 to 3 cm above the SCJ often provide useful information. Additional biopsies are obtained based on clinical findings. Four quadrant biopsies at 2-cm intervals should be taken in the presence of Barrett esophagus. Carditis, manifest as inflamed cardiac mucosa at the gastroesophageal junction, is believed to be an early marker of GERD.

Esophageal Motility Testing

Both muscular and bolus transport function of the esophageal body can now be assessed quantitatively via esophageal manometry and impedance testing. The primary aims of esophageal manometry are to:

1. Detect the presence of a primary or secondary esophageal motility disorder.
2. Assess the structural integrity of the lower esophageal sphincter.
3. Determine the contractile and bolus transport function of the esophageal body.
4. Identify the position of the lower esophageal sphincter (LES) in order to allow accurate placement of a pH probe for ambulatory esophageal pH monitoring.
5. Stratify the severity of GERD and motor diseases by assessment of the competency of the LES and adequacy of esophageal peristalsis.

Stationary Manometry

Stationary esophageal manometry assesses the muscular function of the esophageal body and its upper and lower sphincters. It is important to remember that the procedure measures contractile function and/or sphincter relaxation, not bolus transport. As it is most commonly performed, three separate analyses are included:

- Physiology of the LES, including resting pressure, abdominal and total length, relaxation, and residual pressures.
- Esophageal body function, including contractile pressures at 3 to 5 levels and wave propagation and forms.
- Upper esophageal sphincter resting pressure, relaxation, and coordination.

Each is assessed using water-perfused or solid-state systems using a transnasal catheter. The catheter consists of electronic pressure transducers or five or more water-perfused tubes bound together.

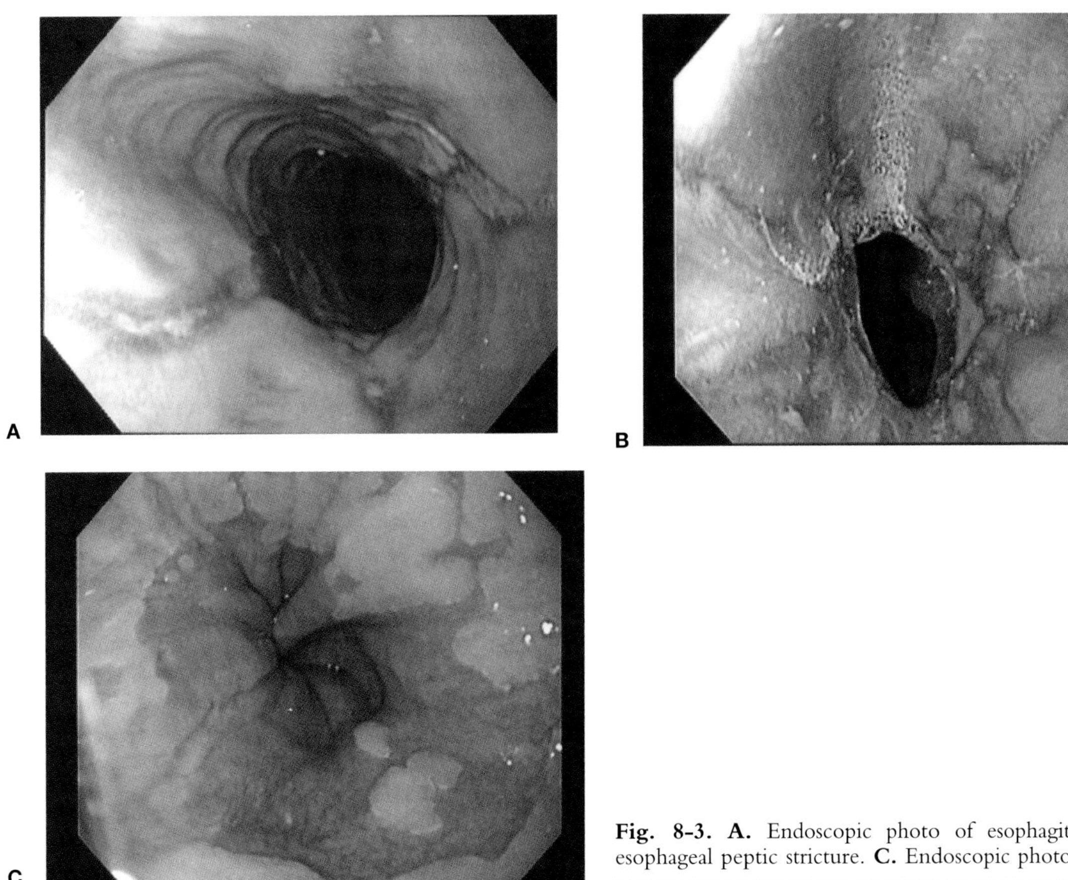

Fig. 8-3. A. Endoscopic photo of esophagitis. **B.** Endoscopic photo of esophageal peptic stricture. **C.** Endoscopic photo of Barrett esophagus.

The transducers or lateral openings are placed at 5-cm intervals from the tip and oriented radially at 72 degrees from each other around the circumference of the catheter. Special catheter configurations can be utilized for more sophisticated analyses.

As the pressure sensor is brought across the gastroesophageal junction, a rise in pressure above the gastric baseline signals the beginning of the LES. The respiratory inversion point is identified when the positive pressure of the abdominal cavity changes to negative deflections with breathing in the thorax. The respiratory inversion point serves as a reference point at which the amplitude of LES pressure and the length of the sphincter exposed to abdominal pressure are measured. As the pressure sensor is withdrawn into the body of the esophagus, the upper border of the LES is identified by the drop in pressure to the esophageal baseline. From these measurements, the pressure, abdominal length, and overall length of the sphincter are determined (Fig. 8-4). To account for the asymmetry of the sphincter, the

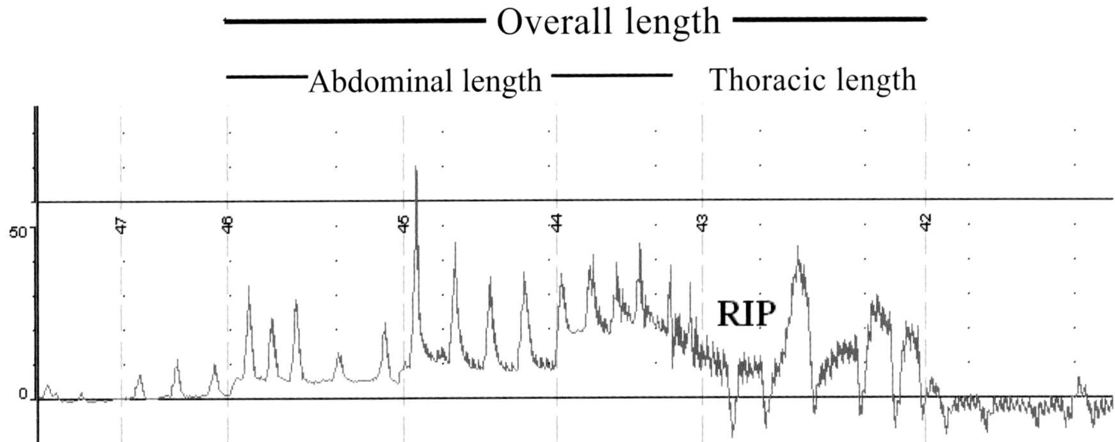

Fig. 8-4. Determination of lower esophageal sphincter (LES) length on conventional manometry. A rise in pressure above the gastric baseline signals the beginning of the LES (lower border). The respiratory inversion point (RIP) is identified when the positive excursions that occur in the abdominal cavity with breathing change to negative deflections in the thorax and it is the point at which the length of the sphincter exposed to abdominal pressure is measured. The upper border of the LES is identified by the drop in pressure to the esophageal baseline.

TABLE 8-2. REFERENCE VALUES FOR CONVENTIONAL MANOMETRY

Normal manometric values of the distal esophageal sphincter, n = 50

Parameter	Median value	2.5th percentile	97.5th percentile
Pressure (mmHg)	13	5.8	27.7
Overall length (cm)	3.6	2.1	5.6
Abdominal length (cm)	2	0.9	4.7

From DeMeester TR, Stein HJ. Gastroesophageal reflux disease. In: Moody FG, Carey LC, et al., eds. *Surgical Treatment of Digestive Disease*. Chicago: Year Book Medical, 1989.

pressure profile is repeated with each of the five radially oriented transducers and the average values calculated.

Table 8-2 shows the values for motility parameters in 50 normal volunteers without subjective or objective evidence of a foregut disorder.

To assess the relaxation and postrelaxation contraction of the LES, a pressure transducer is positioned within the upper portion of the high-pressure zone, with a distal transducer located in the stomach and the proximal transducer within the esophageal body. Ten wet swallows (5 ml water each) are performed. The resting pressure of the LES should drop to the level of gastric pressure during each wet swallow. Assessment of LES relaxation can be among the most difficult portions of the procedure, in part due to relative movement of the esophageus and manometry catheter. Esophageal shortening often results in the catheter moving into the stomach and a "pseudo-relaxation." This can be recognized by its briefness and the lack of post-relaxation hypercontraction. Careful technique (positioning the relevant measuring point high in the LES), sleeve sensors, and high resolution manometry help avoid these problems.

The function of the esophageal body is assessed with pressure transducers located in the esophagus. The positioning of the catheter should be standardized, either with the most proximal pressure transducer 1 cm below the lower border of the cricopharyngeal sphincter or the most distal one 3 cm above the upper border of the LES; normal values have been established for each method. This allows a pressure response throughout the length of the esophagus to be obtained on one swallow. Ten wet swallows are recorded. Amplitude, duration, and morphology of contractions following each swallow are calculated at all recorded levels of the esophageal body (Fig. 8-5). Both the power (contraction amplitude) and coordination (peristalsis) of the esophageal wave are assessed. Swallows are manometrically classified as: (1) normal, if contraction amplitudes at 5 and 10 cm above the LES are each greater than or equal to 30 mmHg and distal onset velocity is less than 8 cm/sec; (2) ineffective, if either of the contraction amplitudes at 5 and 10 cm above the LES are less than 30 mmHg; or (3) simultaneous, if contraction amplitudes at 5 and 10 cm above the LES are each greater than or equal to 30 mmHg and distal onset velocity is greater than 8 cm/sec. Such data are used to classify motor disorders of the esophagus (Table 8-3).

The position, length, and pressure of the cricopharyngeal sphincter are assessed with techniques similar to that used for the LES. The manometric catheter is withdrawn in 0.5-cm intervals from the upper esophagus through the upper esophageal sphincter region into the pharynx. The relaxation of the upper

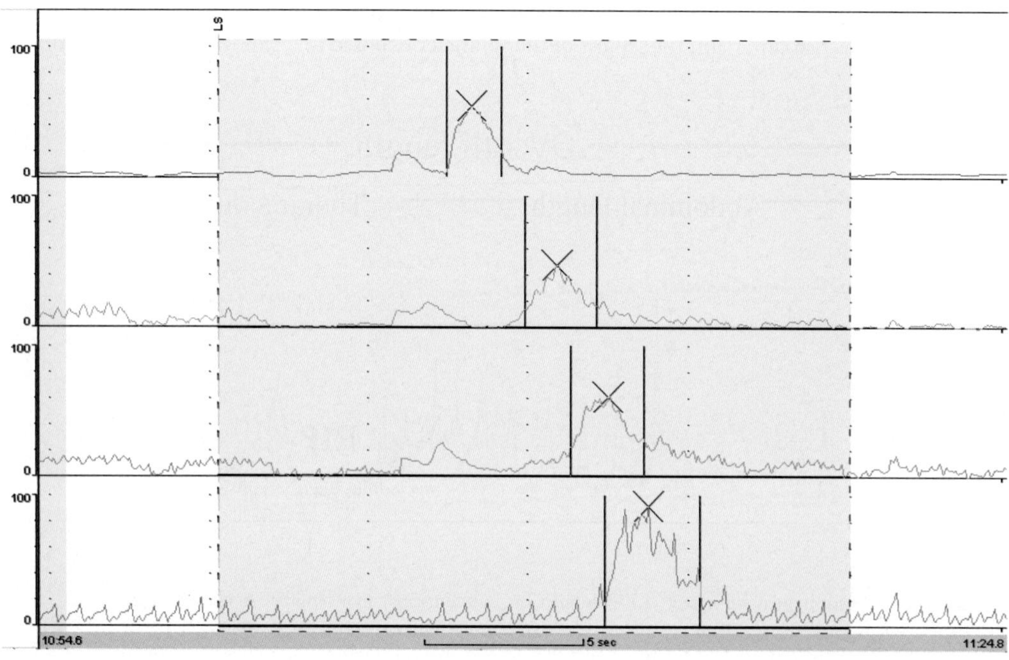

Fig. 8-5. Esophageal body assessment on conventional manometry. Amplitude (X), duration (bars), and morphology of contractions following each swallow are measured. LS, liquid swallows.

TABLE 8-3. MOTOR DISORDERS OF THE ESOPHAGUS

Inadequate LES relaxation	Classic achalasia
	Atypical disorders of LES relaxation
Uncoordinated contraction	Diffuse esophageal spasm
Hypercontraction	Nutcracker esophagus
	Isolated hypertensive LES
Hypocontraction	Ineffective esophageal motility

LES, lower esophageal sphincter.

esophageal sphincter is best studied by straddling eight pressure transducers 1 cm apart across the sphincter, so that some are in the pharynx and some in the upper esophagus. High-speed graphic recordings (50 mm/s) are necessary to obtain an assessment of the coordination of cricopharyngeal relaxation with hypopharyngeal contraction (Fig. 8-6). It is difficult to consistently demonstrate a motility abnormality in patients with pharyngoesophageal disorders. After surgical treatment, manometry is useful to evaluate patients with postoperative dysphagia or obscure anatomical abnormalities. In this case, assessment of the length, pressure, and relaxation of the lower esophageal sphincter and especially the quality of the esophageal body peristalsis are essential (Fig. 8-7, page 74).

Esophageal Function Testing via Multichannel Intraluminal Impedance and Manometry

Conventional esophageal manometry measures the contractile function of the esophagus but not bolus transport. Unfortunately, the presence or absence of dysphagia correlates poorly with mild to moderate contractile abnormalities and the ability of patients with ineffective esophageal motility patterns to tolerate the outflow resistance created by a 360-degree fundoplication. Quantification of bolus transport via multichannel intraluminal impedance (MII) measurement combined with conventional pressure manometric assessment has recently been developed in the hope of overcoming these limitations.

Esophageal bolus transport can be quantified using impedance (measurement of electrical resistance in ohms) between a series of sequentially placed electrodes during the passage of a bolus through the esophagus. Impedance is the ratio of voltage to current at a given measuring frequency and is inversely proportional to the electrical conductivity of a hollow organ and its contents. Air has a very low electrical conductivity and therefore high impedance. Saliva and food cause an impedance decrease because of their increased conductivity. Luminal dilatation results in a decrease in impedance, whereas luminal contraction yields an impedance increase.

An intraluminal electrical impedance catheter has been developed for the measurement of gastrointestinal function (Sandhill Scientific; Highlands Ranch, CO). The probe measures impedance between adjacent electrodes, yielding 4 to 5 measuring segments across the length of the catheter. An extremely low electric current of 0.00025 microwatts (μW) is transmitted across the electrodes at a frequency of 1-2 kHz and is limited to 8 μA. This is below the stimulation threshold for nerves and muscles and is three orders of magnitude below the threshold of cardiac stimulation. A standard pH electrode is also located 4 cm from the distal tip.

Investigations to date have established the impedance waveform characteristics that define esophageal bolus detection (Fig. 8-8, page 74). This allows for the characterization of both esophageal motility and gastroesophageal reflux. When a person swallows, a peristaltic wave develops, pushing air and bolus material ahead of it. This wave can be divided into four phases. During the resting phase 1, the esophageal wall is relaxed, coated with a thin film of saliva, and opposed together. In phase 2 the walls are distended by the bolus. Phase 3 consists of a fully contracted esophageal wall. In phase 4, the esophagus returns to its relaxed state and the saliva film, which had been removed with the bolus, reaccumulates. Gastroesophageal reflux produces the same characteristic wave, except it travels in a retrograde direction.

Simultaneous intraluminal impedance and barium fluoroscopy has shown that impedance waves correspond well with actual bolus transport. Preliminary studies comparing standard manometry with impedance in healthy volunteers has validated that esophageal impedance

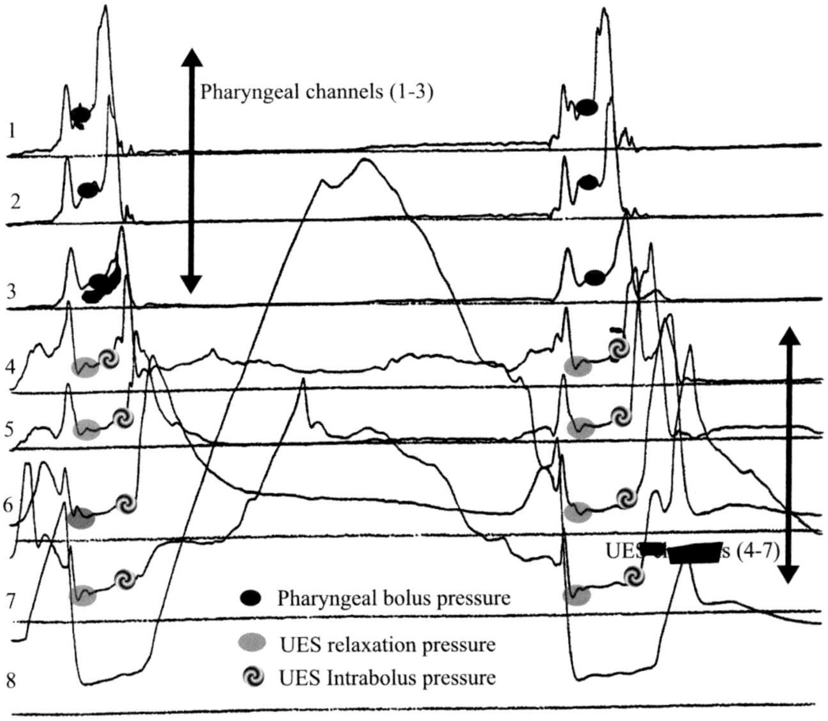

Fig. 8-6. Assessment of the coordination of cricopharyngeal relaxation with hypopharyngeal contraction. UES, upper esophageal sphincter.

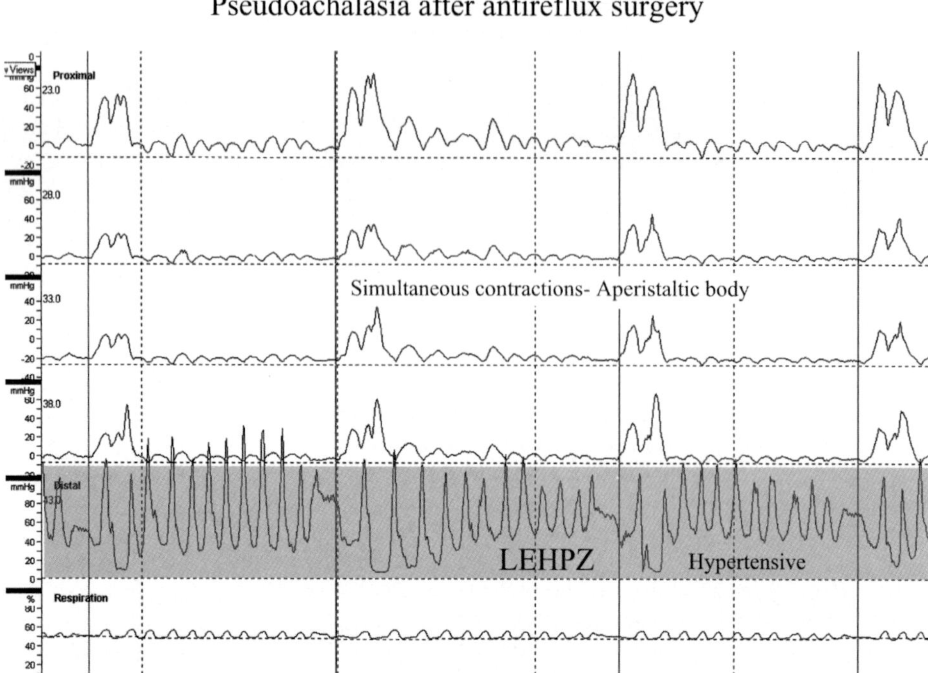

Fig. 8-7. Manometric tracing of pseudoachalasia after antireflux surgery (fundoplication). LEHPZ, lower esophageal high pressure zone.

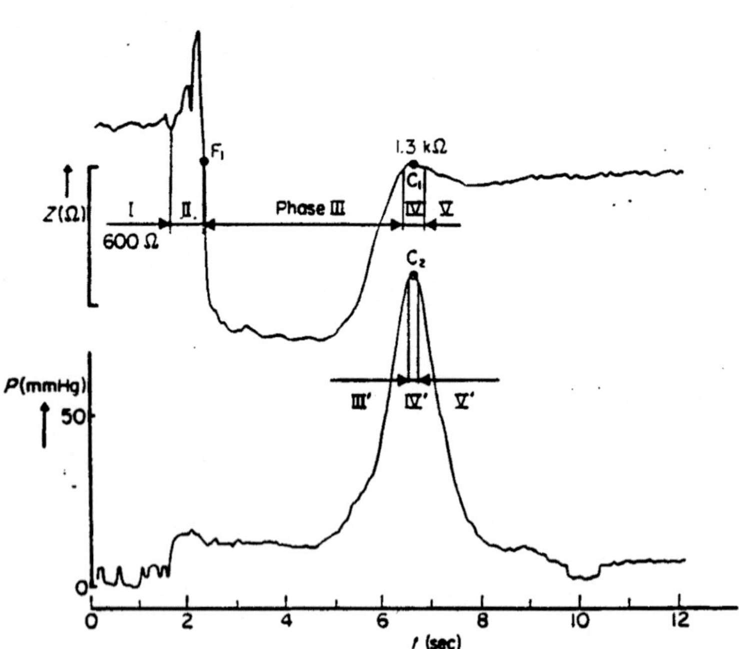

Fig. 8-8. Impedance changes observed during bolus transit over a single pair of measurement rings separated by 2 cm. A rapid increase in resistance is noted when air traveling in front of the bolus head reaches the impedance-measuring segment, followed by a drop in impedance once higher conductive bolus material passes the measuring site. Bolus entry is considered at the 50% drop in impedance from baseline relative to nadir, and bolus exit at the 50% recovery point from nadir to baseline. Lumen narrowing produced by the contraction transiently increases the impedance above baseline. Correlation is seen between esophageal impedance and peristaltic wave contractions.

correlates with peristaltic wave progression and bolus transport. The use of impedance technology is still early in its development but has the potential to add understanding to both normal and abnormal esophageal physiology.

Impedence catheters include two circumferential pressure sensors at 5 and 10 cm from the tip and three unidirectional pressure sensors at 15, 20, and 25 cm. Impedance measuring segments consist of pairs of metal rings placed 2 cm apart and centered at 10, 15, 20, and 25 cm from the tip. The catheter is inserted transnasally to a depth of 60 cm. The LES is identified using a standard stationary pull-through technique. Esophageal body function is assessed with the distal sensor placed in the LES high-pressure zone. Patients are given ten swallows of 5 cc saline and ten swallows of 5 cc of a standard viscous (applesauce-like consistency) material while in the semirecumbent position. Each swallow is 20 to 30 seconds apart.

Impedance parameters include: (1) total bolus transit time (TBTT), counted as the time elapsed between bolus entry at 20 cm above LES and bolus exit at 5 cm above LES; (2) bolus head advance time (BHAT), or the time elapsed between bolus entry at 20 cm above LES and bolus

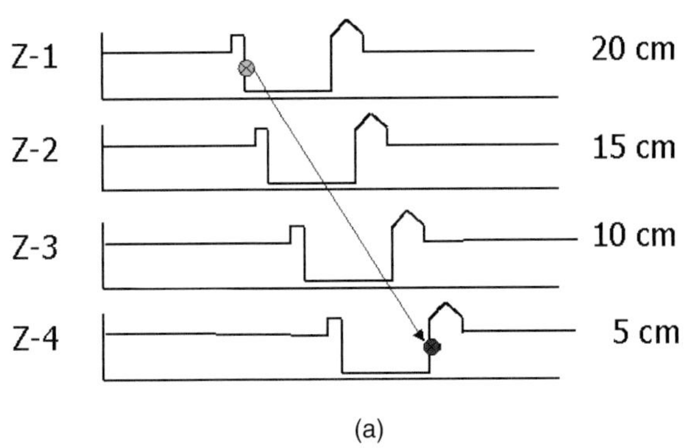

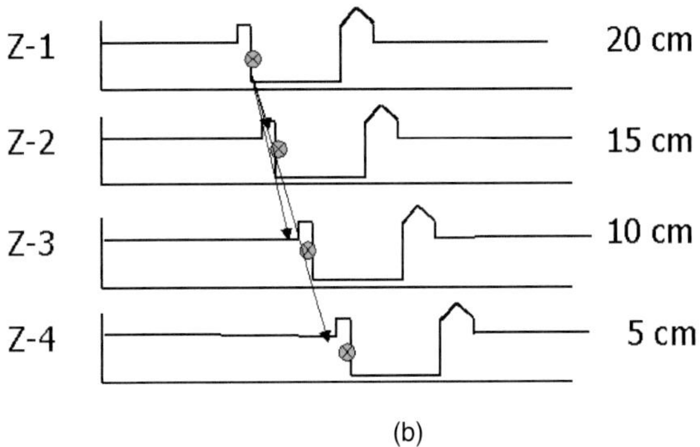

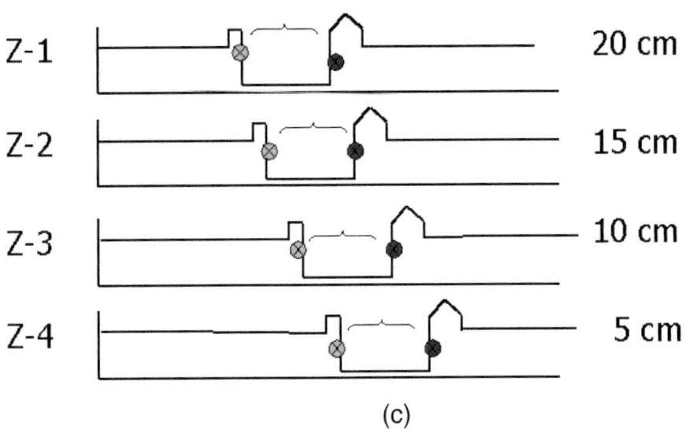

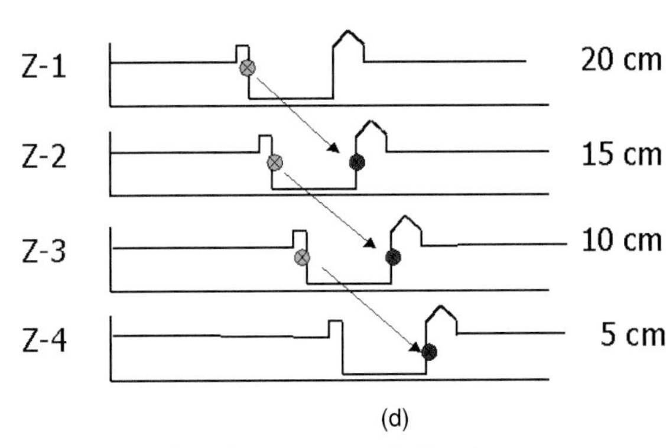

Fig. 8-9. Impedance parameters in the multichannel intraluminal impedance and esophageal manometry. **A.** Total bolus transit time (TBTT) as time elapsed between bolus entry at 20 cm above LES and bolus exit at 5 cm above LES. **B.** Bolus head advance time (BHAT) as time elapsed between bolus entry at 20 cm above LES and bolus entry at 15, 10, and 5 cm above LES. **C.** Bolus presence time (BPT) as time elapsed between bolus entry and bolus exit at each impedance measuring site (5, 10, 15, and 20 cm above LES). **D.** Segment transit time (STT) as time elapsed between bolus entry at a given level above LES and bolus exit at the nearby lower level.

entry at 15, 10, and 5 cm above LES; (3) bolus presence time (BPT), or time elapsed between bolus entry and bolus exit at each impedance measuring site (5, 10, 15, and 20 cm above LES); and (4) segment transit time (STT), or time elapsed between bolus entry at a given level above LES and bolus exit at the next lower level (Fig. 8-9).

Swallows can be classified by MII as showing: (1) complete bolus transit, if bolus entry at the most proximal site (20 cm above LES) and bolus exit points were recorded in all three distal impedance-measuring sites (15, 10, and 5 cm above the LES) and (2) incomplete bolus transit if bolus exit was not identified at any of the three distal measuring sites.

The combination of MII and esophageal manometry allows the identification of four swallow patterns:

1. Peristaltic waves (based on manometry) and complete bolus clearance (based on impedance);
2. Peristaltic waves but with poor bolus clearance;
3. Nonperistaltic or ineffective waves but still with bolus clearance;
4. Nonperistaltic or ineffective waves without bolus clearance (bad).

Normal values have been established and published from several centers around the world. Values from a U.S. multicenter study are shown in Tables 8-4 and 8-5 (page 76).

MII findings in 350 patients with a wide range of esophageal diseases showed that complete bolus transit was present in 96% of manometric normal swallows, in 53% with simultaneous waves, and in 33% with manometrically ineffective waves. The values for viscous swallow were 93%, 59%, and 31% respectively. Furthermore, distal esophageal amplitude was higher in patients with complete bolus clearance, as expected. The addition of viscous swallows to the analysis did not change the sensitivity for the diagnosis of achalasia, scleroderma, and hypotensive LES, but it changed the numbers for other diseases and conditions.

Whether the addition of impedance data adds relevant clinical information to standard motility studies remains unclear. Patients with achalasia and scleroderma almost always have abnormal bolus transit, rendering impedance unnecessary in most instances. Conversely, virtually all patients with primary peristalsis have normal bolus transit. The greatest utility of impedance esophageal function testing may be for patients with motility disorders in which bolus transport is variable. Data suggest that roughly half of such patients will have normal bolus transit and half abnormal. Tutuian and Castell have analyzed bolus transport in 70 patients manometrically classified as having ineffective esophageal motility (IEM) and concluded that the current manometric definition of IEM of >30% manometrically ineffective swallows is too sensitive and does not distinguish patients with abnormal bolus transport. Utilizing the transport of both liquid and

TABLE 8-4. IMPEDANCE PARAMETERS FOR LIQUID AND VISCOUS SWALLOWS

	Liquid swallows (N = 499)		Viscous swallows (N = 495)		
	Mean ± SEM	**95th percentile**	**Mean ± SEM**	**95th percentile**	**p-value**
Bolus head advance time (sec)					
20–15 cm	0.3 ± 0.0	0.7	1.1 ± 0.0	2.4	<0.001
20–10 cm	0.7 ± 0.0	1.7	3.3 ± 0.1	5.0	<0.001
20–5 cm	1.9 ± 0.1	4.9	5.0 ± 0.1	7.4	<0.001
Bolus presence time (sec)					
at 20 cm	2.4 ± 0.1	6.5	2.3 ± 0.1	4.9	0.743
at 15 cm	4.5 ± 0.1	9.9	3.8 ± 0.1	6.1	<0.001
at 10 cm	5.9 ± 0.1	10.1	3.9 ± 0.1	7.7	<0.001
at 5 cm	6.0 ± 0.1	9.6	3.5 ± 0.1	6.5	<0.001
Segment transit time (sec)					
20–15 cm	4.7 ± 0.1	10.3	4.9 ± 0.1	7.5	0.317
15–10 cm	6.3 ± 0.1	11.1	5.9 ± 0.1	10.6	0.024
10–5 cm	7.1 ± 0.1	11.3	5.3 ± 0.1	8.5	<0.001
Total bolus transit time (sec)					
	7.9 ± 0.1	12.3	8.5 ± 0.1	12.4	<0.001

SEM, standard error of measurement.

viscous material they found that approximately one third of patients actually had normal transport of both. These findings are consistent with the observation that many patients with IEM tolerate a complete 360-degree fundoplication without an increased incidence of dysphagia.

High-Resolution Manometry

High-resolution manometry is a variant of conventional manometry in which more recording sites are used, thus creating a "map" of esophageal contractions. Multiple pressure sensors are placed along a 4.2-mm catheter. Catheter designs typically include 36 individual circumferential sensors spaced 1 cm apart. Although solid-state catheters are commonly used, water-perfused systems are also available.

The procedure is similar to but simpler than conventional manometry. The system is first calibrated and then positioned transnasally in a position that allows simultaneous visualization of both sphincters and fixed in that position during the entire study. Because all data are acquired simultaneously, no movements of the catheter (pull-through) are necessary and the test is finished after ten 5-cc swallows of water.

The vast amount of data generated is processed via sophisticated software analysis and presented in traditional linear plots or as a visually enhanced spatiotemporal video tracing. Analysis software can generate both isobaric contour plots in a scale of colors or conventional real-time manometric tracing. The sphincters are easily recognized due to their resting pressure. After swallows, progression of the peristaltic wave in the esophageal body can also be intuitively visualized (Fig. 8-10A).

Simultaneous acquisition of data regarding the pharynx, upper esophageal

TABLE 8-5. PERCENTAGE OF INDIVIDUALS HAVING COMPLETE BOLUS TRANSIT

	% Swallows with complete bolus transit	Individuals (N = 50) %	Cumulative %
Liquid			
	90+	76.0	76.0
	80	14.0	90.0
	70	10.0	100.0
Viscous			
	90+	78.0	78.0
	80	8.0	84.0
	70	8.0	92.0
	60	6.0	98.0
	50	2.0	100.0

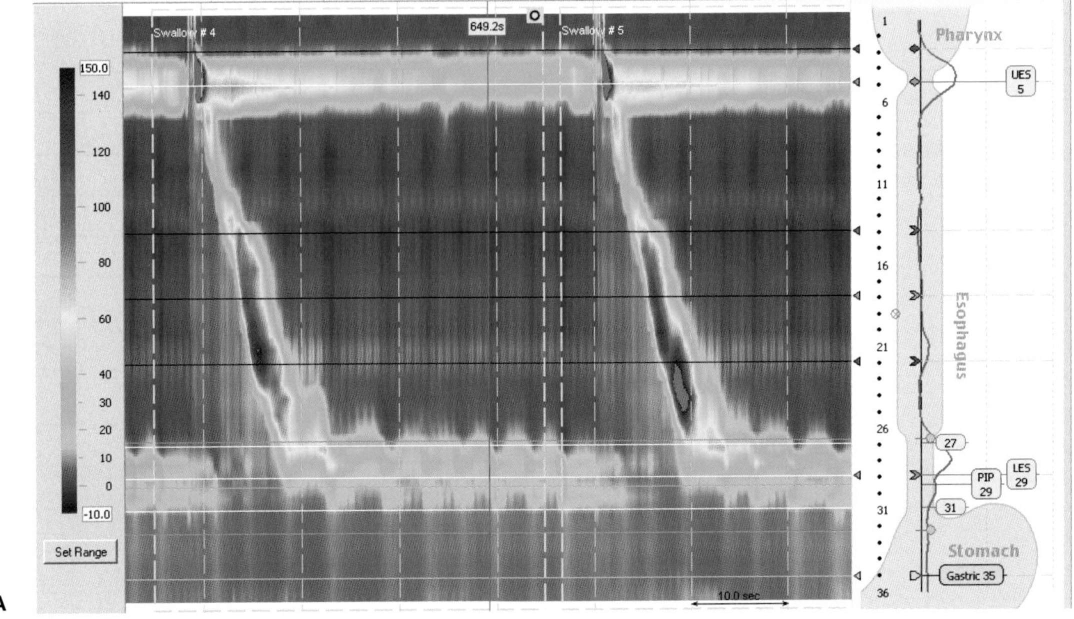

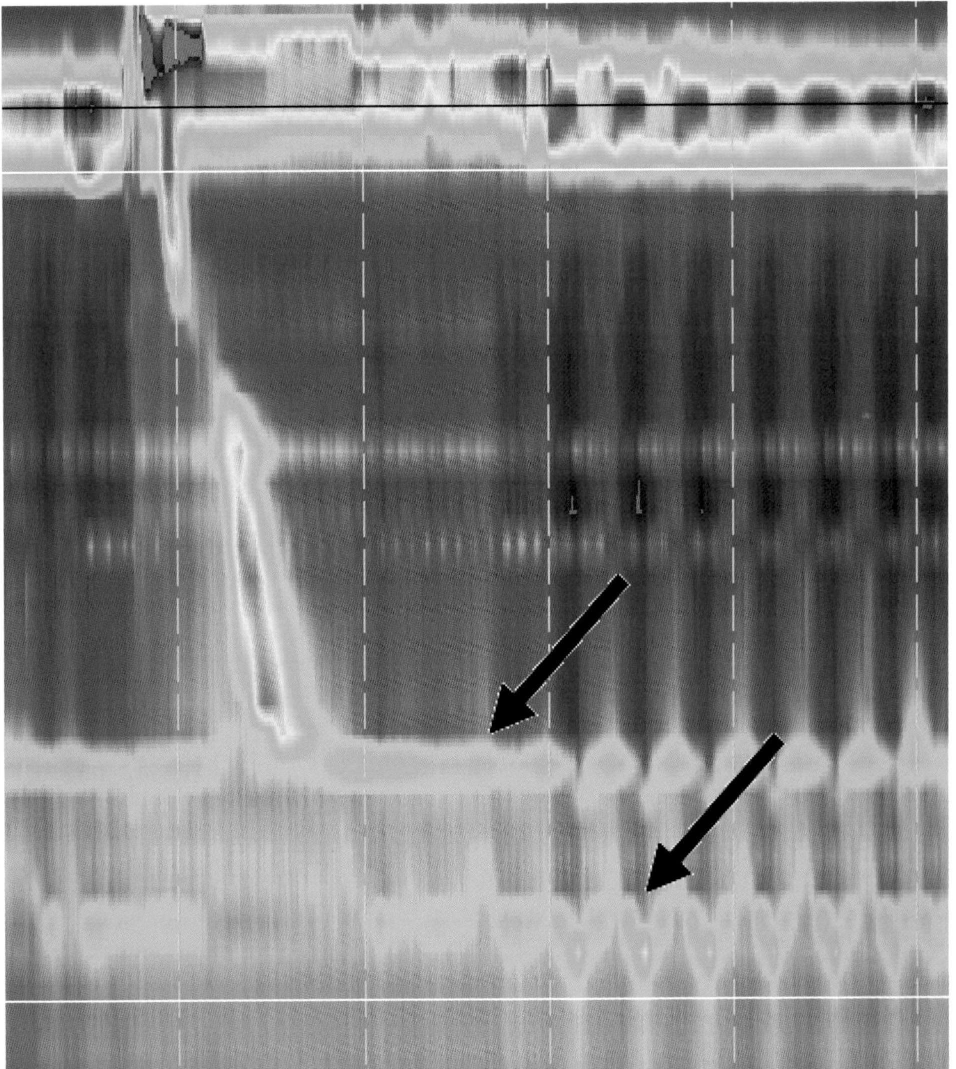

Fig. 8-10. A. Normal high-resolution manometry. **B.** Detection of a hiatal hernia with high-resolution manometry. Two high-pressure zones (arrows) are seen, corresponding to the lower esophageal sphincter (proximal) and the diaphragm (distal).

sphincter, esophageal body, LES, and gastric pressure is a new resource for research and has clinical advantages. The highly visibile sphincter landmarks assist probe placement and data interpretation. High resolution minimizes movement artifacts and decreases study time, improving patient comfort during the test. The performance of the study is easier to reproduce, the analysis visually intuitive, and segmental motility abnormalities readily recognized. While the benefits of high-resolution manometry are unknown as yet, possible advantages include: better detection of transient LES relaxation and hiatal hernia and postfundoplication abnormalities, as well as understanding the effects of esophageal shortening and obesity (Fig. 8-10B, page 77). Normal values have been established for the three key components of the study, namely the upper and lower esophageal sphincters and the esophageal body (Table 8-6).

Ambulatory Assessment of Gastroesophageal Reflux

Objective testing for gastroesophageal reflux is arguably the most important study prior to antireflux surgery. It helps to establish the link between the patient's symptoms and the presence of pathology. Studies have shown that an abnormal 24-hour pH study is the single strongest predictor of success (as measured in symptom relief) in patients with both typical and atypical symptoms of gastroesophageal reflux. Despite these important observations, it is all too often omitted in the evaluation of patients prior to esophageal surgery.

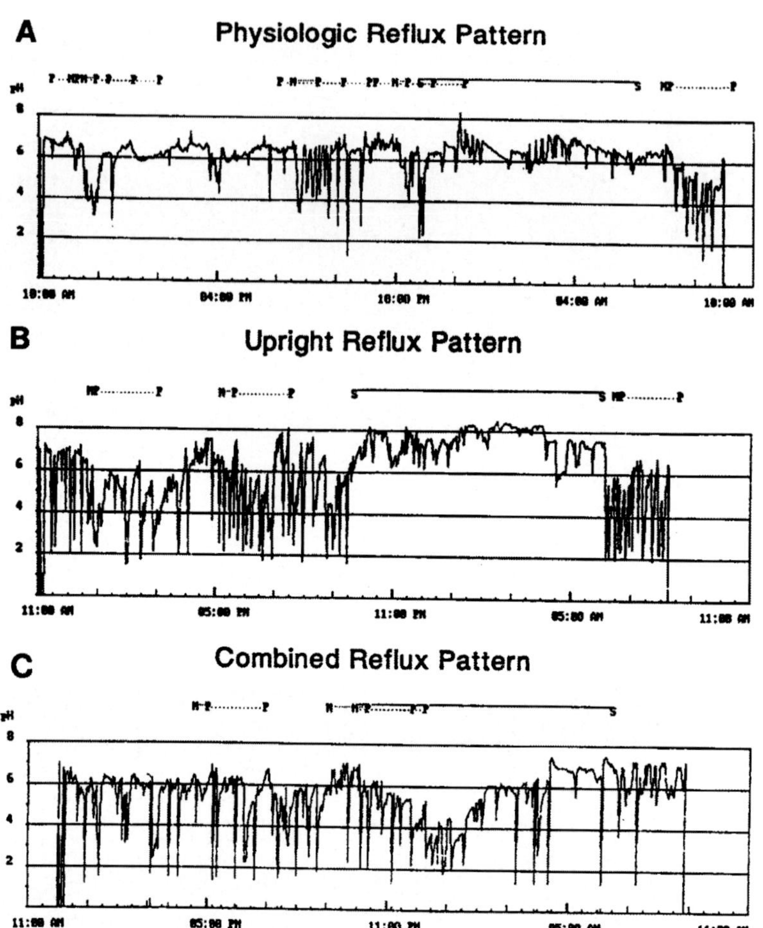

Fig. 8-11. Patterns of reflux: **(A)** physiologic esophageal acid exposure; **(B)** upright reflux; and **(C)** combined upright and supine reflux.

Catheter-Based 24-Hour Esophageal pH Studies

The most direct method of measuring increased esophageal exposure to gastric juice is by an indwelling pH electrode. Monitoring of esophageal pH is most commonly performed by placing a catheter-based pH probe 5 cm above the manometrically measured upper border of the distal sphincter and monitoring the patient for 24 hours off all acid suppression. Esophageal pH values are recorded many times per second (4 to 50). The study quantifies the time the esophageal mucosa is exposed to gastric juice, measures the ability of the esophagus to clear refluxed acid, and correlates esophageal acid exposure to the patient's symptoms. A 24-hour period is ideal to allow measurements to be made over one complete circadian cycle, including the effects of physiological activities such as working, eating, or sleeping on the presence of acid reflux (Fig. 8-11). Measurements are expressed by the time the esophageal pH is below a given threshold (generally pH <4) during the 24-hour period. In addition, units used to express esophageal exposure to gastric juice are: (1) time the esophageal pH is below a chosen threshold expressed as the percent of the total, upright, and supine monitored time; (2) frequency of reflux episodes, expressed as number of episodes per 24 hours; and (3) duration of the episodes expressed as the number of episodes greater than 5 minutes per 24 hours and the time in minutes of the longest episode recorded. Normal values for these six components were established at the 95th percentile using pH = 4 as the threshold. The normal values for the six components are shown in Table 8-7.

TABLE 8-6. REFERENCE VALUES FOR HIGH-RESOLUTION MANOMETRY

LES basal pressure*	LES relaxation pressure*	Proximal esophageal amplitude**	Proximal esophageal duration**	Distal esophageal amplitude**	Distal esophageal duration**
5.0–31.6 mmHg	0–10.1 mmHg	53.7–185.3 mmHg	1.2–4.8 seconds	47.2–216.8	0.6–6.6 seconds

LES, lower esophageal sphincter.
* 5th and 95th percentiles
** Two standard deviations

TABLE 8-7. Reference values for pH monitoring

Normal Values for Esophageal Exposure to pH <4 (n = 50)			
Component	**Mean**	**Standard deviation**	**95th percentile**
Total time pH <4	1.51	1.36	4.45
Upright time pH <4	2.34	2.34	8.42
Supine time pH <4	0.63	1.0	3.45
No. of episodes	19.00	12.76	46.9
No. >5 minutes	0.84	1.18	3.45
Longest episode	6.74	7.85	19.8

From DeMeester TR, Stein HJ. Gastroesophageal reflux disease. In: Moody FG, Carey LC, et al., eds. *Surgical Treatment of Digestive Disease.* Chicago: Year Book Medical, 1989.

To combine all six of the components into one expression of the overall esophageal acid exposure, a pH score was calculated by using the standard deviation of the mean of each of the six components measured in 50 normal subjects (the Johnson-DeMeester score).

When evaluated in a test population with an equal distribution of normal healthy subjects and patients with the classical reflux symptoms and a defective sphincter, 24-hour esophageal pH monitoring had a sensitivity and specificity of 96%. Based on this data, 24-hour esophageal pH monitoring has been used as a gold standard for the diagnosis of GERD.

Dual-channel pH studies provide important information about the proximal extent of acid reflux and may be useful in the assessment of patients with extraesophageal manifestations of GERD. The site for proximal probe placement has included the trachea, the pharynx, and the proximal esophagus. One probe is positioned in the distal esophagus and the other at a more proximal location, usually either 20 cm above the upper border of the LES (15 cm proximal to the distal sensor), 1 cm below the upper esophageal sphincter (UES), or in the hypopharynx. Normal values have been established for each (Table 8-8). Whether probe placement should be relative to the upper or lower esophageal sphincter is unclear.

Wireless pH Monitoring

Catheter-free pH monitoring was developed to prevent the discomfort associated with transnasal catheters. The device consists of a small capsule (6 × 5.5 × 25 mm) with an antimony pH sensor, a reference electrode, a radio transmitter, and a battery. The capsule is pinned to the esophageal mucosa via a removable delivery system, which uses suction to suck the mucosa inside a tiny well located in the capsule and deploy a fixing pin. pH information is sent wirelessly to a receiver within 6 feet of the patient. Data are recorded every 6 seconds. Currently, the only available system is the Bravo pH Monitoring System (Medtronic; Shoreview, MN).

The delivery device can be passed transnasally or transorally using manometric measurements or at the time of upper endoscopy based upon endoscopic landmarks. Transnasal delivery has the advantage of precise positioning based upon manometric measurement of the upper border of the LES but the disadvantage of necessitating the passage of a relatively large capsule through the nose, which can cause significant nosebleeds. The capsule is placed 5 cm above the LES, similar to the pH catheter. A more comfortable transoral placement can also be done but requires a correction factor of 4 cm or so to compensate the difference in length between the nasoesophageal and the oroesophageal routes. When placed endoscopically, the capsule is placed 6 cm above the squamocolumnar junction. Because the squamous-columnar transition is on average 1 cm proximal to the manometrical border of the LES, this 1 cm "correction factor" positions the capsule 6 cm rather than 5 cm above the endoscopic esophagogastric junction (EGJ). Endoscopic placement is complicated in patients with Barrett esophagus or large hiatal hernias, where the recognition of the EGJ is difficult. In these circumstances, the proximal gastric folds have been used to correct identify the EGJ.

Contraindications to placement include patients with a history of bleeding diathesis, strictures, severe esophagitis, varices, pacemakers, or implantable cardiac defibrillators. Some authors also add previous surgery of the upper gastrointestinal tract.

Three groups of normal values have been reported. Wenner et al. found the 95th percentile for the total time pH <4 of 3.3% in day 1, 6.0% in day 2, and 4.4% for both days. Streets et al. compared the simultaneous placement of the pH capsule and catheter-based pH monitoring in volunteers and compared asymptomatic with symptomatic patients. They concluded that the composite score (DeMeester score) is a reliable method to discriminate between normality and abnormality by both the conventional technique and for the Bravo. Pandolfino et al. studied 44 normal volunteers where the 95th percentile for the total time pH <4 was 5.3%. Des Varannes et al. placed

TABLE 8-8. PUBLISHED REFERENCE RANGES FOR pH MONITORING AT DIFFERENT SITES

			% of time spent at pH <4		
Author	**Probe location**	**# Controls**	**Total**	**Upright**	**Supine**
Distal to the UES					
Gustafsson (1990)	15 cm above LES	28*	0.6	0.7	0.8
Dobhan (1993)	20 cm above LES	26	0.9	1.3	0
Vaezi (1997)	1 cm below UES	11	1.1	1.7	0.6
Proximal to the UES					
Wiener (1989)	2 cm above UES	12	0	0	0
Contencin (1992)	Oropharynx	6*	0	0	0
Paterson (1994)	1 cm above UES	13	0	0	0
Kuhn (1998)	2 cm above UES	11	0	0	0

#, indicates the sample size; LES, lower esophageal sphincter; UES, upper esophageal sphincter.
* pediatric study population

both a conventional catheter and Bravo in 40 patients. Using a cutoff value of pH <4 above 4.2% for the catheter-based study they reported a corresponding value of 2.9% for the capsule-based system.

A theoretical advantage of the capsule-based system is the routine collection of data for 48 consecutive hours. Previous reports of repeat studies with standard pH monitoring showed significant day-to-day variability in the results. Consequently, a longer recording time might improve detection of gastrointestinal reflux (GER) and increase the ability to correlate symptoms with actual GER episodes. Reports have suggested that a 24-hour study would have missed actual reflux in 10% to 27% of patients. Interestingly, discordance between day 1 and day 2 (i.e., one day is a positive study and the other one is a negative) ranges from 23% to 44%, a finding similar to the results of the catheter-based pH monitoring. Some authors argue that acid exposure is higher in day 1 due to the endoscopy, associated premedication, and more time in supine position. Others claim that acid exposure is higher in day 2 due to return to routine life and increased food intake.

Studies have shown that catheter-based pH monitoring detects as many as three times more episodes of reflux that the capsule-based systems. That is, the capsule underrecords acid exposure. This is likely due to the lower sampling rate (every 6.25 seconds, compared to 4 times per second) of the capsule system, the fixed position of the wireless capsule preventing dips lower into the esophagus or stomach during swallows, and inaccuracy in calibration of the capsule. The clinical significance of these observations is not clear. Wong et al. randomized 50 patients to either conventional catheter or catheterless pH monitoring. Patients with the catheterless technique experienced less nose pain, throat pain, and throat discomfort and fewer runny noses and headaches, but more chest pain compared to the catheter group. Overall satisfaction and less interference with daily activities, sleeping, and eating were also greater for the catheterless group.

Serious complications related to the placement of the capsule have not been reported. However, nosebleeds are common when the transnasal route is used. In a percentage of patients (ranging from 0.5% to 20%), the capsule fails to attach to the esophageal mucosa. This may happen due to problems with the device itself or movement of the patient (gagging) while the vacuum is applied. Patients can experience a foreign body sensation, especially when eating. On occasion this sensation is painful, probably due to spasm, which has been documented by concomitant manometry. The pain can be severe, and removal of the capsule may be necessary in 2% to 5% of the patients. Nausea has been occasionally reported (6%). Younger age, female gender, normal acid exposure, and nonerosive GER have been associated to these capsule-related symptoms.

In 2% to 12% of placements, data collection fails. Reasons include failure of the capsule or the receiver, interference due to other wireless devices, placement of the receiver too far from the patient, and premature detachment of the capsule. The capsule is designed to detach in 3 to 7 days and to be passed in the stool. But premature detachment can occur in 2% to 5.5% of placements and is readily noted on the uploaded pH tracing (Fig. 8-12). In

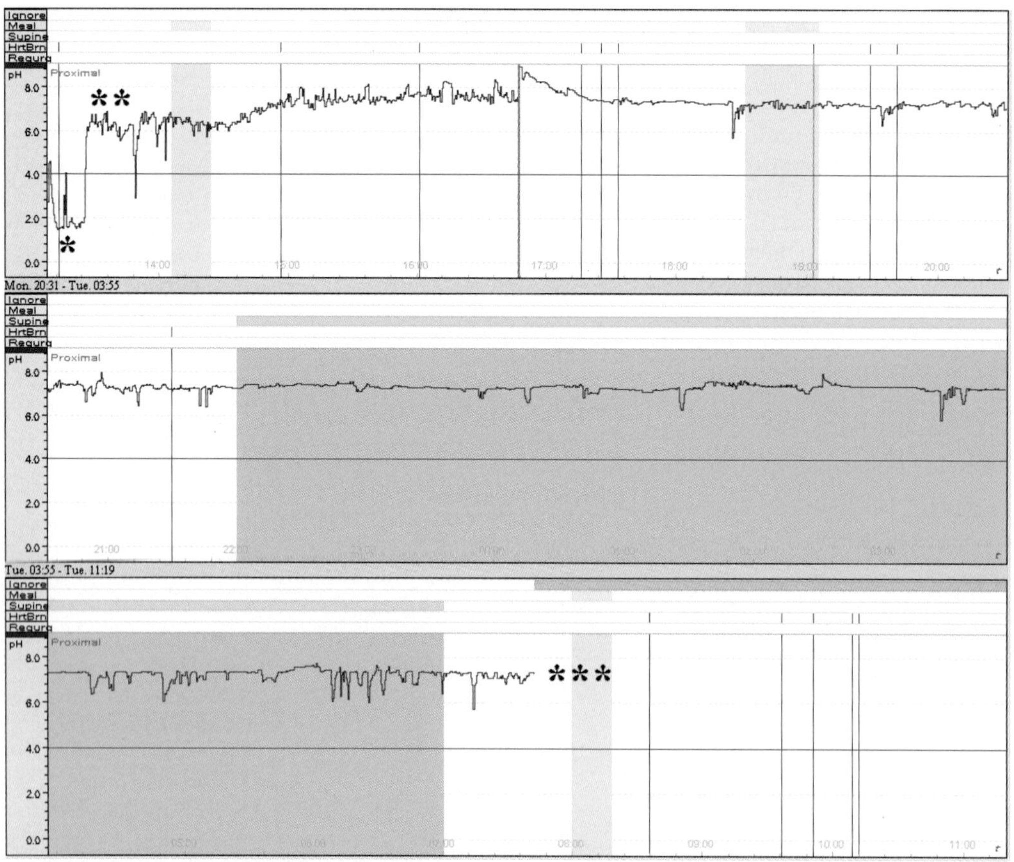

Fig. 8-12. Premature detachment of the wireless capsule. pH tracing shows a sharp drop in pH *, denoting the detachment of the capsule and its position inside the stomach, followed by a sustained raise in pH **, denoting its presence in the small bowel. Absence of data *** is noticed after the patient had a bowel movement and expelled the capsule.

contrast, nondetachment of the capsule after 15 days, requiring endoscopic removal, has also been reported.

Multichannel Intraluminal Impedance–pH

Conventional pH monitoring is restricted to abnormal esophageal acid exposure. In contrast, multichannel intraluminal impedance and pH monitoring (MII-pH) is able to determine: (1) the physical characteristics of the refluxate (liquid, gas, or mixed); (2) the direction of the flow (oral or aboral); (3) the acidity of the refluxate; (4) non-acidic GER; (5) indirect estimation of the refluxate volume; and (6) the height of the GER.

A reflux episode is defined as lumen substances that propagate aborally in at least two proximal sensors (Fig. 8-13). Simultaneous detection of an episode of reflux by the pH sensor and the impedance sensors denotes an *acid reflux*. Detection of an episode of reflux only by the impedance sensors denotes a *nonacid reflux*. These criteria were proposed in a consensus conference and are used by most authors.

Studies have shown that in normal volunteers 81% of distal reflux episodes are acidic, while 25% of proximal episodes are acidic, due to neutralization of the refluxate as it rises in the esophagus. The height of GER has also been studied using the MII-pH technology. Again in normal volunteers, 70% of reflux episodes reach the upper esophagus and, surprisingly, 10% reach the pharynx. Because most episodes were nonacid, they would be undetected by regular pH monitoring. As expected, gas reflux reaches the upper esophagus more easily than liquid reflux.

Re-reflux and weakly acid reflux are new concepts defined by MII-pH. Re-reflux (or superimposed reflux) is characterized by reflux episodes detected at impedance in a background pH <4 after the initialization of a primary reflux event. Weakly acid reflux is an episode of reflux detected at the impedance that causes a drop in pH between 4 and 6.5. Clinical significance of these phenomena is still undetermined. Clinical studies have shown that the number of reflux episodes is the same for GERD and control patients; however, GERD patients have a higher rate and a longer duration of acid reflux. Similar to controls, liquid, gas, and mixed reflux were noticed in 40%, 23%, and 36% of the cases, respectively.

It has been demonstrated that MII-pH improves the ability to correlate symptoms with episodes of reflux, as a significant number of symptoms may occur during nonacid episodes. Different studies showed that heartburn is more commonly experienced in acid reflux, while regurgitation and cough are symptoms most associated to nonacid reflux (from 30% to 50% of the cases).

The effect of antisecretory drugs on the composition of GER has also been investigated in volunteers and in patients. The results showed that proton pump inhibitors did not change the number and duration of reflux episodes, only the pH of the refluxate. Moreover, symptoms may correlate with nonacid reflux in patients with persistent symptoms despite the use of proton pump inhibitors.

Tests of Duodenogastric Function

Esophageal disorders are frequently associated with abnormalities of the stomach and duodenum. Delayed emptying of the gastric reservoir or increased gastric acid secretion can be responsible for increased esophageal exposure to gastric juice. Reflux of alkaline duodenal juice, including bile salts, pancreatic enzymes, and bicarbonate, is thought to have a role in the pathogenesis of esophagitis and Barrett esophagus. Furthermore, functional disorders of the esophagus are often associated with functional disorders of the rest of the foregut, meaning the stomach and duodenum. Tests of duodenogastric function include gastric emptying studies, gastric acid analysis, and the use of cholescintigraphy for the diagnosis of pathologic duodenogastric reflux. 24-hour gastric pH monitoring can be used to identify gastric hypersecretion and imply the presence of duodenogastric reflux and delayed gastric emptying.

Gastric emptying studies are performed with radionuclide-labelled meals. Emptying of solids and liquids can be assessed simultaneously when both phases are marked with different tracers. After ingestion of a labelled standard meal, gamma camera images of the stomach are obtained in 5 to 15 minute intervals for 1.5 to 2 hours. After correction for decay, the counts in the gastric area are plotted as percentage of total counts at the start of the imaging. The resulting emptying curve can be compared to data obtained in normal volunteers. In general, normal subjects will empty 59% of a meal within 90 minutes.

Indications for these other tests include: (1) symptoms of GERD in patients for whom the primary investigations are normal; (2) equivocal findings that may or may not explain patient's symptoms; (3) inconsistent results from other tests; and (4) primary gastric or pharyngeal

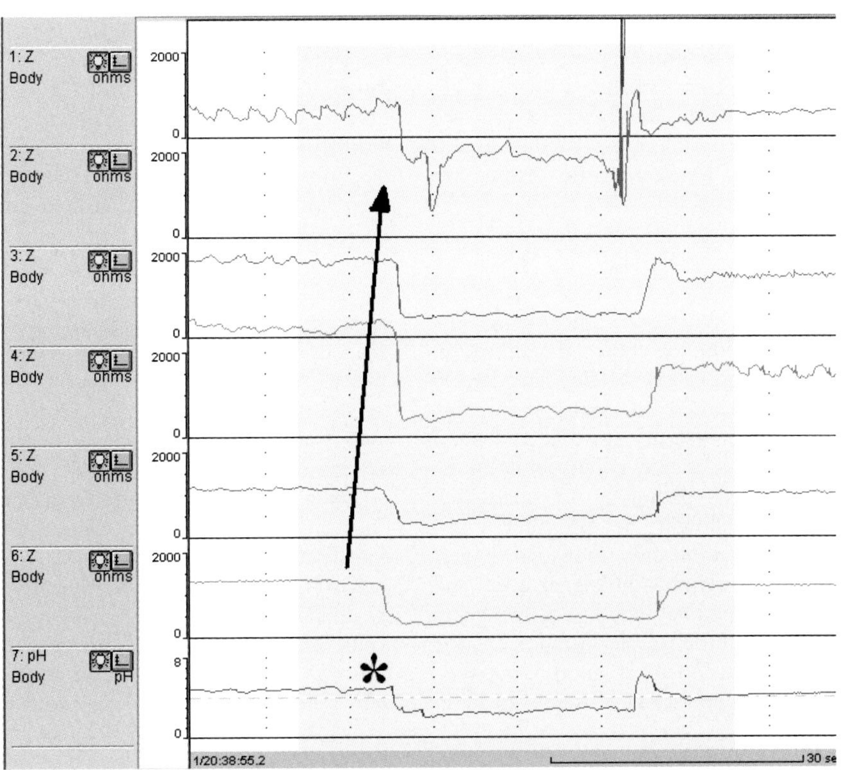

Fig. 8-13. Episode of gastroesophageal reflux detected by multichannel intraluminal impedance pH. Note the drop in pH* and the retrograde bolus direction (arrow).

symptoms. Due to their specific use, these tests will not be further described.

An empiric trial of acid suppression is a popular method among gastroenterologists to diagnose GERD. It is sometimes described as a definitive method for diagnosis of GERD. Although it is cheap and easy, it is nonspecific for GERD as it also treats non-related symptoms such as those caused by gastric or duodenal ulcer, functional dyspepsia, etc. It may also miss an important diagnosis, such as Barrett esophagus.

SUGGESTED READING

Botoman VA, Rao S, Dunlap P, et al. Bill Coding and RVU Committee, American Motility Society. Motility and GI function studies billing and coding guidelines: a position paper of the American Motility Society. *Am J Gastroenterol* 2003;98(6):1228–1236.

Chotiprashidi P, Liu J, Carpenter S, et al. Technology Assessment Committee, American Society for Gastrointestinal Endoscopy. ASGE Technology Status Evaluation Report: wireless esophageal pH monitoring system. *Gastrointest Endosc* 2005;62(4):485–487.

Fox M, Hebbard G, Janiak P, et al. High-resolution manometry predicts the success of oesophageal bolus transport and identifies clinically important abnormalities not detected by conventional manometry. *Neurogastroenterol Motil* 2004;16(5):533–542.

Ghosh SK, Pandolfino JE, Zhang Q, et al. Quantifying esophageal peristalsis with high-resolution manometry: a study of 75 asymptomatic volunteers. *Am J Physiol Gastrointest Liver Physiol* 2006;290(5): G988–997.

Jamieson JR, Stein HJ, DeMeester TR, et al. Ambulatory 24-h esophageal pH monitoring: normal values, optimal thresholds, specificity, sensitivity, and reproducibility. *Am J Gastroenterol* 1992;87(9):1102–1111.

Mittal RK, Bhalla V. Oesophageal motor functions and its disorders. *Gut* 2004;53(10): 1536–1542.

Pandolfino JE, Ghosh SK, Zhang Q, et al. Quantifying EGJ morphology and relaxation with high-resolution manometry: a study of 75 asymptomatic volunteers. *Am J Physiol Gastrointest Liver Physiol* 2006;290(5): G1033–1040.

Pandolfino JE, Kahrilas PJ. American Gastroenterological Association. AGA technical review on the clinical use of esophageal manometry. *Gastroenterology* 2005;128(1): 209–224.

Pandolfino JE, Richter JE, Ours T, et al. Ambulatory esophageal pH monitoring using a wireless system. *Am J Gastroenterol* 2003; 98(4):740–749.

Shay S. Esophageal impedance monitoring: the ups and downs of a new test. *Am J Gastroenterol* 2004;99(6):1020–1022.

Shay S, Tutuian R, Sifrim D, et al. Twenty-four hour ambulatory simultaneous impedance and pH monitoring: a multicenter report of normal values from 60 healthy volunteers. *Am J Gastroenterol* 2004;99(6): 1037–1043.

Sifrim D, Castell D, Dent J, et al. Gastro-oesophageal reflux monitoring: review and consensus report on detection and definitions of acid, non-acid, and gas reflux. *Gut* 2004; 53(7):1024–1031.

Tutuian R, Castell DO. Combined multichannel intraluminal impedance and manometry clarifies esophageal function abnormalities: study in 350 patients. *Am J Gastroenterol* 2004; 99(6):1011–1019.

COMMENTARY

Esophageal physiology tests are a critical component of the treatment schema for foregut problems. As is detailed by Drs. Herbella and Peters, such testing appears straightforward (when used as a screening tool to determine who should have surgery) but, in actuality, is increasingly sophisticated in its ability to measure detailed physiological parameters of esophageal function both before and after surgery.

So, what is absolutely necessary to obtain before surgery and what is of more interest to the esophageal researcher? Upper GI X-rays were once the screening procedure of choice for almost all swallowing problems. They have largely been supplanted by upper endoscopy, which is universally available and often preferred, as it allows therapeutic interventions if pathology is identified. Barium swallow studies can still be a useful tool to aid in difficult diagnoses, particularly in defining difficult anatomy and in evaluating pharyngeal swallowing and functional esophageal clearance. As the authors stress however, good X-ray studies require consistent protocols to be in a collaborative effort between the radiologist and surgeon.

Upper endoscopy is the most mandatory assessment tool before contemplating surgery. Disease severity grading, mapping of anatomy, documentation of disease-related complications, and biopsies for premalignant and malignant conditions are some of the critical functions of endoscopy. Increasingly, endoscopic therapies are available as a less invasive alternative to surgery; this will only increase as evolving technologies permit endoluminal excisions and suturing. For these reasons, surgeons who operate on the upper digestive system should be able to perform upper endoscopy and, for the most part, always perform their own studies on pre- and postsurgical patients.

Likewise, surgeons who deal with functional abnormalities of the esophagus should always look at the original data from motility studies. Interpretations by others can sometimes gloss over clinically important information, and the built-in computer interpretation software is notoriously inaccurate, which can lead to bad operative planning. Recent findings indicating that the majority of reflux patients will tolerate a 360-degree fundoplication have led some to propose eliminating preoperative manometry, but we would disagree with this. There is still a place for a tailored approach in severe primary motility disorders, and mistakenly wrapping an achalasia patient is a disaster for all.

pH studies are also frequently avoided but they remain the single best (most specific) test to determine the presence and severity of reflux disease. The addition of impedance has further strengthened the usefulness of this tool. Arguments for routinely obtaining pH studies for all reflux patients include the growing awareness of the poor correlation of reflux symptoms with disease severity. Also, we know that even in the best of hands, some fundoplications will fail or have problems. In this case a pH test is an important evaluation, but without a preoperative exam to serve as a baseline, the meaning of postoperative results will be difficult to interpret.

LLS

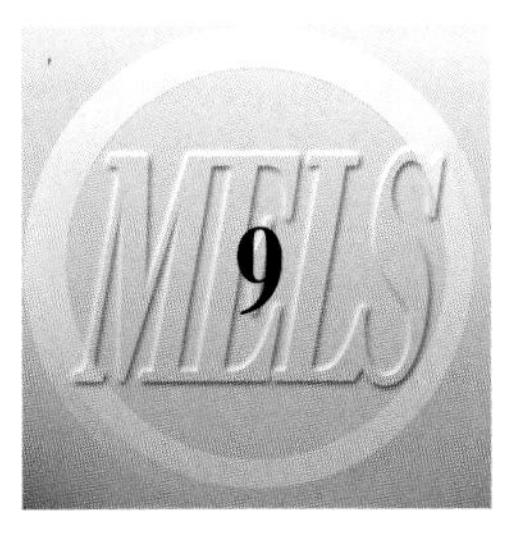

Endoluminal Treatments of GERD

ALFONSO TORQUATI AND WILLIAM RICHARDS

INTRODUCTION

Gastroesophageal reflux disease (GERD) is very common, with approximately 10% of the U.S. population on daily medication for GERD symptoms. These symptoms can compromise the patient's quality of life to a greater degree than even chronic diseases such as congestive heart failure. Medical treatment of GERD with proton pump inhibitors (PPIs) is highly successful in relieving heartburn and healing erosive esophagitis, but once the PPI therapy is discontinued symptoms return in 75% to 90% of patients. In addition, some patients don't tolerate PPI therapy, either because of intolerable side effects or simply because they are in the small minority of patients for whom the medication doesn't work. Also lifelong treatment with these expensive medications adds a significant financial burden to the patient or on the third party paying the bills. In 1999, more than 90 million prescriptions were written for antisecretive medications with an average cost of $218 for a 60-day supply and a total cost of $8.5 billion. PPIs have been shown to reduce esophageal acid exposure, but studies have shown that they do not decrease the total number of reflux episodes and may actually increase the amount of nonacid refluxate.

On the other hand, laparoscopic fundoplication (LF) has been shown to be effective and durable with a success rate over 90% in most published series. Surgery is effective because it reverses most of the defects that contribute to the underlying pathophysiology of severe GERD, including inadequate lower esophageal sphincter (LES) pressure, transient inappropriate LES relaxations (TLESRs), and the presence of sliding hiatal hernia. LF, by correcting the mechanical defects causing GERD, reduces all components of GERD including nonacid refluxate. However, LF is a surgery with potential for operative complications and even death. In addition, 15% to 50% of patients must resume PPI therapy and a smaller number of patients develop disabling symptoms. In some studies, up to 7% of patients undergoing fundoplication develop problems with postoperative dysphagia that requires esophageal dilatation, which has its own unpleasant side effects such as gas bloat, nausea, and diarrhea. Although the laparoscopic approach decreases incisional pain, hospital stay, and recovery time, its intrinsic surgical nature as an "invasive treatment" and the fairly significant alteration of gastric anatomy reinforces arguments against its use, particularly for patients with mild symptoms.

Why is endoluminal treatment of GERD appealing? Medical therapy alone does not change the underlying pathophysiology of GERD, and surgical therapy, even laparoscopic, is seen by many physicians and patients as too invasive and having too many side effects. Endoluminal therapy has a promise of correcting the underlying pathophysiology of GERD while reducing the invasiveness and potentially reducing the side effects of surgery, including gas bloat and dysphagia. It may be time for a paradigm shift in the treatment of medically refractory GERD, asking the the esophageal physician to tailor the invasiveness of the procedure according to the degree of pathology. As shown in Figure 9-1, patients with small hiatal hernias, normal LES pressures, and who do not have Barrett esophagus or pulmonary complications should be considered potential candidates for endoluminal therapy.

If carefully selected, many patients will enjoy a high degree of satisfaction with endoluminal therapy. In this chapter, we will review, with a critical eye, the technique, mechanisms of action, efficacy, safety, and durability of currently available procedures. We will also review and comment on the failures of endoluminal procedures.

Endoluminal Procedures for GERD

Endoscopic treatment of GERD dates back to the 1980s, when Donahue et al. attempted to increase the competence of the LES by sclerosing the gastric cardia. These early efforts were not terribly successful; the "true" era of endoscopic GERD therapy started only in 2000 when two new endoscopic treatments for GERD were approved by the FDA. Since then, several other endoscopic treatments have been introduced into the market. Overall these endoscopic treatments can be categorized into three approaches: tissue approximation (using sutures or staples), radiofrequency therapy, and injection therapy (injecting inert material into the LES).

Endoscopic Full-Thickness Plication System

This device, manufactured by NDO Surgical (Mansfield, MA), relies on taking full-thickness bites, which opposes serosa to serosa creating a durable union and restoring in a single bite the valvular mechanism of the GE junction. The system was FDA-approved in April 2003 after it showed safety and efficacy in animal and human subjects.

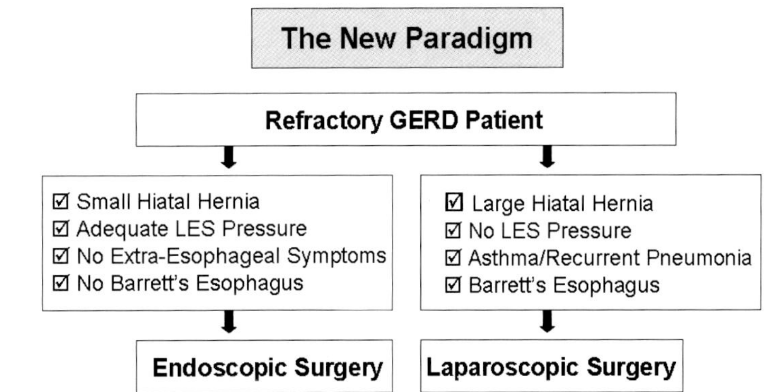

Fig. 9-1. The New Paradigm.

Procedure

After endoscopic evaluation of the gastroesophageal anatomy region, the suturing system device is introduced over a Savary guidewire, and a slim 6-mm gastroscope is inserted through the side channel of the 20-mm device. The rest of the procedure is performed under direct vision provided by retroflexion of the endoscope. The goal is to create a full-thickness plication in the fundus at the GE junction as shown in Figure 9-2. The GE junction is identified, and the plication site is selected (within 1 cm of the GE junction on the lesser curvature of the gastric wall) and the tissue retractor (a 3-mm metal "corkscrew") is advanced through the layers of the gastric wall at the chosen site until it reaches the serosal layer (full-thickness bite), which is verified by observing noticeable tenting of the tissue around the entry point of the helical retractor. This full-thickness gastric fold is pulled toward the open jaws of the instrument, and then the arms are closed. Next, the implant is deployed to create a full-thickness pledgeted plication. Subsequently, the tissue retractor is disengaged from the gastric wall, and the device is removed (Fig. 9-3). The implant used for fixation of the transmural plication consists of pretied suture (standard USP size 2–0 polypropylene), two bolsters made of ePTFE, and two titanium retention bridges, all of which are biocompatible and intended to be permanent.

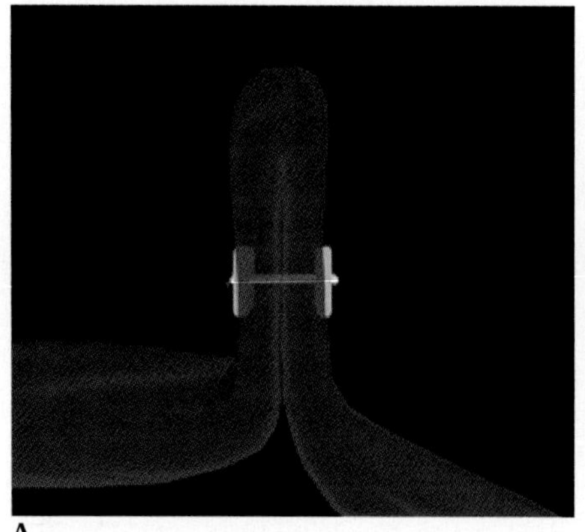

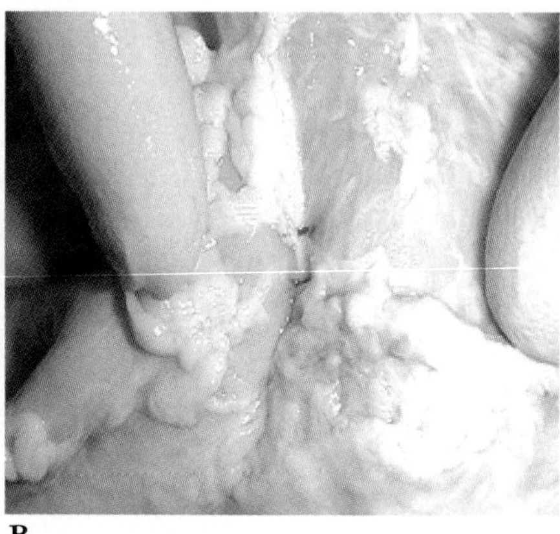

A **B**

Fig. 9-3. Cross section of the GE junction showing the full-thickness NDO plication. **A.** An artist's conception of the plicator placement. **B.** An actual photo of an implant *in situ*. (Courtesy of NDO Surgical.)

Mechanism of Action

Animal studies have shown that the gastric yield pressure is significantly increased in pigs undergoing such a full-thickness plication. While this argues for some sort of augmentation of the GE junction barrier to reflux of gastric contents, the specifics of its action on the lower esophageal sphincter, transient LES relaxations, or other components of the barrier are unclear. Neither the randomized sham-controlled nor the open label trial were able to demonstrate a significant change in LES pressure after full-thickness plication. Other potential mechanisms include alteration of the angle of His and reduction of the compliance of the cardia and fundus, which might reduce the incidence of transient LES relaxations (TLESRs).

Clinical Studies and Efficacy

Chuttani et al. documented ex vivo efficacy by measuring pressures at which the intragastric content leaks back through a plicated GE junction (yield pressure). In the stomachs of 22 pigs, the average gastric yield pressure at the onset (drip) and the severe reflux (steady flow) increased more than eightfold after plication. The human feasibility study done by Chuttani included six men with 12-month follow-up. All had chronic heartburn and pathologic reflux requiring maintenance PPI therapy (twice daily in four patients). Excluded were those with a significant hiatal hernia of more than 2 cm, grade 3 or 4 esophagitis, or Barrett esophagus. A single full-thickness plication was applied in the gastric cardia in a mean time of 21 minutes. At 6 months, five of six patients were off PPI therapy, and the patient who did not improve went on to undergo laparoscopic Nissen fundoplication with no improvement in that case either. Twelve months after the procedure, mean gastrointestinal symptom rating scale (GSRS) and the Gastroesophageal Reflux Disease-Health Related Quality of Life (GERD-HRQL) instrument scores improved in more than 75% of patients, with endoscopic documentation of improvement in esophagitis grade in two patients (plications were found on endoscopy to be intact in all six patients at 12 months).

After this trial, an open-label multicenter study led by Pleskow enrolled 64 patients; follow-up surveys were available for 41, and pH and manometry studies were performed for 35. Inclusion and exclusion criteria were similar to those used in the pilot study. The average off-medication GERD-HRQL scores improved by 63%

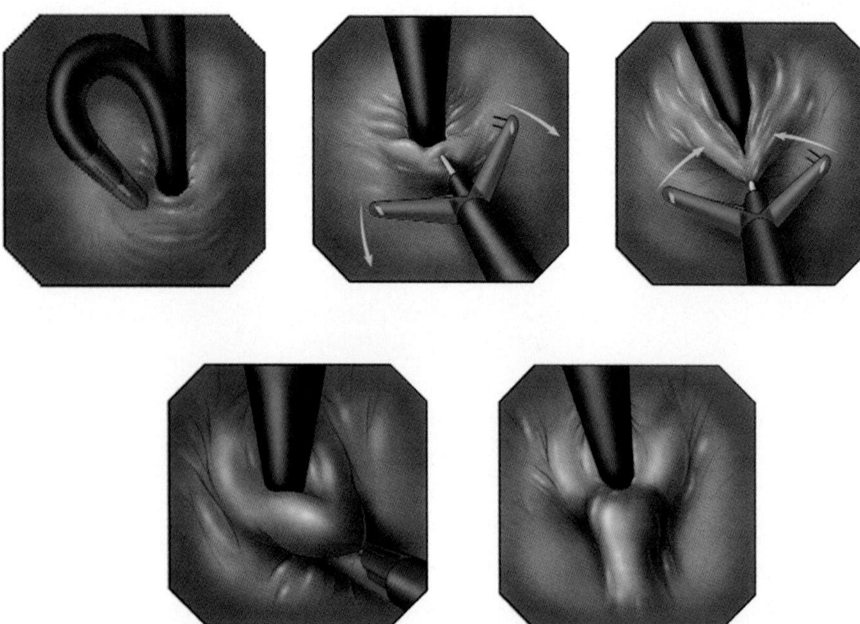

Fig. 9-2. Artist rendition of the placement of the full-thickness NDO plication. (Reprinted with permission from Springer. Originally published by Lutfi R, et al. In: *Surgical Endoscopy* 2004;18:1299–1315.)

(20.1 vs. 6.9), and, interestingly, postprocedure scores were also lower than baseline on-medication GERD-HRQL scores (12.6 vs. 6.9). Of the 41 patients, 34 (83%) were off daily PPIs at 6 months. Manometry and pH studies were performed on 35 patients and documented a 20.7% decrease in mean acid exposure time, with complete normalization of pH achieved in 31% of patients studied. No changes, however, were found in manometric measurements.

A recent randomized controlled trial comparing sham treatment to the full-thickness plication is by far the most conclusive and persuasive study that documents endoscopic plication effectiveness. Full-thickness plication significantly reduced GERD symptom scores and esophageal acid exposure compared to a group of patients undergoing sham treatment. The primary end point of the study was the percentile of patients with greater than 50% reduction in GERD-HRQL (responders) after the procedure. Fifty-six percent of the patients in the treatment group were responders compared to 18.5% of responders in the sham procedure group. Twenty-four hour pH studies showed that percent time acid exposure in the distal esophagus went from 10% to 7% in the treatment group while in the sham group there was no change. The authors of this multicenter randomized controlled trial concluded that the NDO full-thickness plication was a safe and effective procedure that reduced GERD symptoms, PPI use, and distal esophageal acid exposure in the treated group 3 months after the procedure.

The cumulative evidences from the two trials, illustrated with a forest plot in Figure 9-4, show that there is a significant decrease in distal esophageal acid exposure after endoscopic full-thickness plication.

Durability

Intact plication sutures were seen on endoscopy in all patients in the human pilot study at 12 months. In animal studies, pathologic examination performed 3 weeks after the procedure revealed serosa-to-serosa union and no abdominal abscesses or other complications. Pleskow et al. did a 3-year follow-up of the 64 patients undergoing full-thickness plication during the open label trial and were able to obtain follow-up in 29 of the 64 patients. GERD-HRQL median scores were still decreased (from 19 to 8) 36 months after plication. Preoperatively, 28 of the 29 patients utilized daily PPIs for treatment of symptoms, while at 3 years only 14 of 29 required the use of daily PPIs. Responders to therapy were deemed to have greater than or equal to 50% GERD-HRQL score improvement. One year after plication 59% of the patients were responders while at 3 years they had slipped only slightly to 55%. This data suggest that the full-thickness plication may be durable up to 3 years; however, less than half of the patients had complete follow-up, which significantly reduces the strength of these conclusions.

Safety

Studies assessing the safety of the procedure were performed in pigs by performing the endoscopic plication in different areas of the GE junction. No changes were documented in the pigs' behavior, eating habits, posture, respiratory rate, or vocalization. Subsequent endoscopy showed plication stability and no evidence of tissue damage. There were no complications or deaths. Laparoscopy was performed in one pig and confirmed serosa-to-serosa tissue opposition and no injury to surrounding organs.

Human pilot studies documented mild epigastric discomfort in two patients, with eructation difficulty in one, all resolving spontaneously within 1 week. Other studies showed pharyngitis to be the most common adverse event (41% of patients). More serious complications have been noted in prospective studies. These were primarily incidences of pneumothorax and pneumoperitoneum that fortunately resolved without any operative intervention. Pneumomediastinum and fever are usually treated with intravenous antibiotics and resolve without any other intervention. One patient had a gastric perforation seen at the time of endoscopy that was closed with endoscopic clips and required no other intervention. The only long-term complication described was a patient

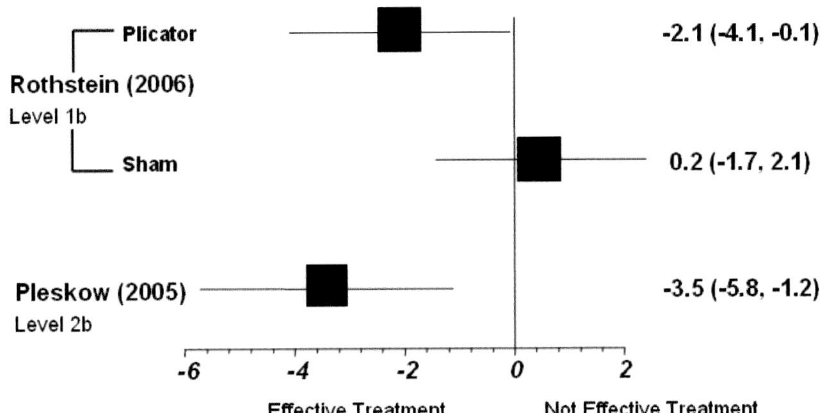

Fig. 9-4. Forest plot of weighted mean differences in % of the time pH <4 after endoscopic plication. Box dimensions are in proportion to the sample size of the trial; horizontal bars are 95% confidence intervals. Statistical significance is achieved when the confidence interval bar is clear of the "0" vertical line. (Reprinted with permission from Springer. Originally published by Torquati A et al. In: *Surgical Endoscopy*, 2007.)

who developed persistent epigastric and chest pain 3 months after the endoscopic plication. He underwent diagnostic laparoscopy, removal of the plication, and laparoscopic fundoplication, which resulted in complete resolution of his pain.

Early clinical studies suggest that the procedure is safe in expert hands but that it must be performed with attention to detail to reduce the incidence of pneumoperitoneum, pneumomediastinum, and gastric perforations. Prophylactic antibiotics are certainly necessary because of the full-thickness nature of the sutures that may result in some contamination of the peritoneum.

Summary

The early results of this technique are very promising. Because the subjective evidences of improvement (quality-of-life scales and medication requirements) are supported by objective data (improved endoscopic findings and reduced esophageal acid exposure), this procedure became the leading endoluminal technique for GERD treatment by 2007. Safety has been a concern because of a few serious complications reported in the clinical trials, including pneumomediastinum, pneumothorax, and gastric perforation. Additional experience will show whether reproducible results can be achieved by newly trained physicians with the same complication rate. This will better define the future role of this technique.

Endoscopic Plication

The EndoCinch Suturing System (C.R. Bard, Inc.; Murray Hill, NY) was cleared by the FDA in April of 2000 for endoscopic suture plication of the GE junction for treatment of GERD.

Procedure

The device is fitted onto the end of a standard diagnostic endoscope and advanced to the level of the GE junction, where typically 2 to 4 plications of gastric mucosa are created. As shown in Figure 9-5, once the site is selected, the physician activates a suction mechanism that pulls the target tissue into the chamber of the device and then deploys the suture. The device is then pulled through the tissue outside of the patient and reloaded with the same suture and redeployed to the target where another bite of tissue is obtained. Then, using a second endoscope, the suture is pulled out of the patient and tied extracorporally using a mechanical crimping device to securely hold the plication in place.

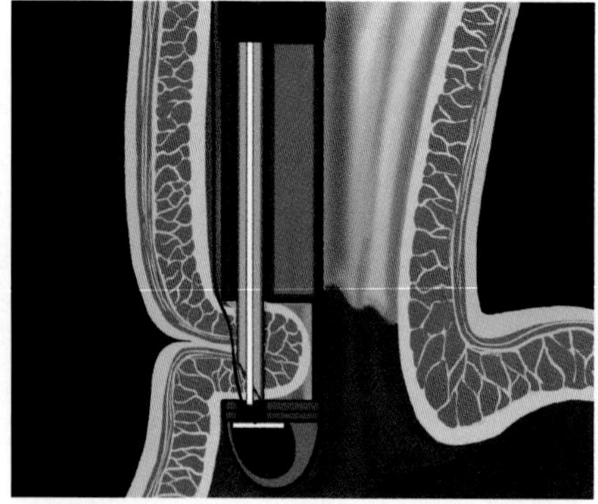

Fig. 9-5. The EndoCinch device at the GE junction placing plications. (Reprinted with permission from Springer. Originally published by Lutfi R et al., in *Surgical Endoscopy* 18: 1299–1315, 2004.)

Mechanism of Action

The proposed mechanism of action is that the EndoCinch improves the anti-reflux barrier at the GE junction by augmenting the LES or by decreasing compliance of the gastric cardia. In the multicenter U.S. trial, however, there was no significant difference in LES pressure 3 months after the procedure. There has in fact been no study that definitively demonstrates either improvements in LES pressure, LES length, or reductions in transient LES relaxations. One problem is the tremendous variability in the procedure as reported in the literature. Variability includes the number of plications, which vary from two to three, and their placement, in either vertical, spiral, or horizontal patterns.

Clinical Studies and Efficacy

In the 6 years since the procedure was first introduced in the U.S., there have been two randomized controlled trials that compared the EndoCinch plication against sham treatment. These two studies showed that EndoCinch plication of the GE junction is no better than sham treatment in reducing distal esophageal acid exposure. Montgomery et al. reported on 46 patients enrolled in a single-center study who were randomized to either sham or EndoCinch plication. One year after the procedure, there was no difference between the sham and the EndoCinch groups in the use of PPIs or total time of acid exposure in the distal esophagus. However there was a significant improvement in the GERD-related quality of life as assessed by GSRS in the treated at group compared to sham at 3 and 12 months postprocedure. Another single-center randomized controlled trial of EndoCinch plication versus sham treatment was carried out by Schwartz et al. Sixty patients were randomly assigned to EndoCinch plication, sham procedure, or observation. Acid exposure in the distal esophagus was reduced slightly in the EndoCinch plication group and in the patients undergoing the sham procedure. There was however no significant difference between the sham and the EndoCinch plication with regard to the amount of acid exposure. Interestingly while there was no objective improvement, there was a significantly greater percentage of patients who had reduced drug use by more than 50% in the treatment group compared to either the sham or observation groups.

Most prospective clinical studies on the efficacy of the EndoCinch procedure have failed to show a significant difference in distal esophageal acid exposure after the procedure. Schiefke reported 54 patients with 24-hour pH monitoring after EndoCinch and found that there was no significant change in acid exposure. Mahmood studied 22 patients and found the same lack of significant difference 12 months after the EndoCinch procedure. The multicenter U.S. trial reported by Filipi showed only a slight change in acid exposure, from 9.6% to 9.3% total time acid exposure in the distal esophagus 3 months after the procedure (Fig. 9-6). One study that did show a significant reduction in acid exposure was that of Arts et al., who enrolled 20 GERD patients who were refractory to high-dose PPI treatment. They found a significant reduction in the percent time of pH less than 4 in the distal esophagus from 17.0% to 9.8%. Seven out of the 20 patients had normal pH studies 3 months after the procedure. These investigators were able to stop PPI use in 13 of the 20 patients 3 months after the procedure, but after 12 months only 6 patients were off PPI use. This is the study that shows the most clinically significant reduction in acid exposure 3 months after the Endocinch procedure. However, they did note an increase in the use of PPIs 12 months after the procedure, suggesting a lack of procedure durability.

Durability

In the Filipi study, patients who experienced treatment failure had separation of the plication or complete loss of sutures, suggesting that the procedure may not be durable. More recently, Schiefke documented sutures remaining in place only in 12 of 70 patients (17%), while absolutely no sutures could be detected in 18 out of 70 (26%). The authors concluded that the

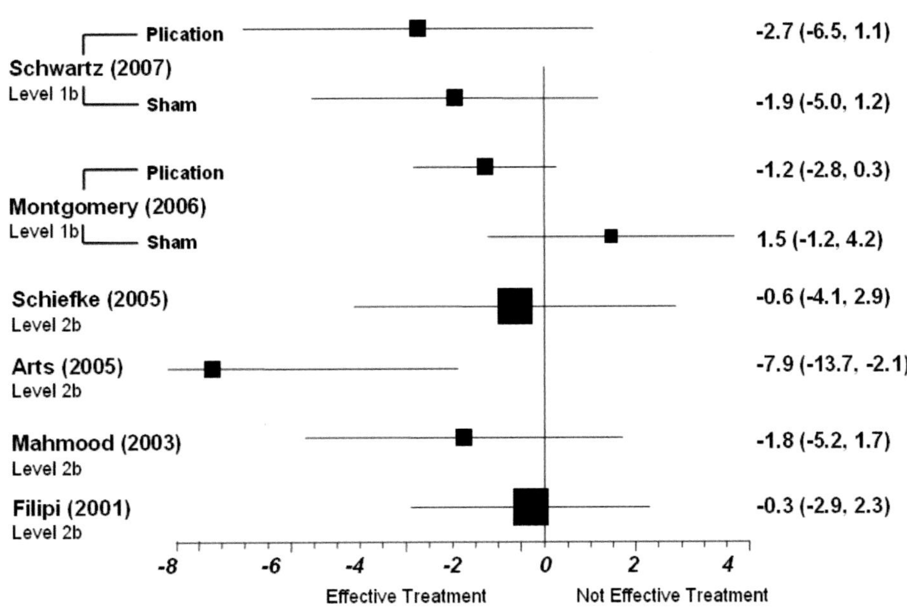

Fig. 9-6. Forest plot of weighted mean differences in % of the time pH <4 after endoscopic plication (Bard EndoCinch). Box dimensions are in proportion to the sample size of the trial; horizontal bars are 95% confidence intervals. Statistical significance is achieved when the confidence interval bar is clear of the "0" vertical line. (Reprinted with permission from Springer. Originally published by Torquati A et al. In: *Surgical Endoscopy*, 2007.)

EndoCinch provides reasonable short-term results, but that long-term outcomes are disappointing, probably due to suture loss in the majority of patients.

Safety

EndoCinch plication for GERD appears to be the safest endoscopic treatment of GERD, with very few reports of serious complications either in the literature or on the FDA website. In the U.S. multicenter trial, one patient required hospitalization for pain, mediastinal air, and fever, but recovered uneventfully. One other study reported two patients who developed GI hemorrhage requiring transfusion. The FDA website reports only one major adverse event of a patient who required two units of blood.

Summary

The initial enthusiasm for this procedure has faded considerably since the early reports of GERD symptom improvement and PPI reduction. Two well-designed trials demonstrated no objective improvement in esophageal acid exposure compared to sham treatment. Furthermore, multiple studies have shown that the majority of the plications were no longer visible nor even present 12 months after the procedure. While the procedure is safe, further development to improve efficacy and durability must be made before it can be recommended for routine clinical use.

RADIOFREQUENCY TREATMENT OF THE GE JUNCTION

Radiofrequency (RF) treatment of the GE junction, known as the Stretta procedure (formerly marketed by Curon Medical, Inc.; Sunnyvale, CA), was approved by the FDA in April 2000.

In this procedure, RF energy similar to that used every day in the operating room, is delivered to the muscle layer of the GE junction while the mucosa is cooled with water irrigation to prevent injury to the mucosa. The RF energy is delivered through 4 needles mounted on a balloon inflated to 2.5 PSI and controlled to a target temperature using a computerized generator. The delivery of RF energy is performed at multiple locations in the distal esophagus and in the gastric cardia. Placement of multiple lesions within the muscularis will theoretically cause scar contraction and enhance the antireflux barrier of the LES (Fig. 9-7).

Mechanism of Action

Initial animal studies demonstrated an increased gastric yield pressure. This increase in the gastric yield pressure is thought to be caused by collagen contraction and subsequent improvement in the antireflux barrier. Human studies have shown no change in fasting LES pressure but a significant postprandial increase in LES pressure, from 5.2 mmHg to 8 mmHg, 6 months after the Stretta procedure. Other studies in human and animal subjects show that transient LES relaxations are significantly reduced in frequency after Stretta procedures.

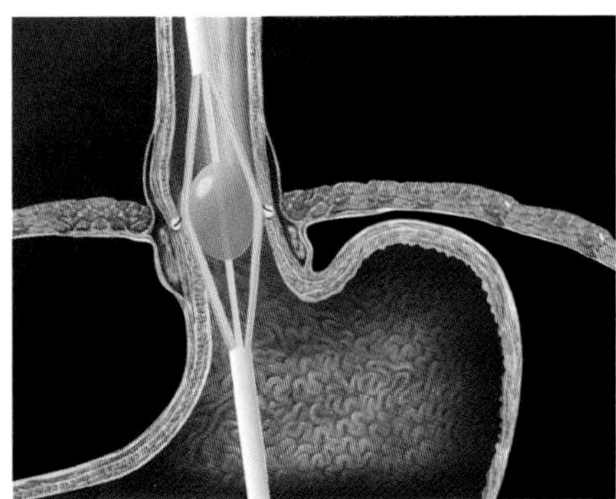

Fig. 9-7. The Stretta catheter in position with the four 5.5-mm needle electrodes delivering radiofrequency energy to the muscularis of the GE junction. (Reprinted with permission from Springer. Originally published by Lutfi R et al. In: *Surgical Endoscopy* 2004;18: 1299–1315.)

Clinical Studies and Efficacy

The clinical data on this procedure are very conflicting. There is only one randomized controlled trial comparing Stretta to a sham procedure. This study randomized 29 patients to sham treatment and 35 patients to Stretta. Patients who underwent treatment with Stretta had significant improvement in GERD-HRQL scores, which was the primary outcome measured. Twenty of the sham patients then elected to undergo Stretta 6 months after the initial randomization. These patients had a significant improvement in GERD-HRQL scores 6 months after undergoing Stretta. While it was concluded that there was a significant improvement in GERD symptoms in the Stretta group compared to sham, the distal esophageal acid exposure was not significantly reduced in the treatment group 6 months after the procedure. This is similar to most other endoluminal trials, in which the treatment group had significant improvement in GERD symptoms but no significant decrease in esophageal acid exposure. This dichotomy in symptom relief but without decrease in esophageal acid exposure is difficult to reconcile.

Most of the prospective trials of Stretta show at least some reduction in esophageal acid exposure. In the multicenter U.S. prospective trial, the Stretta procedure reduced distal esophageal acid exposure from 10.2% to 6.4% in 118 patients at the 1-year follow-up. Tam et al. reported a similar reduction in acid exposure from 10.6% to 6.3% in 20 patients, 12 months after the Stretta procedure. Both studies also documented a significant reduction in GERD-HRQL scores after Stretta. DiBaise and colleagues found that there were no change in esophageal acid exposure time 6 months after the Stretta procedure in 18 patients. Although there was no change in acid exposure time, there was a significant improvement in GERD HRQL scores in the study. In a study performed at Vanderbilt, 65 patients undergoing Stretta were compared to 75 patients undergoing fundoplication. Both the Stretta and the Nissen patients had a significant improvement in their GERD symptoms as assessed by the Quality of Life in Reflux and Dyspepsia (QOLRAD) instrument. Twenty-two out of the 65 Stretta patients returned for 24-hour pH studies, which showed a significant decrease in esophageal acid exposure from 8.2% to 4.4%.

Durability

Data from Vanderbilt suggest that there is a durable treatment effect at a mean of 27 months after the Stretta procedure. While no 24-hour pH studies were performed, long-term patient satisfaction, GERD-specific symptom scores, and PPI use remained improved. Fifty-eight percent of the patients were completely off PPIs at short-term follow-up, while 56% of the patients remained off PPIs at the long-term follow-up.

Safety

Published reports of the Stretta procedure indicate only mild complications, including minor GI bleeding, aspiration pneumonia, fever, leukocytosis, sedation-associated hypotension, or superficial mucosal injury. In these trials there have been no reports of death, esophageal perforation, or other serious adverse events except for several patients that developed transient gastroparesis that appeared to resolve. Review of the FDA website for serious postmarketing adverse events reveals that there had been at least five events, including two deaths, related to cardiac arrhythmia and aspiration pneumonia. Esophageal perforation requiring thoracotomy and repair has also been reported. One patient with prolonged gastroparesis has also been reported to the FDA.

Summary

The data for the Stretta procedure is both conflicting and controversial. The forest plot in Figure 9-8 perfectly depicts the extreme variability in 24-hour pH data. The randomized clinical trial does not show any objective improvement in acid exposure compared to sham treatment, while the majority of prospective trials suggests that there is a significant reduction in acid

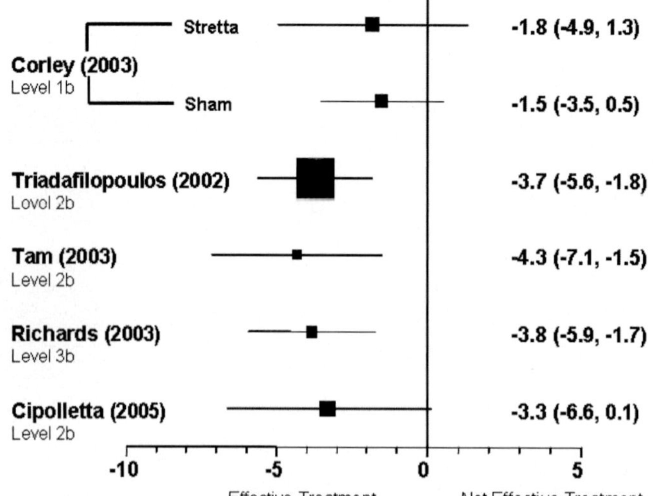

Fig. 9-8. Forest plot of weighted mean differences in % of the time pH <4 after radiofrequency treatment (Stretta procedure). Boxes dimension are in proportion to the sample size of the trial; horizontal bars are 95% confidence intervals. Statistical significance is achieved when the confidence interval bar is clear of the "0" vertical line. (Reprinted with permission from Springer. Originally published by Torquati A et al. In: *Surgical Endoscopy*, 2007.)

exposure. All the clinical trials present evidence for improvement in GERD-specific symptom scores after Stretta. However, as is well known, frequently patients have a modest symptom response to even a sham treatment. More randomized controlled trials are needed to fully assess the efficacy of the Stretta procedure. The Stretta device is not currently being marketed anywhere in the world as the parent company, Curo Medical, Inc., declared bankruptcy in 2006.

OTHER ENDOLUMINAL PROCEDURES FOR GERD

Currently there are more failed procedures for endoluminal GERD treatment than there are unqualified successes. Injectable "bulking" agents have been a particular disappointment. The Enteryx procedure (formerly marketed by Boston Scientific Corporation; Natick, MA) utilized a liquid biocompatible polymer that was injected into the wall of the GE junction, where it formed a spongy semisolid mass within the tissues (Fig. 9-9). The theory was that the polymer would augment the antireflux barrier. Early clinical results showed significant improvements in distal esophageal acid exposure and GERD symptoms. These results, along with a good safety profile during the clinical studies, won the procedure FDA approval in 2003. When the procedure was released to practicing physicians, however, reports of serious complications, including embolus of the polymers to the kidneys and aortoenteric fistulas resulting in several deaths, began to appear. These complications seemed related to experience. In September, 2005 the company voluntarily withdrew the product from the market place.

The Enteryx experience raises multiple questions: (1) How much training in these procedures is needed? (2) What is the learning curve for the safe and efficacious application of endoluminal GERD treatments? (3) How should these techniques be taught?

A similar failed procedure is the Gatekeeper Reflux Repair System (Medtronic; Minneapolis, MN), which also relied on the injection of a bulking polymer at the GE junction in order to reduce GE reflux. This system used an application device that enabled a more reliable placement of the biocompatible cylindrical prosthetics, composed of polyacrylonitrite hydrogel placed into the submucosal area of the distal esophagus as shown in Figure 9-10. After implantation, the small hydrophilic cylinders would enlarge. Unlike the Enteryx system, which was designed to be implanted into the muscular layer of the esophagus, the Gatekeeper system was meant to be placed in the submucosal area. The U.S. multicenter clinical trial failed to demonstrate efficacy of the procedure. Some preliminary reports suggested that many of the Gatekeeper implants were simply missing 6 to 12 months after the procedure. Many also question the theory behind the use of these submucosal implants, as they did nothing to increase LES pressure or to change any the parameters of the GE junction reflux barrier. Another important lesson learned from the failure of the Gatekeeper to achieve clinically important improvements in control of acid exposure is the demonstration of a significant sham effect on GERD symptoms and use of PPIs. It is sobering to realize that in one prospective study of patients taking daily doses of PPIs, physicians were able to wean 39% of patients off their medication using a step-down algorithm. As there appears to be such a significant sham or placebo effect in GERD treatment, it appears that either objective measurements of esophageal acid exposure or well-controlled studies need to be employed in order to scientifically gauge effectiveness of endoluminal treatments for GERD.

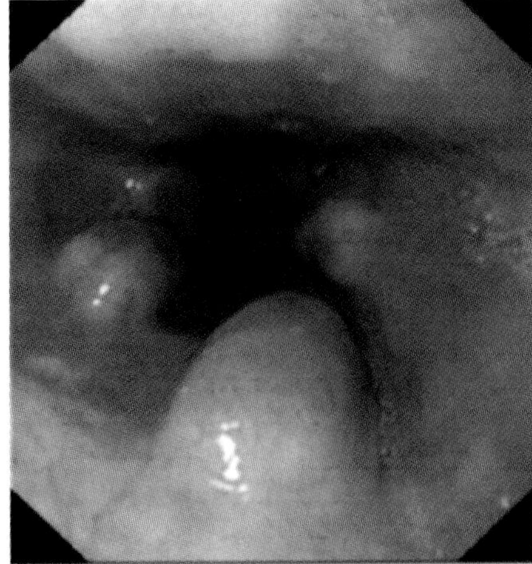

Fig. 9-10. Endoscopic view of the distal esophagus showing Gatekeeper implants within the submucosa of the distal esophagus.

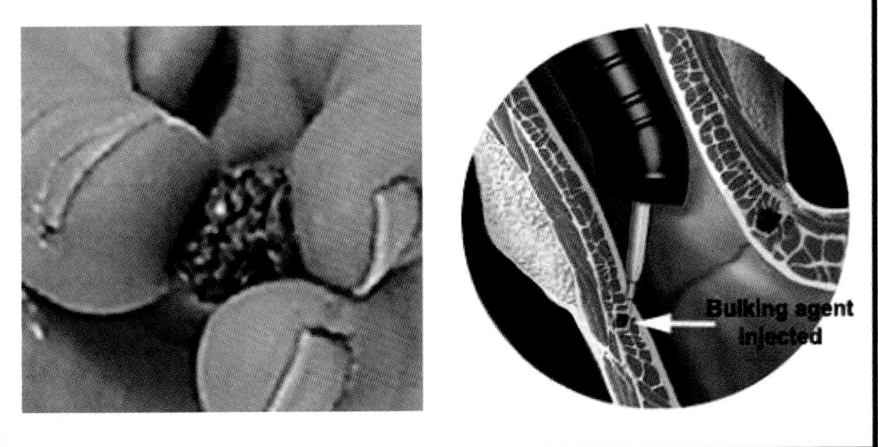

Fig. 9-9. The Enteryx polymer (left) and technique of injection (right). (Courtesy of Boston Scientific.)

FUTURE DIRECTIONS

Treatment of esophageal reflux has changed dramatically since the first description of the Nissen fundoplication. Notable was the contribution by Donahue et al., which changed the long tight Nissen with its unacceptable postoperative rate of dysphagia and gas bloating to the current gold standard antireflux procedure: the short floppy Nissen. Since that time, the open approach has been replaced with laparoscopic fundoplication, and tens of thousands of minimally invasive procedures have been performed in the U.S. In April of 2000, the FDA released to the public two of the procedures discussed in this chapter. Clearly the many refinements of the Nissen fundoplication, which has taken many years, have made the procedure far better than the one originally described by Rudolf Nissen. At the present time, we are going through a similar development phase of endoluminal procedures. This process will most likely take many more years. Large, well-designed randomized sham controlled trials have now shown that several of these endoscopic treatments of GERD provide outcomes superior to the sham treatment. Additional refinements of the procedures discussed and others as yet undisclosed are poised to change the surgical armamentarium in the near future.

SUGGESTED READING

Arts J, Lerut T, Rutgeerts P, et al. A one-year follow-up study of endoluminal gastroplication (Endocinch) in GERD patients refractory to proton pump inhibitor therapy. *Dig Dis Sci* 2005;50:351–356.

Corley DA, Katz P, Wo JM, et al. Improvement of gastroesophageal reflux symptoms after radiofrequency energy: a randomized, sham-controlled trial. *Gastroenterology* 2003;125: 668–676.

Donahue PE, Sugitani A, Carvalho P. Endoscopic control of gastroesophageal reflux: a status report. *World J Surg* 1992;16: 343–346.

Filipi CJ, Lehman GA, Rothstein RI, et al. Transoral, flexible endoscopic suturing for treatment of GERD: a multicenter trial. *Gastrointest Endosc* 2001;53:416–422.

Montgomery M, Hakanson B, Ljungqvist O, et al. Twelve months' follow-up after treatment with the EndoCinch endoscopic technique for gastro-oesophageal reflux disease: a randomized, placebo-controlled study. *Scand J Gastroenterol* 2006;41:1382–1389.

Pleskow D, Rothstein R, Kozarek R, et al. Endoscopic full-thickness plication for the treatment of GERD: long-term multicenter results. *Surg Endosc* Dec 16;2006; [Epub ahead of print].

Pleskow D, Rothstein R, Lo S, et al. Endoscopic full-thickness plication for the treatment of GERD: 12-month follow-up for the North American open-label trial. *Gastrointest Endosc* 2005;61:643–649.

Richards WO, Houston HL, Torquati A, et al. Paradigm shift in the management of gastroesophageal reflux disease. *Ann Surg* 2003;237: 638–647; discussion 648–649.

Rothstein R, Filipi C, Caca K, et al. Endoscopic full-thickness plication for the treatment of gastroesophageal reflux disease: A randomized, sham-controlled trial. *Gastroenterology* 2006;131:704–712.

Schiefke I, Zabel-Langhennig A, Neumann S, et al. Long term failure of endoscopic gastroplication (EndoCinch). *Gut* 2005;54:752–758.

Schwartz MP, Wellink H, Gooszen HG, et al. Endoscopic gastroplication for the treatment of gastro-oesophageal reflux disease: a randomised, sham-controlled trial. *Gut* 2007; 56:20–28.

Tam WC, Schoeman MN, Zhang Q, et al. Delivery of radiofrequency energy to the lower oesophageal sphincter and gastric cardia inhibits transient lower oesophageal sphincter relaxations and gastro-oesophageal reflux in patients with reflux disease. *Gut* 2003;52:479–485.

Torquati A, Houston HL, Kaiser J, et al. Long-term follow-up study of the Stretta procedure for the treatment of gastroesophageal reflux disease. *Surg Endosc* 2004;18:1475–1479.

Torquati A, Richards WO. Endoluminal GERD treatments: critical appraisal of current literature with evidence-based medicine instruments. Accepted for publication: *Surg Endosc* 2007;21(3); 439–444.

COMMENTARY

It is easy for surgeons and gastroenterologists to succumb to a simplistic philosophy of treating gastroesophageal reflux disease (GERD). For gastroenterologists this involves treatment with PPIs for anything remotely sounding like reflux, escalating the dose as breakthrough occurs and performing endoscopic treatment for complications. For surgeons it can involve a laparoscopic fundoplication on anyone who has symptoms and has been on medications. Considering the complexities of etiology and physiology involved in GERD, both approaches are patently absurd and reductionist. Patients suffering from reflux have both a reduced quality of life but also a high incidence of complications such as Barrett metaplasia and strictures. They deserve a comprehensive evaluation and a tailored therapeutic plan. Dr. Richardson has long been a staunch defender of a new paradigm for GERD treatment that includes a comprehensive evaluation, triage to appropriate therapy, and careful long-term follow-up.

Deciding the appropriate therapy calls for the recognition that there is no single perfect choice: medication is great for many but not all and surgery, while effective at restoring damaged anatomy and treating severe positional reflux, remains invasive. This leaves a large pool of patients who are early in their disease process, perhaps too early to appreciate the trade-off of side effects for the reflux relief given by surgery, and yet who won't take medication. This refusal may be for philosophical or financial reasons or simply that they are part of the 15% of the population who does not respond to PPIs. Endoluminal treatments offer a solution for this large grey area of patients who fail or refuse medical therapy but for whom surgery would be overly aggressive. All the therapies described by the authors have similar results—high patient satisfaction, moderate reflux score improvement, but only 30% to 40% normalization of pH scores. These results have been confusing to physicians and have led to the identification of endoluminal therapies as having "bad results." In fact, endoluminal GERD treatments work well for exactly the patients left uncovered by surgical and medical treatment. A recent review of the raw data shows that when endoluminal treatments are used for early, mild disease (DeMeester score <30; LES pressure >15 mmHg) pH normalization is achieved in almost 90% of patients!

As endoluminal GERD treatments evolve and flexible endoscopy becomes a more universal surgical tool, these treatments will find their place in comprehensive treatment protocols for esophageal reflux.

LLS

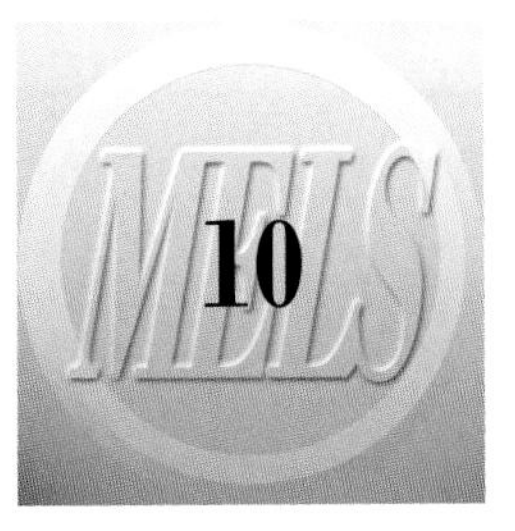

Laparoscopic Nissen Fundoplication

CEDRIC S. F. LORENZO AND NATHANIEL J. SOPER

INTRODUCTION

In 1955, Rudolf Nissen performed one of the first open antireflux operations by plicating the fundus of the stomach around the distal esophagus. Variations of this procedure have become the most commonly performed operations for gastroesophageal reflux disease (GERD). Laparoscopic antireflux surgery (LARS) has recently assumed a major role in the treatment of GERD. This minimally invasive technique for the treatment of GERD has lowered the threshold for surgical treatment and renewed interest in the pathophysiologic features and treatment outcomes for this disease. Most operations for GERD involve plicating the gastric fundus around the distal esophagus. The most commonly performed fundoplication in the United States is the Nissen 360-degree fundoplication, which results in approximately 90% long-term control of reflux symptoms. Other fundoplications that have become eponymous (e.g., Hill, Belsey, Toupet, Guarner, and Lind) have been developed, applied, and reported, but have not achieved the same degree of acceptance as the Nissen procedure.

A randomized trial comparing "open" Nissen fundoplication with medical therapy in patients with complicated GERD proved surgical therapy to be more effective. Despite these findings, many patients and physicians opted instead for lifelong medication and significant lifestyle limitations until 1991, when the first laparoscopic Nissen fundoplications (LNF) were reported from separate centers by Dallemagne and Geagea. Although LNF follows the same surgical principles as the open operation, the laparoscopic approach reduces postoperative pain and shortens hospitalization and recuperation with a functional outcome similar to that of the open operation. Because of this, there has been a rapid increase in antireflux surgery, with LNF gaining acceptance as the current gold standard for the surgical treatment of GERD.

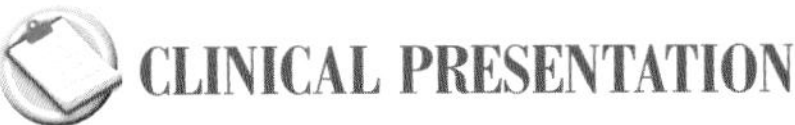

CLINICAL PRESENTATION

GERD symptoms are common in the general population, affecting more than 40% of Americans at least once per month, 20% once per week, and 7% daily. Patients with GERD may exhibit typical or atypical symptoms (Table 10-1). GERD usually presents as heartburn and regurgitation and can progress to dysphagia, odynophagia, and chest pain. Although typical of GERD, these symptoms may also be caused by other entities that must be included in the differential diagnosis, such as cardiopulmonary disease, esophageal motility disorders, gastritis/peptic ulcer disease, and gallbladder disease.

PATHOPHYSIOLOGY

Gastroesophageal reflux (GER) occurs physiologically in all healthy individuals to a limited degree. Frequent and repeated episodes of reflux lead to esophageal mucosal damage. Barriers to GER include the lower esophageal sphincter (LES), the presence of an intraabdominal segment of esophagus, the diaphragmatic crura, the phrenoesophageal membrane, and the angle of His, but the LES and hiatal crura seem to be the major barriers (Fig. 10-1).

TABLE 10-1. SYMPTOMS OF GASTROESOPHAGEAL REFLUX DISEASE

Typical symptoms
• Heartburn
• Regurgitation and aspiration
• Water brash
• Chest pain
• Dysphagia
Atypical symptoms
• Chronic nausea
• Asthma
• Cough
• Hoarse throat
• Dental erosions

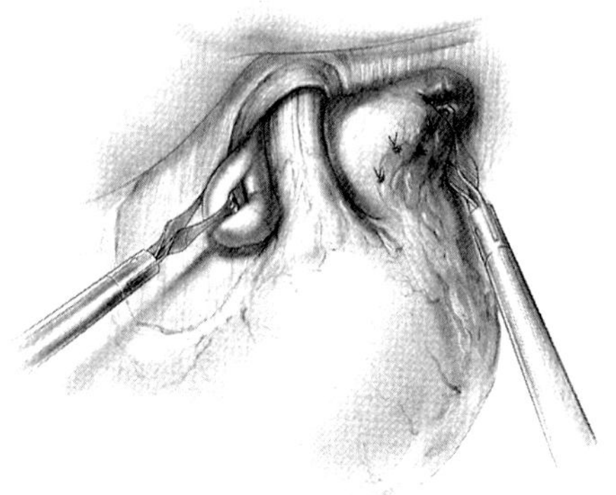

Fig. 10-1. Physiologic features controlling gastroesophageal reflux disease (GERD).

The LES separates two adjacent lower-pressure zones and normally remains tonically contracted except during swallowing, when it relaxes in advance of the peristaltic wave. LES contraction receives important amplification during inspiration and conditions in which the abdominal pressure is increased by contraction of the crural diaphragm. Reflux events in healthy individuals normally result from transient relaxation of the LES complex in which spontaneous, nonswallow-initiated events permit GER by obliterating the high-pressure zone through a vagally mediated mechanism, which is usually initiated by gastric or pharyngeal stimulation. Patients with GERD have reflux more frequently and for longer periods of time than healthy individuals. Reflux events may occur by three primary mechanisms:

1. Accompanying transient LES relaxations.
2. Stress reflux associated with a weakened LES.
3. A nonfunctional LES that cannot maintain competency, resulting in spontaneous GER.

The severity of esophagitis assessed by endoscopic appearance of the esophageal mucosa has been classified by Savary and colleagues as grade I (mild erythema), grade II (isolated ulcerations), grade III (confluent severe ulcerations), and grade IV (secondary complications including Barrett esophagus and stricture). Although a significant number of patients with clinical GERD have normal-appearing esophageal mucosa at endoscopy, patients with longstanding GERD may develop Barrett esophagus, a metaplastic columnarization of the esophageal mucosa that is associated with an increased risk of adenocarcinoma. Barrett esophagus is estimated to occur in approximately 10% of patients with chronic GERD, with these patients having more than 40 times greater risk of developing adenocarcinoma of the distal esophagus than those without Barrett esophagus. After LNF, most patients exhibit an increase in LES pressure, increased esophageal contractile pressure, and a resulting decrease in esophageal acid exposure.

DIAGNOSIS

Factors other than a defective LES may contribute to GERD. The esophageal body plays an important role in clearing acid present within its lumen. Esophageal peristaltic dysfunction is directly related to the degree of mucosal disease, and many patients with Barrett esophagus exhibit abnormalities of esophageal motor function. Abnormalities of the gastric reservoir may also predispose to GER, including gastric dilatation and delayed gastric emptying. Antireflux operations are designed solely to correct a functionally defective reflux barrier; therefore, tests that assess the function of the LES, esophageal body, and stomach may be appropriate in patients with GERD symptoms.

PREOPERATIVE TESTING

Many diagnostic modalities are available for studying patients in whom GERD is suspected (Table 10-2). A history of recurrent heartburn alone is usually adequate to establish the clinical diagnosis of GERD and initiate empiric medical therapy. However, investigations should be performed in patients with persistent symptoms or symptoms and signs indicating significant tissue injury (e.g., dysphagia, anemia, and guaiac positive stools) and in patients in whom the diagnosis is uncertain. Individuals who are being considered for antireflux surgery require additional tests of the anatomic and physiologic features of the stomach and esophagus.

In patients with typical symptoms of GERD, the minimal diagnostic evaluation is esophagogastroduodenoscopy (EGD). Esophageal manometry should be performed in all patients preoperatively to assess LES function and the adequacy of esophageal peristalsis. It may be helpful to perform 24-hour pH testing, but this is not mandatory in patients with typical symptoms if esophagitis is present. It does, however, provide a baseline that may be useful in postoperative follow-up. Patients without erosive esophagitis, with atypical symptoms of GERD, or with an atypical response to medical therapy require more detailed preoperative investigation.

TABLE 10-2. DIAGNOSTIC TESTS FOR GASTROESOPHAGEAL REFLUX DISEASE

Anatomic delineation
• EGD (+/− biopsy) • Contrast radiographs (barium swallow, upper gastrointestinal series)
Physiologic examinations
• 24-hr pH testing • Esophageal manometry • Impedance testing • Scintigraphy (esophageal/gastric emptying)

EGD, esophagogastroduodenoscopy.

ANATOMIC DELINEATION

EGD is an essential part of the evaluation of patients being considered for antireflux surgery. Barrett esophagus (metaplastic columnar epithelium) usually appears as salmon-colored mucosa extending up into the distal esophagus and is confirmed by biopsy. Given the increasing incidence of esophageal adenocarcinoma and the association between long-standing heartburn and adenocarcinoma, the gastroesophageal mucosa should be assessed endoscopically at least once in all patients with persistent or severe symptoms of GERD. If Barrett esophagus with high-grade dysplasia is discovered by biopsy, the patient should be considered for esophageal resection rather than antireflux surgery because of the high incidence of adenocarcinoma in these cases. Treatment of patients with Barrett esophagus with low-grade dysplasia is controversial. There is some evidence that a fundoplication can minimize the risk of dysplasia progression, and up to 40% of patients who have undergone Nissen fundoplication exhibit regression of dysplasia, particularly with short segment Barrett.

Contrast radiographs of the upper gastrointestinal tract may be helpful to assess the size of any associated hiatal hernia, to localize precisely the gastroesophageal junction in relation to the esophageal hiatus, and to qualitatively assess the adequacy of esophageal peristalsis and gastric emptying.

PHYSIOLOGIC EXAMINATIONS

The gold standard to confirm the presence of GER is a 24-hour esophageal pH assessment quantifying the number and duration of episodes of acid reflux into the esophagus. Furthermore, this test correlates subjective symptoms with reflux events and differentiates between upright and supine GER. This test requires prolonged cessation of proton pump inhibitors and usually an indwelling nasoesophageal catheter in an outpatient setting, which is uncomfortable, time-consuming, and relatively expensive. False-negative tests may result from patients refraining from normal dietary and physical activities during the time the nasoesophageal catheter is in place. Alternatively, a 24- to 48-hour esophageal pH assessment can be made using a wireless capsule (Bravo pH Monitoring System; Medtronics: Minneapolis, MN) that is attached to the distal esophagus endoscopically and transmits data to a monitor carried by the patient. After several days, the capsule disengages and passes through the gastrointestinal tract in about 5 to 7 days. This wireless system avoids the discomfort of a catheter-based system, allowing patients to resume their normal activities and diet during the study, and is therefore thought to collect more representative data on esophageal acid exposure.

Esophageal manometry should be performed in all patients before antireflux surgery is considered. With this test, the length, location, and pressure of the LES are assessed along with the ability of the LES to relax during swallowing. In addition, and more importantly, both the amplitude and efficacy of swallowing-induced peristalsis of the esophageal body are measured. Esophageal manometry may identify the rare individual with a primary motility abnormality (e.g., achalasia or scleroderma). The degree of peristaltic failure caused by GERD can also be assessed. The surgeon may ascertain whether a 360-degree fundoplication will likely result in significant dysphagia, thereby allowing a tailoring of the antireflux operation.

INDICATIONS

Virtually all patients should receive a short-term (2-month) trial of intensive medical therapy before considering an antireflux

TABLE 10-3. LIFESTYLE MODIFICATIONS FOR GASTROESOPHAGEAL REFLUX DISEASE

- Weight loss
- Alteration of diet
  - ⋆ Avoid chocolate, peppermint, fats, onions/garlic, alcohol, caffeine, and nicotine
  - ⋆ Nothing by mouth for 2–3 hours before bedtime
- Elevation of head of bed 6–10 inches
- Limit potentially precipitating activities, such as bending over or strenuous exercise

TABLE 10-4. INDICATIONS FOR OPERATION

Objective evidence of GERD plus:
- Complications of GERD not responding to medical therapy (e.g., esophagitis, stricture, recurrent aspiration or pneumonia, Barrett esophagus)
- GERD symptoms interfering with lifestyle, despite medical therapy
- Paraesophageal hernia with GERD
- Need for continuous drug treatment in a patient desiring discontinuation of medical therapy (e.g., financial burden, noncompliance, intolerance to medication, lifestyle choice, young age)

GERD, gastroesophageal reflux disease.

operation. Modern medical treatment of reflux disease is aimed at decreasing gastric acidity and reducing esophageal exposure to gastric contents with the goal of healing the injured esophageal mucosa, eliminating symptoms, and preventing or treating the complications of GERD. The primary tenets of GERD management include lifestyle modifications (Table 10-3), medical therapy to control symptoms, and attempts to convert to maintenance therapy. Unfortunately, recommended lifestyle changes are usually ignored, and although most patients with GERD can be managed adequately with proton pump inhibitors, many eventually require escalating doses over time, relapse quickly when medication is stopped, or desire to be free of medications and their significant expense. There is also a small group of patients who experience intolerable side effects of proton pump inhibitors, such as headaches or diarrhea. It is this group of patients who may benefit greatly from LARS.

Some features of preoperative testing predict a poor response to long-term acid suppression therapy and should be considered as the rationale for referral to surgical therapy earlier in the course. These features include diminished contractility of the esophageal body (contraction amplitudes <30 mmHg), markedly hypotensive LES, severe erosive esophagitis that is poorly responsive to antacid therapy, and, perhaps, Barrett esophagus.

Before considering a surgical approach to GERD, the diagnosis of GERD and its cause must be clearly established. For a patient with typical symptoms (heartburn or regurgitation), at least one additional piece of objective evidence of reflux must be present. For patients with atypical symptoms, two pieces of corroborative evidence of GERD should be required. In addition to objective evidence of GERD, the most common indications for performing antireflux surgery can be summarized as follows (Table 10-4): (1) complications of GERD not responding to medical therapy; (2) GERD symptoms interfering with lifestyle despite medical therapy; (3) GERD associated with paraesophageal hiatal hernia; and (4) chronic GERD requiring continuous proton pump inhibitor therapy in a young patient.

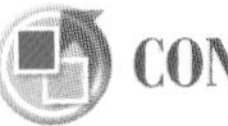

CONTRAINDICATIONS

There are few absolute contraindications to LARS. These include the inability to tolerate a general anesthetic or laparoscopy and an uncorrectable coagulopathy. Numerous conditions, however, render LARS more difficult and should be considered relative contraindications. These factors include previous upper abdominal surgery, particularly operations around the diaphragm or esophageal hiatus, and severe obesity. In obese patients, the omentum and gastrosplenic ligament may be bulky and difficult to retract adequately, and fatty infiltration of the left lateral section of the liver may make exposure of the esophageal hiatus problematic. It is thought that a higher failure rate of LARS in the morbidly obese stems from an increased intraabdominal pressure creating tension on the fundal wrap and crural repair. Consideration should be given to performing a gastric bypass, which may be equally effective in reducing GERD symptoms while also attacking the underlying problem of morbid obesity. Esophageal shortening secondary to stricture can prevent mobilization of the distal esophagus 2 to 3 cm below the diaphragm and the creation of a tension-free intraabdominal gastric wrap.

SURGICAL TECHNIQUE

Laparoscopic antireflux operations are advanced laparoscopic procedures requiring skills that are best developed and practiced in a nonclinical setting to facilitate efficiency and improved technical performance in the operating room. Technical principles common to all fundoplications include the following: (1) Dissection should be performed away from the esophagus, and the esophagus should never be directly grasped or manipulated with traumatic instruments. (2) All dissection must be performed under direct vision. (3) The fundus, rather than any other part of the stomach, must be plicated around the esophagus, rather than around the proximal stomach. (4) There must be no tension present at the conclusion of the fundoplication, either axial (tending to pull the repair up through the hiatus into the mediastinum) or rotational (pulling the fundus counterclockwise back to the left, creating a twist of the lower esophagus). As with most other operations, many technical variations have been described by various authorities on LARS. In the following narrative, the authors describe their practice at the Northwestern University Feinberg School of Medicine and comment on common alternative approaches.

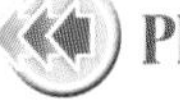

PREOPERATIVE PLANNING

During the preoperative office visit, the expectations and risks of LARS are discussed with the patient. Patients are counseled that if at any point a laparoscopic approach cannot be continued safely, the operation will be converted to an open procedure. Gastric or esophageal perforation; injury to the vagus nerves, spleen, or other abdominal viscera; pneumothorax; dysphagia; and bloating are all delineated as potential complications. Disruption of the crural repair or wrap, as well as migration of the fundoplication into the mediastinum, may require reoperation. Healthy patients are admitted the day of surgery after an overnight fast.

Patient Positioning and Equipment

The patient must be carefully positioned to protect both the patient from injury and the surgeon from undue muscular fatigue (Fig. 10-2). The surgeon stands between the patient's abducted legs facing directly forward during the operation. The legs are abducted on flat padded boards, which allow the knees to be extended and minimize the potential for lower extremity neurovascular traction injury. Video monitors are positioned at the head of the table to allow ergonomically neutral visualization by the surgeon and assistants. The patient must be firmly affixed to the operating table and padded in the appropriate locations because the table is generally maintained in a steep heads-up position to allow gravity to displace the abdominal viscera from the subdiaphragmatic region. The authors' practice is to use a vacuum beanbag mattress that provides gentle support around the patient's sides and perineum to prevent intraoperative movement.

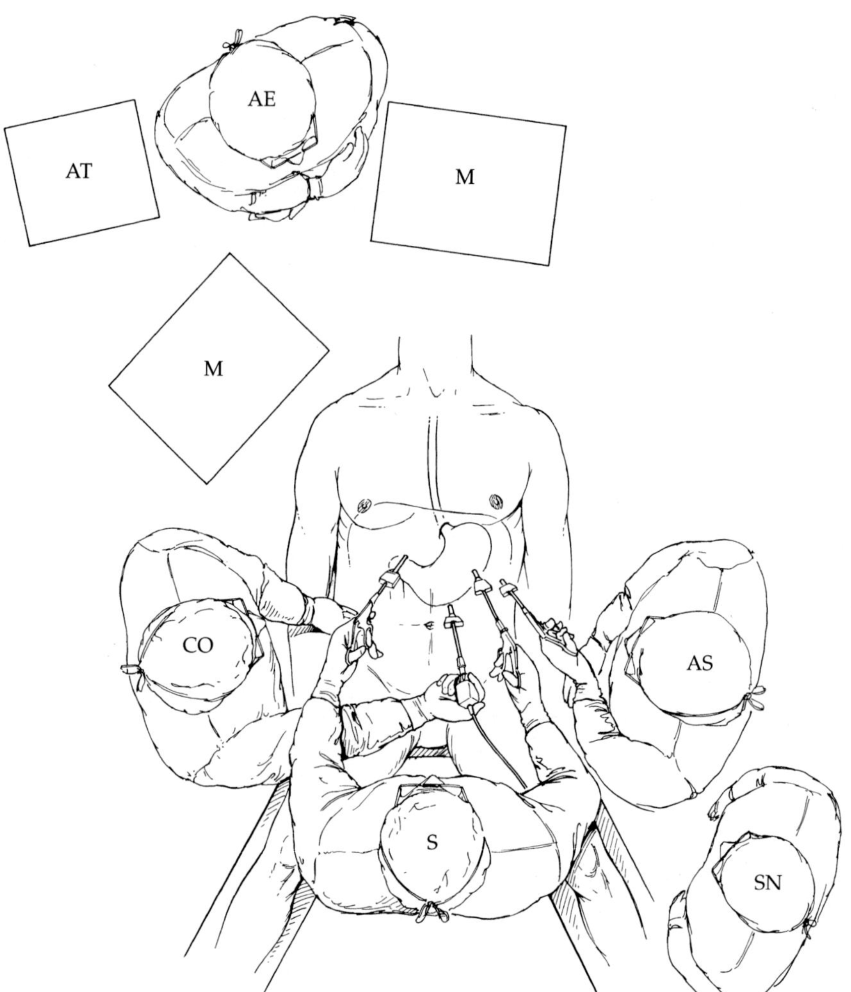

Fig. 10-2. Operating room layout. In this case the camera operator sits on the patient's left and the assistant stands to the patient's right.

Several basic varieties of instrumentation are recommended to facilitate the performance of LARS. These include angled laparoscopes (either 30 or 45 degrees) that allow alternative views of the operative field and adequate visualization of the retrogastric and retroesophageal regions. An adequate, atraumatic liver retractor is imperative to allow the left lateral section of the liver to be elevated for prolonged periods without capsular injury. We use a self-retaining device to hold the liver retractor in an immobile position throughout the operation. Atraumatic grasping instruments should be available, including Babcock-type forceps. Appropriate instrumentation for achieving hemostasis and dividing tissues bloodlessly should be used. These instruments include bipolar or monopolar electrosurgical devices, and ultrasonic coagulation and cutting devices. Also, a flexible endoscope should be available to allow intraluminal evaluation of the esophagogastric region should the need arise.

Abdominal Access and Port Placement

An open or closed technique may be used to access the peritoneal cavity. The laparoscope is inserted, and a visual exploration of the abdominal cavity is performed with particular attention paid to the area immediately posterior to the initial trocar insertion site. The patient is then positioned in a steep heads-up position, and the accessory ports are placed under direct vision. We generally use 5-mm diameter ports for all positions except for the surgeon's right hand and often for the laparoscope port. Surgeon preference and instrument use pattern dictate the size of the port used for the surgeon's right hand. We continue to use a 10-mm port because an SH-size needle can be inserted through the valve, whereas if a 5-mm port is used, straight or "ski" needles must be used for suturing.

The esophageal hiatus is usually located directly posterior to the xiphoid process. Laparoscopic instruments are generally 30 to 35 cm in length. Ideally, the instrument midpoint should be located at the level of the abdominal wall (fulcrum) during critical portions of advanced laparoscopic procedures to maximize its range of motion during tissue manipulation and to establish a 1:1 ratio between external hand movements and internal instrument tip translations. The ports are thus positioned in an arc between 10 and 15 cm inferior to the xiphoid process and costal arch. Because the esophagus generally enters the abdomen from a slightly right-to-left orientation and the falciform ligament and liver limit the right lateral placement of the port for the surgeon's left hand, we generally place the laparoscope to the left of the midline in a supraumbilical location approximately 12 to 15 cm caudal to the xiphoid process

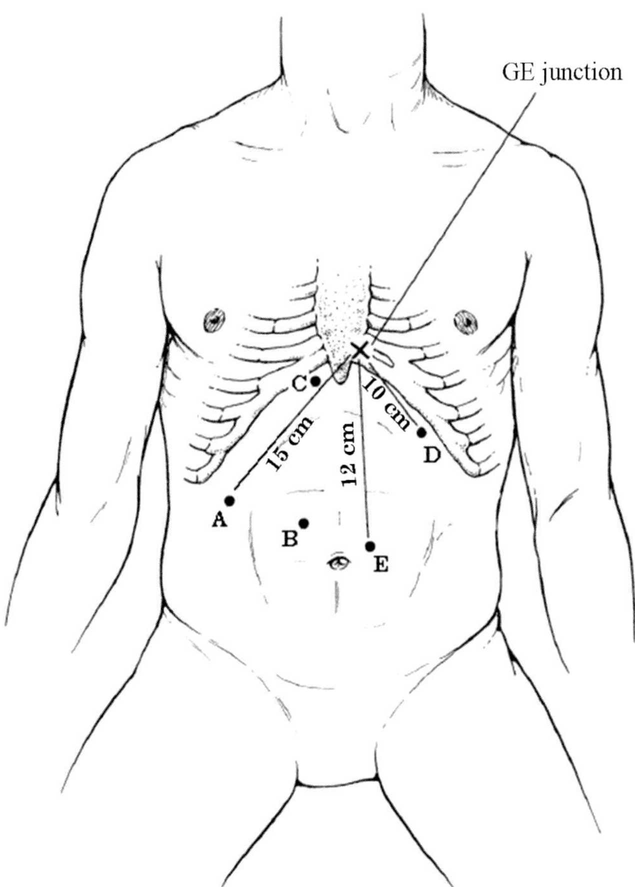

Fig. 10-3. Port placement. A. Liver retractor port. **B.** Assistant port. **C.** Surgeon's left-hand port. **D.** Surgeon's right-hand port. **E.** Camera port.

(Fig. 10-3). This is nearly always superior to the umbilicus. A periumbilical port site is generally too far inferior on the abdominal wall for operations at and around the esophageal hiatus. For optimal visual orientation, the working instruments should be entering the operative field from a 30- to 60-degree angle on either side of the laparoscope. With the camera port to the left of the midline, the surgeon's right-hand port is generally 10 cm from the xiphoid and two finger breadths below the left costal margin, and the surgeon's left hand position is generally just inferior and to the right of the xiphoid process beneath the right subcostal margin. With the laparoscope directed between the operating hands, the surgeon works straight ahead, avoids the problem of the video "mirror image" caused by working back toward the camera, and maximizes visual cues allowing accurate perception of the three-dimensional relationships. The liver retractor port is placed in the right of the abdomen 15 cm from the xiphoid in the subcostal region. This port should enter below the right liver edge to avoid liver injury during the passage of instruments. The assistant's port is placed in the right midrectus region approximately midway from the liver retractor port and camera port. We usually place the port for the surgeon's left-hand instruments last. The precise location of this last port depends to an extent on the size and location of the retracted liver and the shape of the liver retractor itself. A Veress needle can be used to "sound out" potential sites on the abdominal wall for this port before the incision is made and the final trocar and sheath are inserted.

Other surgeons have described alternative techniques in which the assistant stands to the left of the patient and manipulates tissue through a port placed in the left subcostal region. Others prefer the laparoscopic camera port to be placed in a midline position. Both of these alternative and port positions are valid, and the individual surgeon must decide the optimal positioning of his or her operating team.

Initial Dissection

The gastroesophageal fat pad is grasped by the assistant and pulled caudally and to the patient's left, placing traction on the gastrohepatic omentum. The gastrohepatic omentum is divided using the ultrasonic shears, beginning just superior to the hepatic branch of the vagus nerve (Fig. 10-4, page 96). The surgeon must be wary of aberrant left hepatic arteries running beside this nerve. Although these arteries are encountered in less than 5% of patients, they may comprise the majority of arterial inflow to the left lateral section of the liver. The hepatic branch of the vagus nerve generally does not need to be divided to gain adequate visualization as long as one is using an angled laparoscope. The gastrohepatic omentum is divided up to the level of the right crus of the diaphragm, and the phrenoesophageal membrane is divided in a transverse direction, with care taken to divide only the most anterior portion to prevent injury to the underlying esophagus and anterior vagus nerve. The gastric fundus is then pulled inferiorly and to the right. The gastrophrenic ligament is divided to mobilize the gastric cardia.

A meticulous dissection is then undertaken around the esophageal hiatus (Fig. 10-5, page 96). During the hiatal dissection, the assistant grasps the epiphrenic fat pad and retracts inferiorly to place tension on the distal esophagus. With the phrenoesophageal membrane already divided, it is generally easy to insinuate a blunt-tipped instrument just medial to the right crus of the diaphragm and to establish a plane between the esophagus and the right crus. The surgeon's left-hand instrument grasps or pushes the crus to the patient's right while the right-hand instrument gradually and gently sweeps the esophagus and periesophageal tissue to the left to bluntly mobilize the distal esophagus. The posterior vagus nerve is generally clearly seen and is swept along with the esophagus to the left. This mobilization continues in an orad direction as far as possible and then distally to the level of the crus. The tissue attached to the medial border of the base of the right crus is divided until the origin of the right crus from the left crus is visualized from the right side of the esophagus.

Once the right side of the esophagus has been mobilized, the surgeon's right-hand instrument sweeps anterior to the esophagus and elevates the anterior crural arch while gently pushing the esophagus posteriorly with the blunt side of the left-hand instrument. The posterior-medial aspect of the left crus is visualized, and all of the periesophageal tissue is swept posteriorly to develop the plane to the left of the esophagus. Generally, the anterior vagus nerve and left pleura are visualized at

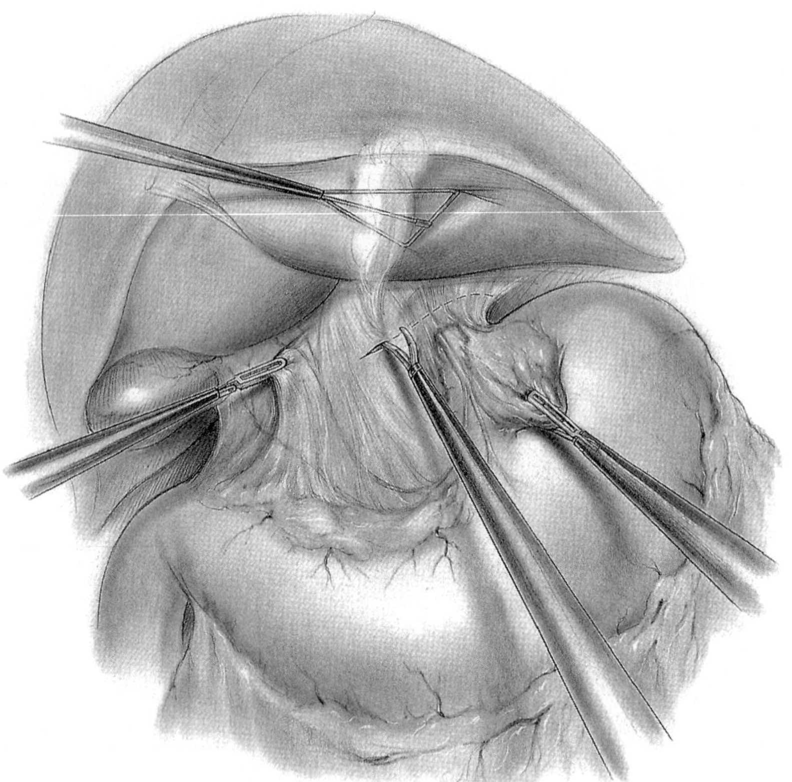

Fig. 10-4. Initial dissection: division of gastrohepatic ligament superior to the hepatic branch of the vagus nerve.

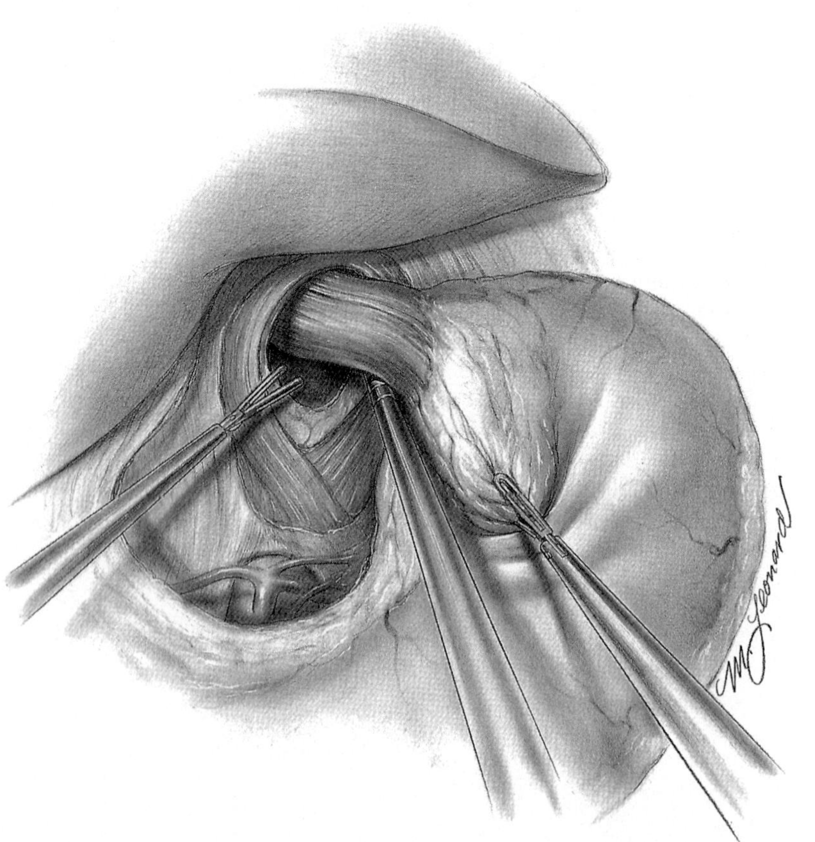

Fig. 10-5. Retraction of the fat pad, blunt dissection, and creation of a window posterior to the esophagus.

this time. The initial dissection of the mediastinum is therefore completed, freeing the esophagus from the pleura, aorta, and lateral crural attachments. The anterior and posterior vagus nerves are clearly identified and maintained alongside the esophagus to avoid injury. If the pleura is inadvertently lacerated during the dissection, the surgeon must communicate with the anesthetist that this event has occurred. With the assumption that the lung parenchyma is not injured, the carbon dioxide pneumothorax generally poses no serious complications to the patient. The anesthetist can increase the airway pressure while the surgeon slightly decreases the insufflator's pressure limit, and adequate ventilation and perfusion can usually be maintained.

The gastric fundus is then mobilized. The left lateral border of the fundus is grasped, elevated, and retracted to the right while the gastrosplenic ligament is grasped, elevated, and retracted to the left. Division of the short gastric vessels is started at a point 10 to 15 cm inferior to the angle of His (Fig. 10-6). The precise location is different with each patient, and there may be difficulty in creating a "floppy" wrap if an inadequate length of fundus is mobilized. We select a point orad to the most proximal gastroepiploic vessels, which are identified by their caudally directed orientation. At this site, a short gastric vessel is identified visually, and a "window" is made between the short gastric vessel and the gastric wall. With the use of a small amount of blunt dissection, entry can usually be made into the free lesser sac, identified by visualizing the space bounded medially by the posterior gastric wall. Once entry into the lesser sac has been gained, traction on the stomach and countertraction on the gastrosplenic ligament is maintained to align the greater curvature of the stomach with the visual axis of the laparoscope. The short gastric vessels and all other posterior attachments to the fundus are then divided sequentially, proceeding from distal to proximal until the entire fundus has been mobilized.

Division of this tissue may be performed with individually placed clips and sharp division, ultrasonic shears, or bipolar electrosurgery. Prospective randomized trials have shown the ultrasonic shears to perform this task more rapidly and more cheaply than clipping and sharp division. All structures tethering the fundus, including the short gastric vessels, posterior gastric vessels, and gastrosplenic and gastropancreatic ligaments, are divided

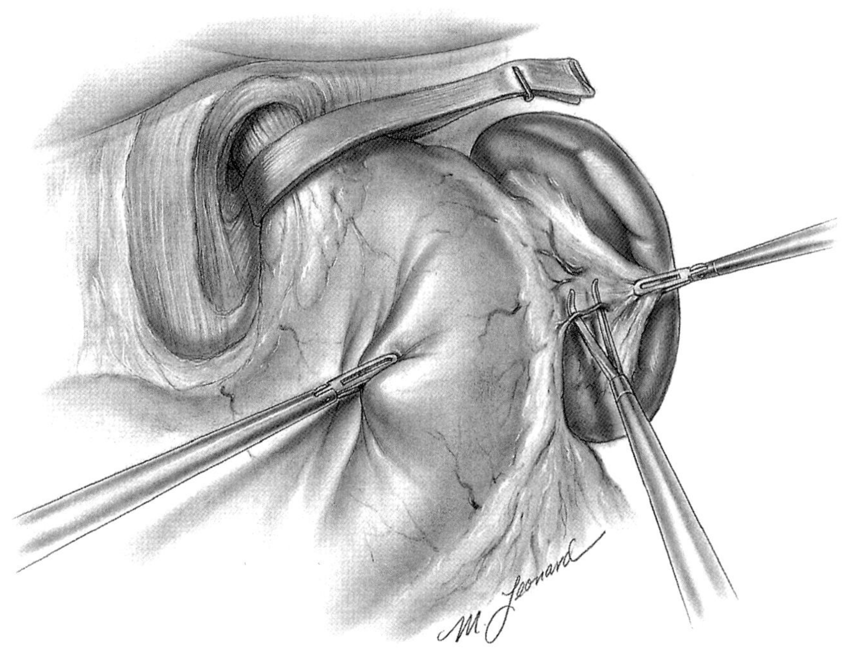

Fig. 10-6. Division of the short gastric vessels to the base of the left crus to allow complete fundic mobilization.

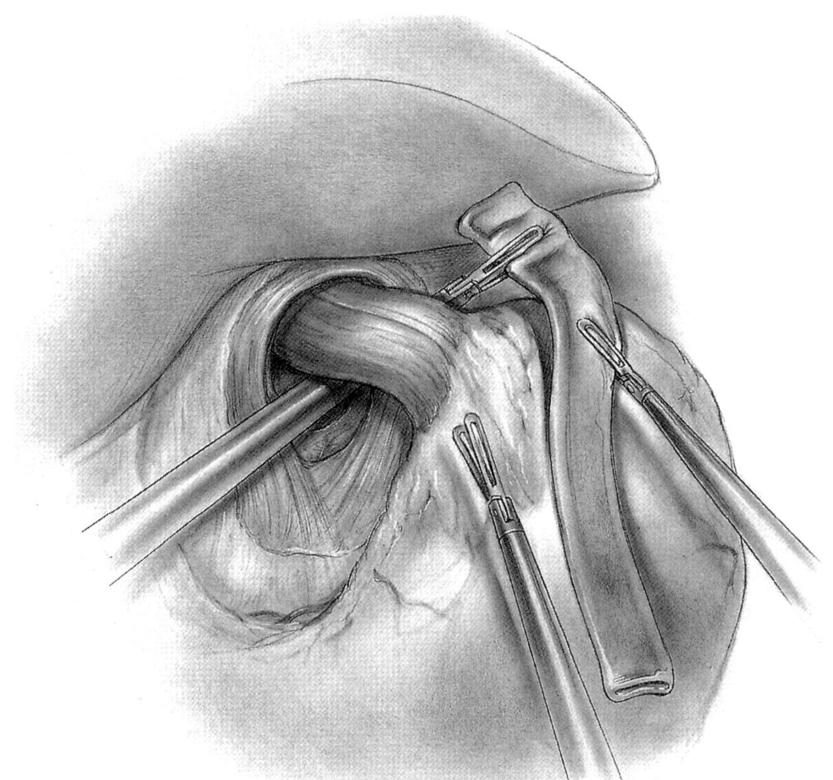

Fig. 10-7. A Penrose drain is placed around the esophagus or the gastric fundus is pulled posterior and to the right of the esophagus to provide inferior retraction.

up to the angle of His. We and others have shown an improved outcome with regard to dysphagia and wrap disruption when the fundus is fully mobilized. Division of the short gastric vessels is necessary in certain anatomic situations to allow a tension-free fundoplication. Increased skill and confidence are developed by performing this maneuver routinely. Dividing the short gastric vessels enhances visualization of the high retrogastric space, which facilitates division of the gastropancreatic ligaments and the posterior gastric vessels. The sites of insertion of the short gastric vessels also pinpoint the lateral border of the fundus, which will later be used for the fundoplication. For all of these reasons, we advocate full mobilization of the fundus during all fundoplications.

After complete fundic mobilization, the retroesophageal space is visualized from the anatomic left side. The medial border of the left crus of the diaphragm is dissected back to its junction with the right crus, joining the plane previously begun from the right side. A large window is thereby created posterior to the esophagus and proximal stomach and anterior to both crura. Once the window is created, many surgeons place a Penrose drain loop for inferior traction on the gastroesophageal junction (Fig. 10-7). This is a useful maneuver and should be encouraged if traction is difficult to achieve by other means. We generally skip this step and use the gastroesophageal fat pad or fundus for inferior traction. A grasper is placed through the retroesophageal window from right to left, which grasps the apex of the fundus and pulls it back through the window to the right side of the esophagus. With caudad traction placed on the wrapped fundus itself, the gastroesophageal junction and distal esophagus can be brought further into the abdominal cavity.

Once the fundus has been pulled to the right behind the esophagus, it is checked for rotational tension and torsion. To assess rotational tension, the wrapped fundus is released and observed. If it retracts back around the esophagus to the left, there is tension that must be eliminated by dividing more fundic attachments. To check for a twist or entrapment of the wrapped fundus in the posterior window, the "shoeshine" maneuver is performed (Fig. 10-8, page 98). The leading edge of the fundus that has been passed behind and to the right of the esophagus is grasped, along with the fundus to the left of the esophagus. The fundus is then retracted back and forth to make sure that it slides easily and is not twisted.

Before closing the crura and constructing the fundoplication, the length of intraabdominal esophagus is assessed. The esophagus must be mobilized to allow at least 3 cm to reside within the abdomen

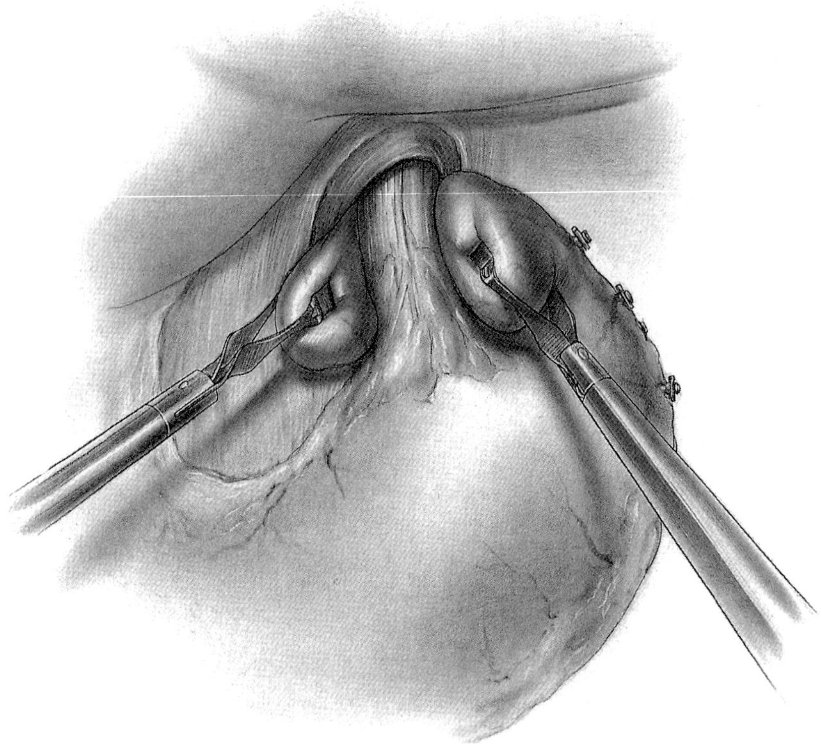

Fig. 10-8. The "shoeshine" maneuver.

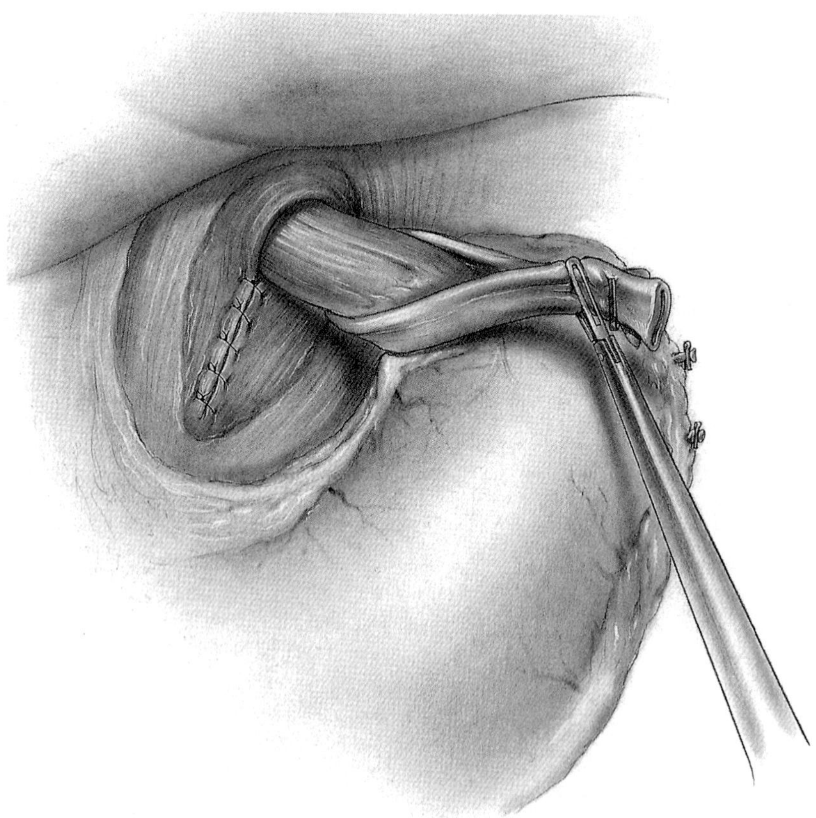

Fig. 10-9. Closure of the crural opening posterior to the esophagus with interrupted, nonabsorbable suture.

when the traction is released. If this is not evident, further esophageal mobilization must be performed within the mediastinum. If the length of esophagus below the diaphragm is less than 3 cm, an esophageal-lengthening procedure should be performed.

After adequate esophageal mobilization, the crura are reapproximated posterior to the esophagus. Inferior and lateral traction is maintained on the proximal stomach either by an atraumatic grasper on the wrapped fundus or with the Penrose drain sling. Interrupted sutures are used to close the crura posterior to the esophagus (Fig. 10-9). We generally use 2-0 gauge, nonabsorbable, braided polyester sutures on an SH needle for this purpose. If there is a large hiatal hernia or if the crural closure appears to be under tension, pledgets are used to reinforce the crural sutures. The intraabdominal crural fascia is incorporated in the sutures rather than the muscle body alone. The crura are closed, beginning posteriorly near the crural junction and then proceeding anteriorly toward the esophagus, until they lightly touch the empty esophagus. Once the closure is completed, it should be possible to pass an instrument between the esophagus and the crura. Esophageal dilators stiffen the esophagus and make it difficult to retract the esophagus anteriorly for adequate visualization of the posterior crural closure and are therefore not used during crural closure. Occasionally, there may be a large crural defect anterior to the esophagus that may require repair. Similar to posterior crural closure, anterior crural closure should begin near the crural arch and then proceed toward the esophagus, with the surgeon making sure to incorporate crural fascia. The completed closure should also lightly touch the empty esophagus and allow the passage of an instrument between the esophagus and crura.

Fundoplication

Most authors advocate placing an indwelling bougie dilator during creation of the wrap. It is probably not imperative that a dilator be inserted as long as the surgeon has adequate experience in placing the sutures, understands the three-dimensional relationships, and avoids excessively narrowing the gastroesophageal junction. We serially pass 50F and 60F Maloney dilators and suture the fundoplication with a 50F to 60F dilator in place. Great care must be taken during the passage of the dilators to prevent inadvertent perforation of the esophagus or stomach. The gastroesophageal junction should be maintained in a nonangulated position by the surgeon and assistant. The dilators are placed under direct vision, and clear and constant communication is maintained between the individual inserting the dilator and the surgical team. The two sides of the fundus are then abutted around the distal esophagus to ascertain whether a tension-free wrap may be achieved.

The lateral edge of the fundus to the left of the esophagus is then sutured to the leading edge of the wrapped fundus to the right of the esophagus. Three 2-0 gauge, nonabsorbable, braided polyester sutures on SH needles are used, taking deep seromuscular suture bites in the fundus to the left and right of the esophagus (Fig. 10-10). At least two of these sutures incorporate anterior muscularis of the esophagus to the right of the anterior vagus nerve. The first suture opposes fundus to fundus, without incorporating the esophageal wall. After this first suture is tied, the location and orientation of the wrap are checked and the fundoplication may be slid up or down the esophagus and positioned just proximal to the gastroesophageal junction. Great care must be taken during knotting of the sutures to prevent anterior traction, which could cause a tear of the esophageal wall. The sutures may be tied either with intracorporeal or extracorporeal knotting techniques. The dilator is then removed, and the wrap is checked for degree of laxity by passing a 5-mm diameter instrument between the left side of the wrap and the esophagus. The length of the fundoplication should be less than 2 cm and it must be situated around the esophagus rather than inferiorly on the proximal stomach. The gastroesophageal fat pad is not excised in most patients unless it is so large that it interferes with the ability to perform an adequate fundoplication. The fat pad functions as a handle and is a visual marker of the angle of His. The suggested orientation of the wrap (the point on the esophagus at which the two sides of the fundus are joined) varies in different centers. Some surgeons advocate that this junction be placed at the right lateral position of the esophagus, presumably to prevent lateral traction. We tend to place the sutures to the right of the anterior midline of the esophageal wall, with the esophagus sutures placed just to the right of the anterior vagus nerve.

With the "short, floppy" wrap completed, the liver retractor is removed, and the undersurface of the liver is examined for capsular tears or bleeding. The upper abdomen is aspirated and checked for hemostasis. The ports are then removed under direct vision. Any port larger than 5 mm in diameter and located below the costal margin on exsufflation of the abdomen should have its fascia closed with heavy-gauge suture. We perform this approximation using a fascial closure device under direct vision rather than attempting to suture the deep fascia through the small skin incision after removing the laparoscopic instruments. The abdomen is exsufflated, the ports are removed, and each incision is infiltrated with local anesthetic.

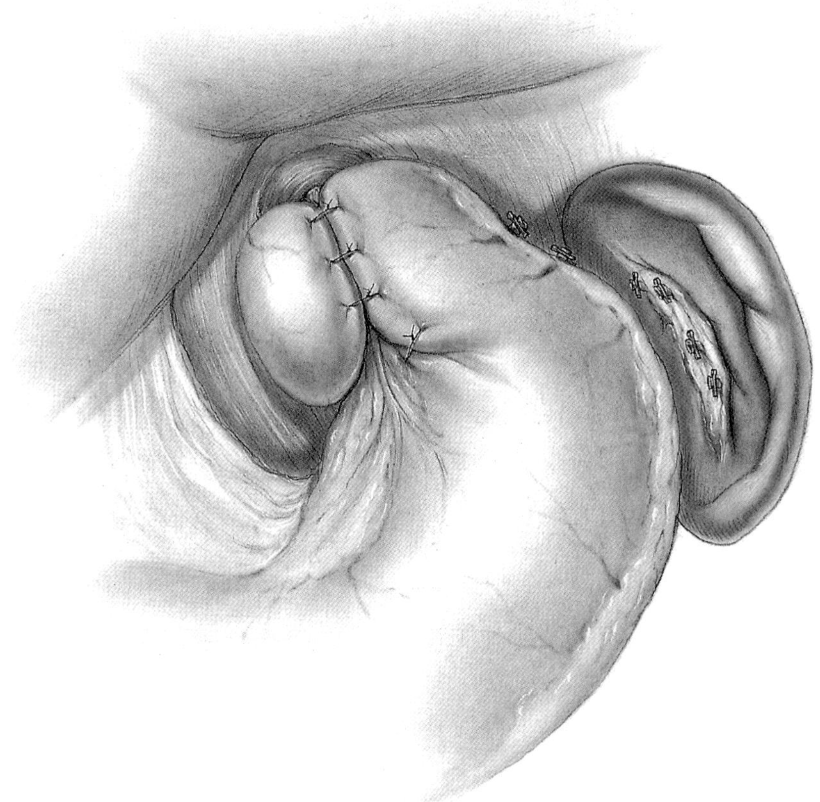

Fig. 10-10. Creation of a 2-cm wrap with three interrupted sutures approximately 5 to 8 mm apart.

 COMPLICATIONS

Pleural injury and pneumothorax are the result of inadvertent entry into the pleura when the esophagus is dissected in the mediastinum. Clinically significant pleural injuries rarely occur. In our experience, the incidence of pleural tears during LNF is 10%. The most common complications from pleural tears occurring during laparoscopic esophageal operations are hypotension and, rarely, increased airway pressures or postoperative pneumothorax. The balance between positive airway pressure and pneumoperitoneum pressure may be adjusted if necessary. Dissection close to the esophagus may prevent pleural injury. At the conclusion of the procedure when a pneumothorax has occurred, suction is applied transhiatally to the mediastinum while the anesthetist administers vital capacity breaths to allow venting of the pneumoperitoneum through the trocar sites. A postoperative chest radiograph is obtained only if the patient experiences respiratory distress. Bleeding (short gastric vessels) is an uncommon complication, which can be managed with the harmonic scalpel or a clip. Splenic injury and liver injury during retraction and dissection can occur. An atraumatic retractor and gentle, meticulous technique will in general prevent significant hemorrhage. Most hepatic bleeding can be stopped by high-wattage cautery, direct pressure, or topical hemostatic agents. Esophageal perforation occurs in less than 1% of cases. Patients with severe periesophageal inflammation are at greater risk for injury given that tissue planes are less clear. Prevention of injury includes circumferentially dissecting the esophagus under direct vision with an angled laparoscope and not directly grasping the esophagus for retraction. Simple perforations are repaired by placing fine dissolvable interrupted sutures with coverage by the fundoplication.

POSTOPERATIVE MANAGEMENT

Before leaving the operating room, the patient is administered intravenous ketorolac and ondansetron. A nasogastric tube is rarely placed. The patient is allowed sips of water and ice chips the afternoon of the operation, clear liquids the following morning, and then a soft diet for lunch the afternoon after the operation. The patient is discharged if this meal is tolerated. We admit patients to the hospital after the operation, but some groups have performed true outpatient LARS. The patient receives scheduled ketorolac and ondansetron intravenously through the first 12 to 18 hours after the operation to minimize the need for narcotics and to diminish the chance of postoperative vomiting, which can lead to disruption of the crural closure and migration of the wrap into the chest. Because of perifundoplication edema narrowing the esophagus in the early postoperative interval, the patient is maintained on a soft diet for the first 2 to 4 weeks. Should the patient experience pain out of proportion to what is expected, or if the patient vomits in the early postoperative period, a water-soluble contrast swallow radiograph is obtained to evaluate for disruption or displacement of the wrap or unrecognized mucosal perforation. The patients are seen in the outpatient office at 2 to 4 weeks after the operation. Although rapid resumption of full activity is encouraged, activities requiring diaphragmatic straining, such as heavy lifting, are discouraged for 4 to 6 weeks after the operation.

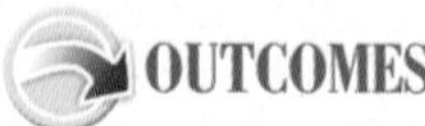

OUTCOMES

Results of LNF have shown low rates of perioperative morbidity and mortality. Conversion from a laparoscopic to an open procedure is higher early in a surgeon's experience with the operation, but in most series the conversion rate is well below 5%. The operative time averages 1 to 3 hours, with a clear learning curve. The duration of postoperative hospitalization is usually less than 2 days with anecdotal reports of outpatient LARS. Patients experience minimal postoperative pain and have few respiratory and wound complications. Perioperative complications requiring reoperation, such as esophageal perforation and wrap migration into the chest, occur in less than 1% of patients.

Common postoperative complaints include dysphagia, abdominal bloating, an inability to belch, and increased flatulence. Dysphagia is a common problem early after the operation but diminishes over time, such that only 10% to 15% of all patients will experience occasional mild dysphagia and only 1% to 2% of patients will require esophageal dilatation. Many patients with GERD develop the habit of swallowing frequently to promote esophageal clearance of acid, leading to aerophagia. With a tight fundoplication, an inability to belch with bloating may occur but often resolves over time.

At long-term follow-up, typical GERD symptoms are markedly reduced after LNF. Recent studies looking at outcomes 5 to10 years after LARS prove long-term durability, continuing efficacy, improved quality of life and patient satisfaction.

Biertho et al. demonstrated long-lasting increase in esophageal contractile pressures in patients who had preoperative esophageal dysmotilty. Patients who preoperatively had normal esophageal motility continued to have normal esophageal function after LNF.

A study comparing LARS and proton pump inhibitor (PPI) therapy after 7 years demonstrated that although both means of therapy are efficacious, there are a number of patients suboptimally treated with PPIs. Those patients who were eventually treated with LARS were able to achieve greater symptom-free improvement and patient satisfaction when compared to those maintained on PPIs alone. In a cohort of patients who underwent LARS studied by Dallemagne et al, 93% and 89.5% of patients reported significant freedom from reflux symptoms at 5 and 10 years respectively. In addition, patients undergoing LARS showed significantly better quality of life scores at 10 years when compared to matched patients on long-term PPI therapy. These and similar studies also showed 5% to 19% of patients were using PPIs at long-term follow-up after LARS, which is in stark contrast to data previously reported by Spechler and colleagues.

The learning curve for LARS is approximately 30 to 50 operations and is reflected by decreasing operative time and diminishing rates of complications and anatomic failures. Failed fundoplications can take several forms (Fig. 10-11). Postoperative dysphagia may be attributable to excessively tight closure of the esophageal hiatus, a tight wrap, or tension on the wrap causing twisting of the lower esophagus. A fundoplication-associated complication after LARS is the migration of the wrap through the hiatus into the mediastinum. This is often heralded by new-onset substernal or epigastric pain rather than reflux symptoms. The wrap itself may disrupt or migrate down onto the stomach (the so-called "slipped" Nissen), but this complication was more frequent after open Nissen fundoplication than after laparoscopic fundoplication. We have reviewed our experience with anatomic fundoplication failure. Fundoplication disruption or migration is associated with surgical inexperience and the shortcomings of the surgical technique, presence of a large hiatal hernia, and occurrence of diaphragmatic stressors. To prevent fundoplication failure, the surgeon must carefully select patients, perform the operation with specific attention to full mobilization of the fundus and esophagus, and close the crura around the esophagus adequately. The management of the fundoplication failures after LARS is complex and discussed in Chapter 13.

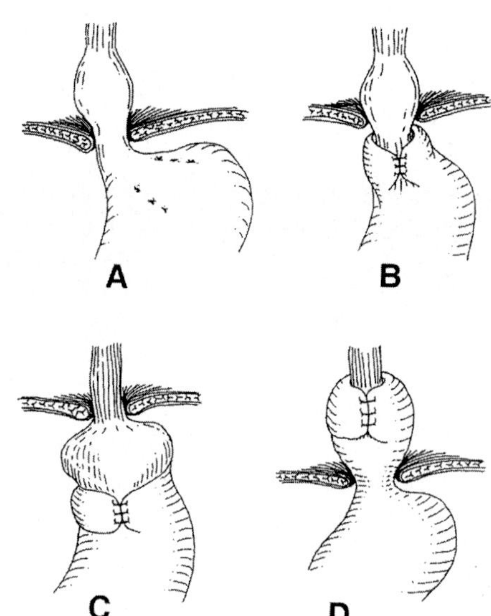

Fig. 10-11. Types of fundoplication failures: **A.** Disrupted wrap. **B.** Sliding hiatal hernia with wrap in abdomen. **C.** "Slipped" fundoplication onto proximal stomach. **D.** Intrathoracic migration of the fundoplication.

CONCLUSION

Advances in surgical instrumentation and techniques have allowed the majority of patients requiring surgical therapy of GERD to undergo a laparoscopic procedure that maintains the principles established over many years with open fundoplication. The minimally invasive approach and the excellent outcomes reported with short- and long-term follow-up have lowered the threshold for surgical intervention and have established the LNF as the gold standard for surgical management of GERD. Laparoscopic Nissen fundoplication provides for a durable cure of GERD and has been shown to be a safe option with similar results to its open counterpart. Furthermore, greater long-term patient satisfaction and improved quality of life are achieved when comparing patients undergoing LARS versus life-long medical therapy. These results justify the vital role of LARS in the paradigm of GERD management and the rationale for its early utilization in the treatment of patients with severe GERD.

SUGGESTED READING

Biertho L, Sebajang H, Anvari M. Effects of laparoscopic Nissen fundoplication on esophageal motility. *Surg Endosc* 2006;20:619–623.

Dallemagne B, Weerts J, Markiewicz S, et al. Clinical results of laparoscopic fundoplication at ten years after surgery. *Surg Endosc* 2006;20:159–165.

DeMeester TR, Bonavina L, Albertucci M. Nissen fundoplication for gastroesophageal reflux disease: evaluation of primary repair in 100 consecutive patients. *Ann Surg* 1986;204:9–20.

DeVault KR, Castell DO. Guidelines for the diagnosis and treatment of gastroesophageal reflux disease. Practice Parameters Committee of the American College of Gastroenterology. *Arch Intern Med* 1995;155:2165–2173.

Hunter JG, Swanstrom L, Waring JP. Dysphagia after laparoscopic antireflux surgery. The impact of operative technique. *Ann Surg* 1996;224:51–57.

Hunter JG, Trus TL, Branum GD, et al. A physiological approach to laparoscopic fundoplication for gastroesophageal reflux disease. *Ann Surg* 1996;223:673–687.

Lagergren J, Bergstrom R, Lindgren A, et al. Symptomatic gastroesophageal reflux as a risk factor for esophageal adenocarcinoma. *N Engl J Med* 1999;340:825–831.

Mehta S, Bennett J, Mahon D, et al. Prospective trial of laparoscopic Nissen fundoplication versus proton pump inhibitor therapy for gastroesophageal reflux disease: seven-year follow-up. *J Gastrointest Surg* 2006;10:1312–1317.

Nissen R. Gastropexy and "fundoplication" in surgical treatment of hiatal hernia. *Am J Dig Dis* 1961;6:959–961.

Peters JH, DeMeester TR, Crookes P, et al. The treatment of gastroesophageal reflux disease with laparoscopic Nissen fundoplication: prospective evaluation of 100 patients with "typical" symptoms. *Ann Surg* 1998;228:40–50.

Soper NJ, Dunnegan DL. Anatomic fundoplication failure after laparoscopic antireflux surgery. *Ann Surg* 1999;229:669–676.

Spechler SJ. Comparison of medical and surgical therapy for complicated gastroesophageal reflux disease in veterans. The Department of Veterans Affairs Gastroesophageal Reflux Disease Study Group. *N Engl J Med* 1992;326:786–792.

Terry M, Smith CD, Branum GD, et al. Outcomes of laparoscopic fundoplication for gastroesophageal reflux disease and paraesophageal hernia. *Surg Endosc* 2001;15:691–699.

Trus TL, Laycock WS, Waring JP, et al. Improvement in quality of life measures after laparoscopic antireflux surgery. *Ann Surg* 1999;229:331–336.

COMMENTARY

The senior author (NJS) of this chapter is one of the true international authorities in the treatment of gastroesophageal reflux disease (GERD). As an editor and surgeon who performs these procedures regularly I continue to learn from the writing of these authors. The approach taken by the senior author in breaking the procedure into specific components for the learner to master portions prior to performing the entire procedure has been implemented at my institution and facilitates taking a surgeon from novice to expert in a logical manner.

Mastery of the laparoscopic Nissen fundoplication procedure involves more than technical mastery of maneuvers or an understanding of proper patient selection. True mastery takes the "cookbook" performance of the operation to a procedure that is tailored to the individual based upon preoperative symptoms, objective studies, patient expectations, and surgeon experience. This is a procedure where the differentiation between the science and art of medicine becomes manifest.

Many areas of controversy persist in the treatment of GERD. Some gastroenterologists and internists refuse to refer patients for antireflux surgery due to personal bias or personal experience with patients who have experienced poor outcomes from antireflux operations. One who practices evidence-based medicine and possesses access to a high quality laparoscopic surgeon should readily admit the appropriate role for this operation in the management of GERD patients. The degree to which Barrett esophagus stabilizes or regresses after fundoplication also remains an area of intense discussion. The lack of a good animal model for the study of treatment modalities in the management of Barrett contributes to the controversy.

The role of laparoscopic Nissen fundoplication in the management of the patient with pulmonary complications from GERD has become increasingly important. Many patients who have adult-onset reactive airway disease (asthma) have dramatic responses to antireflux operations. Additionally, patients who have undergone lung transplantation and are experiencing deterioration of pulmonary function unrelated to rejection should be tested for GERD, as antireflux surgery has been shown to result in marked improvement when reflux is the source of what has been deemed to be bronchiolitis obliterans in the transplant patient.

Laparoscopic Nissen fundoplication currently has a very significant role in the management of the patient with GERD. Future endoluminal therapies have the potential to minimize the role of these operations, but for the immediate future this operation is of great importance.

LLS

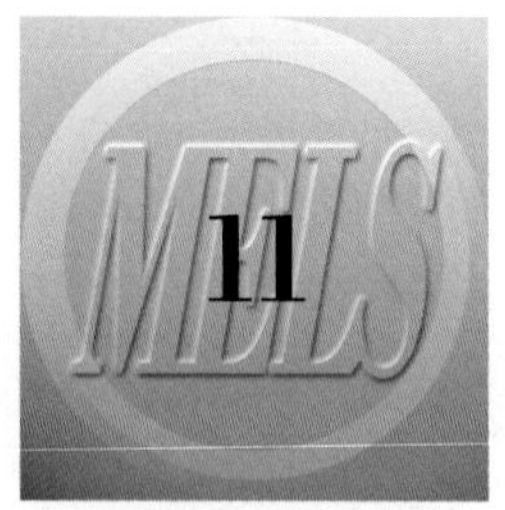

11 Laparoscopic Partial Fundoplication

LEE L. SWANSTRÖM

BACKGROUND

Rudolf Nissen discovered that by completely wrapping the lower esophagus with the fundus of the stomach, one could virtually stop gastroesophageal reflux disease (GERD). This was discovered by serendipity, and it was only years later that the complex physiology of normal swallowing and reflux prevention became understood. As the role of esophageal peristalsis (or the lack of it), the lower esophageal sphincter (LES) structure and function, the gastric reservoir and, finally, learned behaviors became known, it became clear that Nissen's original procedure was not optimal for all patients complaining of reflux. A variety of modifications of fundoplications and other new procedures were developed in an attempt to improve clinical outcomes and to tailor the physiology to a wide spectrum of patients. Partial fundoplications are the most common alternative to the contemporary, "short and floppy" version of the Nissen repair popularized by Donahue and DeMeester. Partial wraps are advocated by some as a superior, more "physiologic" repair for all GERD patients and by others as an alternative to the 360-degree fundoplication for patients with poor esophageal motility. The introduction of laparoscopic fundoplication in 1991 has led to a dramatic increase in the number of antireflux procedures being performed. The laparoscopic Nissen fundoplication remains the most common operation performed and has a high success rate (approximately 90% at 10 years). Laparoscopic versions of most of the partial wraps are also widely used with the same, or better, success as the corresponding open version.

Many different forms of partial fundoplications have been described, mostly differing in the technical details of the wrap construction, but all designed to restore intraabdominal esophageal length and to reinforce the LES to prevent reflux (Table 11-1). The proposed physiologic benefit relates to the partial enclosure of the lower esophagus, which decreases outflow resistance by "hinging" open during bolus passage (Fig. 11-1). Although the procedures have both changed since their original descriptions, the names Dor and Toupet have come to generically represent anterior and posterior fundoplications, respectively, and will be used as such in this chapter.

TABLE 11-1. DESCRIPTIONS OF EPONYMIC PARTIAL FUNDOPLICATIONS

Partial fundoplications	Year of description	Description of repair
Belsey Mk IV	1967	270-degree anterolateral wrap
Dor	1962	180-degree anterior wrap
Toupet	1963	180-degree posterior wrap
Lind	1965	270-degree anteroposterior wrap
Thal	1965	90-degree anterior wrap
Guarner	1966	120-degree posterior wrap
Gastropexy procedures		
Hill	1967	90 to180-degree anterior wrap and posterior esophagogastropexy
Watson	1991	120-degree anterolateral wrap and esophagogastropexy

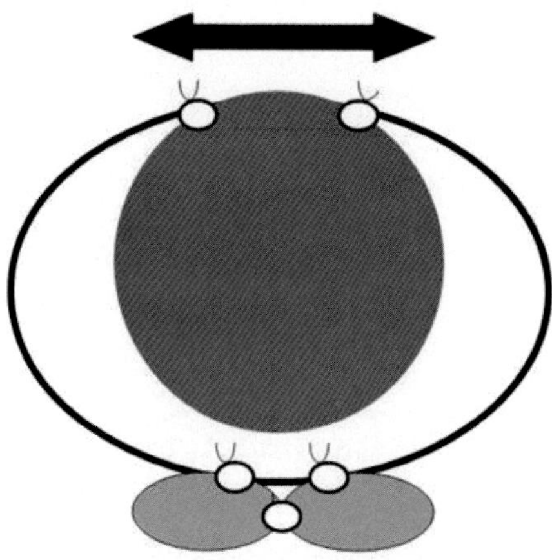

Fig. 11-1. The mechanism of the partial fundoplication requires an incomplete circle of reinforcement to allow the distal esophagus to "hinge" open during food bolus passage.

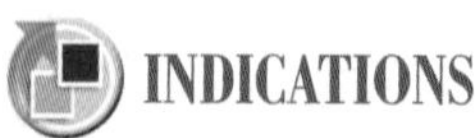

INDICATIONS

Standard indications for GERD surgery apply to the use of partial wraps. These include documented reflux secondary to a defective LES, failure of medical and conservative measures, or development of complications related to reflux in spite of maximal medical treatment.

Specific indications for a partial fundoplication as opposed to a laparoscopic Nissen include but are not limited to the following:

- Patients with esophageal motility disorders in addition to GERD
- As an antireflux procedure in patients undergoing transabdominal Heller myotomy
- Patients unable to tolerate a 360-degree wrap; that is, those who have already undergone a Nissen procedure that caused significant postoperative symptoms
- Patients with severe aerophagia
- As an institutional preference

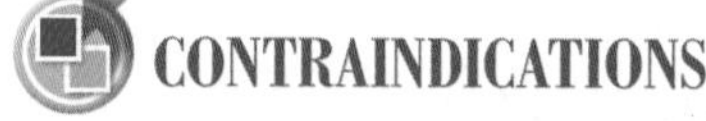

CONTRAINDICATIONS

Absolute contraindications to laparoscopic partial fundoplication are the same as for any laparoscopic surgery and include the inability to tolerate a general anesthetic, severe carbon dioxide retaining pulmonary disease, uncorrected coagulopathy, and the inability to give informed consent.

Although having undergone previous upper abdominal procedures, including

TABLE 11-2. CONTRAINDICATIONS TO A LAPAROSCOPIC PARTIAL FUNDOPLICATION

Absolute contraindications	Relative contraindications
Inability to tolerate general anesthesia	Previous upper abdominal surgery
Severe COPD	Morbid obesity
Uncorrected coagulopathy	Shortened esophagus
Inability to give informed consent	Early pregnancy
Advanced pregnancy	Irreducible hiatal hernia
	Delayed gastric emptying
	Severe reflux disease?

COPD, Chronic obstructive pulmonary disease.

past antireflux surgery, increases the likelihood of conversion to an open procedure, this remains a relative contraindication as long as the surgeon is experienced in reoperative laparoscopy. Other relative contraindications include early pregnancy, morbid obesity, a shortened esophagus, an irreducible hiatal hernia, and delayed gastric emptying (Table 11-2).

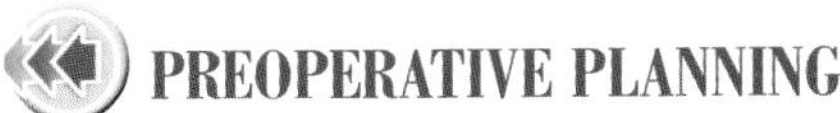

PREOPERATIVE PLANNING

Routine testing should be performed in advance of the day of operation and include standard laboratory tests and other indicated preoperative studies, for example, pulmonary or cardiac as dictated by the patient's presenting condition and comorbidities. In addition, all patients who are being considered for a laparoscopic antireflux procedure should undergo upper endoscopy, esophageal manometry, and 24-hour pH testing as a minimum assessment.

- Barium swallows or upper gastrointestinal (GI) studies are useful evaluations in patients complaining of dysphagia. Radiographs are also useful to assess for pharyngeal dysfunction, esophageal dilatation, and the size and configuration of any hiatal hernias.
- Upper esophagoduodenoscopy should be performed in all patients, particularly those with swallowing difficulty. The degree of esophagitis, presence of Barrett esophagus, length of the esophagus, type of hiatal hernia, and evidence of poor emptying of the esophagus or stomach should be noted. It is important to closely assess and biopsy any mucosal lesions because occult cancers of the gastroesophageal junction can present as dysphagia. Any strictures that are discovered should be aggressively treated before surgery (maximal acid suppression and dilatation).
- Esophageal manometry is a critical test for most patients being considered for a fundoplication. This will show the presence and severity of body motility disorders, define the status of the LES, and provide forewarning of the possibility of esophageal shortening. The actual tracings of the study should be read by the surgeon, because computer interpretations frequently miss subtle changes that can identify sporadic symptom correlations and determine whether dysmotility is secondary to reflux or an intrinsic disorder.
- An important test, which is argued against as a routine study by some, is the 24-hour pH study. This provides valuable preoperative information including whether the patient actually has acid reflux, how severe it is, and how it relates to the presenting symptoms. This information can alter or even obviate the surgical approach. It also permits counseling the patient regarding realistic expectations for outcomes. Finally, preoperative 24-hour pH testing establishes a baseline in these patients to permit accurate postoperative assessment of their results, an important consideration because symptoms alone have been shown to be highly nonspecific.
- Other foregut physiology tests are obtained as dictated by clinical scenarios. Gastric emptying studies may need to be performed if there is a history of early satiety or diabetes. Acid provocation tests, studies for non-acid reflux such as with a Bilitec probe (Medtronics, Inc.; Minneapolis, MN) or impedance/pH testing), serum gastrin levels, and other tests are used on rare occasions to complete the diagnosis.

Once again, it is important for surgeons who deal with a more complex reflux population, particularly with foregut motility problems, to comprehensively test their patients before surgery and *to read the actual studies themselves*. This optimally includes performing the upper endoscopy themselves to obtain maximum information.

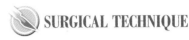

SURGICAL TECHNIQUE

Preoperative Preparation

The patient normally enters the hospital on the day of surgery, having fasted for 8 to 12 hours preoperatively. After general anesthesia is induced, the patient is positioned on a split-leg table with his or her legs extended and separated. Patients must be secured to the table in some fashion because they will be placed in significant reverse Trendelenburg position during the procedure. Antithrombotic compression devices and an orogastric tube are placed. A urinary catheter is not used unless an unusually long procedure is anticipated. A single dose of a first-generation cephalosporin is given as prophylaxis.

Instrumentation

Adequate and appropriate instruments are required as they are for any advanced procedure. These should include:

- Atraumatic liver retractor
- Angled laparoscope (30 or 45 degree)
- Atraumatic graspers
- Safe energy source
  - Ultrasonic
  - Bipolar
- Curved-tip needle holders

Most laparoscopic instruments are 5 mm in diameter, so the majority of ports can also be 5 mm. Imaging equipment should be well maintained because good visualization is of primary importance. A high-flow insufflator and a good suction/irrigator are very useful.

Dissection

The surgeon usually operates from the patient's left with the camera operator between the legs and the assistant on the patient's right side. Alternatively, the surgeon can be positioned between the legs with the camera operator to the patient's left, although this compromises the camera operation, which may slow the surgery. The

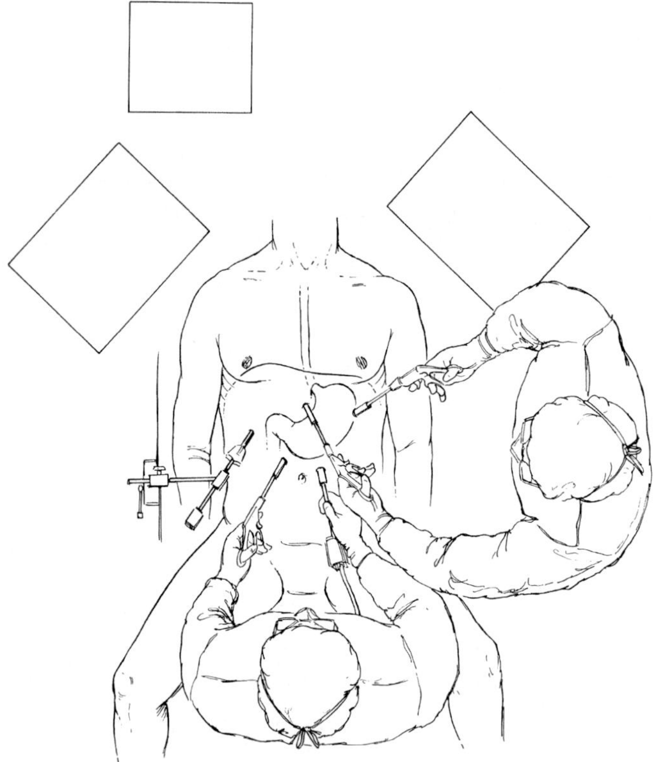

Fig. 11-2. Patient position and room setup for laparoscopic partial fundoplication.

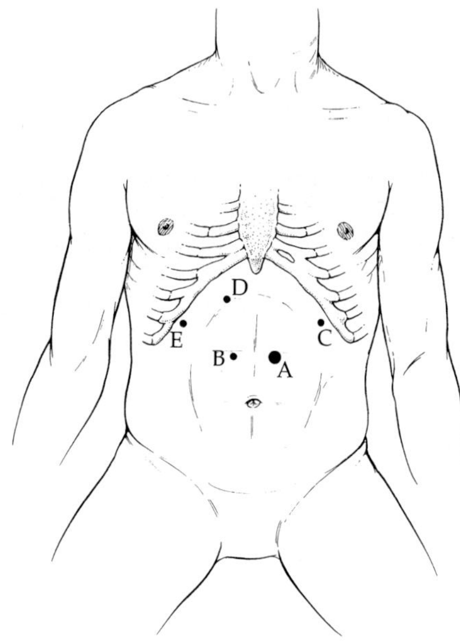

Fig. 11-3. Five ports are placed as shown.

monitors are at the patient's head, to the left and right (Fig. 11-2).

The initial access is placed high in the left upper quadrant at the site of the camera port. In the uncomplicated abdomen, the Veress needle is used for creation of the pneumoperitoneum, or, alternatively, the Hasson direct-access trocar can be used if that is the surgeon's preference. A total of five ports is used. The 5- or 10-mm camera port is placed approximately 15 cm from the xiphisternum, well above the umbilicus and 3 cm to the left of the midline. A 30- to 50-degree laparoscope is inserted in the abdomen, and all additional ports are placed under direct vision. All port sites are infiltrated with bupivacaine before the skin incision is made. The four 5-mm ports are placed in the left upper quadrant (the surgeon's right hand), the right upper quadrant (the liver retractor), the right mid-abdomen (the assistant's ratcheted grasper), and to the right of the epigastrium after the liver has been retracted (for the operating surgeon's left hand), as seen in Fig. 11-3). Low-profile ports are used, with at least one being a soft plastic disposable variety because that will allow the entry of a standard curved GI suture needle. Alternatively, one of these ports may be replaced with a 10-mm trocar to facilitate the passage of suture material and needles, or the needles can be inserted through a 10-mm camera port.

The left lobe of the liver is retracted using an atraumatic 5-mm articulated liver retractor that is secured to the table with a table-mounted retractor holder. The reverse Trendelenburg position of the operating table is increased until the intraabdominal organs fall away from the esophageal hiatus.

The assistant grasps the body of the stomach with a 5-mm Babcock-type grasper and retracts it caudally and to the left. This puts the gastrohepatic ligament on tension. The ligament is then opened with the ultrasonic coagulating shears, starting in the clear area approximately halfway down the lesser gastric curvature. Approximately 15% of patients will have a significant accessory left hepatic arterial branch arising from the celiac trunk or left gastric artery and running through the hepatogastric ligament (Fig. 11-4). These should be preserved if they are larger than 2 to 3 mm to reduce the risk of bleeding and the rare complication of hepatic ischemia. The phrenoesophageal ligament is then carefully incised at the apex of the hiatus, and atraumatic graspers are used to bluntly open the space anterior to the esophagus. The right crus is bluntly retracted away from the esophagus, and the crossing fibers of the phrenoesophageal ligament are divided with the ultrasonic coagulating shears. This right crural dissection is continued downward to its junction with the left crus. With the use of an angled laparoscope and operating from the right side of the esophagus, the surgeon creates a retroesophageal window by incising through the posterior fat pad until the posterior fundus of the stomach can be identified. During this dissection, the assistant is retracting both the esophagus and posterior vagus anteriorly and caudally to expose and protect these structures (Fig. 11-5). After a generous posterior window is established, attention is turned to the left crural mobilization. We do not typically surround the esophagus with a Penrose drain as is commonly described; instead, the assistant grasps the anterior epiphrenic fat pad and retracts it inferiorly and to the patient's right, which places the left side of the phrenoesophageal membrane on stretch. The surgeon can divide the membrane along the left crus while sweeping the anterior vagus to the right with his left grasper. As the phrenoesophageal ligament is being divided, care should be taken to avoid stripping or disturbing the peritoneal covering on the crura because this provides the strength for the subsequent hiatal closure. Mediastinal dissection is performed by using blunt and ultrasonic dissection to

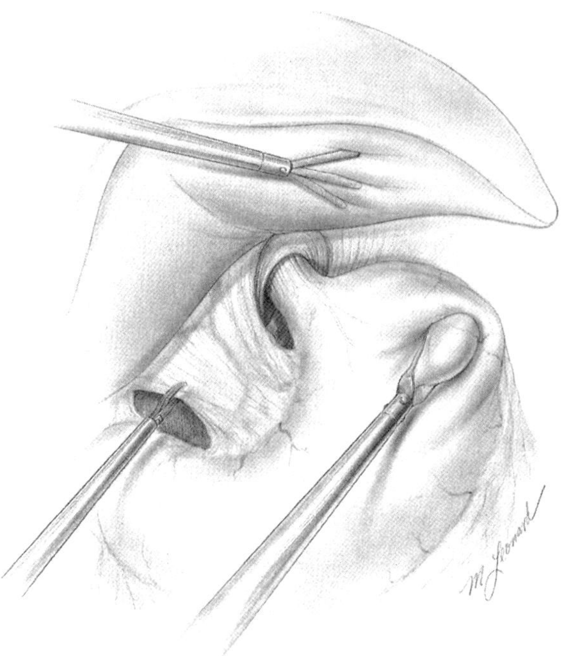

Fig. 11-4. An accessory left hepatic artery is encountered in the hepatogastric ligament in 15% of cases.

ensure that there are at least 3 cm of intraabdominal esophagus around which to place the wrap. Failure to bring enough esophagus into the abdomen is likely to lead to wrap slippage and subsequent failure of the antireflux procedure.

The short gastric vessels should always be mobilized to minimize any chance of tension on the repair. They are easily divided by using the ultrasonic shears, with the assistant retracting the greater curvature omentum inferiorly, and the surgeon pulling the stomach to the midline to create tension. Care must be taken during this dissection to not injure adjacent structures such as the pancreas or splenic hilum. This starts approximately one-third of the way down the greater curve and is the same whether an anterior or posterior partial fundoplication is planned. Retrogastric attachments are exposed for division by progressively rolling the stomach to the patient's right. The upper fundus is then carefully dissected free of its attachments to the left hemidiaphragm and left crus, once again taking care not to strip the peritoneum from the crus. Any posterior attachments of the esophagus are dissected free to enlarge the retroesophageal window. Finally, the intraabdominal esophagus is once again checked for adequate length, and, if needed, additional mediastinal dissection is performed.

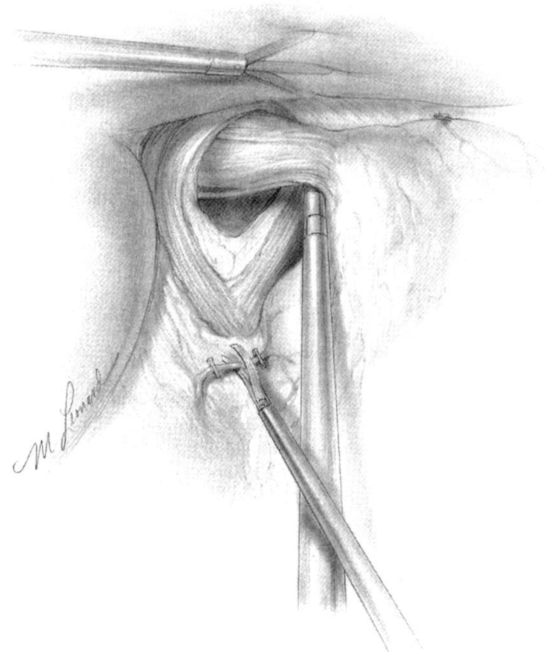

Fig. 11-5. A retroesophageal window is created by dissecting from the patient's right. Direct visualization is obtained with an angled laparoscope.

The Repair

Toupet

To perform a posterior Toupet fundoplication after the completed dissection, the mobilized fundus is placed in the left upper abdomen, and while the esophagus is carefully elevated, it is grasped from the right through the retroesophageal window. While the assistant maintains caudal traction on the epiphrenic fat pad, the surgeon "walks" the fundus around until an appropriately "floppy" portion is identified. This segment is grasped directly on the area of the divided short gastrics with the surgeon's left hand. The right grasper is used to grasp the left side of the wrap, once again directly on the greater curvature as marked by the divided short gastric vessels. A "shoeshine" maneuver is performed by sliding the grasped fundus back and forth behind the esophagus. This movement ensures that the wrap is held at the correct spots, lies without twisting, and is neither too redundant nor too tight (Fig. 11-6, page 106). The assistant is asked to hold the right side of the wrap, using it to distract the esophagus to the left to expose the posterior hiatal opening.

The crura are reapproximated while retracting the esophagus with the fundus. Interrupted sutures of 2-0 woven polyester on a curved tapered GI needle are cut to 6 inches in length and placed by using an intracorporeal suturing technique, which is less likely to tear through tissues. Each of these posterior sutures incorporates some of the posterior fundic wrap as well as the crura (Fig. 11-7, page 106). A typical crural closure requires three or four

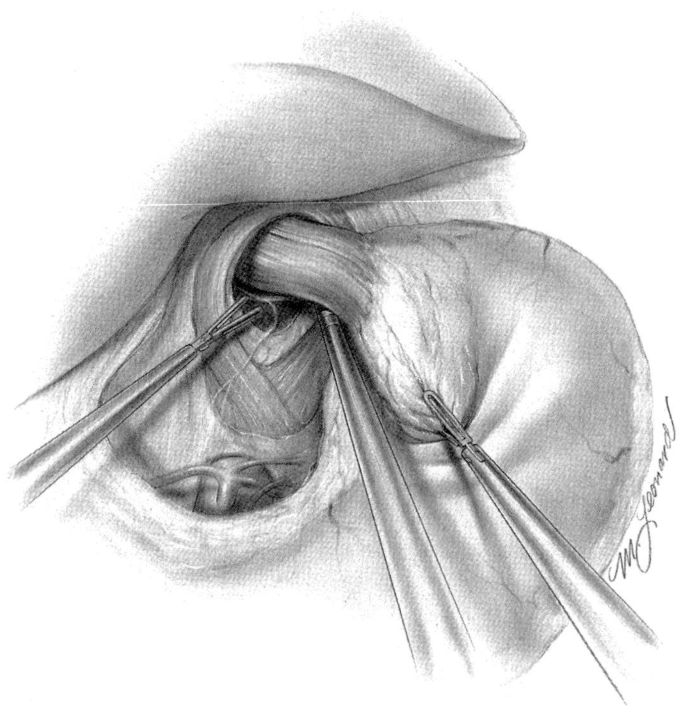

Fig. 11-6. The "shoeshine" maneuver ensures that the correct portion of the fundus is used and that there are no twists or redundancies to the wrap.

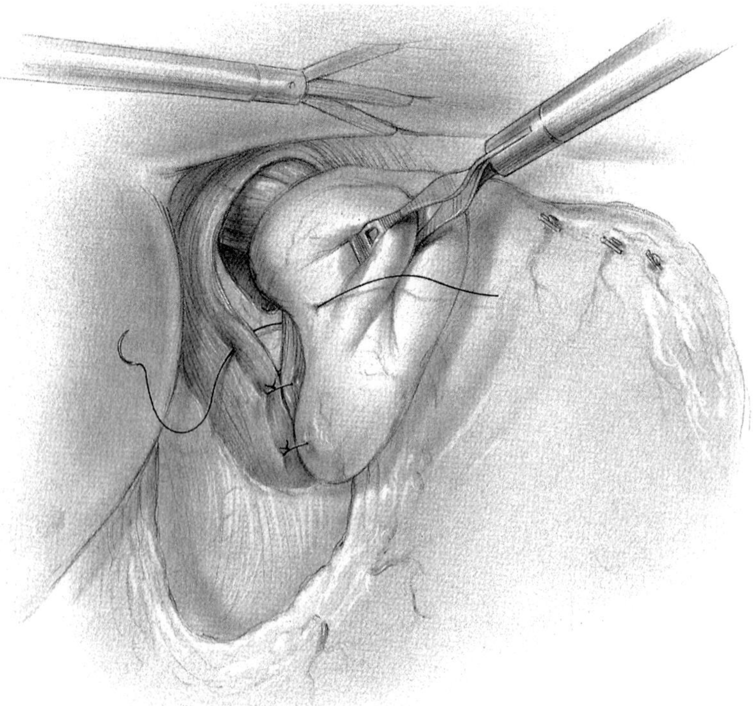

Fig. 11-7. Posterior hiatal closure is accomplished with interrupted, intracorporeally tied sutures, each of which includes a bite of the posterior wall of the wrap.

such sutures. The crura are reapproximated without the placement of a bougie, but it is important in a partial fundoplication that the closure is not too tight around the esophagus. After the hiatal closure, additional sutures are placed from the right wrap to the right crus. The final suture on this side is to the very top of the right crus. These crural sutures are repeated on the left side, still using intracorporeally tied polyester sutures (Fig. 11-8).

Before suturing the anterior portion of the wrap, a 56F esophageal dilator is inserted into the esophagus after removing the orogastric tube. This helps to gauge the location where the sutures need to be placed to create the partial wrap. The right side of the wrap is then sutured to the right-hand side of the esophagus at the ten o'clock position, and the left side of the wrap is sutured to the esophagus at the two o'clock position. The goal is a wrap of at least 270 degrees (even more wrap is preferable) around the esophagus and 3 to 4 cm in length (Fig. 11-9).

If the posterior fundoplication is performed in conjunction with a Heller myotomy, the esophageal sutures are taken to the edges of the myotomy, which has the added benefit of holding open the myotomy.

Dor

An anterior or Dor type of fundoplication is most commonly performed in conjunction with a Heller myotomy, for which it seems to be an adequate antireflux procedure. It is not commonly used as a primary antireflux procedure.

The repair follows the same dissection as has been described. Fundal mobilization is performed, although this does not need to be as extensive as for a Nissen or Toupet wrap. In fact, some authorities have had good results performing the procedure without dividing the short gastric vessels, although there is the danger of performing the wrap with some torsional tension, which can lead to refractory postoperative dysphagia.

The crura are loosely reapproximated while retracting the esophagus laterally to expose the posterior decussation. Once again interrupted, intracorporeally tied sutures of woven polyester are used, taking care to obtain large bites of the crus including the peritoneal covering. A typical loose crural closure requires three or four sutures.

The greater curvature of the fundus 3 cm distal to the angle of His is sutured to the midpoint of the left crus, and a row of three or four sutures is placed from the gastric fundus to the left side of the esophagus. This maneuver accentuates the angle of His and establishes intraabdominal length to the esophagus (Fig. 11-10, page 108). A 56F esophageal dilator is carefully advanced into the stomach. The greater curvature of the stomach is brought anteriorly over the esophagus with sequential sutures to the

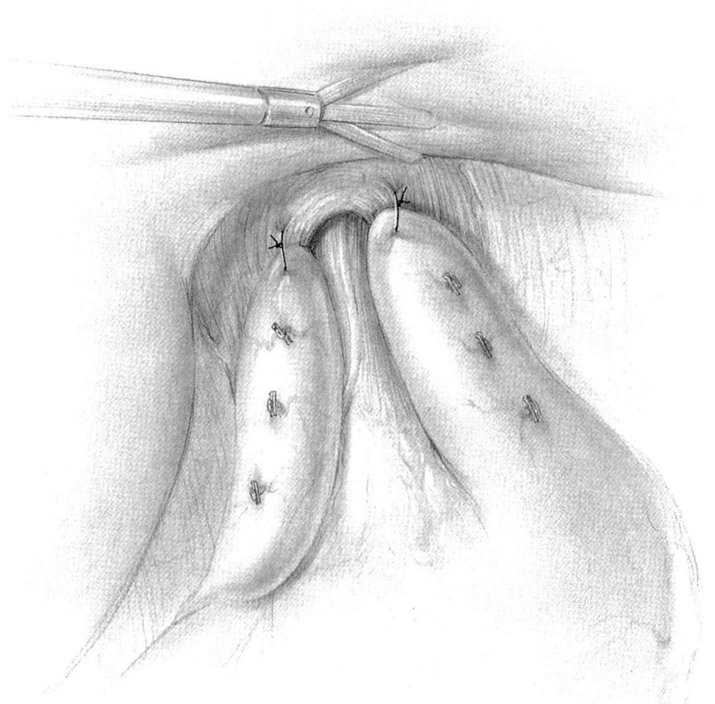

Fig. 11-8. The Toupet repair is securely fixed to right and left crura, which takes the tension off of the esophageal sutures.

anterior rim of the hiatus. A second row of sutures is then placed from the greater curvature of the fundus to the right side of the esophagus (Fig. 11-11, page 108).

When the Dor is used with a Heller myotomy, the sutures that create the wrap are fixed along the myotomy edges. These sutures must be placed very carefully so the myotomy is not reapproximated as the fundus is rolled over the anterior esophagus. Also, after a myotomy, one will often eliminate the step of posterior crural dissection because it may predispose to reflux by increasing the chances of posterior herniation and subsequent loss of this portion of the antireflux mechanism.

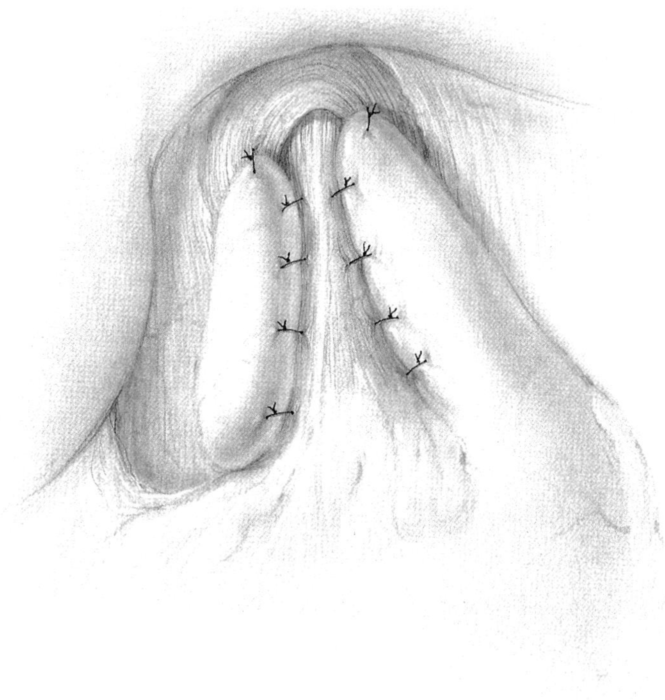

Fig. 11-9. Completed 270-degree "plus" fundoplication.

Completion of the Procedure

Once the repair is finished, the abdomen is carefully inspected for any evidence of bleeding and irrigated to remove any residual blood. The instruments are removed and the trocars are withdrawn under direct vision. If trocars larger than 5 mm in diameter have been used, and if they were not dilating type trocars, the fascia at this site should be closed either externally or internally with a closure device using an absorbable suture. The skin is closed with subcuticular absorbable sutures.

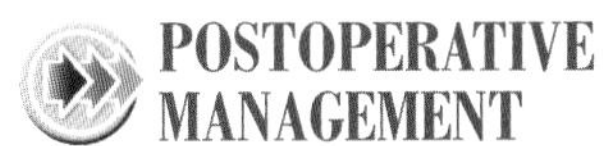

POSTOPERATIVE MANAGEMENT

If the partial fundoplication is a primary procedure, routine postoperative swallowing assessments are not usually ordered. Antiemetics are used liberally in the postoperative period to prevent retching and vomiting, which is associated with early wrap herniation and failure. Once the patient is free of nausea, he or she is started on liquids and gradually advanced to a pureed diet before discharge, typically on postoperative day 1. If the repair was a reoperative procedure or associated with a myotomy, a closed suction drain is placed and sometimes a Gastrografin swallow is obtained on the day after surgery. The drain fluid is routinely sent for evaluation of salivary amylase on the morning after surgery because this has been found to be the most sensitive test for leaks. If the amylase and swallow results are normal, the patient is started on liquids and subsequently advanced as for a primary procedure. These patients typically go home on the second postoperative day.

Patients remain on a pureed diet for 2 weeks, at which time they are assessed in the outpatient setting. We prefer to specify a "pureed" diet rather than a "post-Nissen" or "full liquid" diet to eliminate variations between hospitals and dietitians. They are also instructed to crush all medications or to switch them to a liquid form. The patients are counseled to expect some early dysphagia and are told specifically to

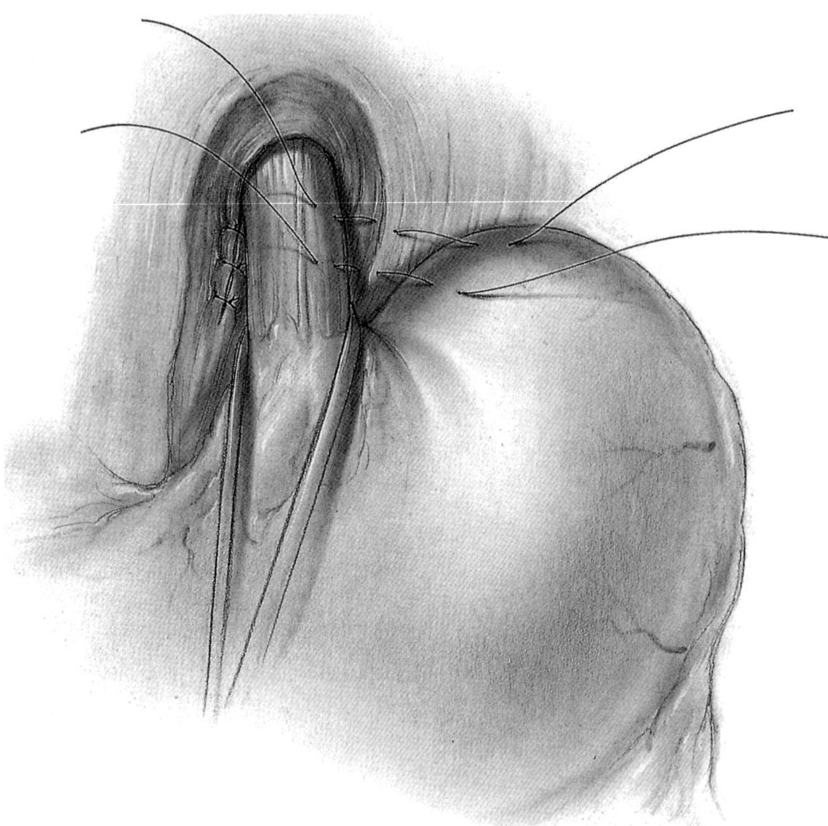

Fig. 11-10. The left-sided sutures of the Dor repair secure the esophagus within the abdomen and accentuate the angle of His.

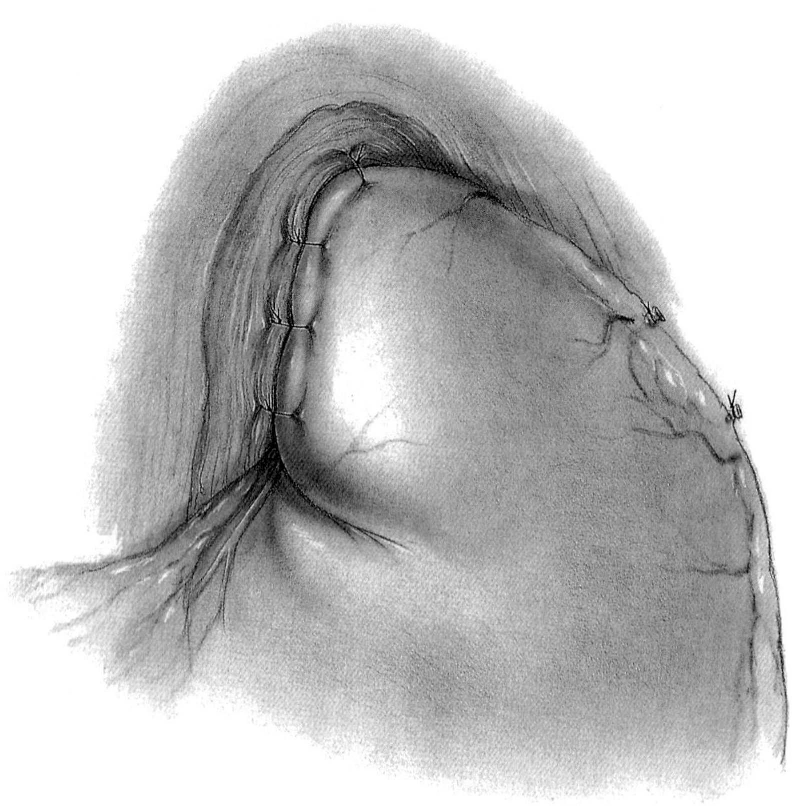

Fig. 11-11. The completed Dor fundoplication.

avoid all breads, meats, and large pills until they are able to tolerate everything else. Patients are encouraged to eliminate chewing gum and carbonated beverages from their diet permanently.

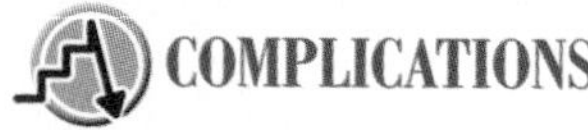

COMPLICATIONS

Intraoperative

Intraoperative complications can result from access problems, injury during dissection, bougie perforations, or bleeding (Table 11-3). Rarely, patients will have anesthetic problems related to the physiology of the carbon dioxide (CO_2) pneumothorax. These are almost always reversed when the CO_2 is evacuated. Access injuries are rare unless the patient has undergone previous upper abdominal surgery; in that case, however, they can occur whether Veress or Hasson techniques are used. The important issue with access injuries is recognizing them at the time they occur and aggressively addressing them, which sometimes requires conversion to an open procedure. Dissection injuries happen most commonly to the stomach, sometimes to the gastroesophageal junction, and rarely to the esophagus. They result from either traumatic retraction or from loss of the tissue planes during dissection. Appropriately atraumatic instruments should be used along with a minimum use of grasping the actual stomach or esophagus. Gastric perforations are easily oversewn and seldom cause problems. If one occurs in an area of extensive dissection and the surrounding tissue looks rough, an endoscopic stapler can be used to excise the whole area. If the perforation is esophageal, it should be assessed with a flexible endoscope before attempting a repair. A laparoscopic repair should be attempted only if the surgeon is very skilled at endoscopic suturing; otherwise conversion to laparotomy or thoracotomy should be performed. The repair should include both the mucosa and muscle layers; closure of the mucosa alone will often lead to an esophageal diverticulum later.

The complication that causes the most apprehension is perforation during insertion of the esophageal dilator. This occurs in as many as 1% of antireflux procedures and is more likely if there is significant anatomic distortion or scarring either as a result of esophagitis or previous nonsurgical treatments such as balloon dilatation, bougienage, or botulinum toxin injection. These perforations occur most frequently at the gastroesophageal junction, where they are

TABLE 11-3. COMPLICATIONS RELATED TO LAPAROSCOPIC PARTIAL FUNDOPLICATIONS

Intraoperative	Early postoperative	Late postoperative
Access injuries	Delayed perforation	Reflux recurrence
Vascular	Stomach	Wrap herniation
Hollow viscus	Esophagus	Wrap disruption
Physiologic reaction	Deep venous thrombosis	Incompetent wrap
CO_2 absorption	Pulmonary complications	Dysphagia
Pneumothorax	Dysphagia	Poor motility
Vaso-vagal response	Early wrap herniation	Tight wrap
Dissection injuries		Twisted wrap
Stomach		Nausea
Esophagus		Vagal injury
Vagus nerves		Delayed gastric emptying
Bleeding		Idiopathic
Aorta, vena cava		Diarrhea
Short gastrics		Vagal injury
Aberrant arteries		Idiopathic

obvious, but can happen in any part of the esophagus and may be unnoticed if mediastinal or cervical. The surgeon should communicate with whoever is advancing the dilator and suspect a perforation if there is any resistance to passage. If a perforation is suspected, instillation of methylene blue into the esophagus or esophagoscopy may help in identifying the site. If technically feasible, it is preferable to suture the perforation laparoscopically with a single layer of intracorporeally tied sutures and by draining the involved space. If the fundoplication can be properly performed to cover the perforation, it will add an extra layer of protection. Obviously, consideration should be given to converting to an open procedure in order to repair the laceration. In all cases of perforation, one should leave a drain in situ and measure the drain fluid amylase on the first postoperative day.

Prevention of these injuries is preferable to treatment and is best done by communicating clearly with the anesthesiologist, making sure that all other esophageal tubes are removed, and retracting the esophagus caudally to allow easy passage of the bougie, which is carefully and slowly advanced under direct vision as much as possible.

Bleeding can arise from injury to the accessory left hepatic vessels, short gastric vessels, or damage to the liver or spleen. Bleeding can normally be controlled laparoscopically by using one or more of the following: ultrasonic coagulating shears, direct pressure and hemostatic materials, 5- or 10-mm clips, or suture ligation with endoloops or stick ties. A scrupulous technique is the best defense against bleeding complications. Very rarely, conversion to an open procedure is required to control bleeding or to perform splenectomy if the spleen is badly torn.

Postoperative

Significant pain, fever, or tachycardia in the postoperative period should prompt a thorough search for a delayed presentation of a leak. If a drain was left because of intraoperative concern it can be checked for drain amylase, the presence of which is the most sensitive test for a leak. A water-soluble contrast swallow or contrast-enhanced computed tomography scan can help localize such a leak. Treatment should be immediate return to the operating room.

Rarely, bleeding can be a problem in the postoperative period, in which case it could be from any of the sources mentioned previously as well as from trocar sites, especially if the inferior epigastric vessels have been injured. Treatment should be directed at the source but may also necessitate a return to the operating room.

Respiratory insufficiency is uncommon, but in those with a significant degree of chronic obstructive pulmonary disease it may be a problem requiring either extended ventilatory support to help wash out the CO_2 or oxygen therapy in the postoperative period. Postoperative pneumothorax, or capnothorax, is rare and can usually be managed expectantly because CO_2 reabsorbs within hours. More troublesome is subcutaneous emphysema that, although not dangerous, can be uncomfortable for the patient and of concern for the nursing staff. Reassurance and observation will usually be all that is required.

Dysphagia is one of the most common problems encountered after surgery, particularly after partial fundoplications because they are frequently performed for esophageal dysmotility. Transient dysphagia is to be expected and is related to edema of the distal esophagus from operative dissection. In most cases this resolves within 2 weeks, during which time the patient is maintained on a semisolid diet. Dysphagia beyond this period is more problematic to deal with and is more likely to be caused by technical reasons related to the fundoplication. Endoscopy should be performed if dysphagia persists more than 6 weeks to assess for strictures or distortion of the fundoplication. A Savary or balloon dilatation should be performed regardless of the findings because sometimes this will solve the problem. Persistent dysphagia should be evaluated by esophageal motility and 24-hour pH testing, particularly if there are reflux symptoms. In rare cases, reoperation may be necessary and would usually be recommended based on results of the physiology testing, recreating the partial wrap if motility is still bad or converting to a Nissen if motility improves. If the partial wrap is intact but the patient is having some documented reflux through it, another option is an endoluminal antireflux salvage procedure.

OUTCOMES

Results after partial fundoplications vary dramatically according to the indications for the surgery. Results of the Dor or Toupet fundoplication after a Heller myotomy are good or excellent in 85% to 90% of cases. Results when the partial fundoplications are used for other motility disorders are not as good (75% to 90%), but these are complex procedures, and patients could not be expected to do as well after any surgery. There is more controversy regarding the appropriateness of partial fundoplications as a primary antireflux operation. Several large clinical series of partial fundoplications, including prospective comparisons with total fundoplications, have suggested the symptomatic outcomes to be excellent. The experience of many in the U.S., including this author, is markedly different, showing a high symptom and objective failure rate, which has slowly increased with time (Fig. 11-12, page 110). It should be noted, however, that 88% of our patients remain satisfied with their surgery and would repeat it again.

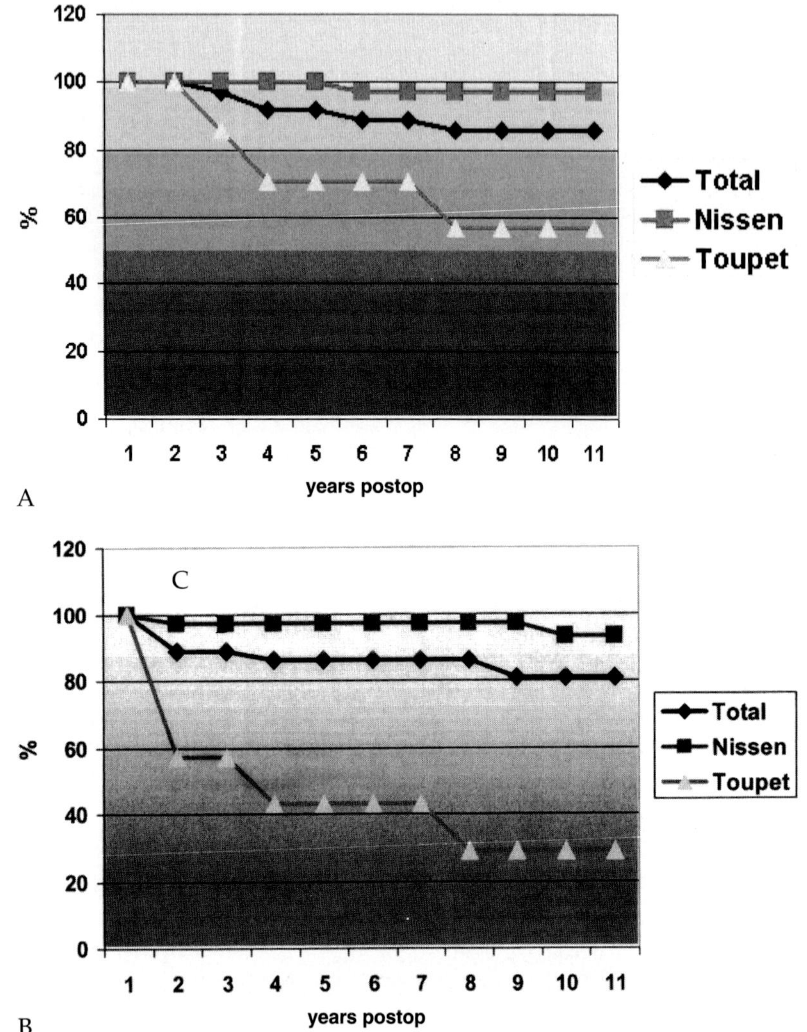

Fig. 11-12. Long-term outcome after partial fundoplication: the author's experience. **A.** Symptomatic outcomes. **B.** Objective outcomes.

CONCLUSION

Although the majority of laparoscopic antireflux procedures are 360-degree Nissen repairs, alternative procedures such as the partial fundoplications have a definite place in the repertoire of the laparoscopic esophageal surgeon. The primary indication is for primary motility disorders, in which case they provide good protection from reflux without increasing dysphagia. The use of partial fundoplications for all patients with primary reflux remains more controversial, and the results of more prospective, randomized long-term trials are awaited to determine the best uses of partial and total fundoplications.

SUGGESTED READING

Chrysos E, Athanasakis E, Pechlivanides G, et al. The effect of total and anterior partial fundoplication on antireflux mechanisms of the gastroesophageal junction. *Am J Surg* 2004;188(1):39–44.

Fernando HC, Luketich JD, Christie NA, et al. Outcomes of laparoscopic Toupet compared to laparoscopic Nissen fundoplication. *Surg Endosc* 2002;16:905–908.

Hagedorn C, Jonson C, Lonroth H, et al. Efficacy of an anterior as compared with a posterior laparoscopic fundoplication: results of a randomized, controlled clinical trial. *Ann Surg* 2003;238:189–196.

Hunter JG, Swanstrom L, Waring JP. Dysphagia after laparoscopic antireflux surgery. The impact of operative technique. *Ann Surg* 1996; 224:51–57.

Jobe BA, Wallace J, Hansen PD, et al. Evaluation of laparoscopic Toupet fundoplication as a primary repair for all patients with medically resistant gastroesophageal reflux. *Surg Endosc* 1997;11:1080–1083.

Krysztopik RJ, Jamieson GG, Devitt PG, et al. A further modification of fundoplication: 90 degrees anterior fundoplication. *Surg Endosc* 2002;16:1446–1451.

Lindbloom MA, Ringers J, Straathof JW, et al. Effect of laparoscopic partial fundoplication on reflux mechanisms. *Am J Gastroenterol* 2003;98:29–34.

Ludeman R, Watson DI, Jamieson GG, et al. Five-year follow-up of a randomized clinical trial of laparoscopic total vs. anterior 180 degree fundoplication. *Br J Surg* 2005;92(2): 240–243.

Patti MG, Molena D, Fisichella P, et al. Laparoscopic Heller myotomy and Dor fundoplication for achalasia: analysis of successes and failures. *Arch Surg* 2001;136: 870–877.

COMMENTARY

Dr. Swanstrom describes the potential indications for performing partial fundoplications and the technical aspects of the two most commonly performed partial wraps. Although most American surgeons perform complete (360 degree or Nissen) fundoplications for the majority of their patients, many surgeons in other countries advocate partial fundoplications for their reflux patients. There have been a few prospective randomized trials comparing total and partial fundoplications for GERD, and most have shown equivalent symptomatic outcomes. Generally, it is believed that partial fundoplications do not control reflux as well as total fundoplications but have fewer postoperative sequelae such as gas-bloat syndrome. Several U.S. studies have suggested that partial fundoplications do not eliminate reflux in up to half of the patients, and that subsequent failure is more frequent than following a Nissen. Furthermore, the incidence of dysphagia following a Nissen fundoplication in patients with GERD-related esophageal dysmotility is not greater than in patients undergoing a partial wrap. We therefore use partial fundoplications very selectively, primarily in patients with named motility disorders and the rare patient with other considerations such as those listed in Table 11-3.

When a partial fundoplication is to be performed, the technical details bear reinforcement. The fundus should be adequately mobilized to prevent torsional tension. Multiple sutures should be used to fix the wrap in position, particularly when sewing to the esophageal wall itself. There is a natural reluctance among surgeons to place stitches deep into the muscularis of the esophagus, and thus extra points of apposition are probably merited. Tissue handling is of critical importance; atraumatic grasping instruments should be used and the esophagus itself should never be directly grasped. Close attention to the patient's postoperative course is important in order to diagnose and treat complications as early as possible. Finally, because ongoing reflux may occur following partial fundoplications, patients may benefit from the use of postoperative acid-reducing drugs.

NJS

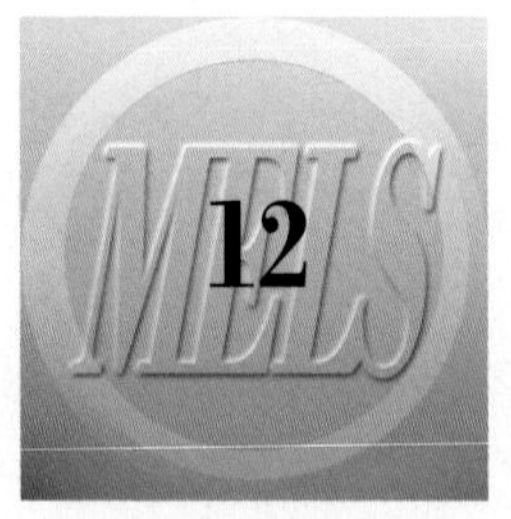

Laparoscopic Antireflux Surgery: Esophageal Lengthening Procedures

COREY E. VAN HOVE, JOHN HUNTER, AND KYLE PERRY

BACKGROUND

The syndrome of the short esophagus and its relationship to longstanding gastroesophageal reflux disease was first described by Norman Barrett, an Australian-born British surgeon, in 1950. Axial shortening of the esophagus is thought to be the end result of chronic esophagitis with subsequent transmural inflammation and ultimately scar formation. A technique to lengthen the esophagus as an adjunct the treatment of reflux disease was first described by John Collis, an English surgeon, in 1957, with variants of his original technique still performed today. Collis performed his esophageal lengthening procedure through a left thoracoabdominal incision. Two clamps were placed in parallel at the angle of His and the stomach divided in between them to create a gastric tube in continuity with the esophagus. The technique has since evolved with the advent of minimally invasive surgery and surgical staplers to include numerous laparoscopic and thoracoscopic variations. While the pathophysiology of shortened esophagus may be less common today due to improved and widespread medical therapies for GERD, it remains critical to recognize this condition when performing fundoplication in order to create a tension-free repair.

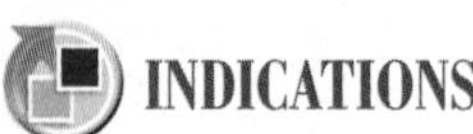

INDICATIONS

A Collis gastroplasty should be considered in any patient undergoing fundoplication with insufficient esophageal length to create a wrap without axial tension. If after extensive mediastinal mobilization, at least 2.5 cm of esophagus does not rest in the abdominal cavity without active retraction, a gastroplasty should be performed.

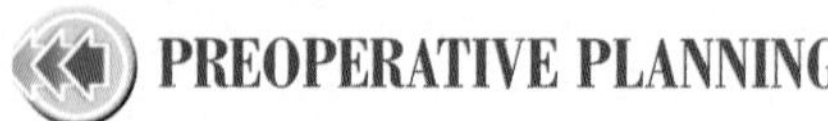

PREOPERATIVE PLANNING

The vast majority of patients who ultimately undergo Collis gastroplasty will have had multiple radiologic studies and other tests of esophageal function in preparation for surgical repair of their gastroesophageal reflux disease. While tests such as esophagram, manometry, and endoscopy may indicate possible esophageal shortening, they are notoriously poor at predicting esophageal length with any accuracy. Preoperative findings that strongly suggest a short esophagus include a hiatal hernia more than 5 cm in length, an esophageal stricture that has been documented by endoscopy, a Type III paraesophageal hernia, the presence of Barrett esophagus, or a previously failed repair. Ultimately, however, the diagnosis of a short esophagus can only be made in the operating room after the esophagus has been dissected free from the mediastinum and diaphragmatic crura in preparation for fundoplication.

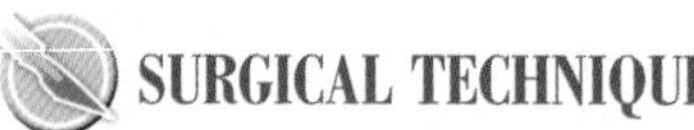

SURGICAL TECHNIQUE

Numerous modifications of Collis's original procedure have been described using open and laparoscopic techniques from the abdomen, chest, or a combination of the two, usually done in conjunction with a fundoplication procedure. Below we describe a completely laparoscopic approach using articulating endoscopic staplers to create a "wedge" Collis gastroplasty, also known as a "wedge fundectomy."

The patient is placed supine on a split-leg table and general anesthesia induced. The legs are separated and the patient should be securely strapped to the operating table to accommodate steep reverse Trendelenburg. Pneumatic compression stockings or subcutaneous heparin should be used depending on the patient's risk for thrombosis.

Access, trocar placement, and the initial operative dissection are identical to those used for Nissen fundoplication, to which this procedure is typically an adjunct. Before the decision to perform a Collis gastroplasty can be made, the gastroesophageal junction (GEJ) must be thoroughly mobilized and its relationship to the diaphragm defined. Dissection of the GEJ begins at the pars flaccida of the gastrohepatic ligament using ultrasonic coagulating shears. A large hiatal hernia is usually associated with a shortened esophagus, and if so the hernia sac should be carefully dissected away from both diaphragmatic crura and the sac reduced into the abdomen. The short gastric vessels are divided to the inferior border of the spleen as are the posterior gastrophrenic attachments, including the posterior gastric artery. A retroesophageal window is created, and a Penrose drain placed around the esophagus for retraction. At this point it is critical to define the true GEJ in order to assess its distance from the hiatus—any redundant hernia sac should be removed from the GEJ, taking care not to injure either vagus nerve, and the epiphrenic fat pad should be dissected away from the angle of His. To accomplish this, the surgical assistant grasps the fat pad immediately to the left of the anterior vagus nerve and elevates it anteriorly. The operating surgeon retracts the stomach with his left hand and divides the fat pad with the harmonic scalpel. The dissection proceeds down to the angle of His and posteriorly around the back of the esophagus, clearing the left-most 180 degrees of the GEJ. The fat located to the right of the esophagus should be left undisturbed, as removal risks injury to both vagal trunks, which deviate to the right just distal to the GEJ. If a large hiatal hernia has been reduced, the proximal stomach may have a tubular appearance and may be mistaken for the distal esophagus, causing an overestimation of esophageal length. If there is any doubt regarding the true position of the GEJ, intraoperative upper endoscopy should be performed and the GEJ transilluminated and marked on the outside for reference.

Once the true GEJ has been identified, any nasogastric tubes or dilators should be removed and the esophagus and stomach should be left in a natural position with no axial tension. The diaphragmatic crura are then held together and the intraabdominal esophagus is measured with a laparoscopic grasper of predetermined length. If this distance measures less than 2.5 cm, then more extensive circumferential mediastinal dissection of the esophagus should be done, using ultrasonic coagulating shears and the previously placed Penrose drain for traction. The mediastinal esophagus can be dissected free to the

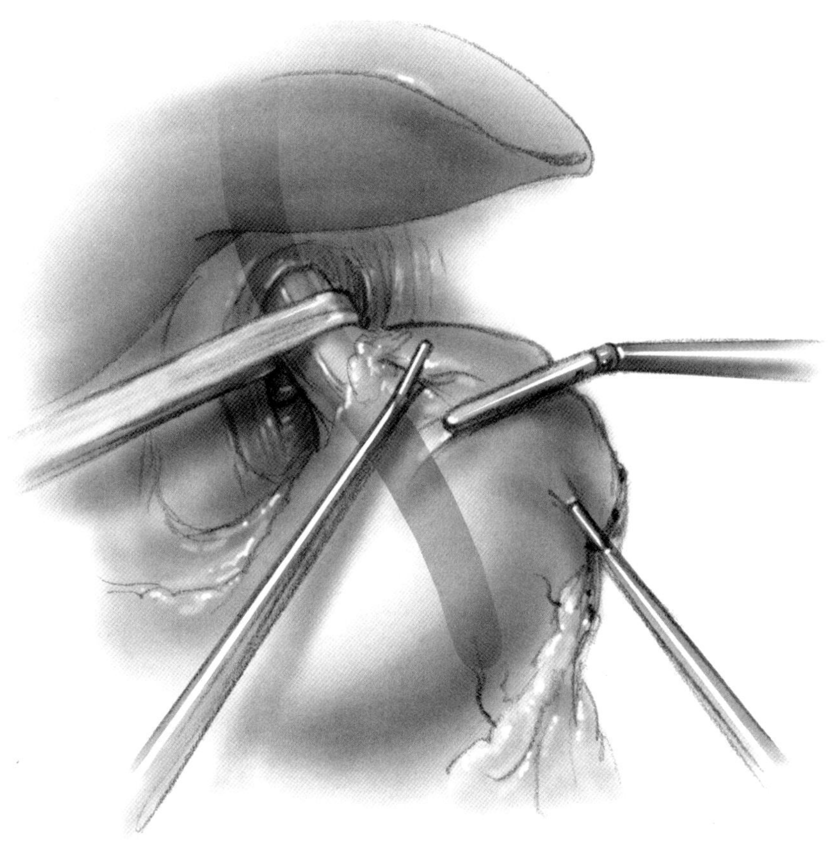

Fig. 12-1. First staple firing of wedge fundectomy.

level of the carina if needed, but 4 to 6 cm of additional exposure is usually adequate. The intraabdominal esophagus should be measured again using the technique described above. If it remains less than 2.5 cm even after extensive mediastinal dissection, a Collis gastroplasty should be performed.

Prior to performing the gastroplasty, a 48F dilator should be placed in the esophagus, past the GEJ, under direct vision. A point 2.5 cm inferior to the angle of His and 1 cm lateral to the recently placed dilator is then marked with a brief tap of electrocautery. This will mark the inferior end of the staple line used to create the neoesophagus, and there is usually more than enough additional length to allow a short, floppy fundoplication. The 10 mm left subcostal port located at the midclavicular line that was placed at the beginning of the operation should then be replaced with a 12-mm trocar to accommodate an articulating stapler. A 45-mm articulating endostapler loaded with 3.8-mm staples, or a "blue load," is introduced into the abdomen and maximally flexed to the left. A 60-mm load may be used, but is usually too cumbersome to manipulate in the tight confines of the upper abdomen. The surgical assistant should grasp a point on the greater curvature of the stomach 5 cm from the angle of His and retract anteriorly as the surgeon elevates the angle of His with his or her left hand and positions the stapler below the assistant's grasper, pointing toward the spot previously marked with electrocautery (Fig. 12-1). The staple is then fired in sequence across the stomach until the dilator is reached. With subsequent firings, the surgeon should grasp the superior staple line and lift it anteriorly while the assistant retracts the inferior staple line. This step usually requires two or three firings, with the final stapling visibly pushing the esophageal dilator out of its jaws. If the staple line does not reach the dilator, a boggy, oversized gastric tube will result. The stapler is then reintroduced through the left subcostal port and articulated in the opposite direction. A vertical staple line is then created parallel to the dilator; the stapler is placed across the remaining wedge of fundus abutting the dilator and fired sequentially until it is amputated (Fig. 12-2, page 114). It is important to staple, rather than cut, small bridges of tissue as the gastric remnant is removed, in order to minimize the risk of postoperative leak. The assistant should place lateral traction on this portion of stomach during the stapling. A 3- to 4-cm tube of stomach distal to the GEJ, or neoesophagus, should be visible. The esophageal dilator is then removed, a nasogastric tube is placed in the stomach under direct vision, and 250 ml of methylene blue is instilled in the stomach to test for leaks from the staple line.

Following the gastroplasty, a tension-free fundoplication is created. The diaphragmatic crura are closed posterior to the esophagus using interrupted sutures. The "new" fundus of the stomach is passed behind the GEJ and secured anteriorly for a traditional 360-degree fundoplication (Fig. 12-3, pages 114–115). If the patient was shown to have poor esophageal motility prior to surgery, a posterior partial fundoplication may be performed instead. The staple line created during the gastroplasty should appose the stomach wall when forming the wrap, effectively burying it and limiting contamination if any leak occurs. The apex of the staple line should be located at the middle fixation stitch and "buried" as the suture is tied. When positioning the wrap, it is crucial to ensure that the superiormost suture fixes it on the true esophagus, cephalad to the GEJ. The neoesophagus should therefore be completely buried by the wrap. This ensures that there is no gastric mucosa above the high-pressure zone of the fundoplication. Failure to place the wrap high enough may also cause the neoesophagus to dilate above this new high-pressure zone, causing a "slipped wrap" appearance, which in this case is actually due to an appropriate wrap causing dilatation of the atonic neoesophagus lying between it and the normally functioning "true" esophagus (Fig. 12-4, page 115).

Following creation of the wrap, the esophageal dilator should be removed and the patient taken out of the reverse Trendelenburg position to assess the native location of the wrap in the abdomen. The space just below the diaphragm should be filled by the fundoplication. If there is obvious extra esophagus or neoesophagus visible, the wrap may have been placed too low.

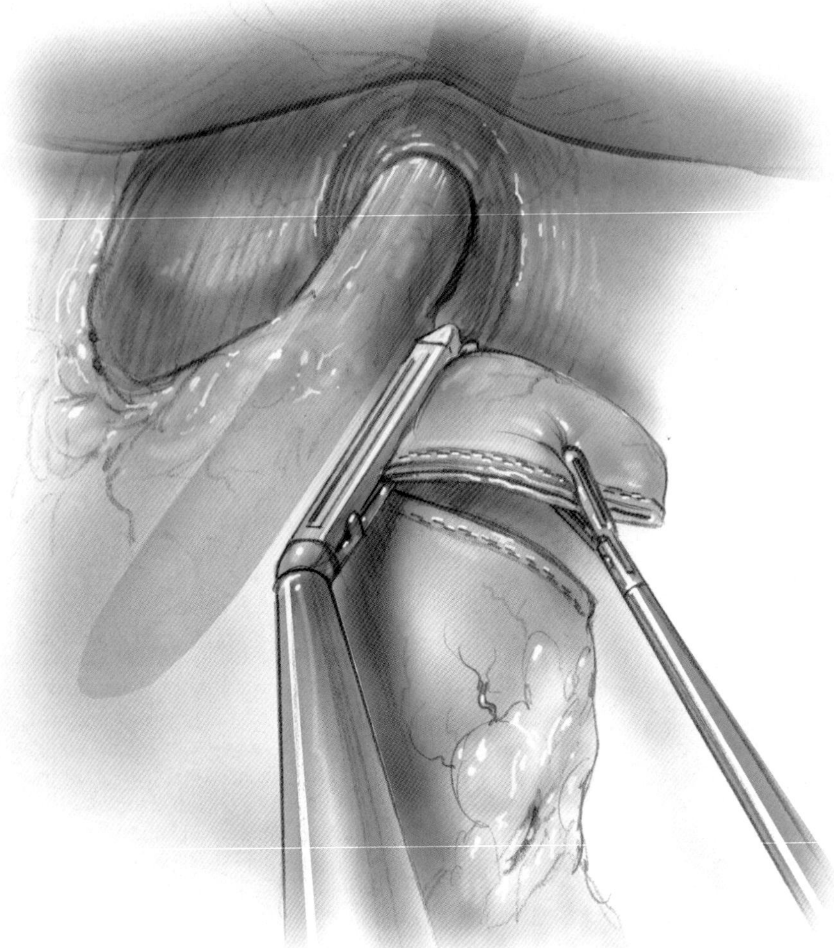

Fig. 12-2. Second staple firing of wedge fundectomy.

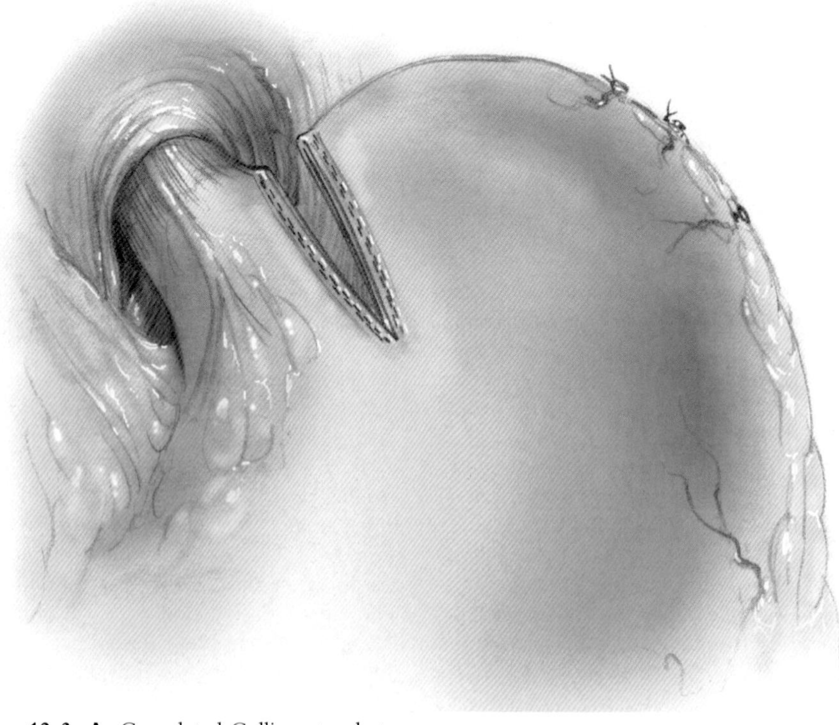

Fig. 12-3. A. Completed Collis gastroplasty.

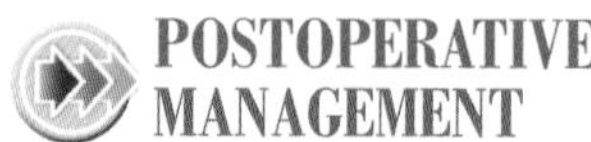

POSTOPERATIVE MANAGEMENT

The patient is kept NPO (*non per os*, or "nothing by mouth") overnight and a Gastrografin swallow study is obtained the morning after surgery. A nasogastric tube is rarely needed postoperatively. If no leak is seen on the esophagram, and contrast passes readily into the stomach, the patient is advanced to a liquid diet and is usually discharged the following day on a pureed diet. Edema of the lower esophagus, a common phenomenon following this surgery, may slow the clearance of contrast, but if complete obstruction is seen on Gastrografin swallow, reexploration is mandated.

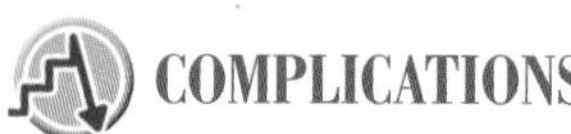

COMPLICATIONS

Collis gastroplasty is usually performed on patients with late-stage gastroesophageal reflux disease; consequently, clinical outcomes for these patients are not as good as for those undergoing an uncomplicated Nissen fundoplication. In most clinical series studying this procedure, a relatively high percentage of patients complain of persistent reflux or dysphagia postoperatively. In experienced hands, however, few patients experience major mechanical complications, such as paraesophageal herniation or wrap slippage, from this operation. Collis patients should be maintained on acid-suppression therapy postoperatively as the patients have been shown to have ectopic acid production and delayed clearance by pH probe studies.

CONCLUSION

While the presence of a true short esophagus in patients undergoing laparoscopic fundoplication may be rare, affecting only 3% to 5% of cases, it is critical to recognize this clinical entity in order to prevent paraesophageal herniation or slippage of the repair following surgery. A fundoplication performed around too little intraabdominal esophagus places too much tension on the repair as the GEJ migrates to its natural resting place above the diaphragm, ultimately leading to wrap failure or herniation. Patients who require esophageal lengthening in addition to fundoplication have higher rates of dysphagia and persistent esophagitis, due to the nonphysiologic nature of the Collis, than those undergoing fundoplication alone. These outcomes seem acceptable, however, when compared

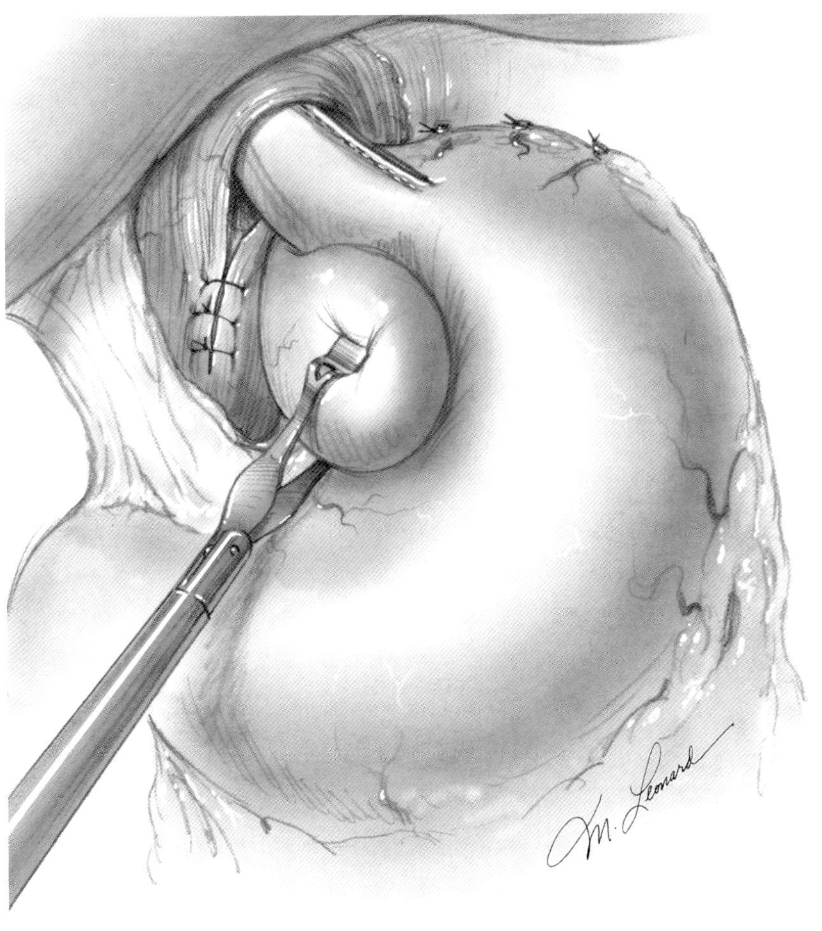

Fig. 12-3. Continued. **B.** Creation of Nissen fundoplication around the neoesophagus.

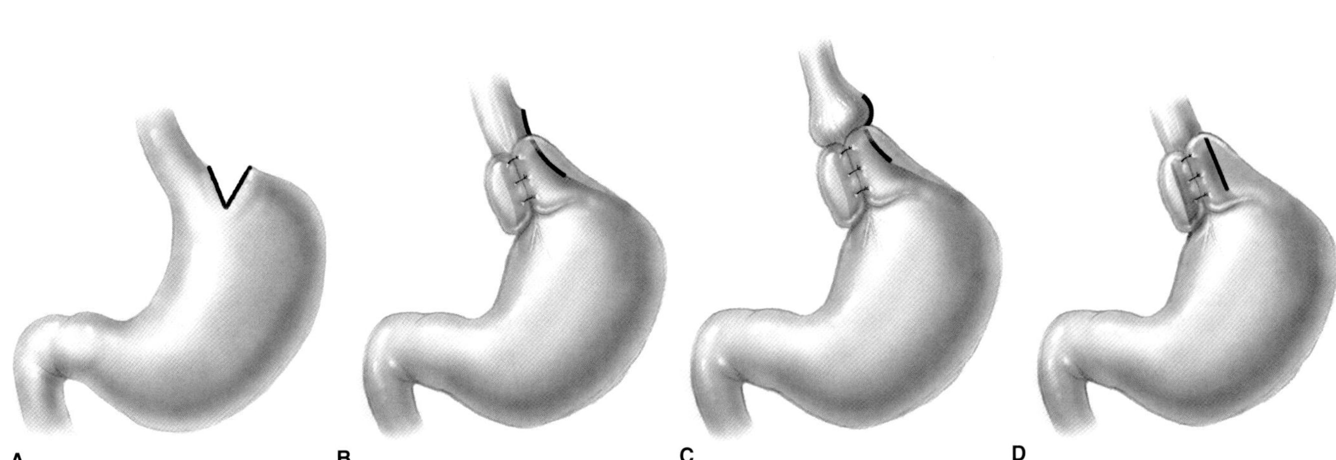

Fig. 12-4. A. Appearance of the gastric fundus after the final stapling. **B.** Placement of the fundoplication wrap too low on the "neoesophagus." **C.** Correct placement of the fundoplication wrap with complete coverage of the gastric staple lines. **D.** Proximal dilatation of the neoesophagus causing the appearance of a "slipped" Nissen.

to esophagectomy, which was the only feasible treatment of end-stage reflux disease prior to the development of this procedure.

SUGGESTED READING

Awad ZT, Filipi CJ, Mittal SK, et al. Left side thoracoscopically assisted gastroplasty: A new technique for managing the shortened esophagus. *Surg Endosc* 2000;14(5):508–512.

Awad ZT, Mittal SK, Roth TA, et al. Esophageal shortening during the era of laparoscopic surgery. *World J Surg* 2001;25(5):558–561.

Ellis FH, Jr, Leonardi HK, Dabuzhsky L, et al. Surgery for short esophagus with stricture: An experimental and clinical manometric study. *Ann Surg* 1978;188(3):34–350.

Gastal OL, Hagen JA, Peters JH, et al. Short esophagus: Analysis of predictors and clinical implications. *Arch Surg* 1999;134(6):633–636; discussion 637–638.

Hoang CD, Koh PS, Maddaus MA. Short esophagus and esophageal stricture. *Surg Clin North Am* 2005;85(3):43–451.

Horvath KD, Swanstrom LL, Jobe BA. The short esophagus: Pathophysiology, incidence, presentation, and treatment in the era of laparoscopic antireflux surgery. *Ann Surg* 2000; 232(5):630–640.

Jobe BA, Horvath KD, Swanstrom LL. Postoperative function following laparoscopic collis gastroplasty for shortened esophagus. *Arch Surg* 1998;133(8):867–874.

Johnson AB, Oddsdottir M, Hunter JG. Laparoscopic collis gastroplasty and Nissen fundoplication. A new technique for the management of esophageal foreshortening. *Surg Endosc* 1998;12(8):1055–1060.

Mittal SK, Awad ZT, Tasset M, et al. The preoperative predictability of the short esophagus in patients with stricture or paraesophageal hernia. *Surg Endosc* 2000;14(5):464–468.

O'Rourke RW, Khajanchee YS, Urbach DR, et al. Extended transmediastinal dissection: An alternative to gastroplasty for short esophagus. *Arch Surg* 2003;138(7):735–740.

Spivak H, Lelcuk S, Hunter JG. Laparoscopic surgery of the gastroesophageal junction. *World J Surg* 1999;23(4):356–367.

Stirling MC, Orringer MB. Continued assessment of the combined collis-nissen operation. *Ann Thorac Surg* 1989;47(2): 224–230.

Swanstrom LL, Marcus DR, Galloway GQ. Laparoscopic collis gastroplasty is the treatment of choice for the shortened esophagus. *Am J Surg* 1996;171(5):477–481.

Terry ML, Vernon A, Hunter JG. Stapled-wedge collis gastroplasty for the shortened esophagus. *Am J Surg* 2004;188(2): 195–199.

Yau P, Watson DI, Jamieson GG, et al. The influence of esophageal length on outcomes after laparoscopic fundoplication. *J Am Coll Surg* 2000;191(4):360–365.

COMMENTARY

The increase in the numbers of antireflux surgeries being performed over the last 10 to 20 years (from 8000 per year in the United States and Canada in the early 1990s to 60,000 or so annually today) has brought some long forgotten controversies into the spotlight once again. The short esophagus certainly is one such eternal subject of debate, not just regarding the best treatment for it but even whether it truly exists as a clinical finding. Prominent esophageal centers are on record claiming a zero incidence of the short esophagus while others advocate the need for a Collis in 30% to 40% of their cases. The vast majority of high-volume centers however, would agree with Drs. Hunter and Van Hove that around 3% to 4% of fundoplications will require a lengthening procedure. While this may sound like a trivial number, perhaps not even worth bothering about, it should be kept in mind that numerically it represents a third to a half of the commonly reported failure rate of fundoplications. The authors stress that the fundoplication surgeon must be prepared to deal with this finding at the time of surgery, as it is difficult to predict before surgery. Most have seen spectacularly shortened esophagi on preoperative evaluations that easily accordion down into the abdomen during dissection, while other times, a 2-cm hiatal hernia can be as noncompliant as a stick and fail to reduce. It is clear that "cheating," by pulling hard on the stomach or placing the wrap "just a little low," are short-term solutions and not in the patient's best interest considering the added cost, risk, and poorer outcomes of reoperations.

The "wedge fundectomy" technique described has certainly become the most commonly used and has the advantage of requiring only abdominal access and upsizing to a 12-mm port. Another technique, that of cutting a circular staple hole in the stomach with a circular stapler and then applying a linear stapler, has largely been abandoned as difficult and costly. We continue to use a transthoracic application of an articulating linear cutting stapler as it is quick, requires only one staple load, and doesn't resect any stomach. Both techniques have similar outcomes and surgeons should choose whichever they are more familiar and comfortable with. Still, as stressed by the authors, Collis gastroplasty is not a very physiologic procedure, with many patients requiring long-term acid suppression and at risk for distal esophageal dilatation and dysphagia. It should be thought of only as an alternative to esophagectomy for severe end-stage disease.

LLS

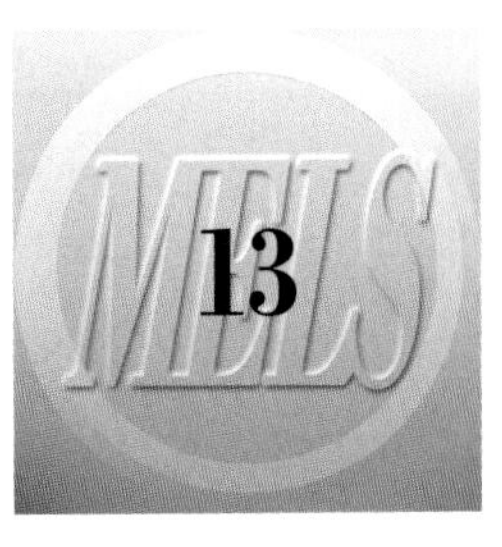

Laparoscopic Antireflux Surgery: Reoperations at the Esophageal Hiatus

C. DANIEL SMITH AND KENT R. VAN SICKLE

INTRODUCTION

Antireflux surgery (ARS) is appropriate and effective management for patients with gastroesophageal reflux disease (GERD) refractory to medical management, on lifelong acid suppression, or suffering from side effects of the medical management. Over the past two decades the operations have evolved from predominantly open thoracic approaches to a predominantly laparoscopic abdominal approach with similar, if not better, outcomes. As the procedures have evolved and patterns of failure and complications have been better characterized, morbidity and mortality have decreased 2.1% and 0.3% respectively, with long-term symptomatic success rates of over 90%.

Despite these excellent outcomes, there remains a small subset of patients who after ARS continue to suffer from persistent or recurrent GERD or develop new symptoms such as dysphagia or chest pain. Although many of these patients respond to nonoperative medical and endoscopic therapies, a small percentage, from 2% to 16%, ultimately undergo revisional ARS.

Reoperation after ARS, like most reoperative surgery, is technically challenging and fraught with potential complications. Additionally, success rates are typically lower than with the primary procedure. Therefore, an understanding of the potential early and late complications following ARS, the patterns of failure, the necessary preoperative workup, and appropriate patient selection are critical in maintaining low morbidity while achieving reasonable success with redo ARS.

The need to reoperate after a laparoscopic antireflux procedure can best be discussed when categorized as those problems arising in the immediate postoperative period, early postoperative period, and late postoperative period.

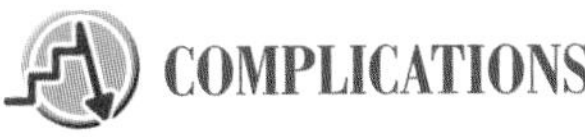

COMPLICATIONS

IMMEDIATE POSTOPERATIVE ISSUES

Major surgical complications immediately after primary ARS occur in 2% to 3% of patients. These include leaks from esophageal or gastric perforations (1%), acute wrap herniation (0.5%), and bleeding (0.2%). The most important predictors of favorable outcome with these complications are early diagnosis and timely operative intervention.

Leaks

Etiology

The most clinically significant immediate postoperative complication is a perforation leading to a leak. This can result from a delayed perforation caused by inadvertent electrocautery injury to the esophagus or stomach or ischemia of the gastric wall due to close cauterization of a short gastric vessel. Additional causes may include unrecognized perforation while performing a difficult dissection during mobilization of the cardia or esophageal hiatus, while passing an instrument around the esophagus, or while passing the esophageal dilator into the stomach.

Diagnosis and Workup

An unrecognized leak can be life-threatening. We commonly perform intraoperative endoscopy if dissection is particularly difficult or a leak is suspected. In the procedure, the esophagus and stomach are distended with air while submerged under water and air bubbles are sought. Some advocate injecting methylene blue through a nasogastric tube in the distal esophagus; in the authors' experience, there are cases where this technique failed to identify a perforation that was subsequently found with endoscopic insufflation as described. Postoperatively, signs of sepsis such as fever, leukocytosis, oliguria, and tachycardia should not be dismissed and must be thoroughly evaluated. An early Gastrografin swallow may help establish the diagnosis when otherwise clinically equivocal. If a leak is suspected, there is no role for diagnostic or therapeutic endoscopy in the early postoperative setting.

Management

If a leak is found or suspected, early reoperation is essential. This can be achieved laparoscopically with a relatively low conversion rate. If minimal or no contamination is found, a primary repair covered by a fundoplication, periesophageal fat patch, or fibrin glue is reasonable. In this setting, a deep drain and gastrostomy tube are also necessary to control the esophagogastric secretions. If excessive inflammation or contamination is encountered, surgical drainage with diversion and a venting/feeding gastrojejunostomy tube may be the safest immediate solution.

Acute Wrap Herniation

Etiology

Another technical complication, usually requiring immediate reoperation, is acute transdiaphragmatic wrap herniation (0.5% to 1.3%). The cause of an acute wrap herniation is usually mechanical or technical in nature. Issues such as incomplete crural closure, closure under tension, or suture disruption may be etiologic. Most commonly, the acute herniation is preceded by a sudden increase in intraabdominal pressure secondary to coughing or postoperative nausea and vomiting.

Diagnosis and Workup

This may present as a sudden severe, unrelenting midepigastric pain associated with nausea, vomiting, and dysphagia. It can also present more subtly as new dysphagia following an episode of retching. Workup should include a Gastrografin swallow, which would be diagnostic. Again, an upper endoscopy is rarely indicated in this acute setting.

Management

The best management of this problem is prevention with careful hiatal reconstruction and aggressive use of perioperative antiemetics. If patients retch in the immediate postoperative period, they should immediately undergo a contrast swallow. If wrap herniation is detected early (within 7 days), reoperation is indicated. Here, the hernia is reduced and the esophageal hiatus reconstructed. However, if wrap herniation is identified more than 7 days postoperatively, it is usually best to avoid redo ARS for at least 6 weeks because of the potential for dense adhesions and a very difficult repair. Reports have been made of tension-free crural repairs for both primary and reoperative paraesophageal herniation using different prosthetic biomaterial; however, this still remains controversial mostly due to a lack of long-term data pertaining to the risks of esophageal erosion and/or obstruction.

Bleeding

Etiology

Postoperative hemorrhage is unusual (0.2% to 0.75%) and most often from the result of an iatrogenic injury to the spleen or the short gastric vessels. Upper GI bleeding from missed peptic ulcer, severe esophagitis, or acute gastritis has been described but is very rare.

Diagnosis and Workup

Diagnosis of the acute intraabdominal hemorrhage is predominantly a clinical one based on the patient's hemodynamics and serial hematocrit measurements.

If the presenting problem is an acute upper GI bleed, the initial evaluation should include an upper endoscopy to localize and possibly address the lesion therapeutically. If bleeding is not localized endoscopically, the source should be considered to be inside the fundal wrap.

Management

If the patient is returned to the operating room, one can start with a laparoscopic exploration only if the patient is stable, and the surgeon is skilled in advanced laparoscopy.

In case of the unremitting upper GI bleed that is not controlled by endoscopic measures, reoperation may also be warranted. In this setting, one can undo the fundoplication and perform intraoperative endoscopy to manage a bleeding site within the wrap.

Once the patient is beyond the immediate perioperative period and discharged to home, the subsequent complications are usually divided into the categories of early problems (less than 6 weeks) and late problems (beyond 6 weeks).

EARLY POSTOPERATIVE PROBLEMS

The early morbidity associated with antireflux surgery can range from benign gas bloating to dysphagia and food impaction. It is important to recognize that more than half of the patients develop some degree of new "transient" symptom or symptoms that will resolve with time. Reoperation in this early postoperative period is extremely rare.

Dysphagia and Food Impaction

Presentation

The most common of the early complications is transient dysphagia, seen in over half of the patients and most commonly due to postoperative edema or a tight wrap. The onset is typically about the tenth postoperative day and should resolve by three weeks. Most patients will complain of difficulty swallowing solids and, in severe cases, intolerance of liquids. This postoperative edema accompanied by dietary indiscretions and consumption of solid foods (patients should not consume solids for one month after surgery) can lead to food impaction.

Diagnosis and Workup

The diagnosis in this setting is primarily based on clinical presentation alone. Contrast swallow will document the narrowing of the distal esophagus or the slow transit of contrast into the stomach. In most cases an upper endoscopy is not indicated for diagnostic purposes. However, if the symptoms don't resolve with conservative treatment, an endoscopic evaluation may be useful to ensure the wrap is not severely twisted and causing obstruction, or that an ulcer hasn't developed within the wrap.

Management

Reassurance and continuation of a soft food/liquid diet is the primary management. Early dilatation is rarely indicated, and risks early wrap disruption and recurrent GERD. Early dilatation is reserved for the small subgroup of patients with dysphagia persistent more than 6 weeks or with high-grade food impaction. If dilatation becomes necessary, serial dilatation with Savary or Maloney dilators is preferred over balloon dilatation because the sudden inflation pressures of the balloon dilators can lead to acute wrap disruption.

Gas Bloating or Aerophagia

Presentation

Other symptoms such as early bloating and aerophagia, or "air swallowing," with postprandial discomfort can also occur. This is most commonly seen with a tight wrap or excessive edema in a patient who preoperatively had symptoms of bloating or delayed gastric emptying (DGE).

Diagnosis and Workup

The most important element of the workup here is documenting a preoperative gastric emptying study. Patients who initially present with bloating associated with their GERD symptoms are more likely to have bloating complications postoperatively. These patients should undergo a gastric emptying study as part of their preoperative evaluation. If DGE is identified prior to surgery, a concurrent pyloroplasty or venting gastrostomy may help avoid the postoperative symptoms.

Management

The majority of the symptoms of gas bloating, pain, and aerophagia will resolve without specific intervention. However if the symptoms persist, and the gastric emptying study suggests DGE, the intervention will depend on the degree of DGE. If the half life (T½) of the study is abnormally long but less than twice the upper limit of normal, a recent comparative study has shown that a temporizing venting percutaneous endoscopic gastrostomy (PEG) can successfully relieve the symptoms without the need for a surgical pyloroplasty. However if the T½ is prolonged by more than twice the upper limit of normal, the patient will likely need a pyloroplasty, which often times can be performed laparoscopically.

LATE POSTOPERATIVE PROBLEMS

Antireflux operations are performed to eliminate pathologic gastroesophageal reflux. Late failure in this setting is defined as either not successfully controlling the reflux or creating new problems as a result of the anatomic alterations of the surgery. In spite of the variability in the primary antireflux operations performed in the U.S. such as the Nissen fundoplication, the Hill posterior gastropexy, or the Belsey Mark IV repair, all repairs seem to have a similar long-term failure rate of 5% to 15%.

In our earlier series of 1000 consecutive patients undergoing laparoscopic antireflux surgery for GERD and paraesophageal hernias, we found a 3.6% reoperation rate at 7 years follow-up. The rate was similar between the GERD and the paraesophageal hernia subgroups. However, the patients with more severe reflux as evidenced by esophageal stricture and Barrett esophagus had a higher rate of revisional surgery than those with uncomplicated GERD (8% vs. 3.6%). Over 90% of the revisional operations after laparoscopic fundoplication were performed within the first two years of follow-up.

Etiologies or Patterns of Failure

Patterns of failure for laparoscopic ARS differ from open ARS. Nonetheless, they can all be classified in one of the categories of anatomic or physiologic failure (Table 13-1). Over the years, as the patterns of failure have been better defined, many authors have identified important intraoperative technical factors that may contribute to failures (Table 13-2). (See also Figs. 13.1 and 13.2.) Careful attention to these critical steps of the procedure may help reduce this failure rate and in fact explain some of the differences between failure rates at different institutions.

The reason to emphasize these mechanisms of failure is that the prevention of failure is by far a much more effective and reliable measure of long-term success than any subsequent attempt at medical, endoscopic, or surgical intervention.

Workup

Before undertaking revisional ARS, a thorough evaluation is essential. This should include a complete history and physical and adjunct studies of barium swallow, upper endoscopy, esophageal physiologic studies of manometry and PH testing, and a gastric emptying study. The history should specifically seek and document symptoms of heartburn, regurgitation, and dysphagia and compare these with the patient's preoperative symptomatology. Specifically, asking

TABLE 13-1. ANATOMIC AND PHYSIOLOGIC PATTERNS OF FAILURE OF ANTIREFLUX SURGERY

Anatomic patterns of failure (see Figs. 13-1 and 13-2)

1. Complete or partial wrap disruption
2. Misplaced or slipped wrap
3. Transdiaphragmatic wrap herniation
4. Wrap too tight or too long
5. Twisted wrap
6. Tight crural closure

Physiologic patterns of failure

1. Incorrect initial diagnosis (e.g., achalasia)
2. Unrecognized associated foregut problem (e.g. delayed gastric emptying, esophageal body dysfunction, peptic ulcer disease)

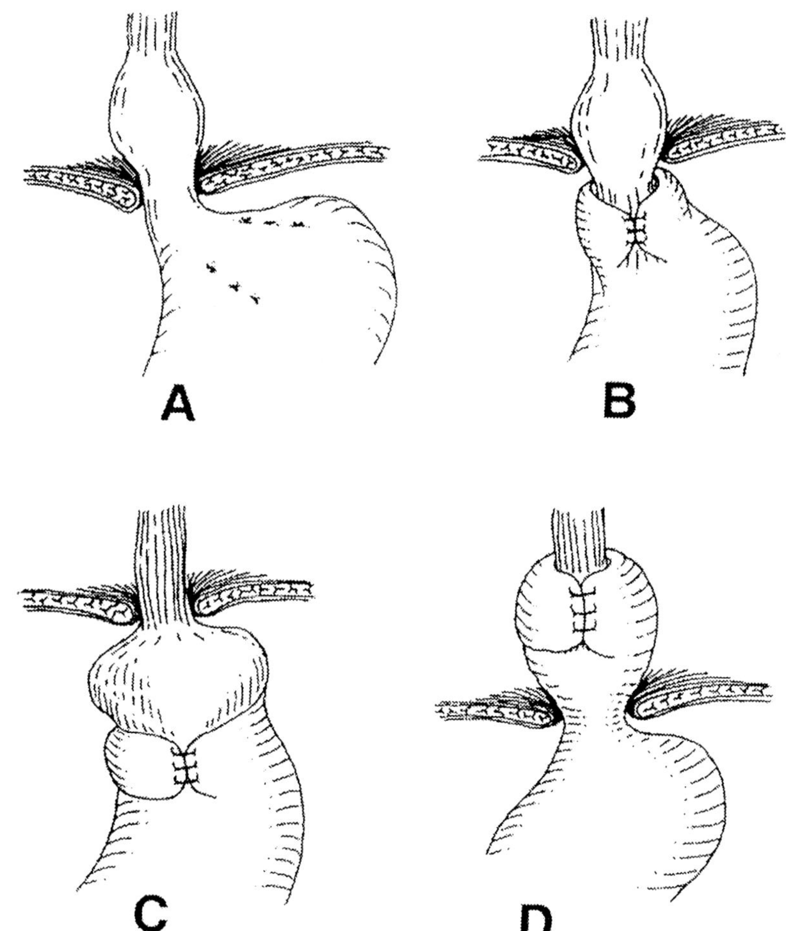

Fig. 13-1. Four types of surgical failure of Nissen fundoplication. A. Wrap disruption. **B.** Gastric herniation above the wrap. **C.** "Slipped" Nissen. **D.** Wrap herniation. (Used with permission from Hinder RA: Gastroesophageal reflux disease. In Bell RH Jr, Rikkers LF, Mulholland MW (eds): *Digestive Tract Surgery: A Text and Atlas*. Philadelphia, Lippincott-Raven Publishers, 1996, p. 19.)

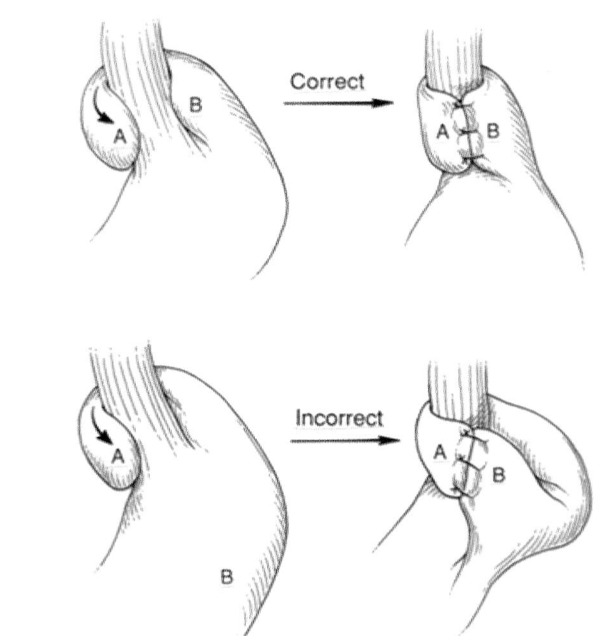

Fig. 13-2. Another failure mechanism: the "twisted" wrap, in which the gastric body rather than the fundus is used to perform fundoplication.

TABLE 13-2. INTRAOPERATIVE TECHNICAL ERRORS LEADING TO LATE SURGICAL FAILURE

1. Inadequate esophageal mobilization
2. Placing the fundic wrap too low onto the stomach or choosing the body of the stomach for the wrap
3. Inadequate fixation of the fundic wrap
4. Inadequate takedown of the short gastric attachments (Rossetti-Nissen fundoplication), which can lead to a twisted wrap
5. Inadequate closure of the crura or primary suture closure under tension
6. Inadequate hiatal dissection +/– incomplete reduction of paraesophageal hernia and hernia sac

about early postprandial bloating will help identify those most likely to have delayed gastric emptying. A copy of the previous operative report may help delineate any potential problems in the first operation that may have led to an anatomic failure and serve as a road map in the reoperation.

An upper endoscopy is the single most useful test for identifying and characterizing anatomic failure, especially wrap twisting, misplacement, or transdiaphragmatic herniation. Barium swallow is often only confirmatory. Esophageal function tests with PH monitoring and manometry are also necessary to assess recurrent GERD or motility problems. Manometry is critical in assessing esophageal clearance both to ensure that the proper operation was performed previously, but also to base the type of reoperative fundoplication on the status of the esophageal motility, sphincter pressures, and clearance.

Medical and Endoscopic Management

Recurrent Reflux

If the failure is secondary to recurrent reflux symptoms, a trial of medical management with proton pump inhibitors (PPIs) is indicated. However, both the patient and the physician should realize that success of medical management is lower in operated than nonoperated patients. At the least, a trial can allow for esophagitis, ulcerations, and edema to resolve prior to further intervention. Furthermore, symptom control with PPIs may also predict favorable response to revisional ARS.

If the workup does not reveal an obvious anatomic or technical etiology for the recurrence of symptoms but documents pathologic gastroesophageal reflux, endoscopic antireflux procedures may be considered. Radiofrequency ablation (RFA) of the lower esophageal sphincter has been shown to be effective in 70% to 85% of patients with primary GERD, although this has not yet been studied in those who have failed ARS. In a recent animal model, we demonstrated that this technique can be performed with reasonable accuracy and efficacy after previously failed ARS using fluoroscopic guidance. The clinical experience in this setting is extremely limited; however, in our recent study of RFA in eight patients after failed fundoplication, seven were documented to have shown improvement in GERD symptoms at a one-year mean follow-up.

Other endoscopic techniques such as the submucosal injection of an expanding biopolymer or utilizing an endoscopic suturing device may also be an alternative to reoperation for a loose wrap or hypotensive lower esophageal sphincter. All such endoscopic therapies are currently approved as primary therapy for GERD; none have any significant data from use in revisional ARS.

Dysphagia

If failure is secondary to new or progressive dysphagia, the usual etiology is an intact but misaligned, misplaced, or herniated wrap. With dysphagia in the absence of a paraesophageal hernia or a slipped, misplaced, or twisted fundoplication, a nonoperative trial of dilatation can be attempted. Balloon dilatation is usually not recommended because the sudden inflation pressures can potentially disrupt the wrap. However serial dilatations with Savary or Maloney dilators may be successful in resolving the problem of an otherwise uncomplicated tight or long wrap.

Reoperative Management

As mentioned earlier, the key predictors of positive surgical outcomes are patient selection and operative technique. Regarding patient selection, those patients who present with recurrent or new symptoms of reflux or dysphagia and have a corresponding anatomic abnormality experience the best results with revisional ARS.

Regarding operative technique, the experience of the surgeon with reoperative ARS is key in determining the outcome of these operations. Revisional ARS is technically challenging; experience and skill with reoperative abdominal surgery along with an understanding of the esophagogastroduodenal physiology and anatomy are imperative in achieving the best functional result. Historically, reoperative antireflux surgery has been approached through an open laparotomy or thoracotomy, which was determined largely by whether the primary procedure was abdominal or thoracic. With increasing skill and experience in laparoscopic techniques, laparoscopic revisional ARS has been shown to be safe and efficacious. However, if the patient has had multiple open foregut procedures, laparoscopic reoperation may not be feasible, and a thoracotomy may then be the safest alternative. In particular, reconstruction of the hiatus in the case of recurrent paraesophageal hernia or esophageal shortening may best be managed through a thoracic approach. Irrespective of the approach, the operation should be crafted to the pathophysiology and anatomy identified in the preoperative workup. For example, if the manometry documents a severe motility disorder, then the wrap should be taken down and redone with a 270-degree (Toupet or Dor) fundoplication. Or, in the case of esophageal shortening, an esophageal lengthening procedure such as a Collis gastroplasty may be needed.

Regardless of the reason for failure, some general principles apply to all revisional ARS, as listed in Table 13-3.

TABLE 13-3. GENERAL PRINCIPLES IN THE CONDUCT OF REVISIONAL ANTIREFLUX SURGERY

1. Perform a complete hiatal dissection and esophageal mobilization well into the mediastinum.
2. Specifically ensure adequate fundic mobilization and take down additional short gastric vessels if necessary.
3. Always take apart the previous fundoplication.
4. Use intraoperative endoscopy to assess esophageal length and integrity of esophagus and stomach (identifying perforations).
5. Calibrate wrap over esophageal dilator.
6. Use gastrostomy tube liberally if concerned about potential esophagus or stomach injury, delayed return of GI function, or ability to eat.
7. Aggressively prevent postoperative nausea and retching with prophylactic antiemetics in all patients.

RESULTS OF REOPERATIVE ANTIREFLUX SURGERY

Most series report acceptable results for revisional ARS. These usually range in the 70% to 85% success rate, as opposed to the success rates of 85% to 95% for primary operations. In the late 1990s, Jamieson reported a 79% success rate in a meta-analysis of 564 redo patients from 14 series. The success rate falls to 66% and 50% respectively with third and fourth reoperations. Morbidity and mortality are also higher in this reoperative group. Morbidity rates range from 2% to 46% and mortality rates are reported anywhere between 0.5% to 17%. In our own series of 251 reoperative cases, overall morbidity and mortality were 14% and 0.4% respectively.

As mentioned earlier, these redo patients can be highly complex and technically challenging, and the operations inherently carry a high complication rate and lower success rates. Therefore, before considering a patient for reoperative anti-reflux surgery, one must carefully determine the cause of failure, assess the severity of their symptoms, and ultimately weigh these factors against the risks of a redo operation in order to determine the necessity for intervention and the likelihood of its success.

SUGGESTED READING

Morganthal CB, Lin E, Shane MD, et al. Who will fail laparoscopic Nissen fundoplication? Preoperative predication of long-term outcomes. *Surg Endosc* 2007;21(11):1978–1984.

Smith CD, McClusky DA, Rajad MA, et al. When fundoplication fails: redo? *Annals of Surg* 2005;241(6):861–869; discussion 869–881.

COMMENTARY

Reoperative anti-reflux surgery can be extremely challenging. Complication rates are clearly documented to be higher than initial procedures. Average operative times are longer than initial operations, and the technical expertise required to provide reasonable outcomes from reoperative anti-reflux operations is greater. Some experts report perforation rates for gastric or esophageal perforations as 25% for second (redo) laparoscopic Nissen fundoplication and up to 50% for a third revision.

The authors have appropriately emphasized the need for extensive evaluation to determine the most likely cause of failure of the initial operation. A revision performed without such a workup and a reasonable determination of the cause of failure is likely to lead to a repeat failure.

Management of complications is described in detail in this chapter. Recent reports have indicated that temporary endoscopic stent placement at the site of esophageal or gastroesophageal junction leaks can lead to healing and avoid reoperation in selected patients.

The patterns of failure described are important for the surgeon to know and fully comprehend when caring for this patient population. This characterization of the type of failure aids in planning an effective reoperation. Additionally, describing wrap failures in these terms allows for a reasonable comparison of outcomes from various reoperation techniques or centers.

WSE

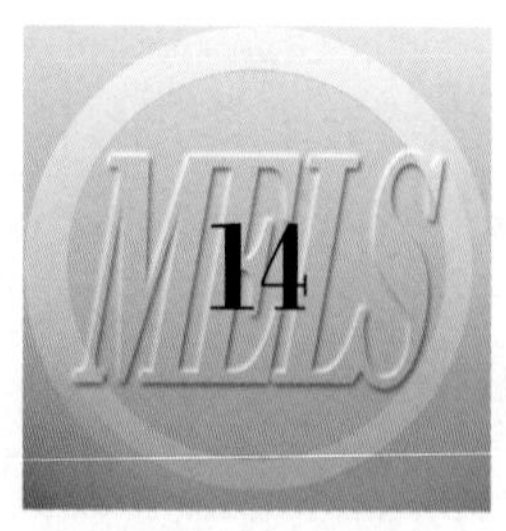

Laparoscopic Repair of Paraesophageal Hernias

SAJIDA AHAD AND BRANT K. OELSCHLAGER

INTRODUCTION

Henry Ingersoll Bowditch published the first description of hiatal hernia in 1853. However, it wasn't until 1926 that Ake Akerlund first used the term *hiatus hernia* and classified it into the three types still used today. When the diaphragmatic hiatus aperture enlarges, it can allow the stomach and other viscera to herniate into the thorax. While this can predispose a patient to gastroesophageal reflux disease (GERD), it can also result in a partial or complete volvulus and substantial morbidity and mortality from complete gastric obstruction, strangulation, and mucosal ischemia. Therefore, most paraesophageal hernias (PEHs) are surgically repaired, most commonly using a laparoscopic approach.

CLINICAL PRESENTATION

Most PEHs are thought to start as small hiatal hernias that over time lead to a further weakening of the phrenoesophageal membrane and development of a much larger defect. The phrenoesophageal membrane is formed by the fusion of endothoracic and endoabdominal fascia. The latter is a continuation of the transversalis fascia and attaches intimately to the esophageal adventitia. This membrane anchors the distal esophagus circumferentially within the diaphragmatic hiatus. Through congenital or acquired weakness, this membrane is progressively stretched and becomes attenuated. Known risk factors for the development of hiatal hernias are conditions that increase intraabdominal pressure like obesity, pregnancy, chronic constipation and chronic obstructive pulmonary disease. The incidence of this type of hernia increases with age, as these hernias are unusual before the sixth decade of life.

Hernias of the esophageal hiatus are classified according to the position of the gastroesophageal junction and extent of herniated stomach. Type I or "sliding" hiatal hernias occur when the gastroesophageal junction (GEJ) extends axially above the diaphragm and may slide into and out of the posterior mediastinum. This is by far the most common type, accounting for approximately 95% of hiatal hernias and usually associated with GERD. Other types of hiatal hernias in which the stomach extends alongside the esophagus are grouped and classified as paraesophageal hernias. In Type II hernias, the fundus of the stomach extends cranially through the hiatus, with the GEJ remaining in its normal, intraabdominal position (Fig. 14-1). When the GEJ is herniated with the stomach, it is a Type III hernia, which is much more common than type II hernias. A Type IV hiatal hernia sometimes refers to a paraesophageal hernia that also contains other viscera, such as spleen or colon, herniated along with the stomach in the sac.

While some patients with PEHs are asymptomatic, most PEHs cause symptoms. Like Type I hernias, PEHs may be associated with GERD and its constellation of symptoms. However, patients are just as likely to present with obstructive symptoms related to compression or volvulus of the stomach within the mediastinum resulting in chest pain, dysphagia, postprandial fullness, or early satiety. Many patients will present with iron deficiency anemia. Chronic ulceration of the gastric mucosa at the hiatus may cause Cameron ulcers, and can be associated with chronic blood loss. Even in the absence of these ulcers, one should assume that a PEH is the cause of anemia in the absence of more likely sources. In most cases, this anemia will resolve after repair. Occasionally, an acute volvulus occurs, resulting in complete obstruction and possibly vascular compromise. The triad of epigastric pain, inability to vomit, and failure to pass a nasogastric tube into the stomach, also known as Borchardt's triad, heralds gastric volvulus and warrants prompt intervention.

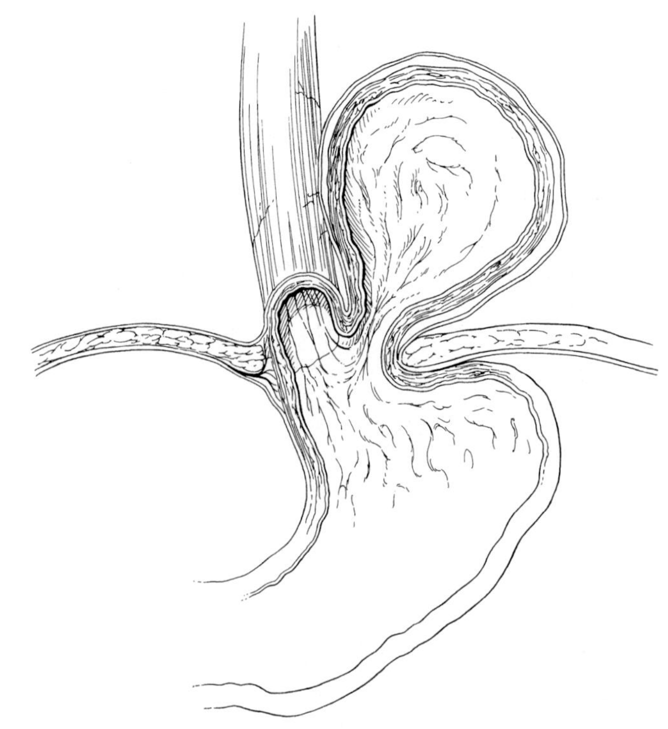

Fig. 14-1. Type II paraesophageal hernia.

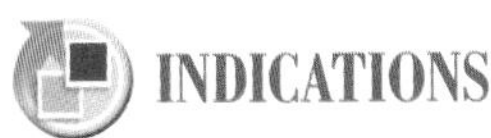

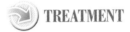

INDICATIONS

Until recently, the advice given to all patients with a paraesophageal hernia was to undergo surgical repair, based on earlier reports of a high risk of gastric incarceration and strangulation. Hill reported a 30% incidence of incarceration and strangulation in 10 of 29 patients managed expectantly without operation, and the resulting mortality for the emergent operation was 50%. Around the same time as Hill's report, Skinner and Belsey reported their experience with treating 21 of a cohort of PEH 82 patients nonoperatively. Of these 21 patients, six (28%) died from complications of strangulation, perforation, exsanguinating hemorrhage, or acute dilatation of herniated intrathoracic stomach. Because of these two reports, surgeons for decades treated the presence of a PEH as an indication for repair. More recent experience and studies have estimated the risk of life-threatening complications to be much lower. Stylopoulos et al. used a Markov-based Monte Carlo decision analytic model and administrative data to estimate this risk and found it to be approximately 1.1% per year for a 65-year-old patient. Moreover, in a review from the Mayo Clinic, Allen et al. managed 21 minimally symptomatic or asymptomatic patients with PEH expectantly; at a median follow-up of 78 months, 19 of these patients reported no worsening of their symptoms, and none experienced strangulation or acute symptoms. Not only is the risk of acute volvulus lower than previously reported, but the overall lifetime risk of death in expectantly managed patients is more likely closer to 1%. Thus for many patients, especially the elderly and those with severe comorbidities, it is not beneficial to offer routine repair of all paraesophageal hernias in the absence of symptoms. Nevertheless, most patients who present with a PEH are symptomatic and warrant consideration of repair in the absence of prohibitive risk factors.

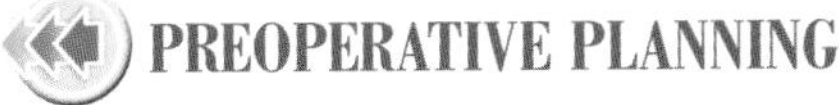

PREOPERATIVE PLANNING

Many hernias first show up on a lateral chest x ray as a retrocardiac bubble, though most are discovered during workup for symptoms. A barium esophagram is the best study to confirm the diagnosis and to delineate the anatomy of the esophagus, stomach, and position of the GEJ. All patients should undergo endoscopy to evaluate the upper gastrointestinal tract for ulcers, esophagitis, gastritis, or neoplasms. While a CT scan can incidentally diagnose a paraesophageal hernia, it is not routinely obtained preoperatively. While it rarely changes management, esophageal manometry is useful to evaluate the lower esophageal sphincter and esophageal body peristalsis. Because many institutions such as the University of Washington Medical Center routinely perform a fundoplication with repair, pH testing may not alter operative decision making. However, for groups using a selective approach to fundoplication with PEH repair, 24-hour pH testing becomes an important part of preoperative planning. In addition, patients should have appropriate medical workup as dictated by their clinical situation.

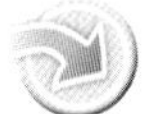

TREATMENT

Classically, PEHs have been treated with either a thoracotomy or laparotomy, but increasingly the laparoscopic approach is preferred. The first laparoscopic PEH repair was reported in 1991, and many subsequent publications have demonstrated the technical feasibility of laparoscopic paraesophageal hernia repair. There are advantages to both thoracotomy and laparotomy, though the laparoscopic approach incorporates many of the advantages of both.

The transthoracic approach offers the advantage of direct visualization and dissection of the esophagus, intrathoracic stomach, and hernia sac, allowing a tension-free reduction of the herniated stomach. Moreover, if a short esophagus is indeed encountered, a Collis gastroplasty can be easily reconstructed through the thorax. Some authors have suggested that a short esophagus is common in PEHs. For example, Swanstrom et al. reported a 20% incidence of short esophagus and subsequent need for an esophageal lengthening procedure in their patients with PEH. Indeed, there are institutional reports with good outcomes of the transthoracic approach, such as Maziak et al., who reported the results of 94 patients with PEH treated surgically with a transthoracic repair. In their hands, the approach seemed justified as a gastroplasty was added in 80% of cases because of clearly defined or presumed short esophagus. In addition, their long-term outcomes were good, with 80% of patients reporting excellent results at median follow-up of 72 months. Most of the downsides to the thoracic approach are associated with the incision, including pain, need for a tube thoracostomy, increased length of hospital stay, increased risk of pulmonary complications, and higher cost, all of which make the transthoracic approach less appealing than others. Finally, if one agrees that a fundoplication is necessary, it is much more difficult to fashion one through the chest.

Laparotomy offers an advantage in emergent operations as it can be performed in a more expeditious and possibly safer manner. However, like thoracotomy, it has substantial morbidity associated with the incision. In addition, visualization and operating in the mediastinum are very difficult via laparotomy, perhaps increasing the risk of inadvertent injury to viscera or surrounding structures during hiatal dissection in a tight space. This is especially more challenging in the obese patient.

The burgeoning enthusiasm for laparoscopic surgery, especially for GERD, has led to an increasing number of centers using laparoscopic repair for large paraesophageal hernias. Laparoscopy takes advantage of the benefits of laparotomy (easier access) and thoracotomy (superior visualization of hiatus and mediastinum), combining them in a much less morbid operation. Because most patients with a PEH are elderly, a laparoscopic procedure is even more appealing, as it decreases the morbidity and mortality in a high-risk population. Several nonrandomized comparisons of PEH repaired by laparoscopy or laparotomy have demonstrated significantly less blood loss, intensive care unit stay, ileus, hospital stay, and overall morbidity with the laparoscopic approach. Morbidity with laparoscopic paraesophageal hernia repairs (LPEHR) ranges from 0% to 14%, with mortality around 0.3%. In contrast, an open approach is associated with morbidity rates of 5% to 25% and mortality of 1% to 2%. Although no randomized trial exists, it seems logical that LPEHR is associated with decreased morbidity and faster recovery, compared to its open counterpart. Patient satisfaction and quality of life are also very high with the laparoscopic approach, greater than with laparotomy.

There are also many technical advantages inherent in laparoscopy that makes it an ideal approach for operating on the hiatus. Angled scopes provide superior visualization and greatly facilitate mediastinal dissection. Through a standard laparotomy incision, this dissection is much more difficult and poorly visualized. At the same time, the higher morbidity of a larger incision, tube thoracostomy, and the lung collapse associated with transthoracic approach are avoided. The operative time, hospitalization, and conversion rate to laparotomy are higher in inexperienced surgeons, but all improve with the learning curve.

Recurrence rates following LPEHR have been a common criticism: early reports from several institutions noted significant recurrence rates. Most of these were radiographic and not symptomatic recurrences, but they underscored the importance of developing new methods of avoiding postoperative failure. The addition of an antireflux procedure, a gastrostomy, and the use of mesh to reinforce hiatal closure are all techniques used in an attempt to decrease recurrence and will be discussed in more detail in ensuing sections. At the University of Washington, we believe that laparoscopy offers a minimally invasive, safe, and durable means to repair PEH, and it is our procedure of choice.

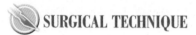

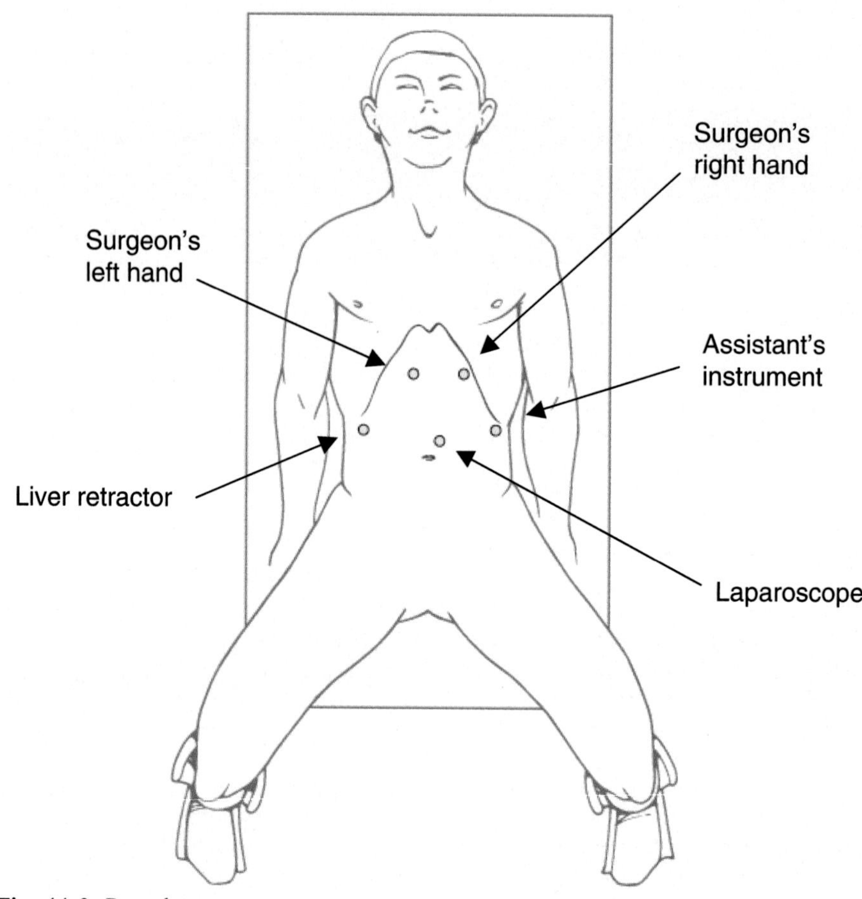

Fig. 14-2. Port placement.

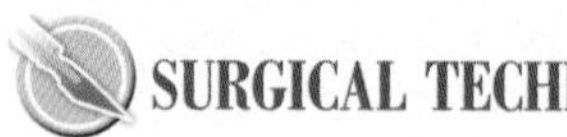

SURGICAL TECHNIQUE

It is our practice to perform this operation with the patient in a modified low lithotomy position. A beanbag creates a "seat" for the patient, which along with straps is used to avoid patient slippage when placing the patient in steep reverse Trendelenburg position. As a result, the surgeon is able to stand between the patient legs and operate in the ideal ergonomic position, while the assistant stands on the left side of the patient.

A 1-cm transverse incision is made over the left costal margin lateral to the midclavicular line. A Veress needle is introduced through this incision, and a carbon dioxide pneumoperitoneum established followed by an optical trocar that is advanced through the different planes of the abdominal wall. Four additional ports are placed as noted in Figure 14-2. The principles of a PEH repair are the same as the repair of any hernia in the body; that is, tension-free repair and closure of the defect. The distinct steps described below accomplish this.

Reduction of Hernia Sac and Assessment of Esophageal Length

Adequate mobilization of the hernia contents, including circumferential dissection of the distal esophagus, is necessary for achieving a successful repair (Fig. 14-3, page 125). Failure to do so may result in a short esophagus, which is likely a major reason for recurrence. While the exact incidence of a short esophagus is unknown, all surgeons recognize the concept. A recent meta-analysis suggested the rate to be about 12% for patients with PEH, 10 times higher than the overall incidence of short esophagus in patients undergoing a fundoplication for GERD. The combination of reflux esophagitis, stricture formation, adhesions within the hernia sac, and chronic position of the stomach and GEJ within the mediastinum probably all contribute to short esophagus. Unfortunately, no preoperative study accurately predicts the problem. An esophagram has a sensitivity of 66% and a positive predictive value of 37%, whereas manometric length had a sensitivity of 43% and a positive predictive value of 25% for the diagnosis of short esophagus. The preoperative endoscopic finding of either a stricture or Barrett esophagus was the most sensitive test for predicting the need for a lengthening procedure. Hernia size is also not a reliable predictor of short esophagus. Ultimately, the surgeon can only make this diagnosis in the operating room after all attempts at achieving an adequate esophageal length fail. It is important to have at least 2.5 to 3 cm of intraabdominal esophagus to decrease the chances of recurrence. In our institutional experience, we have found that adequate dissection and mobilization of the mediastinal esophagus, sometimes up to the carina, decreases the finding of short esophagi substantially. Other authors have reported a similar experience. Madan et al. described 628 fundoplications, with 351 requiring hiatal hernia repair. After appropriate esophageal mobilization was performed, no further lengthening procedure was necessary. In the rare instance when esophageal mobilization fails, the surgeon performs a Collis gastroplasty.

Another less discussed option for the short esophagus is vagotomy. Division of one or, if needed, both vagii can lengthen the esophagus by several centimeters, potentially avoiding the need for gastroplasty. While this theoretically has the potential for causing symptoms of delayed gastric emptying and dumping syndrome, we have studied numerous patients with a vagotomy during PEH repair and have

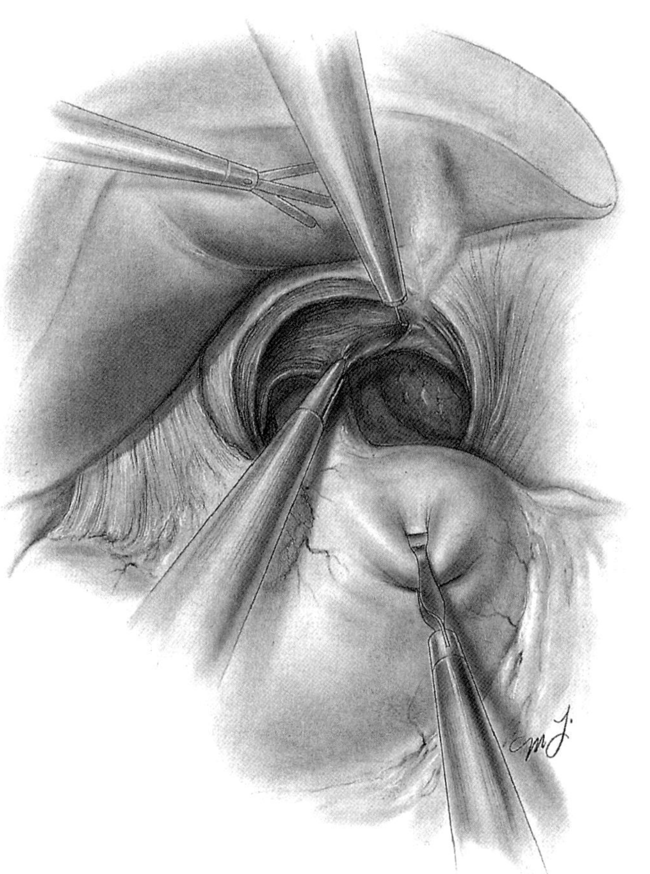

Fig. 14-3. Dissection of hernia sac off the hiatus and right crus.

Reapproximation of the Hiatus

Tension-free closure of the hiatus is a crucial step in the repair of PEH, but one that is quite challenging for many reasons. First, the crura are not static structures and are continually under significant tension and stress. Over time, even durable repairs may wear down and lead to hernia recurrence. Secondly, with a PEH the muscles of the crura are stretched and attenuated, making it difficult to get proper purchase with sutures. Finally, the sheer size of the hernia creates a large gap between the crura. Primary crural repair places undue tension on the crura, with a higher risk of disruption. Not surprisingly, simple suture closure is associated with a higher failure rate. Therefore, many strategies have been developed to assist in closure. Some authors have used pledgets to decrease the direct injury of suture on crural muscle. Others have described the use of a relaxing incision in the right crus to decrease tension on the crura. The use of prosthetic mesh for hiatoplasty has also gained acceptance. Mesh, discussed in more detail below, has shown promise in reducing hernia recurrence rates. The crural repair is performed by placing interrupted sutures between the right and left crura posterior to the esophagus and sometimes anterior to the esophagus if needed (Fig. 14-5).

found no difference in gastric emptying compared to patients with PEH repair and intact vagii. Therefore, we generally prefer a vagotomy to Collis in the unusual case of the short esophagus.

Excision of the Hernia Sac

Complete excision of the hernia sac is necessary for several reasons. First, the hernia sac tends to exert upward traction on the stomach and esophagus, and removing this relieves the tension on the newly reduced hernia. Second, leaving the sac behind also impairs visualization of the hiatus and the gastroesophageal junction (GEJ). Because the sac is connected to the GEJ, the intrathoracic stomach cannot be completely reduced without complete sac excision. It may also compromise crural approximation. According to one comparison, not removing the hernia sac is associated with a recurrence rate of up to 20% compared to a 0% recurrence rate when the sac is excised. The hernia sac is dissected circumferentially from the hiatal and mediastinal structures (Figs. 14-3 and 14-4). The sac is then everted over the GEJ and excised.

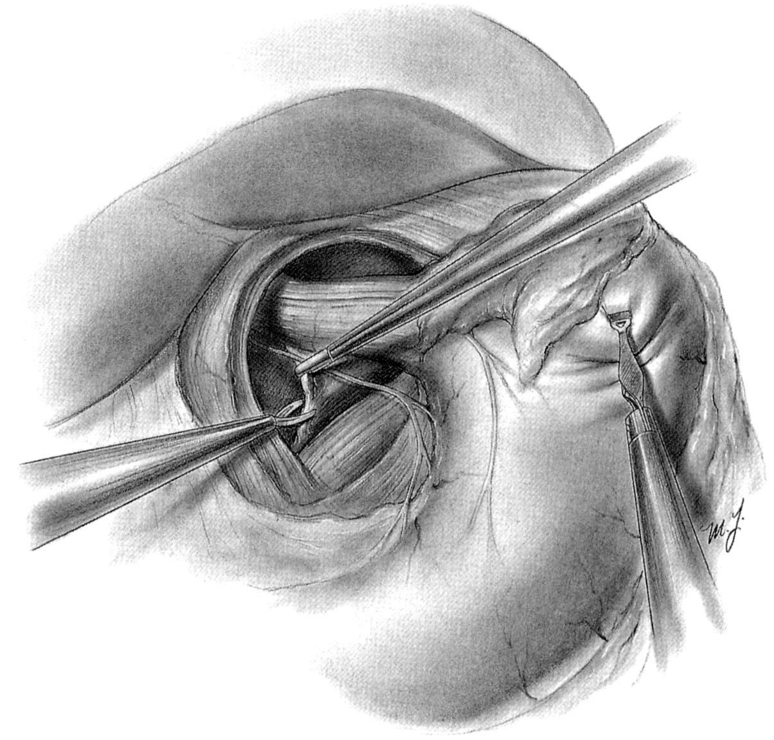

Fig. 14-4. Posterior dissection of the hernia sac and esophagus within the mediastinum. The posterior vagus nerve is identified and preserved.

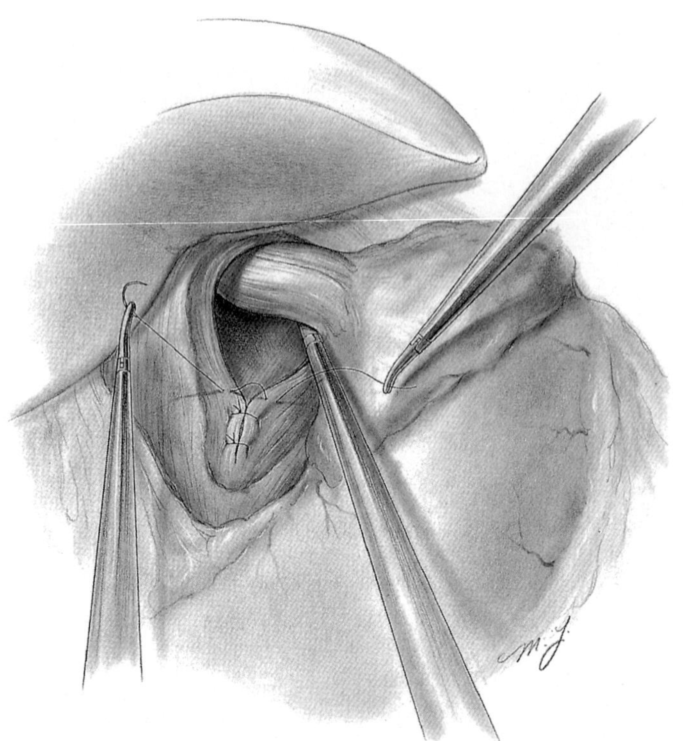

Fig. 14-5. Posterior crural repair.

Fundoplication

Subdiaphragmatic anchoring of the stomach is an important step in repair of PEH. In the past, gastrostomy and gastropexy were commonly use to accomplish this. Although no prospective randomized trials prove that anterior gastropexy or gastrostomy reduces reherniation rates, several authors advocate their use. A surgeon can rapidly accomplish a simple gastropexy. It is, however, associated with relatively higher recurrence rates. Gastrostomy is felt to be superior to gastropexy in preventing recurrences mainly because the former serves as an anchoring point to prevent failure of repair. It also helps to keep the stomach decompressed and prevent acute gastric distention in the early postoperative period, as this potentially reduces the risk of early postoperative reherniation. However since the stomach is quite pliable and can stretch over time, both gastropexy and gastrostomy by themselves are associated with higher recurrence rates.

The role of fundoplication in patients with paraesophageal hiatal hernia remains controversial. Some suggest that in Type II hernias the lower esophageal sphincter is located within the abdomen and is therefore likely to be competent, making fundoplication unnecessary. The other argument against routine fundoplication is that it adds to operative time, a factor that could prove detrimental to fragile patients with multiple comorbidities. As we have gained understanding of the pathophysiology of fundoplication and reflux, fundoplication has gained more acceptance. We routinely perform a Nissen fundoplication on all patients with PEH, because careful preoperative questioning shows that 30% to 85%

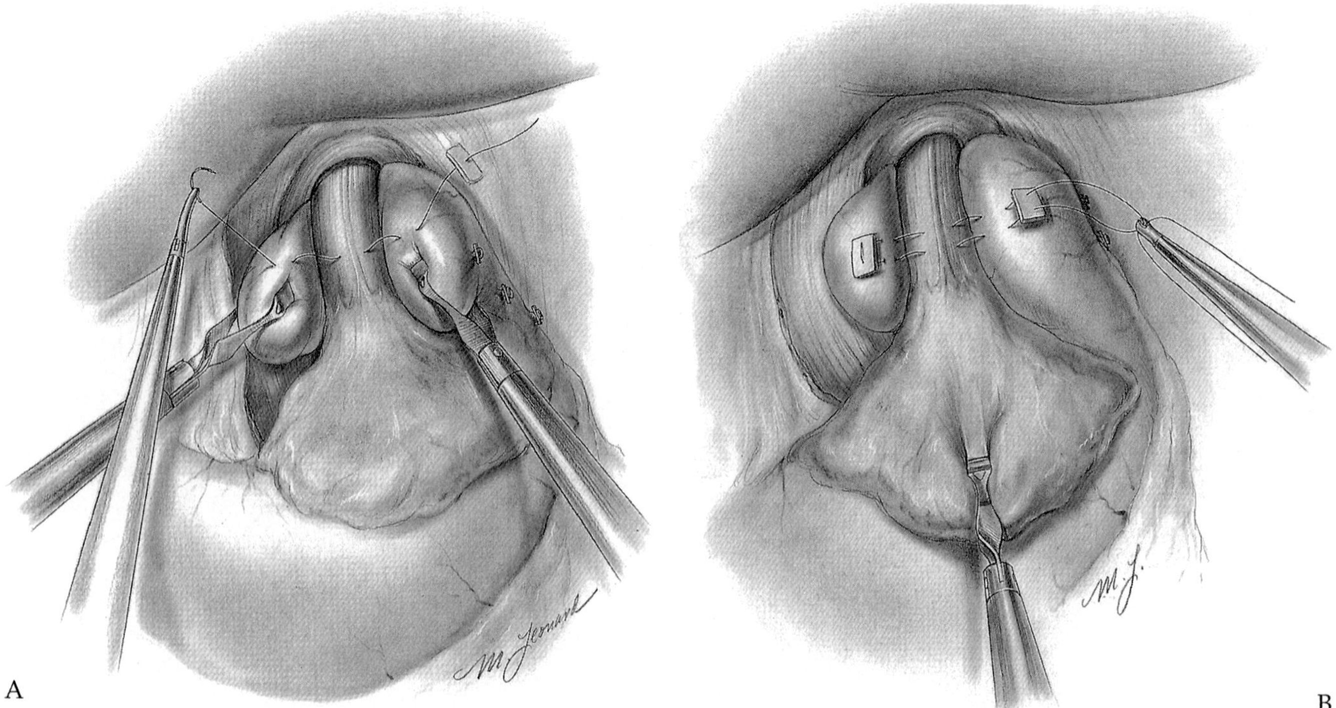

Fig. 14-6. **A** and **B**. A 360-degree fundoplication.

of these patients have reflux symptoms. If 24-hour pH studies and manometry are performed in these patients preoperatively, 60% to 100% of them will have GERD and/or low LESP (lower esophageal sphincter pressure). Furthermore, the extensive dissection essential to reduce the hernia and gain sufficient esophageal length results in disruption of the normal anatomy of the LES, predisposing to postoperative reflux. Studies have shown that up to 65% of patients who do not receive an antireflux procedure as part of the repair go on to manifest reflux symptoms after the operation. Finally, fundoplication helps to anchor the stomach below the diaphragm, thus potentially reducing recurrence. We routinely use four to five sutures to fix the fundoplication to the diaphragm and esophagus (Fig. 14-7).

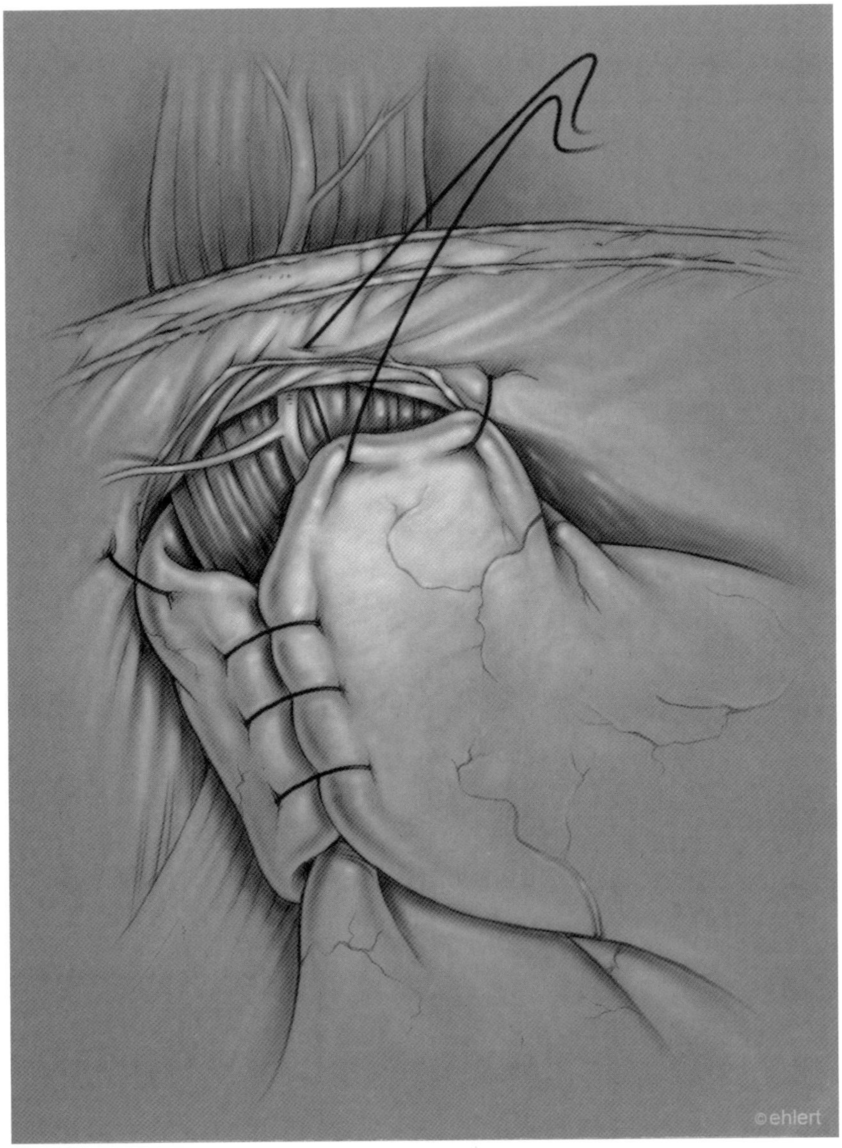

Fig. 14-7. The fundoplication is anchored to the diaphragm and crura. (Used with permission from the University of Washington. © Drawn by David Ehlert.)

Mesh

Over the past several years, solid randomized data show a clear superiority of tension-free meshed hernia repairs for both inguinal and ventral hernias. The immediate clinical outcome of laparoscopic PEH repair is highly satisfactory, but the recurrence rate is higher than expected (up to 42%). Similarly, while Mattar et al. showed a high level of patient satisfaction (90%) with LPEHR, 33% of patients had anatomic recurrence on esophagrams. One of the likely reasons for the failure of the hernia repair is failure of the crural closure. Therefore, it is not surprising that using prosthetic material either as an interposition repair or as an onlay reinforcement of the hiatus effectively decreases the recurrence more than it does for most other hernias.

There is no consensus on the best prosthetic material to use in LPEHR. The most commonly used mesh materials are polypropylene and polytetrafluoroethylene (PTFE). The technique for placing these prosthetic materials is also variable, and both posterior and anterior onlay repairs as well as interposition mesh have been described. Most surgeons prefer primary sutured repair of the hiatus followed by an onlay of prosthetic material. The overall objective remains the same: namely making the hiatal repair as tension-free as possible.

There have been several randomized trials suggesting that use of prosthetic material decreases the recurrence rate following laparoscopic repair of PEH. However, the hiatus is a dynamic anatomic structure in which the esophagus moves during respiratory excursion of the diaphragm; thus the use of prosthetic mesh is linked with potential problems of mesh erosion, ulceration, stricture, and dysphagia. As a result, few surgeons use synthetic mesh materials during hiatal repairs, unless the hiatus is unclosable.

Because of the risk of mesh and the high recurrence rate, there is an interest in the use of biomaterials in PEH repair. These modern biomaterials serve as a temporary extracellular matrix by design, acting as a temporary scaffold for tissue remodeling. The resultant tissue is stronger than normal healing, and because the mesh is absorbable, it avoids complications such as erosions and stricture. In 2003, we reported our pilot results with use of a bioprosthetic small intestinal submucosa (SIS) mesh for hiatal reinforcement in LPEHR. In our initial series of nine patients, eight had follow-up at a median of 8 months, with barium esophagram, endoscopy, or both. Based on these results a recent multicenter prospective randomized trial of repair of PEH using bioprosthesis was completed with 108 patients. Ninety-five patients completed an upper gastrointestinal X-ray at 6-month follow-up with a statistically significant reduction in recurrence rate: 9% in patients with mesh vs. 24% in patients without mesh. While this trial clearly shows that the use of SIS reduces the rate of short-term (within 6 months) recurrences, it is unclear whether this will confer long-term protection against recurrence. Because most recurrences of PEH occur early, one would expect to see recurrences within 6 months after PEH repair. Furthermore, SIS is rapidly remodeled so that the strength of the native mesh deteriorates within the first week, which

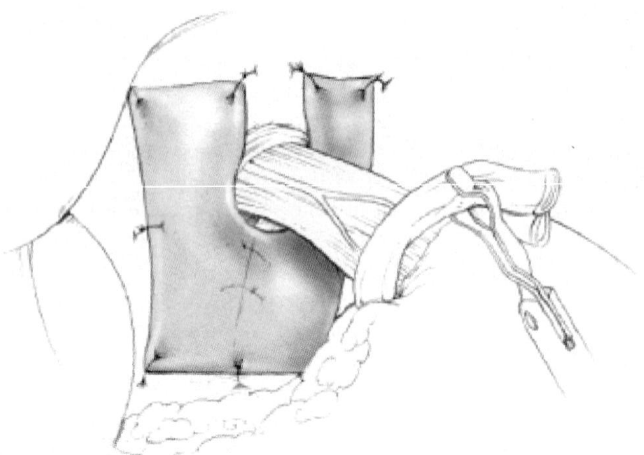

Fig. 14-8. SIS-reinforced hiatal repair. (Used with permission from the University of Washington. © Drawn by David Ehlert.)

again favors recurrences manifesting themselves in the first 6 months. Long-term follow up data is needed to establish the validity of this assumption.

Our technique uses an onlay technique. After hiatal closure with interrupted sutures, a U-shaped piece of 4-ply 7 × 10 cm Surgisis soft tissue graft (Cook Medical Inc; Bloomington, IN) is placed on the posterior hiatal closure and sutured to the diaphragm (Fig. 14-8).

CONCLUSION

Paraesophageal hernia is a difficult problem that usually requires surgical repair. Both a meticulous workup and a careful surgical technique are important for achieving optimal results. A laparoscopic approach is associated with reduced morbidity and, if combined with the use of biologic mesh, provides relief of symptoms and a durable repair.

SUGGESTED READING

Hill LD. Incarcerated paraesophageal hernia. A surgical emergency. *Am J Surg* 1973; 126(2):286–291.

Stylopoulos N, Gazelle GS, Rattner DW: Paraesophageal hernias: Operation or observation? *Ann Surg* 2002;236:492–500.

Schauer PR, Ikramuddin S, McLaughlin RH, et al. Comparison of laparoscopic versus open repair of paraesophageal hernia. *Am J Surg* 1998;176(6):659–665.

Draaisma WA, Gooszen HG, Tournoij IA, et al. Controversies in paraesophageal hernia repair: A review of literature. *Surg Endosc* 2005;19: 1300–1308.

Targarona EM, Novell J, Vela S, et al. Mid term analysis of safety and quality of life after the laparoscopic repair of paraesophageal hiatal hernia. *Surg Endosc* 2004;18(7):1045–1050.

Edye M, Salky B, Posner A, et al. Sac excision is essential to adequate laparoscopic repair of paraesophageal hernia. *Surg Endosc* 1998; 12(10):1259–1263.

Walther B, DeMeester TR, Lafontaine E, et al. Effect of paraesophageal hernia on sphincter function and its implication on surgical therapy. *Am J Surg* 1984;147(1):111–116.

Trus TL, Bax T, Richardson WS, et al. Complications of laparoscopic paraesophageal hernia repair. *J Gastrointest Surg* 1997;1: 221–228.

Oelschlager BK, Pellegrini CA, Hunter J, et al. Biologic prosthesis reduces recurrence after laparoscopic paraesophageal hernia repair: a multicenter, prospective, randomized trial. *Ann Surg* 2006;244(4):481–490.

COMMENTARY

The laparoscopic repair of paraesophageal hiatal hernias (PEHs) can be one of the most challenging operations done by the general surgeon and should be performed only by those with extensive experience in laparoscopic esophageal procedures. Not only is the operation technically challenging, but the patients themselves typically have comorbidities, complicating perioperative management. The mean age of these patients exceeds 60 years and they frequently have heart and lung ailments, kyphoscoliosis, and hernias in other locations (either simultaneously or sequentially). Laparoscopic PEH operations generally take almost twice as long as an otherwise uncomplicated laparoscopic Nissen fundoplication, and the complication rate is two to three times greater than for the standard fundoplication.

There has been a number of reports suggesting the recurrence rate for laparoscopic PEH repair exceeds that done by thoracotomy or laparotomy; unfortunately, prospective randomized trials have not compared these various approaches. Most patients with recurrent hiatal abnormalities following laparoscopic repair of PEH exhibit asymptomatic and small Type I (sliding) hiatal hernias rather than a full-blown recurrence, and the reoperation rate in most series is less than 5%. It is generally felt that the lower morbidity attendant to a laparoscopic operation is probably worth this recurrence rate and that we as surgeons must try to improve our laparoscopic techniques.

There are several potential reasons for the recurrences. These include the possibility that there is less intraabdominal scarring as a result of the laparoscopic approach, that a shortened esophagus is not adequately recognized or treated, and that a tension-free repair of the hiatal defect is difficult without the use of prostheses. In most cases, the esophagus can be mobilized well into the mediastinum from below to allow an adequate length of esophagus to remain below the diaphragm without axial tension. In the unlikely event that an esophageal lengthening procedure is necessary, various techniques can be used and are detailed in Chapter 12. A number of surgeons have championed the use of prosthetic material to bridge the hiatal defect and close it without tension. The use of a patch for this makes intuitive sense, as the rate of inguinal hernia recurrence drops from approximately 30% to less than 5% with the use of tension-free repairs. Because the diaphragm is stressed on a regular basis and moves independently of the esophagus at least 15 times a minute, a tension-free repair of the diaphragmatic defect would be ideal. However, there are several anecdotal reports of prosthetic material (both polypropylene and polytetrafluoroethylene) eroding into the stomach or esophagus; thus, many surgeons are hesitant to use these patches. A recent multicenter prospective randomized trial demonstrated the use of a bioprosthesis to buttress a primary PEH repair resulted in a markedly reduced incidence of recurrent hiatal hernias. To date, there has been no report of this bioprosthetic material eroding into the esophagus, and chronic canine studies have shown that native tissue completely replaces the bioprothesis within a year of the procedure. For that reason, our group now routinely uses a bioprosthetic patch in all patients undergoing laparoscopic repairs of large hiatal hernias.

NJS

B. Benign Disorders

Motility Disorders

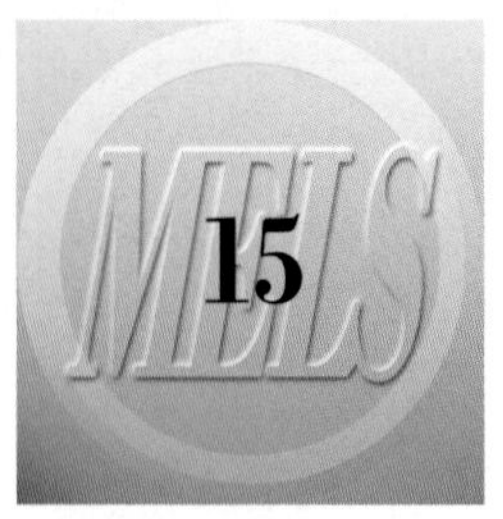

Esophageal Achalasia

MARCO G. PATTI AND PIERO M. FISCHELLA

INTRODUCTION

In the 1970s and the 1980s pneumatic balloon dilatation was considered the primary form of treatment for esophageal achalasia. During that period, only a few myotomies were performed every year, even in tertiary care hospitals, and these were mostly for patients whose dysphagia did not improve with balloon dilatation or whose esophagus had been perforated during the procedure. Because many studies had clearly shown the superiority of the Heller myotomy over dilatation, it was probably a bias on the part of gastroenterologists, along with the patient's fear of a long hospital stay and painful postoperative recovery, that relegated the role of surgery to a remedial form of treatment for the failure of pneumatic dilatation.

In 1991 minimally invasive surgery was first applied to the treatment of esophageal achalasia. Initially the operation was performed through a left thoracoscopic approach, replicating the technique popularized over the years by Ellis, with a 7-cm myotomy extending onto the gastric wall for 5 mm only, without an antireflux procedure. Over the following 3 years it was shown that the operation was feasible and safe, that patients' recovery was much shorter and smoother than after either a thoracotomy or a laparotomy, and that swallowing status was improved in 85% to 90% of patients. However, some shortcomings of this approach slowly surfaced, and it became clear that: (1) the anesthesia was more cumbersome (single-lung ventilation with a double lumen endotracheal tube); (2) the exposure of the gastroesophageal junction (GEJ) was inadequate due to the left hemidiaphragm; (3) most of the postoperative discomfort after thoracoscopic myotomy was due to the chest tube; (4) the incidence of postoperative reflux was high (60% of patients tested postoperatively by pH monitoring); and (5) it was not possible to correct pre-existing reflux due pneumatic dilatation. These were the key reasons that prompted the switch to a laparoscopic myotomy and partial fundoplication, in the attempt to find a balance between relieving dysphagia and avoiding postoperative reflux. In addition, the experience gained by antireflux surgery for the treatment of gastroesophageal reflux disease had clearly shown that the laparoscopic approach determined an excellent exposure of the lower esophagus, the GEJ, and the stomach, allowing a longer myotomy onto the gastric wall and the addition of a partial fundoplication.

Today, a laparoscopic Heller myotomy and partial fundoplication is considered the treatment of choice for esophageal achalasia, as many studies from centers all over the world have shown that the operation is safe and effective in most patients. These results have changed the treatment algorithm of esophageal achalasia, relegating pneumatic dilatation to the few patients who have persistent or recurrent dysphagia after the operation.

The following chapter describes the preoperative evaluation, the operative treatment, and the postoperative management of patients with esophageal achalasia.

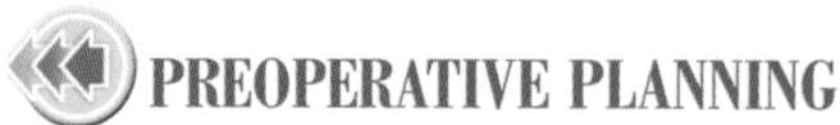

PREOPERATIVE PLANNING

All patients who are candidates for a laparoscopic Heller myotomy should undergo a complete preoperative evaluation.

Symptomatic Evaluation

In the preoperative evaluation, patients are questioned regarding the presence of dysphagia, regurgitation, chest pain, heartburn, and weight loss. Every patient has some degree of dysphagia. About 70% to 80% of patients have regurgitation, and 50% complain of chest pain. Heartburn is present in about 50% of untreated patients, due to stasis and fermentation of food in the distal esophagus. It is also present in 25% to 50% of patients after pneumatic dilatation. It is important to know if a patient has undergone previous treatment with either pneumatic dilatation or intrasphincteric injection of botulinum toxin, as fibrosis at the level of the GEJ can develop as a consequence of these treatment modalities. Unfortunately, the consequent loss of anatomic planes usually makes the operation more difficult and the outcome less predictable.

Barium Swallow

Distal esophageal narrowing is often present. In addition, a barium swallow shows the diameter and shape (straight vs. sigmoid) of the esophagus (Figs. 15-1A and 15-1B, page 131). This information is very important, as the degree of dilatation and the presence of a sigmoid esophagus increase the complexity of the operation and may affect its outcome. In addition, it helps in differentiating achalasia from other motility disorders such as diffuse esophageal spasm (Fig. 15-1C, page 131).

Endoscopy

Endoscopy should be performed in all patients to rule out the presence of a cancer of the GEJ, which can sometimes mimic the radiological and manometric picture of achalasia (pseudo-achalasia). This is particularly important in elderly patients with recent onset of dysphagia (<6 months) and excessive weight loss (>20 pounds). An endoscopic ultrasound and a CT scan should be performed if the presence of a cancer is suspected.

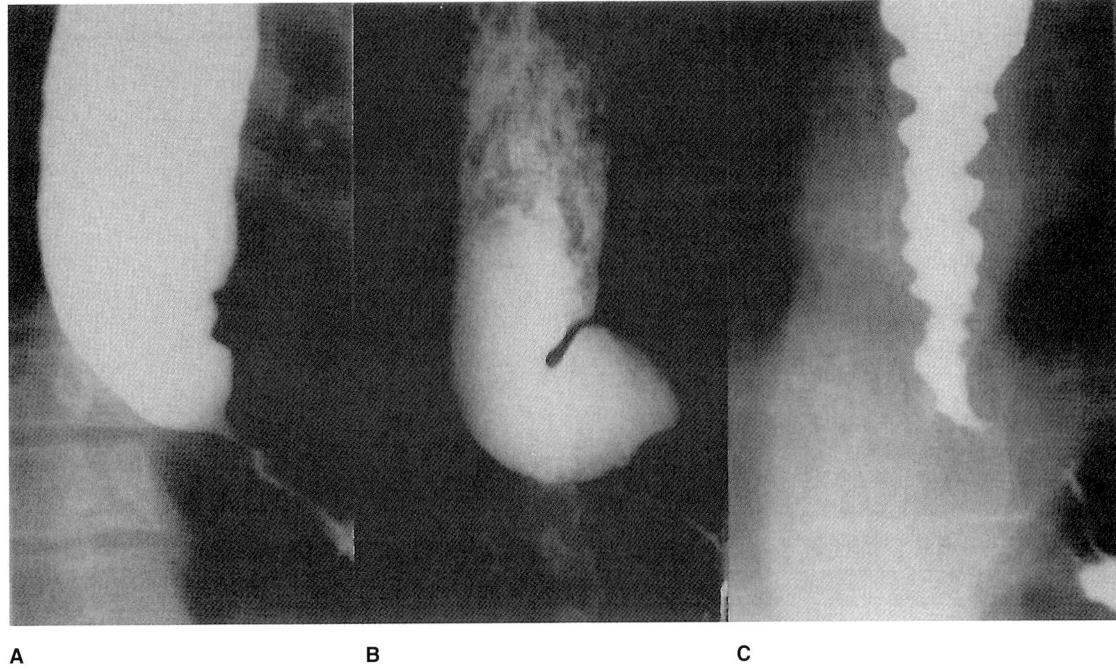

Fig. 15-1. A. Esophageal achalasia: distal esophageal narrowing, air-fluid level. **B.** Esophageal achalasia: dilated and sigmoid esophagus. **C.** Diffuse esophageal spasm: corkscrew esophagus.

Esophageal Manometry

Esophageal manometry is the key test for establishing the diagnosis of achalasia. The classic manometric findings are the absence of esophageal peristalsis and a lower esophageal sphincter (LES) that fails to relax appropriately in response to swallowing. The LES is hypertensive in about 50% of patients only.

Ambulatory pH Monitoring

This test should be performed preoperatively in patients who complain of heartburn and in those who have undergone previous treatment (such as balloon dilatation) to determine if abnormal reflux is present. Review of the pH monitoring tracing is important to distinguish between *real* reflux due to acid reflux from the stomach into the esophagus and *false* reflux due to stasis and fermentation of food secondary to poor esophageal emptying (Fig. 15-2). After myotomy and partial fundoplication, abnormal reflux is present in about 10% to 30% of patients, often being asymptomatic. Therefore, ambulatory pH monitoring should be routinely performed postoperatively (even in the absence of symptoms), particularly in young patients. Reflux should be treated aggressively with acid-reducing medications even when asymptomatic, because it can cause Barrett esophagus and the development of a distal esophageal stricture (a known cause of late failure and recurrent dysphagia).

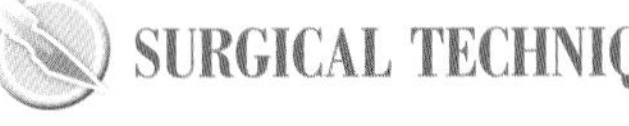

SURGICAL TECHNIQUE

Positioning of the Patient

After induction of general anesthesia with a single-lumen endotracheal tube, the patient is placed in low lithotomy position with the legs extended on stirrups. Pneumatic compression stockings are applied to the lower extremities as prophylaxis against deep vein thrombosis. To avoid sliding when the patient is placed in a steep reverse Trendelenburg position, a bean bag (secured to the table with Velcro and C-clamps) is inflated under the patient with the lower part of the bag folded under the patient's perineum in order to create a "saddle." The surgeon stands between the patient's legs and views the operation on a monitor above the patient's head. The first and second assistants stand on the right and left side of the operating table (Fig. 15-3).

Insertion of Trocars

Five trocars are used for the operation (Fig. 15-4, page 132).

- **Port 1** is placed in the midline, 14-cm distal to the xiphoid process. It is used for the camera (30-degree scope).
- **Port 2** is placed in the left midclavicular line at the same level of port 1. It is used for inserting a Babcock clamp for traction on the GE and for inserting an instrument to take down the short gastric vessels.
- **Port 3** is placed in the right midclavicular line at the same level of ports 1 and 2. A fan retractor is used through this port to lift the left lateral segment of the liver to expose the GEJ. This retractor is held in place by a self-retaining system fixed to the operating table.
- **Ports 4** and **5** are placed under the right and left costal margin, about 6 cm from the midline so that their axes form an angle of about 120 degrees. These ports are used for the insertion of graspers, electrocautery, and suturing instruments.

A common mistake is to place the trocars too low. If this happens, both the dissection and the suturing become very difficult, as the instruments might not reach. If the angle between ports 4 and 5 is less than 60 degrees, suturing becomes almost impossible. A 0-degree scope should rarely be used, but a 45-degree scope is sometimes useful.

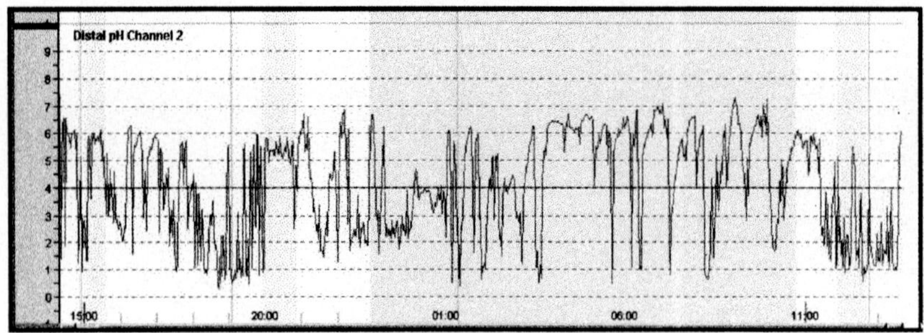

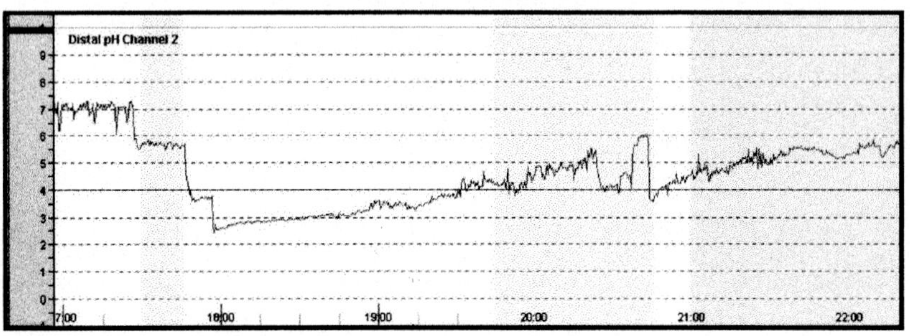

Fig. 15-2. Esophageal achalasia. Preoperative ambulatory pH monitoring can differentiate between true reflux and regurgitation. **A.** Real GER, or gastroesophageal reflux. **B.** False reflux.

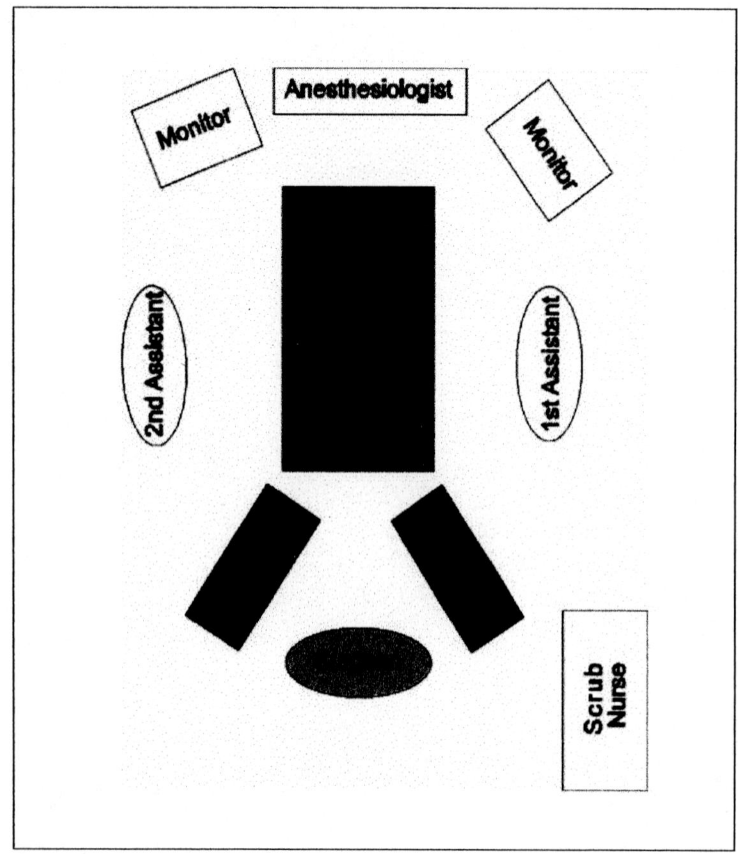

Fig. 15-3. Surgeon and monitor placement.

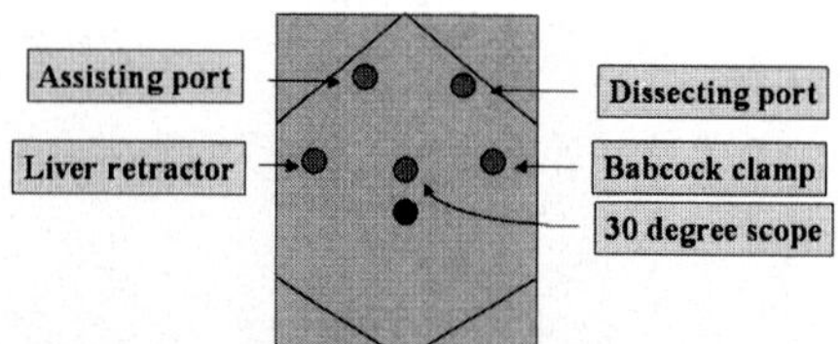

Fig. 15-4. Placement of port sites.

Dissection

The gastrohepatic ligament is divided toward the diaphragm until the right pillar of the crus is encountered. The dissection is started over the caudate lobe of the liver, where the ligament is thinner. The right pillar of the crus is separated from the esophagus by blunt dissection, and the posterior vagus nerve is identified. If an anterior fundoplication is used after the myotomy, no posterior dissection is necessary (unless a hiatal hernia is present). Subsequently, the peritoneum and phrenoesophageal membrane above the esophagus are divided, and the anterior vagus nerve is identified. The left pillar of the crus is then dissected away from the esophagus. Blunt dissection is finally performed in the posterior mediastinum in order to have about 5 to 6 cm of the esophageal wall well exposed to perform the myotomy. This maneuver is particularly important when dealing with a dilated and sigmoid esophagus.

Division of the Short Gastric Vessels

The short gastric vessels are divided, starting from a point midway along the greater curvature of the stomach. No posterior dissection is necessary if an anterior fundoplication is used.

Myotomy

The fat pad should be removed in order to get better exposure of the GEJ. Traction is then applied with a Babcock clamp, grasping below the GEJ and pulling toward the left in order to expose the right side of the esophagus. The myotomy is performed in the 11 o'clock position using a hook cautery. The proper submucosal plane is found by blunt dissection and using the cautery, about 3 cm above the GEJ. Once the mucosa is exposed, the myotomy is extended proximally for about 6 cm above the GEJ and distally for 2 to 2.5 cm onto the gastric wall (Fig. 15-5, page 133). Intraoperative endoscopy is rarely necessary, as it is easy

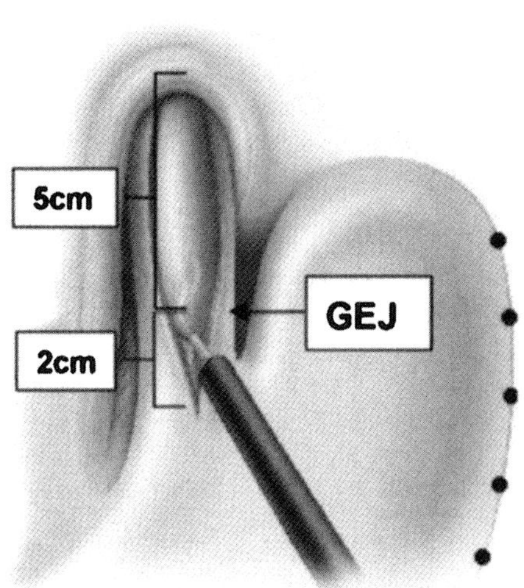

Fig. 15-5. The Heller myotomy is extended 6 to 7 cm proximally and at least 2 cm onto the anterior stomach. GEJ, gastroesophageal junction.

to identify laparoscopically the landmarks between the gastric and the esophageal musculature (Fig. 15-6).

If bleeding occurs from the cut muscle edges, pressure should be applied with a dry sponge. Use of the cautery can damage the mucosa and cause an immediate or delayed mucosal perforation.

Once the mucosa is exposed, a Maryland dissector should be used to separate the mucosa from the circular muscle fibers before the cautery is used again. Be aware that the myotomy can be technically more difficult in patients who have been previously treated with intrasphincteric injections of botulinum toxin. In some patients an inflammatory reaction can in fact occur at the level of the GEJ, with consequent fibrosis and loss of the normal anatomic planes.

If a perforation is suspected, air should be insufflated by an endoscope or an orogastric tube and the esophagus covered with water to identify the hole. Alternatively, diluted methylene blue can be injected through an orogastric tube. Any perforation should be repaired using 5-0 absorbable suture materials on a small needle.

Dor Fundoplication

A partial fundoplication (anterior or posterior) should always be used after a myotomy to limit the incidence of postoperative reflux.

The Dor fundoplication is a 180-degree anterior fundoplication. Two rows of sutures are used (2-0 silk). The first row, on the left side of the patient, has 3 stitches. The uppermost stitch incorporates the esophagus, the fundus of the stomach, and the left pillar of the crus (Fig. 15-7A). The lower two stitches incorporate only the stomach and the esophageal wall (Fig.15-7B). Subsequently, the fundus is folded over the exposed mucosa so that the greater curvature is next to the right pillar of the crus. Similar to the first row, the uppermost stitch incorporates the stomach, the esophageal wall, and the right pillar of the crus (Fig. 15-8A). The second and the

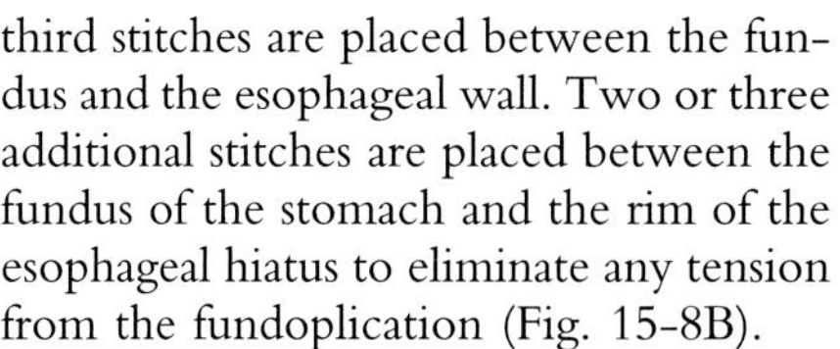

third stitches are placed between the fundus and the esophageal wall. Two or three additional stitches are placed between the fundus of the stomach and the rim of the esophageal hiatus to eliminate any tension from the fundoplication (Fig. 15-8B).

We favor an anterior fundoplication. An effective antireflux operation, it is simple to perform (no posterior dissection) and it gives nice protection to the exposed mucosa.

Posterior Fundoplication

A posterior fundoplication, such as a Toupet fundoplication, is also frequently used. It has been suggested that it might prevent recurrent dysphagia by keeping the edges of the myotomy apart and it might be more effective than an anterior fundoplication in preventing reflux.

The posterior fundoplication requires the creation of a posterior window between the left pillar of the crus, the stomach, and the esophagus followed by the passage of the gastric fundus under the esophagus. The hiatus is usually loosely closed posterior to the esophagus. Subse-quently, each side of the wrap is attached to the esophageal wall lateral to the myotomy with three stitches. The resulting wrap measures about 220 degrees (Fig. 15-9, page 135).

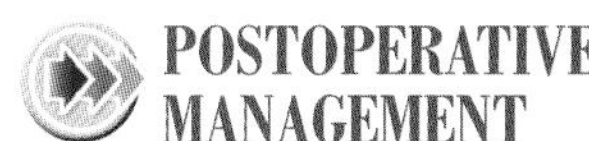

POSTOPERATIVE MANAGEMENT

The orogastric tube and the urinary catheter are removed at the end of the operation and patients are fed the morning of the first postoperative day. We do not obtain an esophagogram routinely before starting feedings. About 90% of patients are discharged within 48 hours and resume normal activity within 2 weeks.

COMPLICATIONS

Perforation

A delayed esophageal or gastric perforation is the most feared postoperative complication. In this scenario, patients usually develop fever and chest pain, and a chest X-ray often shows a pleural effusion. An esophagogram should be immediately obtained. Treatment depends on the time of the diagnosis and the size and location of the leak. Small early leaks can be repaired primarily through either a laparotomy (if at the level of the GEJ) or through a left thoracotomy (if the leak is more proximal). Extensive damage not amenable to primary repair may require an esophagectomy.

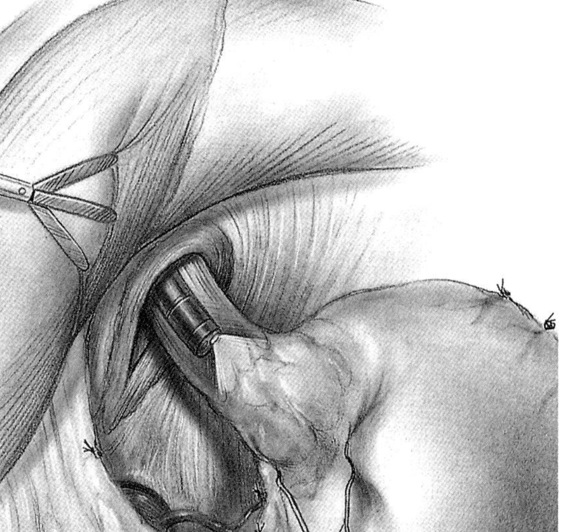

Fig. 15-6. In the rare instance that the landmarks between the gastric and esophageal musculature are not easily identified, intraoperative endoscopy can prove helpful.

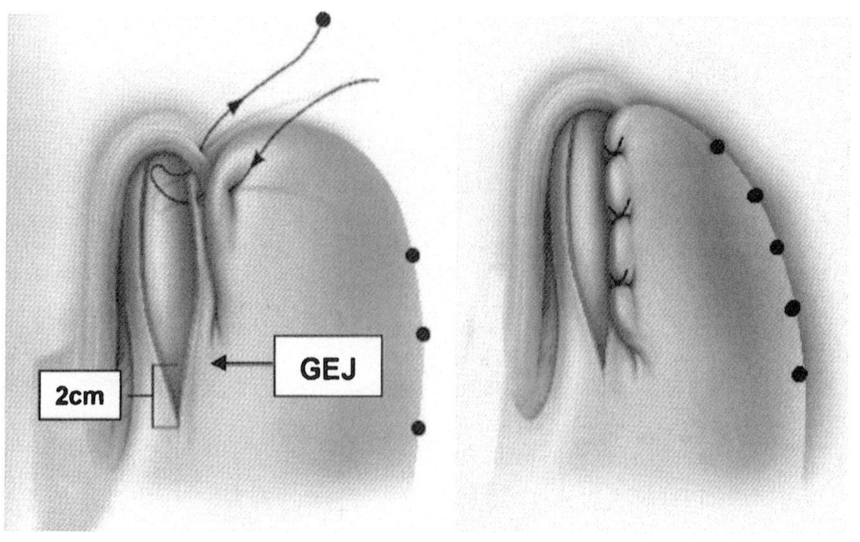

Fig. 15-7. Dor fundoplication: left row of sutures. **A.** The first stitch. **B.** The second and third stitches.

A

B

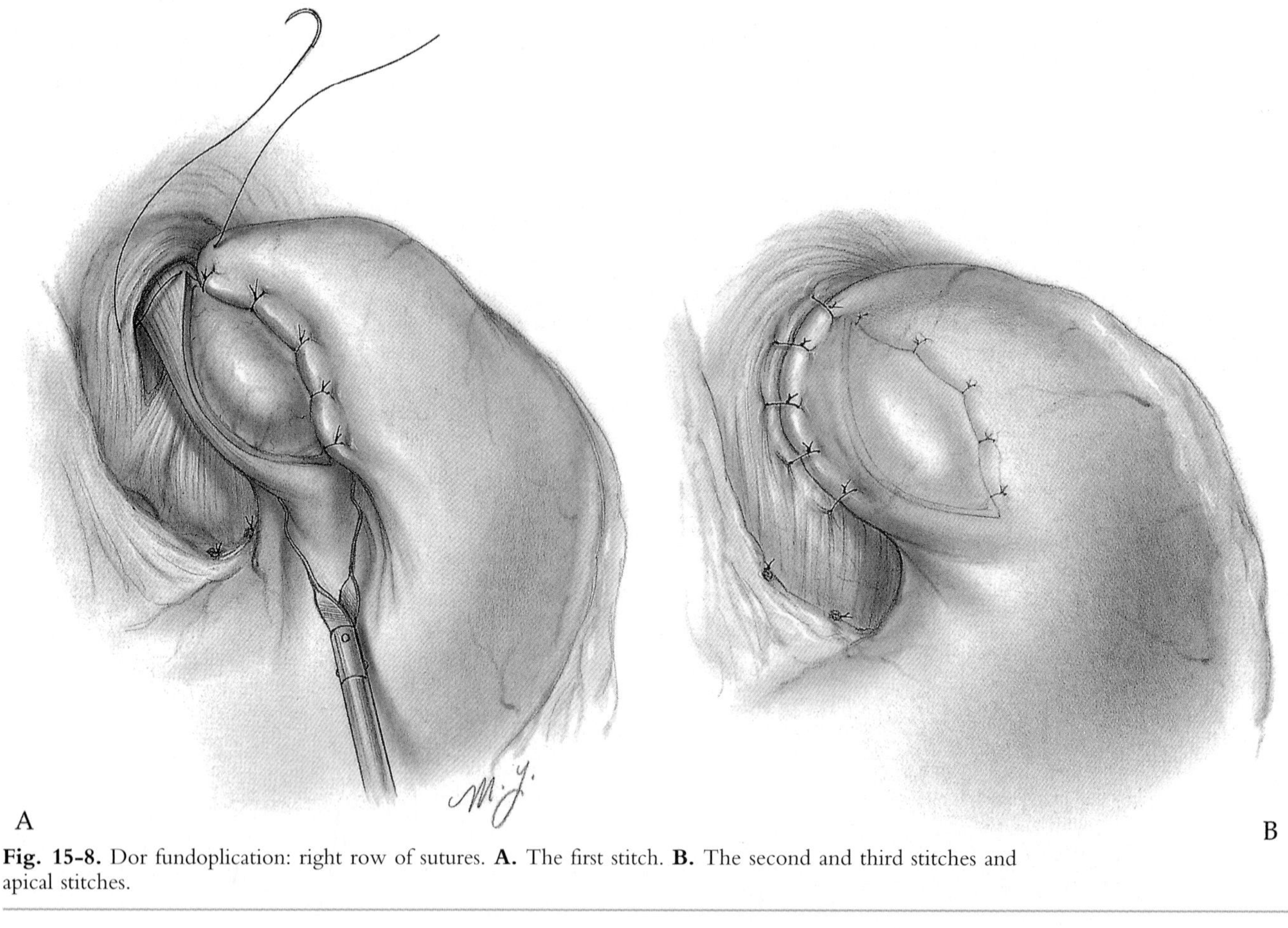

Fig. 15-8. Dor fundoplication: right row of sutures. **A.** The first stitch. **B.** The second and third stitches and apical stitches.

Dysphagia

If dysphagia persists or recurs after a symptom-free interval, a complete workup is necessary to identify the cause. We repeat the barium swallow, the endoscopy, the manometry, and the pH monitoring (in case of recurrent dysphagia). In addition, it is very useful to review the movie of the first operation. A short myotomy and a wrong orientation of the Dor fundoplication are the most common causes of postoperative dysphagia. This can be treated by pneumatic dilatation or may require a second operation.

Gastroesophageal Reflux

Abnormal gastroesophageal reflux is found in 10% to 30% of patients studied postoperatively by ambulatory pH monitoring. As half of these patients are asymptomatic, it is important to perform

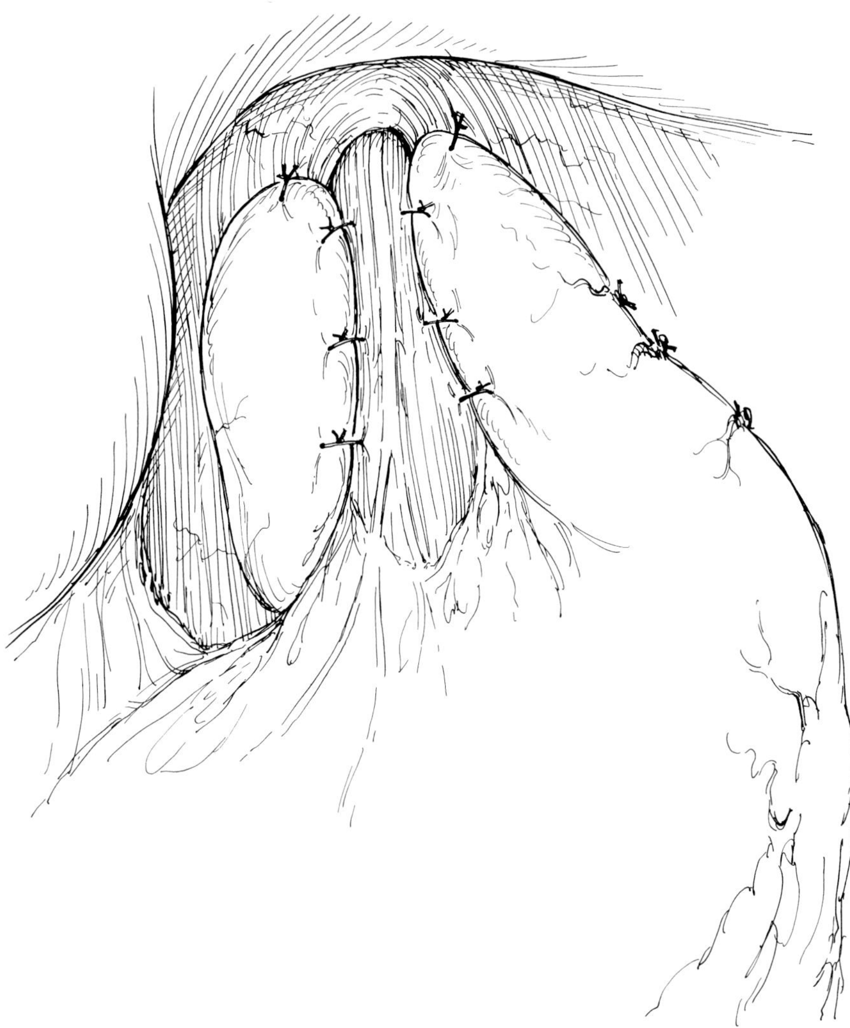

Fig. 15-9. Heller myotomy and posterior partial fundoplication.

this test in all patients, particularly if they are young. Because peristalsis is absent in patients with achalasia, esophageal acid clearance is very slow, and prolonged contact of gastric refluxate with the mucosa can cause strictures, Barrett esophagus, and even adenocarcinoma. Patients in whom gastroesophageal reflux is present should be treated with acid-reducing medications, regardless of their symptomatic status.

CONCLUSION

A laparoscopic Heller myotomy and partial fundoplication is considered today the preferred surgical approach for esophageal achalasia as it gives relief of dysphagia in more than 90% of patients. As the surgical technique has evolved during the last 10 years with further improvement of the outcome, it has become clear that the results of the other forms of treatment for achalasia (botulinum toxin and pneumatic dilatation) are inferior to those of surgery. As a consequence we have observed the following trends

Referral for Surgery

Since 1991, we have witnessed a 15- to 20-fold increase in the number of patients referred for surgery, from one to two patients per year in the 1980s to 25 to 35 patients per year today.

Minimally Invasive Surgery as Primary Treatment Modality

The gradual increase in the number of patients referred for surgery and the improvement in the outcome has been paralleled by a similar trend in the number of patients referred without previous treatment. Before the advent of minimally invasive surgery it was extremely rare that a gastroenterologist or a patient chose surgery over pneumatic dilatation. Today, more than 75% of the operations we perform are in patients never before treated. Minimally invasive surgery has therefore caused a shift in the classic treatment algorithm of esophageal achalasia, whereby today a laparoscopic Heller myotomy is considered the primary treatment modality, and pneumatic dilatation reserved for the treatment of the few failures of this operation.

SUGGESTED READING

Eckardt VF, Gockel I, Bernhard G. Pneumatic dilation for achalasia: late results of a prospective follow up investigation. *Gut* 2004;53: 629–633.

Khajanchee YS, Kanneganti, Leatherwood AEB, et al. Laparoscopic Heller myotomy with Toupet fundoplication. Outcome predictors in 121 consecutive patients. *Arch Surg* 2005;140:827–834.

Oelschlager BK, Chang L, Pellegrini CA. Improved outcome after extended gastric myotomy for achalasia. *Arch Surg* 2003; 138:490–497.

Patti MG, Feo CV, Arcerito M, et al. Effects of previous treatment on the results of laparoscopic Heller myotomy for achalasia. *Dig Dis Sci* 1999;44:2270–2276.

Patti MG, Fisichella PM, Perretta S, et al. Impact of minimally invasive surgery on the treatment of esophageal achalasia. A decade of change. *J Am Coll Surg* 2003;196:698–703.

Patti MG, Diener U, Molena D. Esophageal achalasia: preoperative assessment and postoperative follow-up. *J Gastrointest Surg* 2001; 5:11–122.

Patti MG, Gorodner MV, Galvani C, et al. Spectrum of esophageal motility disorders. Implications for diagnosis and treatment. *Arch Surg* 2005;140:442–449.

Patti MG, Molena D, Fisichella PM, et al. Laparoscopic Heller myotomy and Dor fundoplication for achalasia: analysis of successes and failures. *Arch Surg* 2001;136:870–877.

Pellegrini CA, Wetter LA, Patti MG, et al. Thoracoscopic myotomy. Initial experience with a new approach for the treatment of achalasia. *Ann Surg* 1992;216:291–299.

Richards WO, Torquati A, Holzman MD, et al. Heller myotomy versus Heller myotomy with Dor fundoplication for achalasia: a prospective randomized double-blind clinical trial. *Ann Surg* 2004;240:405–412.

Smith CD, Stival A, Howell DL, et al. Endoscopic therapy for achalasia before Heller myotomy results in worse outcomes than Heller myotomy alone. *Ann Surg* 2006; 243:579–586.

Zaninotto G, Costantini M, Portale G, et al. Etiology, diagnosis, and treatment of failures after laparoscopic Heller myotomy for achalasia. *Ann Surg* 2002;235:186–192.

Zaninotto G, Annese V, Costantini M, et al. Randomized controlled trial of botulinum toxin versus laparoscopic Heller myotomy for esophageal achalasia. *Ann Surg* 2004;239: 364–370.

COMMENTARY

Patients presenting with esophageal problems of various etiologies often have multiple and overlapping symptoms. Not infrequently, those with achalasia present initially with symptoms suggesting gastroesophageal reflux. Performing a standard 360-degree fundoplication in a patient who ultimately is found to have achalasia leads to predictably poor outcomes, and is one of the reasons why many esophageal surgeons feel that all patients presenting with reflux symptoms should undergo a comprehensive physiologic evaluation. Drs. Patti and Fischella have outlined the necessary preoperative evaluation for patients with achalasia. We do not generally perform preoperative 24-hour pH testing, as the results of that test may be inaccurate and misleading and furthermore do not modify our treatment algorithm. However, pH testing at an interval of 3 to 6 months postoperatively probably is of value to rule out asymptomatic reflux. This has been reported to occur in approximately 10% of patients who have undergone the combined Heller/Dor procedure.

The authors have a large experience in laparoscopic Heller myotomy and partial fundoplication. Their technique emphasizes the anterior dissection of the distal esophagus and performance of a Dor fundoplication. The authors state that a posterior dissection is not required except in the presence of a hiatal hernia. Our protocol and technique differ slightly from those of Dr. Patti's group; we routinely perform both an anterior and posterior dissection of the distal esophagus. Not infrequently, a small hiatal hernia is present, and there is often a component of tortuosity of the esophagus that a full mobilization may help to correct. Because the anterior vagus nerve crosses the proposed line of myotomy from left to right, we routinely mobilize the distal anterior vagus nerve away from the esophageal wall to facilitate the myotomy and potentially minimize the risk of damage to the vagus itself. We, too, primarily use the hook cautery for dividing the muscles themselves. However, the circular muscle layer should be lifted well away from the underlying submucosa to prevent thermal injuries. Bleeding from the cut edges of the muscle is rarely a major problem; the use of a dry sponge or a pledget soaked in a dilute epinephrine solution may diminish this occurrence.

The most likely location that full thickness perforations occur is at the GEJ. Great care must be taken in this region to dissect the sling fibers away from the underlying mucosa and prevent injury. We also routinely perform intraoperative endoscopy for two reasons: First, the end-on view through the gastroscope from the distal esophagus will assure that the GEJ is widely patent and that the dissection has been carried out onto the gastric wall itself. Second, we routinely insufflate the esophagus under water to rule out a subclinical perforation. Finally, our group preferentially performs a Toupet fundoplication rather than the Dor fundoplication following the myotomy. Sometimes the geometry of the Dor fundoplication can be difficult to recreate technically, potentially leading to twisting of the GEJ and postoperative swallowing difficulties. With a Toupet fundoplication, the fundus is sewn to the cut edge of the myotomy on both sides of the esophagus, with the top stitches incorporating the crura on both sides. The precise location for suture placement in a Toupet fundoplication is readily visualized and may be slightly easier to perform by surgeons with less experience than Dr. Patti's group. At this time, whether to perform a Dor or Toupet fundoplication is the surgeon's choice. There is currently a multicenter prospective randomized trial comparing partial anterior and posterior fundoplications following myotomy in patients with achalasia.

It must be kept in mind that treatment of achalasia is simply a palliative procedure. The underlying neuromuscular disorder is currently idiopathic and irreversible. The surgeon must strive to achieve a balance between the relief of dysphasia and the creation of new problems such as reflux or recurrent dysphagia caused by either an inadequate myotomy or a malpositioned fundoplication.

The treatment algorithm for patients with achalasia has changed over the last decade. Laparoscopic Heller myotomy and partial fundoplication has now become the preferred primary approach by most practitioners for this disorder. Referring gastroenterologists are coming to the realization that treatment with Botox or esophageal dilatation may lead to complications or decrease the effectiveness of a subsequent myotomy. However, poor surgical results could easily change the current "surgery friendly" atmosphere. Thus, surgeons who care for patients with achalasia will benefit from Dr. Patti's description of his group's approach to this uncommon disorder.

NJS

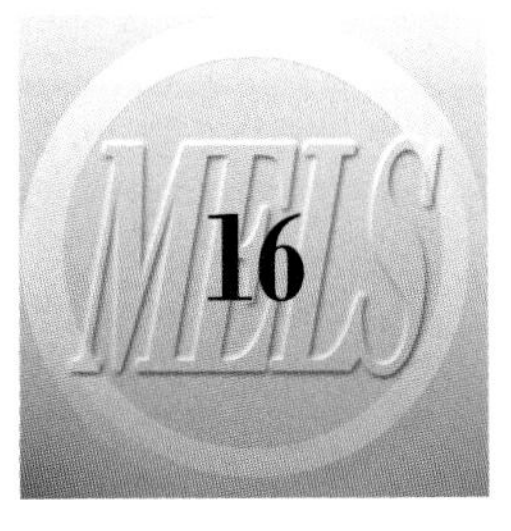

Other Esophageal Motility Disorders and Diverticula

GLYN G. JAMIESON AND SARAH K. THOMPSON

Esophageal Motility Disorders

INTRODUCTION

Esophageal motility disorders range from the common, acquired hypomotility seen with reflux to rare neurogenic spastic disorders, including diffuse esophageal spasm, nutcracker esophagus (also referred to as high-amplitude peristaltic contractions), hypertensive lower esophageal sphincter (LES), and ineffective esophageal motility. We will refrain from discussing ineffective esophageal motility because the therapy for this is primarily medical in nature; if these patients do eventually progress to surgery, the procedure of choice is an antireflux procedure (see Chapter 10). Likewise, achalasia is discussed in Chapter 15.

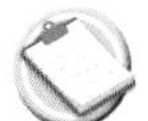

CLINICAL PRESENTATION

In patients with a presumed esophageal spasm disorder, the correct diagnosis is of the utmost importance. This is first and foremost a *clinical* diagnosis, one that is made only when other more common entities have been ruled out. The clinical and manometric findings for each of these spastic motility disorders are outlined in Table 16-1. Figure 16-1 demonstrates the manometric differences between the three conditions, as proposed by Spechler and Castell in 2001. Diffuse esophageal spasm (Fig. 16-1A) is characterized by simultaneous contractions associated with >10% of wet swallows and a mean simultaneous contraction amplitude of >30 mmHg. Nutcracker esophagus (Fig. 16-1B) is diagnosed when manometry shows a mean distal esophageal peristaltic wave amplitude >180 mmHg. This is measured at 3 and 8 cm above the LES and is averaged over 10 consecutive swallows. Long-duration contractions (>6 seconds) are seen commonly but are not required for diagnosis. It should be noted that there is not always a correlation between the patient's symptom of chest pain

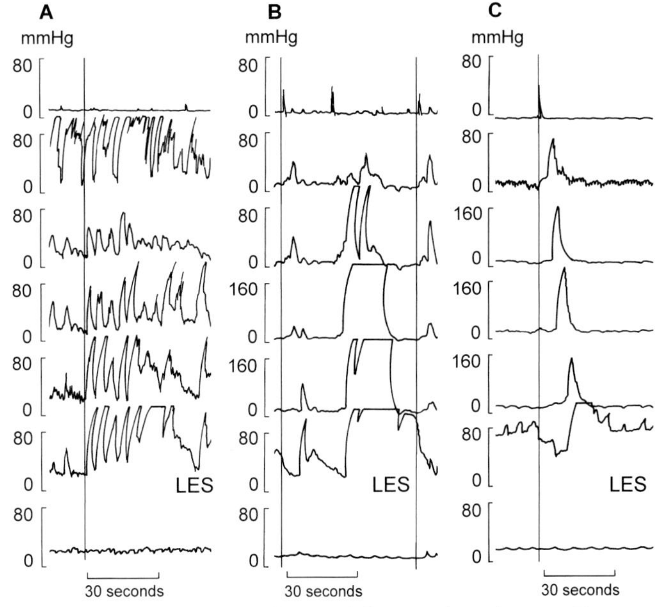

Fig. 16-1. Typical manometry tracings for: **A.** diffuse esophageal spasm; **B.** nutcracker esophagus; and **C.** and hypertensive LES. LES, lower esophageal sphincter. (Courtesy of Jenny Myers, Esophageal Function Laboratory, Royal Adelaide Hospital, Australia.)

TABLE 16-1. ESOPHAGEAL SPASM SYNDROMES

Condition	Symptoms	Manometric findings
Diffuse esophageal spasm	Chest pain/dysphagia	>10% tertiary nonpropulsive waves Mean amplitude of 3 degree waves >30 mmHg Repetitive contractions (>3 peaks) Normal LES relaxation
Nutcracker esophagus	Chest pain	High-amplitude peristaltic contractions (>180 mmHg) Long-duration contractions (>6 sec) Normal LES relaxation
Hypertensive LES	Dysphagia/heartburn	Mean basal LES pressure (>45 mmHg) Normal LES relaxation

LES, lower esophageal sphincter.

and high-amplitude contractions. Finally, isolated hypertensive LES syndrome (Fig. 16-1C) is diagnosed when there is a mean resting LES pressure of >45 mmHg (mid-respiratory) but with normal LES relaxation. One should note that some patients may have features of both nutcracker esophagus and a hypertensive LES on manometry.

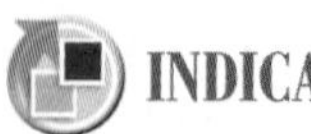

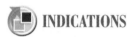

INDICATIONS

Attempts to treat all three of the above conditions are best done by medical and/or endoscopic means (pneumostatic dilatation). Gui et al. published a review article looking at endoscopic botulinum toxin injections for diffuse esophageal spasm. They reported on two series with a small number of patients in whom this therapy had been performed. They found good initial symptomatic relief; however, this did not last past a few months. We do not believe this is a good option in this patient population, because it is not a definitive treatment and may complicate future operative intervention. It may, however, be a useful diagnostic tool for certain cases.

In the uncommon situation where a patient suffers a mechanical complication (see next section on "Midesophageal and Epiphrenic Diverticula") or severe refractory symptoms from their spastic motility disorder, a long myotomy is the procedure of choice. It cannot be stressed enough that operative treatment should be the *last resort* in this patient population. A long myotomy succeeds in only about 50% of patients (and even this estimation may be overgenerous), and seldom is long-term relief achieved.

PREOPERATIVE PLANNING

Assessment

All patients should undergo a comprehensive cardiology examination to exclude myocardial ischemia as a cause of their chest pain. In addition, we feel patients warrant investigation and treatment of any underlying psychiatric component to their symptoms. Additional mandatory and optional diagnostic tests are listed below.

Mandatory Diagnostic Testing

Upper endoscopy is critical to exclude an abnormality at the gastroesophageal junction (GEJ), whether it be a segment of Barrett esophagus, uncontrolled esophagitis, a peptic stricture, or a malignancy. An ambulatory 24-hr pH study should be done to exclude reflux disease, especially in patients with a presumed esophageal spasm disorder, because their symptoms could be due to uncontrolled reflux rather than a primary esophageal motility disorder. This is particularly true in patients with a hypertensive LES on manometry. A radiologic contrast study may show a characteristic corkscrew esophagus in a patient with diffuse esophageal spasm. This should be performed with video fluoroscopy in order to evaluate esophageal motility at the same time. A barium swallow will also identify complications of an esophageal motility disorder, such as an epiphrenic diverticulum (see "Midesophageal and Epiphrenic Diverticula" section below).

Optional Diagnostic Testing

Optional (yet helpful) preoperative testing includes radionuclide transit studies using liquid and solid markers to quantify esophageal retention and a gastric emptying study to evaluate gastric motility, as gastric dysfunction is more frequent in patients with an esophageal motility disorder.

LONG MYOTOMY

SURGICAL TECHNIQUE

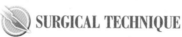

Patient Preparation and Mobilization of the Esophagus

This procedure can be done either through a left-sided thoracotomy incision or with a thoracoscopic approach; we will describe the thoracoscopic approach in this chapter. There are two approaches that can be used.

For the first approach, the patient is placed in a right lateral decubitus position with rolls under the axilla and between the legs. Port placement has the camera port placed in the fifth intercostal space in the posterior axillary line (Fig. 16-2). Working and retraction ports are added as required. A double-lumen endotracheal tube is used to allow exclusion and retraction of the left lung following division of the inferior pulmonary ligament. The mediastinum is opened over the esophagus from the aortic arch to the diaphragm. The esophagus is mobilized with hook electrocautery and/or the harmonic scalpel. Although some authors do not advocate the use of traction loops around the esophagus in the thoracoscopic technique, we feel that vascular tapes encircling the esophagus both proximally and distally facilitates mobilization.

The second approach, which we favor, has the patient placed in the prone position. This has the great advantage that there is rarely a need to collapse the left lung as it falls forward, away from the posterior mediastinum. Port placement is shown in Figure 16-3.

Myotomy

Myotomy is undertaken by a combination of endoshears and the hook diathermy. It is helpful to use a curved instrument, such as a Mixter or Maryland clamp, which helps to separate the mucosa from the muscle, and, by gently spreading the jaws of

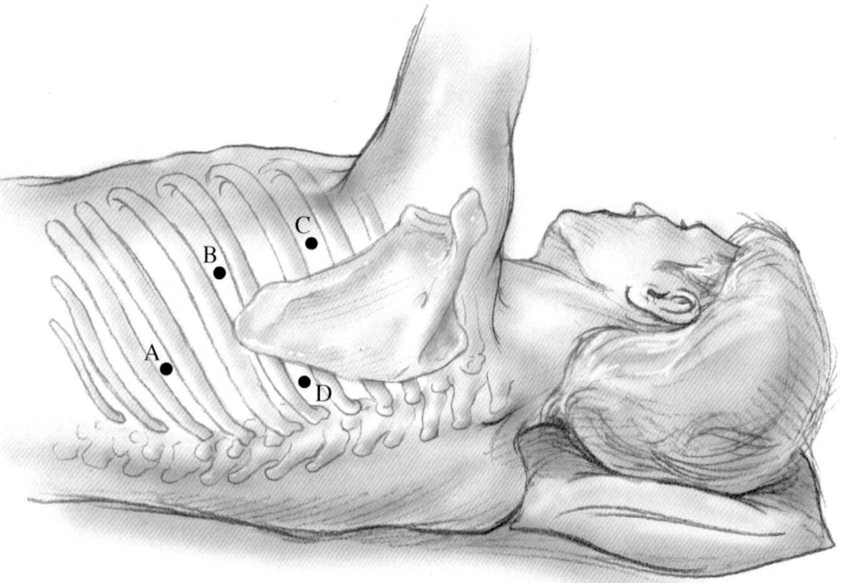

Fig. 16-2. Patient position and port placement for the left-sided thoracoscopic approach for long myotomy.

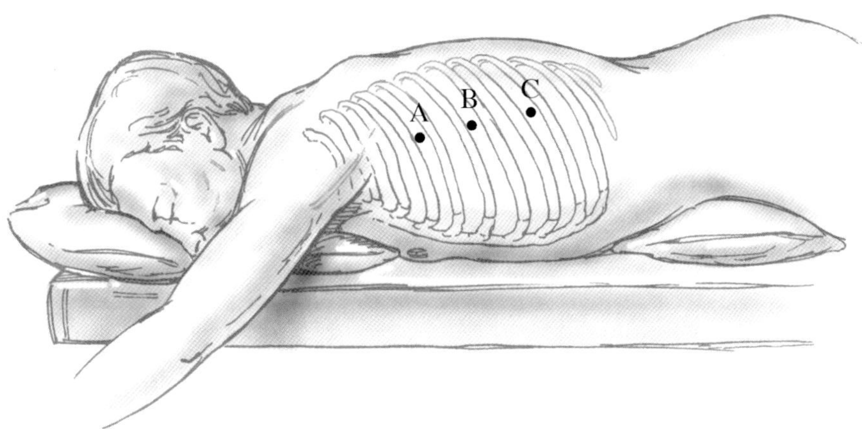

Fig. 16-3. Patient position and port placement for the prone approach for long myotomy.

the instrument, puts the muscle under tension for division with the diathermy hook or scissors (Fig. 16-4). This should be performed over either a 48F bougie or an endoscope. An endoscope is more useful in confirming an adequate myotomy and in checking for mucosal perforation (to be discussed later), so this is our preference. The mucosa will protrude as the myotomy is extended both proximally and distally. The myotomy should be extended proximally as needed, depending on the specific manometric diagnosis. We then extend the myotomy for 1 to 2 cm onto the gastric wall to ensure complete division of the LES. We believe that this decreases the pressure buildup and retention that may lead to a postoperative leak and reduces progressive dilation over the long term. As well, we think there is a high association of LES dysfunction in this patient population. The myotomy is then checked for leaks by submerging the field in saline and gently filling the esophagus with air through the replaced endoscope. If a leak is found, it is usually small and closed with a 5-0 Prolene suture, with intracorporeal suturing.

Having divided the muscle, we think it is important to now suture the longitudinal layer together again with two to four sutures. This is done to prevent pseudodiverticulum formation, which is a problem over the long term if the myotomy is left with mucosa pouting out over a long area.

Partial Fundoplication

A two-thirds fundic wrap of the Belsey type is then carried out using 2-0 Prolene sutures. Two sutures anchor the fundoplication on each side of the myotomized esophagus at two levels (Fig. 16-5, page 140). The two layers of muscle are transfixed from outside to inside to evert the muscle while anchoring the seromuscular layer of the fundus to the esophageal wall. This is done to prevent reflux and any closure of the myotomy at the GEJ. A chest drain is inserted, the lung is reinflated, and the skin incisions are closed with staples.

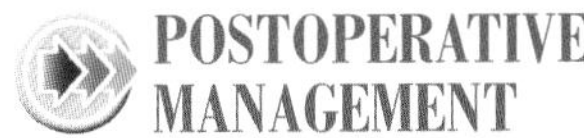

POSTOPERATIVE MANAGEMENT

We do not advise routine nasogastric drainage. Most patients are extubated immediately, and the chest tube is placed on underwater sealed drainage. A contrast swallow is obtained on the first postoperative day, and, if satisfactory, the patient is allowed a liquid diet. The chest tube is usually removed on the first postoperative day, and the patient is discharged on the second or third postoperative day with instructions to slowly introduce soft foods until he or she is reviewed 14 days later.

Midesophageal and Epiphrenic Diverticula

INTRODUCTION

Diverticula arising from the esophageal body are usually pulsion diverticula as a result of abnormal motility, which leads to pressurization of the body of the esophagus. Such diverticula occur most frequently in the lower esophagus near the hiatus and are called epiphrenic diverticula. The motility disorder associated with a diverticulum does not always affect the LES, but this is usually the case.

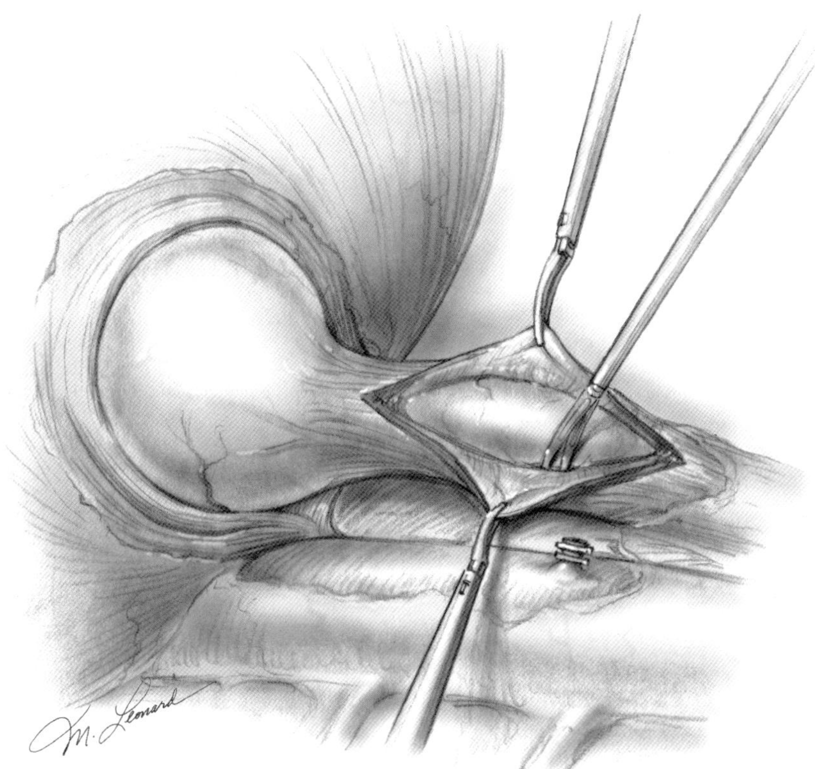

Fig. 16-4. Long myotomy using endoshears through a thoracoscopic approach.

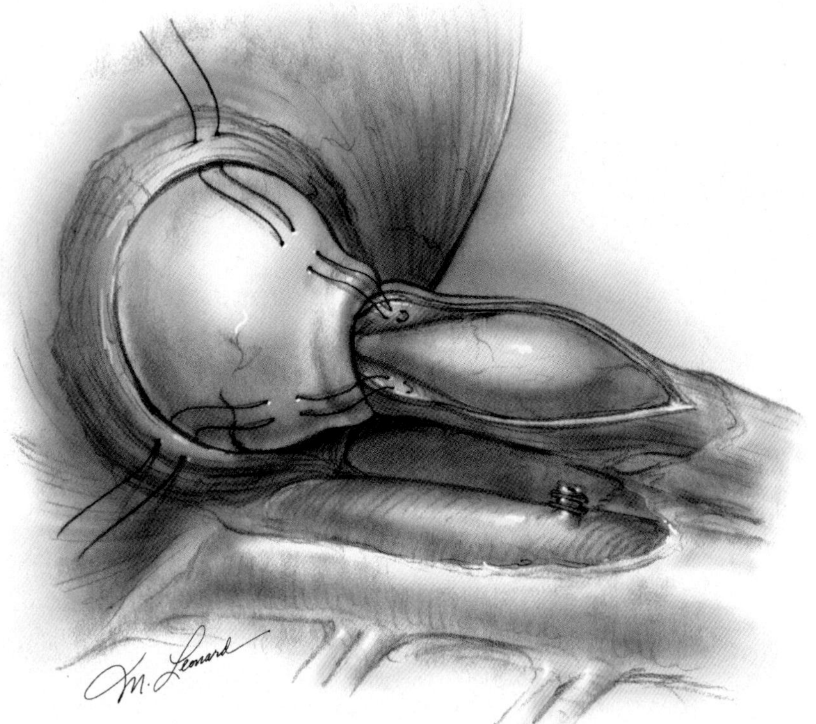

Fig. 16-5. A two-thirds Belsey fundic wrap is created using 2-0 Prolene sutures.

CLINICAL PRESENTATION

The diagnosis of a diverticulum is best established with a contrast swallow. Upper endoscopy will sometimes locate the diverticulum, but, not infrequently, the diverticulum can be missed if the opening is small or hidden in a mucosal fold near the distal high-pressure zone. If dysphagia is part of the symptom complex, however, an endoscopy is mandatory to rule out other causes of dysphagia.

We advocate esophageal manometry in all patients, although it is a controversial point whether it is absolutely mandatory. If the surgeon believes that all patients should have a myotomy, it can be argued that manometry is not necessary. Nevertheless, not all patients have involvement of the LES, and if it appears uninvolved, a myotomy can stop short of the last 2 cm of the esophagus. This knowledge can only be gleaned from esophageal manometry.

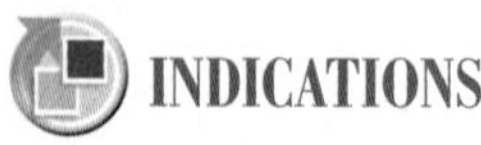

INDICATIONS

The mere presence of a diverticulum is not usually regarded as an indication for treatment, although there are dissenters to this view. The justification for operation in a patient with an asymptomatic diverticulum is that sometimes the diverticulum leads to regurgitation and laryngeal spillover symptoms and possibly even respiratory problems. In fact this seems to happen infrequently, and the only symptom the diverticulum itself is likely to cause is regurgitation of undigested food some time after the food has been swallowed. Because most of these diverticula are widemouthed, it is only when they become very large and dependent that this becomes a problem. It should probably be assumed that small- and moderate-sized diverticula alone do not cause symptoms. For instance, pain and dysphagia will almost always have another cause. Pain may be due to gastroesophageal reflux or the diffuse esophageal spasm associated with a diverticulum, and dysphagia should always be assumed to be the result of a malignancy until proven otherwise by endoscopy. Of course, it may also be associated with the underlying motility disorder.

THE MINIMAL ACCESS APPROACH

When planning for a minimal access approach to a diverticulum, there are two possible approaches: thoracoscopy (also referred to as video-assisted thoracic surgery, or VATS) or laparoscopy. If the diverticulum is in the midesophagus, our preference is for a right-sided thoracoscopic approach. If the diverticulum is epiphrenic (i.e., in the lower third of the esophagus), our preference is a laparoscopic approach. Epiphrenic diverticula are almost always attainable through an abdominal approach, as it is feasible to mobilize the lower third of the esophagus through the esophageal hiatus. This approach has therefore now replaced the thoracoscopic approach as the standard of care.

PREOPERATIVE PLANNING

If a diverticulum is large and dependent, food and debris often occur within the diverticulum. In such a case, an endoscopy should be performed preoperatively to make sure the diverticulum is empty, because debris can lead to problems intraoperatively.

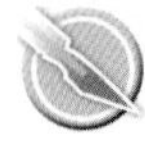

SURGICAL TECHNIQUE

RIGHT THORACOSCOPIC MIDESOPHAGEAL DIVERTICULECTOMY

Position of the Patient

The patient is intubated with a double-lumen endotracheal tube. As most diverticula being operated on are large, the aspiration risk in these patients is substantial and preventative care is required during induction. The patient is then placed either in the full left lateral decubitus position or the fully prone position (Fig. 16-6), which is our preference. The advantage of the fully prone position is that the lung falls away from the esophagus and only minimal insufflation gas pressure is needed to push the right lung from the operative field.

Trochar Placement

A small amount of gas at 5 mmHg pressure is then introduced into the right hemithorax. This can be done with a Veress needle or by the introduction of a 10-mm round-ended rod placed blindly through a 1-cm cut, followed by the introduction of a 10- to 11-mm trochar over the rod. Two other trochars (10 to 11 mm) are placed under direct vision in the sites shown in Figure 16-6, with the middle site for the camera. It is not usually necessary to deflate the right lung, although if it obscures the view it can be collapsed.

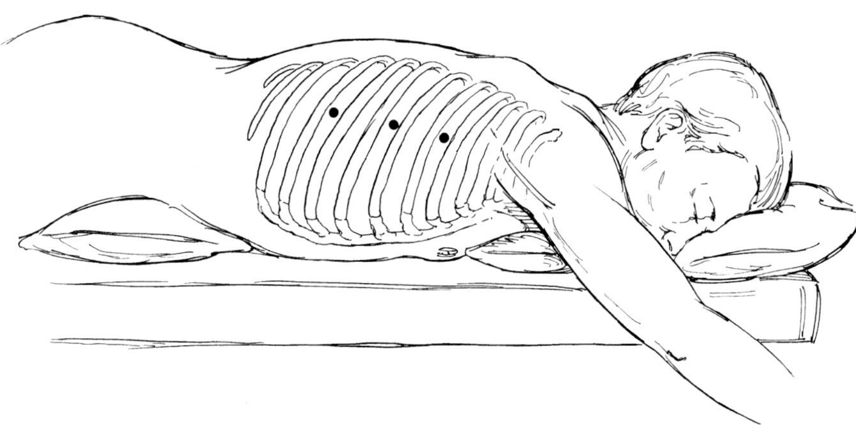

Fig. 16-6. Patient position and port placement for a right thoracoscopic midesophageal diverticulectomy in the prone position.

Esophageal Exposure

Identification of the esophagus is facilitated by introducing a flexible endoscope into the esophagus with the light of the endoscope making it easy to identify the esophageal body. The pleura over the esophagus is picked up and incised longitudinally, using endoscissors, with the incision passing the whole length of the esophagus up to the azygos vein. Sharp and blunt dissection is then used to mobilise the distal esophagus. Particular care needs to be exercised in the region of the diverticulum, as it is frequently associated with peri-diverticular inflammation, making dissection of the diverticulum difficult. The esophagus itself is not usually difficult to dissect from its bed, although the most difficult maneuver is getting around the esophagus with a curved instrument in order to place a tape or a piece of Penrose drain. We usually use a tape that is brought out through one of the port sites. Next, the diverticulum is dissected out in its entirety, using a mixture of blunt and sharp dissection with scissors. It may be necessary to rotate the esophagus so that the neck of the diverticulum can be clearly displayed (Fig. 16-7).

Diverticulectomy

Both intraluminal (through the endoscope) and extraluminal (through the thoracoscope) views can help to provide a complete demonstration of the anatomy of the diverticulum. Sometimes it can prove helpful to use an additional port if those already in place do not give optimal access, particularly for the stapling instrument. An Endo GIA stapler (U.S. Surgical) or its equivalent with an articulating head is then introduced. The endoscope is removed and a 52F bougie is passed down the esophagus. The neck of the diverticulum is then stapled across (Fig. 16-8, page 142), the diverticulum is removed, and the longitudinal muscle of the esophagus is approximated across the staple line, using several sutures of either 5-0 monofilament or braided suture (Fig. 16-9, page 142).

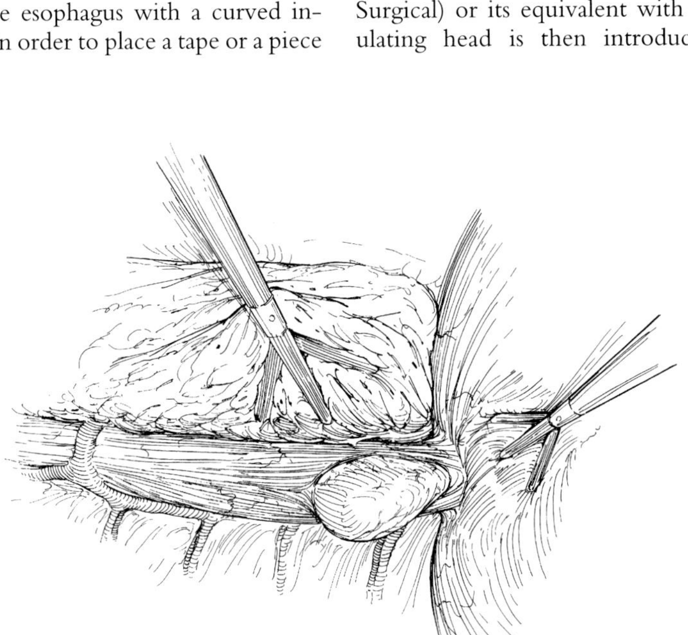

Fig. 16-7. Right thoracoscopic view of the exposed esophagus after incising the mediastinal pleura.

Myotomy

Myotomy is performed at a different site from the staple line in the esophagus, preferably at a site 90 to 180 degrees away from the staple line. The technique has been described in the previous section (see "Long Myotomy"). The proximal extent of the myotomy should be just above the proximal extent of the neck of the diverticulum. The distal extent is directed by manometric findings, but in any case it should always be taken well below the diverticulum. The diverticulectomy and myotomy sites are then checked for leaks as described in the previous section (see "Long Myotomy Technique"). The myotomy is closed loosely using several interrupted sutures in the longitudinal muscle layer of the esophagus. This is done to prevent herniation of the mucosa at a later date through the myotomy site. The skin wounds are closed in standard fashion, and a chest drainage tube is brought out through one of the trochar sites.

LAPAROSCOPIC APPROACH FOR EPIPHRENIC DIVERTICULA

Mobilization of the esophagus is performed using a standard approach for a fundoplication (see Chapter 10). The only difference is that the mobilization is taken more proximally in the posterior mediastinum and the diverticulum is dissected free in its entirety. Once again, intraoperative endoscopy is very helpful. A 52F bougie is then passed, and the diverticulectomy is carried out using an Endo GIA or similar stapler passed across the hiatus. We advocate the use of 2.5-mm staples (vascular cartridge) for this step. It is not unusual to require more than one application of the stapler to transect the entire neck of the diverticulum sac. As with the thoracoscopic approach, several tacking sutures of a fine Prolene are used to close the muscle defect where the neck of the diverticulum has been stapled. We then close the diaphragmatic hiatus posteriorly with 2-0 Prolene

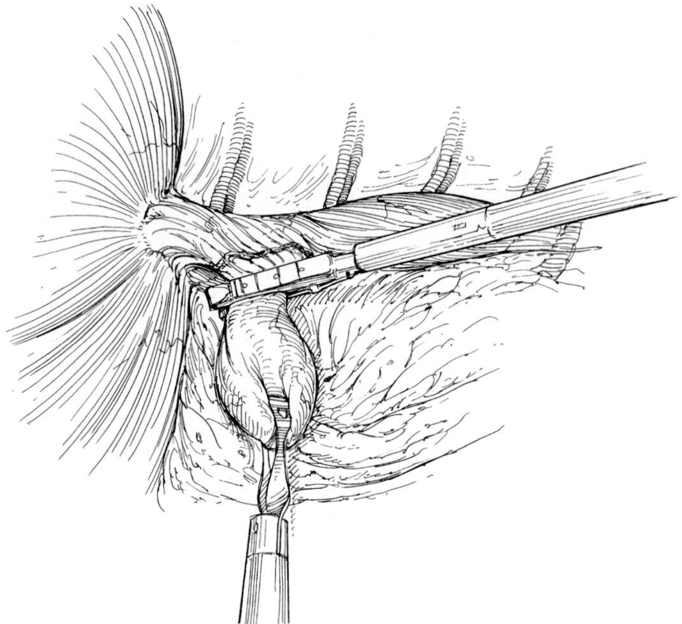

Fig. 16-8. Mobilization of the esophagus allows the diverticulum to be rolled into the operative field, where the neck can be completely dissected free.

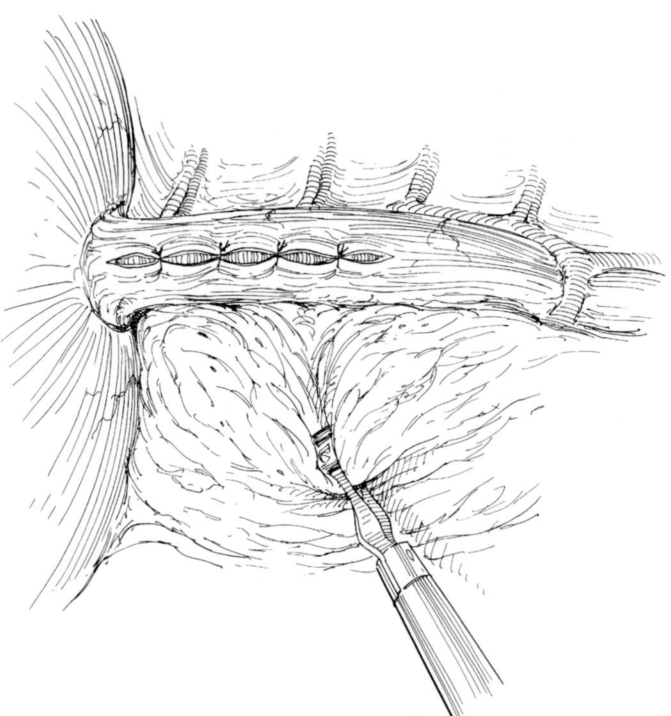

Fig. 16-9. The longitudinal muscle should be loosely reapproximated over both the staple line and the distal myotomy.

sutures. Next, a myotomy is carried out in a different plane from the diverticulectomy, using the same principles as with the thoracoscopic myotomy (see "Long Myotomy"). If the myotomy is taken down through the GEJ and onto the stomach, a Dor partial fundoplication, which acts as a patch, should be added to the procedure. Again we believe that it is important to close the longitudinal muscle layer of the esophagus above any patch (Fig. 16-10).

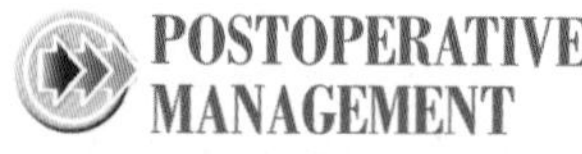

POSTOPERATIVE MANAGEMENT

Postoperative care is the same as described in the previous section (see "Long Myotomy").

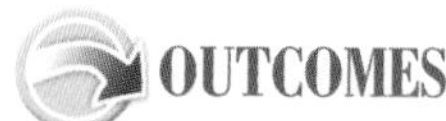

OUTCOMES

Esophageal diverticulum is not a common problem, so experience with the minimal access approach to its management has been slow to accumulate. Nevertheless, from recent publications on the subject, several points have emerged. First, there is an 80% to 90% association of motility disorders with esophageal diverticula. In a series of 21 patients with epiphrenic diverticula, Tedesco et al. found an associated motility disorder of achalasia (9%), diffuse esophageal spasm (24%), nutcracker esophagus (24%), and nonspecific esophageal motility disorder (24%). Second, in patients with an esophageal spasm syndrome plus an epiphrenic diverticulum, their clinical symptoms and esophageal function improved substantially after a long myotomy when compared to patients with pure spastic disorders.

Third, the laparoscopic approach for epiphrenic diverticula has completely superseded the thoracoscopic approach for these patients. In one of the largest series reported to date, Fernando et al. present 20 patients who were treated for esophageal diverticula. The morbidity of the procedure was reported at 45%, and good or excellent results were achieved in 83% of patients. However, the most striking finding of their paper was an esophageal leak rate of 20%, which is more than three times higher than those of reported open series. The reason why the leak rate is higher than with open surgery is not altogether clear, except that this is a very technically challenging procedure and is therefore only indicated for those patients with symptomatic large diverticula.

It is clear that the minimal access approach should only be used in centers experienced with minimally invasive esophageal surgery. Patients should also be fully informed that the possibility of leakage is higher than with the open approach. Nevertheless, the gains of minimal access surgery for this condition are so undeniably greater when the patient's course is uncomplicated that there seems little doubt the procedure will establish a place in the treatment of this condition.

Zenker Diverticulum

The treatment of a pharyngeal pouch (Zenker diverticulum) through the mouth and pharynx has been undertaken for many years, notably by H.A. Mosher in 1917,

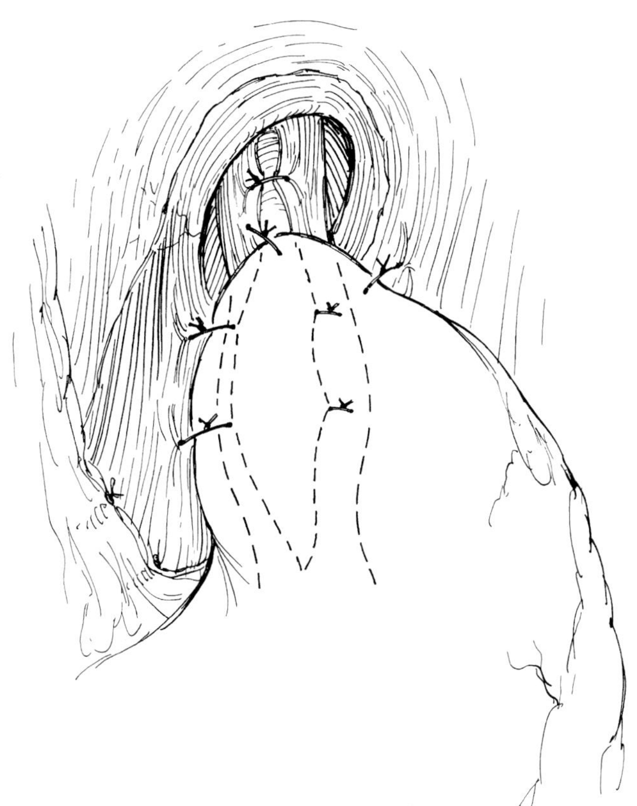

Fig. 16-10. If the distal myotomy crosses the gastroesophageal junction, a Dor fundoplication should be added to minimize postoperative reflux.

who introduced the concept of using an endoscope to divide the common wall between the diverticulum and the pouch. However, one of his patients died of mediastinal sepsis, and the technique was not widely accepted until F.A. Dohlman and his colleagues published their 30 years of experience with endoscopic-assisted diverticulostomy in 1960. Dohlman et al. used electrocautery to divide the common wall; subsequently J.J.M. van Overbeek published a modification using a CO_2 laser. In 1993, Collard et al. described the use of an endoscopic stapler to divide the common wall, and the procedure has gained in popularity since.

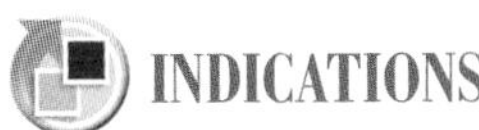

INDICATIONS

Indications for Treatment of a Zenker Diverticulum

The diverticulum is treated if it is producing symptoms that are spoiling the patient's enjoyment of life ("Food is an important part of a balanced diet!"—Fran Lebowitz) or threatening the patient's life either because of inanition or recurrent aspiration pneumonia associated with spillover from the pouch. The diagnosis is nearly always made by endoscopy (the endoscope often passes preferentially into the pouch) or by a radiological contrast swallow. Patients are often elderly and infirm, and it is not unusual that a patient with a known diverticulum is referred for treatment only when the diverticulum is threatening the patient's life, which is the likely reason that surgical treatment is associated with a higher mortality rate than might be expected with what is essentially a minor operation.

Indications for Endoscopic Treatment by Stapling

The diverticulum needs to be of moderate size (>2 cm) for the limb of the stapler to easily enter it. There are strategies that can be used in smaller pouches (see "Endoscopic Stapling Technique"), but many surgeons prefer to use an open approach with a small diverticulum.

Such patient features as retrognathia, short neck, fixed cervical kyphosis, and prominent front teeth can make passage of the diverticuloscope difficult and serve as relative contraindications to the procedure. All other patients are suitable candidates, including those with diverticular recurrence after previous pouch surgery. Indeed, in patients who have undergone pouch surgery or other forms of neck surgery, the endoscopic approach may be regarded as the preferred approach, because it is simpler and safer.

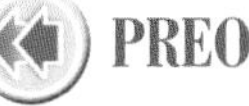

PREOPERATIVE PLANNING

In addition to a careful history and physical examination, preoperative testing for the majority of patients with a pharyngeal pouch is minimal. A barium swallow or endoscopy has confirmed the diagnosis, and the surgeon has assessed the patient's suitability for the endoscopic procedure. The procedure is best done under general anesthesia, but it is very quick and carries minimal morbidity in fit patients.

Equipment

The equipment required for endoscopic diverticulostomy is quite simple. A double-lipped Weerda diverticuloscope (Karl Stortz; Tuttlingen, Germany) is needed to expose the diverticulum, a chest support is required to hold the diverticulosope in place, and a 5-mm 0-degree telescope will project the procedure on screen. The telescope should have a 300-watt light source coupled with a high-resolution monitor. Additional instruments needed include a laparoscopic stapler with a vascular 40-mm staple load, a suction device, an endostitch, and a long grasper to remove any retained food.

SURGICAL TECHNIQUE

The surgery is performed under general anaesthesia with the patient supine and the neck extended. A roll is placed beneath the patient's shoulder blades in order to elevate the esophagus and create a straight line for placement of the diverticuloscope. The Weerda diverticuloscope is introduced to expose the esophageal lumen, pharyngeal pouch, and cricopharyngeal bar and common wall, which lie between the lumen and the pouch (Fig. 16-11, page 144). The introduction of the diverticuloscope is similar to the introduction of a rigid esophagoscope.

Once the common wall between the diverticulum and the esophagus has been visualized (Fig. 16-12, page 144), the diverticuloscope is fixed and held in place by means of a chest support. In order to obtain a magnified view of the common wall, a 5-mm 0-degree telescope is inserted through the diverticuloscope and connected to a cold light source and video camera, so that the

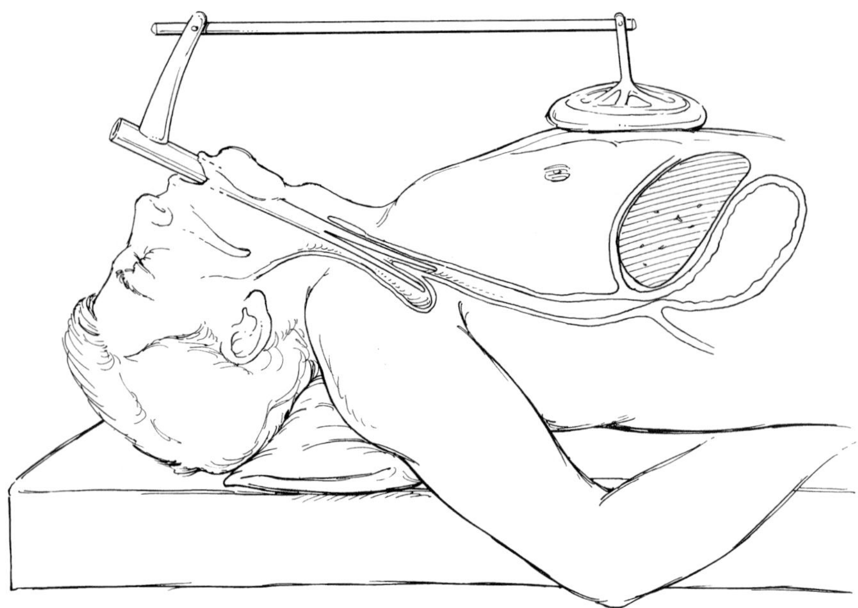

Fig. 16-11. The operative setup for stapled Zenker diverticulectomy showing the rigid diverticulectomy scope in position and the exposure of the common wall of the diverticulum.

procedure is viewed on the screen. After inspection of the pouch, to exclude mucosal abnormalities or retained food, an Endo GIA 30 stapler (Autosuture; Norwalk, CT) is passed under endoscopic vision, placing the longer of the two cartridge limbs into the esophageal lumen and the other limb into the pouch, thus straddling the common wall, including the cricopharyngeal bar. When fired, the cricopharyngeal bar and common wall are cut, and a double row of staples is inserted on either side to seal the wound edges (Fig. 16-13). Additional firings of the stapler are performed as needed. This results in a cricopharyngeal myotomy and makes the lumen of the sac continuous with the lumen of the esophagus. Although not exactly physiologic, this does allow emptying of the pouch into the esophagus. Introduction of the stapler into small pouches is difficult, and conversion to open surgery may be required. One useful strategy for small pouches is to apply an endostitch on either side of the cricopharyngeal bar and elevate it toward the mouth. This artificially deepens the pouch and may allow successful application of the Endo GIA. Some surgeons have suggested the removal of the protective extension of the stapler to facilitate deeper access and more complete myotomy. Advantages of the stapling technique over the Dohlman procedure are that it is quicker, with less risk of bleeding and postoperative leak, as the edges of the wound are sealed by a staple line.

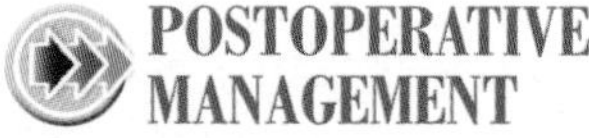

POSTOPERATIVE MANAGEMENT

Patients are fed clear liquids the morning of the first postoperative day. In the absence of worrisome symptoms or signs (pain, fever, tachycardia), we do not advise a routine contrast study following endoscopic diverticulostomy. Patients are advanced to a soft diet, and most are discharged within 24 to 48 hours following surgery.

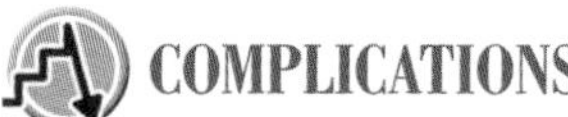

COMPLICATIONS

Table 16-2 summarizes complications after endoscopic stapling. Although theoretically leak is less of a concern compared to other techniques, there is an overall leakage rate of 1.4% in the literature. The cause of these has been such things as direct instrumental perforation and leakage from the staple line. Differences in stapler type may play a role. Other minor morbidities reported in the literature include gingival or mucosal laceration, dental damage, neck and throat pain, and hematoma in various sites. Temporary vocal cord paralysis has been reported, despite the fact that avoidance of this problem is theoretically an advantage endoscopic treatment offers over open surgery.

As the pouch is not removed in this technique, it seems that symptomatic pouch recurrence may necessarily be more of a problem than with open repair. Time will tell whether this holds true.

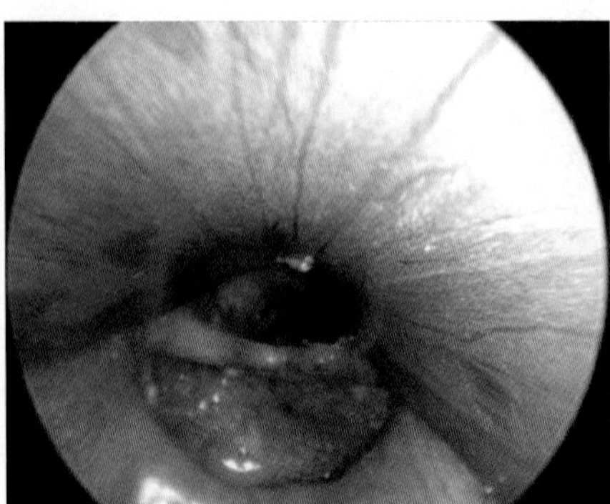

Fig. 16-12. The endoscopic appearance of a pharyngeal pouch showing the cricopharyngeal bar between the pouch (posterior) and the esophageal lumen (anterior). (Courtesy of Peter G. Devitt, Royal Adelaide Hospital, Australia.)

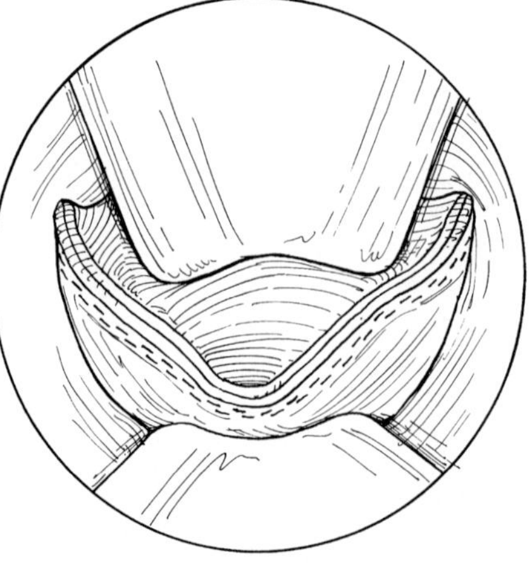

Fig. 16-13. A view through the diverticulectomy scope after the stapler has been fired.

TABLE 16-2. COMPLICATIONS AFTER ENDOSCOPIC STAPLE DIVERTICULOSTOMY FOR ZENKER DIVERTICULUM

Complications
Leak and/or development of fistula
Temporary vocal cord paralysis
Gingival or mucosal laceration
Dental damage
Neck and throat pain
Hematoma
Carcinoma
Recurrence
Retained foreign body/bezoar in residual pouch

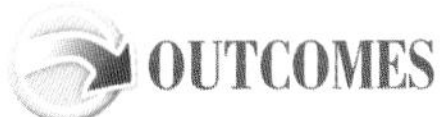

OUTCOMES

The success of endoscopic stapling in achieving the desired outcome is dependent on two key elements. The first is that sufficient division of the cricopharyngeus occurs (that is, an adequate myotomy is produced). This remains controversial in the current literature. However, a well-written editorial by DeMeester and Bremner states that "... although the results of diverticulectomy only give reported good results of about 92%, the results of myotomy with diverticulectomy (...) appear marginally better, with reported excellent results in nearly 100% of patients." We also believe that a myotomy is necessary and should be incorporated into any open operation for pharyngeal pouch.

The second element is that the septum between the pouch and the esophageal lumen is adequately divided, so that emptying from the pouch into the esophagus is facilitated. This has been verified radiologically by Ong et al., who studied seven patients with complete symptomatic improvement after endoscopic stapling. They demonstrated that the pouch was still present postoperatively and could not be distinguished from preoperative static images. However, dynamic fluoroscopy revealed rapid emptying from the pouch. It is important to warn the patient of this preoperatively, because if they have further radiological contrast studies at a later date the radiologist will report the presence of a pouch.

CONCLUSION

The endoscopic treatment of Zenker's diverticulum is another of the minimal access operations that has a firmly established place because of its advantages compared with open surgery. These include a shorter operating time, less morbidity, shorter hospital stay, more rapid resumption of oral intake, and a shorter convalescence. Nevertheless, it is important to realize that it has not completely supplanted open surgery, and it is best seen as a very useful addition to operations available to treat this condition.

SUGGESTED READING

Aly A, Devitt PG, Jamieson GG. Evolution of surgical treatment for pharyngeal pouch. *Br J Surg* 2004;91:657–664.

Chang CY, Payyapilli RJ, Scher RL. Endoscopic staple diverticulostomy for Zenker's diverticulum: review of literature and experience in 159 consecutive cases. *Laryngoscope* 2003;113:957–965.

Collard JM, Otte JB, Kestens PJ. Endoscopic stapling technique of esophagodiverticulostomy for Zenkers diverticulum. *Ann Thorac Surg* 1993;56:573–576.

DeMeester T, Bremner CG. Editorial: Selective cricopharyngeal myotomy for Zenker's diverticulum. *J Am Coll Surg* 2003;196:451–452.

Fernando HC, Luketich JD, Samphire J, et al. Minimally invasive operation for esophageal diverticula. *Ann Thorac Surg* 2005;80: 2076–2081.

Gui D, Rossi S, Runfola M, Magalini SC. Review article: botulinum toxin in the therapy of gastrointestinal motility disorders. *Aliment Pharmacol Ther* 2003;18: –16.

Heitmiller RF, Moore LJ. Esophageal Spasm Syndromes. In: Cameron JL, ed. *Current Surgical Therapy*, 8th ed. Philadelphia: Elsevier Mosby, 2004;19–22.

Hoffman HT. Clinical Review: Cricopharyngeal spasm and Zenker's diverticulum. *Head & Nec*, 2003;25:681–694.

Jamieson GG, Duranceau W, Payne WS. Pharyngo-esophageal diverticulum. In: *Surgery of the Esophagus*. Churchill Livingstone, 1988; 435–443.

Nastos D, Chen LQ, Ferraro P, et al. Long myotomy with antireflux repair for esophageal spastic disorders. *J Gastrointest Surg* 2002;6: 713–722.

Ong CC, Elton PG, Mitchell D. Pharyngeal pouch endoscopic stapling: are postoperative barium swallow radiographs of any value? *J Laryngol Otol* 1999;113:233–236.

Sen P, Kumar G, Bhattacharyya AK. Pharyngeal pouch: associations and complications. *Eur Arch Otorhinolaryngol* 2006;263:463–468.

Spechler SJ, Castell DJ. Classification of oesophageal abnormalities. *Gut*, 2001;49: 145–151.

Tedesco P, Fisichella PM, Way LW, et al. Cause and treatment of epiphrenic diverticula. *Am J Surg* 2005;190:902–905.

Van Overbeek JJM. Meditation on the pathogenesis of Zenkers diverticulum and a report of endoscopic treatment in 545 patients. *Ann Otol Rhinol Laryngol* 1994; 103:178–185.

COMMENTARY

Patients with esophageal motility disorders often present a diagnostic and therapeutic problem to the GI practitioner. This is true whether or not the disorder is characterized by hypomotility or by spasticity. Either condition can be symptomatic or totally asymptomatic and is often associated with other foregut disorders such as GERD and/or delayed gastric emptying. As discussed by Drs. Jamieson and Thompson, the hypomotility disorders are often the result of chronic peptic damage and, if so, will usually improve after an antireflux surgery removes the noxious stimuli. However, on rare occasions there can be a primary neuromotor degenerative disease, which can progressively deteriorate even after a fundoplication and lead to refractory dysphagia. The clinician must always be aware of this possibility and aggressively move to reverse the fundoplication if progressive dysphagia and esophageal dilation happens.

The spastic disorders are even more difficult to address. Many patients with spastic disorders have no symptoms and symptoms that do occur are often difficult to directly tie to the spasms. As Dr. Jamieson stresses, the best place to start with these patients is with medical treatment (PPI, calcium channel blockers, or nitroglycerin). Vigorous dilatation with a large dilator is sometimes beneficial as well. We would advocate a trial of endoscopic Botox injection if possible and feel somewhat better about recommending surgery if the patient had symptom improvement post-Botox. Short of this, the patient with noncardiac chest pain can be a surgical slippery slope—we have seen cases with no improvement with distal myotomy and fundoplication, still no improvement with a long myotomy, and still with incapacitating pain after an esophagectomy!

The treatment of esophageal diverticula can be deceptively simple on paper and yet very difficult in actuality. The authors appropriately stress the need to carefully and thoroughly dissect the diverticulum off of the esophagus, to which it is typically closely adherent. As noted, the simultaneous use of an endoscope inside the esophagus is useful and even mandatory for complete dissection and to check for leaks. When at all possible a

(continued)

single firing of the stapler should be done as opposed to multiple applications, as the latter dramatically increases the possibility of a leak. Finally, a distal myotomy including ablation of the sphincter below the diverticulum (cricopharyngeal for Zenker and the LES for diverticula of the esophageal body) is always necessary to prevent recurrence.

The wide distribution of presenting symptoms of these significant motor disorders points out yet again how critical it is to obtain esophageal physiology studies before considering surgery. Motility testing can differentiate between the different types of dysmotility and provide a road map for surgical ablation, and 24-hour pH testing will ensure that the patient's symptoms actually have some connection to the spasm.

LLS

C. Premalignant and Malignant Diseases

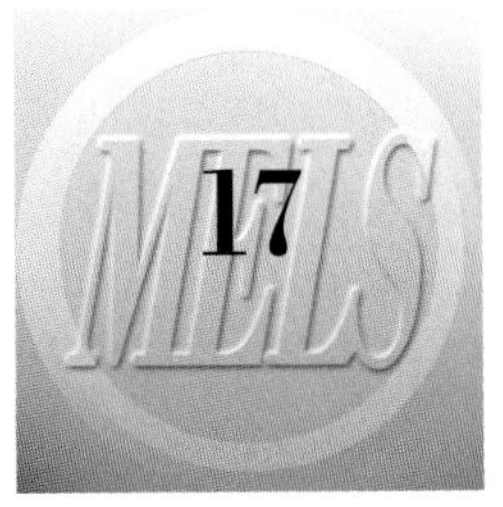

Endoscopy for Diagnosis, Screening, and Staging of Premalignant and Malignant Diseases of the Esophagus

JOSH WALKER, BRUCE MACFADYEN, AND JOHN MELLINGER

INTRODUCTION

Flexible upper gastrointestinal endoscopy plays a major role in the diagnosis and surveillance of gastroesophageal reflux disease, Barrett esophagus, and esophageal malignancy. Endoscopy is currently the primary diagnostic tool, based on its capacity to provide tissue confirmation in settings of suspected malignancy or Barrett changes. Major technological advancements over the last decade have provided many tools that have decreased the expected morbidity and mortality of patients with these disorders. Patient education and outcomes have benefited from these noninvasive modalities and therapeutic strategies.

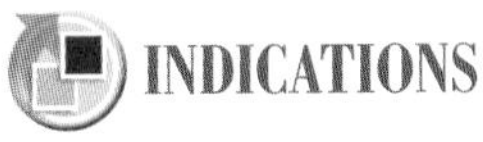

INDICATIONS

Esophagogastroduodenoscopy (EGD) is generally indicated when its results will lead to change in management. It is also an alternative to radiographic studies as an initial method of diagnosis. However, there are settings in which a contrast study is helpful before an EGD. These situations include stricture, preoperative planning, possible perforation, and high risk for sedation. Table 17-1 shows a list of the indications for upper endoscopy. Certain symptoms such as dysphagia along with weight loss are very concerning for malignancy.

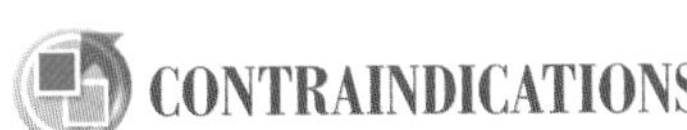

CONTRAINDICATIONS

Contraindications to EGD include an unwilling patient, inexperienced personnel, poor cardiorespiratory status, coagulopathy (relative), and perforated viscus. These contraindications are all relative depending on the indication for endoscopy.

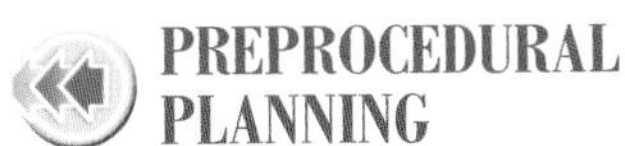

PREPROCEDURAL PLANNING

Once the indication for EGD is confirmed, informed consent should be obtained explaining the full nature of the procedure and extent of potential complications. The history and physical should be thorough, including any anticoagulation medications (including antiplatelet therapy), bleeding tendencies, or history of vascular disease. There are no data to support an increased risk of bleeding during diagnostic EGD while on aspirin, but elevated bleeding risk continues to be present during therapeutic endoscopy. If the patient is on short-term anticoagulation, the procedure should be delayed if possible. If chronic anticoagulation is necessary, then stopping Coumadin for 3 to 5 days or correcting the coagulopathy with fresh frozen plasma (FFP) if necessary to an international normalized ratio (INR) of >2 is adequate. Vitamin K is not recommended for correction of warfarin therapy for a procedure, as appropriate anticoagulation postprocedure may be difficult to obtain. Antibiotic prophylaxis is not indicated in most patients, but it is

TABLE 17-1. INDICATIONS FOR ESOPHAGOGASTRODUODENOSCOPY

Indication	Example
Symptoms	Dyspepsia Gastroesophageal reflux disease (GERD) Dysphagia/odynophagia Nausea/vomiting Chest pain (noncardiac)
Surveillance	Barrett epithelium Lye-induced strictures Plummer-Vinson syndrome Gastric polyps Familial adenomatous polyposis (FAP) Esophageal ulcer Gastric ulcer Postgastrectomy ulcer
EUS specific	Pancreatic disease Biliary disease Submucosal abnormalities Varices Cancer staging FNAC/core biopsy guidance
Miscellaneous	Bleeding Radiographic abnormalities Malabsorption Caustic ingestion Varices

EUS, endoscopic ultrasound.

indicated in patients at high risk for endocarditis. Transient bacteremia may occur during diagnostic endoscopy, but more often happens during therapeutic procedures. High-risk patients include those with prosthetic valves, a history of endocarditis, surgically constituted shunts or conduits, or synthetic vascular grafts within the last year. Defibrillators should be deactivated if electrocautery is to be used, but no intervention is necessary for pacemakers. The patient should not have any solids for 6 hours and no liquids for 4 hours. Essential medications should be taken with sips of water. Standard monitoring and conscious sedation is usually obtained with a benzodiazepine (midazolam or diazepam) and a narcotic (meperidine or fentanyl).

In the United States, most EGDs are performed with the patient under conscious sedation, which is a state of moderate sedation and analgesia in which the patient maintains both ventilatory and cardiovascular function and should respond purposefully to a verbal or nonpainful tactile stimulus. The minimal level of sedation required to perform a procedure is patient- and procedure-specific and should be governed by patient comfort and safety. The two factors that are of utmost importance when determining sedation are patient characteristics and difficulty and anticipated duration of the procedure. Some patient characteristics are associated with tolerance of EGD with little or no sedation. Transnasal esophagoscopy, ultrathin endoscopes, and capsule esophagoscopy are procedures that employ minimal or no sedation. Patients that require minimal sedation are usually older men without a history of abdominal pain or anxiety. Even cultural background may play a role in sedation requirements. Other characteristics predict difficulty with sedation. These are prior difficulty with sedation, prescribed benzodiazepine or opiates, and heavy alcohol use. Difficulty has been described in up to 30% of such patients. These particular patients may be good candidates for droperidol, propofol, or general anesthesia. In the U.S., propofol is currently being used in approximately 25% of flexible endoscopies. The major drawback of its use is respiratory depression, which can be decreased if used as a balanced anesthetic with fentanyl and Versed. For this reason, the use of propofol has been limited to anesthesiologists in most gastrointestinal centers in the U.S. The use of conscious sedation for outpatient diagnostic EGD is decreasing because of increased cost as well as the inconvenience to the patient.

Instrumentation

The modern era of endoscopy began with the development of fiber-optic instruments in the 1960s, which for most purposes have been supplanted by video chip endoscopes that were developed in the 1990s. Thus, there are two types of flexible endoscopes: fiber-optic and video-imaging. In the former, viewing bundles of a standard fiber endoscope are 2 to 3 mm in diameter and contain 20,000 to 40,000 fine glass fibers, each fiber measuring approximately 10 μm in diameter. Light focused onto the face of each fiber is transmitted by repeated internal reflections. Accurate transmission of an image depends upon the spatial orientation of the individual fibers being the same at both ends of the bundle (a "coherent" bundle). Videoendoscopes are mechanically similar to fiber endoscopes, with a charged couple device (CCD) "chip" and supporting electronics mounted at the tip, along with wiring replacing the optical bundle and other electronic instrumentation and switches occupying the site of the ocular lens on the upper part of the control head. The CCD chip camera transmits digital images back to the processor that produces capable video imaging. This technology allows for a reduced outer diameter of the working shaft, superior optical resolution, increased durability, increased magnification, and a better quality image.

Most endoscopes have a standard set of controls consisting of two knobs and two buttons arranged ergonomically around a grip. The larger inner knob produces up and down deflection, while the smaller inner knob controls left and right sideways deflection. Each deflection control has a locking mechanism. Two forward-facing buttons are operated by the index finger. The upper button is for aspiration and is activated by depression of the button. The lower button has two roles. When this button is occluded, it serves as an air insufflator, and when depressed, the button serves as an irrigating lens cleaner. The accessory port for diagnostic and therapeutic instruments is located distal to the lower button on the anterior aspect of the shaft. The control section of the endoscope is connected to the light source, water, suction, compressed air, and an image-processing computer through the computer to a monitor. A photo of an endoscopy cart is shown in Figure 17-1.

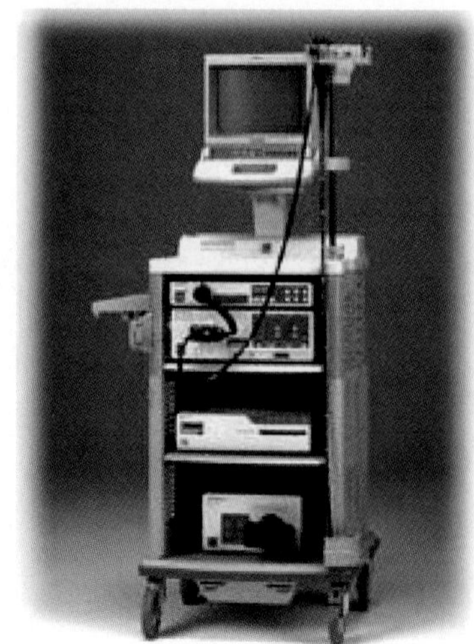

Fig. 17-1. Endoscopy cart.

Ultrathin endoscopes with a miniaturized CCD chip camera at the tip of the endoscope have an outer diameter as small as 5.3 mm and a single 2-mm accessory channel that can accommodate a 1.8-mm biopsy forceps. These endoscopes are especially useful for passing through areas of stenosis and for transnasal procedures in the unsedated patient. However, they are not stiff enough to use for viewing the distal duodenum. Image quality, lavage suction, and biopsy capabilities are slightly inferior to conventional endoscopes.

Dedicated ultrasound endoscopes have additional piezoelectric transducers at the tip in a linear or radial array that use frequencies of 5 to 30 MHz to generate ultrasonic images of internal organs, in addition to video or fiber-optic endoscopy of the bowel lumen. This frequency is much higher than the standard transabdominal ultrasounds, which operate at 3.5 to 5 MHz. As the frequency of the ultrasound probe is increased, the resolution is increased but the penetration is decreased.

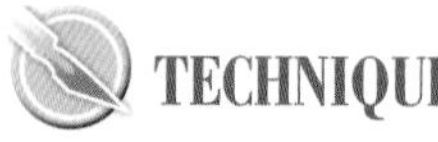

TECHNIQUE

During upper endoscopy, the patient should be positioned in the left lateral decubitus position. A bite block is inserted to protect the endoscope immediately after sedation is administered, and the endoscopist stands facing the patient at the patient's head. An assistant positioned behind the patient should monitor the respiratory and cardiovascular parameters and help with instrumentation, suctioning, and endoscope stabilization.

The headpiece of the endoscope is held in the left hand with the flat side toward the palm and the grip held by the last three fingers. The weight of the endoscope is balanced by the umbilical shaft, which lies over the base of the thumb. The index finger depresses the air/water and suction buttons. The larger wheel produces upward and downward deflection of the tip. The smaller outer knob produces left/right deflection, and by locking the tip of the endoscope either left or right out of the neutral position, rotation of the endoscope clockwise or counterclockwise will turn the tip right and left, respectively. This rotational technique enables the endoscopist to steer with the left hand alone while the right hand controls the working shaft and advances the tip. Although one-handed steering is very efficient, when fine adjustments are necessary it is still sometimes necessary to use two hands to control the deflection of the tip, with the right hand controlling the smaller knob.

A water-soluble lubricant should be applied to the distal end of the endoscope, staying just short of the tip so that the lens does not get obscured. There are several methods to advance the lubricated endoscope through the posterior pharynx and insert it into the esophagus. This maneuver is a challenging part of the EGD examination, and it is important to be familiar with all the methods. If one method should fail, switching to another may prove successful.

The safest method is using direct vision with the light source on and the right hand holding the shaft 20 to 30 cm from the tip. This length allows passage through the cricopharyngeal muscle without releasing and re-grasping the shaft. Holding the shaft further away from the tip may cause it to buckle. The shaft should be rotated such that downward deflection of the tip by the left thumb's manipulation of the large knob moves the tip inferiorly in the patient's sagittal plane. The tip should then be straightened and passed through the bite block, over the tongue and past the uvula until the posterior pharynx is in view. Holding the shaft in the midline, the downward deflection of the tip is repeated. The base of the tongue and epiglottis should be visible anteriorly, corresponding to 6 o'clock on the monitor. The vocal cords diverge from the midline anteriorly toward the arytenoid cartilages posteriorly (Fig. 17-2). The opening to the first part of the esophagus is a slit in the midline, immediately posterior to the arytenoids. The opening may be seen at 6 o'clock on the monitor, when the cricopharyngeal sphincter momentarily relaxes. On either side of the arytenoids lie the pyriform sinuses; perforation of these can easily occur if the tip of the endoscope is deflected laterally and excessive pressure is applied. It is, therefore, important to keep the endoscope in the midline as one attempts to enter the esophagus and to keep the tip inferiorly deflected to prevent excessive gagging by impingement on the posterior wall. Momentary relaxation of the cricopharyngeus muscle during swallowing facilitates passage of the endoscope into the esophagus. The presence of the endoscope and some air insufflation may initiate a swallow; otherwise, asking the patient to swallow will relax the sphincter, and the endoscope can then be advanced under vision into the esophagus.

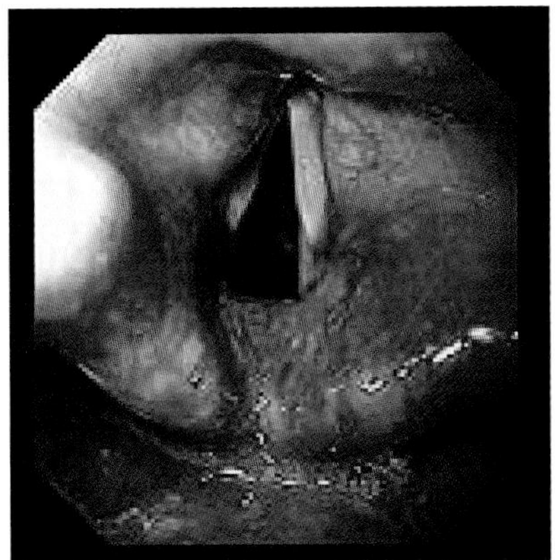

Fig. 17-2. Vocal cords. (With permission from Atlanta South Gastroenterology, P.C.)

An alternate technique in a responsive patient capable of swallowing is blind tip manipulation. The shaft of the endoscope is held as described previously, and the tip is passed over the tongue in the midline until it reaches the back of the mouth. The tip is then deflected posteriorly in the sagittal axis, and slight forward pressure is applied. The patient is asked to swallow when the 20 cm mark on the endoscope is at the level of the incisors. As the cricopharyngeus muscle relaxes, there is a loss of resistance, and the endoscope enters the esophagus.

The third method involves placing two fingers of the left hand in the patient's mouth, posterior to the tongue, to guide the endoscope with the right hand between them. This helps to keep the endoscope in the midline. There is a risk of the endoscopist's left hand being bitten by the patient, so this technique is best used in the anesthetized patient. When the endoscope's 20-cm mark passes the incisors, successful entry into the esophagus is marked by a sudden loss of resistance as the endoscope passes the sphincter. If the patient has had endotracheal intubation, the balloon may need to be deflated to permit the endoscope's passage. Throughout the procedure, the endotracheal tube should be held in position to prevent accidental extubation.

Once in the esophagus, the lumen is located by gentle air insufflation and limited circular movements of the tip. The endoscope should be advanced slowly under direct vision, using rotational torque on the endoscope. Small corrections are made with the thumb on the up/down control to keep the lumen in the visual field at all times. This maneuver is important to prevent perforation. If the luminal view is lost (a "red out"), insufflating a small amount of air and withdrawing the endoscope slightly or repeating the circular movements of the tip often helps to identify it. If the wall is still in view, deflecting the tip in the opposite direction may locate the lumen.

While advancing the endoscope down the esophagus, it is important to observe the peristaltic activity, distensibility, points of normal extrinsic compression (cricoesophageal sphincter, aorta, left bronchus, the diaphragmatic hiatus, and the lower esophageal sphincter), and mucosal appearance. The esophagus is normally lined by a pale-pink, smooth, and flat mucosa, which is a nonkeratinized, stratified squamous epithelium. By visualizing the esophageal mucosa during advancement, one can easily differentiate true esophagitis from scope trauma. The gastroesophageal junction (Z-line) is normally visible as a distinct zone where the pale pink squamous esophageal mucosa abruptly transitions to a salmon color, which is columnar gastric mucosa. This zone of transition is typically 38 to 40 cm from the incisors and normally approximately 1 to 2 cm above the diaphragmatic hiatus. In severe anemia, it may be difficult to discern. Alterations in these measurements may give the examiner an indication that some pathology exists in this area. The diaphragmatic hiatus can be identified by asking the patient to sniff when the endoscope is slightly above the Z-line. The diaphragm contracts and produces luminal occlusion or narrowing by external compression. The physiologic lower esophageal sphincter (Fig. 17-3, page 150) is usually just below the diaphragmatic hiatus, and although frequently closed on examination, it normally allows the endoscope to pass through easily into the cardia of the stomach with some air insufflation. A description of the technique for examining the stomach and duodenum is provided in Chapter 23.

The normal anatomy of the foregut may be altered by surgical intervention.

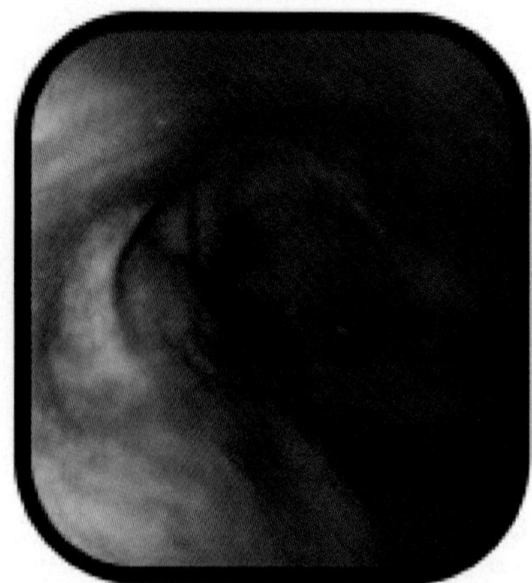

Fig. 17-3. Lower esophageal sphincter (With permission from Jackson Siegelbaum Gastroenterology.)

The endoscopist needs to be aware of the type of surgery and be able to anticipate and adapt to the difficulties that a particular operation presents to a complete endoscopic examination. It is beneficial to review operative reports from previous surgeries and obtain contrast studies before proceeding with endoscopic procedures in such settings. The basic maneuvers need not change, and simply repositioning the patient to shift fluid or blood away from an area of concern or to place an area of interest in a nondependent position may allow for a successful examination.

DIAGNOSTIC PROCEDURES

Endoscopy provides unparalleled minimally invasive visual access to the gastrointestinal (GI) mucosa. Magnified visualization of lesions in the stomach that show minor differences in color and shape from normal mucosa may identify microvascular patterns that are associated with intramucosal cancer. Enhanced magnification endoscopy approaches 100% sensitivity for detecting specialized intestinal metaplasia. In this method, 1.5% acetic acid is sprayed on the esophageal mucosa, enhancing the architecture of glandular epithelium and causing a whitish discoloration of the normal, squamous epithelium.

Chromoscopy techniques are useful to improve the detection of early GI cancer and pre-neoplastic changes involving the mucosa, particularly when used with endoscopic magnification and endoscopic ultrasound (EUS). Lugol's iodine applied endoscopically as a 1% to 2% solution stains the glycogen brown in normal esophageal epithelial cells, whereas inflamed, dysplastic, or neoplastic tissue will not stain. Mucosal areas with Barrett esophagus, squamous dysplasia, or esophageal carcinoma become well-defined targets for biopsy. The use of Lugol's iodine solution is 96% sensitive and 63% specific in detecting high-grade dysplasia or invasive cancer. The blue color of indigo carmine, applied as a 0.1% to 0.4% solution, increases mucosal contrast by accumulating in mucosal crevices and depressions. It outlines the borders of lesions and enhances superficial irregularities on their surfaces. A 0.5% to 1% solution of methylene blue applied after a mucolytic agent (10% acetylcysteine) identifies intestinal metaplasia, which selectively absorbs it. The sensitivity and positive predictive value of methylene blue in detecting intestinal metaplasia in Barrett esophagus has been reported as 72% and 89%, respectively. However, some patients may experience vomiting during the procedure, which increases procedure time. Magnification chromoendoscopy with methylene blue may play a role in the surveillance of patients at high risk for gastric cancer by detecting intestinal metaplasia and dysplasia, which are associated with gastric cancer.

Other diagnostic procedures can enhance the utility of endoscopy beyond inspection alone. Using the brush and touch techniques, cytology specimens can be obtained and are useful for diagnosing malignancy and fungal, viral, and bacterial infections. In the brush technique, a sheath with a retractable brush is deployed through the accessory channel of the endoscope and positioned near the lesion. The brush is unsheathed and rubbed over the surface of the lesion, capturing cells and organisms in its bristles. The brush is resheathed to prevent loss of the specimen while being retracted through the working channel of the endoscope and removed. The brush contents are rolled on a slide and a fixative is applied. If required, the specimen-laden brush can be cultured. Brush cytology is often used to obtain specimens from strictures (Fig. 17-4) where a biopsy would be difficult. Used alone, brush cytology is 79% sensitive and 98.5% specific in diagnosing foregut malignancies, and when used together with a biopsy it can add almost 10% to the diagnostic yield from these lesions. If both brushing and biopsy need to be performed, the brushing should be performed second; otherwise, bleeding caused by the cytology brush may obscure the field for accurate biopsy forceps placement. Touch cytology is also useful in investigating for infectious organisms. In this technique, a standard biopsy specimen is touched on a slide, which is then fixed and stained for cytologic examination.

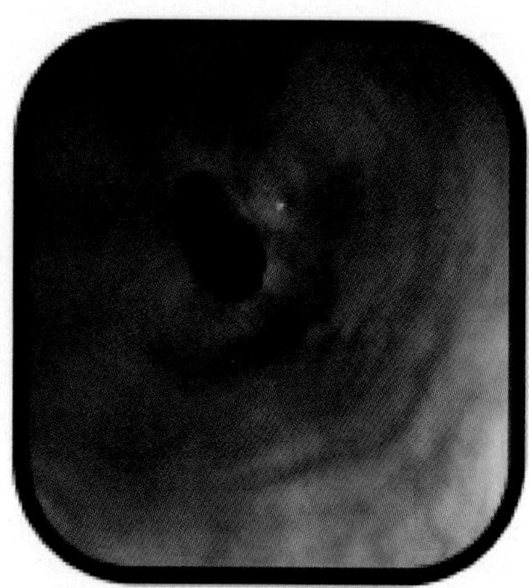

Fig. 17-4. Esophageal stricture. (With permission from Jackson Siegelbaum Gastroenterology.)

Aspirates are likewise easily obtained by instillation of sterile saline through the working channel and subsequent aspiration. To avoid any contamination by other material previously aspirated, the fluid should be collected in a clean container with a trap attached to the suction apparatus. The aspirate can be cytologically examined or cultured.

Standard biopsy forceps provide a high diagnostic yield if the pathology involves the mucosa (sensitivity 88.3% and specificity 99.9%). The endoscope is positioned as perpendicular as possible to the area to be biopsied. The biopsy forceps are passed through the working channel with the jaws closed. Once the tip is visible, the jaws are opened, thrust into the tissue, closed tightly, and quickly pulled back bringing with them an adequate specimen. The specimen is actually cut by pulling the forceps back against the tip of the endoscope. Another recommended approach is the "turn and suction" technique, using suction to pull the mucosa toward the tip of the endoscope and then grasping it with the biopsy forceps.

Biopsy forceps (Fig. 17-5) come in many shapes and sizes, but there are two general categories. The first is the spiked forceps, which has a small, needle-like spike between the jaws allowing them to retain multiple specimens without being removed from the endoscope after each bite. An added benefit is that by virtue of their firm grasp on tissue, spiked forceps are useful in obtaining biopsies from

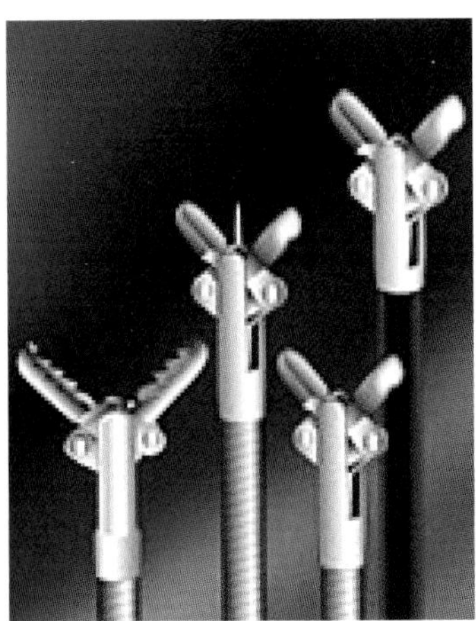

Fig. 17-5. Biopsy forceps.

targets that present tangentially to the endoscope. The second category of forceps is the jumbo or large cupped forceps. These forceps require a 3.7-mm internal diameter working channel and cannot be used to biopsy submucosal lesions but can deliver large mucosal specimens. Larger specimens do not necessarily lead to increased diagnostic efficacy. Diagnostic yield increases when multiple well-targeted biopsies are taken. Typical lesions evaluated by biopsy include esophageal strictures and mass lesions. Lesions suspected of being a varix should not be biopsied, because this can lead to significant bleeding.

If a lesion is suspicious for malignancy, eight to ten biopsies should be obtained from the tumor margins as well as from an ulcer base. The margins contain a transition zone between the ulcer and surrounding mucosa that most likely contains increased mitotic activity if the lesion is indeed malignant. Using standard biopsy forceps, the biopsy of submucosal masses or tissues with a great deal of superficial necrosis may have low yield, because of the inability of the forceps to penetrate deeply. Several biopsies from the same location may improve the diagnostic yield in submucosal tumors but may also lead to weakening and possible perforation of the esophagus, stomach, or duodenal wall.

DIAGNOSIS AND SCREENING OF BARRETT ESOPHAGUS

The most common premalignant esophageal condition encountered during EGD is Barrett esophagus. (An esophageal adenocarcinoma within an area of Barrett esophagus is shown in Figure 17-9, page 152.) This esophageal mucosal change is considered to be responsible for the profound increase in the incidence of adenocarcinoma of the esophagus seen in the Western world over the past several decades. Barrett esophagus is the presence of columnar epithelium lining the esophagus that histologically resembles specialized intestinal epithelium with metaplasia. The presence of goblet cells is required for the diagnosis, and there is a 30- to 50-fold increased risk of carcinoma in Barrett esophagus. Once the diagnosis is made, aggressive attempts to decrease acid exposure should be made, with frequent surveillance to observe any progression of the intestinal metaplasia to dysplasia or malignancy. There is evidence that curtailing alkaline (duodenal) as well as gastric acid is necessary to diminish or completely eliminate the tendency toward dysplastic and/or malignant degeneration of existing Barrett epithelium. Therefore, controversy exists over the need for surveillance of alkali exposure in patients with Barrett esophagus.

The identification of Barrett esophagus begins with the careful inspection of the mucosa surrounding the gastroesophageal junction in patients with gastroesophageal reflux disease (GERD). Confirmation of the characteristic salmon-colored, erythematous appearance requires tissue sampling (Figs. 17-6 and 17-7). The standard technique for obtaining the diagnosis consists of a four-quadrant biopsy every 1 cm in areas of metaplastic changes, along with additional biopsies of any other suspicious lesions. Esophagitis (Fig. 17-8) or erythema of the esophagus can be confused with Barrett. Therefore, biopsy is essential. Some studies have even shown the presence of Barrett on biopsy without visual cues. If either of these conditions is diagnosed by biopsy, then reendoscopy should be performed after acid suppression therapy to rule out intestinal metaplasia. A variety of other techniques can be used for recognition of Barrett esophagus. One of these methods includes magnification endoscopy. Topical stains such as Lugol's iodine, toluene blue, indigo carmine, and methylene blue can also be used to assist in identifying areas of concern that require biopsy.

The presence and grade of dysplasia determines the interval for surveillance endoscopy (Table 17-2, page 152). The cytological and architectural changes associated with dysplasia represent the best current indicator of the cancer risk. The most recent guidelines for surveillance from the American College of Gastroenterology recommend a 3-year interval for endoscopic examination and biopsy if no dysplasia is noted on two

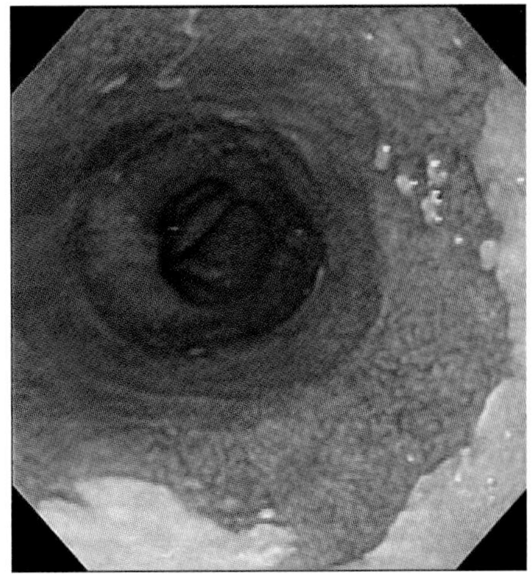

Fig. 17-7. Another view of Barrett esophagus.

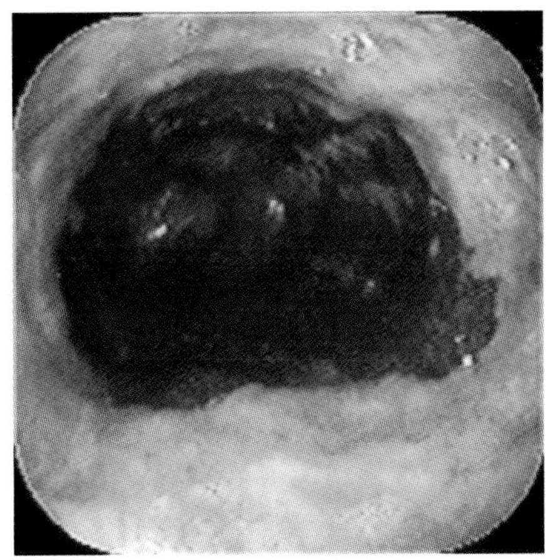

Fig. 17-6. Barrett esophagus.

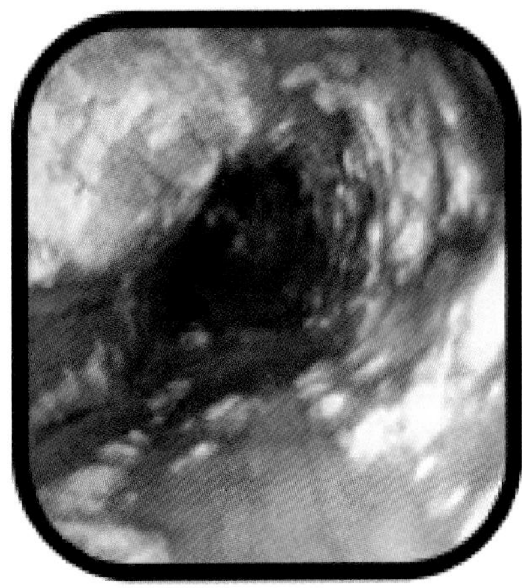

Fig. 17-8. Candida esophagitis. (With permission from Jackson Siegelbaum Gastroenterology.)

TABLE 17-2. GRADED DYSPLASIA AND PROPOSED SURVEILLANCE

Dysplasia	Documentation	Follow-up endoscopy
None	Two EGDs with biopsy	Every 3 years
Low-grade	Highest grade on repeat	Yearly until no dysplasia
High-grade	Repeat EGD with biopsy to rule out cancer and document high-grade dysplasia. Expert pathologist confirmation.	Focal: every 3 months
		Multifocal: intervention
		Mucosal irregularity: EMR

EGD, esophagogastroduodenoscopy; EMR, endoscopic mucosal resection.

successive examinations. In patients with low-grade dysplasia, yearly endoscopy is recommended until there is no dysplasia on biopsy. High-grade dysplasia requires a repeat endoscopy with biopsy every 6 to 12 months to rule out cancer with expert pathological confirmation. This type of dysplasia is further categorized into focal, multifocal, and mucosal irregularities. The recommendations are the same for short-segment and long-segment Barrett esophagus.

OTHER PREMALIGNANT AND MALIGNANT CONDITIONS

The incidence of esophageal cancer is increased in several other conditions besides Barrett esophagus. Adenocarcinoma may be present in an area of Barrett esophagus such as shown in Figure 17-9. Another premalignant condition is achalasia. The incidence of esophageal cancer has been reported to be 33 times higher in achalasics than expected in the general population. Squamous cell carcinoma is the most common type and usually occurs in the middle third of the esophagus. Chronic esophagitis is another condition considered to be premalignant. A third premalignant disease is tylosis. This disease is an autosomal inherited defect of keratinization associated with a 95% risk of squamous cell carcinoma of the esophagus by the age of 65. Although hyperkeratosis of the palms and soles is a clinical characteristic of this disease, the esophageal epithelium does not usually manifest significant abnormalities of keratinization. Plummer-Vinson Syndrome represents another inherited defect that carries an increased risk of esophageal cancer. This syndrome is characterized by cervical esophageal webs, iron deficiency anemia, stomatitis, pharyngitis, and dystrophic changes of the nail bed. There is an increased risk of cervical esophageal cancer and a possible link to various nutritional deficiencies implicated in the disorder. A final condition recognized for the propensity to undergo malignant degeneration in the esophagus is a history of caustic injury and strictures, specifically from lye ingestion. However, the latency period prior to cancer formation may be as long as 40 years. Formal recommendations have not been agreed upon for the surveillance of these conditions, but regularly scheduled endoscopy every 2 to 5 years should be performed in efforts to diagnose early stage esophageal cancer.

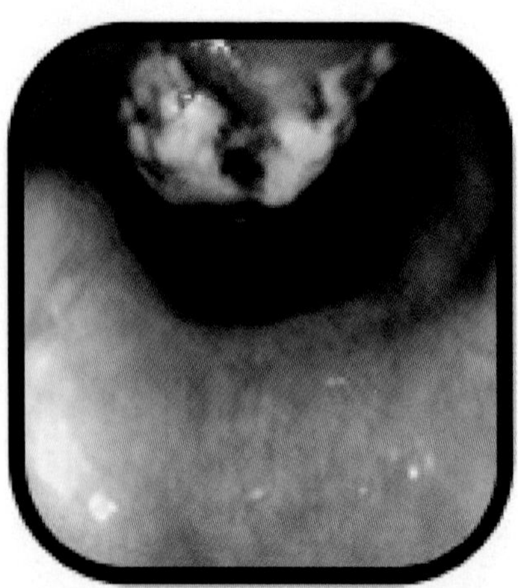

Fig. 17-9. Esophageal adenocarcinoma in Barrett esophagus. (With permission from Jackson Siegelbaum Gastroenterology.)

ENDOSCOPIC ULTRASOUND

Endoscopic Ultrasound (EUS) has emerged over the last decade as an extremely useful modality in the staging of esophageal cancer. Once the diagnosis of malignancy has been confirmed with biopsy, a computerized axial tomography (CAT) scan of the chest and abdomen should first be performed. EUS is considered an adjunct rather than a substitute to such a CAT scan. The current recommendations from the American Journal of Gastroenterology are that CAT scan should first be used to evaluate for distant disease, and EUS should be used to evaluate for tumor depth (T) and regional disease (N). Therefore, EUS provides better T and N staging and also allows tissue sampling of nodes. The combination of EUS-guided biopsy and CAT scan leads to greater accuracy in staging and diagnosis when compared with CAT scan alone. However, EUS staging has not been shown to improve the overall mortality of patients with esophageal cancer when compared with staging using only CAT scan.

EUS uses high frequency ultrasound transducers (7.5 MHz), to provide detailed images of the esophageal layers and structures up to 5 cm from the esophagus. Increased frequency can be used for higher resolution with the price of decreased depth of penetration. The greatest advantages of EUS are the visualization of the esophageal wall layers as well as a guided biopsy of the specimen. The determination of the depth of tumor invasion using EUS produces a five-layer image of the esophageal wall: the first layer represents the superficial mucosa, the second layer corresponds to the mucosa, the third layer to the submucosa, the fourth layer the muscularis propria, and the fifth layer the adventitia. Esophageal cancer is often visualized as a hypoechoic disruption of the wall layers. Figure 17-10 shows the layers of the esophageal wall using the staging criteria for esophageal cancer. Figures 17-11 through 17-13 (pages 153–154) show ultrasound photos of these esophageal wall layers and the depth of tumor invasion. The overall accuracy of EUS for staging depth of tumor invasion (T) is 85% when compared with surgical pathology. For staging regional lymph node metastasis (N), the accuracy is 75%.

Regional disease can be evaluated by assessing lymph nodes. Lymph nodes >10 mm in diameter on CAT scan are considered to be metastatic; Figure 17-14 (page 154) shows a metastatic lymph node visualized by EUS. Similar EUS measurements are used to assess the lymph nodes, but additional criteria are also used to distinguish malignant nodes from benign nodes. Malignant lymph nodes are uniformly hypoechoic and may be enlarged,

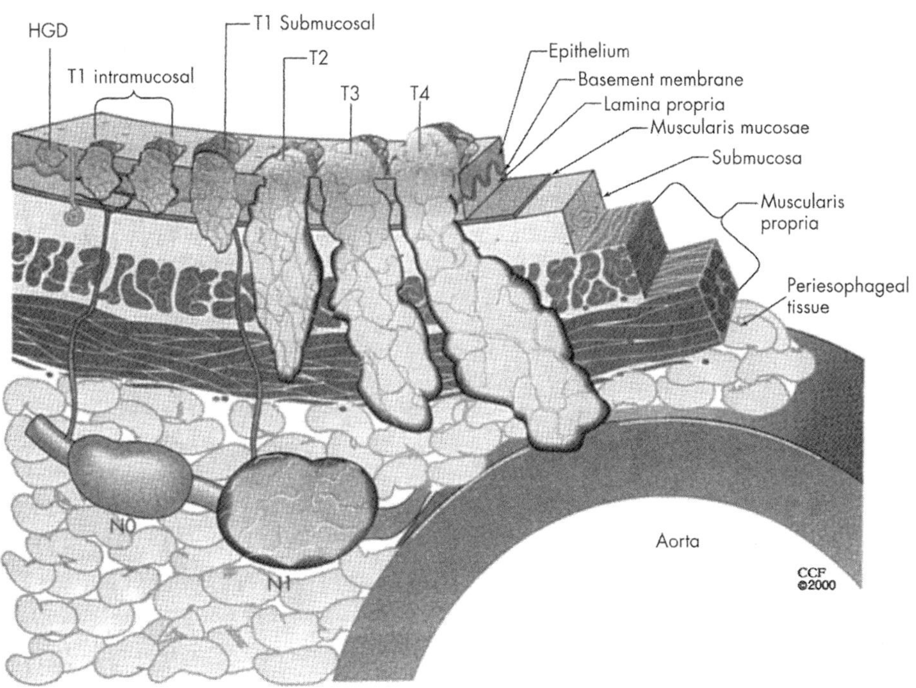

Fig. 17-10. EUS *u*T and *u*N staging of the esophageal wall. EUS, endoscopic ultrasound; HGD, high-grade dysplasia. (With permission from Cameron JL. *Current Surgical Therapy, 7th ed.* St. Louis: Mosby, 2001)

rounded, and sharply demarcated from surrounding fat. On the other hand, benign nodes are often elongated with distinct cortical and medullary areas and are more hyperechoic with less distinct borders. EUS combined with fine needle aspiration for cytology may help to improve specificity for staging if suspicious nodes are present. EUS tends to overstage tumors if preoperative chemotherapy and radiation have been performed. Fibrosis and inflammation cannot be distinguished from residual primary tumor or nodal metastasis. Therefore, EUS for staging purposes should be performed before chemotherapy and radiation for the most reliable results.

Another problematic area where EUS may be beneficial is in the detection of submucosal invasion in patients with cancer in Barrett esophagus. In the absence of submucosal invasion or regional disease, nonoperative therapy with Endoscopic Mucosal Resection (EMR) may be curative. By detecting unsuspected submucosal invasion, EUS may change the therapeutic options in a significant number of patients with Barrett esophagus. Benign tumors and cystic lesions can also be assessed for resectability by employing EUS.

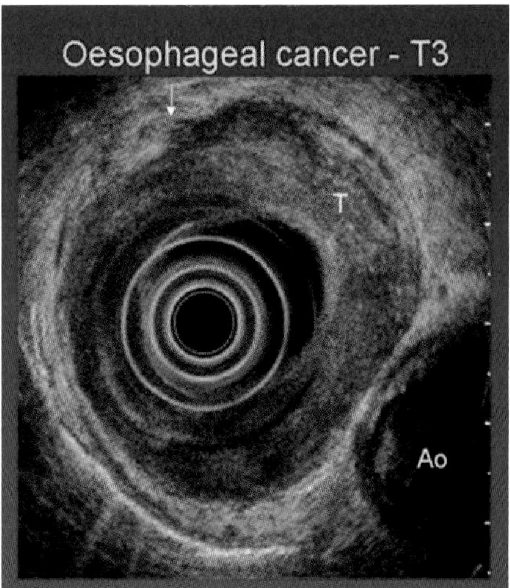

Fig. 17-12. EUS photo of T3 lesion. EUS, endoscopic ultrasound. (With permission from MUSC Digestive Disease Center Clinical Atlas.)

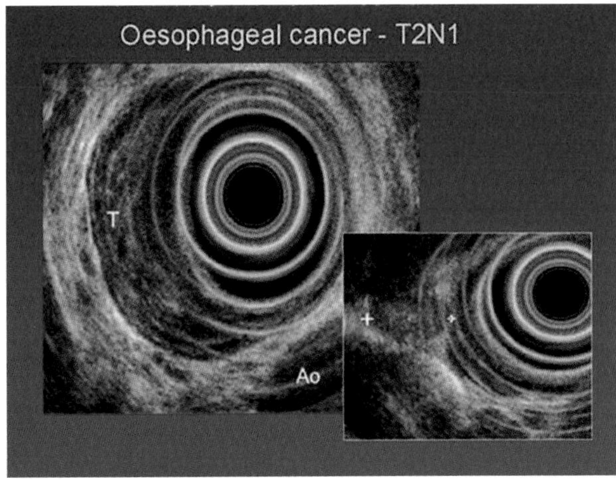

Fig. 17-11. EUS photo of T2 lesion. EUS, endoscopic ultrasound. (With permission from MUSC Digestive Disease Center Clinical Atlas.)

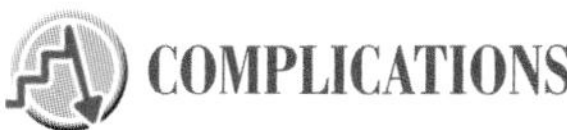

COMPLICATIONS

Estimates of complication rates during diagnostic EGD are often based on a 1974 survey, in which a complication rate of

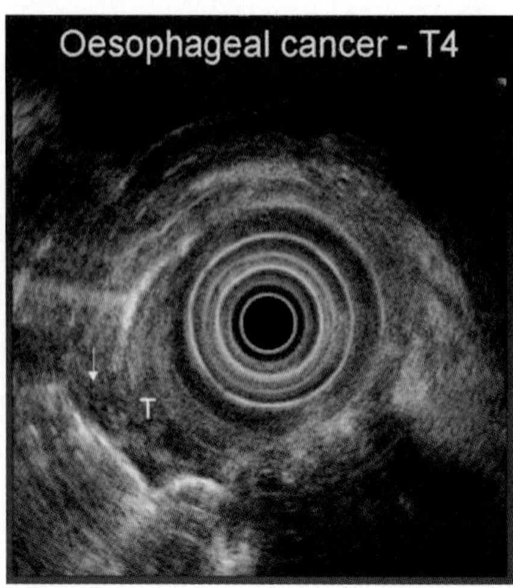

Fig. 17-13. EUS photo of T4 lesion. EUS, endoscopic ultrasound. (With permission from MUSC Digestive Disease Center Clinical Atlas.)

0.13% and an associated mortality rate of 0.004% were reported in more than 200,000 cases. More recent data from a large prospective survey of German gastroenterologists indicates a complication rate of 0.009%, a significant hemorrhage rate of 0.002%, a perforation rate of 0.0009%, and a mortality rate of 0.0009%. Overall, complications during EGD can be divided into four categories: those related to sedation, infectious complications, perforation, and bleeding.

Sedation and analgesia have been reported to cause up to 40% of the complications that occur during EGD. Mild to moderate oxygen desaturation detected by pulse oximetry is the most common complication, although it is often clinically insignificant. Serious complications include severe respiratory depression, myocardial infarction, hypotension, shock, and death. Midazolam has fewer cardiorespiratory complications than diazepam. The correct management of a complication during sedation centers on life support and the administration of appropriate reversal agents, namely flumazenil for benzodiazepines and naloxone for opiates. These particular agents have a shorter half-life than the drugs they are reversing, so redosing may be necessary. Sporadic cases of life-threatening methemoglobinemia have been reported with pharyngeal sprays using benzocaine, and some endoscopists do not use it for local anesthesia. Cyanosis is the most striking physical finding of methemoglobinemia, but seizures, coma, acidosis, and dysrhythmias can also occur. Direct measurement of methemoglobin with multiple wavelength co-oximeters is diagnostic, but pulse oximetry is unreliable in this condition. Treatment is supportive with supplemental oxygen along with methylene blue, which reduces methemoglobin. Some data has shown that pharyngeal spray adds little if sedation is being used.

Infectious complications as the result of the EGD procedure are extremely rare. In the German study, more than 110,000 EGDs were conducted without an infectious complication. Infections may be transmitted autologously, exogenously, or between patients and health care providers. Mucosal trauma may allow the patient's endogenous microbes to penetrate into the mucosa and submucosa, allowing autologous infection. The overall incidence of transient bacteremia after a diagnostic EGD with or without biopsy is approximately 4%. This number can be higher with injection therapy or other invasive procedures. Although probably not very significant, there is one documented case of EGD-associated prosthetic valve endocarditis and one case of meningococcemia after EGD in a child. Retropharyngeal and retroesophageal abscesses occasionally occur in patients who have had traumatic intubations.

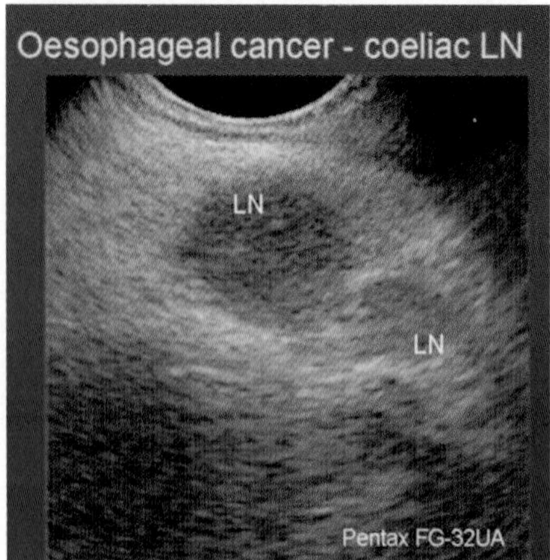

Fig. 17-14. EUS photo of lymph node metastasis. EUS, endoscopic ultrasound; LN, lymph node. (With permission from MUSC Digestive Disease Center Clinical Atlas.)

Exogenous infection can occur by transmission of pathogens from patient to patient by contaminated endoscopic equipment. According to the Spaulding classification, developed by Earle Spaulding in 1968, flexible GI endoscopes have a semi-critical level of risk (contact with intact non-sterile mucosa or non-intact skin) and require high-level chemical disinfection if sterilization is not possible. Flexible endoscopes are heat labile and cannot withstand the heat of steam sterilization. The Food and Drug Administration (FDA) has mandated that flexible GI endoscope reprocessing methods must achieve high-level disinfection, defined as the destruction of all microorganisms with the exception of high levels of bacterial spores. The FDA has instructed endoscope manufacturers to provide detailed instructions of at least one method of reprocessing validated for their products. After a mechanical cleansing, most endoscopes undergo a high-level disinfection with a chemical agent such as glutaraldehyde. Ethylene oxide gas sterilization is an option, but it requires an overnight cycle. Endoscope sterilization, although desirable, is required only for use in a sterile operative field.

Transmission of infectious disease during EGD has been estimated at 1 in 1.8 million cases and usually results from a failure to adhere to current reprocessing guidelines, which include flushing all channels immediately after each procedure, inspecting for leaks or broken parts, and the meticulous mechanical cleaning and rinsing of all surfaces and channels with a brush. The endoscope must then be immersed in an effective liquid chemical germicide at an appropriate concentration and duration, rinsed again, flushed with 70% alcohol, dried with forced air, and hung on a rack to prevent moisture accumulation and contamination. Automated endoscope reprocessors (AERs) are available, but their capabilities must be carefully matched to the endoscope manufacturer's reprocessing recommendations. All the steps of mechanical cleaning must be performed before using an AER. The elevator channel in duodenoscopes must be manually cleaned, because it has a very small lumen that cannot be effectively cleaned by AERs. The advantages of AERs include reduced staff exposure to chemical germicides, standardization of reprocessing, and efficiency.

When reprocessing guidelines for endoscopes are correctly followed, mechanical cleaning alone achieves a 4 log reduction of mycobacterial contamination. The FDA has cleared 2% glutaraldehyde (Cidex, Rapicide), 0.2% peracetic acid (Steris 20), 7.5% hydrogen peroxide (Sporox), 0.08% peracetic acid/1% hydrogen peroxide, and 0.55% ortho-phthalaldehyde for use as liquid chemical disinfectants for reprocessing flexible GI endoscopes. Immersion in 2% glutaraldehyde for 20 minutes at 20°C after mechanical cleaning achieves a total reduction of 8 to 10 log of mycobacterium under worst-case conditions, more than the FDA-mandated 6 log reduction. Endoscopic accessories such as biopsy forceps can be disposable or sterilized and should be reprocessed by cleaning with an enzymatic agent, ultrasound cleaning (40°C, 30 minutes, 47 Hz), rinsing/neutralization, drying, and sterilization (134°C for 5 minutes).

Transmission of infection by EGD has been associated with the following:

1. Inadequate mechanical cleaning before disinfection
2. Contaminated irrigating fluid or water containers
3. Improper use of AERs
4. Substandard disinfectants
5. Incomplete drying of the channels before endoscope storage

Bacterial spores (*Bacillus* and *Clostridium*) are the most resistant organisms: If they are eliminated, most other organisms are as well. In descending order, resistance is seen in mycobacteria, nonlipid viruses, vegetative fungi, and bacteria. Lipid-containing viruses such as hepatitis B virus, hepatitis C virus, and human immunodeficiency virus are highly sensitive to germicides. No documented case of transmission of these three viruses has occurred when current reprocessing guidelines have been followed, although hepatitis B virus and hepatitis C virus transmission have been documented because of improper reprocessing. *Salmonella* species and *Pseudomonas aeruginosa* are the most frequent causes of transmitted infection because of contaminated endoscopes.

A sheathed, disposable endoscope (Endosheath; Vision-Sciences, Inc.; Natick, MA) is now available and may prevent transmission of infection and improve turnaround times. Essentially, it consists of two components: a reusable part and a disposable part. The reusable part contains the optical bundle, control cables, and electronic processor. The disposable part consists of a sterile sheath, which incorporates all the contamination-susceptible elements (the working channel and water, air, and suction channels). The disposable sheath fits over the reusable part much like a condom, and initial reports are promising.

Perforation during an EGD occurs from blind passage of the endoscope or forceps. It is uncommon, although when it occurs it can be associated with considerable morbidity and mortality. An iatrogenic esophageal laceration pictured in Figure 17-15 may lead to perforation. All levels of the upper GI tract are vulnerable, but it occurs most commonly in the cervical and distal esophagus. Anterior cervical osteophytes, esophageal strictures, malignancies, and a Zenker's diverticulum are predisposing patient factors. Immediate pain is the usual indicator of a perforation; however, if the perforation occurs in the stomach or duodenum, the immediate pain may be less pronounced. Diagnosis may be delayed until the patient exhibits signs of mediastinal, retroperitoneal, or peritoneal irritation. Fever, chest pain, crepitus, or pleural effusions may alert the endoscopist to the presence of this complication. If there is a suspicion of perforation during the procedure, it should be terminated, and a chest X-ray film and abdominal series obtained. Plain films may show air dissecting into the neck, chest, mediastinum, peritoneum, or retroperitoneum. A water-soluble contrast X-ray study should be obtained first. An inconclusive study can be followed with a barium contrast study or CAT scan. Negative studies do not rule out a perforation if the clinical suspicion is strong. In larger perforations or in cases when diagnosis is delayed, emergency surgical intervention is indicated. In select patients who receive diagnoses in a timely fashion, conservative management with intravenous antibiotics, nasogastric aspiration, and intravenous hyperalimentation may suffice. Patients that meet criteria for nonoperative management include the elderly, those who exhibit no signs of sepsis at initial presentation, or those with multiple comorbidities. Other requirements include minimal pleural soilage, isolation of lesion within the mediastinum, the absence of malignancy or stricture, lack of enteral intake since perforation, minimal symptoms, and either recent perforation or well-circumscribed perforation.

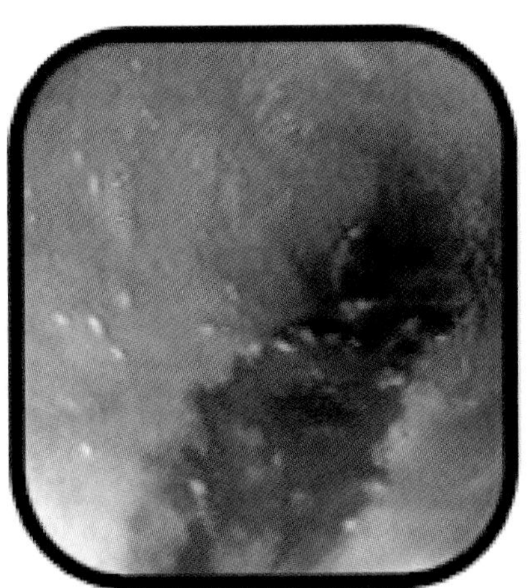

Fig. 17-15. Esophageal laceration. (With permission from Jackson Siegelbaum Gastroenterology.)

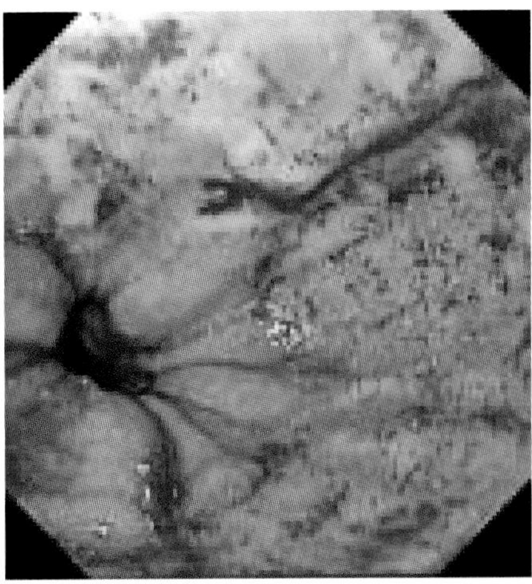

Fig. 17-16. Mallory-Weiss tears. (With permission from Jackson Siegelbaum Gastroenterology.)

Excessive bleeding occurs infrequently after an EGD with biopsy if the guidelines of patient preparation outlined previously have been followed. Endoscopic mucosal resection (EMR) and polypectomies are more frequently associated with bleeding. In less than 0.1% of EGD procedures, Mallory-Weiss tears (Fig. 17-16) occur, although they may cause significant bleeding, which is typically self-limited.

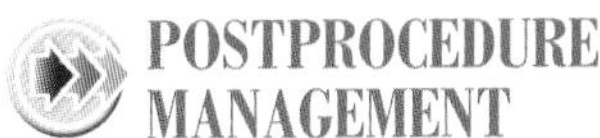

POSTPROCEDURE MANAGEMENT

After the EGD procedure is completed, patients should be monitored until the sedation has worn off, or for 1 hour, whichever occurs later. Hemodynamic and respiratory monitoring should continue until patients are fully awake and the effects of the sedation have sufficiently resolved. Signs of abdominal discomfort may be caused by excess air left in the stomach or may be an indication of perforation, which deserves rapid attention. When patients are ready for discharge, an instruction sheet should be given to the patient indicating diet, further follow-up, and a phone number to call in case of any questions. The patient will need to be driven home by an attendant.

FUTURE DIRECTIONS

High magnification techniques allow "virtual biopsies" by detecting patterns on the surface of the mucosa that are indicative of the underlying histology. This has the advantage of being relatively simple and inexpensive compared with spectroscopic techniques. However, cardiorespiratory movement makes it difficult to maintain focus on the mucosal surface.

Spectrometric principles are finding applications in endoscopic diagnosis. Spectroscopy uses a standard endoscope in addition to expensive equipment such as a specialized light source that emits a photon beam, spectrograph, and multifiber accessory probe. The incident photon beam is directed to the tissue of interest by the multifiber probe, which is close to or in contact with the tissue. Depending on the nature of the tissue, incident photons are absorbed, reflected (reflectance spectroscopy), or scattered (light scattering spectroscopy) or they cause the tissue to emit its own photons (fluorescence endoscopy). Oxyhemoglobin maximally absorbs photons at 420 nm, whereas fluorophores (nicotinamide adenine dinucleotide, flavin adenine dinucleotide, and porphyrins) absorb the energy of the incident photons and emit their own fluorescent beams. Exogenously administered fluorophores are concentrated in the mucosa and submucosa of neoplastic tissue. The interactions between the tissue and the photons are analyzed point-by-point in real time in areas of 1 mm^2. The vascularity, concentration of fluorophores, cell size, and crowding of nuclei can be determined by trimodal spectroscopy. This advanced spectroscopic technique can detect areas with no dysplasia, low-grade dysplasia, and high-grade dysplasia. Infrared spectrometry has also been used to study the vascularity of tumors with an intravenous injection of indocyanine green.

Optical coherence tomography (OCT), although similar to ultrasound, has three important differences. OCT forms images from back-reflection of infrared photons instead of sound, has a real-time resolution limit of 10μ compared with 100μ for EUS, and does not require tissue contact or acoustic coupling. In OCT, a photon beam is split into two beams, one directed at the target tissue and another at a mirror placed at a known distance. The difference in phase of the reflected beams is detected by a Michelson interferometer. Successive layers of the GI wall can be defined by minute displacements of the mirror. The depth of penetration is up to a maximum of 4 mm, enabling evaluation of mucosal histology in vivo and in real time. Ultra-high resolution OCT has achieved 1.1μ resolution on in vitro tissue. Spectroscopic OCT can identify minute areas of differential light scattering and further improve tissue resolution, identifying the nuclei within single cells.

Optical biopsy or optical diagnostics is a technique whereby light energy is used to obtain information about the structure and function of tissues without disrupting them. In fluorescence spectroscopy, light energy (provided by laser) is used to excite tissues, and the resulting fluorescence provides information about the target tissue. Its major GI application has been in the evaluation of colonic polyps, in which it can reliably distinguish malignant from benign lesions. Optical coherence tomography (OCT) may be used to identify preneoplastic conditions of the GI tract, such as Barrett epithelium and dysplasia, and evaluate the depth of penetration of early-stage neoplastic lesions. Imaging of the pancreatic and biliary ductal system could improve the diagnostic accuracy for ductal epithelial changes and the differential diagnosis between neoplastic and nonneoplastic lesions.

CONCLUSION

The use of the flexible endoscope for accurate diagnostic purposes continues to improve. Newer instruments and techniques have the potential to allow the endoscopist to perform the procedure more efficiently and accurately with lowered risk of complications. As endoscopists continue to increase their knowledge and skill, more products such as Barrx (Barrx Medical, Inc.; Sunnyvale, CA) will emerge. This particular product circumferentially ablates Barrett to a controlled depth (>1 mm). Currently, Barrx can be used to treat noninvasive Barrett esophagus. With evolving modalities available, an expanding therapeutic potential exists for endoscopy. Therefore, it is imperative for the endoscopist to be skilled in these areas in order to optimize patient care.

SUGGESTED READING

Altorki N. Carcinoma of the Esophagus. In: *Surgical Oncology*. Bland K, ed. McGraw-Hill; 2001;609–623.

Deb SJ, et al. Esophageal Tumors. In: *Current Surgial Therapy*. Cameron J, ed. Mosby 2004; 44–49.

Greene, et al. Flexible Endoscopy in Barrett's Esophagus and Esophageal Cancer. In: Soper N, ed. *Mastery of Laparoscopic and Endoscopic Surgery*. LWW 2005;231–236.

Guelrud M, Herrera I, Essenfeld H, et al. Enhanced magnification endoscopy: a new technique to identify specialized intestinal metaplasia in Barrett's esophagus. *Gastrointest Endosc* 2001;53:559–565.

Gupta N and Macfadyen B. Diagnostic Upper Gastrointestinal Endoscopy. In: Soper N, ed. *Mastery of Laparoscopic and Endoscopic Surgery*. LWW 2005;163–174.

Larghi A, et al. EUS followed by EMR for staging of high-grade dysplasia and early cancer in Barrett's esophagus. *Gastrointest Endosc* 2005 Jul;62(1):16–23.

Lightdale C. Practice Guidelines for Esophageal Cancer. *Am J Gastroenterol* 1999;94(1):20–27.

Mellinger JD. Diagnostic Upper Gastrointestinal Endoscopy. In: Scott-Conner CEH, ed. *The SAGES Manual*. New York: Springer, 1999; 422–437.

Sampliner, Richard E. Updated Guidelines for the Diagnosis, Surveillance, and Therapy of Barrett's Esophagus. *Am J Gastroenerol* 2002; 97(8):1887–1892.

Schrager, et al. Endoscopic Ultrasound: impact on survival in patients with Esophageal Cancer. *Am J Surg* 2005 Nov;190(5):682–686.

Scotiniotis IA, et al. Accuracy of EUS in the evaluation of Barrett's esophagus and high-grade dysplasia or intramucosal carcinoma. *Gastrointest Endosc* 2001 Dec;54(6):689–696.

Shami VM, et al. Clinical impact of conventional endosonography and endoscopic ultrasound-guided fine-needle aspiration in the assessment of patients with Barrett's esophagus and high-grade dysplasia or intramucosal carcinoma who have been referred for endoscopic ablation therapy. *Endosc* 2006 Feb;38(2):157–161.

Society of Gastroenterology Nurses and Associates, Inc. Guideline for the use of high-level disinfectants and sterilants for reprocessing of flexible gastrointestinal endoscopes. *Gastroenterol Nurs* 2000;23:180–187.

Waring JP, et al. Guidelines for conscious sedation and monitoring during gastrointestinal endoscopy. *Gastrointest Endosc* 2003;58:317.

Zhang X, et al. Endoscopic Ultrasound for preoperative staging of esophageal carcinoma. *Surg Endosc* 2005 Dec;19(12):1618–1621.

COMMENTARY

Drs. Walker, MacFadyen, and Mellinger discuss the techniques of endoscopic assessment of the esophagus for patients with premalignant and malignant diseases. In this well-illustrated chapter, the technique of endoscopy of the proximal foregut is clearly described. The potential risks and complications of these procedures, although uncommon, must be acknowledged and identified as soon as possible for optimal outcomes. In patients with premalignant disease, various techniques can be used to highlight the dysplastic or metaplastic lesions, including the use of Lugol's iodine. Other newer techniques on the near horizon for generalized use include spectroscopy, fluorescence endoscopy, and optical coherence tomography. Ultimately, a true histologic diagnosis may be made by simple visualization. The authors also describe the technique and advantages of the use of endoscopic ultrasound for the diagnosis of esophageal malignancy. Endoscopic ultrasound has rapidly been incorporated into the routine staging algorithm for esophageal malignancies. Clearly, flexible endoscopy has come a long way over the last 30 years. Additional technological advances will undoubtedly be seen over the next few years, and surgeons must be aware of those advances that have a great impact on surgical therapy of esophageal disorders.

NJS

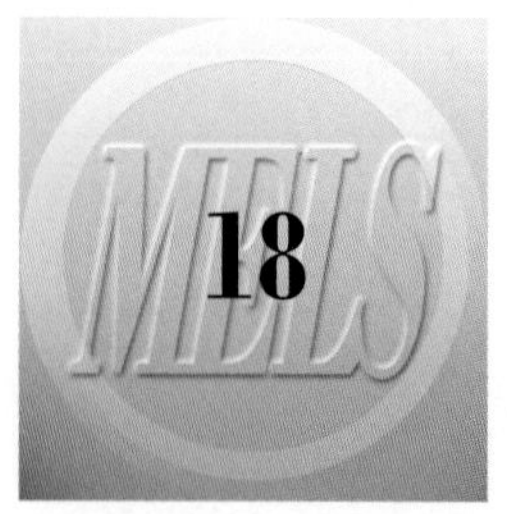

Laparoscopy and Laparoscopic Ultrasound for Staging Foregut Cancers

KEVIN C. CONLON AND DESMOND P. TOOMEY

INTRODUCTION

The arsenal of investigations for staging foregut cancers has increased over the last decade in line with increasingly sophisticated treatment algorithms. These rely on accurate staging at their foundation. Understaging subjects the patient to unnecessary surgery and the associated morbidity, while overstaging excludes patients from potentially curative treatment regimes. Staging laparoscopy (SL) is now a widely accepted replacement for open exploration, while the development of laparoscopic ultrasound (LUS) has added a sensitive tool for imaging solid tissues and tumor masses.

Despite the many preoperative staging modalities available, such as CT/CAT, MRI, PET, and endoscopy/endoscopic ultrasound (EUS), there often exists a small but significant margin of error between preoperative stage and findings at laparotomy. Minimally invasive surgery (MIS) would seem to be an ideal tool to bridge this diagnostic gap. The aim of laparoscopic staging is to mimic open exploration, allowing patients with resectable disease to proceed to laparotomy with a high likelihood of resection and avoiding open surgery for the group of patients who would not benefit (Table 18-1). In this chapter we will discuss the role of SL and LUS in the staging of foregut neoplasms and show how they complement other diagnostic modalities.

TABLE 18-1. POTENTIAL BENEFITS AND RISKS OF STAGING LAPAROSCOPY

Potential benefits	Potential risks
Shorter hospitalization	No individual benefit if resectable
Decreased morbidity	False negative rate
Less delay of adjuvant therapy	No prophylactic palliation
Reduced hospital cost	Port site recurrence
Improved quality of remaining life	

Esophageal Carcinoma

In 2007, approximately 15,560 patients were expected to be diagnosed with esophageal cancer in the United States, a figure that is increasing by 5% to 10% per annum. The relative incidence of adenocarcinoma, located in the lower esophagus and at the gastroesophageal junction, as opposed to squamous cell carcinoma (SCC) of the mid to upper esophagus, has increased in Western practice. The overall prognosis is poor, with 5-year survival rates of 14%. However, neoadjuvant chemoradiotherapy has positively impacted on the prognosis of locally advanced tumors, and resection may effectively treat early disease. Thus, accurate staging is essential before embarking on a treatment regime, especially as distant metastases, which preclude curative therapy, are often undetected by conventional imaging.

 PREOPERATIVE PLANNING

Endoscopy is the gold standard for diagnosis of premalignant and malignant lesions. Apart from allowing biopsy it also enables the operator to perform balloon dilation, stent placement, or laser ablation to relieve obstruction and palliate symptoms. The addition of EUS allows detailed imaging of the esophageal wall, local lymph nodes, and neighboring structures. This makes it an ideal tool for both T- and N-staging of locoregional disease, although it is operator-dependant, may not pass through tight strictures, and is less efficacious at imaging more distant nodes, especially those obscured by air-containing structures.

Computed tomography (CT) of the thorax and abdomen allows visualization of both the primary tumor and metastatic disease. However, its accuracy for T-staging and predicting lymphatic and peritoneal spread remains approximately 60%, 45% to 60%, and 60% to 80% respectively. Although CT recognizes nodes greater than 1 cm, it may not distinguish between inflammation and tumor involvement, whereas EUS uses a number of other criteria, including shape, pattern, and demarcated borders, to assess metastatic potential. Thus EUS is superior for locoregional staging with documented accuracy rates of 85% to 95% for T-staging and 65% to 85% for detecting nodal disease. In addition to this, EUS also facilitates fine needle aspirate cell (FNAC) examination of suspicious lymph nodes and liver lesions. Overall, combined CT and EUS evaluation has been documented to under- or overstage as many as 30% of esophageal tumors.

Fluorodeoxyglucose-positron emission tomography (FDG-PET) has a higher specificity (89% vs. 67%) but lower sensitivity (33% vs. 81%) than EUS for detecting nodal disease, and its accuracy is superior to CT for detecting nodal (76% vs. 45%) and distant (84% vs. 63%) metastases. It upstages approximately 15% to 30% and downstages 10% of cases. Some of the limitations of PET, namely differentiating local lymph nodes from the tumor mass, recognizing metastases from reactive lymphadenopathy, and masking by physiological hot spots, are being addressed by the introduction of PET/CT.

This combination of the two modalities facilitates better anatomic identification of hot spots and allows consideration of morphological features during the "benign or malignant" decision making process. Although still in its infancy the results are encouraging. Accuracy for detection of distant metastases is superior to that of sequential CT and EUS examination (86% vs. 62%), it decreases false positives by 53%, and allows separation of local nodes from the tumor mass in 64% of cases. Overall many authors agree that currently the maximal diagnostic yield is obtained from combination of EUS, CT, and PET (or PET/CT where available).

Despite this increasingly sophisticated diagnostic algorithm, up to 20% of patients have occult disease not currently detectable by preoperative imaging, although the full impact of PET/CT remains to be determined. Laparoscopy has been advocated as a means to detect peritoneal, nodal, or liver metastases and thus exclude this group of patients from costly and potentially ineffective treatment regimes that are associated with high morbidity.

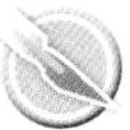

SURGICAL TECHNIQUE

We recommend that staging laparoscopy is performed under general anaesthesia and that carbon dioxide pneumoperitoneum is established via an open approach. A 30-degree angled laparoscope is used to assess the peritoneal cavity and two 5-mm accessory ports are generally placed in the right and left upper quadrants (Fig. 18-1). Obvious metastatic disease is biopsied (Fig. 18-2). The liver, gastroesophageal junction, hepaticoduodenal ligament, and infrahepatic space are examined, and an additional trocar is often placed in the epigastric angle to facilitate retraction of the left lobe of the liver and division of the gastrohepatic omentum. This latter maneuver gains entry into the lesser sac. Nodes within the left gastric pedicle can be seen and biopsied as required. LUS can also be performed to scan the liver, regional nodes, and primary tumor, if it is located in the distal esophagus.

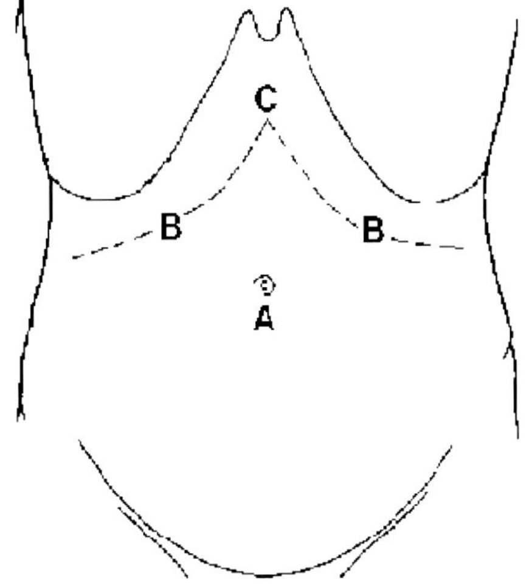

Fig. 18-1. Diagram of port site placements. **A.** 10-mm camera port; **B.** 5-mm instrument ports; **C.** Extra 5-mm port for retracting left lobe of liver.

Value of Laparoscopic Staging

In esophageal cancer, the value of the SL is higher in adenocarcinoma than SCC. Occult disease is demonstrated in one quarter to one third of patients with adenocarcinoma but in less than 5% of those with SCC. Both thoroscopy and laparoscopy can be incorporated into the staging algorithm, although some centers utilize laparoscopy alone. The CALGB 9380 prospective, multicenter trial (n = 107; 69% adenocarcinoma; 31% SCC) found that combined thoroscopic and laparoscopic staging was both feasible and safe. They identified positive lymph nodes in 56% of patients, 27% of which had been missed by noninvasive imaging. Furthermore, unsuspected T4 or M1 disease was detected in 8 and 2 patients respectively.

We perform laparoscopy in isolation; to maximize the yield we restrict it to T3-T4 adenocarcinoma of the lower esophagus. It is reported that 75% of these distal adenocarcinoma metastasize to coeliac lymph nodes, and so the operator should concentrate on the coeliac axis, hepatoduodenal ligament, and the paraaortic area, which account for 40% of positive findings during SL. Our policy is supported by results from Krasna et al. (n = 76; 2002). In a retrospective study they found that 32% of patients had abdominal and 12% had mediastinal nodal disease, and that positive abdominal nodes were more likely in lower esophageal lesions, adenocarcinoma, or T3-T4 tumors (Table 18-2). Overall staging laparoscopy has been shown to have an accuracy of 81% to 94% for determining metastasis status.

Combined SL and LUS has been shown to be more accurate (81% vs. 72%) and specific (100% vs. 90%) for the detection of intraabdominal metastases than CT. Other benefits include the imaging of stenotic tumors that don't allow EUS and the placement of jejunostomy feeding tubes in those being considered for multimodal therapy. SL may also be performed as the initial step in a minimally invasive esophagectomy.

In summary, the role of MIS staging in esophageal cancer is mainly focused on better stratification of patients to improve treatment selection and prevent unnecessary surgery. Current published data show that laparoscopic staging is indicated for most patients presenting with T3-T4 lower esophageal adenocarcinoma, particularly if a multimodal approach is contemplated. Despite the advance of PET/CT, both SL and LUS should remain a valuable tool in esophageal cancer for staging high-risk cases or those where ambiguity remains.

Gastric Carcinoma

Gastric carcinoma is the second most common cancer worldwide, after lung cancer. Although its incidence in Western countries is lower than in Far Eastern countries such as Japan, China, and Korea, 80% of Western cases present at an advanced stage. Complete resection of the tumor and involved lymph nodes, with or without neoadjuvant chemotherapy for downstaging, is the only proven curative treatment. Even so, "curative resection" still carries a disease-related mortality of 50%.

This poor outcome is partly related to a combination of late onset of presentation and inadequacies in the accurate staging and subsequent selection for surgery. Traditionally every patient with gastric carcinoma underwent open surgery either for

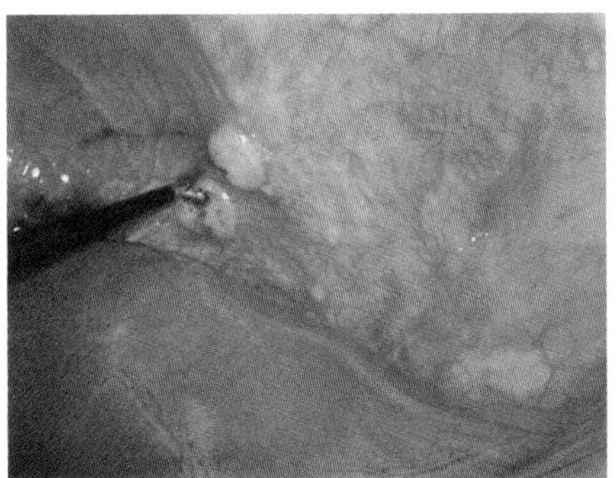

Fig. 18-2. Biopsy of metastatic deposit.

TABLE 18-2. BENEFIT OF SL IN LOWER ESOPHAGEAL ADENOCARCINOMA

	All tumors n = 76 (%)	Cases with positive abdominal nodes n = 24 (%)
Lower esophageal tumor	58	71
Adenocarcinoma	61	75
Clinical T3-T4	67	83

SL, staging laparoscopy.
Source: Krasna et al.; 2002.

cure or palliation. With the development of multidisciplinary approaches to the disease and the establishment of less invasive palliative algorithms, however, there is no longer a need for operative intervention in all cases. Staging laparoscopy may identify tumor metastases in lymph nodes, liver, or on the peritoneal surface that are not detectable by noninvasive imaging; therefore it has been recommended that all patients being considered for curative gastrectomy undergo staging laparoscopy to identify those patients suitable for neoadjuvant treatment and those who will not benefit from extensive surgery.

As with esophageal cancer, endoscopy and biopsy are the gold standard for diagnosis of the primary tumor. EUS is the best means of determining T stage, with high levels of accuracy of 78% to 94%, especially for gastroesophageal junction gastric tumors, where it is also effective in diagnosing nodal deposits. CT is inferior to EUS for T-staging; however, new advances utilizing thin slices, optimum contrast material enhancement, and multiplanar reformation have shown promising increases in accuracy.

CT is the noninvasive modality of choice for determining nodal status despite its limited ability to detect nodal malignancy less than 1 cm in diameter and to differentiate, in some cases, between reactive hyperplasia and tumor deposits. CT may also detect larger hepatic metastases, but small volume liver, peritoneal, omental, and ovarian seeding are easily missed as they fall below the CT's resolution threshold.

The uptake of FDG-PET by gastric tumors varies depending on the cell type, but as a general rule is inversely proportional to tumor mucous production. Where there is uptake by the primary lesion, it hinders N-staging in low N stage disease due to masking of signals arising in the N1 and N2 nodes. A recent study by Yun et al. has suggested accuracies for PET of 56%, 72%, and 95% and for CT of 69%, 69%, and 95% in N1, N2, and N3 disease, respectively, although the sensitivity of PET for N1 and N2 disease was only 34%. Similar to CT, even widespread, small volume, peritoneal deposits can be missed due to the modality's resolution. However, most studies suggest that FDG-PET is the most sensitive, noninvasive modality for detecting distant lymphatic and extralymphatic metastases. The possible role of PET/CT in gastric cancer has yet to be assessed (Fig. 18-3).

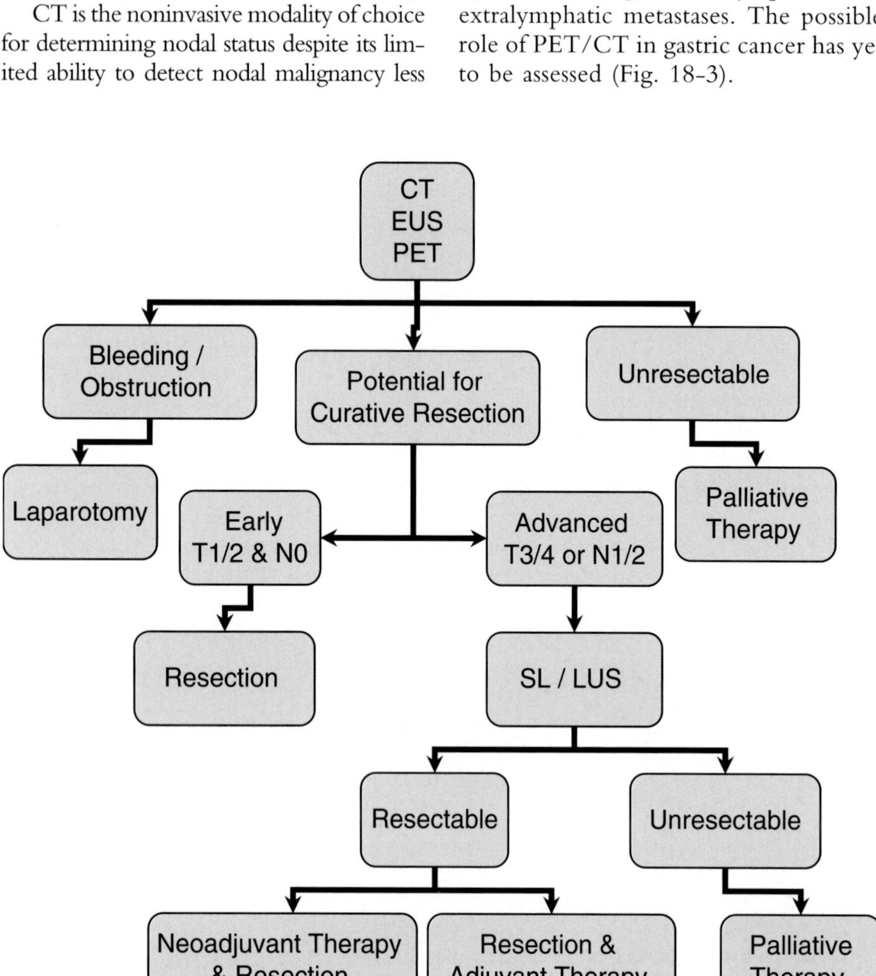

Fig. 18-3. A gastric cancer diagnostic algorithm.

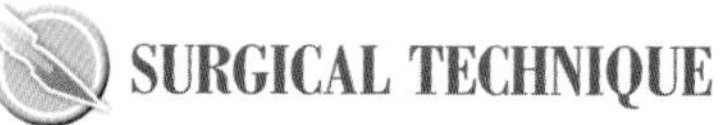

SURGICAL TECHNIQUE

Following induction of anaesthesia, our preferred method of establishing pneumoperitoneum is via the Hassan open technique. Secondary ports (usually 5 mm) are then placed in both upper quadrants along the line of a possible bilateral subcostal incision. A full examination of the peritoneal cavity is performed. If present, ascites is sampled. Particular attention is paid to the primary tumor, liver, pelvis, and omentum (Fig. 18-4). The patient is then placed in a slight anti-Trendelenburg position, which facilitates the inspection of the fourth part of the duodenum, ligament of Treitz, and small bowel mesentry. Diagnostic lavage cytology is then taken from both upper quadrants and pelvis after 200 ml of saline is placed into the peritoneal cavity. It is important to gently agitate the abdomen before aspirating the fluid. In addition, specimens should be taken from both the upper abdomen and pelvis because this increases the yield for the test.

Assessment of the liver can be difficult because of the lack of tactile sensation during laparoscopy. We have developed a technique using a suction device and dissecting forceps to palpate the liver in a sequential fashion (Fig. 18-5). Further examination is facilitated by LUS. Small intraparenchymal lesions can be seen (Fig. 18-6) and biopsies can be obtained under LUS control. LUS is also useful in determining the T stage of the primary tumor. To do this, the stomach is filled with 500 to 750 ml of warmed saline. The probe is then brought slowly over the serosal surface. Excellent images can be obtained. However, technical constraints such as near field loss limit the utility of this technique.

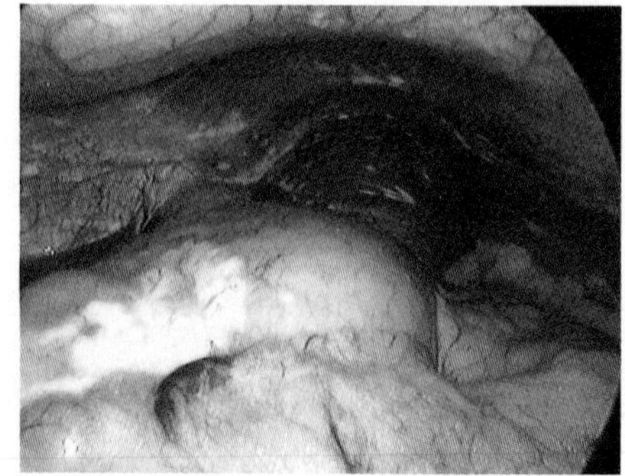

Fig. 18-4. A primary gastric tumor with peritoneal metastases.

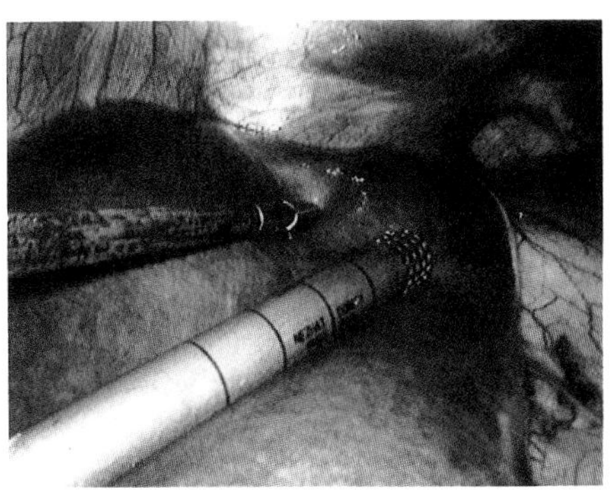

Fig. 18-5. A two-instrument technique for palpating the liver surface.

TABLE 18-3. SUITABILITY CRITERIA FOR SL IN GASTRIC CANCER

Existing inclusion criteria
Advanced gastric cancer
Absence of hemorrhage or obstruction
Medically fit for gastrectomy
M0 by preoperative staging
Additional exclusion criteria suggested by MSKCC study
All intraabdominal nodes less than 1 cm on spiral CT
Tumor does not involve the GE junction or "whole stomach"

SL, staging laparoscopy; MSKCC, Memorial Sloan-Kettering Cancer Center; GE, gastroesophageal.

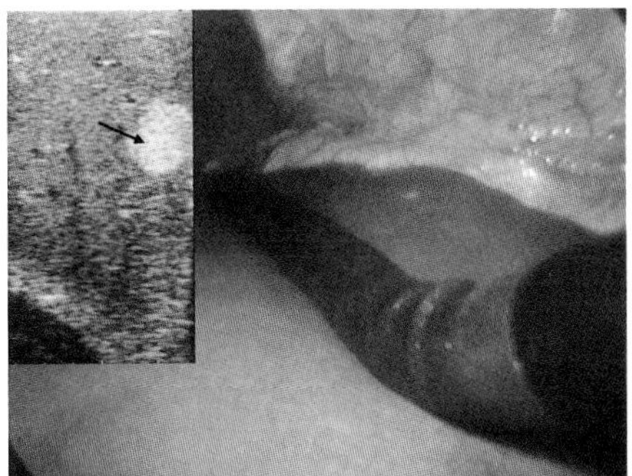

Fig. 18-6. Laparoscopic ultrasound (LUS) of the liver with an intraparenchymal deposit (arrow).

Value of Laparoscopic Staging

When limited to patients with potentially resectable T3 or T4 lesions with no other indication for laparotomy (obstruction, bleeding, etc.) and M0 (no distant metastases) radiological staging, SL will prevent laparotomy in 21% to 44% of patients. However, 8% to 13% will be found to be unresectable at laparotomy. This false negative rate may be partly explained by an absolute reliance on histology for diagnosing unresectability in many studies in order that false positives are avoided. The reported accuracy of LUS in nodal staging varies widely from 60% to 90%, but again it has not been extensively investigated and may be due to the requirement of the 1997 TNM classification for 15 nodes to accurately define N stage. However LUS is also of benefit for detecting M1 disease and may upstage a further 8% of patients following negative laparoscopy.

The rise of complex laparoscopy in many types of abdominal surgery has produced a generation of surgeons for whom SL is a relatively routine procedure; complication rates of 1% to 3% should now be the norm. Critics of SL refer to a need for open palliation in patients with gastric cancer. However a recent study that followed 97 patients who were upstaged to M1 by SL revealed that only 12% underwent a subsequent laparotomy: 8% for gastrostomy, jejunostomy, or gastrojejunostomy, 1% for gastric perforation, and 3% for distal bowel obstruction. The remaining 88% were successfully palliated by endoscopic or percutaneous techniques.

Previous criteria for selecting patients who would benefit from SL include (1) advanced gastric cancer, (2) the absence of hemorrhage or obstruction, (3) medical fitness for gastrectomy, and (4) M0 by preoperative staging. Refinements to these have been suggested by a recent large study (n = 657) from Memorial Sloan Kettering Cancer Center (MSKCC). This study concluded that patients with intraabdominal nodes less than 1 cm on spiral CT and tumors that do not involve the GE junction or "whole stomach" are significantly less likely to demonstrate M1 disease and so could be excluded from SL (Table 18-3). However, these have not been prospectively tested, and clinical discretion in individual cases is advised. Furthermore, many neoadjuvant schemes require a negative staging laparoscopy for inclusion.

Pancreatic Carcinoma

Despite improvements in preoperative, operative, and postoperative care, the prognosis of pancreatic cancer remains bleak. Actual 5-year survival is less than 5% with surgical resection, the only chance of cure, and it is a viable option in only 20% of cases. Even then, up to 30% of noninvasively staged patients will be found to be unresectable at laparotomy. The traditional paradigm of surgical exploration and biliary/gastric bypass has been outdated by improvements in nonoperative and laparoscopic staging and palliation.

The current noninvasive staging modality of choice is multidetector 3D CT (MDCT) scan that allows acquisition of three-dimensional data and imaging of the entire pancreas in a single breath hold. Although some studies (Ellsmere; 2004) report specificity as low as 33%, CT has been shown to predict resectability in up to 96% of cases with 94% sensitivity and specificity for detecting vascular invasion. Despite technological advances, small yet devastating hepatic and peritoneal metastases are missed on CT, and it may not distinguish between reactive lymphadenopathy and nodal malignancy. EUS has been shown to have a diagnostic role and can be very useful for determining local vascular invasion and peripancreatic lymph node involvement, with results similar to MDCT. Results vary between studies, possibly due to its dependence on operator skill. Other modalities such as ERCP, MRI, and angiography are useful in specific cases but overall are inferior to CT for staging pancreatic cancer.

The low spatial resolution of PET scans renders it of little use in T-staging and in detection of local nodal metastases, with sensitivity and specificity reported as 46% to 71% and 63% to 100% respectively. The results of M-staging are more encouraging, especially in the detection of liver metastases. However the problem remains of small volume peritoneal deposits being below the resolution threshold of the modality. Furthermore, many patients with pancreatic disease have disordered glucose metabolism, resulting in increased risk of a false negative result. Overall the sensitivity of PET for staging of pancreatic cancer varies from 68% to 84%. There are only limited studies investigating the

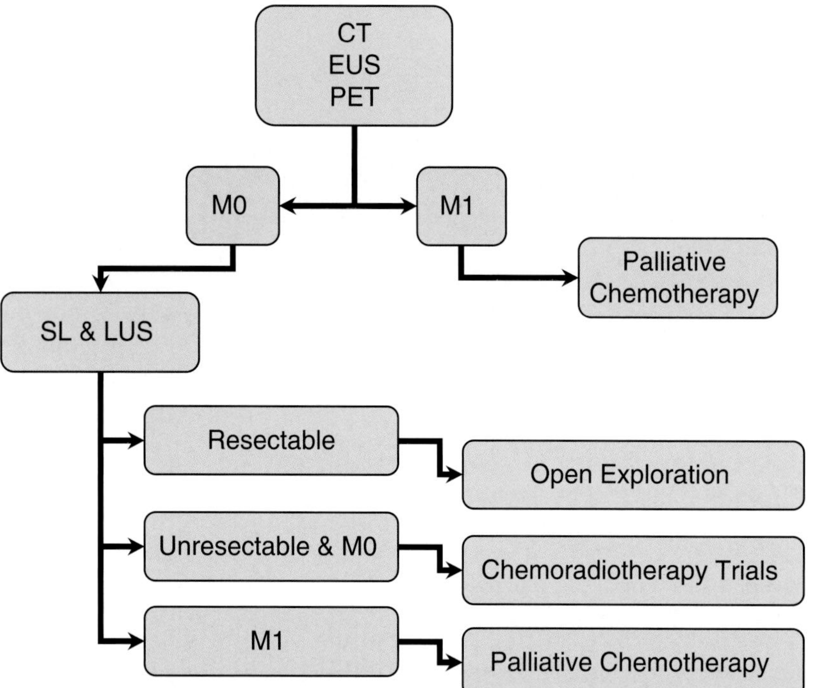

Fig. 18-7. A pancreatic cancer diagnostic algorithm.

value of PET/CT in pancreatic cancer. It has been shown to detect CT occult metastases in 16% of patients, although guided biopsy and staging laparoscopy are still often required to clarify the nature of abnormalities detected (Fig. 18-7).

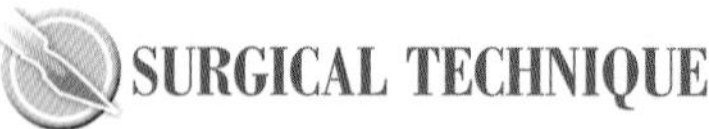

SURGICAL TECHNIQUE

As with other upper gastrointestinal tumors a multiport technique, with ports placed in the right and left upper quadrants along the line of a proposed bilateral subcostal incision, allows for a thorough examination of the peritoneal cavity. Biopsy of suspicious peritoneal or hepatic lesions can be readily performed, and, if positive, the procedure may be terminated. In the absence of obvious metastatic disease, peritoneal washings can be taken for cytology and a sequential examination of the liver, hepaticoduodenal ligament, pancreas, transverse mesocolon, ligament of Treitz, and lesser sac can be performed. Finally LUS is used to systematically evaluate the liver and the pancreas to assess the tumor's relationship to the major peripancreatic vessels (Fig. 18-8).

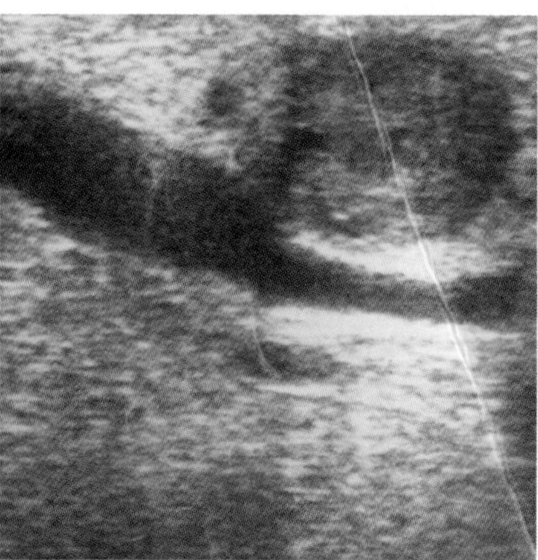

Fig. 18-8. A laparoscopic ultrasound (LUS) showing vascular encroachment.

Patients are considered to have unresectable disease if histologic proof is obtained of (1) metastases (serosal, hepatic, or peritoneal) (Fig. 18-9), (2) extrapancreatic tumor extension, (3) coeliac or high portal node involvement, (4) invasion or encasement of the coeliac or hepatic artery, or (5) involvement of the superior mesenteric artery (portal or superior mesenteric vein involvement is a relative contraindication depending on the degree and extent of involvement).

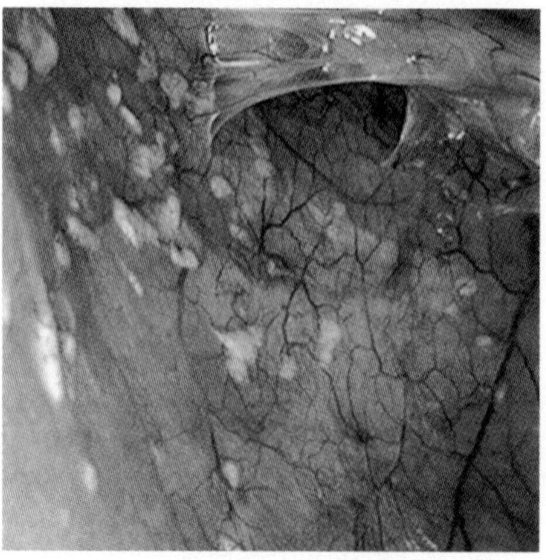

Fig. 18-9. Widespread carcinomatosis.

VALUE OF LAPAROSCOPIC STAGING

Despite recent advances, CT continues to overestimate resectability of pancreatic cancers; thus SL remains a valuable staging tool. SL not only predicts unresectability but also filters out patients who are unsuitable for radiotherapy.

Several large studies from MSKCC during the 1990s have validated SL. In two separate studies, SL correctly identified resectable disease in 91% of patients and unresectable disease in 100% of patients. The dominant missed diagnosis in cases found to be unresectable at laparotomy was small hepatic metastases. Overall the accuracy of SL approaches 94%, and subsequent studies have suggested sensitivities as high as 97%. In contrast, a large series from Johns Hopkins (Barreiro et al.; 2002; n = 188) extrapolated that 35.3% of pancreatic body or tail but only 2.5% of head of pancreas adenocarcinoma would have been saved a laparotomy by SL. However, this analysis assumes that SL is only capable of detecting unresectability in M1 disease (not vascular invasion, etc.) and does not incorporate LUS into the algorithm. It is worth noting that, in this study, the resection rate for head of pancreas tumours was 59.7%, the majority of patients were surgically bypassed (pylorus and/or bile duct) rather than utilizing less invasive techniques, and the criteria for determining need for bypass were not defined.

The addition of LUS aids the detection of small, intraparenchymal, hepatic metastases and allows examination of the porta hepatis, portal vein, and superior mesenteric vessels, an area where it is particularly effective, thus increasing the accuracy of SL to as high as 98%. LUS after SL can provide information that will alter patient management in 14% to 28% of cases. Furthermore, Jimenez et al. demonstrated that the addition of peritoneal lavage cytology to SL increased their yield from 24% to 31% and that tumours of the body and tail of the pancreas are twice as likely to have M1 disease at SL than those in the head. Several studies have verified the MSKCC results, reporting that the resection rate at laparotomy following SL is 74% to 91%. Factors that may explain the variability in these rates include use of LUS, the extent of laparoscopic dissection, and differing thresholds for exploratory laparotomy (histologically unproven vascular invasion). Overall, 11% to 41% of potentially resectable patients who staged by SL/LUS are spared an unnecessary laparotomy. In addition, Jimenez, Liu, and Shoup have all shown that SL can upstage, to M1, 34% to 37% of known locally advanced cases, excluding them from radiotherapy that would not benefit them and preventing dilution of clinical radiotherapy trials.

It was traditionally thought that up to 25% of patients would require subsequent bypass for gastric outlet obstruction, strengthening the argument for open exploration and prophylactic palliation. In a prospective randomized trial from Johns Hopkins (n = 87; 1999), patients who were unresectable at laparotomy (no SL) and deemed not to need an immediate gastric outlet bypass were randomized to gastrojejunostomy or not. The author concludes that prophylactic bypass should be performed in all cases, because 19% of the group that did not receive gastrojejunostomy required subsequent reoperation, which carries a higher complication rate. However, we would maintain that if the other 81% had been found unresectable by SL, then they would never have needed a laparotomy at all. Large studies from MSKCC and Massachusetts General Hospital strengthen this argument, having determined that only 3% and 5% of patients found unresectable at SL later required open surgical intervention. This discrepancy may be due, in part, to aggressive endoscopic stenting, laparoscopic bypass, (Fig. 18-10) and increased recognition of gastric dysmotility as a differential diagnosis for gastric outlet obstruction (Table 18-4).

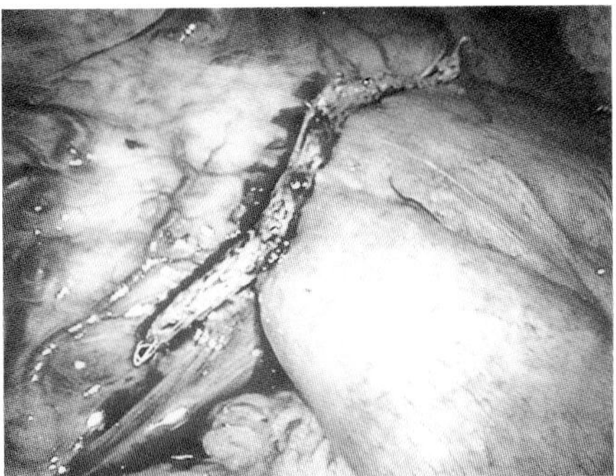

Fig. 18-10. Completed laparoscopic gastrojejunostomy in patient with duodenal outlet obstruction secondary to pancreatic cancer.

Endoscopic and percutaneous stenting techniques for biliary obstruction and guided analgesic nerve blocks are viable alternatives to operative intervention. If required, laparoscopic gastroenterostomy is straightforward and successful in 90% of cases. Laparoscopic Billroth I and II gastrectomy are also feasible, while both laparoscopic cholecystoenteric and choledochoenteric bypass are options if more conservative measures fail. This wealth of minimally invasive intervention that is available for palliation when complications arise obviates the need for prophylactic surgical intervention in the majority of cases.

Most of the published studies to date concentrate on pancreatic adenocarcinoma. For other cell types, including neuroendocrine tumors, intraductal papillary mucinous neoplasm, and cystadenocarcinoma, the data are sparse. However, nonfunctioning islet cell tumors also may lead to small volume metastatic disease ideally suited to laparoscopic diagnosis. There is evidence that the addition of SL to CT staging in these cases raises the predictive value for resection from 74% to 96%. Brooks et al. (MSKCC; 2002) demonstrated that SL spared only 2% to 4% of patients with duodenal or ampullary tumors an unnecessary laparotomy due to high resectability and surgical bypass rates. Although developments in stenting technology will improve this yield in the future, it is unlikely that SL will become important in this scenario. In contrast patients with distal bile duct tumors seem to benefit from laparoscopic staging both in terms of determining resectability and avoiding unnecessary surgery.

TABLE 18-4. LATE LAPAROTOMY FOR GASTRIC OUTLET BYPASS IN PANCREATIC CANCER

	Johns Hopkins	Massachusetts General Hospital	MSKCC
Year	1999	2000	1999
n	44	39	155
Inclusion criteria	Unresectable at laparotomy and not in need of immediate gastrojenunostomy and randomized to no gastrojejunostomy	M0 on CT and M1 at subsequent SL*	Potentially resectable patients found unresectable at SL/LUS
Late open bypass	19%	<5%	2%

MSKCC, Memorial Sloan-Kettering Cancer Center.
*Includes patients with locally advanced disease undergoing SL prior to radiotherapy

Hepatobiliary Malignancy

Surgical resection remains, in most cases, the most effective modality for primary and metastatic disease of the liver and for extrahepatic biliary carcinoma. Hepatocellular carcinoma (HCC) is a common solid tumor worldwide, and resection is the treatment of choice when possible. However, studies report that despite preoperative imaging 35% of tumors are unresectable at laparotomy, in many cases because of extensive cirrhosis, extrahepatic spread, or multifocal disease. Considering the treatments available for nonoperative management of HCC and the general lack of need for open surgical palliation, SL should play a valuable role in assessing these tumors. Similarly, 25% to 50% of extrahepatic biliary tumors are unresectable at laparotomy, many of which could be palliated by radiologically placed stents.

CT, MRI, and PET are all useful modalities for noninvasive staging of these tumors. The role of PET in staging of HCC is limited, due to variable tumor uptake and background interference from liver activity. Its sensitivity and specificity for detecting extrahepatic metastases is low (63% and 60%, respectively) but remains superior to MRI. In extrahepatic biliary carcinoma, fluorodeoxyglucose (FDG) uptake is dependant on tumor subtype, and sclerosing cholangitis, granulomatous disease, and stents can all mimic malignancy. There has been only limited investigation in these conditions; the results are not encouraging. It is, however, expected that PET/CT will have a positive impact on staging, with an early study showing an accuracy of 100% for diagnosing distant metastases from gallbladder cancer.

SURGICAL TECHNIQUE

Many of these patients will have had prior abdominal surgery; thus an open cut down is again the preferred means of access to the peritoneal cavity. The initial incision is usually placed along the line of a subcostal incision in the right upper quadrant. Subsequently two additional ports are inserted. Adhesions can be divided under direct vision, and extra ports can be inserted as required. The peritoneal cavity is examined as before, and LUS is useful for examining the hepatic parenchyma. A systematic approach minimizes the potential for missing small lesions. Segments I, II, and III are best viewed from the anterior surface. Segment IV is viewed from the right of the falciform ligament, and segments V to VIII are likewise viewed in a stepwise fashion.

VALUE OF LAPAROSCOPIC STAGING

The benefits of MIS staging for hepatobiliary cancer are similar to those seen in other tumors: more accurate assessment, avoidance of unnecessary laparotomy, decreased hospital stay, decreased morbidity, and quicker initiation of adjuvant therapies.

The benefit of SL in hepatocellular carcinoma was evaluated by Weitz et al. (MSKCC; 2004). SL was found to increase the resection rate from 68% to 89% and to have an accuracy of 74% for determining unresectability. The study suggests that the overall low yield (22%) could be increased by selecting patients with evidence of cirrhosis and bilobar tumors for SL. These figures are consistent with several previous studies, although some report laparotomy sparing rates of up to 54%, differences that may be explained by advances in preoperative imaging. The addition of LUS may provide clinically useful information in 5% to 20% of cases.

The role of SL in extrahepatic biliary carcinoma has been assessed by a study from MSKCC. Overall SL had an accuracy of 51% in detecting unresectability for hilar cholangiocarinoma and gall bladder carcinoma (42% and 58% respectively). SL detected most cases of peritoneal metastases (87%) but failed to identify any locally advanced tumors. They also found no benefit from utilizing LUS, although it was only used in selective cases. The study concludes that the yield may be increased by only laparoscoping high T stage tumors.

SUMMARY

Laparoscopy is no longer a tool of limited use and now has widespread indications within surgical oncologic practice. It is of proven benefit in the detection and staging of foregut malignancies and, despite improvements in radiological imaging, still spares a significant number of patients with unresectable disease from unnecessary laparotomy. The role of laparoscopic palliation may still be limited, but, together with medical, radiological, and endoscopic advances, it minimizes the need for open palliation, thus firmly cementing staging laparoscopy as a vital tool of the surgical oncologist.

SUGGESTED READING

Brooks AD, Mallis MF, Brennan MF, et al. The value of laparoscopy in the management of ampullary, duodenal and distal bile duct tumors. *J Gastrointest Surg* 2002;6:139–146.

Espat NJ, Brennan MF, Conlon KC. Patients with laparoscopically staged unresectable pancreatic adenocarcinoma do not require subsequent surgical biliary or gastric bypass. *J Am Coll Surg* 1999;188(6):654–657.

Jimenez RE, Warshaw AL, Rattner DW, et al. Impact of laparoscopic staging in pancreatic cancer. *Arch Surg* 2000;135:409–415.

Krasna MJ, Xiaolong J, Sonett JR, et al. Thoroscopic and laparoscopic lymph node staging in esophageal cancer: Do clinicopathological factors affect the outcome. *Ann Thorac Surg* 2002;73:1710–1713.

Lehnert T, Rudek B, Kienle P, et al. Impact of diagnostic laparoscopy on the management of gastric cancer: prospective study of 120 consecutive patients with primary gastric adenocarcinoma. *Br J Surg* 2002;89:471–475.

Lillemore KD, Cameron JL, Hardacre JM. Is prophylactic gastrojejunostomy indicated for unresectable periampullary cancer. *Ann Surg* 1999;230(3):322–330.

Michl P, Pauls S, Gress T. Evidence based diagnosis and staging of pancreatic cancer. *Best Prac Res Clin Gastroenterol* 2006;20(2):227–251.

Patel AN, Buenaventura PO. Current staging of esophageal carcinoma. *Surg Clin N Am* 2005; 85:555–567.

Sarela AI, Miner TJ, Karpeh MS, et al. Clinical outcomes with laparoscopic M1, unresected gastric adenocarcinoma. *Ann Surg* 2006;243(2): 189–195.

Shoup M, Winston C, Brennan MF, et al. Is there a role for staging laparoscopy in patients with locally advanced, unresectable pancreatic adenocarcinoma? *J Gastrointest Surg* 2004; 8:1068–1071.

Smith A, Finch MD, John TC, et al. Role of laparoscopic ultrasonography in the management of patients with esophagogastric cancer. *Br J Surg* 1999;86:1083–1087.

Taylor AM, Roberts SA, Manson JM. Experience with laparoscopic ultrasonography for defining tumor resectability in carcinoma of the pancreatic head and periampullary region. *Br J Surg* 2001;88:1077–1083.

Weber SM, DeMatteo RP, Fong Y, et al. Staging laparoscopy in patients with extrahepatic biliary carcinoma. *Ann Surg* 2002;235(3): 392–399.

Weitz J, D'Angelica M, Jarnagin W, et al. Selective use of diagnostic laparoscopy prior to planned hepatectomy for patients with hepatocellular carcinoma. *Surgery* 2004;135(3): 273–281.

COMMENTARY

Drs. Conlon and Toomey outline the rationale for and results of the use of laparoscopy and laparoscopic ultrasound in the staging process for cancers of the foregut. As the resolution of computed tomography has improved over the last decade, the indications for staging laparoscopy have likely decreased slightly; however, this modality remains an important tool in the armamentarium of surgeons caring for patients with cancer of the GI tract. It is intuitive that a nontherapeutic laparotomy in a patient with unresectable cancer will lead to a shortening of his or her functional lifetime. The ability to provide a laparoscopic bypass procedure or insert a feeding tube laparoscopically, as outlined in other chapters, is an obvious additional advantage should an unresectable disease be apparent on the staging laparoscopy.

The authors have provided algorithms for the staging of gastric and pancreatic carcinoma. They also address the commonly held belief that patients who have unresectable pancreatic cancer require a laparotomy in order to perform a prophylactic double bypass procedure. There are now several studies suggesting that it is rare for an unresectable patient to require a subsequent laparotomy or bypass of the duodenum or bile duct. They have also pointed out the accuracy of staging laparoscopy and laparoscopic ultrasound in foregut cancers. Laparoscopic ultrasound may be valuable in several of these cancers to examine the parenchyma of the liver, to assess for enlarged lymph nodes that may be sampled using ultrasound guidance, and to assess for involvement of major vascular structures that would preclude resection.

One issue that the authors do not discuss is whether the staging laparoscopy should be done during the same anesthetic as the planned resection. The problem with the simultaneous approach is that if unresectability is documented, inefficiencies in the operating schedule will become manifest. Many surgeons today will first schedule the staging laparoscopy and laparoscopic ultrasound and wait for the results of the final histology from biopsies and cytology from peritoneal washings before scheduling the definitive laparotomy. Should unresectable disease be discovered, consideration should be given to applying palliative procedures by laparoscopic or endoscopic techniques.

NJS

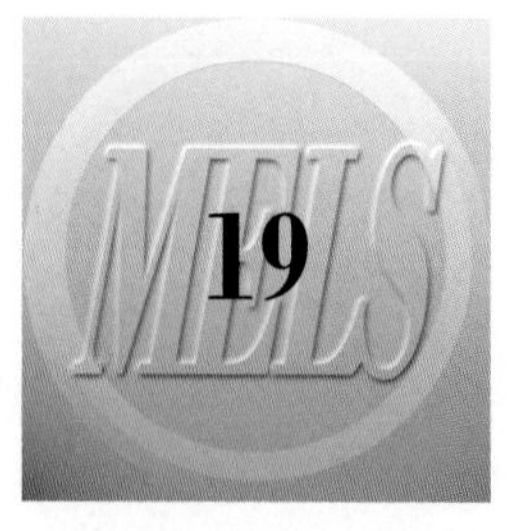

19 Endoscopic Therapies for Barrett Esophagus

BRIAN J. DUNKIN

INTRODUCTION

Barrett esophagus (BE) is an alteration of the type of cells lining the esophagus, in which they transform from normal squamous epithelium to a columnar epithelium similar to that seen in the intestine. It is also called intestinal metaplasia or IM and was first described by Norman Barrett (1903–1979), an Australian-born British surgeon, at St. Thomas' Hospital in London in 1950. The condition is thought to be an adaptive response to gastroesophageal reflux.

CLINICAL PRESENTATION

Barrett esophagus is a known risk factor for the development of esophageal adenocarcinoma (EAC). Some studies have shown that, overall, a patient with BE has a 30-fold increased risk of developing esophageal cancer when compared to a patient without BE. The risk of progressing from BE to esophageal cancer is further defined by the degree of dysplasia (low or high) and the length of the Barrett segment. While there is general agreement that BE with dysplasia carries a significantly increased risk of EAC when compared to nondysplastic BE, there remains some debate on the significance of the risk of carcinoma in patients without dysplasia.

Sharma et al. followed 618 patients who had a new diagnosis of BE without dysplasia for 4 years. During that time, 16.1% developed low-grade dysplasia (LGD), 3.6% high-grade dysplasia (HGD), and 2% adenocarcinoma. When you consider that the current standard of care for patients in the U.S. with BE containing HGD or carcinoma is esophagectomy, Sharma's data argues that there is a 1.4% chance per year of a BE patient progressing to a state where esophagectomy will be recommended to them. To put this in perspective, a colon polyp carries a 0.58% incidence per year of progressing to colon cancer, which is a significantly lower chance than BE progressing to HGD or carcinoma. The standard of care for colon polyps, however, is screening, surveillance, and removal, whereas the standard for BE with no dysplasia is to do surveillance endoscopy and biopsy every 2 to 3 years (Table 19-1). This type of comparison has led some practitioners to wonder if it would be advantageous to ablate the esophageal epithelium containing the BE before it has a chance to progress. This chapter explores the various endoscopic modalities used to treat BE.

TREATMENT

The ideal endoscopic therapy for BE would allow for complete removal of the metaplastic or dysplastic tissue down to, but not through, the muscularis mucosa. This would avoid stricture formation or transmural injury (Fig. 19-1) and also prevent regrowth of metaplastic mucosa either from continuation of the initiating insult or from a "buried" gland—residual intestinal metaplasia that grows beneath a normal appearing squamous epithelium. Finally, the ideal therapy would be reliable enough to remove the patient from the surveillance cycle, inexpensive, and easy to administer and it would lead to minimal complications.

With this ideal therapy as a background, one can assess the various endoscopic treatment modalities that have been used to ablate BE. Because none of the currently available technologies completely meet this ideal, their use, for the most part, has been focused on BE with dysplasia or early carcinoma in nonsurgical candidates. The available ablation modalities fall into three categories: thermal, cryogenic, and mechanical.

Thermal

The majority of the endoscopic therapies for treating dysplastic BE fall into this category. They include multipolar electrocoagulation (MPEC), argon plasma coagulation (APC), laser photodynamic therapy (PDT), and a newer balloon-based bipolar radiofrequency ablation.

Multipolar Electrocoagulation

The probe for this modality is 7F or 10F and is attached to an electromechanical energy source similar to those used in the operating room. It is essentially bipolar energy conducted between adjacent wire wraps on the tip of the catheter. These wires are gold in color, resulting in the commonly used term "gold probe" (Fig. 19-2). One advantage of this technique is that it uses a readily available energy source that is familiar to gastrointestinal and surgical endoscopists. The typical energy settings are between 15 and 20 watts.

In a review of published MPEC data done by Sampliner, 292 patients with nondysplastic BE and four with LGD were treated. On average, 92% of patients had resolution of their BE, with a range of 72% to 100%. This variability may be

TABLE 19-1. RISK OF TRANSFORMATION TO CANCER: COLON POLYP VS. BARRETT ESOPHAGUS

	Colon cancer	Esophageal cancer
U.S. incidence	106,370	14,250 (~ 60% adeno)
U.S. deaths	56,730	13,300 (~ 8000 adeno)
Risk of precursor transformation to cancer (and HGD) in cases per patient years	5.8 cases/1000 pt years (0.58% incidence)	14 cases/1000 pt years (1.40% incidence)
Current management	Polypectomy	Watch and wait
Intervention risk reduction	80%	Not yet available

HGD, high-grade dysplasia.

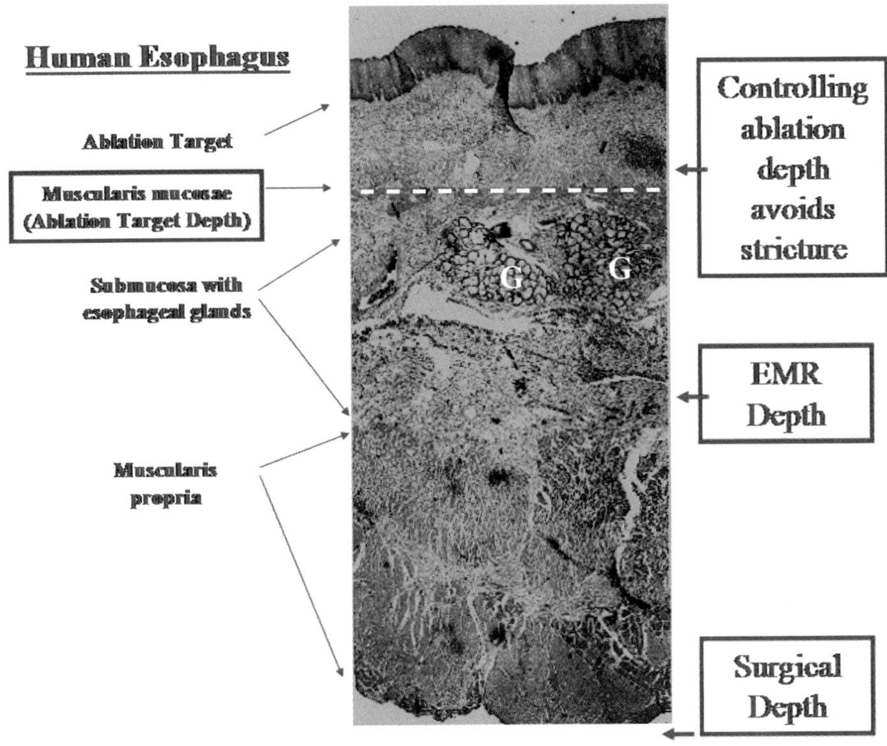

Fig. 19-1. The histology of esophageal ablation. EMR, endoscopic mucosal resection.

a result of different biopsy techniques in the follow-up surveillance, different treatment protocols, varying dosage of acid suppression, or varying length of follow-up. Two strictures developed in this group and complications were mostly minor but included transient fever, chest pain, and odynophagia. Application of this technique is also somewhat tedious because of its "point-and-shoot" nature. Other studies have shown a significant rate of "buried" glands in patients treated with MPEC. Buried glands are residual islands of intestinal metaplasia that remain after treatment and are covered with normal appearing squamous epithelium. It probably results from inconsistent application of cell-destroying energy, either from technique difficulties or from shielding from carbonization. The development of buried glands creates a worse situation than the original problem because subsequent direction of surveillance biopsies becomes impossible. The presence of buried glands is a significant problem in most endoscopic therapies for Barrett esophagus as these glands have been shown to have the capacity to progress to cancer. MPEC is currently used only in combination with another modality such as photo dynamic therapy, which has the ability to rapidly treat larger areas of BE, leaving the MPEC for the clean-up of residual areas on follow-up endoscopy.

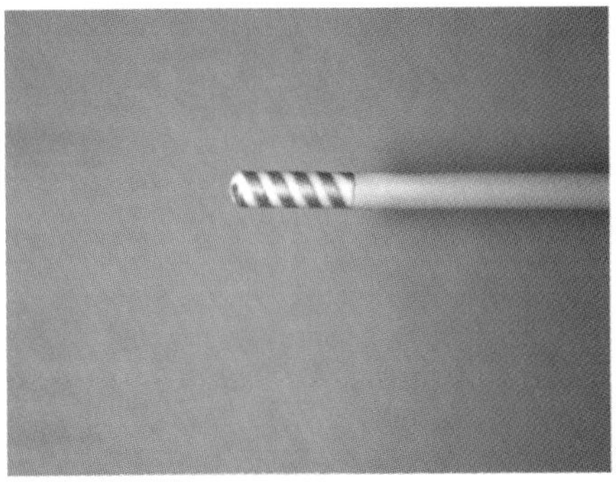

Fig. 19-2. A multipolar electrocoagulation (MPEC) probe.

Argon Plasma Coagulation

Argon plasma coagulation (APC) is a modality familiar to most surgeons. It is simply high-frequency monopolar electromechanical energy delivered to the target tissue using argon gas as a conductor. It is not much different than the energy used for the Bovie pen in the operating room, except that instead of using metal as a conductor, it uses argon gas. The gas, when electromechanically energized, becomes a plasma that directly transfers that energy to the target tissue. The advantage of using a gas as a conductor is that the probe can deliver energy without touching any tissue, thus avoiding fouling with coagulum (Fig. 19-3). The broader gas pattern also allows the operator to "paint" larger surfaces more quickly and the depth of thermal energy to be fairly well controlled at 1 to 3 mm. The APC probe is a 7F- or 10F-catheter that has either a forward firing or side firing tip. It is passed down the working channel of the endoscope and used under direct endoscopic vision. Typical energy settings for the generator are 30 to 90 watts and an argon gas flow rate of 1 to 2 liters per minute. Lower energies cause less penetration of the thermal energy into the tissues. The flow of argon gas must be as low as possible, as it can easily overinflate the stomach or bowel and must be frequently aspirated during the conduct of the procedure.

One report of the data for using APC to treat BE is from Franchimont et al., in which nine studies examining ablation of nondysplastic BE in 333 patients are reviewed. One to eight treatment sessions were required, resulting in 55% to 100% of patients obtaining eradication of their BE. This variability again reflects differences in treatment (varying power settings and number of treatment sessions) and acid suppression regimens, the experience of the surgeon, and length of follow-up. Of most concern is that one study demonstrated a 44% incidence of buried glands on follow-up. There were also five perforations and eight strictures reported in this review, with up to 68% of patients in one series relapsing back to BE at 12-month follow-up. In the same review, very little data was found for using APC to treat patients with HGD. Of the eleven such patients reported on, nine achieved ablation of the BE, but the follow-up was limited.

In summary, APC does not seem to be an effective de novo treatment for BE because of a relatively high serious complication rate and the frequent finding of

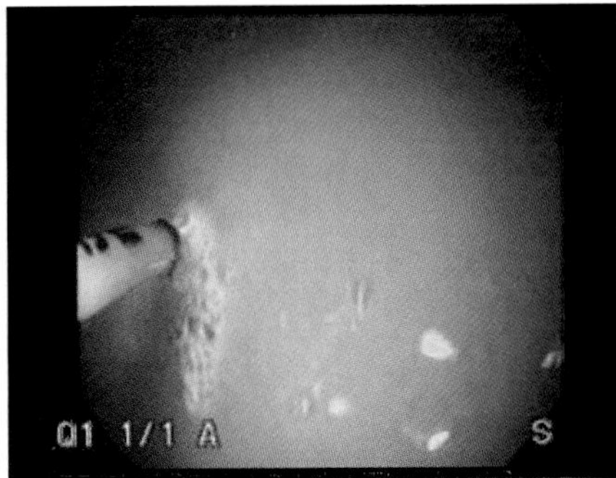

Fig. 19-3. Argon Plasma Coagulation (APC).

buried glands on follow-up. This "point-and-shoot" technology, like MPEC, is mainly used as an adjunct to another treatment modality for clean-up.

Laser

Laser light causes thermal destruction of tissue, the depth of which is determined by the wavelength of light used and the optical properties of the target tissue. Three types of lasers have been studied for the treatment of BE: Nd:YAG, KTP:YAG, and Argon. Nd:YAG has a depth of light penetration of 1.4 mm with tissue damage down to 4 to 6 mm. KTP:YAG lasers at 532 nm wavelength have light penetration of about 0.4 mm. Argon lasers working at 457 nm, 488 nm, and 515 nm have the shallowest depth of light penetration at 0.3 mm.

There are two ways to deliver laser light to the tissue. The most basic is "free fiber," which uses forward- or side-viewing bare laser fibers passed through the working channel of the scope. The target tissue is cooled with CO_2 or water. Keeping the fiber centered in the lumen is very challenging and, as a result, sapphire contact probes have been developed to assist in the laser light delivery. These sapphire tips allow for direct contact to the tissue. Different tip shapes are used to deliver different power densities and different tissue effects such as cutting, coagulation, or vaporization. Forward- or side-firing sapphire contact probes are also available and are backloaded onto the endoscope as their tip is too large to pass down the working channel. Light-absorbing coatings can be added to the sapphire tip to give further focus to the energy density and limit the depth of penetration.

The reported experience with laser therapy for BE is very limited. Nd:YAG, KTP:YAG, and argon lasers have been used to treat nondysplastic BE and LGD. Up to 100% eradication of the BE has been reported, but buried glands have also been found in up to 80% of patients! Only Nd:YAG and KTP:YAG lasers have been reported for treating HGD and only in conjunction with endoscopic mucosal resection (EMR) if dysplasia associated lesions or masses (DALMs) were found. Out of 22 patients treated in three different studies,16 had ablation of all BE, four had down-staging from HGD to LGD, and two had either residual HGD or buried glands.

In summary, laser treatment of BE, even with the modification of a sapphire contact probe, remains technically challenging and is still considered experimental.

Photodynamic Therapy (PDT)

PDT uses a combination of laser light and a photosensitizing agent to effect selective tissue destruction. A number of photosensitizing drugs can be used, but only two are clinically available. Sodium porfimer (Photofrin II; Axcan Pharma Inc.; Montreal, Canada) is the only agent with FDA approval in the U.S. and is administered parenterally. In Europe, 5-amino levulinic acid (5-ALA) is used and can be given orally, but this has not been approved for use in the U.S. Sodium porfirmer is given to the patients 48 to 72 hours before their endoscopy. This photosensitizing drug results in photosensitivity for 30 to 90 days, so these patients must avoid exposure to sunlight for a significant period of time. The photosensitizer is taken up preferentially in abnormal tissue with a higher metabolic activity level, resulting in a degree of selectivity of tissue destruction to the abnormal epithelium.

Within 48 to 72 hours of the administration of the photosensitizing agent, endoscopy is performed to deliver light to the treatment area. Laser light is the only source of photoradiation strong enough to elicit the tissue destruction desired in the gastrointestinal tract. Three lasers are approved for PDT, although only two are currently commercially available: the Laserscope 630XP Dye Module (San Jose, CA) and the Diomed 630 PDT Laser (Cambridge, U.K.). The Laserscope is a tunable dye KTP:YAG laser delivering 7 watts at 630 nm wavelength. The Diomed laser delivers 2 watts at 630 nm. The laser fiber can be positioned manually within the lumen of the esophagus but is usually centered with a positioning balloon for even therapy. PDT therapy has only been approved by the FDA for treatment of BE with HGD. 200 J/cm (joules per centimeter) are delivered for flat HGD while 300 J/cm is used for nodular disease.

The published results for PDT are variable because the data is from single centers using varying techniques. Overholt reported on 84 patients followed for 19 months after PDT: 43% had complete clearance of BE, and 88% cleared their HGD. However, 34% developed strictures, and 6% had buried glands on follow-up biopsy.

The PHO-BAR trial is an ongoing international, multicenter trial with almost 200 patients treated at 30 centers. Patients with BE and HGD were randomized to receiving PDT plus omeprazole, or omeprazole alone. At the 12-month follow-up, 41% of the PDT-treated patients had no residual BE, and 72% had no more HGD. This was statistically better than the omeprazole-only group, which had only a 38.6% resolution of the HGD. The PDT also resulted in a three-fold decrease in the development of esophageal adenocarcinoma in these patients.

In summary, PDT is an effective therapy for clearing BE with HGD but is associated with a significant stricture rate, frequently causes odynophagia, fever, and chest pain, and requires patients to deal with photosensitivity for a significant period of time. It can also result in the development of buried glands. Because of the severe mucosal damage it causes, its use should be reserved for treating BE with HGD.

Bipolar Balloon-Based Radiofrequency Ablation

In December of 2001, the FDA cleared a new device for ablating esophageal mucosa (Fig. 19-4). It is an over-the-wire 3 cm balloon-based radiofrequency electrode array that is inserted under direct vision into the treatment area of the esophagus to ablate the mucosa (HALO^{360}; BÂRRX Medical, Inc.; Sunnyvale, CA). Treatment patients undergo standard esophagoscopy to place a guidewire. A sizing balloon is then inserted over the wire into the esophagus and used to choose the appropriate diameter for the treatment catheter. The sizing balloon inflation and measurement is done automatically with a sophisticated control box. The balloon is then removed and the treatment catheter introduced over the guidewire and alongside the endoscope into the area of planned ablation. When activated, the control box automatically inflates the treatment balloon to 4.5 psi and then delivers an ultra short burst of high power (300 to 350 watts) before deflating. This firing sequence takes approximately 2 seconds and results in a uniform, well-demarcated, circumferential 3-cm ablation of the esophageal mucosa down to the muscularis mucosa (Fig. 19-5). The exact energy density used varies according to the target tissue. BE with HGD is treated at 12 J/cm^2 with two separate applications of the treatment catheter to the area. Nondysplastic BE is treated at 10 J/cm^2. Patients are usually surveyed at 2-month intervals by repeat endoscopy with retreatment until all evidence of BE has resolved. These follow-up treatments often do not require a repeat circumferential ablation; as a result, a smaller, spot-treating bipolar radiofrequency electrode that mounts on the end of the gastroscope was introduced in 2006 (HALO^{90}; BÂRRX Medical, Inc.; Sunnyvale, CA). This device allows treatment of small

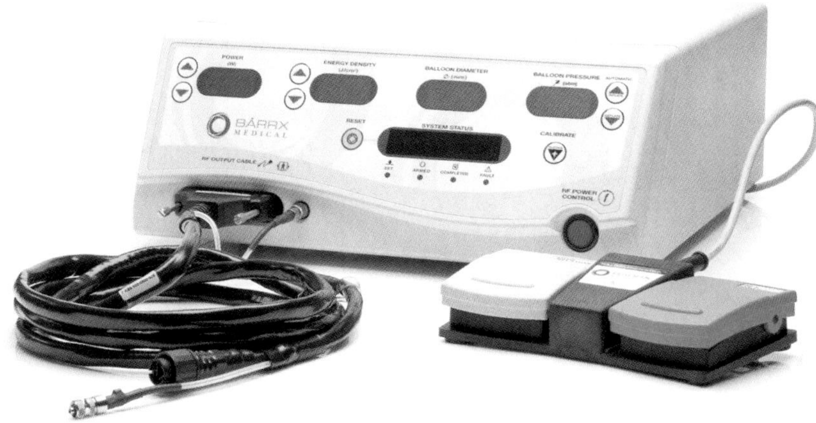

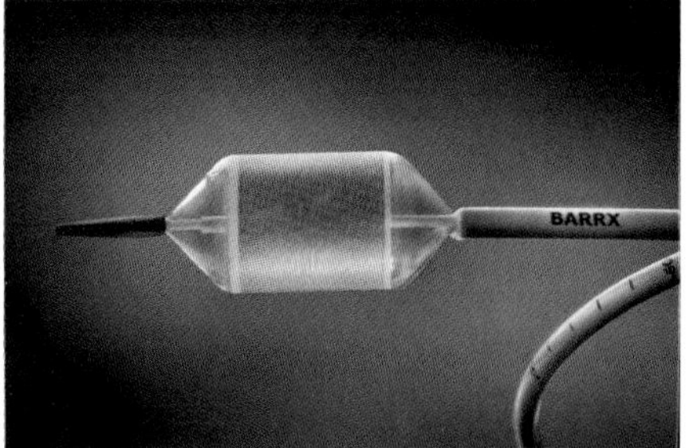

Fig. 19-4. A bipolar balloon-based radiofrequency ablation system. **A.** A microprocessor radiofrequency generator. **B.** A balloon-based 360 ablation catheter.

areas of BE under direct endoscopic vision (Fig. 19-6).

In February 2007, Sharma published the largest series of patients undergoing ablation of nondysplastic BE using the BÂRRX device. It was a multi-institutional prospective study evaluating over 100 patients with a 12-month follow-up. The study had two phases: a dosimetry phase and an effectiveness phase. In the dosimetry phase, 32 patients underwent ablation of their BE using an escalating energy density and were followed with repeat endoscopy and biopsy at 1, 3, and 12 months. One additional treatment was performed at 4 months if the follow-up biopsies showed residual BE. Subsequently, 70 patients had ablation of 2 to 6 cm of nondysplastic BE at a fixed energy density of 10 J/cm^2 and were then followed with repeat biopsies at 1, 3, 6, and 12 months. Again, one additional treatment was performed if the biopsies showed residual BE. The study demonstrated that 70% of the patients had achieved complete remission of their BE at their 12-month follow-up. Even more significant was the fact that all patients were treated under conscious sedation in the outpatient setting with no serious adverse events and no strictures. Also, over 4000 biopsy specimens were looked at blindly by a central pathologist with no finding of buried BE. In the 30% of patients with residual BE post-ablation, the surface area of the residual disease was significantly reduced to only small islands or tongues of IM.

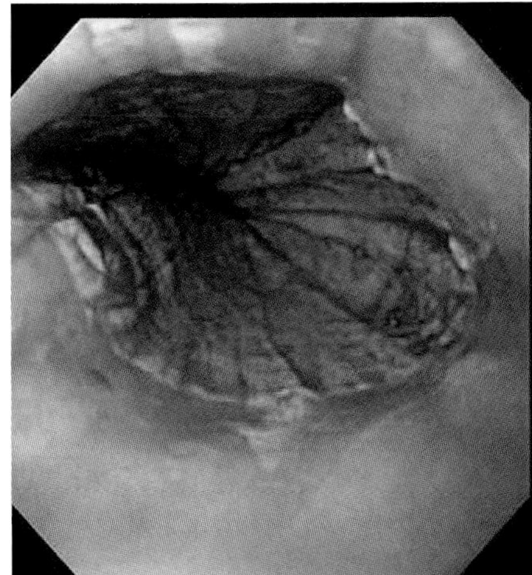

Fig. 19-5. Ablated esophageal mucosa using a bipolar balloon-based radiofrequency catheter.

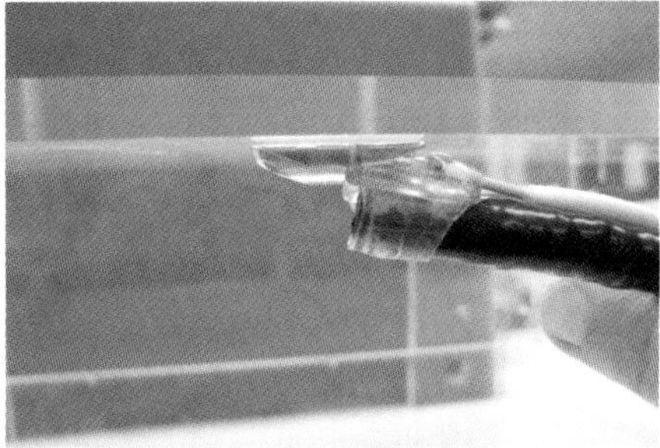

Fig. 19-6. Newer radiofrequency ablation catheters attach directly to the end of the scope and allow ablations under direct vision.

The most obvious target for ablation therapy is BE with HGD. The high risk of this disease progressing to esophageal adenocarcinoma and the significant morbidity associated with total esophagectomy make it an ideal target for endoscopic ablation. In January 2007 Smith published a dosimetry study involving eight patients undergoing treatment of their HGD using the BÂRRX device. These patients were scheduled to have an esophagectomy for definitive therapy; a BÂRRX ablation performed intraoperatively just prior to removal of the esophagus. The treated area was then examined grossly and histologically to determine the effect. The study demonstrated that, as expected, a higher energy density is required to ablate BE with HGD (12 J/cm^2), but that this could be done effectively without causing deep injury to the esophagus. This dosimetry study has paved the way for a multi-institutional clinical trial investigating the use of the BÂRRX device to ablate BE with HGD.

Most proponents of this new endoscopic ablative therapy recommend a "top-down" approach to its study and utilization. That is, to test it in BE with HGD as the first target, and then move to LGD and finally nondysplastic BE. Many questions remain about the long-term efficacy of this device, but the initial clinical results suggest that it is a step closer to achieving the ideal ablative therapy that resolves BE completely and removes the patient from the surveillance cycle.

Cryotherapy

High-pressure nitrous oxide or low-pressure liquid nitrogen can be used to ablate esophageal mucosa. It is sprayed onto the mucosa using a 7F- or 9F-probe connected to a delivery device that has a console for monitoring the cryogen release and a dual-control foot pedal to control delivery and warm the catheter. It is another "point-and-shoot" technology that requires the endoscopist to spray the visualized area of treatment.

The mechanism of injury to the mucosa is distinct from thermal. Cryoablation of the mucosa causes apoptosis and necrosis resulting from transient ischemia and stimulation of the immune system. This distinct ablation mechanism may allow cryotherapy to work on segments of BE that have not responded to other modalities.

There is limited published clinical data on cryotherapy. Johnston reported on eleven patients with Barrett metaplasia ranging from no dysplasia to HGD. Nine of the eleven patients had complete resolution of their BE at the 6-month follow-up. There were, however, two patients found to have buried glands.

Mechanical

Mechanical resection of BE with dysplasia has been accomplished using endoscopic mucosal resection (EMR). There are essentially three techniques for EMR: strip biopsy, the cap technique, and the band technique. For the strip biopsy, a polypectomy-type snare is used to resect the diseased mucosa (Fig. 19-7). This is usually reserved for polypoid lesions and is a technique similar to polypectomy in the colon. If the lesion is flat, solutions can be injected into the submucosa to elevate the area and provide a more polypoid target for resection. The submucosal injection also increases the safety margin in preventing full-thickness injury to the esophagus. Saline alone, saline with epinephrine, or 50% dextrose are common solutions used for the injection. The dextrose is slower to absorb, thus giving a more stable "lift" to the mucosa. Methylene blue is often added to such solutions to better delineate the submucosal layer after resection. It is also common to mark the perimeter of the intended resection area by creating punctuate superficial burns to the mucosa around the margin. This will help maintain orientation during the resection and assure complete removal of the intended tissue.

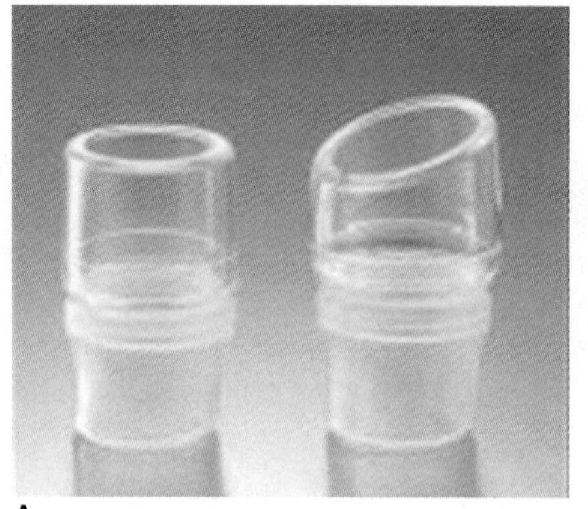

A

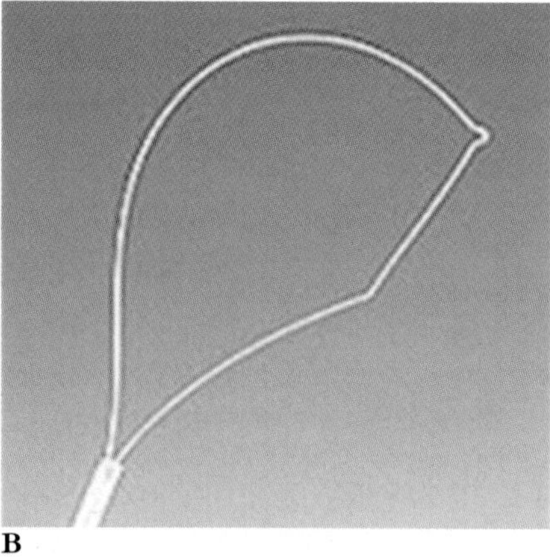

B

Fig. 19-8. Endoscopic mucosal resection: cap technique.

In 1990, Inoue et al. developed the cap technique for EMR. A straight or angled clear plastic "cap" is mounted on the end of the gastroscope, similar to a variceal bander. An asymmetrical snare is mounted on the inside of the cap (Fig. 19-8A and B). Once in position, the mucosa is sucked into the cap exactly like a varix is suctioned into a banding device. The snare is then tightened around the base of the captured tissue, and electrocautery is used to excise it. Submucosal injection is usually added to this technique to decrease the risk of perforation. The cap method makes it easier to excise flat mucosa, and multiple resections can be done quickly and precisely.

A variation of the cap technique is the band technique. A variceal band ligator is used to ligate the tissue intended for resection. A hard-wire snare is then used to excise the pseudopolyp created by the band. The excision can be done above or below the band (Fig. 19-9). A saline lift is helpful for preventing deeper injury. A more recent modification to the variceal band device allows the snare to be introduced directly through the cap of the bander. In this way, multiple resections can be quickly accomplished by placing multiple bands first and then introducing the snare for excision. Studies comparing the cap technique with the band technique have not shown any difference in safety or amount of tissue resected.

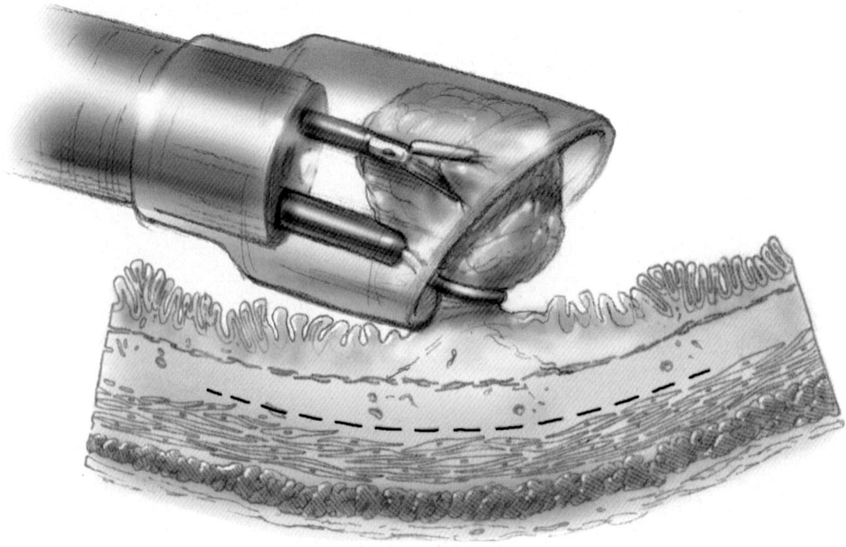

Fig. 19-7. Endoscopic mucosal resection: strip biopsy.

EMR has been reserved mainly for patients with HGD or early Barrett carcinoma who are not candidates for esophagectomy or who refuse surgery. Ell reported in 2000 on 64 patients who underwent EMR for early Barrett carcinoma (n = 61) or HGD (n = 3). Overall, they had complete remission in 82.5% of these patients. When these patients were further stratified into low- and high-risk groups, the low-risk group (non-ulcerated lesions < 20 mm in diameter, with favorable histology) had 97% remission compared to 59% in the high-risk group. There was only one major complication, which was bleeding, and it was controlled endoscopically. At 12 months, 14% of these patients had recurrent or metachronous carcinoma, and all were treated with repeat endoluminal therapy. Other studies have had similar results for remission, but strictures and perforations have been reported.

A more aggressive extension of the EMR technique is endoscopic submucosal dissection (ESD). The Japanese pioneered this technique for managing early gastric cancer, and it has been subsequently used in the esophagus for resecting early Barrett cancers. The lesion is approached as described for EMR by marking the margins and performing a submucosal injection. An incision is then made through the mucosa and into the submucosa using

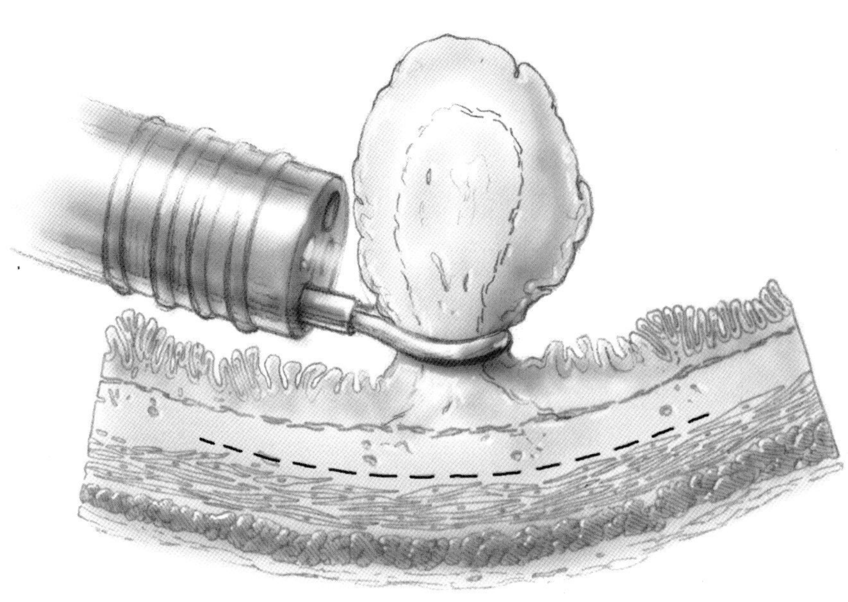

Fig. 19-9. Endoscopic mucosal resection: band technique.

needle-knife cautery. Once access to the submucosal space is gained, the needle-knife is replaced with an insulation-tipped knife (IT-knife). This is essentially a needle catheter with a porcelain ball on the tip. The ball does not conduct energy and, as a result, minimizes the chance of full-thickness perforation. The mucosa is incised circumferentially and sequentially elevated, delivering a full-thickness specimen excised down to the submucosal layer (Fig. 19-10). Full-thickness excisions like this have been done in the esophagus, although there is a significant stricture rate.

Adding ablative therapy to EMR is also of interest. EMR in combination with PDT has been studied in inoperable patients, and early results show a 94% remission rate. This is in contrast to 53% remission seen in this group with PDT alone. Large BE referral centers, such as the Academic Medical Center at the University of Amsterdam, are quite aggressive in the use of combination therapies for managing HGD or early cancer. Their patients are evaluated with visible light gastroscopy, narrow band imaging, autofluorescence endoscopy, and high-resolution ultrasound. If deemed appropriate for endoscopic therapy, the patients then have their nodular mucosa removed with EMR followed by ablation of the remaining BE. This ablation used to be performed with PDT, but more recently it is done with a balloon-based radiofrequency ablation catheter. The EMR yields a pathologic specimen with architecture intact for accurate staging and, if no invasive carcinoma is found, the patients go on to surveillance at 2-month intervals. Any residual BE is further ablated. Early results from this center show excellent remission rates with this approach.

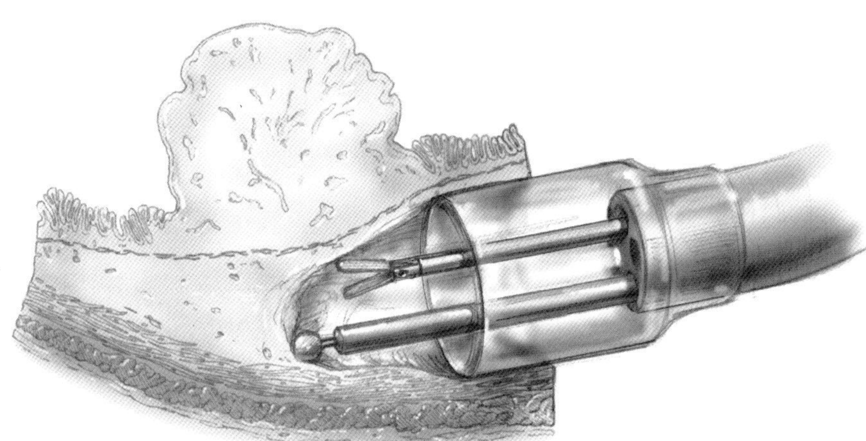

Fig. 19-10. Endoscopic submucosal dissection (ESD) is performed with a clear dissecting cap and a dual-channel endoscope using specialized monopolar dissection instruments. The specimen is removed intact, down to the submucosa.

CONCLUSION

In summary, multiple ablative therapies, either alone or in combination, have been used to treat BE. The diverse body of work in this area is an indication of the problems encountered in managing patients with this disease. The cost of surveillance alone is estimated at $290 million per year in the U.S., and this does not take into account the lost time from work required to undergo surveillance. It also does not account for the psychological impact of living with a condition that is perceived by patients to be a "ticking time bomb" for the development of esophageal cancer. The ideal ablative device would result in 100% remission of the BE with no strictures and no buried glands, allowing the patient to be removed from the surveillance cycle. While newer technologies such as the balloon-based radiofrequency ablation catheter seem to be closer to reaching this ideal goal, the data do not yet support cessation of surveillance after treatment with any ablative device in patients with BE.

Once the disease has progressed to high-grade dysplasia or early carcinoma, the drive to find an endoscopic cure is even stronger. Surgical resection of the esophagus, while offering the most definitive chance for cure, is a morbid procedure with significant risk of death or serious complications. PDT, while effective in these patients, has its own significant morbidity including stricture and problems dealing with photosensitivity. Combination therapy, such as that described by the Amsterdam group, will likely be the solution in this population, and preliminary results seem to show that endoscopic mucosal resection combined with circumferential or spot ablation using a radiofrequency catheter is the most effective endoscopic treatment regimen with the least risk of serious complications or buried glands. With further study, the approach to managing properly selected patients with HGD or early esophageal carcinoma will move away from surgery and toward combination endoscopic therapy.

SUGGESTED READING

Bergman J. Latest developments in the endoscopic management of gastroesophageal reflux disease and Barrett's esophagus: an overview of the year's literature. *Endoscopy* 2006;38:122–132.

Lightdale CJ, Sharma P, eds. *Gastrointestinal Endoscopy Clinics of North America* July 2003; 13(3).

Lopes CV, Hela M, Pesenti C, et al. Circumferential endoscopic resection of Barrett's esophagus with high-grade dysplasia or early adenocarcinoma. *Surg Endosc* 2007 May;21(5):820–824.

Sharma VK, Wang KK, Overholt BF, et al. Balloon-based, circumferential, endoscopic radiofrequency ablation of Barrett's esophagus: 1-year follow-up of 100 patients. *Gastrointest Endosc* 2007;65(2):185–195.

Smith CD, Bejarano PA, Melvin WS, et al. Endoscopic ablation of intestinal metaplasia containing high-grade dysplasia in esophagectomy patients using a balloon-based ablation system (HALO^{360} System). *Gastrointest Endosc* 2007;21(4):560–569.

Soetikno RM, Gotoda T, Nakanishi Y, et al. Endoscopic mucosal resection. *Gastrointest Endosc* 2003;57(4):567–579.

Wolfsen HC. Endoprevention of esophageal cancer: endoscopic ablation of Barrett's metaplasia and dysplasia. *Expert Rev Med Devices* 2005;2(6):1–11.

COMMENTARY

Esophageal reflux disease, and related complications such as Barrett esophagus and esophageal cancer, are experiencing a remarkable increase in frequency throughout the world. Adenocarcinoma of the esophagus (Barrett cancer) is the most rapidly increasing malignancy in North America today and remains highly lethal in spite of advances in chemoradiation and aggressive surgery. The lethality of advanced Barrett cancers has led to a policy of extremely aggressive treatment when premalignant transformation of Barrett is discovered. Offering an esophagectomy has long been considered as the gold standard in patients with high-grade displastic Barret or intramucosal cancers. This results in a prophylaxis or "cure" in almost 100% of patients—if they survive the surgery. Esophagectomy, in spite of advances in technique and postsurgical intensive care, continues to have mortality rates as high as 8% and major morbidity rates of over 50%. A less invasive therapy is clearly indicated. Dr. Dunkin describes the current standing of esophageal mucosal ablation as well as techniques for the "endosurgical" excision of early cancers. This almost certainly represents the future of treatments for dysplastic Barrett and early cancers.

The development of the radiofrequency mucosal ablation technologies has solved many of the issues of mucosal ablation that prevented widespread adoption of PDT or heat-based procedures: they were messy, imprecise, and led a persistent problem with the "buried" glands. Documentation of cancers occurring in these buried glands dramatically curtailed interest in the procedures' use. Results from the balloon-based RFA systems seem to show a more consistent mucosal ablation and an absence of the buried gland phenomenon. Whether this will hold up over the long term remains to be seen. With mucosal ablation, the issue of dealing with nodularity, which compromises the effectiveness of superficial ablations, and the possibility of intramucosal cancers, where ideally a deeper ablation or resection is needed, still remain As described in the chapter, this is an ideal role for endoscopic excisions—whether EMR for small lesions or ESD for more extensive resections. Our current protocol for nodular dysplasia or mucosal cancers involves optical staging and EUS, EMR or submucosal resection for all raised lesions followed by a mucosal ablation 8 weeks later, repeat biopsy and ablation every 3 months until clear, and, finally, an antireflux surgery to prevent recurrence of the Barrett. The risk of a missed invasive cancer with this approach has been shown to be minimal and certainly is less concerning than the mortality of an esophagectomy. It is apparent that the future of early Barrett cancer treatments lies in this direction.

LLS

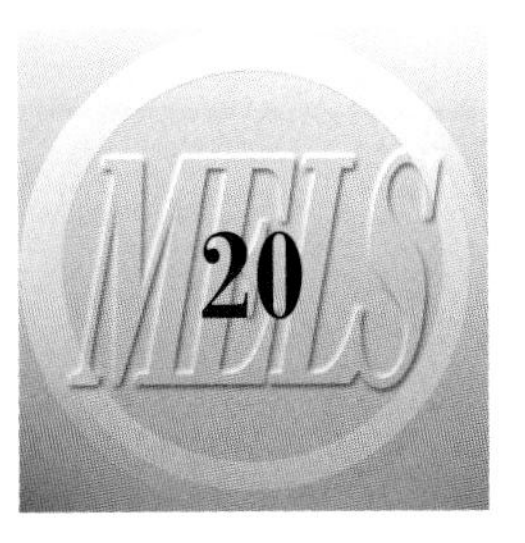

Laparoscopic Transhiatal Esophagectomy: Resection for Curative Intent

AUREO LUDOVICO DE PAULA
AND VLADIMIR SCHRAIBMAN

INTRODUCTION

Esophageal cancer is the ninth most common cancer in the Western world. The incidence of esophageal adenocarcinoma and gastroesophageal junction tumors is documented to have risen dramatically from 1980 to 2000; a disturbing trend that continues today. The overall prognosis of patients with esophageal cancer remains poor, although the combination of neoadjuvant chemoradiation with surgical resection offers hope of some improvement in overall survival. Still, complete surgical excision remains the best hope for most patients.

Esophageal malignancies are frequently associated with significant clinical comorbidities and important nutritional problems that must be addressed. A preoperative risk analysis of patients and staging of the tumor are necessary to identify those patients who will benefit from surgery. Patient-related risk stratification includes an evaluation of cardiac, pulmonary, hepatic, renal, and nutritional functions and associated underlying disorders, such as cirrhosis and chronic pulmonary disease. The most significant prognostic factors in esophageal cancer are resectability, the occurrence of postoperative complications, and the DNA profile of the cancer cells. Analysis of tumor stage and resectability is of utmost importance in relation to survival rate. Preoperative radiotherapy and chemotherapy are also important surgical risk factors. On the other hand, most authors have not observed that the patient's age or the type of tumor has any influence on outcomes. The most frequent causes of postsurgical death include pulmonary complications, anastomotic leak, and hemorrhage.

Esophagectomy has always presented a challenge for surgeons. It is a technically demanding operation, the incidence of complications and mortality is quite high, and the survival rate of patients with esophageal carcinoma is suboptimal. Only half of the patients who present with esophageal cancer have resectable disease, with an overall 5-year survival rate of 10% to 15%.

The type of treatment approach is also related to outcomes morbidity: The Ivor Lewis operation, modified by McKeown, involves the risks associated with thoracotomy and intrathoracic anastamosis as well as those related to the esophageal resection. A right-sided thoracotomy in combination with a laparotomy and thoracic or cervical esophagogastric anastomosis offers the advantage of an excellent exposure of the esophagus, allowing complete esophageal dissection and en bloc resection. In the 1970s, esophagectomy without thoracotomy became more common, particularly for patients with multiple clinical risk factors, especially pulmonary and nutritional problems. The transhiatal approach was initially described by Denk in 1913 and was later popularized by Ferreira, Pinotti, and Orringer. Advocates of the transhiatal approach claim that it is a technically feasible and safe operation associated with a lower incidence of pulmonary complications and blood loss. Survival rates are similar to patients having a standard transthoracic esophagectomy. The transthoracic approach with radical lymphadenectomy, however, offers the opportunity to accurately stage the disease and adequately dissect lesions of the middle and thoracic esophagus, as well as a better 5-year survival rate for some subgroups of patients. Even now there is continuing controversy about which the best approach is and whether resection is even advisable, as both the transthoracic and transhiatal procedures have high complication rates, varying from 40% to 80%. In-hospital mortality rates range from an average of 7.5% to less than 5% in experienced centers. In a meta-analysis comparing transthoracic and transhiatal resections, it was concluded that the 5-year survival rate was approximately 20% after both transthoracic and transhiatal resections. This study documented significantly higher early (pulmonary) morbidity and mortality rates for the transthoracic approaches. A recent prospective randomized study in which en bloc esophageal resections with systematic abdominal and mediastinal lymph node dissection were compared with the transhiatal approach showed that the transhiatal approach results in a lower morbidity rate than the extended en bloc lymphadenectomy. Moreover, median disease-free survival and quality-adjusted survival were not statistically different.

The technical viability of minimally invasive surgery has been demonstrated for the treatment of a number of diseases in and out of the abdomen, even for major procedures such as gastrectomy, pancreatectomy, and esophagectomy. The main goal of the minimally invasive esophagectomy (MIE) is to minimize the incidence of intra- and postoperative complications for benign and malignant esophageal diseases, in spite of the recognition that the approach constitutes only one of the factors that determine the incidence of postoperative complications and survival. Since first described by DePaula in 1993, MIE has demonstrated many patient advantages, including less postoperative discomfort, a rapid recovery, less trauma, shorter hospital stays, and better aesthetic results.

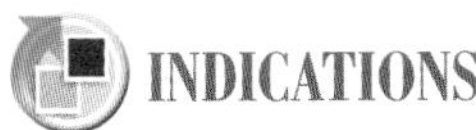

INDICATIONS

The indications for laparoscopic transhiatal esophagectomy include patients with both benign and malignant esophageal diseases. For benign diseases, common indications are: (1) patients with advanced achalasia (sigmoid esophagus); (2) patients with achalasia who have had failed treatment by Heller myotomy; (3) extensive nondilatable esophageal reflux stricture; (4) failed antireflux surgery, especially those patients with end-stage disease and nondilatable stenosis; and (5) caustic strictures.

Esophageal Carcinoma

Selection of patients for minimally invasive cancer resection is more complex and must be individualized for each individual. Thorough preoperative staging, both by imaging and by laparoscopic exploration, is always critical. Triage for neoadjuvant chemoradiation depends on institutional protocols and can also influence the choice of approach. Ideal indications for a laparoscopic approach include:

1. Carcinoma of the cervical esophagus
2. Carcinoma of the lower third of the thoracic esophagus and abdominal esophagus
3. Early esophageal carcinoma
4. Palliative resection
5. Patients with pleural adhesions
6. Higher risk patients, especially those with serious cardiopulmonary diseases

PREOPERATIVE PLANNING

A careful preoperative evaluation has to be performed, as these patients are often elderly, undernourished, and presenting with multiple comorbidities. A risk analysis of the patient and a staging of the tumor are necessary to reduce postoperative mortality and to identify those patients who will benefit most from surgery.

Special emphasis is given to the evaluation of cardiac, pulmonary, hepatic, and renal function. The most important cardiac risk factors are a cardiac output of less than 2 l/min. and a history of coronary heart disease. Pulmonary risk factors include a partial pressure of oxygen in arterial blood (PaO_2) of less than 70 mmHg and a forced expiratory volume in one second (FEV_1) less than 75%. Hepatic risk factors include the diagnosis of cirrhosis and serum protein of less than 5 g.

The diagnosis of esophageal cancer and the type of tumor are confirmed through upper digestive endoscopy and biopsy. Preoperative evaluation includes barium meal, thoracic and abdominal computed tomography (CT) scan, and endoscopic ultrasound. Broncoscopy is selectively indicated. In staging the cancer it is important to determine the extent of wall infiltration, especially above the carina, the presence of lymph node metastases, and, as a result, whether the tumor can be completely resectable.

SURGICAL TECHNIQUE

The necessary instruments for the performance of a laparoscopic transhiatal esophagectomy are listed in Table 20-1.

The procedure is carried out with the patient in supine position on a split-leg operating table. The legs are abducted, and the procedure is performed with the patient in a reverse-Trendelenburg of approximately 30 degrees and with the head

TABLE 20-1. INSTRUMENTS REQUIRED FOR LAPAROSCOPIC TRANSHIATAL ESOPHAGECTOMY

Laparoscopic instruments	30-degree telescope for the mobilization of the stomach 0-degree extra-long telescope for the mediastinal dissection Flexible 10-mm liver retractor 42-cm scissors, bipolar grasper, ultrasonic shears, and graspers to permit an adequate mediastinal dissection Regular laparoscopic instruments including needle holders Linear stapler with 45- or 60-mm "blue" cartridges
Open instruments	Minor instrument set for the cervical dissection Standard cautery Deep self-retaining retractor for neck
Ancillary instruments	Flexible upper endoscope Laparoscopic ultrasound

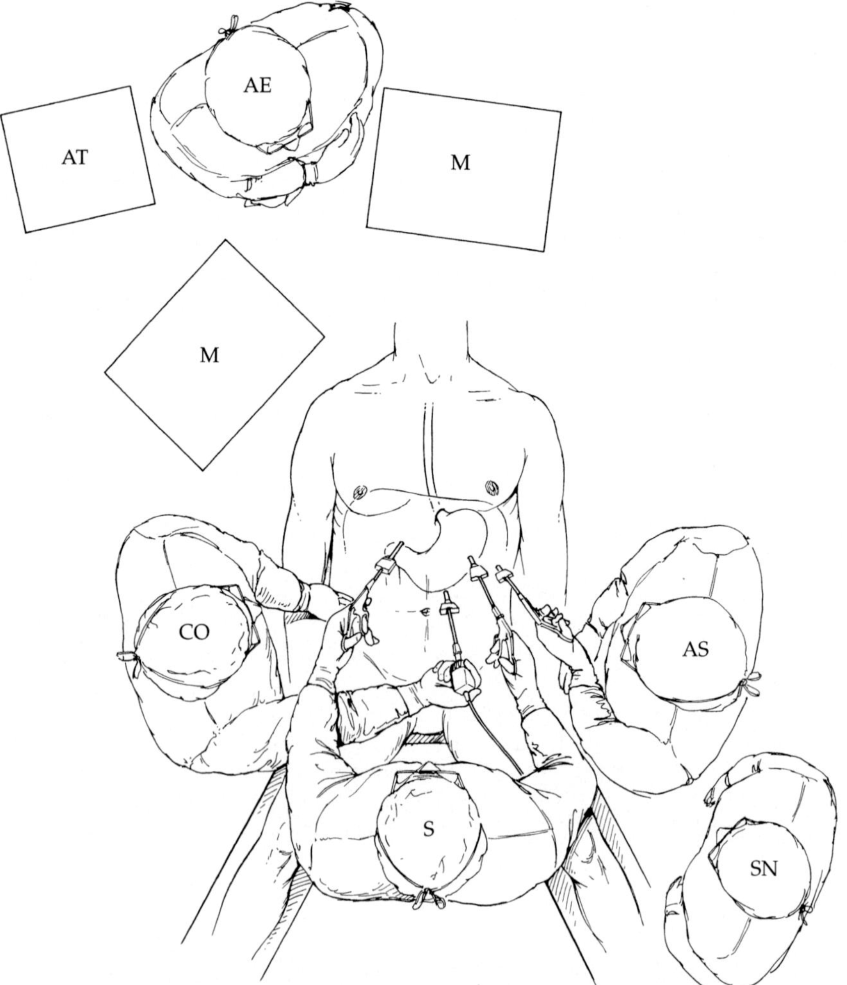

Fig. 20-1. The operating room setup for a laparoscopic transhiatal esophagectomy. S, surgeon; AS, first assistant surgeon; CO, camera operator/second assistant surgeon; SN, surgical nurse; AE, anesthesiologist; AT, anesthesiologist equipment; M, monitor.

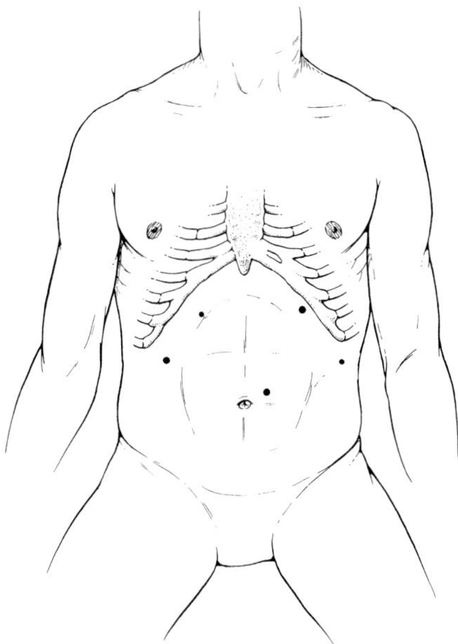

Fig. 20-2. The port placement for a laparoscopic transhiatal esophagectomy.

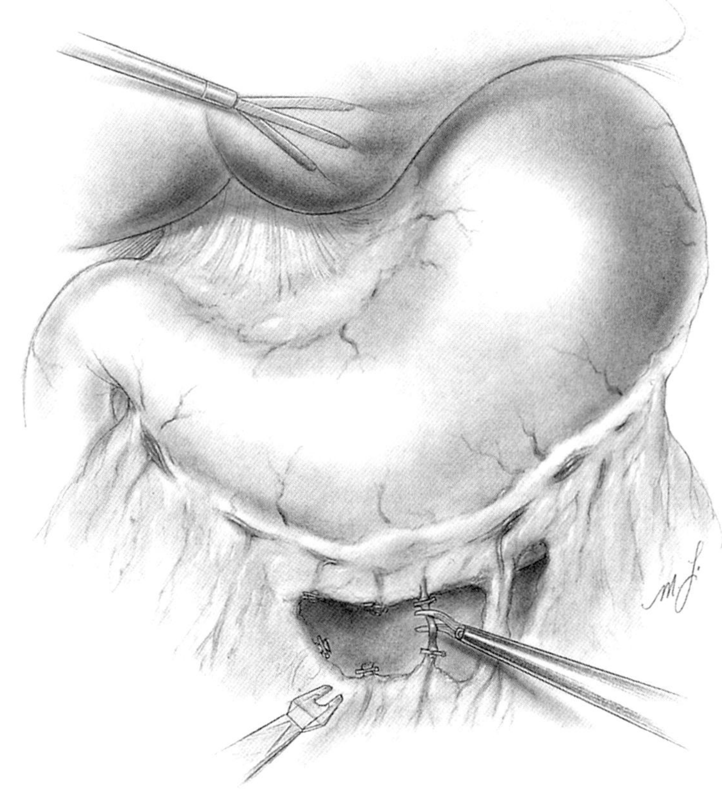

Fig. 20-3. The greater curvature is mobilized by dividing the gastrocolic omentum wide of the epiploic arcade.

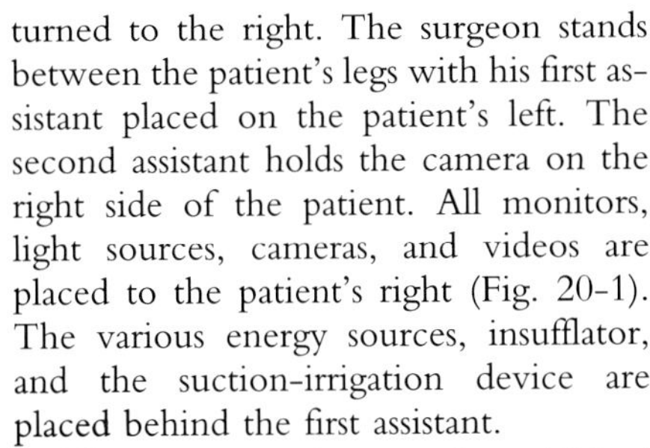

turned to the right. The surgeon stands between the patient's legs with his first assistant placed on the patient's left. The second assistant holds the camera on the right side of the patient. All monitors, light sources, cameras, and videos are placed to the patient's right (Fig. 20-1). The various energy sources, insufflator, and the suction-irrigation device are placed behind the first assistant.

The pneumoperitoneum is established using a Veress needle at the umbilicus. Intraperitoneal pressure is maintained at or below 12 mmHg to minimize pulmonary problems. The first 10-mm trocar is then inserted approximately 3 to 4 cm above and 1 to 2 cm to the left lateral of the midline. This port is used for the 30-degree telescope and camera. Two 5-mm trocars are placed in the right and left subcostal margins at the midclavicular line. A 10-mm trocar is positioned below the xiphoid. The last, a 12-mm trocar, is introduced somewhere between the left subcostal trocar and the 30-degree telescope (Fig. 20-2). Careful exploration of the abdominal cavity to rule out extraesophageal disease is critical. Any suspicious lesions should undergo ultrasound and biopsy to make sure resection is possible and indicated. The first step is to mobilize the stomach. The critical mobilization of the greater gastric curvature, including the vessels of the gastrocolic omentum and short gastric vessels, is performed beginning at the second portion of the duodenum and extending to the angle of His (Fig. 20-3). Preservation of the gastroepiploic arcade is of paramount importance, as the gastric conduit will depend on it for its blood supply. The epiploic vessels are sometimes visible but often hard to detect; laparoscopic ultrasound can be helpful to identify them. This dissection is best done utilizing an ultrasonic scalpel and staying a respectful distance away from the vessels. It is also important for the assistant to avoid grasping either the gastric conduit portion of the stomach or the greater curve vascular pedicle, to prevent crush injuries that may cause later disasters. Blunt retraction is preferred when at all possible.

Retrogastric adhesions to the pancreas are divided while the assistant lifts the stomach anteriorly. This dissection should extend from the duodenal bulb to the origin of the left gastric artery near the base of the right crus (Fig. 20-4, page 176). Sweeping the stomach to the left lower quadrant, the gastrohepatic ligament is exposed and divided close to its insertion with the liver, which exposes the upper portion of the right crus (Fig. 20-5, page 176). Both the right and left crura of the diaphragm are then dissected to open up the mediastinum. For distal esophageal cancers this dissection should be wide, actually removing a portion of the hiatal rim in order to stay clear of the cancer. Next, the left gastric artery and vein are dissected flush with the celiac axis, secured between ligatures and clips, and divided. An extensive lymphadenectomy is performed around the celiac, hepatic, and splenic arteries (Fig. 20-6, page 177). A Kocher maneuver is performed selectively, depending on the length of conduit needed and the mobility of the pylorus. In general, the pylorus should be mobilized enough to be able to be grasped and pushed up to touch the base of the right crus (Fig. 20-7, page 178). A gastric tube of 3 cm is then created based on the greater curvature, starting 2 to 3 cm below the crow's foot and ending lateral

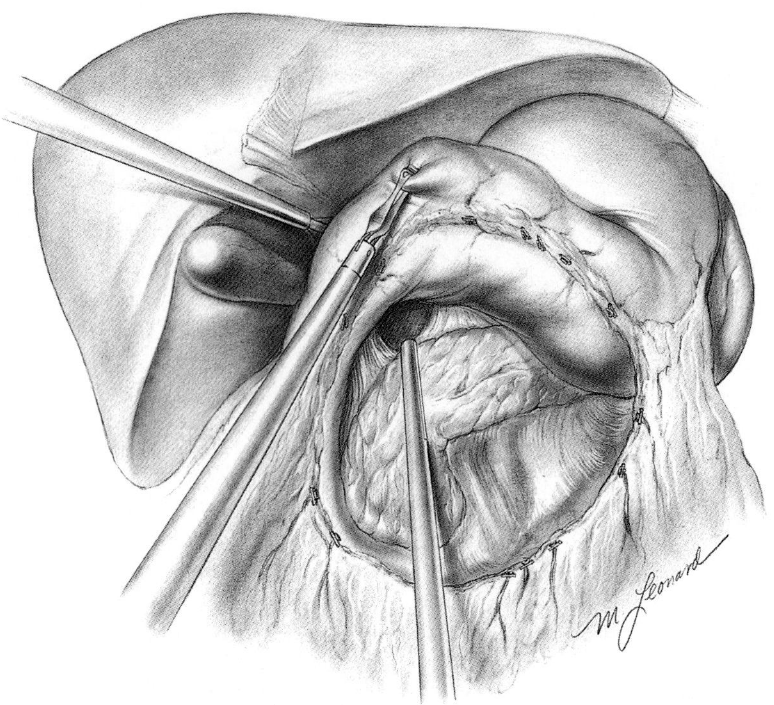

Fig. 20-4. The assistant bluntly retracts the stomach anteriorly to allow division of the filmy adhesions to the pancreas.

to the angle of His (Fig. 20-8, page 178). The division of the stomach is performed with multiple loads of 45-mm or 60-mm long endoscopic linear staplers using the 3.5-mm or "blue" cartridges. A 3-0 prolene interrupted invaginating suture is used to reinforce the staple line. The proximal end of the gastric tube is then sutured to

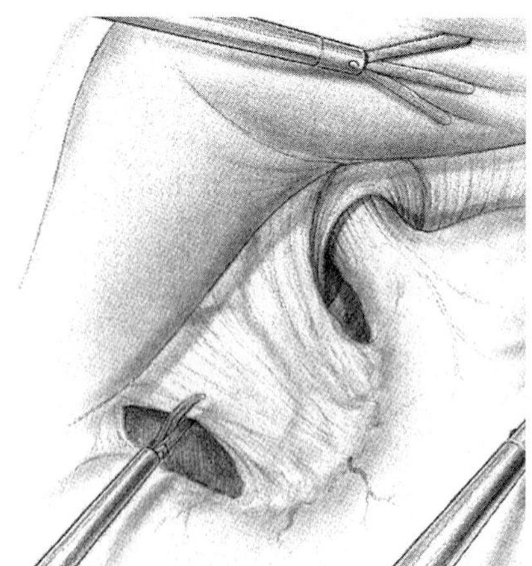

Fig. 20-5. The gastrohepatic ligament is divided close to the liver, extending from the porta hepatis to the right crus.

the proximal end of the transected stomach. As mentioned above, the phrenoesophageal membrane is opened and the esophagus separated from its attachments to the crus. The thoracic esophagus is mobilized using a bariatric length 0-degree telescope and 42-cm instruments passed through the hiatus (Fig. 20-9, page 179). This step largely consists of a blunt dissection but a few small vessels are divided using an ultrasonic coagulating scissors and/or bipolar grasper. The dissection is carried out as far as possible, usually 2 to 3 cm above the trachea bifurcation. It is usually unnecessary to enlarge the esophageal hiatus, but that is an option if visualization is poor.

The cervical dissection is started with a neck incision made parallel to the anterior border of the left sternomastoid muscle. The prethyroid muscles are divided, and the recurrent laryngeal nerve is identified and protected. The cervical and upper thoracic esophagus is bluntly separated from its attachments far enough down to meet the esophageal dissection from below using a sponge stick. At this point, the esophagus should be completely detached from adjacent structures. However, in some patients, remaining lateral and or anterior adhesions around the trachea bifurcation area preclude the complete dissection of the esophagus. When facing this problem, the cervical esophagus can be divided and a Penrose drain sutured to the distal esophagus. Traction on the drain from the cervical incision will invert the esophagus into the mediastinal cavity and allow further laparoscopic dissection of any residual adhesions (Fig. 20-10, page 180). The cervical esophagus is divided to allow specimen extraction through the cervical incision. A plastic camera sleeve is inserted over the esophagus and pulled down into the abdomen laparoscopically in order to protect the incision during retrieval of the specimen. Traction on the esophagus from above pulls the gastric tube up into the mediastinum and into the neck. This should be done under laparoscopic vision to prevent the conduit from twisting. The hiatus is left open, but nonabsorbable sutures are placed between the gastric tube and the rim of the hiatus to prevent visceral herniation. The superior part of the gastric tube is also sutured to the prevertebral fascia. Finally, an end-to-end, two-layer

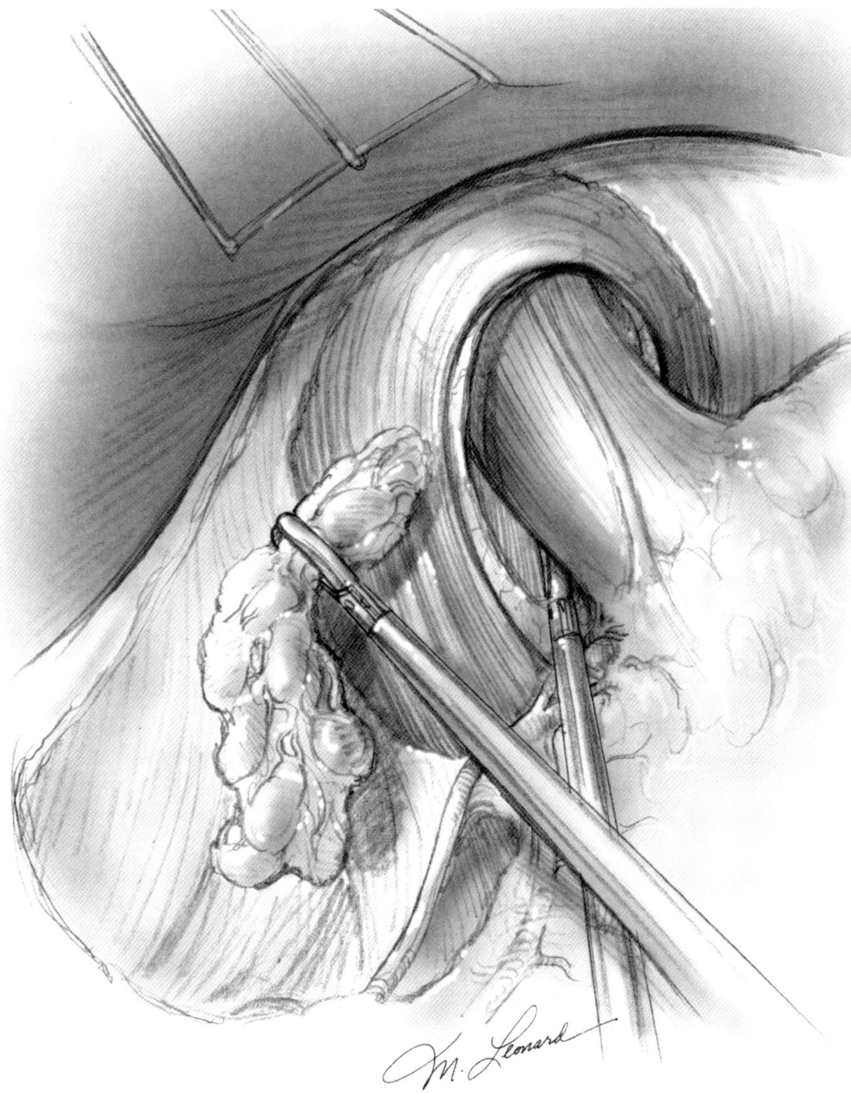

Fig. 20-6. Regional lymphadenectomy is routinely done for cancer cases.

esophagogastric anastomosis is performed using interrupted sutures or, alternatively, a side-to-side anastomosis using an endoscopic linear stapler, as suggested by Orringer et al. Finally, an extramucosal pyloromyotomy or a pyloroplasty is performed (Fig. 20-11, page 180).

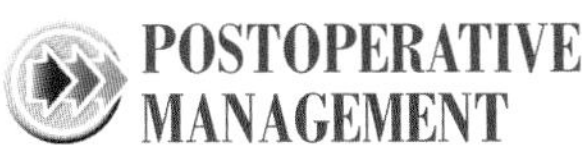

POSTOPERATIVE MANAGEMENT

Postoperatively, patients are routinely admitted to the intensive care unit (ICU) with respiratory support for a variable period of time. After suspension of the respiratory support, respiratory exercises and early walking are stimulated. A nasogastric tube is maintained for 24 to 48 hours for gastric drainage. Chest X-rays and iodine contrast radiography of the upper digestive tract are normally performed in all patients before resumption of oral feeding, usually between the 7th and 10th postoperative day. An aggressive policy of upper digestive endoscopy and early dilatation using a Savary dilator if indicated is performed 1 month after discharge.

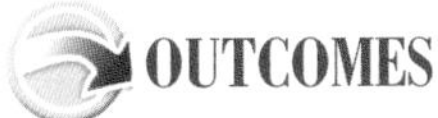

OUTCOMES

The case volume and experience of the centers involved in the performance of esophagectomy is probably more important than the approach itself in relation to postoperative morbidity and mortality. This has been documented in recent reports showing that mortality rates following esophagectomy ranged from 12.2% in low-volume centers to 3% in high-volume centers.

Our own series of 81 patients with esophageal carcinomas who underwent a laparoscopic transhiatal esophagectomy from July 1992 to July 2000 had an overall morbidity of 38.1% and a mortality of 5.9%. Esophagogastric anastomotic leak (14.8%) was the most frequent complication. Mean operative time was 216 minutes. Mean ICU length stay was 36 hours. Only one patient needed blood transfusion. Two required prolonged ventilation. One patient required conversion to open thoracotomy. Mean hospital stay was 7.2 days. Mean number of lymph nodes was 23.1. Overall 5-year survival rate for esophageal adenocarcinoma was 31%. Lesions classified as R0-N0 had a 5-year survival rate of 62%. Locoregional recurrence was 14.7%.

These results are similar to those reported for open resection where total morbidity rates including all minor and major complications are around 60% when reported. Most authors tend to report specific complications, such as the anastomotic leak rate. The series by Orringer et al. of 1085 patients is one of the largest reported. In their series, the overall anastomotic leak rate was 13%, with a perioperative mortality of 4%. Fifty-three percent of patients were discharged by the 10th postoperative day.

CONCLUSION

Esophagectomy remains a challenge for surgeons. In spite of recent advances, such as the minimally invasive approach, morbidity is still high, mortality is significant, and in cases of carcinoma, the 5-year survival rate is still poor. Laparoscopic surgery represents a new alternative for the treatment of esophageal diseases, offering the possibility of applying the same advantages already demonstrated for cholecystectomy to this radical resection. Minimizing surgical trauma is an important aspect of the treatment for malignant and benign esophageal diseases. Laparoscopic transhiatal esophagectomy is technically feasible in the majority of patients with indications for resection. Laparoscopic

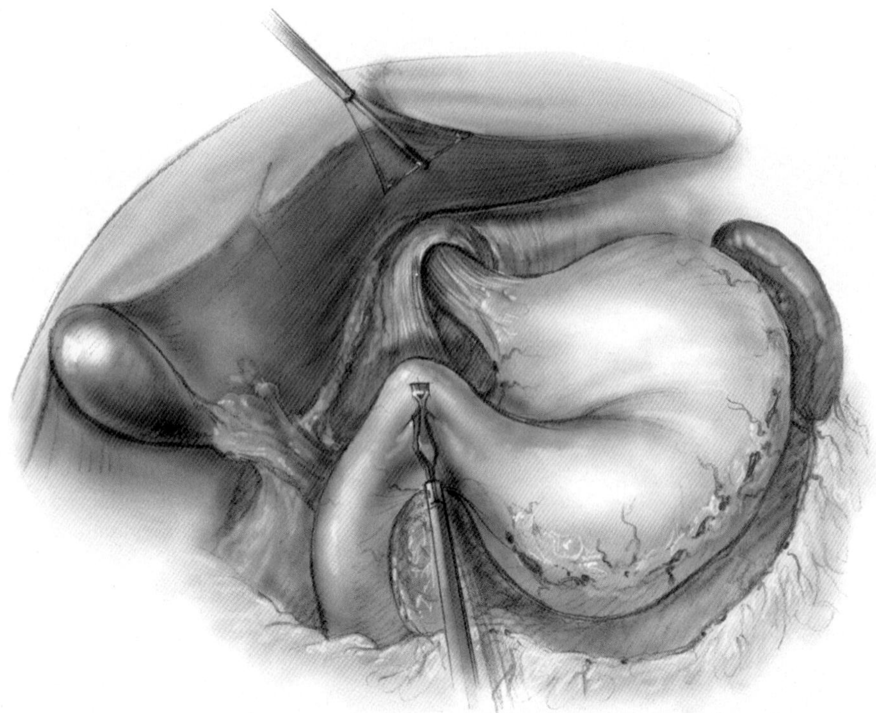

Fig. 20-7. Adequate duodenal mobilization has been attained if the pylorus can be made to touch the right crus.

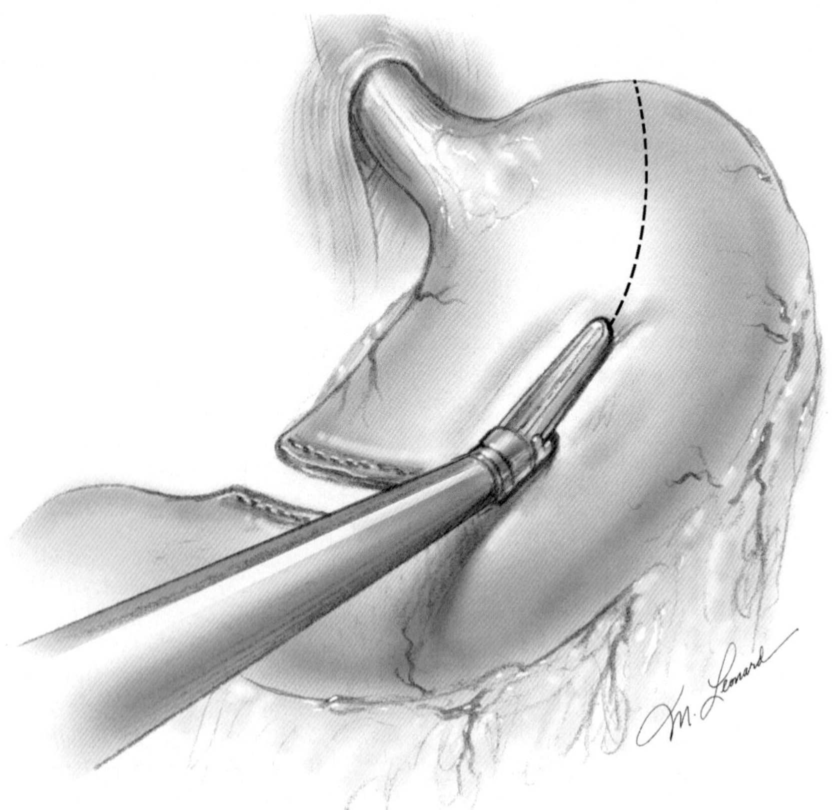

Fig. 20-8. A 3-cm gastric conduit is created based on the greater gastric curvature. Multiple firings of an articulating endoscopic stapler are required.

resection is difficult but offers better definition and precision of the mediastinal dissection, permits adequate mobilization of the stomach, and minimizes morbidity to the patient.

Laparoscopic transhiatal esophagectomy is a minimally invasive operation that can be accomplished safely and precisely in selected patients with esophageal carcinoma.

SUGGESTED READING

Akiyama H, Tsurumaru M, Udagawa H, et al. Radical lymph node dissection for cancer of the thoracic esophagus. *Ann Surg* 1994;220: 364–373.

Buess GF, Becker HD, Naruhn MB, et al. Endoscopic esophagectomy without thoracotomy. *Probl Gen Surg* 1991;8:478–486.

Caracci B, Garvin P, Kaminski DL. Surgical therapy of advanced esophageal cancer: a critical appraisal. *Am J Surg* 1983;146:704.

Dallemagne B, Weerts JM, Jehaes C, et al. Case report: subtotal oesophagectomy by thoracoscopy and laparoscopy. *Minim Invasive Ther Allied Technol* 1992;1:183–185.

De Paula AL, Hashiba K, Ferreira EAB, et al. Laparoscopic transhiatal esophagectomy with

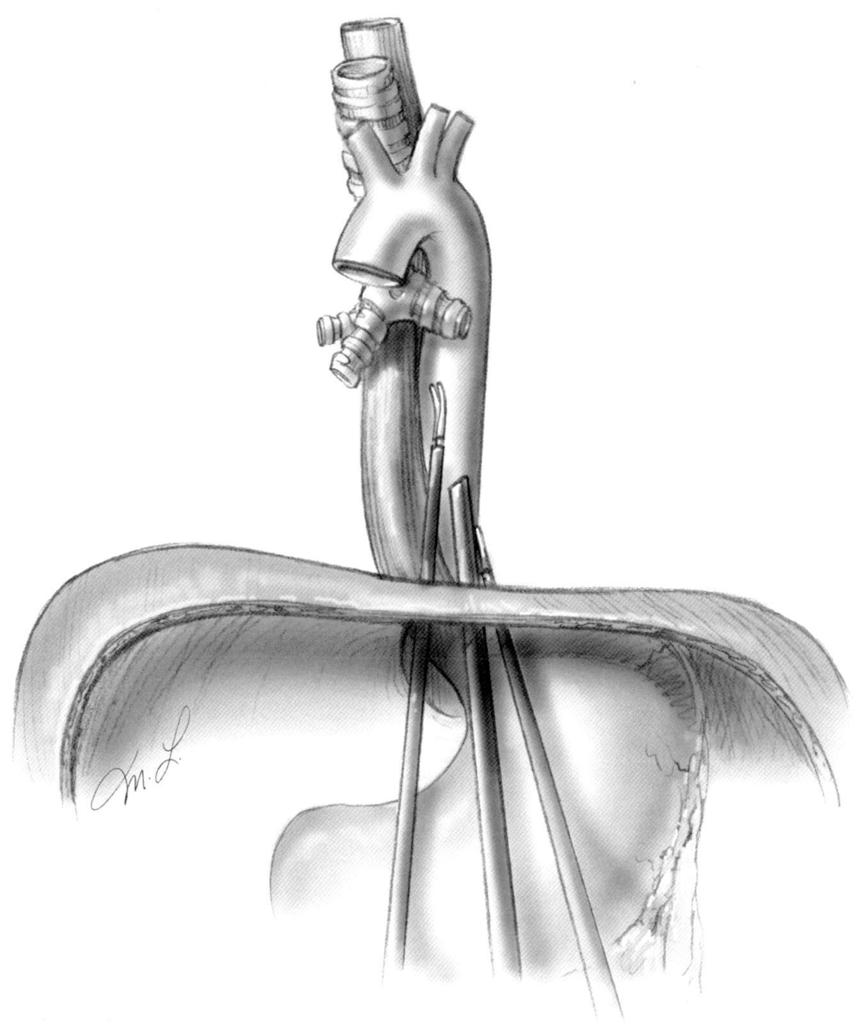

Fig. 20-9. Extra-long instruments and scopes are advanced into the mediastinum to allow direct dissection.

esophagogastroplasty. *Surg Laparosc Endosc* 1995;5:1–5.

Ferreira EAB. Esophagogastroplasty and esophagocoloplasty through the posterior mediastinum without thoracotomy: a preliminary note. *Rev Paul Med* 1974;84:142.

Hagen JA, Peters JH, DeMeester T. Superiority of extended en bloc esophagogastrectomy for carcinoma of the lower esophagus and cardia. *J Thorac Cardiovasc Surg* 1993;106:850–859.

Hankins JR, Safuh A, Coughilin TR Jr, et al. Carcinoma of the esophagus: a comparison of the results of transhiatal versus transthoracic resection. *Ann Thorac Surg* 1989;47:700–705.

Moon MR, Schulte WJ, Haasler, GB, et al. Transhiatal and transthoracic esophagectomy for adenocarcinoma of the esophagus. *Arch Surg* 1992;127:951.

Orringer MB, Stirling MC. Transhiatal esophagectomy for benign and malignant disease. *J Thorac Cardiovasc Surg* 1993;105: 265–267.

Pinotti HW, Zilberstein B, Pollara W, et al. Esophagectomy without thoracotomy. *Surg Gynecol Obstet* 1981;152:344.

Sadanaga N, Kuwano H, Watanabe M, et al. Laparoscopy-assisted surgery: a new technique for transhiatal esophageal dissection. *Am J Surg* 1994;168:355–357.

Skinner DB. En bloc resection for neoplasms of the esophagus and cardia. *J Thorac Cardiovasc Surg* 1983;85:59.

Steiger Z, Wilson RF. Comparison of the results of esophagectomy without thoracotomy. *Surg Gynecol Obstet* 1981;153:653.

Tilanus HW, Hop WCJ, Langenhorst BLAM, et al. Esophagectomy with or without thoracotomy. Is there any difference? *J Thorac Cardiovasc Surg* 1993;105:898–902.

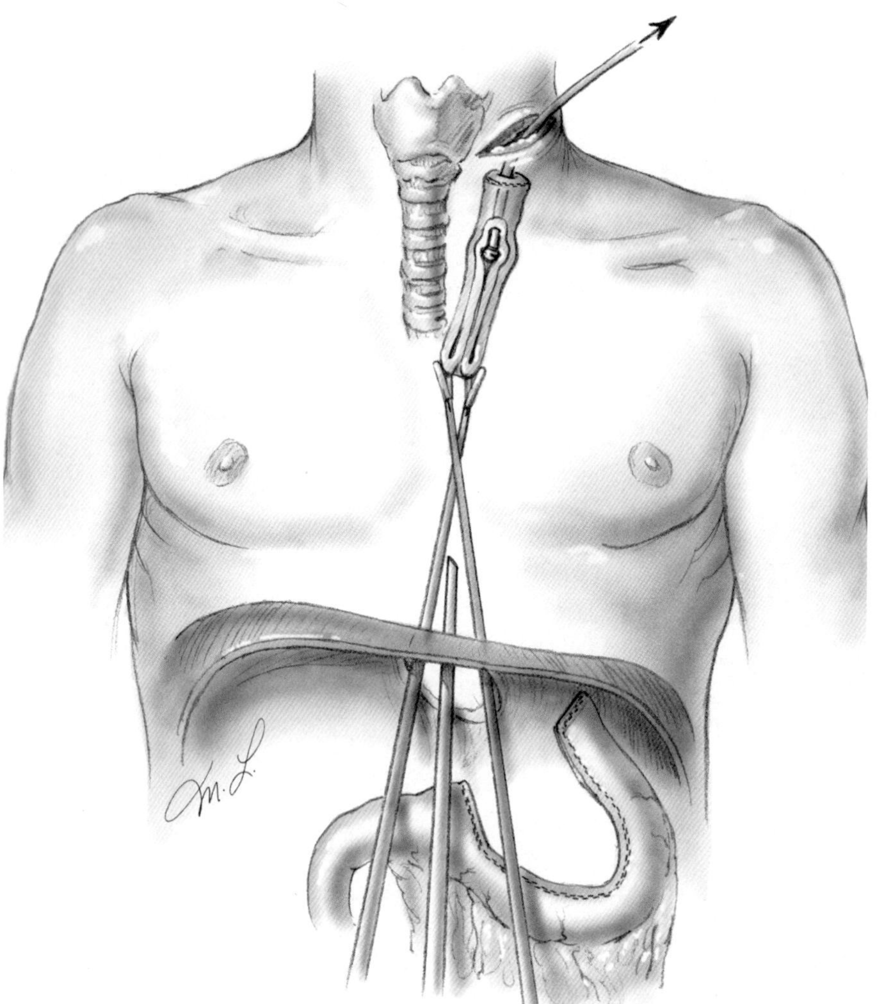

Fig. 20-10. The “inversion technique” is a good way to complete mediastinal esophageal mobilization, as it gives more working room in the mediastinum and makes it easy to identify attachments needing divided.

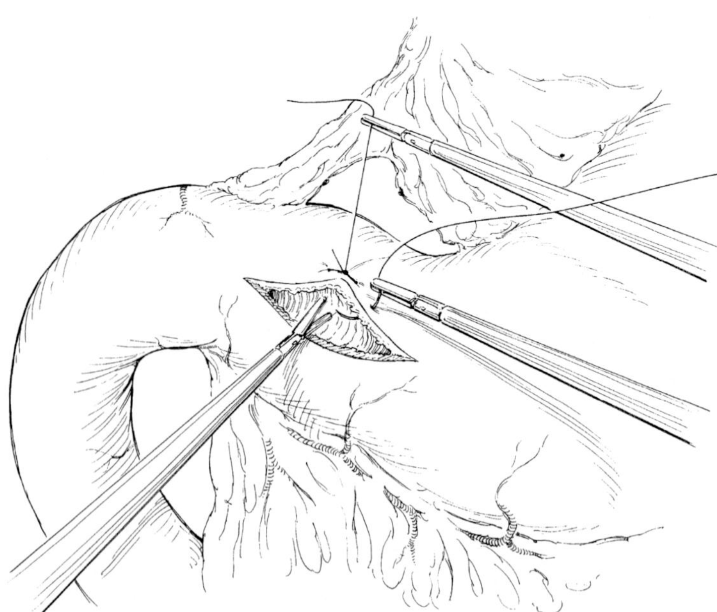

Fig. 20-11. A standard pyloroplasty is easily performed at the end of the procedure.

COMMENTARY

As emphasized by Drs. De Paula and Schraibman, esophagectomy remains a challenge to surgeons no matter what surgical approach is taken. It is clear that the postoperative outcome for patients who undergo esophagectomy is considerably affected by the magnitude of the procedure itself and not necessarily by the approach, as reflected by the significant complications with both the open and laparoscopic approaches. For cancers, in spite of recent advances in staging, adjuvant therapy, and postoperative patient management, morbidity is still high, mortality remains significant, and the 5-year survival rate continues to be poor. This has led to a nihilistic view of surgical resection for cancer in spite of the fact that surgery remains the only chance for a cure. Even for "benign" conditions such as end-stage achalasia, refractory strictures, and failed fundoplications, physicians are resistant to referring patients for esophageal resection because of the perceived morbidity of the operation and poor quality of life following reconstruction. It is therefore critical for surgeons to adopt measures to decrease mortality, minimize morbidity, address quality of life issues, and to adopt a "best treatment" multifactorial approach to esophageal cancer treatment. There are many aspects of this programmatic approach to be considered, including volume concentration through regionalization, multidisciplinary assessment, aggressive staging, post-surgical rehabilitation, early treatment of strictures and nutrition deficits, and treatment algorithms that include surgical arms. The ability to offer a minimally invasive approach to cancer resection is critical as well, as it both truly offers decreased patient morbidity and makes surgical options more palatable to patients and referring physicians.

Whether a laparoscopic transhiatal approach, as described above, or a thoracoscopic/laparoscopic approach is the best remains an unresolved question. The ideal approach for esophagectomy is a highly controversial subject even for open resections. In principle, the main advantage of transhiatal esophagectomy would be lessened morbidity for the patients, who are frequently elderly, debilitated, undernourished, and have a number of concomitant serious clinical conditions. Other advantages include shorter surgical time, less blood loss, and a lower incidence of pulmonary complications. According to most of the open literature, survival rates are similar to those obtained after transthoracic esophagectomy. Its main disadvantages when compared to the transthoracic approach have been the inability to perform en bloc node dissection, which increasingly appears to have some importance in 5-year survival for certain stages of cancers. On the other hand, we have found that the visualization offered by the laparoscope allows an excellent intraabdominal node dissection and even the opportunity for a very thorough node clearance of the lower mediastinum and sampling of the carinal nodes.

Undoubtedly someone will eventually determine which approach is better: transthoracic or transhiatal. This will not be for many years, however, due to the small numbers of cases done and the strong institutional biases. What is sure is that any serious esophageal treatment center increasingly needs to master all methods of esophageal resection—especially minimally invasive options—in order to customize the treatment to the individual patient's needs.

LLS

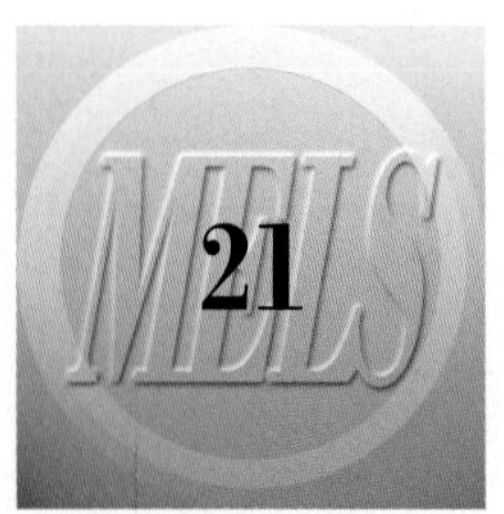

A Minimally Invasive Ivor Lewis Method for Resection of Esophageal Cancer with Curative Intent

NINH T. NGUYEN AND SAMUEL E. WILSON

INTRODUCTION

The most commonly performed open esophagectomy procedures are the blunt transhiatal esophagectomy (popularized by Orringer) and the combined abdominal and right thoracic esophageal resection (Ivor Lewis resection). Esophagectomy is considered by surgeons a complex operation associated with significant morbidity and mortality. Current reports indicate that mortality ranges from 2.5% to 6.3% after blunt transhiatal esophagectomy and from 2.5% to 9.4% after transthoracic esophagectomy. Also, postoperative mortality after esophagectomy has been reported to correlate with the annual hospital volume. Institutions with high volume of esophagectomy cases have the lowest mortality (<5%), whereas centers with a low volume have mortality up to 20%. In an attempt to reduce the morbidity and mortality associated with esophagectomy, selected centers have begun to apply minimally invasive surgical techniques. The first minimally invasive surgical approach to esophagectomy employed thoracoscopic mobilization of the mediastinal esophagus combined with a standard upper midline laparotomy for construction of the gastric conduit. Although feasible, the benefit of this technique was not readily evident.

In 1994, DePaula et al. from Brazil were the first group to describe the total laparoscopic transhiatal esophagectomy technique. Their technique was similar to that of the blunt transhiatal esophagectomy approach, but mobilization of the esophagus was performed by laparoscopic transhiatal technique under direct vision. The middle and distal esophagus was mobilized using laparoscopic instruments placed through the esophageal hiatus. The cervical esophagus was mobilized through a left neck incision. A gastric pull-up was performed with construction of a cervical esophagogastric anastomosis. The main limitation of this laparoscopic technique is the difficulty in mobilizing the midesophagus. Subsequently, Luketich et al. reported the combined thoracoscopic and laparoscopic approach to esophagectomy, otherwise known as the 3-hole technique for resection of the esophagus. The 3-hole technique consists of thoracic esophageal mobilization, laparoscopic construction of the gastric conduit, and a cervical esophagogastrostomy. More recently, Nguyen et al. reported the minimally invasive Ivor Lewis esophagogastrectomy. This approach consists of laparoscopic construction of the gastric conduit and thoracoscopic esophageal resection with thoracic removal of the surgical specimen and construction of a high intrathoracic esophagogastrostomy. This is our preferred approach for patients who have middle and distal esophageal cancer. This chapter discusses the indications for esophagectomy, preoperative planning, our preferred minimally invasive surgical approach to esophagectomy (Ivor Lewis or 3-hole technique), routine postoperative care, and complications associated with minimally invasive esophagectomy.

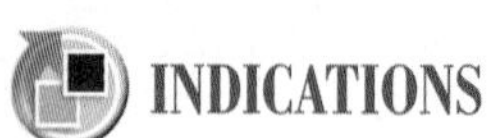

INDICATIONS

Indications for esophagectomy include both benign and malignant esophageal and gastric pathology. Benign pathology of the esophagus requiring esophagectomy includes severe recalcitrant esophageal stricture from complications of gastroesophageal reflux or lye ingestion or end-stage achalasia. The most common condition requiring esophagectomy is esophageal cancer at various stages, from carcinoma in situ to stage IV cancer. Additionally, a small number of patients undergo esophagectomy for Barrett esophagus with high-grade dysplasia. Another major indication for esophagectomy is gastric cardia cancer with involvement of the gastroesophageal junction. In this condition, an Ivor Lewis esophagogastrectomy is often performed to obtain clear proximal and distal margins.

Nonoperative treatment for esophageal cancer should be reserved for patients who refuse surgical intervention, patients who are poor surgical candidates, and patients with stage IV disease. Minimally invasive esophagectomy, although less invasive than open surgery, is rarely performed for palliation because other effective minimally invasive options are available, such as esophageal stenting and photodynamic therapy.

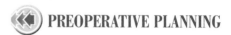

PREOPERATIVE PLANNING

Diagnostic studies for evaluation of patients with esophageal cancer include upper endoscopy with biopsy, upper gastrointestinal contrast study, computed tomography (CT) of the chest and abdomen, endoscopic esophageal ultrasound, and positron emission tomography. Esophagoscopy with biopsy is usually the first diagnostic test to confirm the diagnosis of cancer with pathologic confirmation. Endoscopy provides information on the size and site of the cancer, the presence of circumferential involvement, and the proximal and distal involvement of the cancer. The information obtained from endoscopy is critical for preoperative surgical planning. For example, cancer of the upper esophagus will require a total esophagectomy that can be performed using the minimally invasive 3-hole technique. In contrast, a distal esophagus cancer with involvement of the gastric cardia may be approached with a minimally invasive modification of the Ivor Lewis resection. An upper gastrointestinal contrast study is performed to provide a "road map" of the esophagus and give information on the site of luminal narrowing, degree and length of obstruction, and, in rare cases, presence of a concomitant tracheoesophageal fistula. A CT scan of the chest and abdomen is performed to provide an overall survey for distant metastatic disease and local-regional involvement of the cancer. Endoscopic esophageal ultrasound provides information on the depth of tumor penetration, presence of stage IV disease (involvement of thoracic aorta, trachea, or pericardium), and presence of regional lymphadenopathy. Endoscopic ultrasound can also be used to perform fine-needle aspiration of suspected lymph

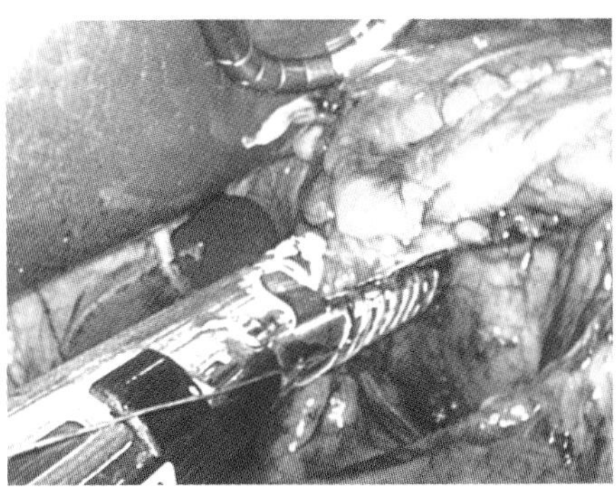

Fig. 21-1. Laparoscopic gastric ischemic conditioning, with division of the left gastric vessels at the time of laparoscopic staging.

node. A positron emission tomography scan is used to evaluate uptake and retention of radionuclides in the primary tumor, lymph nodes, and distant metastatic sites. Other preoperative workup includes pulmonary function test and cardiac stress test or two-dimensional echocardiogram, as indicated.

After completion of these diagnostic tests, laparoscopic staging is done if the patient is considered to be a surgical candidate. Laparoscopic staging consists of diagnostic laparoscopy, placement of a jejunostomy feeding tube, and laparoscopic ligation of the left gastric vessels (Fig. 21-1). Staging laparoscopy is often performed as a separate, outpatient procedure. The primary aim of laparoscopic staging is to identify patients with stage IV cancer as these patients would not benefit from a surgical resection. Additionally, ligation of the left gastric vessels is performed at the time of staging as a gastric ischemic conditioning procedure in an attempt to improve the submucosal gastric collateral blood flow of the gastric conduit. The gastric ischemic conditioning procedure has been shown to improve blood flow for the gastric conduit and may reduce the risk for postoperative anastomotic dehiscence. The jejunostomy catheter is also placed at the time of the staging procedure. Our staging procedure is often performed 1 to 2 weeks before the esophagectomy.

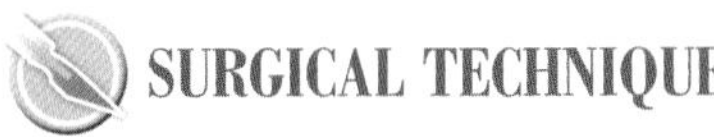

SURGICAL TECHNIQUE

Patient Setup

The patient's operative position facilitates the different minimally invasive approaches. Some surgeons begin the operation with the patient placed in a supine position and later change to a left lateral decubitus position. In contrast, the 3-hole thoracoscopic and laparoscopic esophagectomy procedure is performed first with the patient in a left lateral decubitus position and later switched to a supine position. A double-lumen endotracheal tube is necessary for both procedures and is used for selective ventilation and collapse the right lung during right thoracoscopy. Standard cardiorespiratory monitoring is used in all patients. In addition, central venous and radial arterial catheters are placed for invasive monitoring. A nasogastric tube and Foley catheter are placed, and antibiotic prophylaxis is administered. Sequential compression devices are used for prophylaxis against deep venous thrombosis.

Which Procedure?

Currently, the minimally invasive Ivor Lewis esophagogastrectomy is our preferred approach for patients presenting with benign or malignant stricture of the middle or distal esophagus and gastric cardia cancer with involvement of the gastroesophageal junction. The 3-hole thoracoscopic and laparoscopic esophagectomy technique is reserved for patients presenting with lesions of the upper esophagus requiring total esophagectomy.

MINIMALLY INVASIVE IVOR LEWIS ESOPHAGOGASTRECTOMY

First Stage

The patient is placed in a supine position and the abdomen is sterilely prepped and draped. The surgeon stands on the patient's right side, and the assistant stands on the patient's left. Abdominal insufflation is achieved, and pneumoperitoneum is maintained at 15 mmHg. Five abdominal trocars are placed (Fig. 21-2). The first trocar (11 mm) is placed at the left midclavicular line at the level of the umbilicus for the camera. A 5-mm trocar is placed at the right anterior axillary line below the costal margin and used for retraction of the left lobe of the liver. A 5-mm trocar is placed at the left anterior axillary line below the costal margin and used by the assistant surgeon. The trocars used by the surgeon include a 5-mm trocar placed at the right midclavicular line below the costal margin and a 12-mm trocar placed close to the midline above the umbilicus. The patient is placed in reverse Trendelenburg position to help with exposure by displacing the small

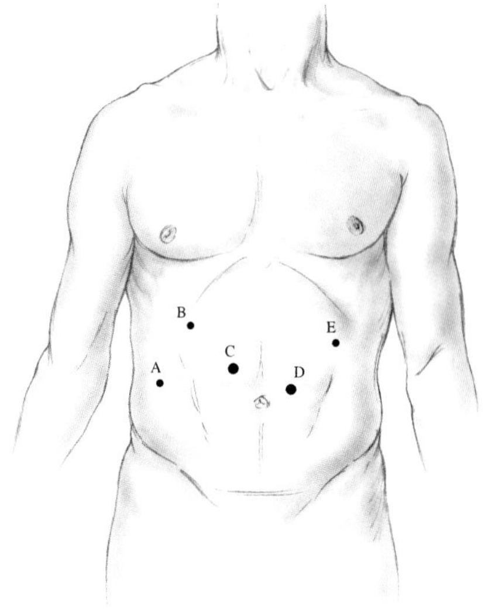

Fig. 21-2. Laparoscopic port position for minimally invasive Ivor Lewis esophagogastrectomy.

bowel and colon toward the pelvis. The operation begins with mobilization of the stomach by dividing the gastrocolic omentum. The greater curvature of the stomach is mobilized toward the first portion of the duodenum with care to preserve the right gastroepiploic vessels. The stomach is also mobilized toward the gastric fundus by dividing the short gastric vessels adjacent to the spleen. Adhesions in the posterior aspect of the stomach are divided. The hepatogastric ligament is also divided to enter the lesser sac. The left gastric vessels should have been divided previously at the time of laparoscopic staging.

Currently we perform neither pyloroplasty nor pyloromyotomy because of the relatively narrow gastric conduit (4 to 5 cm in diameter). Endoscopic linear staplers are used to construct the gastric conduit. A gray stapler (2.0-mm staple height) is used first to divide the branch of the right gastric vessels along the lesser curvature of the stomach. The next stapler is a green (4.8-mm staple height) load and is used to staple the lesser curvature of the stomach, which tends to be thicker than other areas of the stomach. A gastric tube is constructed (5 cm in diameter) based on the greater curvature of the stomach and separated from the gastric cardia near the angle of His (Fig. 21-3). Once the gastric tube is separated from the surgical specimen, the staple lines along the gastric tube are oversewn with a layer of continuous seromuscular suture. The tip of the gastric tube is sutured to the surgical specimen with three

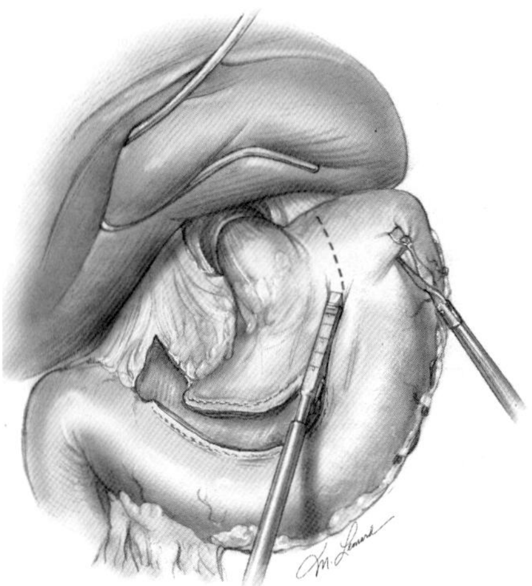

Fig. 21-3. Laparoscopic construction of the gastric conduit.

interrupted sutures (Fig. 21-4). The last portion of the abdominal dissection is mobilization of the distal esophagus through the esophageal hiatus. Once the distal esophagus is circumferentially mobilized for a segment of 5 to 6 cm, a Penrose drain is placed around the esophagus with the two ends stapled together. The Penrose drain is placed high up on the thoracic esophagus above the esophagus hiatus. For bulky esophageal or gastric cardia cancer, a portion of the left and right crus of the diaphragm can be divided to enlarge the esophageal hiatus for delivery of the surgical specimen and gastric conduit.

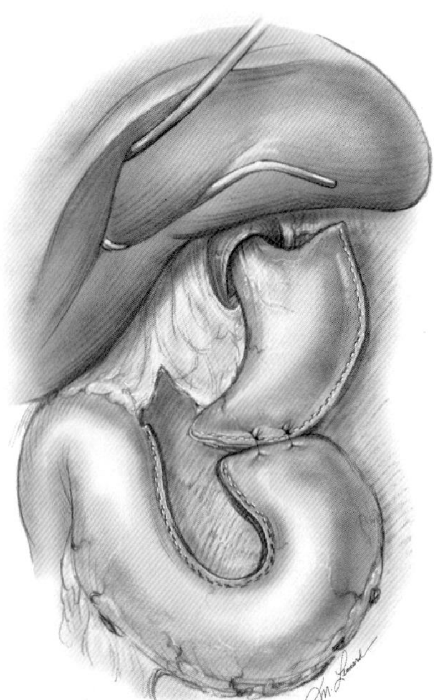

Fig. 21-4. The tip of the gastric conduit is sutured to the gastric cardia (surgical specimen) in preparation for gastric pull-up.

Second Stage

The patient is now positioned in a left lateral decubitus position on a beanbag cushion. The surgeon stands facing the patient's back. Single-lung ventilation is initiated by occluding ventilation to the right lung. A suction catheter is placed in the trachea port of the double-lumen endotracheal tube to further decompress the right lung. Four thoracic trocars are introduced into the right chest. The first trocar (10 mm) is placed at the eighth intercostal space below the tip of the scapula and used for the 30-degree camera (Fig. 21-5). The trocars used by the surgeon require a 5-mm port placed immediately posterior to the scapula and a 4-cm incision placed at the ninth intercostal space, below the posterior axillary line. The 4-cm incision is lined by a self-retractable plastic port. The last trocar (5 mm) is used by the assistant surgeon and placed at the sixth intercostal space at the anterior axillary line. Carbon dioxide insufflation is not used during thoracoscopy.

The 30-degree angled scope is used to inspect the pleural cavity and surface of the lung. A grasper is used to retract the lower lung lobes laterally to expose the inferior pulmonary ligament, which is divided with ultrasonic dissection. The mediastinal pleura overlying the esophagus is divided to expose the distal esophagus. The Penrose drain placed around the esophagus during laparoscopy is retrieved and used for esophageal retraction. The esophagus is mobilized circumferentially toward the azygous vein. The azygous vein is isolated and divided with the endoscopic linear stapler using a gray load (2.0-mm staple height) and staple line reinforcement. The esophagus is completely mobilized above the azygous vein with lymphadenectomy to remain en bloc with the surgical specimen. At the completion of thoracoscopic esophageal mobilization, the gastric cardia is pulled into the right chest, hence also pulling the gastric conduit up into the right chest. The esophageal specimen is separated from the gastric conduit. The esophagus is divided at the level of the azygous vein. A portion of the proximal margin is sent for intraoperative frozen section. The esophageal specimen is removed through the 4-cm port protected with the plastic wound retractor (Fig. 21-6). Upon confirmation of a clear proximal margin, a 25-mm anvil from the circular stapler is placed into the esophageal stump and secured with a purse-string suture. The gastric conduit is positioned with care to avoid twisting. The tip of the gastric conduit is opened with the Harmonic scalpel. The circular stapler is placed into the chest through the 4-cm port and then placed into the gastric conduit. The spike from the circular stapler is positioned through the posterior wall of the gastric conduit and connected to the anvil. A circular esophagogastric anastomosis is constructed (Fig. 21-7). The nasogastric tube is positioned into the gastric conduit under

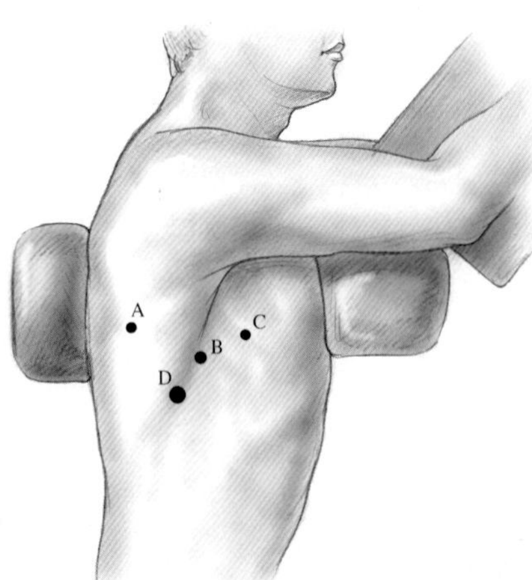

Fig. 21-5. Trocar placement for thoracoscopy during minimally invasive Ivor Lewis esophagogastrectomy.

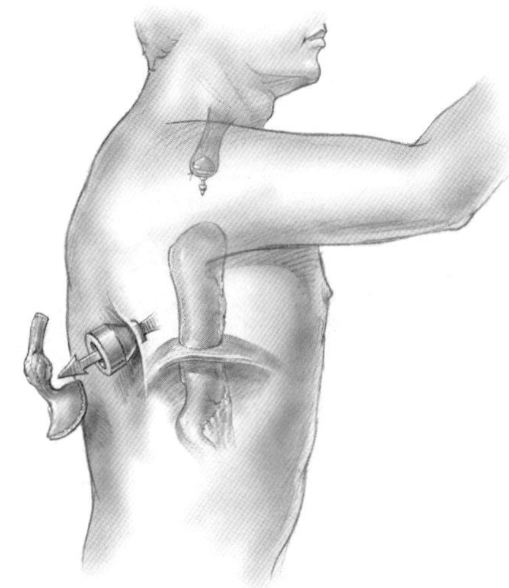

Fig. 21-6. Thoracoscopic resection of the esophagus. The surgical specimen is removed through the 4-cm thoracic port protected with a plastic wound protector. The anvil from the 25-mm circular stapler is placed within the esophageal stump and secured with a purse-string suture.

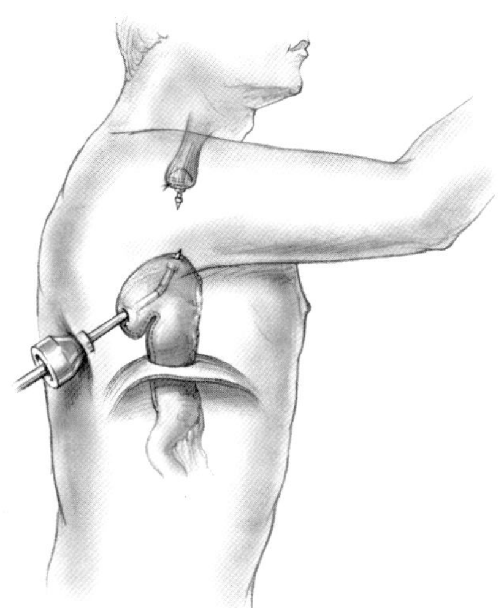

Fig. 21-7. Thoracoscopic construction of an intrathoracic anastomosis using a circular stapler. The stapler is inserted through a gastrotomy at the tip of the gastric conduit.

direct visualization. The tip of the gastric conduit is closed with a linear stapler (Fig. 21-8). The gastric staple lines are oversewn with a second layer of continuous Lembert suture. The esophagogastric anastomosis is also oversewn with multiple interrupted Lembert sutures to relieve the tension on the anastomosis. A 28F chest tube and a 10F flat Jackson-Pratt drain are placed for chest drainage. The muscle fascia is closed with multiple interrupted sutures and the skin is closed with skin staples.

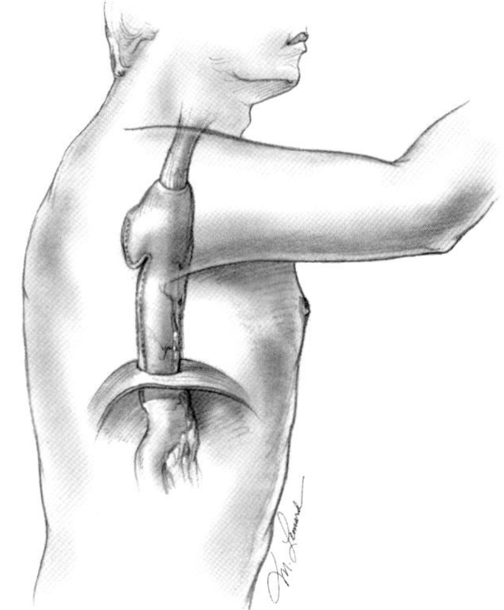

Fig. 21-8. Thoracoscopic construction of an intrathoracic anastomosis using a circular stapler. The gastrotomy at the tip of the gastric conduit is closed with a linear stapler.

Common Variation: A Three-Hole Thoracoscopic and Laparoscopic Esophagectomy

In this technique, thoracoscopy of the right chest is performed in a lateral decubitus position for mobilization of the entire esophagus with lymphadenectomy as the first step. A Penrose drain is placed around the esophagus and pushed into the neck for later retrieval. Upon completion, the chest is drained with a chest tube and closed. The patient is repositioned to a supine position. Laparoscopy is performed for construction of the gastric conduit and mobilization of the distal esophagus. The gastric conduit is sutured to the surgical specimen. A horizontal neck incision is performed above the suprasternal notch. The cervical esophagus is mobilized until the dissection plane in the neck is connected with the dissection plane achieved in the right chest. The Penrose drain placed around the esophagus during the thoracoscopic dissection is retrieved through the neck incision. Under laparoscopic guidance, the esophagus specimen is removed through the neck incision, delivering the gastric conduit into the neck. The esophagus is divided proximally, and the surgical specimen is separated from the gastric tube. A two-layer hand-sewn esophagogastric anastomosis is performed. The nasogastric tube is positioned into the gastric tube. The platysma layer is approximated with interrupted sutures, and the skin incision is approximated with staples. After completion of the neck anastomosis, the laparoscope is reinserted to inspect the abdominal cavity. The gastric conduit at the level of the esophageal hiatus is sutured to the left crus of the diaphragm with a single interrupted suture. The fascia of the 12-mm trocar is closed with interrupted sutures, and the skin is approximated with subcuticular sutures.

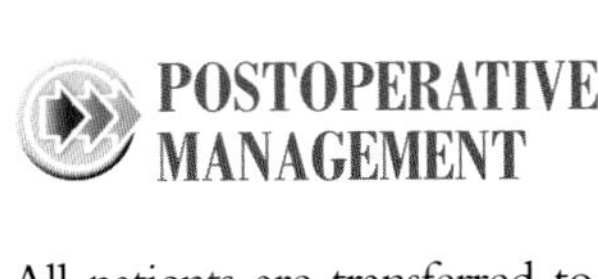

POSTOPERATIVE MANAGEMENT

All patients are transferred to the intensive care unit for observation. The chest and nasogastric tubes are placed to wall suction. Postoperative pain is managed by patient-controlled analgesia. If clinically stable, patients are transferred to the surgical ward on the first postoperative day. The patient is encouraged to ambulate on the first postoperative day. A Gastrograffin contrast study is performed on the fifth postoperative day

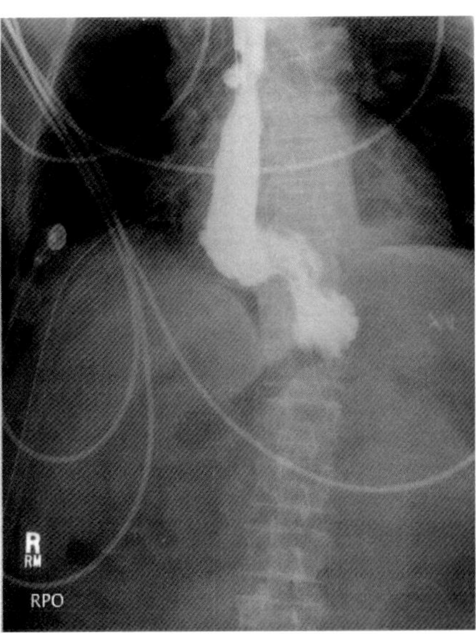

Fig. 21-9. Chest radiograph with upper gastrointestinal contrast outlining the esophagus, the anastomosis at the level of the carina, and the gastric conduit.

(Fig. 21-9). The chest and nasogastric tubes are removed if the contrast study demonstrates no leaks. Jejunal tube feeding is administered on the third postoperative day and maintained for 1 to 2 weeks. Patients are seen at follow-up 1 week after surgery, at 1, 6, and 12 months postoperatively, and yearly thereafter. A 1-year follow-up CT scan of the chest and abdomen and upper endoscopy is obtained for patients with cancer.

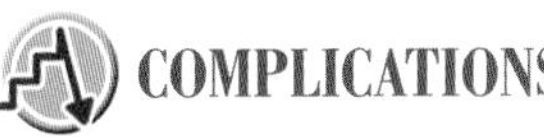

COMPLICATIONS

Intraoperative complications during minimally invasive esophagectomy are divided into complications during thoracoscopy or complications during laparoscopy. Complications during thoracoscopy include bleeding during transection of the azygous vein and potential injury to the pulmonary parenchyma, the pulmonary hilum (particularly, the inferior pulmonary vein), the trachea, and the pericardium. Complications during laparoscopy include bleeding during division of the left gastric vessels and short gastric vessels and inadvertent devascularization of the gastric conduit with interruption of the right gastroepiploic vessels.

Early postoperative complications include postoperative bleeding, atelectasis, respiratory failure, prolonged chest tube air leak, pneumonia, chylothorax, arrhythmia, myocardial infarction, deep venous thrombosis, hoarseness, urinary retention,

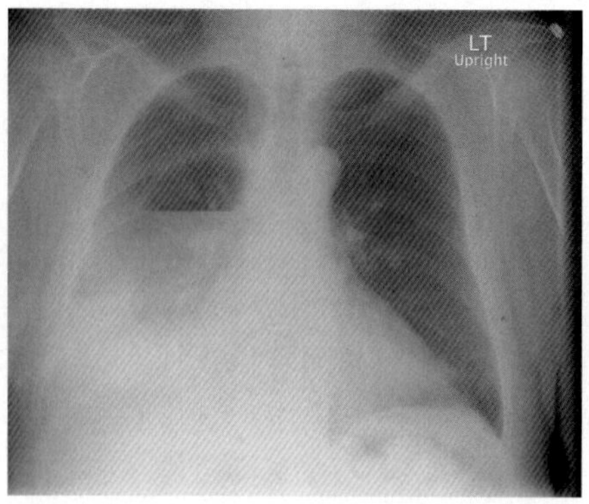

Fig. 21-10. Chest radiograph showing a large pleural effusion consistent with a leak after minimally invasive Ivor Lewis esophagogastrectomy.

anastomotic leak, and gastric conduit staple line failure. Leak is one of the most serious complications after esophagectomy, particularly if it is in the chest. In the neck, anastomotic leaks can be treated by opening of the neck wound and local wound care, whereas leaks in the chest often require complicated treatments (Fig. 21-10). Management of a thoracic leak depends on site and extent of the defect. The option for treatment includes placement of a T-tube drain through the gastrointestinal opening and wide drainage of the pleural cavity or, if a large staple-line dehiscence is encountered, proximal esophageal diversion may be necessary.

Late complications include anastomotic stricture and delayed gastric emptying. Anastomotic stricture is a frequent complication after esophagectomy, and the preferred treatment is endoscopic balloon dilation. Delayed gastric emptying is uncommon but can occur even after a pyloroplasty or pyloromyotomy. Treatment consists of endoscopic dilation of the pylorus.

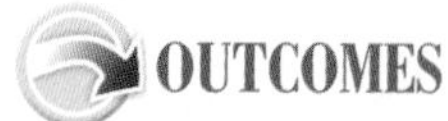

OUTCOMES

Luketich et al. have reported the largest series of minimally invasive Ivor Lewis esophagogastrectomy to date (50 patients). In 35 of the 50 cases, a minithoracotomy was utilized for construction of an intrathoracic anastomosis; the remaining 15 cases were performed using thoracoscopy. A circular stapler was used in all patients. There was one conversion during laparoscopy. Three patients (6%) developed an anastomotic leak, and all were managed nonoperatively. Four patients (8%) developed postoperative pneumonia. There were no recurrent laryngeal nerve injuries. The mortality rate was 6%.

CONCLUSIONS

Minimally invasive esophagectomy is a complex, advanced laparoscopic operation requiring knowledge of open esophagectomy and techniques of thoracoscopy and laparoscopy. There are many variations in the technique, including hybrid operations to total laparoscopic or thoracoscopic operations. Hybrid operations include thoracoscopic esophageal mobilization combined with a laparotomy, laparoscopic gastric mobilization combined with a mini-thoracotomy, or hand-assisted laparoscopic blunt transhiatal esophagectomy. Total minimally invasive esophagectomy procedures include laparoscopic transhiatal esophagectomy, combined thoracoscopic and laparoscopic esophagectomy, and laparoscopic and thoracoscopic Ivor Lewis resection. Selection of a particular minimally invasive procedure depends on the tumor's size and location, the patient's history of prior thoracic or abdominal surgery, and the surgeon's preference.

Minimally invasive esophagectomy may be best performed in centers with a large experience in esophagectomy and by surgeons with thoracoscopic and advanced laparoscopic skills. A future challenge will be exploring training and credentialing issues for surgeons interested in performing minimally invasive esophagectomy.

SUGGESTED READING

Bizekis C, Kent MS, Luketich JD, et al. Initial experience with minimally invasive Ivor Lewis esophagectomy. *Ann Thorac Surg* 2006;82:402–406.

DePaula AL, Hashiba K, Ferreira EA, et al. Laparoscopic transhiatal esophagectomy with esophagogastroplasty. *Surg Laparosc Endosc* 1995;5:1–5.

Luketich JD, Schauer PR, Christie NA, et al. Minimally invasive esophagectomy. *Ann Thorac Surg* 2000;70:906–911.

Nguyen NT, Follette DM, Roberts P, et al. Thoracoscopic management of postoperative esophageal leak. *J Thorac Cardiovasc Surg* 2001;121:391–392.

Nguyen NT, Follette DM, Wolfe BM, et al. Comparison of minimally invasive esophagectomy with transthoracic and transhiatal esophagectomy. *Arch Surg* 2000;135:920–925.

Nguyen NT, Longoria M, Chang K, et al. Thoracolaparoscopic modification of the Ivor Lewis esophagogastrectomy. *J Gastrointest Surg* 2006;10:450–454.

Nguyen NT, Longoria M, Sabio A, et al. Preoperative laparoscopic ligation of the left gastric vessels in preparation for esophagectomy. *Ann Thorac Surg* 2006;81:2318–2320.

Nguyen NT, Schauer PR, Luketich JD. Combined laparoscopic and thoracoscopic approach to esophagectomy. *J Am Coll Surg* 1999;188:328–332.

Nguyen NT, Tran CL, Gelfand DV, et al. Laparoscopic and thoracoscopic Ivor Lewis esophagectomy after Roux-en-Y gastric bypass. *Ann Thorac Surg* 2006;82:1910–1913.

Orringer MB, Marshall B, Stirling MC. Transhiatal esophagectomy for benign and malignant disease. *J Thorac Cardiovasc Surg* 1993;105:265–276.

COMMENTARY

The minimally invasive approach to esophageal resection has been clearly demonstrated to be safe and efficacious in properly selected patients. The senior author is a recognized authority in this area with significant experience with these procedures. Many surgeons rarely encounter a patient who is an appropriate candidate for this approach. However, surgeons who work in centers with high volumes of esophageal and upper gastrointestinal disease patients routinely encounter such patients. In many centers, the procedure is performed through the collaborative efforts of two teams: thoracic surgery and general MIS surgery. The techniques described in this chapter are of help to those who frequently perform MIS esophagectomy as well as a useful guide for the novice.

The authors appropriately emphasize preoperative evaluation and patient selection. Endoscopic esophageal ultrasound has taken on an increasingly important role in the evaluation of the patient with esophageal cancer. The authors present their approach as a staged procedure and describe the logic for their decisions. Staging the operation is a topic of some controversy, with vocal supporters for both sides of the argument.

The authors describe the technique for this procedure well and express strong caution regarding complications. Leakage is one of the most serious complications, and recent reports have indicated that endoscopically placed esophageal stents have resulted in healing of esophageal anastomotic leaks without further intervention. Patients receiving stent coverage of leaks must be carefully monitored for signs of sepsis or clinical deterioration.

WSE

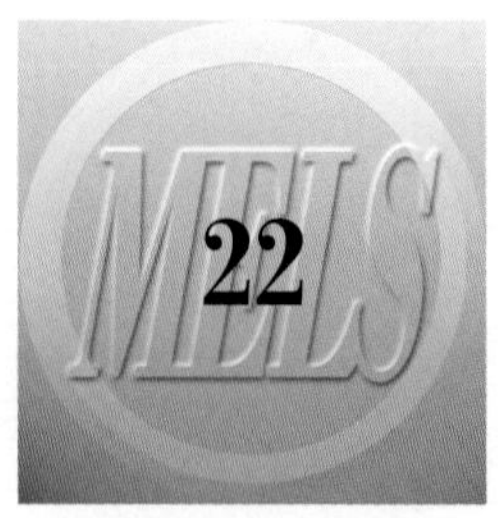

Endoscopic Palliation of Unresectable Cancers of the Esophagus

BRIAN D. LAYTON AND FREDERICK L. GREENE

INTRODUCTION

Flexible gastrointestinal endoscopy plays a major role in the treatment of malignant esophageal stricture and is currently the preferred diagnostic test for patients presenting with suspicious symptoms, having supplanted radiographic studies, which cannot provide tissue confirmation of malignancy. The ability to assess the size and location of an esophageal cancer and to provide video and photographic documentation make flexible endoscopic assessment mandatory in the development of a treatment plan for patients with esophageal cancer (Fig. 22-1). In addition to being a diagnostic tool, the flexible endoscope can be used for palliation of severe dysphagia in patients who eventually will undergo surgical resection or who are nonresectable and are treated nonsurgically using combinations of radiation, chemotherapy, and stenting.

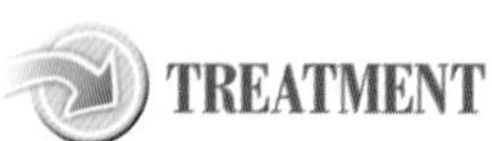

TREATMENT

Because initial symptoms can be vague dysphagia and/or weight loss, esophageal cancer is often diagnosed when advanced. Nearly 50% of patients with newly diagnosed esophageal cancer have distant metastases, and only 20% of these patients will survive 1 year. With over 14,500 new cases and over 13,500 deaths from esophageal cancer annually, it is one of the most lethal malignancies. Despite advances in the treatment of esophageal cancer, little can be done to cure it in its later stages (Fig. 22-2A to C, pages 189–191). Palliation of symptoms for these patients should be a priority of care. The goals of therapy are not based on survival but concentrate on the relief of dysphagia.

Although systemic chemotherapy and external beam radiation have a role in the treatment and palliation of late-stage esophageal cancer, the majority of palliative techniques for esophageal cancer rely on endoscopy. Endoluminal stenting, dilation, photodynamic therapy, brachytherapy, endoscopic ablation, alcohol injection, and argon plasma coagulation all rely on the use of the endoscope.

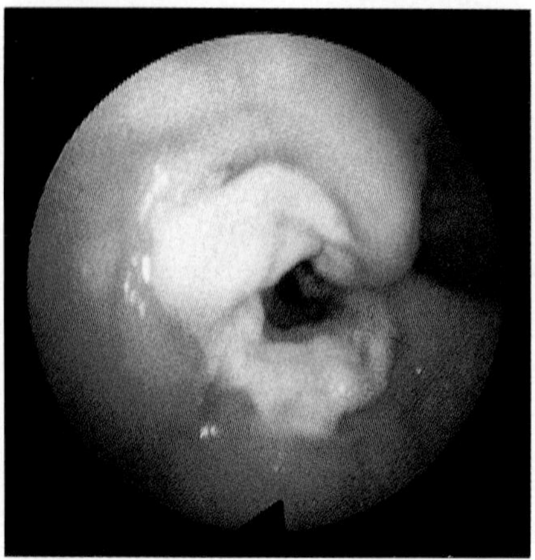

Fig. 22-1. Endoscopic view of squamous cell carcinoma of the thoracic esophagus.

Bougienage

An immediate use of flexible endoscopy during or after diagnosis is bougienage to relieve the dysphagia associated with advanced esophageal cancer. Dilation of the strictured segment may be very helpful. The principle of dilating an esophageal stricture with a bougie was introduced in the 16th century. The initial technique used a wax taper to blindly dilate the narrowed area of the esophagus. The word *bougie,* the French term for candle, is derived from the Arabic name of Boujiyah, Algeria, which was a medieval center known for its wax candle trade. Current principles of endoscopic treatment were developed more than 100 years ago when the English physician J. C. Russell introduced a balloon dilator similar to those used today. Samuel Mixter of Boston developed the concept of passing a bougie over a string, which served as a guide to avoid perforation. The patient initially swallowed the string; when the string became anchored in the small intestine, a dilating bougie was passed. Sir Arthur Hurst introduced the mercury-filled flexible bougie in 1915. More recently, rigid and flexible endoscopy were well suited to adapt the techniques of bougienage and make them safer.

Current advances in dilation include balloon techniques and tapered bougies, known as Savary-Guillard bougies, that can be safely passed over a guidewire (Fig. 22-3A and B, page 192). Strictures can occur in any area of the esophagus, but they are most common in the middle and distal segments. This corresponds to the most common locations of squamous cancer and adenocarcinoma of the esophagus. The use of dilating techniques is also appropriate in patients who have been previously treated with external-beam radiation or intracavitary techniques using high dose-rate brachytherapy, which not uncommonly causes nonmalignant strictures. Flexible endoscopy also serves as an excellent tool for performing biopsies to rule out the presence of ongoing tumors in such treated patients.

Esophageal dilation under direct visualization can be accomplished by a hydrostatic balloon system that is passed directly through the instrument channel of most flexible esophagoscopes (Fig. 22-4, page 192). Dilating balloons are available with diameters of 8 to 20 mm; however, symptom relief usually occurs with dilation to diameters of approximately 12 mm or larger. Balloons are considered safer than blindly placed bougies or even than bougies inserted with the assistance of a guidewire. This is most likely due to the fact that with dilation only radial forces are applied, compared with the fact that both radial and shearing forces occur with bougienage. The major complications remain perforation and bleeding, with complication rates of about 2%. Contrast agents can be used with balloons to confirm the location of the devices radiographically or fluoroscopically. Repeat dilation is usually needed for patients with strictures caused by tumor. Postirradiation strictures may also need redilation if dysphagia redevelops. If multiple dilations are required, one should consider the addition of a self-expanding metal stent, which will prolong the patency rate and decrease visits to the hospital for interventions.

Stenting

Intraluminal stents have been available for several decades for the palliation of esophageal cancer. Originally these stents

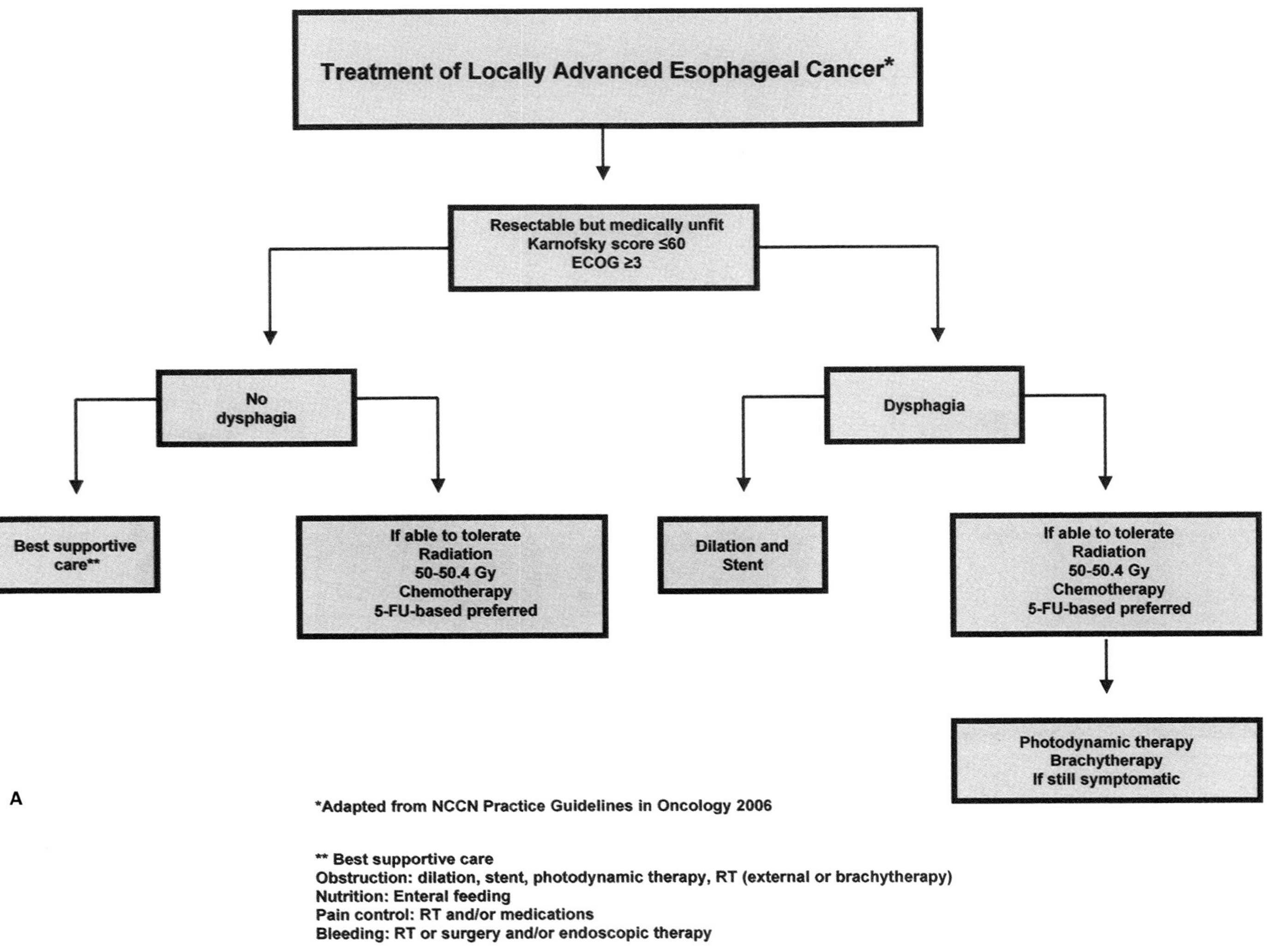

Fig. 22-2. A. Treatment algorithm for resectable locally advanced esophageal cancer when the patient is medically unfit. **B.** Treatment algorithm for locally advanced esophageal cancer. **C.** Treatment algorithm for metastatic esophageal cancer. NCCN, National Comprehensive Cancer network; RT, radiation therapy.

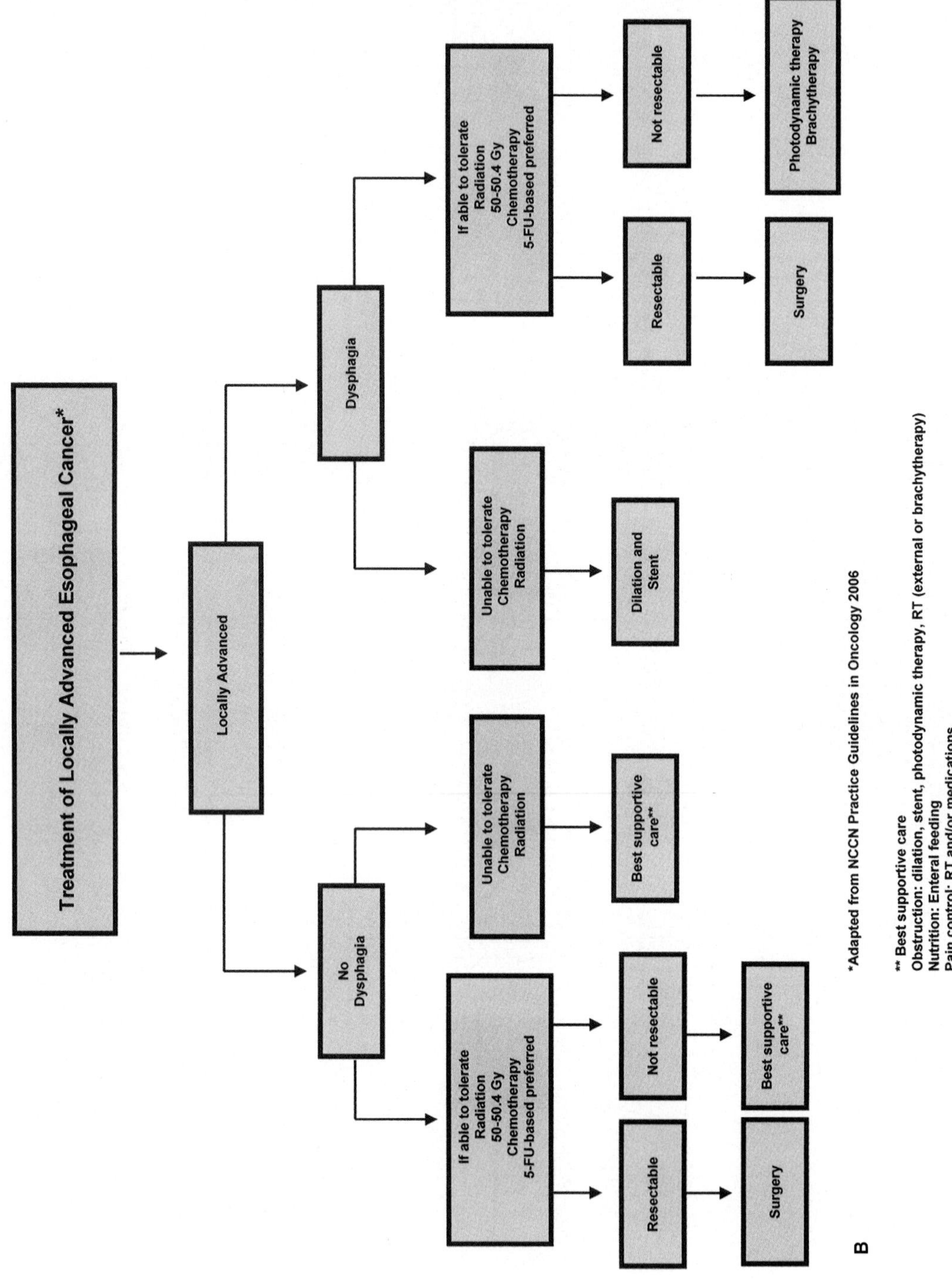
Treatment of Locally Advanced Esophageal Cancer*
Locally Advanced
No Dysphagia
Dysphagia
If able to tolerate Radiation 50-50.4 Gy Chemotherapy 5-FU-based preferred
Unable to tolerate Chemotherapy Radiation
Unable to tolerate Chemotherapy Radiation
If able to tolerate Radiation 50-50.4 Gy Chemotherapy 5-FU-based preferred
Resectable
Not resectable
Best supportive care**
Dilation and Stent
Resectable
Not resectable
Surgery
Best supportive care**
Surgery
Photodynamic therapy Brachytherapy
B
*Adapted from NCCN Practice Guidelines in Oncology 2006
** Best supportive care
Obstruction: dilation, stent, photodynamic therapy, RT (external or brachytherapy)
Nutrition: Enteral feeding
Pain control: RT and/or medications
Bleeding: RT or surgery and/or endoscopic therapy

Fig. 22-2. Continued

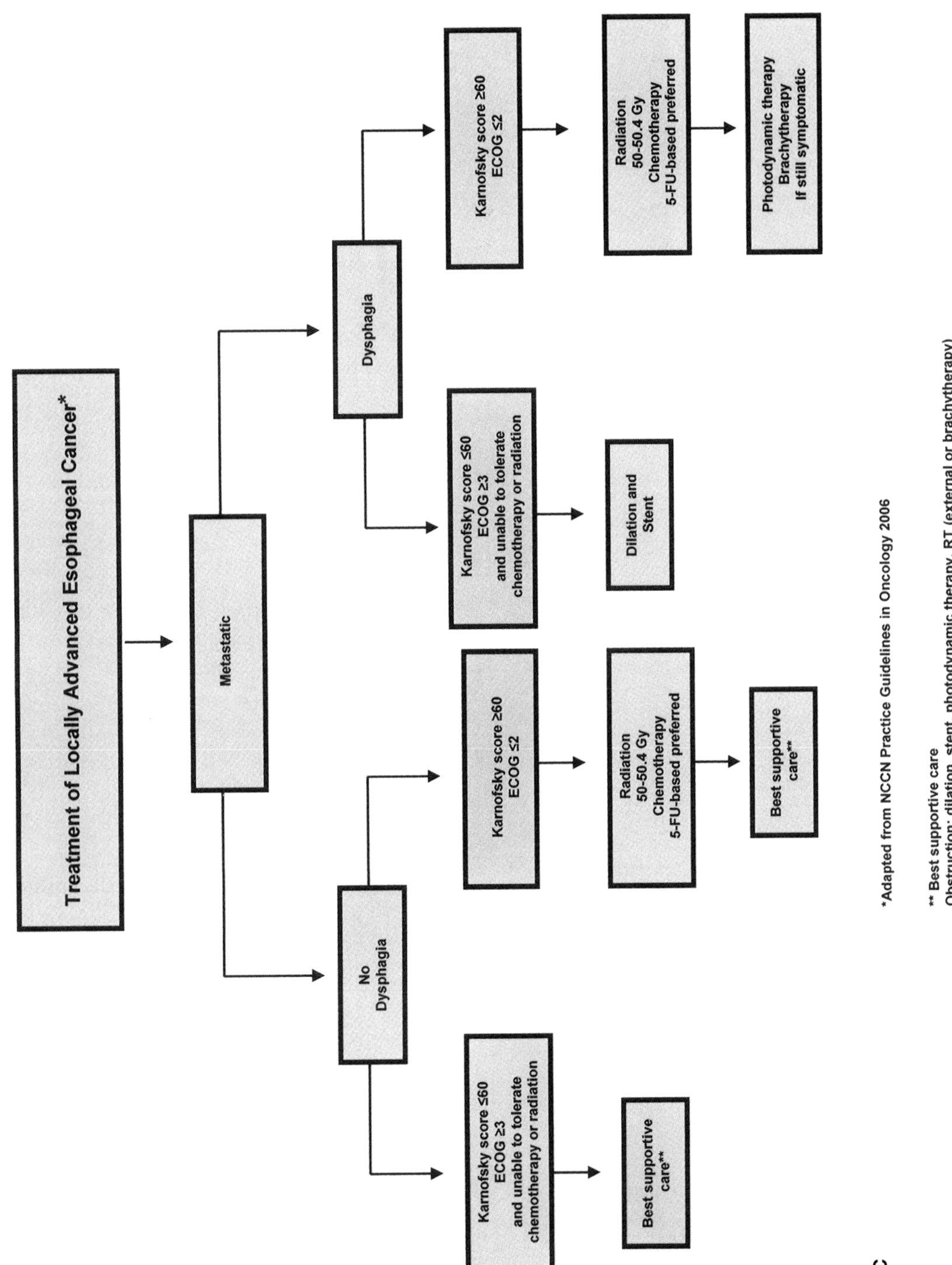

Fig. 22-2. Continued

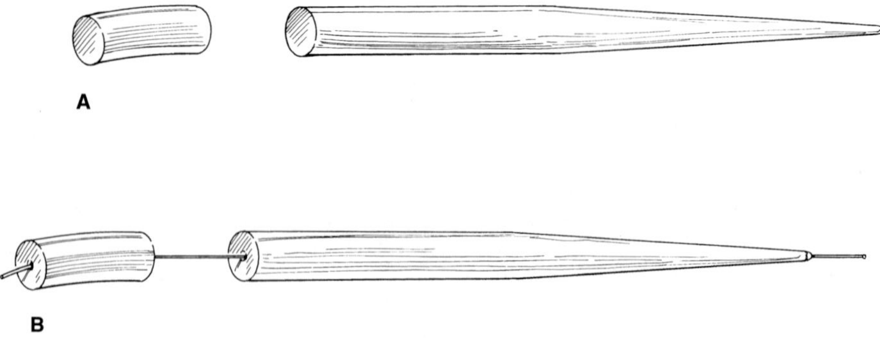

Fig. 22-3. A. A tapered bougie for blind dilation of a malignant stricture. **B.** A Savary-Guillard dilator used over a guidewire.

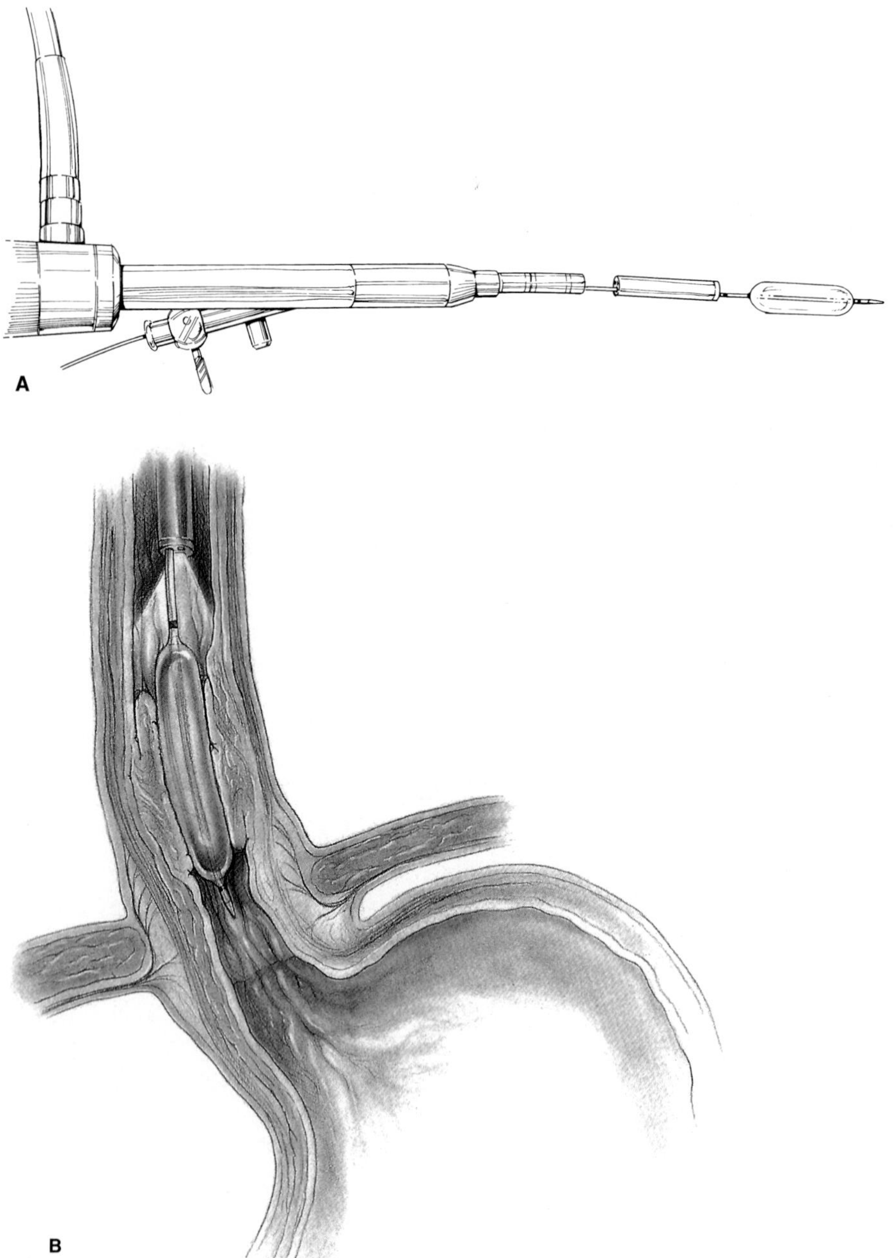

Fig. 22-4. A. A hydrostatic balloon dilator is passed through an endoscope. **B.** An expandable balloon is positioned using flexible endoscopy.

were simple rubber or plastic tubes, such as the Celestin tube. These plastic stents, which were difficult to place and became associated with high rates of perforation and migration, are no longer used. Contemporary intraluminal stents have been developed to allow safe placement utilizing flexible endoscopic techniques. Stents are useful for palliation of obstructing intraluminal tumors or relief of obstruction caused by extraluminal disease. They are packaged in a collapsed form, permitting easy placement across the esophageal tumor (Fig. 22-5). After placement they can be expanded to create a lumen, which will allow a patient to eat at least a soft diet (Fig. 22-6A and B). These stents are self-expanding and are made from metal alloys, usually titanium or nickel titanium. Stents come in either an uncovered or a covered version. Uncovered stents have a low insertion profile but are prone to tumor ingrowth and subsequent loss of the esophageal lumen. Covered stents have a thin, impermeable covering preventing tissue ingrowth. They tend to migrate more than uncovered stents but have low rates of luminal occlusion. The most recent stents are fully covered, which actually permits their endoscopic removal.

All stents are made in variable lengths, ranging from 7 to 15 cm, and a variety of diameters (typically 16 to 22 mm). The endoscope serves as the vehicle for proper stent placement, either enabling placement of a guidewire across the lesion or used adjacent to the stent to permit deployment under direct vision. Traditionally stents were placed under fluoroscopic imaging after first placing an endoscopic guidewire. More recent stents have applicators that are small enough to permit concomitant insertion of the endoscope, which allows deployment under direct vision. Dilation of the obstruction may also be needed to allow the stent deployment catheter to pass the tumor, but overdilation must be avoided as some narrowing is needed to hold the stent in place (Fig. 22-7, page 194). The stent should be of adequate length to span the distance of the stricture or tumor and should have at least 2 cm of proximal and distal overlap. This will allow for some migration and for continued tumor growth. Achieving this overlap, however, can be difficult, especially in the proximal or distal esophagus. Stenting the proximal esophagus can cause a persistent foreign body sensation or even aspiration issues. Stents placed across the gastroesophageal junction (GEJ) induce gastroesophageal reflux and

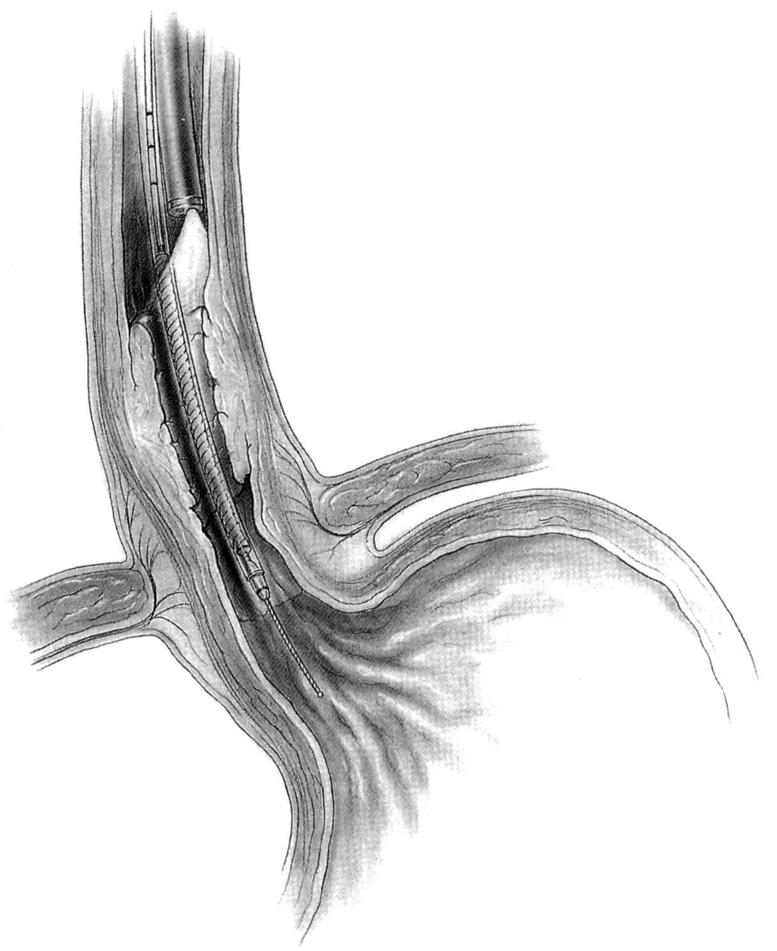

Fig. 22-5. Placement of an expandable esophageal stent with endoscopic confirmation.

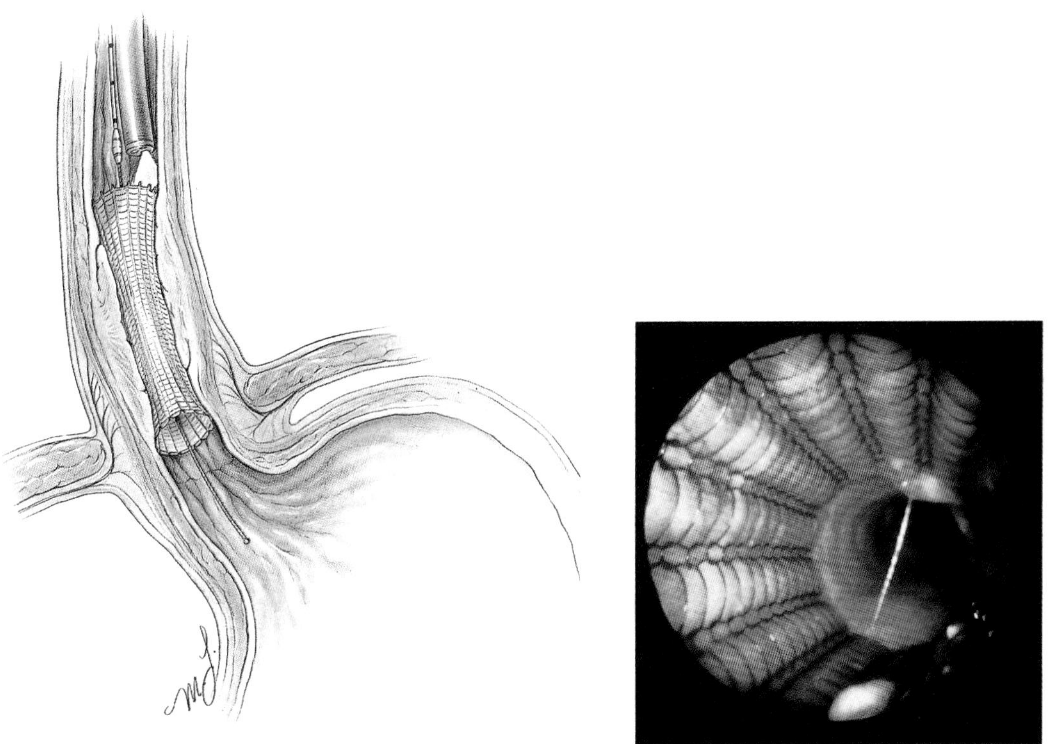

Fig. 22-6. A. Expandable stent in position. **B.** Endoscopic view of deployed metal stent.

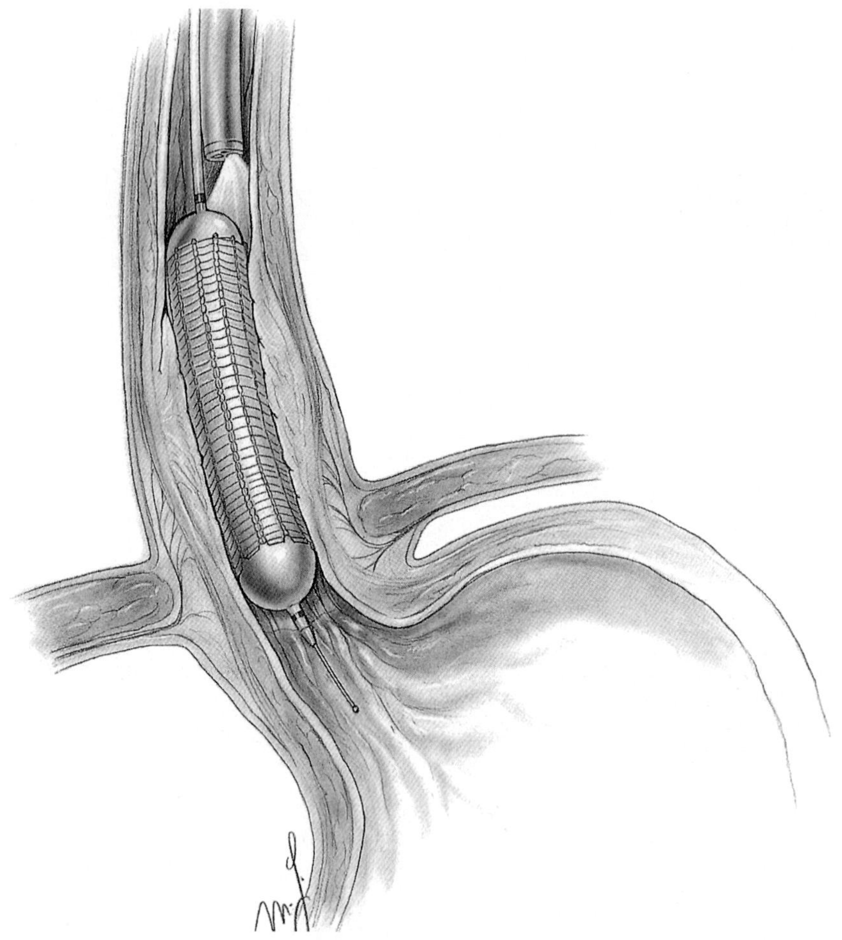

Fig. 22-7. Balloon dilation of a tumor after stent placement.

can also predispose to pulmonary aspiration. To minimize the gastroesophageal reflux caused by stents placed across the GEJ, some systems come with anti-reflux valves (Fig. 22-8). These anti-reflux systems should be considered for distal esophageal malignancies, although definitive data to support their effectiveness are lacking.

Even patients with tracheoesophageal fistulae can have covered stents placed to serve as a buttress between the esophagus and trachea to protect from chronic aspiration and pneumonia. Fistula closure can succeed in 60% to 100% of the cases in which covered stents are used to treat nonmalignant tracheoesophageal fistulae. Covered stents are coated with polyurethane or silicone, which minimizes the tumor ingrowth that can occur through woven metal stents, resulting in longer patency rates. Stenting provides effective treatment relief for malignant esophageal strictures, and, with the advent of removable (fully covered) stents, benign or post-treatment strictures can also be effectively treated, though these stents must be followed for migration and changed every 6 months as they will deteriorate. Also, when adjuvant treatments of esophageal cancer such as chemotherapy and external beam radiation are planned, one should consider alternative therapies such as photodynamic therapy instead of dilation and

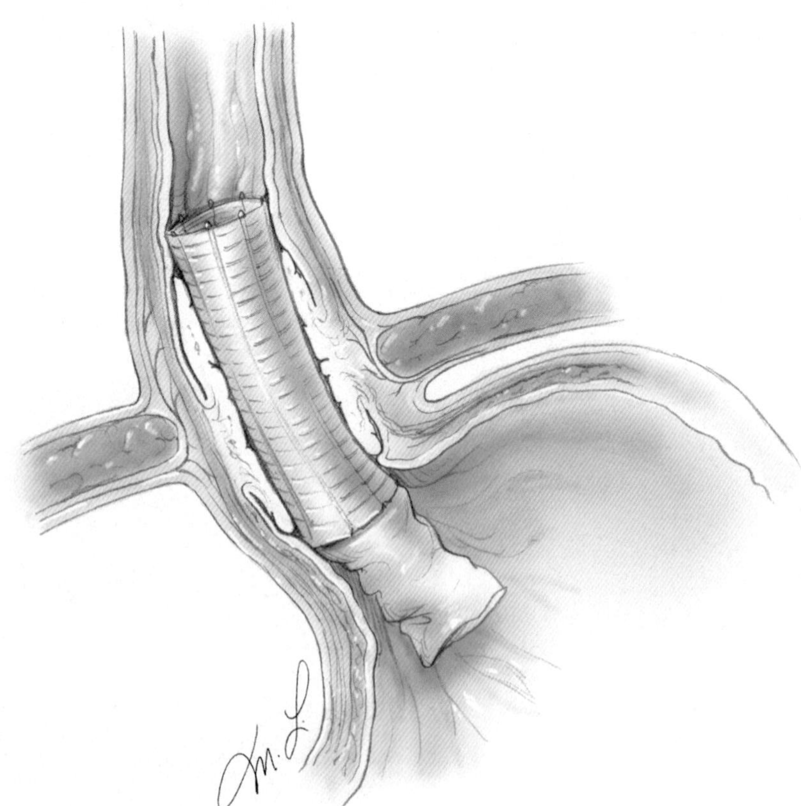

Fig. 22-8. An esophageal stent with antireflux mechanism for distal esophageal placement.

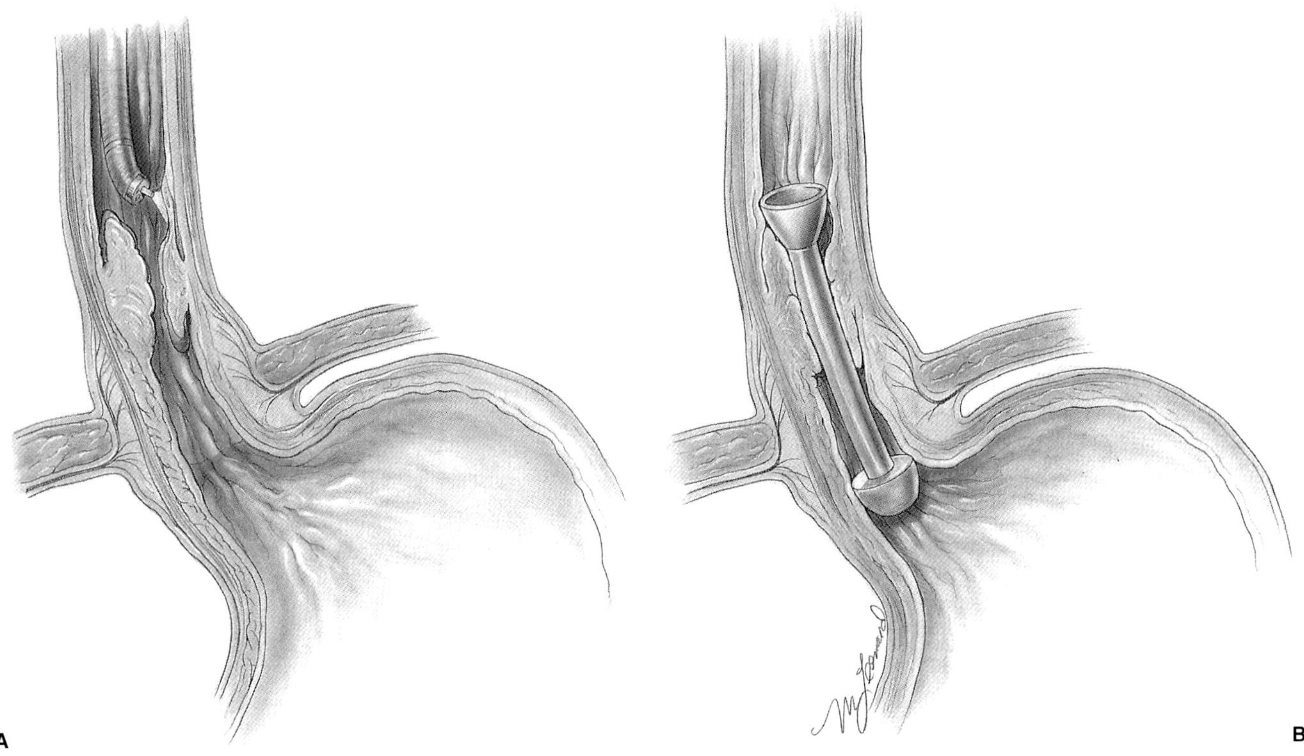

Fig. 22-9. A. Laser ablation of a circumferential esophageal tumor. **B.** A rigid endoluminal esophageal stent is placed using flexible endoscopic technique.

stenting, due to a higher incidence of complications (stent erosion). When stenting is selected following chemotherapy or radiation, several weeks should elapse before attempting to stent the esophageal stricture. Also, if a percutaneous endoscopic gastrostomy tube might be needed for nutrition, it should be placed before the stent, so the gastrostomy tube is not placed through the stent, risking displacement. Endoscopic placement of expandable stents allows patients to be treated in an outpatient setting, improving the overall quality of life for these patients, who have a short life expectancy.

Other Methods of Endoscopic Palliation

Although dilation and endoluminal stenting are the standard treatments for symptomatic strictures, other techniques can be effective for symptom relief. External beam radiation is often used for palliation of locally advanced esophageal cancer; however, median survival is still limited to about 9 months. Even with aggressive radiation fields, only 50% to 60% of patients achieve relief of dysphagia, compared with approximately 80% of those receiving stents. Time to relief is also longer, taking as long as 1 to 2 months, which may result in devastating weight loss.

Flexible upper endoscopy can also serve as a vehicle for both laser tumor ablation and the delivery of endoluminal regional irradiation. Contact ablation using a neodymium:yttrium-aluminum-garnet (Nd-YAG) laser is often effective in relieving malignant obstruction when a patient has an identifiable lumen through which the laser fiber can be passed (Fig. 22-9A). Initially, placement of a guidewire and the dilation of the esophagus may be needed before passing the laser fiber. Several applications of the contact laser may be needed to create an appropriate esophageal diameter to mitigate dysphagia. Nd-YAG lasers used through flexible endoscopes are typically set at wavelengths of 1064 nm for tumor ablation. Short pulses of the laser are used for ablation of the superficial tissue layers and can produce short-term dysphagia relief equivalent to esophageal stenting. For short (less than 5 cm) lesions, laser treatment can even be superior to stenting because of lower morbidity and cost. However, symptom relief can be short, due to tumor regrowth. For longer (greater than 5 cm) lesions, stenting is almost always superior to Nd-YAG laser treatment. Stenting may be used after laser ablation.

Recently, a combined external-beam radiation and endoluminal radiation utilizing flexible endoscopic technique has facilitated palliation of malignant strictures. Patients can generally be treated as outpatients and seldom require general anesthesia. The technique involves placement of a guidewire through the flexible endoscope to guide the passage of a 16F plastic tube. This tube serves as an afterloading receptacle for either iridium or cesium seeds, which can deliver 500 to 1000 rads (5 to 10 Gy) of radiation energy to an isolated area of the esophageal tumor. This technique has the advantage of avoiding radiation effects to adjacent lung tissue and surrounding structures, which are often damaged by external-beam therapy. The endoscopist must work closely with the radiation oncologist to ensure that the afterloading device is placed at the appropriate level to encompass the entire length of the esophageal tumor and to allow calculation of the dosimetry. A postendoscopy chest X-ray must be obtained before application of radiation to ensure appropriate placement of the afterloading device. High-dose brachytherapy is not often used. This treatment requires multiple endoscopies and weekly treatments, has shorter symptom-free survival, and involves longer delays to symptom relief. Side effects such as esophagitis and back pain are common. Strictures, perforation, and fistulae have also been documented following brachytherapy.

Photodynamic therapy, another technique of palliation for malignant strictures, is becoming more widely used as treatment for early esophageal neoplasms and dysplastic Barrett changes, but it also has utility in the symptomatic treatment of advanced esophageal lesions. Photodynamic therapies are ablative techniques that use an oxidative reaction within the cancer cells, which ultimately leads to cytotoxic activity. A photosensitizing agent such as porfimer sodium is administered 48 hours before exposure to short wavelengths of light. The light induces necrosis of the tumor over the next 2 to 3 days. The patient undergoes endoscopy again, and necrotic tissues are debrided. Symptom relief occurs about a week after treatment and can last up to 3 months. Side effects are chest pain, increasing dysphagia, fevers, light sensitivity, and light reactions. To minimize these reactions, patients are cautioned to avoid sunlight and bright lights for several weeks after the administration of the porfimer sodium. The perforation rate is lower with photodynamic therapy than with other treatments, while having similar efficacy and dysphagia-free survival; however, long-term relief is similar to other non-stenting techniques. Photodynamic therapy can also be used to treat tumor growth at the ends of a previously placed esophageal stent or as salvage therapy for recurrent disease after chemoradiation.

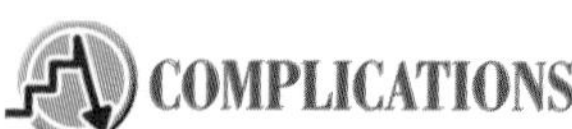

COMPLICATIONS

Palliation of carcinoma of the esophagus using endoscopic techniques has significant risk of complications including perforation, bleeding, migration, stent erosion, fistula formation, obstruction, chronic reflux, and aspiration, particularly when attempted by endoscopists inexperienced in their use. Passage of endoscopes or instrumentation through areas of narrowed friable tumor inevitably risks perforation. Optimally, direct visualization of the lumen is maintained at all times, though this can be difficult with fungating obstructing tumors. Use of dilators also compounds the risk of complication, particularly bleeding or perforation. Dilation with guidewire or balloon dilators is optimal in this high-risk group. Lasers or thermal devices can easily perforate the esophagus, which can be difficult to identify at the time of treatment. These potential complications also apply to endoscopic stent placement. It is important to obtain a chest film following any manipulation of an esophageal tumor to look for air extending outside the esophageal lumen. Fluoroscopy during these procedures and X-ray confirmation following stent placement with or without dilation are mandatory to minimize perforation.

Late recurrence of dysphagia after palliative treatment can be from tumor growth, stent displacement or non-cancer strictures, especially after intracavitary irradiation. Follow-up esophagoscopy will identify the cause and retreatment can be performed to re-establish the patency of the lumen. Even if a stricture appears benign, a biopsy should be performed to exclude the possibility of a local recurrence, which can have a subtle appearance particularly after radiation.

CONCLUSION

The flexible endoscope is an important diagnostic and therapeutic tool, both for assessing patients with esophageal cancer and for palliating obstructive symptoms caused by this disease. In patients who have undergone esophageal resection, endoscopic surveillance of the remaining esophagus or the esophagogastric or esophagocolic anastomosis is appropriate and may identify early recurrent disease. Techniques such as dilation and stenting can be used when anastomotic strictures occur and for palliation for patients with malignant processes.

SUGGESTED READING

Adams DB. Endoscopic management of esophageal stricture. In: Greene FL, Ponsky JL, eds. *Endoscopic surgery*. Philadelphia: WB Saunders, 1994:36–54.

Adler DG, Merwat SN. Endoscopic approaches for palliation of luminal gastrointestinal obstruction. *Gastroenterol Clin* 2006; 35:65–82.

Alexander P, Mayoral W, Reilly HF, et al. Endoscopic Nd:YAG laser with aggressive multimodality therapy for locally advanced esophageal cancer. *Gastrointest Endosc* 2002; 55:674–679.

American Society for Gastrointestinal Endoscopy. Photodynamic therapy for gastrointestinal disease. *Gastrointest Endosc* 2006; 63:927–931.

Christie NA, Patel AN, Landreneau RJ. Esophageal palliation-Photodynamic therapy/Stents/Brachytherapy. *Surg Clin North Am* 2005;85:569–582.

Greene FL, Boulware RJ, Bianco J. Role of esophagogastroscopy in application and follow-up of high-dose-rate brachytherapy (HDRB) for treatment of esophageal carcinoma. *Surg Laparosc Endosc* 1995;5: 425–430.

Jacobson BC, Hirota W, Baron TH, et al. The role of endoscopy in the assessment and treatment of esophageal cancer. *Gastrointest Endosc* 2003;57:817–822.

Tierney W, Chuttani R, Croffie J, et al. Enteral stents. *Gastrointest Endosc* 2006;63: 920–926.

Weigel TL, Frumiento C, Gaumintz E. Endoluminal palliation for dysphagia secondary to esophageal carcinoma. *Surg Clin North Am* 2002;82:747–761.

COMMENTARY

There is no greater gift a surgeon can give to a patient with an incurable gastrointestinal cancer than to provide them with effective palliation. Ideally this would be provided on an outpatient basis and provide for long-lasting relief. For esophageal cancers, palliation is primarily a matter of maintaining the luminal patency of the esophagus, both to allow the patient to continue to eat and to prevent the misery of being unable to control one's secretions. As described in this chapter, flexible endoscopy represents an ideal way to approach these goals—at least for the majority of presentations of endstage esophageal cancers. There are limitations to the palliation that can be provided, though. Obstructive symptoms due to late cancers can be a result of exophytic tumor growth, post-treatment strictures, or extrinsic compression from mediastinal tumor metastases. The latter is certainly the most difficult to treat with endoluminal approaches, although stenting certainly can play a role. For the most part, mediastinal disease is best treated with chemotherapy and radiation when possible. As pointed out by the authors, endoluminal treatments have changed over the last decade: direct ablation has pretty much given way to the use of stents. This is a result of improvements in stent technology including smaller introducers, covered stents, and the latest advance, fully lined ("removable") stents. Removable stents are an important improvement as they allow the stents to be repositioned at the time of placement and to be removed at any time if they are not tolerated. While endoscopic palliation is by far the most commonly used modality, it should be kept in mind that in rare instances esophagectomy offers the best palliation—primarily in cases of uncontrollable bleeding or when the lumen is totally obliterated.

Decisions about palliative care need to take into account the patient's wishes and should always involve the family as well. At some point, the surgeon has to recommend that no further efforts be made even if it is technically feasible. For endoluminal palliation this point often comes when the probability of complications from the intervention, particularly perforation or stent erosion, exceeds the potential for improving the patient's remaining quality of life.

LLS

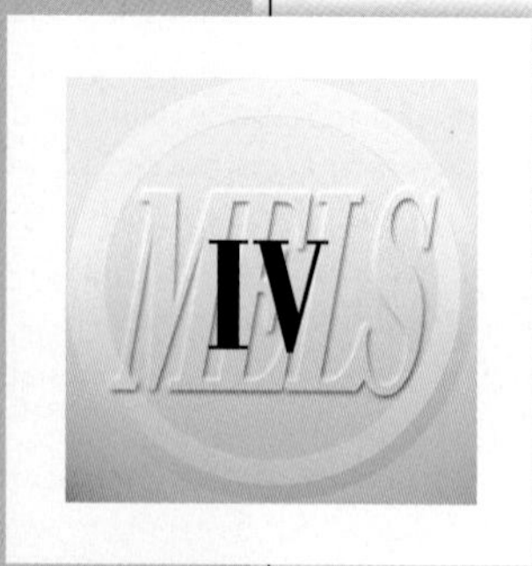

IV Gastric Diseases and Procedures

A. Benign Disorders

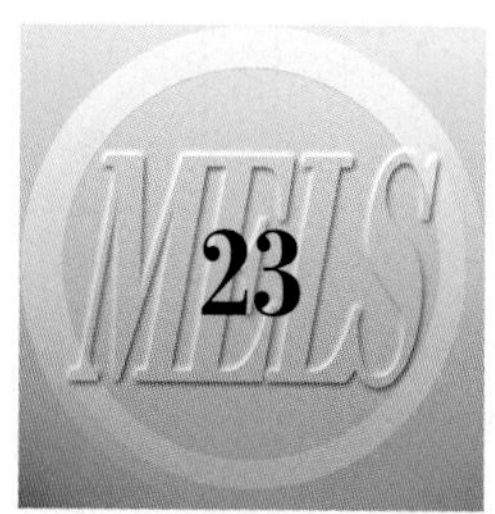

23 Flexible Endoscopy for Diagnosis and Treatment of Benign Gastric Disorders

SAMUEL SZOMSTEIN AND PETER F. LALOR

INTRODUCTION

Flexible endoscopy has dynamically altered the diagnosis and management of gastrointestinal disease in the 21st century and provides the clear foundation for the future of minimally invasive procedures. Esophagogastroduodenoscopy (EGD) screening and intervention is definitively the standard of care for many upper gastrointestinal (GI) disorders. Over 5 million EGDs are performed annually, offering not only an outpatient diagnostic experience but also a potential therapeutic opportunity. EGD is a challenging procedure in which success and safety depend upon a thorough understanding of the instruments and their limitations, the indications and risks of the procedure, and the recognition and treatment of endoluminal pathology.

EGD is a comprehensive tool that, when used in combination with radiological imaging, provides a thorough evaluation of the upper GI tract. Furthermore, EGD allows biopsy and brushings of tissue, foreign body removal, direct control of bleeding, and stricture dilatation, all under direct vision. The experienced endoscopist will develop a personal technique for accessing and navigating the GI tract in a safe and all-inclusive manner. Endoscopic interventional skills are also mandatory in effectively treating a variety of symptomatic GI disorders. Benign disorders of the stomach are commonly encountered during EGD. The knowledge, recognition, and treatment of these findings are vital to every endoscopist's repertoire.

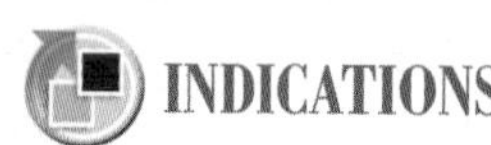

INDICATIONS

Upper endoscopy is a relatively safe procedure, but determining whether or not the examination is appropriately indicated is an important decision. Indications for EGD can be divided into diagnostic, surveillance, and therapeutic (Table 23-1).

Diagnostic EGD is performed for symptomatic patients who have not improved with medical or surgical treatment. These symptoms include heartburn, acid reflux, and epigastric or chest pain, which may reveal peptic or gastric ulcer disease. EGD is also indicated when malignancy is suspected. Symptoms of pain, weight loss, or melena may suggest adenocarcinoma of the foregut. EGD is warranted when there is any evidence of acute or chronic upper GI bleeding manifested by hematemesis, melena, or hematochezia. Localizing bleeding in the upper GI tract is crucial to endoscopic or surgical treatment options. EGD is also indicated for chronic symptoms of dysphagia, odynophagia, pain, malabsorption, or unexplained nausea, vomiting, or diarrhea. Any imaging study demonstrating pathology or studies equivocal for disease in the upper GI tract may indicate EGD evaluation.

Surveillance EGD is generally used to screen for malignancy in high-risk patients, tumor recurrence, and assessment

TABLE 23-1. INDICATIONS FOR ESOPHAGOGASTRODUODENOSCOPY (EGD)

Diagnostic

- Persistent upper abdominal symptoms despite an appropriate trial of therapy
- Refractory gastroesophageal reflux disease (GERD)
- Confirmation and histologic diagnosis of radiologically suspected or demonstrated lesions such as:
  - ⋆ Ulcer
  - ⋆ Neoplasia
  - ⋆ Stricture
- Gastrointestinal bleeding
- Caustic ingestion
- Sampling or biopsy of tissue
- To rule out malignancy

Surveillance

- To rule out malignancy in high-risk patients
- Follow-up after previous medical or endoscopic therapy
- To rule out erosions in gastric band surgery/banded bypass pouch

Therapeutic

- Removal of foreign body
- Removal of selected polyposis lesions
- Dilatation of strictures
- Treatment of bleeding lesions (ulcers, tumors, vascular abnormalities)
- Banding or sclerotherapy for varices
- Placement of feeding tube or drainage tube
- Miscellaneous
  - ⋆ Management of achalasia
  - ⋆ Endoluminal GERD treatment

of therapy. Patients with pernicious anemia, atrophic gastritis, prior partial gastrectomy, or gastric ulcers are at elevated risk for developing gastric adenocarcinoma. Follow-up EGD is recommended for annual evaluation in bariatric patients to assess for gastric band erosions.

Therapeutic upper endoscopy is most commonly utilized in the setting of acute upper GI bleeding where emergent EGD is required. Resuscitation and hemodynamic stability are mandatory prior to endoscopic evaluation. Peptic ulcer disease and acute gastric mucosal lesions account for two-thirds of endoscopically diagnosed bleeding sources. Variceal bleeding may also warrant acute intervention or may be prophylactically addressed in candidates undergoing liver transplant. Stricture dilatation is used to treat achalasia, esophageal strictures, or postsurgical strictures after gastric resection or bariatric procedures with gastrointestinal anastomosis. Any suspicious lesions, ulcers, or polyps should be biopsied or snared.

CONTRAINDICATIONS

EGD should be contraindicated in cases of confirmed or suspected perforation or peritonitis. Severe hypotension, respiratory distress, coagulopathy, hypoxemia, sepsis, or shock are all contraindications for EGD until these conditions are markedly improved or resolved; an inadequate environment such as an uncooperative patient, inappropriate sedation, or lack of trained personnel should preclude the endoscopist from performing an EGD. Other relative contraindications include recent myocardial infarction or upper GI surgery, pregnancy, obstructing lesion, severe trauma, and Zenker's diverticulum. The risk-benefit ratio should always be considered for each patient before attempting an EGD.

EQUIPMENT

There is a variety of flexible endoscopes based on diameter, length, and visualization. A standard upper endoscope has a 0-degree forward view and is 10 mm in diameter and 120 cm in length. Side-viewing endoscopes are usually reserved for visualization of the ampulla of Vater. These endoscopes are advanced blindly during access to the posterior pharynx and through the esophagus, providing limited evaluation. All endoscopes are either video or fiber-optic and have a control head with common components. Fiber-optic instruments contain an eyepiece for direct viewing or may be connected to a video attachment. The shaft of the endoscope is usually 110 to 120 cm in length with a diameter between 5.5 and 11 mm. Therapeutic endoscopes and duodenoscopes are larger and may expand to 12.5 mm in diameter.

The distal tip of the shaft is the most flexible area and is maneuvered by two knobs on the control head. The inner knob produces up and down deflection ranging between 90 and 240 degrees. The smaller, outer knob allows 100-degree deflection in both the right and left direction. Both knobs have a locking mechanism, if necessary. The anterior aspect of the control head also holds two depressible buttons. The top button controls suction, and the lower button adds either air insufflation or saline irrigation. Covering the lower button without pressure provides air insufflation, while depressing the button releases irrigation for clearing the field of view or cleaning the lens tip. All flexible endoscopes require a light source that is either a 300-watt xenon arc lamp or a halogen-tungsten lamp. The light source unit incorporates the video connection as well as the air and water pumps. Insufflation, irrigation, and suction can then be accessed using the control buttons. Video endoscopes also have two smaller buttons on the superior aspect of the control head that may freeze images on the video screen or save images for printing.

Most endoscopes contain a working channel for interventions. Biopsy forceps, cytology brushes, balloon dilators, snares, baskets, and hemostatic instruments can all be passed separately through this accessory channel. The working channel diameter ranges from 2 mm in pediatric endoscopes to 4.2 mm in duodenoscopes. The standard therapeutic gastroscope has a 3.7-mm instrument channel. For advanced therapeutic endoscopy, a double-lumen working channel is also available.

Optimizing hand positioning on the control head and the shaft facilitates a thorough examination. The control head is usually manipulated in the left hand with the thumb managing the up/down inner knob and the first two fingers working the air/water buttons (Fig. 23-1, page 200). The right hand is reserved for advancing, withdrawing, and rotating the flexible shaft. For better control of the deflectable tip, the left hand with control head may be lowered to the mouth and used to stabilize the shaft while the right hand works

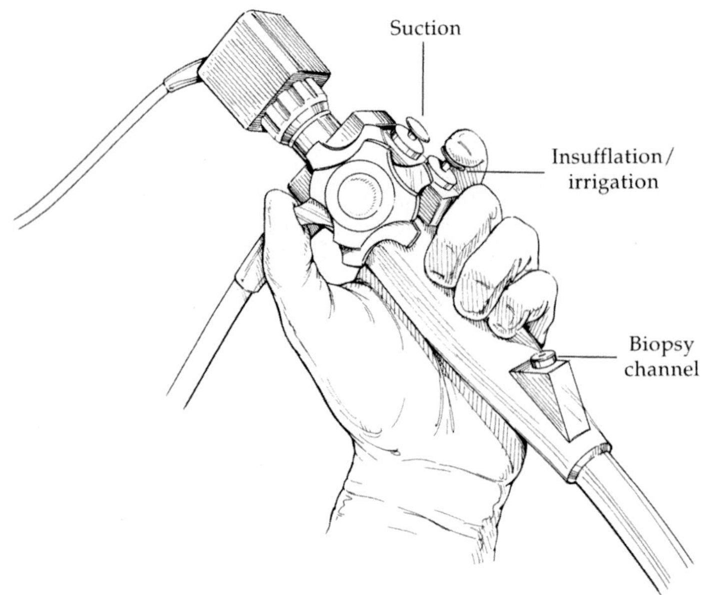

Fig. 23-1. Controls of a modern video upper endoscope.

the outer and inner knobs. Stabilization is not always needed when the endoscope has been far enough advanced.

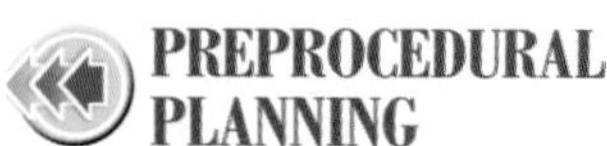

PREPROCEDURAL PLANNING

Every endoscopy begins with a thorough evaluation of indications for the procedure based on a complete assessment of the patient's history and radiological studies. Personal review of any contrast studies may delineate altered anatomy and may warn the endoscopist of any pitfalls, such as tight strictures or an esophageal diverticulum. Ideally, this analysis is performed in the initial office or clinic visit, and the patient's chart and films then arranged to accompany the patient for the EGD.

Written, signed, and witnessed informed consent is obtained after relating possible complications and giving the patient ample opportunity to ask questions. A successful patient-doctor relationship involves fulfilling the patient's expectations of the procedure. Symptomatic patients expect the endoscopist to find the problem and treat it. Thus, it is important to describe the possibility of normal findings in diagnostic procedures, and also the possibility of a failed therapeutic intervention or an inadequate tissue diagnosis from biopsy. Prehospital and postprocedure written instructions should be given to the patient in advance. These include continuing any necessary antihypertensive or antiarrhythmic medications through to the procedure date but restricting any oral food or liquid intake for 8 hours prior to EGD. Diabetic patients should adjust their oral hypoglycemic or insulin regimens to compensate for fasting. Patients should plan on arriving to the hospital at least one hour before the scheduled procedure time. Patients undergoing sedation should always be instructed to bring a companion or family member that can safely escort them home postprocedure.

Laboratory blood work is not routinely indicated for elective endoscopy. Only patients with a history of coagulopathy or taking anticoagulant agents such as warfarin may require a coagulation profile. Patients are instructed to stop taking aspirin, non-sterile anti-inflammatory drugs (NSAIDS), anticoagulants (warfarin, Lovenox) and antiplatelet agents (clopidogrel) for up to 2 weeks prior to the procedure. Any medication that adversely affects hemostasis should be withheld. Injectable prophylactic deep vein thrombosis medications (heparin, low-molecular-weight heparin) have not been shown to increase bleeding complications from EGD and may be continued. Prophylactic antibiotics are not indicated unless cardiac valvular disease is present.

Intravenous access is obtained in all patients prior to arrival to the endoscopic suite. The right hand or arm is used because the patient is usually placed in the left lateral decubitus position for EGD. Noninvasive hemodynamic monitoring is applied to follow blood pressure, heart rate, and pulse oximetry with oxygen accessible. The oral cavity is inspected and the airway may also be assessed. All dentures, prostheses, glasses, contacts, and facial jewelry should be removed. The endoscopy equipment is then tested and confirmed to be functioning properly. The patient is placed in the left lateral decubitus position to reduce the risk of aspiration. Video monitors are arranged behind the patient so the endoscopist is manipulating the endoscope in direct line with the image. The assistant or nurse helps comfort the patient, secures the mouth guard, monitors vital signs, and manages secretions.

Sedation

Prior to the initiation of intravenous sedation, topical local anesthesia can be sprayed to the back of the pharynx to prevent the gag reflex when the endoscope is inserted. Most endoscopists advocate conscious sedation when performing EGD. The goal of conscious sedation is to provide both sedation and analgesia without respiratory compromise. Sedation regimens usually consist of a benzodiazipine and a narcotic, based upon physician preference. The narcotic is usually administered first because it lasts longer and may allow for smaller doses of benzodiazipine to be administered. All of these medications cause some degree of respiratory depression, thus appropriate dosing and close respiratory monitoring is crucial. The sedation medications should be administered in small sequential doses to achieve the desired effect with more caution in the elderly and children, patients with significant comorbidity or those with cardiopulmonary disease. Equipment such as endotracheal intubation, cardiac defibrillation, and reversal agents such as naloxone and flumenazil should always be available at the patient's bedside.

The presence of an anesthesiologist is required during the procedure for complicated patients or when intervention is necessary. Monitoring and drug administration under an anesthesiologist's supervision is optimal, but it is costly and in some institutions may be reserved for specific cases. General anesthesia is commonly implemented in pediatric cases, but rarely indicated in the adult population. Severe trauma, hemodynamic instability, massive GI hemorrhage, complex interventional procedures, super obesity, previous failed attempts at sedation, history of drug or alcohol abuse, or an extremely uncooperative patient would be reasons to induce general anesthesia. Conversely, EGD can be performed without sedation if absolutely necessary.

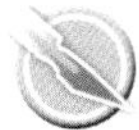

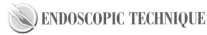

ENDOSCOPIC TECHNIQUE

Developing a system for evaluating the upper GI tract is the key to a consistent and thorough EGD examination. Once the patient is positioned and sedated, a bite block is placed orally to protect the instrumentation and the patient. The endoscopic controls and the quality of the images are tested and the tip lubricated. Placing the lens tip over material with printed lettering conveniently tests the image.

The EGD diagnostic procedure can be divided into four major components: insertion, advancement, stomach examination, and pyloric cannulation. A fifth component can be reserved for intervention. The most difficult aspect of the procedure is intubating the posterior pharyngx and esophagus. Three different techniques have been described for access, and it is important to understand all three should one method fail. The safest technique utilizes direct visualization. The tip of the endoscope is introduced, and the structures of the posterior pharynx are visually identified. The endoscope is advanced carefully over the tongue to its base, and the epiglottis, vocal cords, and cricoarytenoid cartilages are seen. The trachea usually has a triangular shape and will lay on the endoscopist's left if the endoscope is oriented with the patient in the left lateral decubitus position. A slight downward angle of the tip of the endoscope will deflect in the posterior pharyngeal direction. The tip can then be passed below the cricoarytenoid cartilage on either side to the upper esophageal sphincter. With insufflation, the sphincter will relax and open, allowing the endoscope to be advanced into the upper esophagus.

The second technique for EGD insertion is blind tip manipulation. The endoscope is inserted over the tongue to the back of the mouth. The tip is again deflected downward with gentle pressure and the patient is asked to swallow. Resistance is lost as the cricopharyngeal muscle relaxes and the endoscope passes into the esophagus. The last method for access uses finger guidance. The bite block is first placed over the endoscope rather than in the patient's mouth. The instrument is then inserted with the right hand directing the shaft posteriorly and the left hand fingers placed over the tongue to keep the endoscope midline. The left hand fingers are withdrawn and the bite block is slid down into the patient's mouth. The patient is asked to swallow and the endoscope passes into the esophagus as the cricopharyngeal sphincter relaxes. Both of these techniques are potentially dangerous. Blind tip manipulation can be traumatic for the patient's pharynx and the finger guidance method risks the inopportune bite of the endoscopist's fingers prior to bite block insertion.

With the upper esophageal sphincter intubated, the depth of the shaft should read around 20 cm. The endoscope is then advanced under direct vision and air insufflation. Minor adjustments are made using the wheels of the control head to keep the lumen central. The normal esophageal epithelium is a light pink color until it reaches the gastroesophageal junction. This transition zone, or Z-line (Fig. 23-2), is a darker red gastric mucosa followed by the lower esophageal sphincter (LES). It is located approximately 38 to 40 cm from the incisors and 1 cm above the diaphragmatic hiatus. Any discrepancy in distance may suggest abnormal pathology; however, these measurements are an inconsistent guide which do not take into account anatomical variability and later instrumental looping.

The LES is easily passed to access the stomach with air insufflation. We recommend examination upon entry to the stomach before advancing to the duodenum. Minor trauma from the torque of the shaft while examining the postpyloric GI tract may aggravate unseen pathology or irritate gastric mucosa, which would otherwise be described as normal. A systematic approach is mandatory so that no lesions or accessible areas are missed, regardless of which technique is chosen.

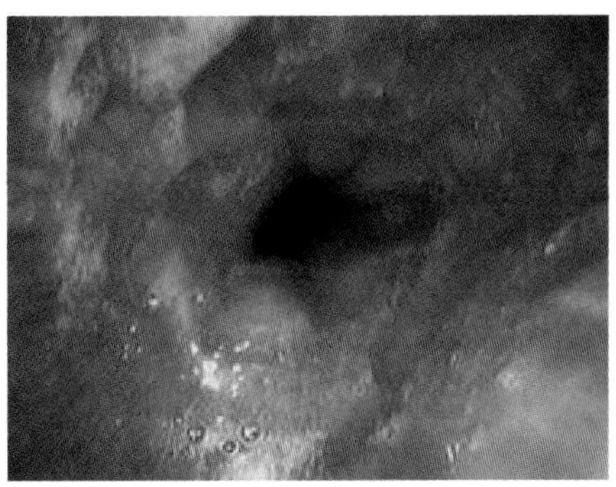

Fig. 23-2. The Z-line delineates esophageal and gastric mucosa.

As the endoscope enters the stomach, the tip angles posteriorly as the lesser curvature comes into view. Care must be taken at this point as this posterior and inferior area to the gastroesophageal junction is where most perforations will occur. These iatrogenic complications can be prevented by advancing under direct vision and avoiding forceful advancement of the scope. Counterclockwise rotation of the shaft and tip deflection to the right will align the smooth surface of the lesser curvature on the right and the rugae of the fundus on the left. The incisura of the lesser curve will delineate the stomach walls and point the endoscopist in the direction of the pylorus. Gastric juices should be aspirated with care to avoid aspiration of the mucosa and the subsequent formation of a "suction polyp," which can later be confused as pathologic. This can be avoided by positioning the endoscope tip at the fluid level rather than complete immersion. Excessive gas bubbles can be managed by irrigating and then suctioning a solution containing simethicone. The antegrade assessment of the stomach includes noting anatomy, pliability and motility of the walls, fold thickness, vascularity, and mucosal characteristics.

As the endoscope is advanced in the direction of the pylorus, the antrum can be inspected. The antrum lacks rugae and may be noted to have peristaltic waves of contraction. These waves may average three times per minute, leading to the view of the pylorus. Prior to cannulation, the endoscope is retroflexed in order to visualize the proximal fundus and cardia. A hiatal or paraesophageal hernia can also be identified by this maneuver. The tip is deflected upward using the control knobs to a complete 180-degree angulation, and the shaft of the endoscope is seen passing through the gastroesophageal junction (Fig. 23-3, page 202). Shaft rotation in a clockwise and counterclockwise direction will allow for complete visualization during retroflexion. Withdrawal of the endoscope will also provide a closer examination of the mucosa. Once gastric inspection is complete, the endoscope is placed in the neutral position and the pylorus is approached.

Pyloric cannulation can be a difficult maneuver when there are multiple sphincter contractions. The tip of the endoscope is placed at the opening, and, as the channel relaxes and opens, the endoscope is quickly advanced. Once the

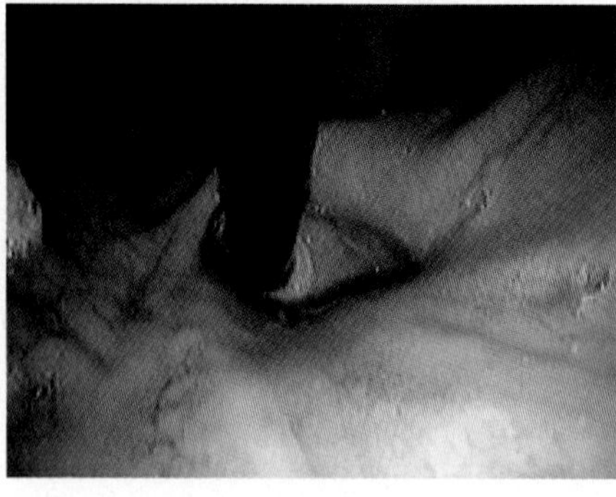

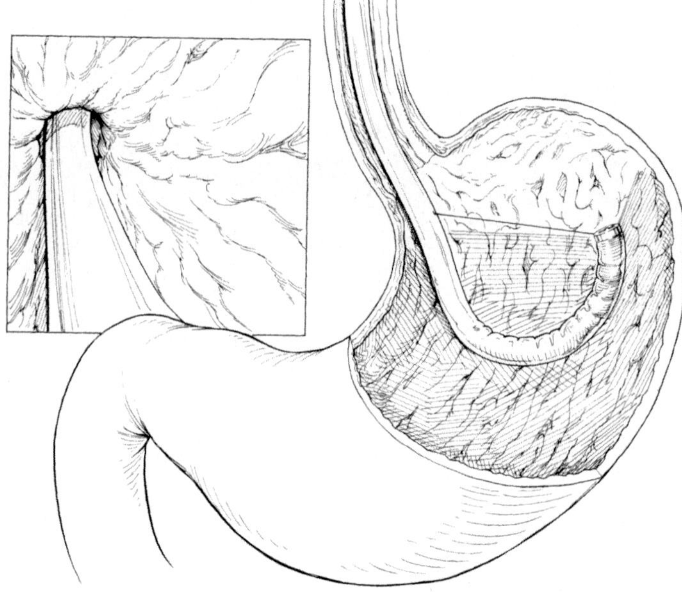

Fig. 23-3. Hiatal hernia identified by an upward retroflexion of 180 degrees.

duodenal bulb is accessed, the shaft is rotated clockwise and the tip deflected to the right and slightly upward. Duodenal advancement of the endoscope may be difficult if the endoscope loops in the stomach. Slow withdrawal of the endoscope will correct the loop and straighten the shaft for better control. Once the endoscopist is satisfied with duodenal inspection, the endoscope is carefully withdrawn to the stomach. Any diagnostic or interventional procedures can now be performed.

After all procedures have been completed, the endoscope is returned to the neutral position at the gastroesophageal junction. All excess air is aspirated to facilitate patient comfort while recovering, and the instrument is withdrawn under direct vision.

Diagnostic Procedures

The evolution of EGD has advanced beyond visual diagnostic capabilities to endoluminal interventional procedures for tissue diagnosis and therapy. Modern endoscopes provide an easily accessible working channel to manipulate endoluminal tissue. In the absence of significant coagulopathy, any nonvascular lesion including strictures, masses, polyps (Fig. 23-4), and ulcers should be liberally biopsied. Biopsies, brushings, and aspirates can be routinely obtained from any suspicious area. Multiple biopsies will also increase diagnostic yield in excess of 90%. We recommend a four-quadrant biopsy approach to ulcers. The base of the ulcer should also be included.

There are many different instruments used with EGD to sample tissue. Biopsy forceps and snare are most frequently used during EGD. The endoscope is placed approximately 1 cm above the area to be sampled, and the forceps are threaded through the working channel coming into view at the bottom corner of the screen. The forceps' jaws are opened and thrust into the lesion. The forceps are then closed and pulled away quickly, tearing the tissue sample from the mucosa wall. The tissue is withdrawn through the endoscope and placed immediately in a fixative solution for histological review. Biopsies can be repeated from the same site, although greater focal tissue loss will increase risk of perforation. Any submucosal lesion can be difficult to reach by biopsy and will have a low diagnostic yield.

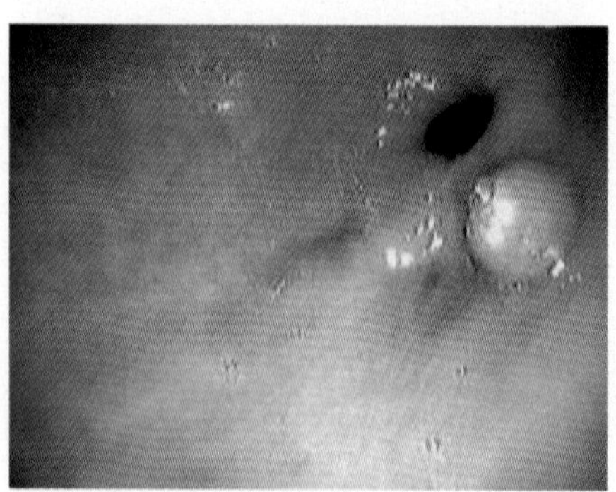

Fig. 23-4. Close-up of a gastric polyp near the pylorus.

Instrument choice to sample potentially malignant polyps depends on size. Minute polyps (<5 mm) are best addressed with hot or cold biopsy forceps while larger polyps will require a snare. The snare is positioned at the base of the polyp, closed, and the lesion is sampled in a piecemeal fashion. Fragments can be removed by forceps or a suction grasper. Any residual bleeding can be controlled by coagulation.

Cytologic brushings and aspirates are easily obtained to rule out malignancy or infection. The brush is passed via the working channel and scraped against the lesion. The brush is then withdrawn and smeared on a slide with fixative solution. Candidiasis and cytomegalovirus would be common pathogens diagnosed with brushings. Aspirates are simply obtained by instilling sterile saline into the area and suctioning the fluid into a clean container trap. The aspirated fluid can be evaluated for cytology and microbiology findings.

ENDOSCOPIC FINDINGS

There is a long list of benign gastric pathology that can be diagnosed by EGD (Table 23-2). These lesions can be further categorized by symptomatology: asymptomatic, associated with bleeding, or associated with pain. In identifying abnormal pathology, a visual understanding of normal mucosa is crucial. Normally the

TABLE 23-2. BENIGN GASTRIC DISORDERS FOUND ON ESOPHAGOGASTRODUODENOSCOPY (EGD)

Asymptomatic lesions

- Hiatal hernia
- Bezoars
- Gastritis

Bleeding lesions

- Esophageal/gastric varices
- Mallory-Weiss tear
- Anastomotic ulcers (marginal)
- Angiodysplasia
- Dieulafoy lesion
- Stress-related gastric injury
- Hemangioma
- Gastric antral vascular ectasia (GAVE)
- Portal gastropathy

Painful lesions

- Gastric/duodenal ulcers
- Gastroesophageal reflux disease (GERD)

LES signifies a single point of constriction that separates the esophagus from the baggy stomach. A sliding hiatal hernia will reveal a small pouch between the esophagus and stomach lined by rugae and gastric mucosa during antegrade inspection (Fig. 23-3). This pouch may extend for several centimeters above the diaphragmatic hiatus. Upon retroflexion, there is normally a tight cuff of gastric mucosa around the shaft of the endoscope at the cardia. In the case of a hiatal hernia, there is no tight cushion of gastric mucosa around the shaft, only a loose and pliable hiatus. A hiatal hernia is commonly associated with gastroesophageal reflux disease (GERD). If a paraesophageal hernia is present, retroflexion will display an outpouching of gastric mucosa into the thorax, juxtaposed to the gastroesophageal junction. Significant paraesophageal hernias may manifest as gastric erosions, gastric volvulus, perforation, or respiratory compromise.

Gastric bezoars are masses of undigested foreign material such as plants (phytobezoars) and hair (trichobezoars). Unusual dietary habits, gastric dysmotility, and prior gastric surgery are risk factors. Bezoars should be differentiated from intrinsic gastric masses by motility on copious irrigation. The underlying mucosa should always be carefully inspected for injury or tumor. Phytobezoars are green or yellow, while trichobezoars are brown or black and covered by mucous. A biopsy forceps can break up the mass, as necessary. Chemical dissolution with meat tenderizer, cellulase, or diet soda has also been effective.

Gastritis is a diffuse mucosal erythema and is a nonspecific finding attributable to a number of gastric pathologies. More commonly, *Helicobacter pylori* infection can cause antral gastritis. *H. pylori* is associated with gastric and duodenal ulcers, and can be diagnosed by tissue biopsy or enzymatic urease test. Treatment includes triple therapy of antibiotics and acid suppression.

Recognizing pathology for lesions that cause bleeding is particularly important in order to determine the appropriate intervention. Gastric varices look similar to esophageal varices except the former tend to occur in clusters and must be carefully distinguished from rugae. They are graded by number, site, extent, and size with air insufflation at a minimum to prevent intraluminal collapse. Varices typically occur in patients with cirrhosis and portal hypertension. Recent hemorrhage is manifested by overlying clots, red spots (wale marks), or hemocystic spots or blisters. Local treatment of bleeding lesions may include banding, sclerosing, or injection. Portal gastropathy may also be associated with varices and portal hypertension. These lesions appear as areas of patchy erythema encircled by thin pale white threads in a "snakeskin" pattern. Portal gastropathy is a diffuse endoscopic finding only amenable to medical or surgical treatment of portal hypertension. Gastric antral vascular ectasia (GAVE), or "watermelon stomach" (Fig. 23-5), occurs most commonly in females and the elderly and may be related to cirrhosis. Its description includes parallel antral folds with linear erthymatous streaks leading to the pylorus, similar to the stripes of a watermelon. Bleeding is self-limiting and even biopsy will only produce slight and easily controllable hemorrhage.

Patients with repeated retching and hematemesis associated with alcohol abuse, diabetic ketoacidosis, or drug-induced vomiting may be susceptible to a Mallory-Weiss tear. These superficial and linear tears are visualized on the gastric side of the gastroesophageal junction; evidence of bleeding may or may not be present. These acute mucosal tears usually heal rapidly within days, without much evidence of fibrosis, vascularity, or exudation. Stress-induced gastritis refers to mucosal breakdown in severe physiologic illness such as severe burns, multisystem trauma, and intracranial bleeding. Patients are usually ventilator-dependent in the ICU, and EGD will reveal diffuse, shallow erosions throughout the stomach. Management includes optimizing oxygenation and blood pressure, avoidance of NSAIDs, and therapy with proton pump inhibitors (PPIs).

A Dieulafoy lesion is an ectatic submucosal artery that usually occurs within 6 cm of the gastroesophageal junction, usually near the lesser curvature. It is described as a clean pigmented vessel stump without surrounding erosion or ulceration. The true Dieulafoy lesion is commonly missed due to size and association with a minute and narrow mucosal defect. Treatment includes coagulation or injection therapy. Hemangiomas are much larger lesions and appear as purple-bluish polypoid lesions. These are rare GI findings associated with Klippel-Trenaunay syndrome or may be isolated lesions. Risk of hemorrhage during endoscopic biopsy is increased, and biopsy should only be performed cautiously.

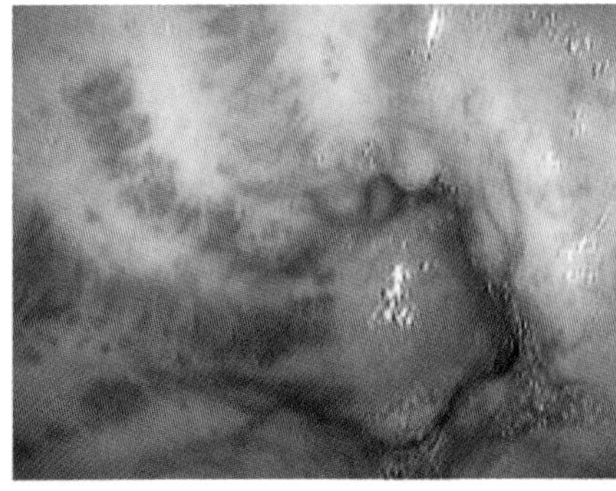

Fig. 23-5. Gastric antral vascular ectasia (GAVE), or "watermelon stomach."

Angiodysplasia may occur anywhere in the alimentary tract and is visualized as a dense red vascular tuft in a starburst pattern. These lesions are small (2 to 8 mm) and occasionally bleed, but can be easily missed on EGD. Angiodysplasia can be confused with fresh blood, endoscopic trauma, suction trauma, or missed under blood or gastric folds. Unless definitive bleeding is noted, any angiodysplasia seen on EGD cannot be implicated as the cause of acute hemorrhage.

Marginal ulcers can occur from days to years after surgery and may be secondary to bile reflux, retained antrum, local ischemia, NSAIDs, and smoking. At EGD the proximal side of the anastomosis should be examined meticulously for inflammation, erosion, friability, or disrupted sutures. For a Bilroth II reconstruction, both afferent and efferent limbs should be thoroughly examined. A low threshold for endoscopic biopsies is appropriate for anastomotic lesions to rule out carcinoma, especially after partial gastrectomy. Treatment may include hemostatic intervention if there is active bleeding, a PPI, and Carafate.

Gastroesophageal reflux is commonly associated with pain. EGD may reveal erythema, hypervascularity, erosion, or exudation of the esophageal mucosa. Reflux injury is best seen above the gastroesophageal (GE) junction and may lead to complications of bleeding, Barrett esophagus, adenocarcinoma, stricture, and even perforation. Current treatment options favor medical management with H2 blockers or PPIs and surgery in severe or refractory cases.

Gastroduodenal ulcers will appear as deep, depressed craters with surrounding exudates and are described by size, site, number, and evidence of recent hemorrhage. Acute ulcers are characterized by erythema, edema, and fibrinopurulent exudate, while chronic ulcers will demonstrate fibrosis and healing. A visible vessel in the ulcer base is prone to rebleeding and thus should be treated as an active source of bleeding using coagulation or injection therapy. With a high incidence of *H. pylori* infection and the possibility of cancer, the presence of gastric ulcers will warrant endoscopic biopsies and a Campylobacter-like organism (CLO) test. Triple therapy with a PPI and antibiotic coverage is the standard of care for *H. Pylori* infection. When ulcers are multiple and in atypical sites such as the esophagus or the second portion of the duodenum, gastrinoma and Zollinger-Ellison syndrome should be considered in the differential diagnosis.

Therapeutic Procedures

FOREIGN BODY REMOVAL

Foreign body ingestion can be a difficult problem based on the age of the patient and the object ingested. Most foreign body ingestions occur unwittingly in children 1 to 5 years of age. Adults with an ingested foreign body usually present with an associated psychiatric disorder, alcohol abuse, or for a secondary gain (e.g., prisoners). Whether intentionally or unintentionally swallowed, up to 90% of foreign bodies will traverse the GI tract without impediment and be spontaneously passed. Most of the remaining 10% cases can be removed endoscopically; only about 1% of cases require surgical extraction.

Urgent intervention to remove foreign bodies is indicated for respiratory compromise, unmanageable secretions, and sharp objects that are at risk for perforation. General anesthesia should be used in all pediatric patients, in the acute setting, and selectively in adults if adequate sedation cannot be achieved; however, airway protection is the first priority in endoscopic foreign body removal. An overtube may be required to protect the esophagus from sharp objects or if the endoscope must be reinserted for multiple retrievals. The Trendelenburg position will also help prevent objects from finding the trachea, if dropped during removal. Larger objects (>2 cm) will generally lodge in the stomach due to the diameter of the pylorus. Retrieval within the stomach allows adequate space for object manipulation; whenever possible extraction rehearsal with a similar object is recommended prior to passing the endoscope.

Coins are the most common foreign bodies ingested by children. The majority of swallowed coins will lodge in the cervical esophagus, but the likelihood of distal migration, respiratory symptoms, and pressure necrosis increases with time. Alligator or tenaculum forceps are most frequently used for endoscopic coin retrieval, yet a polypectomy snare may sometimes suffice. Once the endoscope is carefully advanced to the cricopharyngeus, the coin is usually visible and can be grasped and withdrawn with the endoscope. Failure to see the coin in the cricopharyngeus indicates distal migration or that the coin may be buried in a posterior mucosal fold. Meticulous inspection of the posterior esophageal wall is necessary before proceeding distally. Objects that have migrated can be pushed to the stomach, where they can be easily removed or left to pass spontaneously, if small enough.

The most common problem with foreign body ingestion in adults is meat impaction. A clear history and symptoms of pain, discomfort, and the sensation of something stuck will determine the presence of a foreign body, thus radiological studies are usually unnecessary. Spontaneous passage to the stomach may occur prior to endoscopy, aided by the administration of sedation. EGD is still indicated to inspect for esophageal trauma and to rule out abnormal pathology that is often present. An impacted bolus may be pushed past the point of obstruction distally to the stomach. If removal is necessary, a snare can be used. Large meat impactions can be fragmented and removed with the help of an overtube for multiple reinsertions of the endoscope. Contrary to common perception, meat-tenderizing agents are not beneficial. Bariatric patients may be particularly prone to food bolus impaction at the gastrojenunal anastomosis.

After any offending foreign object is retrieved or fragmented, the esophagus should be carefully inspected for injury or lesion. Objects with sharp edges must always be removed before reaching the pylorus as up to one third of sharp objects will perforate the small intestine. This commonly occurs in the terminal ileum. Removing sharp objects can be dangerous during extraction; thus an overtube is used to protect the esophagus. The object should be extracted with the sharp end trailing. It may be necessary to push the object into the stomach where it can be best manipulated and grasped for removal. Safety pins, large straight pins, and razor blades can be particularly challenging extractions. Packets of drugs such as cocaine swallowed to avoid police detection should not be removed endoscopically due to the risk of rupture. These cases are optimally managed with surgical extraction, although an expectant approach may be considered.

Radiological studies are useful when dealing with foreign body ingestion to help delineate the object and define the site prior to endoscopy. A patient who has completed a difficult extraction with signs and symptoms of perforation should undergo an urgent water soluble contrast study. Acute perforations at any point in the GI tract should be treated expeditiously with broad spectrum antibiotic coverage and/or surgical repair.

BARIATRIC STRICTURE DILATION

The population of patients who have undergone bariatric surgery needs special consideration during endoscopic examination and intervention. Familiarity with the surgical anatomy is vital to a safe and thorough diagnostic and possibly therapeutic procedure. Any patient may undergo endoscopy after Roux-en-Y gastric bypass (RYGB), gastric banding, sleeve gastrectomy, vertical banded gastroplasty (VBG), and other bariatric procedures. Upper endoscopy in the bariatric patient is most commonly indicated for suspected gastrojejunal anastomotic stricture, marginal ulcer, bleeding, or food bolus impaction. It is also used for preoperative evaluation, intraoperative inspection of a fresh anastomosis, and annual screening to identify gastric band erosions.

Anastomotic stricture after RYGB is the most frequent complication requiring bariatric endoscopic intervention. Gastrojejunal stricture rates will vary by technique, ranging from 4.7% to 27%. This rate is acceptable, due to modern endoscopic dilatation capabilities and the difficulty in addressing weight-loss failure in a gastrojejunal anastomosis that was initially created too large.

The appropriate diameter of the gastrojejunal anastomosis after RYGB is approximately 12 to 15 mm. Fibrosis from ischemia and ulcer disease can stricture the gastric pouch outlet, producing symptoms such as dysphagia, nausea, and vomiting. These patients will often require one or more endoscopic balloon dilatations to allow adequate food passage and possibly repeat dilatations to achieve success. The diameter of the anastomosis can be assessed by comparing it to the diameter of the endoscope viewing field. Most endoscopes have a diameter of approximately 10 to 12 mm. If the endoscope cannot be safely advanced through the anastomosis of a symptomatic patient, dilatation is likely required.

Once an anastomotic stricture is recognized, a balloon dilator is passed through the scope and through the stricture under direct vision. After placing the deflated balloon (Fig. 23-6A), it is inflated with water using an injector that monitors inflation pressure (Fig. 23-6B). An excessive inflation pressure can disrupt the anastomosis, leading to acute perforation. The balloon is repeatedly inflated for 3-minute intervals, and balloons of increasing size may be required to achieve an adequate anastomotic diameter. We recommend no more than a slow and gradual 6-mm change in anastomotic diameter in any single procedure. Stretching the anastomosis more than 6 mm at one sitting increases the risk of disruption, bleeding, or perforation. In experienced hands, the risk of perforation is less than 1%; however, a high index of suspicion will optimize the outcome following any of these complications. Postprocedural pain or tachycardia should be taken seriously with a low threshold for water-soluble contrast study. Subcutaneous emphysema is diagnostic. Uncomplicated endoscopic dilatations are performed as an outpatient procedure, and patients are discharged with the possibility for repeat dilatation if necessary in 2 to 4 weeks.

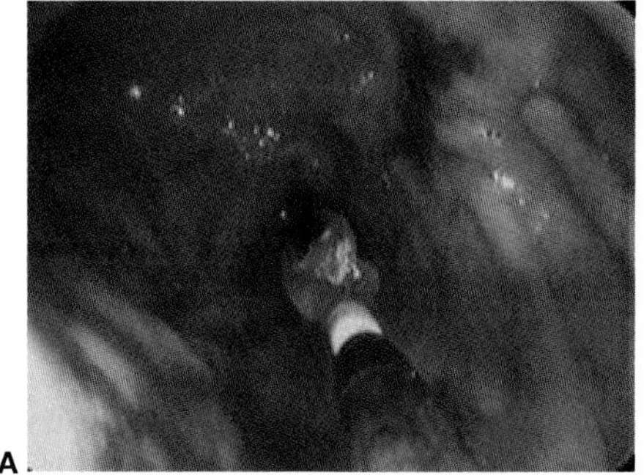

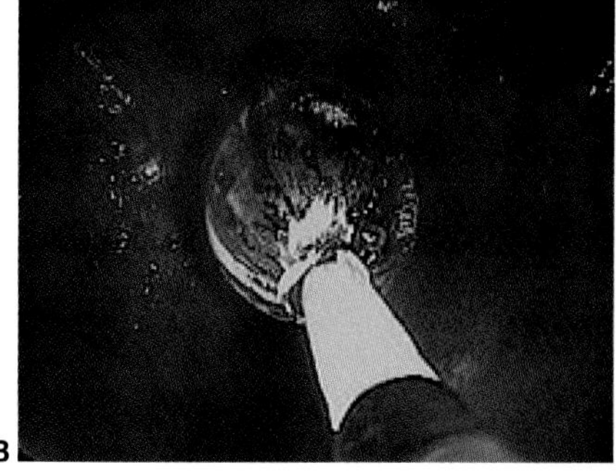

Fig. 23-6. Through-the-scope balloon dilatation of a gastrojejunal stricture after laparoscopic gastric bypass. **A.** Before dilatation. **B.** During dilatation.

NONVARICEAL UPPER GASTROINTESTINAL BLEEDING

Upper GI bleeding can be acute or chronic in nature and is a common indication for upper endoscopy. Before any diagnostic examination or therapeutic intervention is entertained, airway control, definitive intravenous access, and hemodynamic stability via resuscitation must be achieved. The majority of GI bleeds are self-limiting, and it is usually unnecessary to endoscopically identify the source when there is active bleeding. In fact, endoscopy in the face of active bleeding can be a challenging procedure. The nonbleeding period following an acute bleeding episode often provides the best opportunity to identify the source and assess the risk of rebleeding. Peptic ulcer disease and gastric mucosal lesions account for two thirds of upper GI bleeding, with remaining incidents caused mostly by esophageal varices and Mallory-Weiss tears.

Early endoscopic evaluation is advocated in bleeding to determine the need for intervention in persistent, active bleeding, and to identify lesions likely to rebleed. With an acute bleeding episode, when feasible, it is best to first lavage the stomach of clots and blood with a large bore tube prior to EGD to allow optimal visualization. Factors predictive of rebleeding are related to site, size, quantity, and vascular characteristics of the lesion. In lesions that are actively bleeding, 80% to 90% will continue to bleed or rebleed without intervention. Evidence of a sentinel clot or visible vessel in an ulcer bed is also a strong predictor of rebleeding tendency. These findings also require intervention as approximately half of these lesions will rebleed. Proximity to vasculature, such as a posterior duodenal bulb ulcer, will increase the likelihood of further problems without therapy.

Hemostatic intervention is an advanced endoscopic procedure, and there are several options available to the experienced endoscopist. Coagulation can be achieved by thermal energy, chemical injection or topical application, and mechanical means. Electrocautery and injectable sclerosing agents are most frequently employed.

Thermal coagulation implicates tissue protein denaturation and vessel shrinkage using monopolar or bipolar electricity, direct heat, or laser light. Monopolar electrocautery was first used as an energy source in coagulation. A generator transfers electric current through a probe to the tissue and subsequently to a grounding pad. The focal electrical current is converted to heat at the tissue level, providing coagulation. The probe tip is positioned 2 mm from the target in a circumferential fashion and activated repeatedly for 2-second intervals. This technique is successful in more than 80% of cases; however, the depth of thermal injury is difficult to control. Perforation is a serious risk with monopolar electrocautery, and thus safer methods have been developed.

Bipolar or multipolar electrocautery offers a safer alternative. This device passes current between electrodes arranged around the probe tip and limits depth of tissue injury to 2 to 3 mm. The electrical circuit that passes from electrode to electrode also eliminates the need for a grounding pad. The probe uses a foot pedal to control power and irrigation. Up to 50 watts of power is delivered in intervals of 1 to 2 seconds or in a continuous fashion. Larger probes appear to be more successful in attaining hemostasis. Ideally, a 3.2-mm bipolar probe is positioned directly on the lesion and activated at high power for 2-second intervals for coaptive coagulation. Using a lower power for longer duration (5 to 10 seconds) is another hemostatic option for deep heating.

Direct heat conduction is a third alternative for coagulation of bleeding sites. A heater probe can achieve extreme temperatures that conduct heat to the tissue without the transfer of electrical current. A polytef (Teflon)-coated, aluminum-encased heater coil at the probe tip placed into direct contact with the tissue allows coaptive coagulation. Irrigation is used to prevent tissue adherence to the probe tip. The amount of thermal energy and irrigation can both be controlled. Using a heater probe or a bipolar electrocautery, hemostatic success is accomplished in over 90% of cases with a low risk of perforation.

The most advanced thermal coagulation method uses laser light. A quartz probe delivers laser light to the tissue while the tip is cooled with water irrigation or carbon dioxide. Depth of tissue penetration depends on the characteristic of tissue absorption. The devices used for hemostasis of GI bleeding include argon and neodymium:yttrium-aluminum-garnet (Nd:YAG) lasers. The blue-green argon laser is strongly absorbed by tissue hemoglobin, which minimizes depth penetration. These lasers are effective for superficially vascular lesions but are generally inadequate for bleeding within fibrotic ulcers. The infrared Nd:YAG laser is poorly absorbed by tissue and thus results in a wider and deeper target of tissue injury and coagulation. Although both these lasers have equivalent results to thermal coagulation, their cost, size, and training requirements have limited their utilization to specialty roles such as ablating pigmented lesions.

TABLE 23-3. INJECTABLE SCLEROSING AGENTS FOR UPPER GASTROINTESTINAL HEMORRHAGE

Sclerosing agent	Recommended dose (mL)
Absolute ethanol (98%)	0.5–1
Epinephrine (1:10,000)	6–12
+ polidocanol (1%)	5–12 + 5
Hypertonic saline (3.6%)	9–12
+ epinephrine (1:20,000)	
Morrhuate sodium (5%)	3 + 2
+ (thrombin + dextrose [50%])	
Thrombin (100 IU) in 3 mL saline (0.9%)	10–15

Chemical sclerosing injection techniques were originally developed for variceal bleeding, but are commonly used for nonvariceal hemorrhage. There are numerous vasoconstricting, coagulopathic, and sclerosing agents available (Table 23-3). Under direct endoscopic vision, a 23- or 25-gauge retractable 5-mm needle is passed through the working channel. Submucosal injections are administered circumferentially at the lesion and up to 1 cm away from the target. Volume of injection depends on the agent selected and its concentration. No individual chemical has shown superiority as most carry an 85% to 95% success rate with few complications.

Chemical topical agents such as fibrin glues, clotting factors, and collagen compounds are generally inferior to electrocoagulation and injection therapies and have shown variable success. Mechanical devices have advanced to endoscopically applied clips and sutures but are expensive and require advanced training.

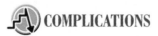

COMPLICATIONS

In the modern era, EGD is a well-tolerated procedure with rare complications. Morbidity from EGD is approximately one complication per 1000 cases with a mortality rate of one per 10,000 cases. Risk factors for complications are most commonly related to underlying patient disease, anesthesia, or operator technique. The most frequent complications are cardiopulmonary, secondary to a combination of underlying cardiac disease and sedation-induced respiratory depression. Aspiration during therapeutic intervention for acute GI bleeding is the most common cardiopulmonary complication.

Perforation from diagnostic EGD occurs in less than 0.1% of patients and usually occurs in the pharynx, esophagus, or just inferior to the gastroesophageal junction. Risk factors for perforation include altered anatomy (diverticulum, malignancy, stricture), an uncooperative patient, and an inexperienced endoscopist. The biopsy forceps is rarely responsible for perforation; modern instruments are flexible and only remove tissue to a mucosal depth. Early recognition of perforation is crucial to optimizing patient survival. Treatment of full-thickness, uncontained perforation is generally surgical; however, occasionally bowel rest, intravenous nutrition, and broad spectrum antibiotics may be considered for a small perforation in the absence of peritoneal signs.

Bleeding most commonly occurs with manipulation of vascular lesions, examination of coagulopathic patients, and in association with dilatation, sclerosing, and polypectomy procedures. EGD-related bleeding is dealt with by endoscopic hemostasis techniques.

Complications for hemostatic interventions are infrequent, and include perforation, tissue necrosis, and induced, delayed, or refractory hemorrhage. Perforation rates range between 1% to 3%, specifically with monopolar electrocautery and Nd:YAG lasers. Tissue necrosis is rare but most commonly associated with ethanolamine oleate injection. Induced bleeding can occur in 5% to 30% of cases, usually from thermal coagulation. Delayed hemorrhage will require repeat endoscopy and intervention, and bleeding refractory to endoscopic therapy will require surgery if a clear source has been delineated.

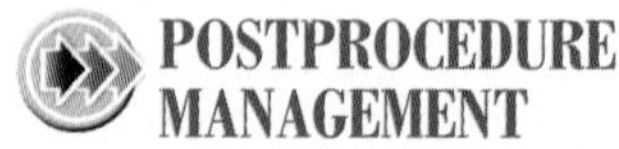

POSTPROCEDURE MANAGEMENT

After diagnostic or therapeutic EGD has been completed, patients should be monitored for at least an hour until fully awake and alert. Any symptoms of pain or discomfort should be seriously considered with a low threshold for reexamining the patient or obtaining X-rays. Abdominal symptoms and tachycardia may simply be due to excess air within the alimentary tract but may also be manifestations of an unrecognized perforation. A plain radiograph of the abdomen and chest in the upright lateral and posterolateral position may delineate free air under the diaphragm or in the mediastinum. In patients unable to stand, a plain film in the left lateral decubitus position should be obtained. Equivocal images should be followed by an oral contrast study of a meglumine diatrizoate (Gastrograffin) esophagram or a CT scan of the chest and abdomen. Early recognition of perforation will optimize outcome. In the absence of complications and once the patient has been cleared for discharge, written and verbal instructions on diet, medications, follow-up visits, and emergency phone numbers are given.

Thorough cleansing of used equipment will help prevent the spread of infection. The endoscope and its channels should be disinfected with a 2% glutaraldehyde solution (Cidex) for approximately 20 minutes and left to dry prior to storage. An intraoperative endoscope utilized in the sterile field should be sterilized with ethylene oxide gas or thoroughly exposed to liquid disinfectant. Disposable instruments used for intervention are the best option to minimize transmission of infection, although reusable instruments, carefully cleaned and sterilized between uses, tend to be more cost-effective. Additional information of endoscope cleaning protocols is provided in Chapter 17.

SUMMARY

Flexible endoscopy is an excellent medium for the diagnosis of upper GI pathology. Technological advances provide the opportunity for endoluminal therapy in many benign gastric conditions. The experienced surgical endoscopist will be familiar with normal and abnormal endoscopic findings, and have the skill set to intervene as necessary for biopsy, bleeding, dilatation, and foreign-body removal. EGD can be particularly challenging in patients with previous gastric or bariatric surgery. Mastering flexible EGD instrumentation and tissue manipulation techniques in the stomach is a stepping-stone to the future of flexible surgical endoscopy.

SUGGESTED READING

Cappell MS, Friedel D. The role of esophagogastroduodenoscopy in the diagnosis and management of upper gastrointestinal disorders. *Med Clin N Am* 2002;86:1165–1216.

Carrodeguas L, Szomstein S, Zundel N, et al. Gastrojejunal anastomotic strictures following laparoscopic roux-en-y gastric bypass surgery: analysis of 1291 patients. *Surg Obes Relat Dis* 2006;2(2):92–97.

Chan MF. Complications of upper gastrointestinal endoscopy. *Gastrointest Endosc Clin N Am* 1996;6:287–303.

Cohen J, Safdi MA, Deal SE, et al. Quality indicators for esophagogastroduodenoscopy. *Gastrointest Endosc* 2006;63(4 suppl):S10–15.

Harris JH Jr, Harris WH (eds). *The radiology of emergency medicine, 4th ed.* Lippincott Williams and Wilkins:Philadelphia, 2000.

Pinto D, Carrodeguas L, Soto F, et al. Gastric bezoar after laparoscopic roux-en-y gastric bypass. *Obes Surg* 2006;16:365–368.

Reed WP, Kilkenny JW, Dias CE, et al. SAGES EGD Outcomes Study Group. A prospective analysis of 3525 esophagogastroduodenoscopies performed by surgeons. *Surg Endosc* 2004;18(1):11–21.

COMMENTARY

Drs. Szomstein and Lalor describe the use of flexible endoscopy for the diagnosis and treatment of benign gastric disorders, including postoperative problems. They give a complete description of the indications and contraindications for EGD, the equipment necessary to perform adequate endoscopy, the preparation of patients, and the detailed technique for endoscopic evaluation of the foregut. Furthermore, they catalogue the more common benign findings seen at the time of EGD. The technique for removal of foreign bodies is detailed, along with the procedure for dilatation of anastomotic strictures. Given the marked increase in the numbers of bariatric procedures being done in the United States, the prevalence of postoperative strictures has also increased accordingly. Surgeons should be willing and able to evaluate their patients postoperatively and provide acute treatment of these benign but lifestyle-altering complications.

Finally, the authors describe the various techniques currently available to control acute upper GI hemorrhage endoscopically. As advances are made in the field of interventional endoscopy, increasing numbers of diseases and disorders previously only treated surgically are now being managed endoscopically. Many of the indications for endoscopic therapy discussed in this chapter were disorders that previously required surgical therapy. In older textbooks of surgery, entire chapters covered the surgical management of upper GI bleeding and invariably discussed the indications for operation, including the location of bleeding vessels, number of units of blood administered, etc. At the current time, operative therapy of proximal GI hemorrhage is generally only mandated when endoscopic techniques are unsuccessful in controlling the bleeding.

NJS

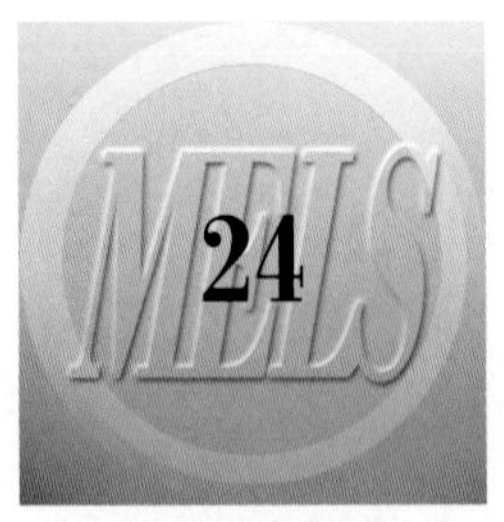

Laparoscopic Treatment of Benign Gastric Disease

KENRIC M. MURAYAMA AND RACQUEL S. BUENO

INTRODUCTION

Gastric surgery, once quite common, has decreased dramatically over the past 30 years. The introduction of the histamine receptor blocker cimetidine, to the US in 1977 revolutionized the treatment of peptic ulcer disease, shifting practice patterns toward nonoperative management. Furthermore, increased understanding of the physiology of acid secretion and the gastric mucosal barrier, as well as the discovery of the role of *H. pylori* in the pathophysiology of peptic ulcer disease, have all contributed to this evolution. Moreover, the changing incidence of gastric cancer has also contributed to the decline in the number of operations performed on the stomach.

By 1987, another paradigm shift in abdominal surgery was beginning. Reports of the first laparoscopic cholecystectomy ushered in a new approach to abdominal operations. Minimally invasive methods offered decreased morbidity, less pain, shorter lengths of hospital stay, quicker recovery, and smaller incisions. A seismic shift in practice patterns occurred as operating suites were rebuilt, new instruments and technologies created, and a nascent subspecialty, minimally invasive surgery, emerged. Predictably, more and more innovative applications for laparoscopic methods were being reported. In the early 1990s, the first laparoscopic approaches to foregut surgery were introduced. As experience increased, technology advanced, and the safety and feasibility of laparoscopic approaches widely reported, the role of laparoscopy in foregut surgery expanded.

Laparoscopic foregut operations, including antireflux procedures, bariatric operations, and esophageal myotomy, are now performed routinely. More recently, laparoscopic techniques have been used to remove benign gastric tumors and to treat peptic ulcer disease, becoming the preferred method in many situations. Reports indicate that laparoscopic resection for benign gastric tumors such as gastrointestinal stromal tumors (GIST) and neuroendocrine lesions is oncologically safe and technically feasible. Although the role of surgery in the treatment of peptic ulcer disease has decreased, it is now feasible when necessary to approach these operations laparoscopically in select situations.

Minimally Invasive Surgical Approaches to Peptic Ulcer Disease

The success of nonoperative therapy for the management of peptic ulcer disease has contributed to the significant decline in the number of operative procedures performed for gastric and duodenal ulcers. The need for elective surgery to treat nonhealing ulcers is currently nearly nonexistent. Emergency operative intervention for bleeding or perforation is required in fewer than 3% of patients. Unfortunately, the limited numbers of procedures has resulted in a diminished comfort level of surgeons in the surgical management of peptic ulcer disease. Interestingly, over the last 15 years, surgical experience with minimally invasive foregut operations (such as antireflux and bariatric operations) has led to an increased comfort level with this technique. While the need for operative management of peptic ulcer disease has decreased significantly, it has not disappeared altogether, and it is the surgeon who is called on to treat patients who are most recalcitrant to nonoperative therapies or who suffer from complications.

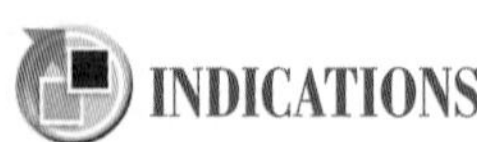

INDICATIONS

Although elective procedures for peptic ulcer disease are uncommon, the traditional indications for operative intervention in peptic ulcer disease are applicable to laparoscopy. Surgery should be considered for patients suffering from intractability to medical management and those with obstruction or perforation. A laparoscopic approach is usually not performed for acute hemorrhage due to difficulties with the control of bleeding and visualization. If, however, the acute situation has been controlled, but a more durable attempt at preventing subsequent re-bleeding is necessary, minimally invasive techniques may be feasible. The procedures outlined here include the management of hemorrhage and perforation, truncal vagotomy with pyloroplasty, highly selective vagotomy, and posterior truncal vagotomy with anterior seromyotomy.

An extensive discussion detailing the clinical presentation and diagnosis of peptic ulcer disease is beyond the scope of this chapter. In acute situations such as perforation, an extensive acid-reducing resective procedure can safely be omitted due to the efficacy of available medications promoting healing of ulcers. A conservative operation is an appropriate option for patients that are likely to comply with medical therapy. A more extensive acid-reducing operation should be considered in patients unable to comply with medical therapy or in whom ulcers are NSAID-induced and cessation of NSAIDs is not possible due to their primary disease process. Important consideration must be given to unusually located ulcers that may indicate a hyperacidic state, such as is present in the Zollinger-Ellison syndrome.

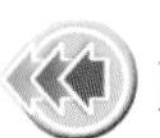

PREOPERATIVE PLANNING

Adequate preoperative preparation is essential for success with minimally invasive techniques. Patients must be able to tolerate general anesthesia and laparotomy. Although the rate of conversion to laparotomy is low, patients must always be made aware of this possibility. The preoperative period is also when a discussion should occur regarding the risks and benefits of the surgical procedure as well as the chosen minimally invasive approach. The patient's history of previous abdominal surgeries may be a factor in the success of a laparoscopic approach. Previous abdominal surgery with resultant adhesions may make a minimally invasive approach difficult, necessitating conversion to laparotomy. Moreover, serious complications such as inadvertent or missed enterotomy and a need for reoperation must be discussed with the patient. The discussion should also include the possible development of post-gastrectomy problems requiring lifestyle and dietary modifications and the potential for recurrent disease and reoperative intervention.

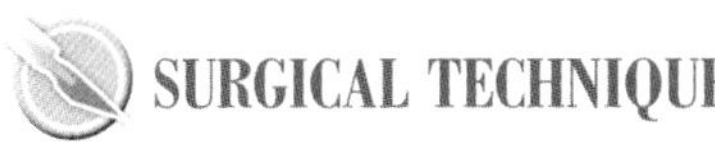

SURGICAL TECHNIQUE

General Considerations

Adequate preparation is essential for minimizing frustration and ensuring not only operative success, but a good outcome. The appropriate antibiotic as well as stress gastritis and venous thrombosis prophylaxis should be considered. Once in the operating room, bilateral lower extremity sequential compression stockings are applied for additional prophylaxis against deep venous thrombosis. Once general anesthesia is induced, placement of an orogastric tube and bladder catheter may be necessary. The lithotomy or split-leg position is generally used for most minimally invasive foregut procedures. Monitors placed directly above the patient's head provide a natural line of sight for the operative surgeon, who is normally positioned between the patient's legs (Fig. 24-1). The patient's arms may be in the abducted or tucked position. Securing the patient with wide tape and safety straps provide added security, and all pressure points need to be padded; a bean bag mattress is helpful to stabilize the patient's position. Checking the extremes of patient positions in steep reverse-Trendelenburg position prior to prepping and draping the patient is an invaluable exercise. Typical trocar positions are as depicted in Figure 24-2.

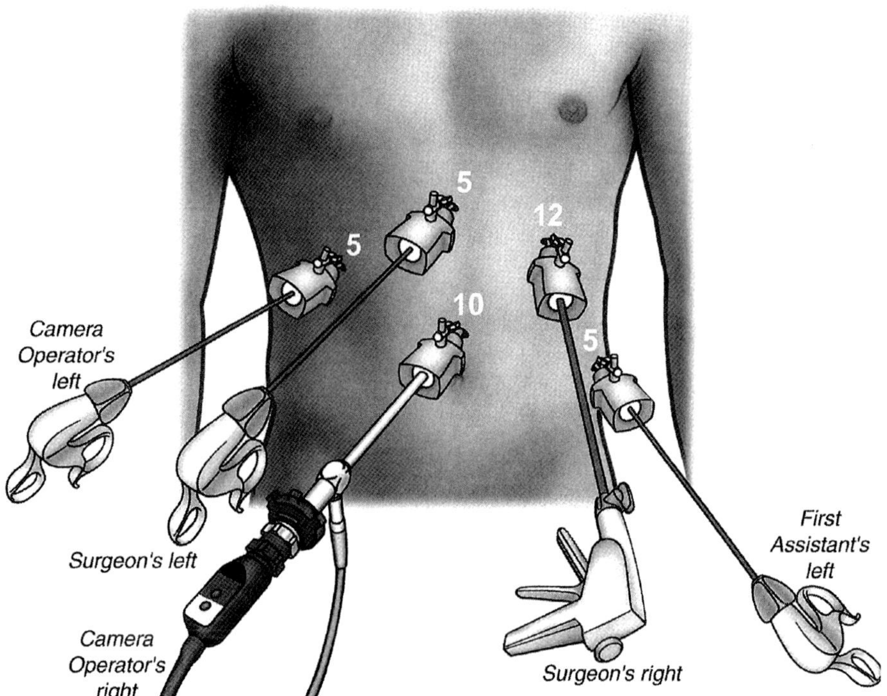

Fig. 24-2. Port placement and instruments for minimally invasive approaches to the stomach. Three 5-mm ports, one 10-mm port, and one 12-mm port are indicated.

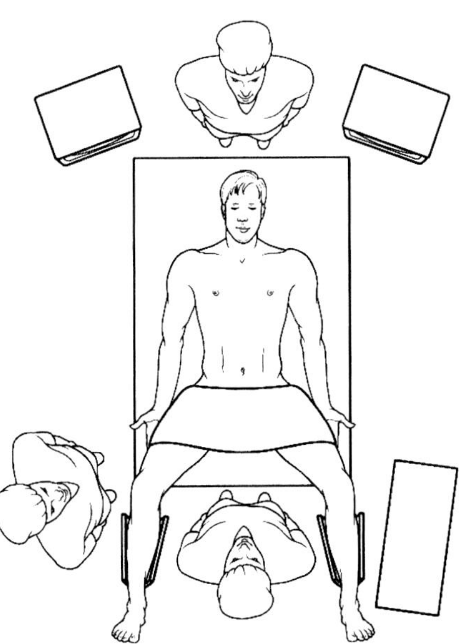

Fig. 24-1. A typical operating room setup for minimally invasive foregut procedures.

SURGERY FOR MANAGEMENT OF PEPTIC ULCER COMPLICATIONS

Hemorrhage

A laparoscopic approach is usually not performed for acute hemorrhage due to difficulties with the control of bleeding and visualization. If, however, the acute situation has been controlled, but a more durable attempt at preventing further rebleeding is necessary, minimally invasive techniques may be feasible. Endoscopic findings such as pulsatile bleeding, a visible clot, a visible vessel, or pulsation at the ulcer base all suggest a higher risk for ongoing or repeat bleeding. Despite initially controlling the bleeding with endoscopic interventional techniques such as coagulation, injection of epinephrine, or sclerosant or laser therapy, the rate of rebleeding approaches 10% to 20% when these findings are present. Once such bleeding is temporarily controlled, attempts at a more definitive repair using minimally invasive techniques are reasonable, provided that the patient is hemodynamically stable and fit for surgical intervention.

The operative approaches are dependent on the location of the bleeding within the stomach. Typically, simply oversewing the site of bleeding is all that is required to assure a lower risk of a recurrent bleeding event. The approaches to the site of bleeding depend on specific locations in the stomach. The approaches described elsewhere in this edition related to accessing nonadenomatous tumors of the stomach can be applied in these situations.

Perforation

Perforation of peptic ulcers most commonly occurs in the first portion of the duodenum (50%), followed by the pylorus (40%), and the stomach (10%). Due to the efficacy of medical treatment for ulcer disease, omental patch repair of the site of perforation followed by aggressive pharmaceutical therapy is appropriate in most cases.

Patients are positioned in modified lithotomy with thighs abducted and minimal flexion at the hips. This allows for comfortable surgeon positioning between the legs and a direct line of sight to the operative field viewed by the monitor placed above the patient's head. Bladder decompression, if a catheter has not been previously placed, is often necessary for appropriate monitoring of the patient's intravascular volume status, as these patients are often volume-depleted. The patient can be secured to the bed with a bean bag, securing straps, and tape, and all pressure points are carefully padded. Access into the abdomen can be achieved with the Veress needle, open technique, or the use of a visualizing trocar system. The laparoscope is placed in the supra-umbilical location to the left of midline. An incision is then made to the left of the xiphoid, and a large clamp is then introduced into the abdomen to create a tract for placement of the Nathanson liver retractor; having the patient in reverse-Trendelenburg assists in the placement of the retractor. A stationary, side-rail-mounted mechanical arm holds the liver retractor in position. The working ports for the surgeon's right and left hands can then be placed on either side of the camera port below the transpyloric line. These working trocars will be slightly cephalad from the umbilicus, usually in the midclavicular line. One working port should be 10 to 12 mm in diameter to accommodate the passage of curved suture needles.

The abdomen is then explored with cultures of any ascites or purulent fluid visualized. Exploration proceeds with a search for the site of perforation. As previously mentioned, ulcers most commonly occur in the antrum, pylorus, and duodenum. Unusual sites should prompt concern for a possible malignant process, and the appropriate biopsies performed. The perforation site is closed transversely to prevent luminal narrowing. Full-thickness bites at the edges of the perforation re-approximate the defect (Fig. 24-3). The tails of the suture are left long after the knots are tied (Fig. 24-4). The long suture tails are then used to secure a healthy tongue of omentum placed over the repair (Fig. 24-5). If re-approximation of the defect edges is not possible due to tissue friability or induration, simple closure via omental patch alone is acceptable. The remainder of the abdomen is then re-explored to ensure the absence of complications or unexpected findings. Several liters of warmed normal saline are used to irrigate the abdomen. The Nathanson liver retractor and all ports should be removed under direct laparoscopic visualization.

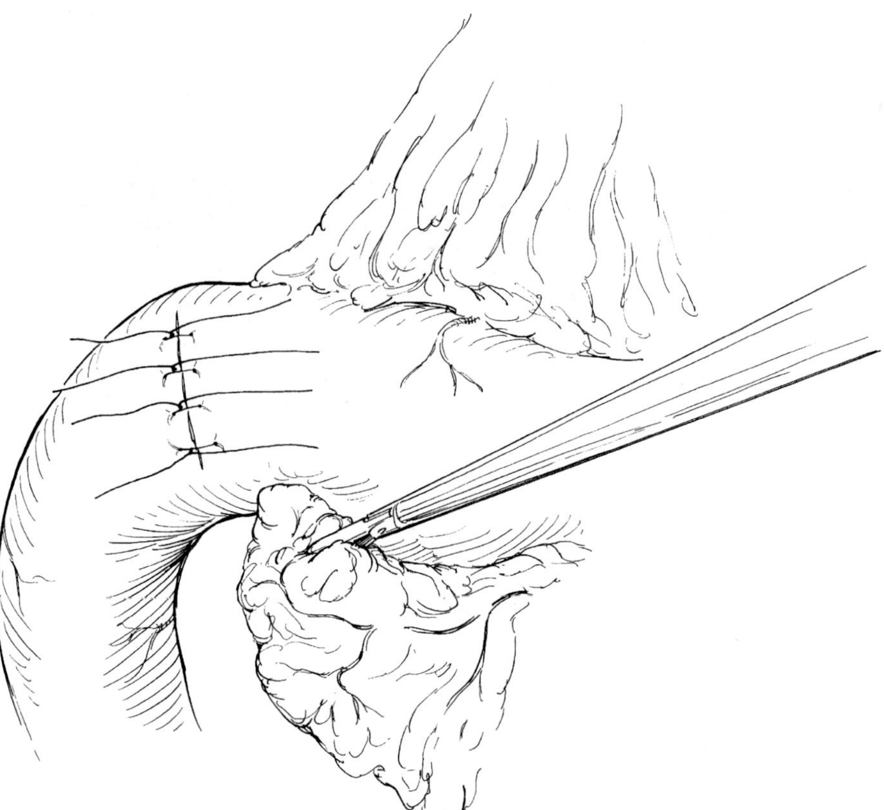

Fig. 24-4. After closure of the perforated ulcer, a tongue of omentum is placed over the knots of the tied suture. Leaving the suture tails long allows for securing the omentum over the repair.

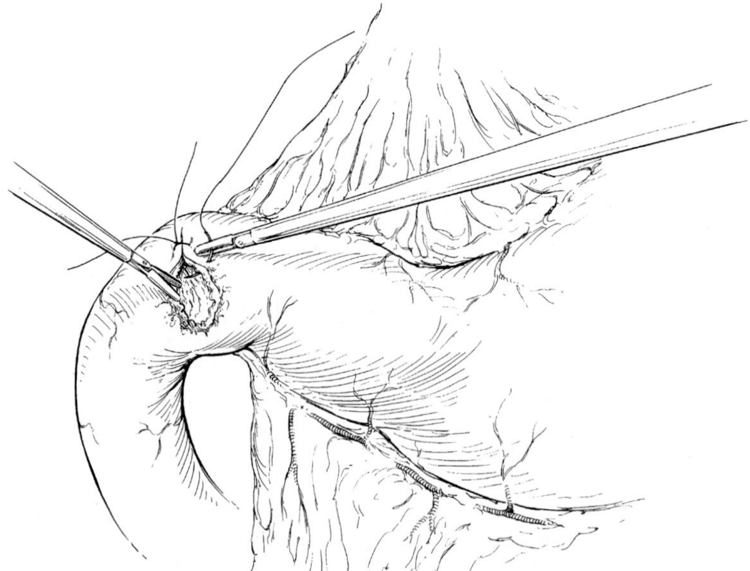

Fig. 24-3. Ulcer closure is performed with a single-layer, full-thickness interrupted technique in a transverse fashion to limit lumen narrowing.

OPERATIONS TO TREAT INTRACTABLE PEPTIC ULCER DISEASE

Although surgical treatment of peptic ulcer disease has decreased significantly with improved medical therapy, it remains essential for surgeons to understand the physiology of ulcer disease and the operations designed to prevent complications and recurrence. While an open operative approach may be indicated in situations of patient instability, a laparoscopic approach can be safely attempted with the expectation of similar outcomes.

The technique for antrectomy is described elsewhere and can be applied along with truncal vagotomy accompanied by a gastroduodenostomy (Billroth I) or gastrojejunostomy (Billroth II) to treat refractory peptic ulcer disease. Herein, we

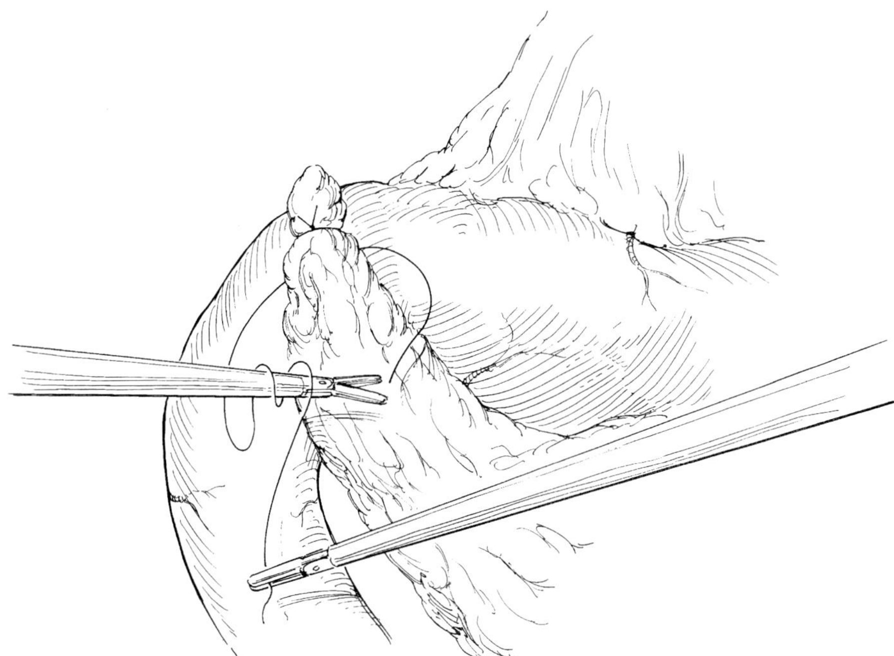

Fig. 24-5. Suture tails are tied over the omental patch to secure it. Tying the sutures with minimal tension prevents complete ischemia of the omental tissue.

describe several other approaches to laparoscopic management of refractory peptic ulcer disease.

Truncal Vagotomy with Pyloroplasty

Truncal vagotomy describes the division of both of the vagus nerves above the first branches to the fundus and stomach. Truncal vagotomy is particularly useful for recurrent ulcer disease. Division of the vagal fibers to the distal stomach results in altered antral function; therefore, a drainage procedure (such as a pyloroplasty) is necessary to prevent delayed gastric emptying.

Once again, the patient is placed in lithotomy to create the most optically correct view of the operative field. The five-port placement scheme previously described is used here as well. Dissection begins at the esophageal hiatus. The pars flaccida is incised and dissection continues until the right crus is seen. The phrenoesophageal ligament is divided, and careful dissection continues toward the left crus to identify the anterior vagus nerve. A minimum of 4 to 5 cm of nerve must be mobilized from the surrounding tissue and esophagus to allow for safe instrumentation. The nerve is clipped proximally and distally, allowing for an approximately 1-cm segment to be resected and sent to pathology for histologic confirmation (Fig. 24-13, page 215).

More dissection may be needed to mobilize the esophagus in order to expose the posterior vagus nerve. The posterior vagus is less adherent to the esophagus; it is located in the loose areolar tissue surrounding the esophagus and can be seen as a bowing, taut structure when the esophagus is retracted downward. Retraction of the stomach toward the left upper quadrant further exposes the posterior esophagus. Similar to the anterior vagus, 4 to 5 cm of the length of the posterior vagus nerve is skeletonized and clipped proximally and distally; a nerve segment should be sent to pathology. With limited dissection, an antireflux procedure can be avoided.

A Heineke-Mikulicz pyloroplasty is the emptying procedure of choice due to its simplicity and effectiveness (Fig. 24-14, page 216). A full-thickness gastrotomy is created in the prepyloric distal stomach. This gastrotomy is extended longitudinally through the pylorus, using ultrasonic shears. The incision through the pylorus is then closed transversely with a running suture. Begin by placing the apical stitch halfway along the length of the longitudinal defect.

Highly Selective Vagotomy

Highly selective vagotomy (HSV) involves division of the gastric branches of the vagus nerves innervating the acid-producing portions of the stomach. This approach is the ideal treatment for intractable disease without gastric outlet obstruction. Each branch of the nerve follows the arterial and venous branches of the left gastric vessels along the lesser omentum. These branch vessels are thin, friable, and easily damaged. Maintaining hemostasis is critical for the dissection as bleeding obscures anatomical planes, increasing the risk for esophageal or gastric perforation.

Patient preparation and positioning and trocar placement should be very similar to positions chosen for other foregut procedures, such as the Nissen fundoplication for the treatment of gastroesophageal reflux. Laparoscopic HSV has the additional advantage of magnification significantly improving the identification of anatomical structures. This operation has been greatly facilitated by the application of the ultrasonic shears, which enable rapid and hemostatic division of all neurovascular input to the lesser curve. The anterior vagus nerve will be identified as being closely adherent to the esophagus. It can be seen as it courses across the GEJ to the left of midline. A marking stitch is placed just to the left of the anterior vagus nerve as it appears at the GEJ. Close inspection of the lesser omentum along the lesser curvature will reveal the anterior nerve of Latarjet (Fig. 24-6, page 212). Each branch of this nerve follows the arterial and venous branches of the left gastric vessels. The pylorus is identified by locating a prepyloric groove in the distal antrum. The distal extent of the pylorus is marked by the pyloric vein of Mayo. Approximately 5 to 6 cm from the pylorus, the most proximal branch of the thin, string-like "crow's foot" can be seen. A second marking stitch is placed at this level and to the left of this first branch of the crow's foot (Fig. 24-7, page 212). The branches to the distal antrum must remain intact to maintain pyloric function. These two stitches mark the upper and lower limits of dissection (Fig. 24-8, page 213). It must be emphasized again that adequate hemostasis is important for safe dissection. Dissection will proceed from the distal stitch and then move in a cephalad direction, working toward the proximal stitch. Dissection will always remain to the left of the sutures and extend over the anterior aspect of the cardia to the angle of His and as far posteriorly as the lateral aspect of the left crus. The gastrohepatic ligament should be completely incised, creating a window above and below each neurovascular bundle. Each vessel with its accompanying nerve is controlled and divided

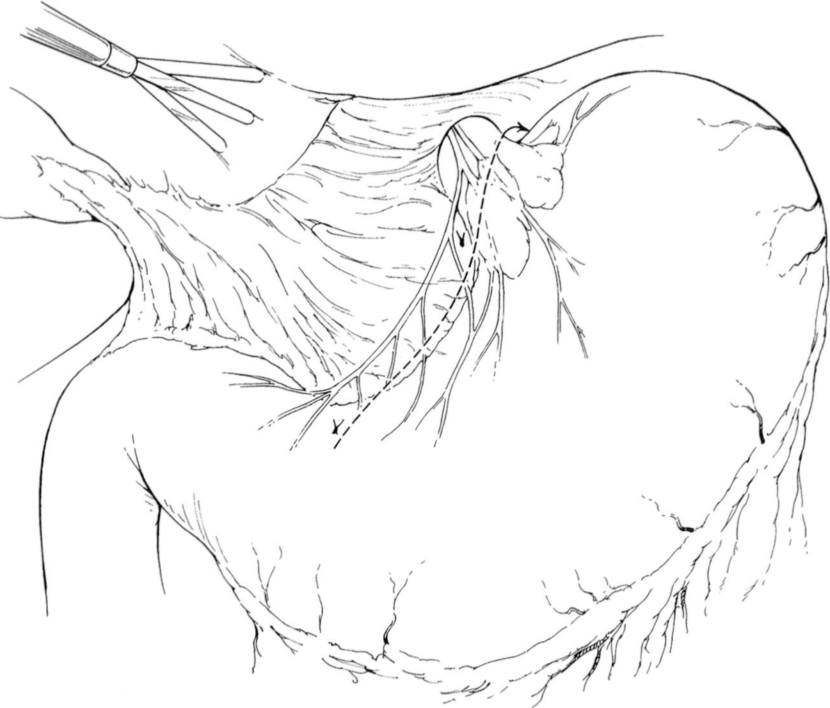

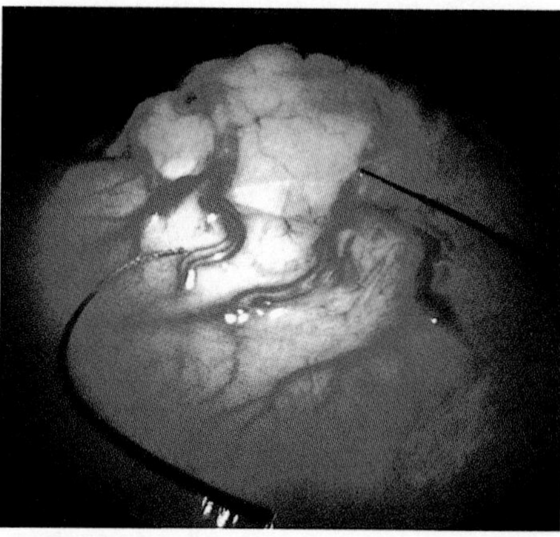

Fig. 24-6. Left: The nerve of Latarjet is identified as a thin, white filament (see arrow) descending on the lesser curve in the lesser omentum. Color inset: The crow's foot is demonstrated by the lowermost blue thread, with accompanying antral branches that must be protected.

using ultrasonic shears. To prevent injury to the vagus nerves in the lesser omentum, it is essential to remain just on the gastric serosa and no deeper. Once all anterior leaflet neurovascular bundles are divided, the anterior leaflet should be completely opened from the crow's foot to the angle of His.

Once the opening of the anterior leaflet is completed, the posterior leaflet can be addressed (Fig. 24-9, page 213). Begin by hugging the lesser curve just above the incisura and bluntly dissecting to create a window into the lesser sac just above the lower limit of dissection of the crow's foot. The greater curve of the stomach can then be elevated. The hanging omentum is incised to enter the lesser sac. The posterior stomach is gently retracted, further elevating the greater curve to expose the posterior crow's foot (Fig. 24-10, page 214). A Penrose drain can then be placed through the window created earlier, encircling the distal stomach at the crow's foot. The position of the Penrose drain marks the distal extent of the dissection (Fig. 24-11, page 214). Proceed in a cephalad direction, controlling the posterior neurovascular pedicles with the ultrasonic shears. Dissection should continue until the left diaphragmatic crus is identified from this position. The back of the stomach should be completely free of retroperitoneal attachments. Once the left crus is visible, a second Penrose drain can be placed around the esophagus. This allows upward traction of the esophagus and dissection of its posterior aspect, controlling the posterior vagal fibers under direct visualization (Fig. 24-12,

Fig. 24-7. A second stitch is placed just after the first branch of the crow's foot.

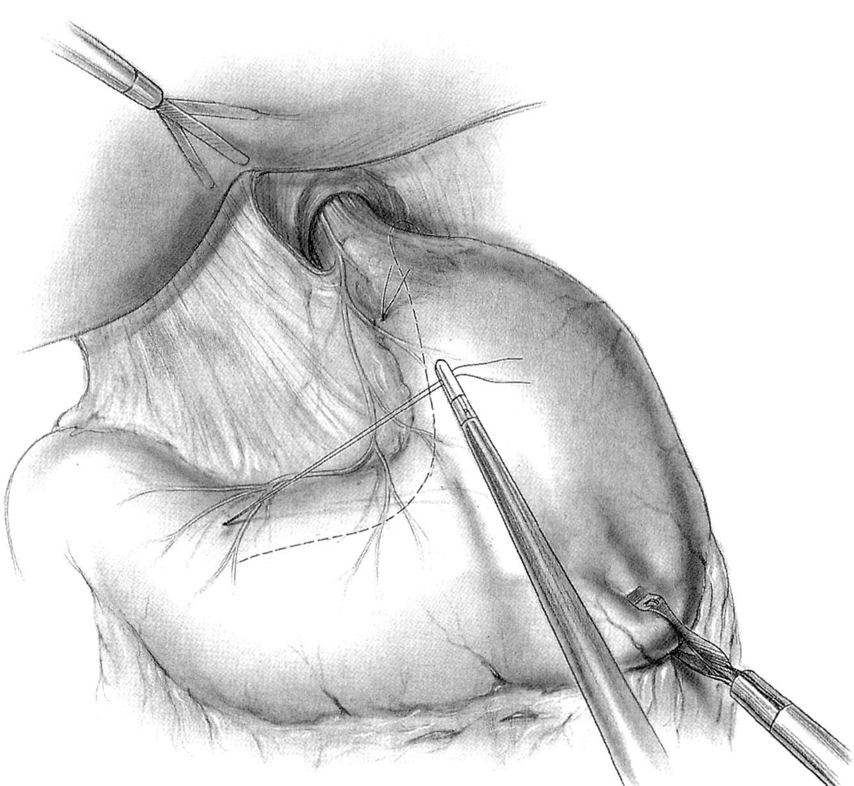

Fig. 24-8. The relative position of the two marking stitches is seen with traction on the stomach. The line of dissection passes from the lower stitch cephalad, hugging the stomach wall and passing to the left of the upper stitch toward the angle of His.

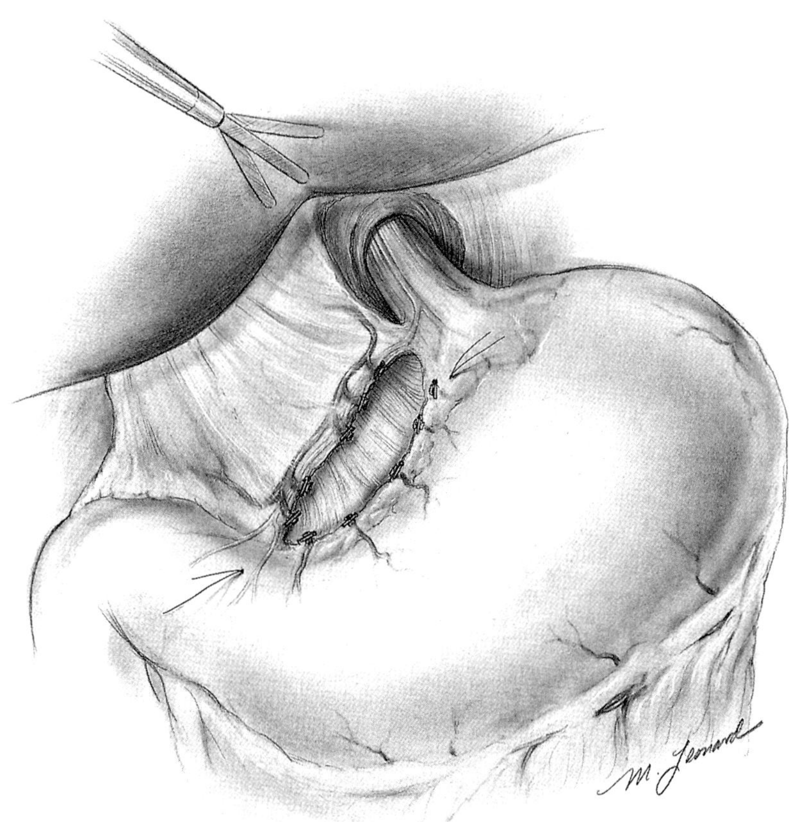

Fig. 24-9. The anterior leaf dissection is complete, leaving the intermediate and posterior leaves (not seen) yet to be dissected.

page 215). Five centimeters of the distal esophagus should be cleared of vagal branches. An antireflux procedure is unnecessary if the crura and hiatal area are not formally dissected. If appropriate sparing of the vagal braches to the antrum has been done, a drainage procedure is unnecessary.

Posterior Truncal Vagotomy with Anterior Lesser Curve Seromyotomy

A modification of the HSV was developed to simplify the tedious dissection involved with the individual isolation of each neurovascular branch prior to availability of ultrasonic technology. This modification involves a posterior truncal vagotomy with an anterior seromyotomy. Port positioning is similar to the five-port method described for HSV. A posterior truncal vagotomy, detailed in the previous section, is then performed. A path along the lesser curve is then delineated. This line begins at a point 5 to 7 cm from the pylorus and continues toward the angle of His. Marking stitches are placed at the proximal and distal extents of this line. The gastric wall is then divided along this path, developing a plane between the gastric serosa and mucosa. Larger neurovascular bundles can be controlled with the ultrasonic shears. After the myotomy is completed and all vagal branches divided, the serosa is closed with a running silk suture.

Further modification involves having marking sutures function as traction sutures delineating a ridge of gastric tissue that may be introduced into a laparoscopic linear cutting stapler. Several loads will be required to continue the path toward the angle of His. Use of the linear cutting stapler in this manner eliminates the need for suturing the serosal defect closed.

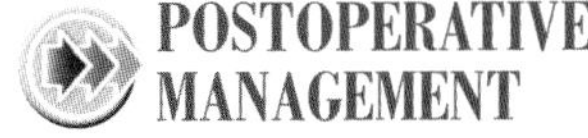

POSTOPERATIVE MANAGEMENT

Patients undergoing elective laparoscopic surgery to treat peptic ulcer disease generally do well and begin ambulating in the immediate postoperative period. Appropriate analgesics are provided. Nasogastric decompression is unnecessary, and NSAIDs should be used sparingly, if at all. Oral intake is advanced appropriately, and patients are usually discharged on the second postoperative day.

Patients presenting with acute perforation tend to be sicker and may require close monitoring in an intensive care unit. Appropriate IV fluid rehydration and

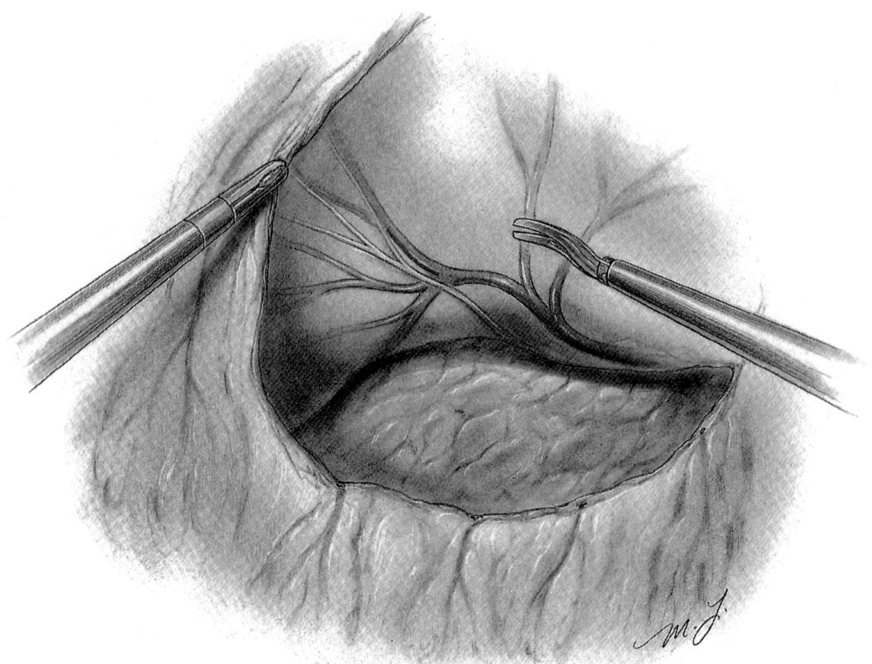

Fig. 24-10. The posterior gastric nerve is visible crossing the arcade of vessels of the posterior crow's foot. This view is achieved by elevating the posterior wall of the stomach.

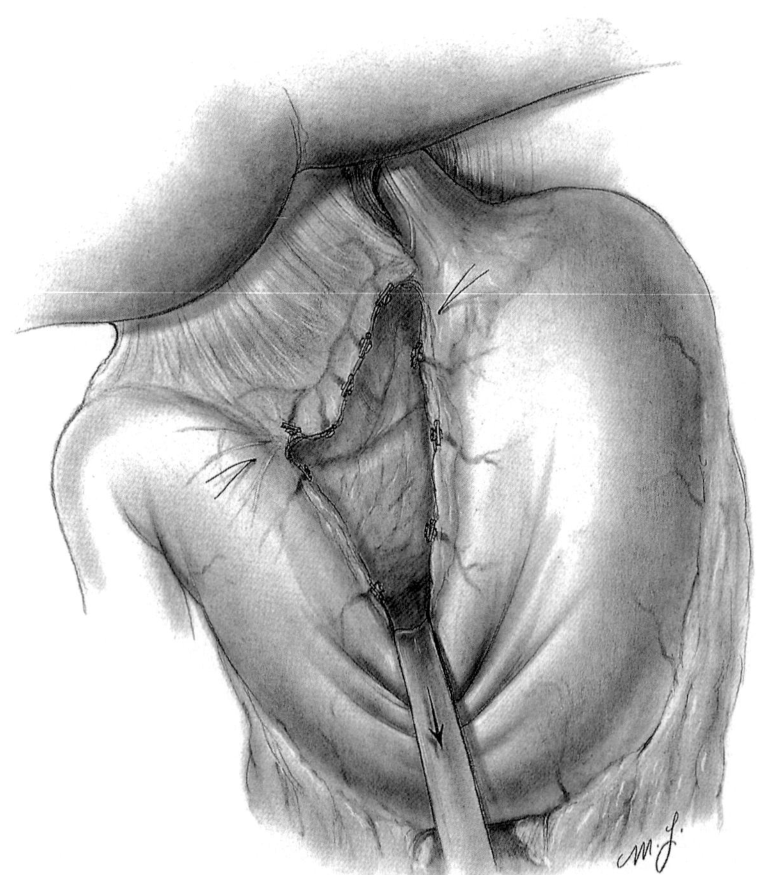

Fig. 24-11. The appearance of the lesser curve with downward traction, using a Penrose drain at the lower limit of the vagotomy dissection.

intravenous antibiotics are imperative. A postoperative paralytic ileus is common, and oral intake is initiated when the patient displays evidence of return of gastrointestinal function.

POSTGASTRECTOMY SYNDROMES

Accompanying the steep decline in the frequency of operations performed for PUD is the surgeon's unfamiliarity with postgastrectomy and postvagotomy syndromes. Disturbed gastric motor function can occur as a direct consequence of upper abdominal surgery, gastric surgery, and particularly vagal nerve disruption. Approximately 25% of patients undergoing gastric surgery will experience postgastrectomy symptoms. Symptoms severe enough to warrant further surgical intervention, however, will persist in only 1% to 3% of the cases. Increased familiarization with these postoperative issues is essential for prevention at the time of the initial operation and for accurate diagnosis when they do occur.

Dumping Syndrome

Dumping syndrome describes the rapid and poorly controlled gastric emptying after meals that patients experience after gastrectomy with vagotomy. With the pylorus being either resected or bypassed, the functional reservoir of the body of the stomach is lost and the pyloric regulatory mechanism no longer exists. Moreover, destruction of the vagal nerve causes a loss of receptive relaxation of the proximal stomach and weakened antral peristaltic contractions. These processes lead to the accelerated emptying of hyperosmolar chyme into the duodenum and small bowel. Patients complain of vasomotor or gastrointestinal symptoms that range in severity from being annoying to debilitating.

Early dumping occurs within 10 to 30 minutes after a meal. This rapid "dumping" of the hyperosmolar chyme into the small bowel precipitates the inappropriate release of vasoactive gut peptides, and fluid shifts from the intravascular space into the small bowel. At this point, patients may complain of postprandial bloating, nausea, and crampy abdominal pain. Tachycardia, palpitations, and lightheadedness may develop as a result of the relative hypovolemia and hypotension. Explosive diarrhea ensues in some.

Late dumping occurs less often and usually develops 2 to 3 hours after meals.

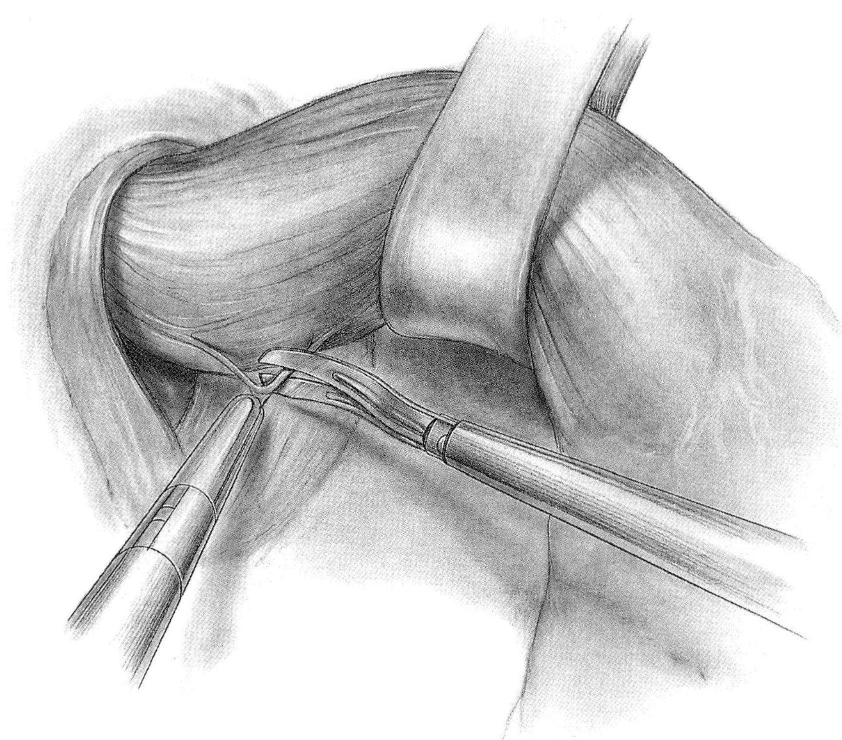

Fig. 24-12. The posterior aspect of the esophagus is carefully cleaned of vagal fibers under direct vision. The esophagus is meticulously dissected for 5 cm of its intraabdominal course to divide any small vagal filaments passing the fascial bands, seen here in the scissors blade.

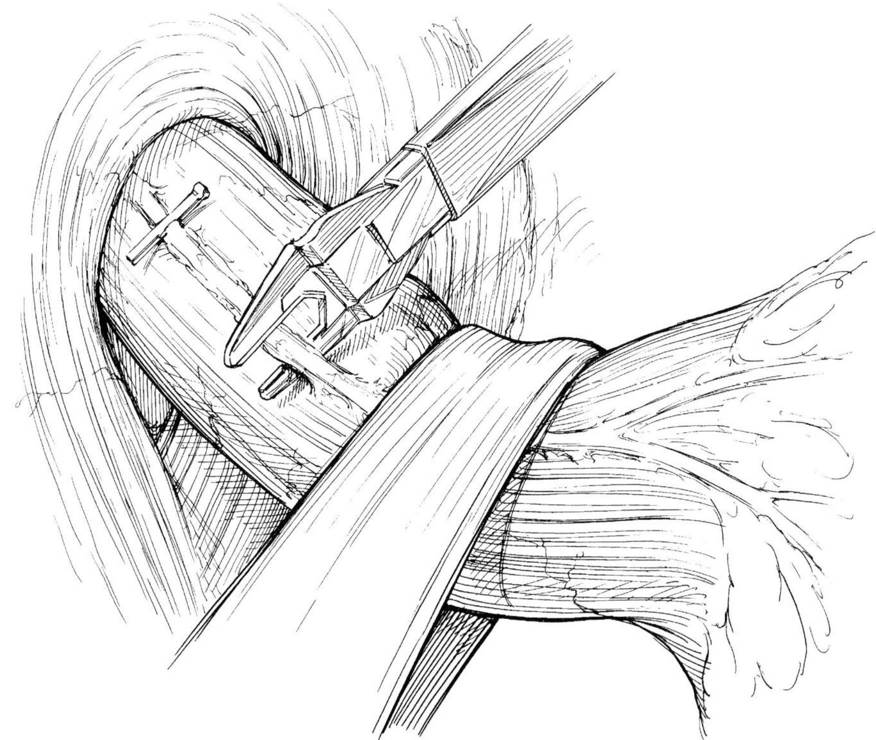

Fig. 24-13. Posterior and caudad retraction of the gastroesophageal junction, with the assistance of a Penrose drain, reveals the anterior vagus nerve. The nerve is skeletonized from the surrounding tissue and clipped proximally and distally. A short segment is removed and sent to pathology postoperatively for confirmation of vagotomy.

This syndrome is a result of reactive hypoglycemia that occurs due to the exaggerated peptide release, including enteroglucagon, triggered by the presence of the initial high carbohydrate load into the proximal small bowel. These peptides sensitize the β-cell to stimulation by blood glucose levels, resulting in excessive insulin release. The patient experiences symptoms similar to the vasomotor symptoms of hypoglycemia in a diabetic with an insulin reaction. These symptoms are usually relieved by the administration of sugar.

The incidence of the dumping syndrome is dependent upon the type of gastric surgery performed. It is uncommonly encountered in patients who have undergone highly selective vagotomy (1% to 3%). After gastrectomy with truncal vagotomy, however, 25% to 50% of patients experience some form of dumping. Fortunately, the overwhelming majority of patients respond to conservative management efforts.

The mainstay of treatment involves dietary and lifestyle modifications. Small, frequent meals, separating the ingestion of solid and liquids, avoiding simple or concentrated carbohydrates, and adding fiber or complex carbohydrates to meals are recommended. The supine position after meals may also slow gastric emptying and increase venous return, thus minimizing symptoms. Octreotide, a somatostatin analogue, may be effective for patients who are refractory to simple dietary modifications. Octreotide acts to slow gastric emptying, inhibit insulin release, and decrease gut peptide secretion.

The overwhelming majority of patients improve with these conservative measures. Surgery for refractory dumping syndrome is rarely ever needed. Multidisciplinary nonsurgical management must be optimized prior to considering a surgical solution, as surgical options have not been met with uniform success.

For patients with a pyloroplasty, the remedial procedure is a pyloric reconstruction. Pyloric reconstruction is amenable to a minimally invasive approach. Patient preparation, positioning, and trocar placement is similar to that previously described. The previous pyloroplasty scar is opened, and the pyloric muscular ring is reapproximated as the incision is closed longitudinally. Approximately 80% of patients report relief of their dumping symptoms.

Patients with a prior distal gastrectomy and gastroduodenostomy (Billroth I) or gastrojejunostomy (Billroth II) reconstruction can be managed with conversion to

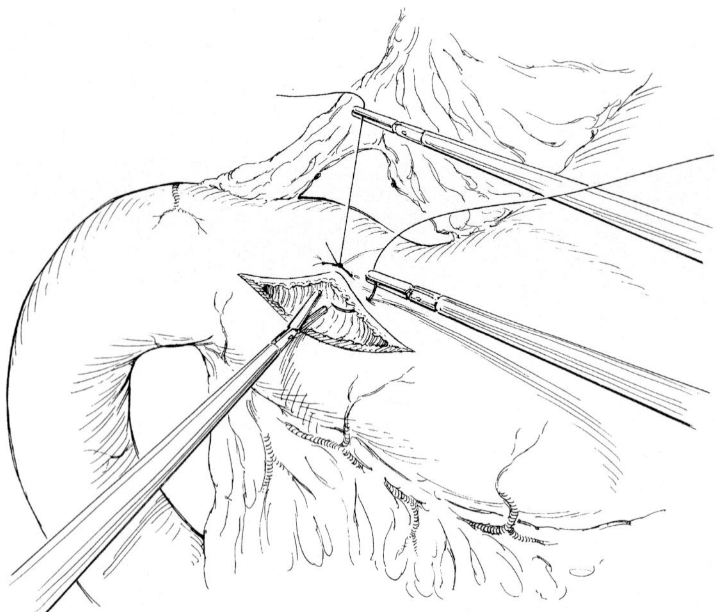

Fig. 24-14. Heineke-Mickulicz pyloroplasty: The gastrotomy must extend to the duodenum distally and the antrum proximally. Transverse closure is performed in a single layer with full-thickness interrupted sutures.

a Roux-en-Y gastrojejunostomy. Patient preparation, positioning, and trocar placement is similar to that previously described. For conversion of a Billroth I to a Roux-en-Y gastrojejunostomy, the prior anastomosis should be resected, and a retrocolic gastrojejunostomy constructed with a 50-cm Roux limb. For conversion of a Billroth II to a Roux-en-Y gastrojejunostomy, the previous anastomosis may be left in place provided that it is satisfactory; the afferent limb is then transected proximal to the stomach and anastomosed to the jejunum at least 50 cm downstream. These procedures are illustrated in Chapter 29, as they pertain to the laparoscopic Roux-en-Y gastric bypass.

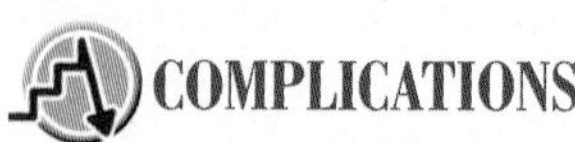

COMPLICATIONS

Postvagotomy Diarrhea

Although approximately 20% of postvagotomy patients complain of diarrhea, fewer than 1% will experience disabling diarrhea. This diarrhea occurs immediately after eating and is not associated with other symptoms. The absence of a constellation of symptoms is important in distinguishing postvagotomy diarrhea from a dumping syndrome. All other potential causes of diarrhea, including bacterial overgrowth, *Clostridium difficile* colitis, malabsorption, laxative abuse, parasites, gluten enteropathy, and inflammatory bowel disease must be ruled out. Most patients respond to nonsurgical management, including dietary and lifestyle changes similar to that suggested for the dumping syndromes, antidiarrheals, cholestyramine to bind bile salts, and octreotide.

Surgical treatment for refractory postvagotomy diarrhea is rarely needed. An appropriate interval, at least 1 year from the onset of symptoms, should be allotted to ensure that all nonsurgical therapies have been appropriately assessed. If surgical intervention has been deemed necessary due to severe, intractable, debilitating diarrhea, the procedure of choice is a 10-cm reversed jejunal interposition placed in continuity 100 cm distal to the ligament of Treitz.

Bile Reflux Gastritis

Pyloric sphincter destruction, removal, or bypass allows for the reflux of duodenal contents into the stomach with resultant inflammation. Symptomatic patients complain of constant burning epigastric pain and nausea with or without vomiting. Determining a causal relationship of the development of symptoms to bile reflux, however, is problematic as asymptomatic patients often experience bile reflux as well. Fortunately, severe symptoms of alkaline reflux gastritis develop only 1% or less of the time. Other problems, such as afferent or efferent loop obstruction, gastric stasis, and small bowel obstruction, must be ruled out before attributing the symptoms to bile reflux gastritis.

Bile reflux is diagnosed using endoscopy with gastric biopsy or with a bile reflux (DISIDA) scan showing significant entry of the radionuclide into the stomach. Once the diagnosis is made, medical therapies are attempted as dietary and behavioral changes are not usually helpful. Options include prokinetic agents, coating agents such as sucralfate, and cholestyramine.

Unlike other postgastrectomy syndromes, the nonsurgical options for the management of bile reflux gastritis are largely disappointing. The best surgical option is conversion to a Roux-en-Y gastrojejunostomy. The Roux limb must be at least 50 cm to prevent pancreaticobiliary secretions from refluxing into the gastric remnant. This resolves symptoms in approximately 80% of those with documented bile reflux gastritis. For patients with a Billroth II reconstruction, the afferent and efferent jejunal limbs can be anastomosed in a side-to-side fashion (Braun enteroenterostomy) to divert the bile/pancreatic juice from the stomach.

Gastric Dysmotility

Gastroparesis is defined as gastric motor dysfunction in the absence of a structural or mechanical obstruction. Gastric stasis may occur after gastric surgery, due to either altered gastric motor function or obstruction. Etiologies other than gastric surgery include diabetes mellitus, idiopathic causes, neurologic disorders, connective tissue diseases, and intestinal pseudo-obstructions. Patients typically complain of early satiety, postprandial epigastric pain, and intractable nausea and vomiting. Weight loss and malnutrition may result. Symptoms may become severe enough to necessitate enteral or parenteral nutritional supplementation.

Evaluation includes upper GI series with small bowel study, EGD, and gastric emptying scan. The imaging and endoscopic studies are necessary to identify strictures or narrowing, searching for a possible site of mechanical obstruction. Gastric scintigraphy, a gastric emptying scan, is the gold standard for diagnosis of delayed gastric emptying. The patient ingests a radio-labeled meal and a gamma camera evaluates the degree of gastric emptying at regular intervals for 2 to 4 hours. Emptying of greater than 50% of the meal by 2 hours is considered normal. Retention of greater than 10% of the meal at 4 hours is considered delayed. The results are typically reported as a T½ for liquid and solid emptying.

Dietary measures, including frequent small meals low in fiber and fat and prokinetic drugs, bring relief to most patients. Metoclopramide is a dopamine antagonist that works on the stomach and also has antiemetic properties. Domperidone, stimulating the stomach and small intestine via cholinergic mechanisms, also displays both prokinetic and antiemetic actions. Erythromycin, a motilin agonist, works on both the stomach and the intestine. Patients with severe nausea and vomiting may benefit from the specific addition of antiemetic medications to their regimen.

A small subset of patients will not respond to these conservative measures and require operative intervention. The initial procedure is often placement of a simple venting gastrostomy tube. This intervention may be performed using the endoscopic-percutaneous approach or laparoscopically. The patient suffering from intractable nausea and vomiting may require enteral access for nutritional support via a jejunostomy feeding tube.

The jejunostomy feeding tube may be placed laparoscopically. For this operation, the patient is usually positioned supine. Once intraperitoneal access is obtained with two trocars positioned along the right abdominal side wall, the anterior abdominal wall is cleared of any adhesions. Great care in dissection and the avoidance of the use of energy is essential for the prevention of an inadvertent enterotomy. The small bowel is then evaluated from the ligament of Treitz to the ileocecal valve. At this point, patient positioning in the right lateral reverse Trendelenburg position may be helpful. The omentum and the transverse colon are then gently manipulated upward to expose the ligament of Treitz. The internal entry site for the feeding jejunostomy tube is selected some distance away from the ligament of Treitz, but still in the proximal jejunum in the left upper quadrant. Various commercially available laparoscopic jejunostomy tube kits are available. These prepackaged items are convenient as all necessary tools are enclosed. The external jejunostomy site is then selected on the anterior abdominal wall, usually to the left of midline. The chosen limb of jejunum is then retracted anteriorly to ensure that it reaches this site without undue tension. Commercially available T-fasteners are then loaded onto the slotted needle. The pneumoperitoneum is decreased to 7 to 10 mmHg to allow the jejunum to be drawn close to the anterior abdominal wall, thus preventing tearing of the small bowel by the T-fasteners. Four T-fasteners are placed through the antimesenteric wall of the jejunum, aligning them in a diamond configuration. After the four T-fasteners are properly positioned, the sutures are pulled to snug the jejunum to the anterior abdominal wall. The jejunum is then accessed with a needle at a 45-degree angle into the jejunal lumen entering at the center of the diamond configuration. Air is injected to confirm placement. The J-guidewire is then passed, J-end first, through the needle into the jejunum. The T-fasteners are then dropped to loosen the jejunum and ensure that the J-guidewire is indeed within the jejunal lumen. A small skin incision is then placed at the J-guidewire entry site. The peel-away sheath/dilator is then placed over the J-guidewire and the path into the jejunum dilated. The jejunostomy tube is inserted into the jejunum using the Seldinger technique. The J-guidewire is removed once it is confirmed that the jejunal feeding tube is in good position with its tip directed in the distal direction. Its position can also be tested by injecting saline into the side feeding port. The T-fasteners are then pulled snug and stabilized, and the J-tube is secured to the skin. A radiologic examination must be performed using contrast medium to confirm positioning and to check for possible extravasation.

If patients continue to have problems with intractable symptoms of gastroparesis in spite of these conservative surgical procedures, a pyloroplasty (described above) or gastrojejunostomy (described in association with antrectomy elsewhere in the text) may be required to drain the stomach.

For patients with previous vagotomy and drainage with refractory postresection gastroparesis, a subtotal (75%) gastrectomy with Billroth II reconstruction and Braun enteroenterostomy may be helpful. Intractable gastroparesis after subtotal gastric resection can be treated with a near-total (95%) or total gastrectomy with a Roux-en-Y reconstruction. If a total gastrectomy is performed, the patient may benefit from the creation of a jejunal reservoir. These procedures are certainly amenable to the minimally invasive approach. Detailed discussions on laparoscopic gastric resection are detailed elsewhere in this edition.

Gastric electrical stimulation, using an implantable gastric electrical stimulator, has been reported to enhance nutritional status and reduce the requirements for supplemental feeds. This device has been approved for use in refractory gastroparesis since March 2000 by the Food and Drug Administration under a humanitarian device exemption. Longer-term controlled trials are needed to help better define patient selection criteria and optimum pacing parameters. Specific details regarding gastric electrical stimulator implantation are addressed elsewhere in this edition.

CONCLUSION

Although the overall numbers of procedures performed for benign gastric disorders are diminishing, a wide range of pathology still requires intervention. Laparoscopic techniques for the management of benign gastric disorders have gained acceptance as being safe and feasible. Increased minimally invasive surgical experience and improved technology have led to increasingly creative ways to surgically treat benign gastric disease. Newer innovations and hybrid procedures combining laparoscopy with endoscopic and robotic techniques portend less invasive methods in the future.

SUGGESTED READING

Ali T, Hasan M, Hamadani M, et al. Gastroparesis. *South Med J* 2007;100(3):281–286.

Eswaran S, Roy MA. Medical management of acid-peptic disorders of the stomach. *Surg Clin North Am* 2005;85(5):895–906.

Hasler WL. Gastroparesis: symptoms, evaluation, and treatment. *Gastroenterol Clin North Am* 2007;36(3):619–647.

Jamieson GG. Current status of indications for surgery in peptic ulcer disease. *World J Surg* 2000;24(3):256–258.

Jones MP, Magani K. A systematic review of surgical therapy for gastroparesis. *Am J Gastroenterol* 2003;98(10):2122–2129.

Kaiser AM, Katkhouda N. Laparoscopic management of the perforated viscus. *Semin Laparosc Surg* 2002;9(1):46–53.

Martin RF. Surgical management of ulcer disease. *Surg Clin North Am* 2005;85(5):907–929.

Millat B, Fingerhut A, Borie F. Surgical treatment of complicated duodenal ulcers: controlled trials. *World J Surg* 2000;24(3):299–306.

Sarosi GA Jr, Jaiswal KR, Nwariaku FE, et al. Surgical therapy of peptic ulcers in the 21st century: more common than you think. *Am J Surg* 2005;190(5):775–779.

Shafi MA, Pasricha PJ. Post-surgical and obstructive gastroparesis. *Curr Gastroenterol Rep* 2007;9(4):280–285.

Siu WT, Leong HT, Law BK, et al. Laparoscopic repair for perforated peptic ulcer: a randomized controlled trial. *Ann Surg* 2002;235(3):313–319.

COMMENTARY

Drs. Murayama and Bueno have summarized the current laparoscopic approach to benign diseases of the stomach. Although elective surgical therapy of peptic ulcer disease has essentially become a thing of the past, treatment of complications and the surgical management of other diseases (such as gastroesophageal reflux) in the presence of an ulcer diathesis may lead to an acid-reducing procedure. Because most of the younger surgeons today have minimal experience with treatment of ulcers, basic principles should be remembered: that is, ulcers of the duodenum, pylorus, and prepyloric region generally are caused by too much acid, whereas ulcers higher in the stomach are usually caused by a defect of gastric mucosal resistance. Furthermore, gastric ulcers may be associated with cancer; thus, resection of the gastric ulcer is often the appropriate initial therapy. Most of the literature dealing with surgical therapy of peptic ulcer disease was generated prior to the era of our understanding the role of *H. pylori* in its etiology.

There have been a few relatively small prospective randomized trials comparing laparoscopic to open management of perforated duodenal ulcers, which generally have found the laparoscopic approach to be associated with fewer complications, shorter operative times, and shorter lengths of hospital stay. When performing laparoscopic repair of perforated duodenal ulcers, the authors have described closing the perforation before performing the omental patch. The original Graham patch technique did not include closure of the hole, but rather simply patched it with the omentum, and this procedure performed laparoscopically is also appropriate.

The authors describe performing the highly selective (proximal gastric) vagotomy using the ultrasonic shears to "control and divide each vessel with its accompanying nerve." The reality is that ultrasonic shears are simply used to totally disconnect the lesser curve of the stomach from the nerve of Latarjet while being absolutely certain to maintain the integrity of both anterior and posterior vagal trunks. Surgeons should remember the experience from open surgery that suggested at least 5 to 7 centimeters of the distal esophagus should also be denervated. When performing a highly selective vagotomy, I usually encircle both vagal trunks with vessel loops to allow gentle traction to be placed on them and ensure that all nervous input to the proximal portion of the stomach is divided. The inclusion of the section describing posterior truncal vagotomy with anterior lesser curve seromyotomy is largely of historical interest. This operation was initially described by Katkhouda et al. prior to the availability of the ultrasonic shears and has largely been supplanted by the use of this very convenient energy device.

Accompanying the decrease in the number of operations performed for peptic ulcer disease is a decrease in the incidence of postgastrectomy syndromes. Patients who have dumping and diarrhea may be very difficult to manage. They should be extensively evaluated to be sure of the diagnosis. Most patients may be managed medically, but occasionally surgical solutions will be required.

NJS

B. Premalignant and Malignant Diseases

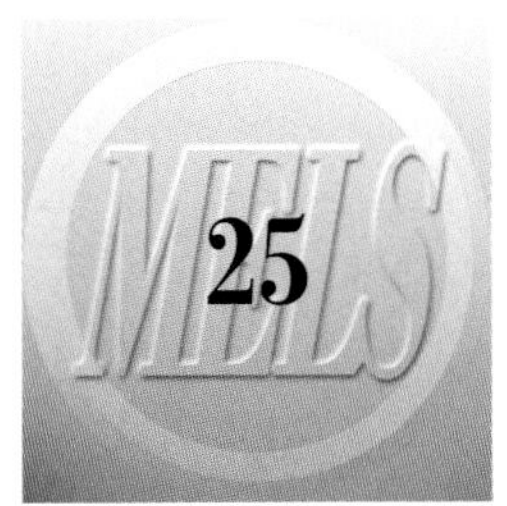

Endoscopic Diagnosis, Staging, and Resection of Premalignant and Malignant Gastric Disease

BRENT WHITE AND EDWARD LIN

INTRODUCTION

Gastric cancer is a prominent cancer in the world, second only to lung cancer in overall cancer mortality statistics. The prevalence of gastric cancer in Asia, South America, and Eastern Europe is high, whereas gastric carcinoma is uncommon in the United States and Canada. The reason for this discrepancy in epidemiology remains unclear.

In Japan, a country where gastric cancer is the most frequently diagnosed malignancy in men, mass population screening programs have been in place since the 1960s. Likely because of this, nearly half of new gastric cancer diagnoses made in Japan are deemed early gastric cancers. Early gastric cancer is confined to the mucosa or submucosa regardless of lymph-node status and is associated with a better than 90% five-year survival rate. In the United States, early gastric cancers account for only 10% of new gastric cancer cases diagnosed. With increasing use of endoscopy in the evaluation of foregut complaints in the U.S., the detection of earlier stage gastric cancer may be increasing. This chapter focuses on the methods for endoscopic resection developed in Japan nearly 20 years ago. These methods are being increasingly utilized in Europe and the United States.

Diagnosis

GASTRIC POLYPS

Gastric polyps include three broadly recognized types: (1) fundic gland, (2) hyperplastic, and (3) adenomatous. These polyps are found infrequently on upper endoscopic procedures and are histologically benign more than 80% of the time. There are no reliable endoscopic "appearance" criteria that can be used to distinguish different gastric polypoid histologies.

The fundic gland polyp is a cystic mucosal elevation composed of normal parietal and chief cells. They are usually 2 to 3 mm in size and appear clustered together in a grapelike fashion within the gastric fundus and body. These polyps generally have no malignant potential but can, in rare cases, be associated with familial adenomatous polyposis (FAP) and/or harbor dysplastic or adenomatous changes.

Hyperplastic polyps can be found throughout the stomach and range widely in size (from millimeters to centimeters), number, and morphology (pedunculated or sessile). While these polyps have little malignant potential they are associated with chronic atrophic gastritis, an entity that may predispose to gastric malignancy.

Adenomatous polyps are the rarest of polyps found within the stomach, but they are premalignant lesions and contain foci of invasive adenocarcinoma as often as 40% of the time. These polyps are generally larger in size than both hyperplastic and fundic gland polyps but can be variable in both size and shape. The risk of invasive adenocarcinoma directly correlates with the size of the polyp.

The use of pinch biopsy forceps, shown in Figure 25-1, affords a simple method of obtaining mucosal tissue for histologic diagnosis for small polyps (<2 cm). Such a biopsy can be performed with either conventional-sized or "jumbo" forceps. While conventional forceps can fit within a standard 2.8-mm endoscopic channel, jumbo forceps require an endoscope with a larger endoscopic working channel (3.6 mm). Larger forceps can provide a sample with greater surface area and less crush artifact.

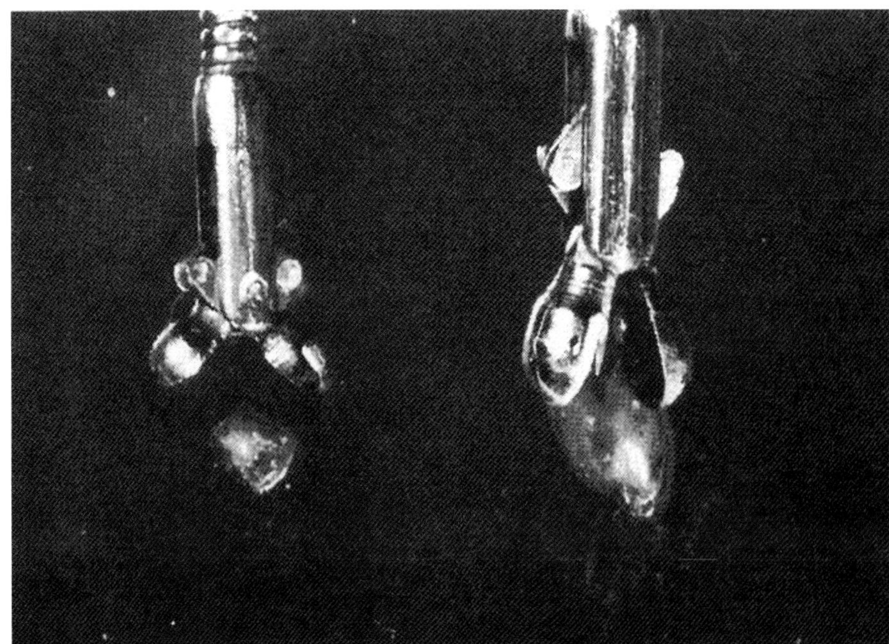

Fig. 25-1. Conventional biopsy forceps on left, jumbo forceps right. (With permission from *Textbook of Gastroenterology*, Yamada et al. eds. Philadelphia: Lippincott Williams & Wilkins, 2003, p. 2827.)

This can make specimen orientation easier and also potentially reduce the chance of an insufficient tissue sample. Regardless of size chosen, forceps biopsies provide larger tissue yields by turning the scope toward the lesion and aspirating mucosa into the open jaws of the forceps (the "turn-and-suction" technique), rather than simply applying the forceps with greater force against the lesion. Forceps biopsies should be obtained from a polypoid lesion until the endoscopist is confident of a representative sample. In addition, biopsies of the mucosa adjacent to the polyp should also be submitted for inspection.

Further management of small gastric polyps should be guided by the histology results from the initial forceps biopsy. For fundic gland polyps, barring any dysplasia or association with FAP, there is no need for further intervention or surveillance. Endoscopic polypectomy can be used for hyperplastic polyps with dysplasia and for adenomatous polyps. After removing adenomatous or dysplastic polyps, endoscopic surveillance is recommended to monitor for either recurrence or the development of cancer.

A complete polypectomy is indicated as the initial procedure for any polyp 2 cm in diameter or larger. For resection of a pedunculated polyp, a wire snare can be used to encircle the pedicle or stalk of the polyp close to its base, and electrocautery applied through the snare as it is tightened. Most snares can be deployed via a 2.8-mm conventional endoscopic channel. If the pedicle or stalk of the polyp is particularly thick, the risk of post-resection bleeding may be increased due to larger feeding vessels. To minimize bleeding, the base or stalk of the lesion can be injected with an epinephrine solution prior to carrying out the snare polypectomy. Another method is to place a *detachable* snare snugly around the base of the stalk prior to performing the snare polypectomy above the snare. Other hemostatic techniques can be applied as well, which can include clipping, sclerotherapy, electrocautery, and argon plasma coagulation (APC).

A polyp can have a sessile configuration, making it difficult to perform a polypectomy with a simple snare procedure. In this case, the snare is placed around the lesion and gently tightened while electrocautery is utilized to transect the lesion from surrounding normal mucosa and deeper normal gastric tissues. Injection of the submucosa with saline or dilute epinephrine prior to snare application facilitates this technique. Depending on the diameter of the lesion, multiple resections, known as "strip biopsy," may be required for complete resection, resulting in a piecemeal polypectomy specimen.

Endoscopic mucosal resection (EMR) is a modification of the original strip biopsy and can be applied to large sessile or flat polyps. The technique consists of converting flat lesions into a more polypoid shape, usually with the use of submucosal injection. The specimen is then transected deep to the mucosa, at the submucosal level, with electrocautery.

ATROPHIC GASTRITIS, INTESTINAL METAPLASIA, AND DYSPLASIA

Chronic atrophic gastritis, defined as the loss of appropriate glands in a given gastric region, has been associated with the development of gastric adenocarcinoma in some patients (Fig. 25-2). Given the lack of clear features (Fig. 25-3) and a frequently patchy distribution throughout the stomach, efforts have been made to standardize biopsy protocols such as the Updated Sydney System (Fig. 25-4).

When atrophic gastritis is found on endoscopic biopsy at the present time, there is no consensus on the need for endoscopic surveillance or follow-up. The presence of *Helicobacter pylori* in this setting is an indication for eradication therapy. Atrophic gastritis with high-grade dysplasia is an indication for resection (endoscopically or surgically) due to the propensity for transformation into invasive adenocarcinoma.

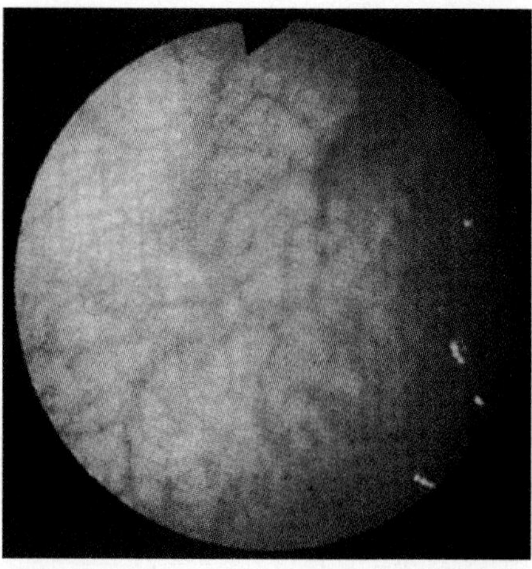

Fig. 25-3. Endoscopic photograph demonstrating the appearance of atrophic gastritis. (With permission from Textbook of Gastroenterology, Yamada et al. eds. Philadelphia: Lippincott Williams & Wilkins, 2003.)

MALIGNANT LESIONS

Gastric cancer can be variable in its endoscopic appearance and morphology, with ulcerated lesions being most commonly

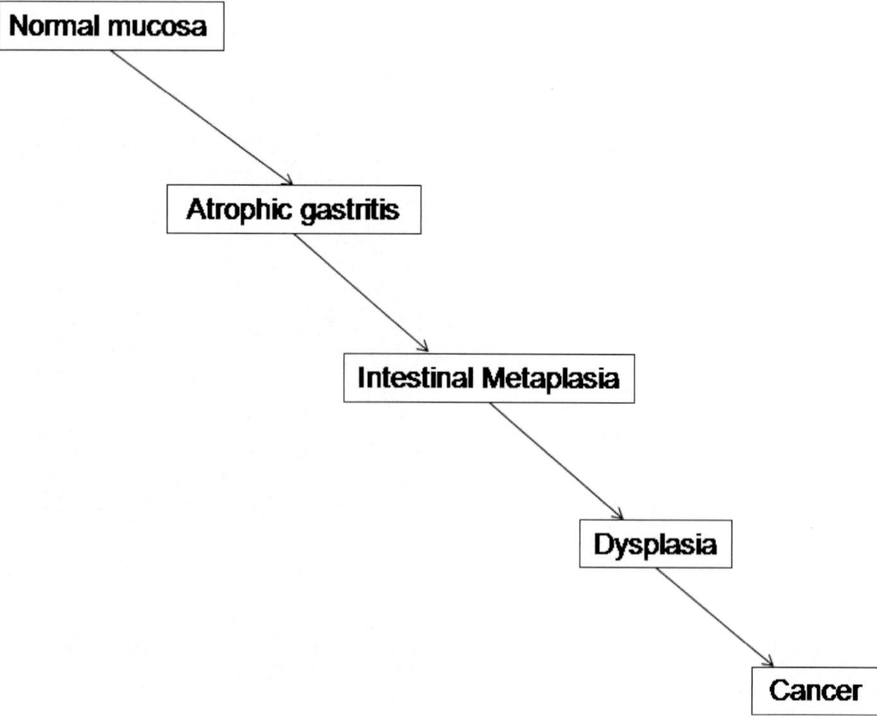

Fig. 25-2. Demonstration of the progression from normal mucosa to intestinal-type adenocarcinoma of the stomach.

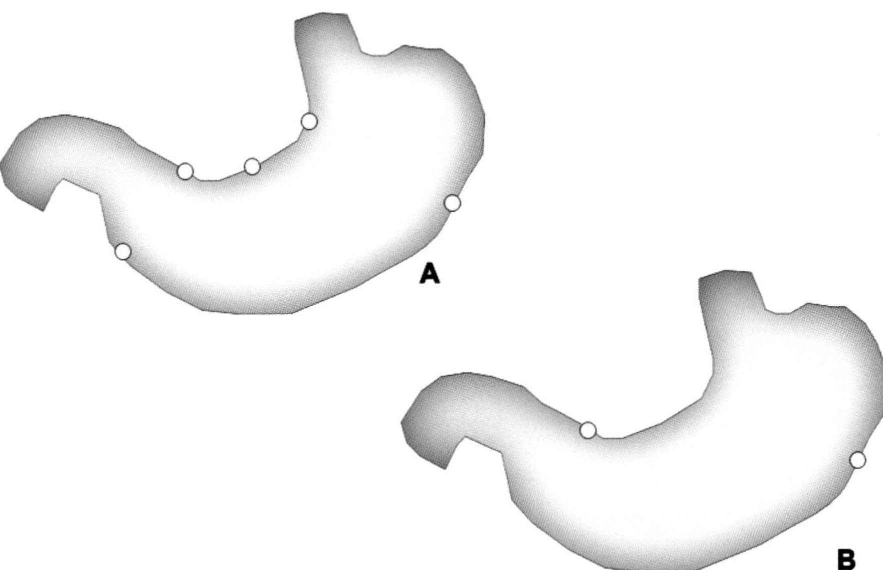

Fig. 25-4. The Updated Sydney Pattern of gastric mucosal biopsy for gastritis or metaplasia with **(A)** two biopsies in the antrum (each 2 cm from pylorus), one biopsy at the incisura, another biopsy midway between incisura and cardia, and a final biopsy along the midportion of the greater curve, compared with **(B)** the typical biopsy pattern for *H. pylori* with one biopsy from the body and another from the antrum.

encountered (Fig. 25-5). In contrast to the endoscopic appearance of advanced lesions, early gastric cancers can be subtle in their endoscopic appearance, sometimes appearing as slight depressions or elevations. Indeed, one Japanese study demonstrated that nearly 20% of early cancers went undetected on upper endoscopy examination. Therefore, endoscopic evaluation for early gastric cancer requires tissue biopsies from all areas of abnormality: discoloration, ulceration, nodularity, or depression. One regimen proposed to improve visualization and detection rates consists of an intramuscular injection of scopolamine ten minutes prior to the planned endoscopy to reduce gastric peristalsis. This is then followed by an oral solution containing dimethylpolysiloxane (simethicone) as well as a standardized amount of pronase, a proteolytic enzyme. This solution assists in reducing the amount of foam bubbles as well as gastric mucus.

Another means of enhancing mucosal lesion detection is chromoendoscopy. Several different chromoendoscopy solutions have been applied in the diagnosis of early gastric cancer. These agents fall into several categories based on their mechanism: (1) vital stains, which are absorbed into certain cell types, (2) contrast stains, which are not absorbed but instead pool in mucosal depressions, thus highlighting subtle topography, and (3) reactive stains, which change appearance when placed in environments with specific conditions. Indigo carmine is a contrast stain frequently used in gastric endoscopy, taking advantage of its blue color pooling in mucosal folds and highlighting subtle abnormal surface topography (Fig. 25-6). Methylene blue, absorbed by abnormal cells but not normal gastric epithelium, is another common stain applied either alone or in tandem with Congo red, a dye that changes from red to dark black if pH is <3. All of these topical solutions are easily applied with an endoscopic spray catheter to deliver a uniform mist onto the mucosa being inspected.

A final means of enhancing mucosal lesion detection is the use of narrow-band imaging (NBI). This technology utilizes differences in the depth of light penetration to provide high-resolution imaging that delineates fine structural changes on mucosal surfaces. Green light, with longer wavelengths, penetrates deeper than blue light. The blue light in NBI has been increased to detect superficial capillary networks characteristic of early mucosal

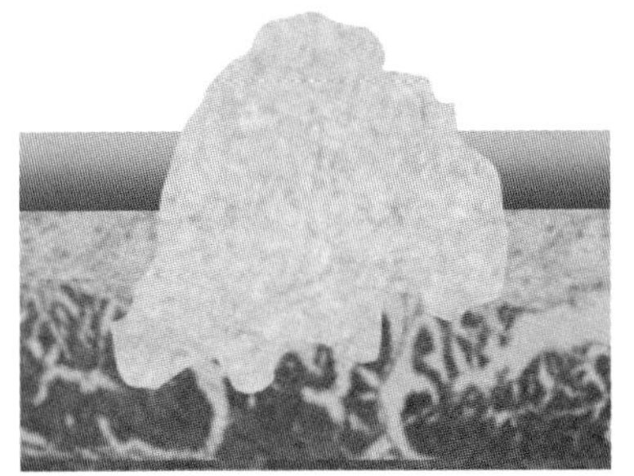

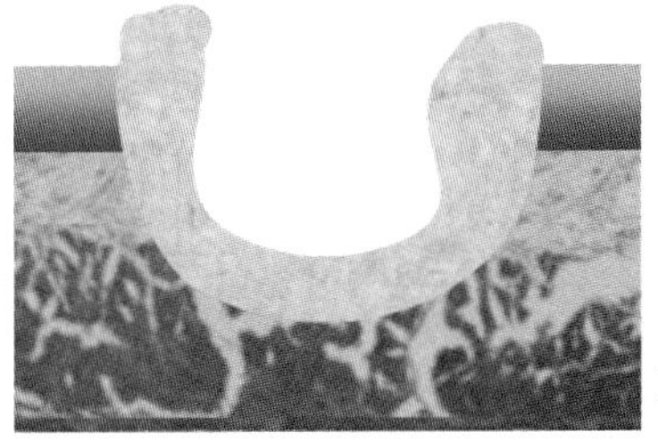

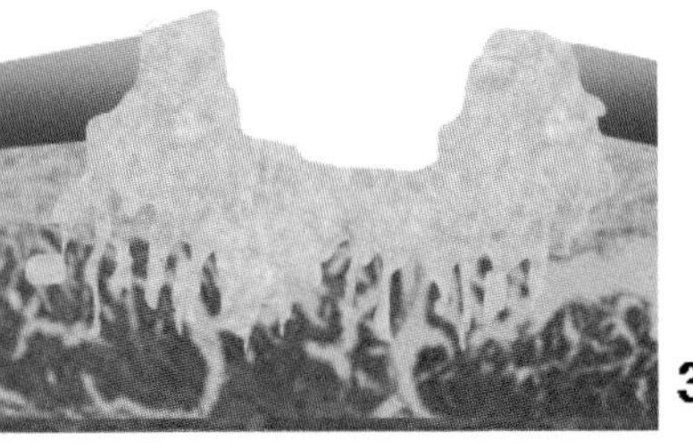

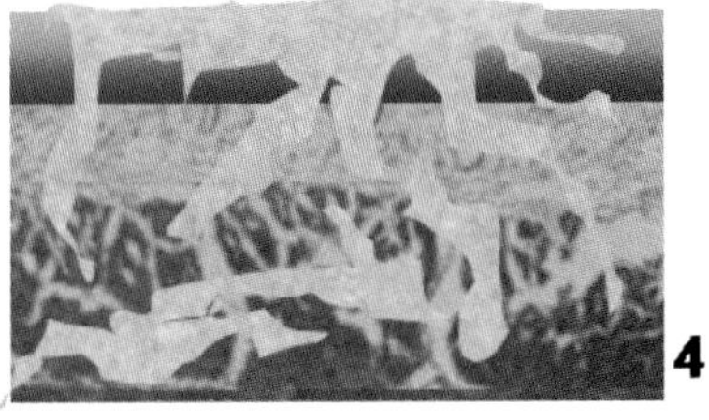

Fig. 25-5. Borrmann classification of macroscopic patterns of advanced gastric adenocarcinoma: (1) polypoid, (2) ulcerated with sharp margins, (3) ulcerated and infiltrating, and (4) diffusely infiltrating.

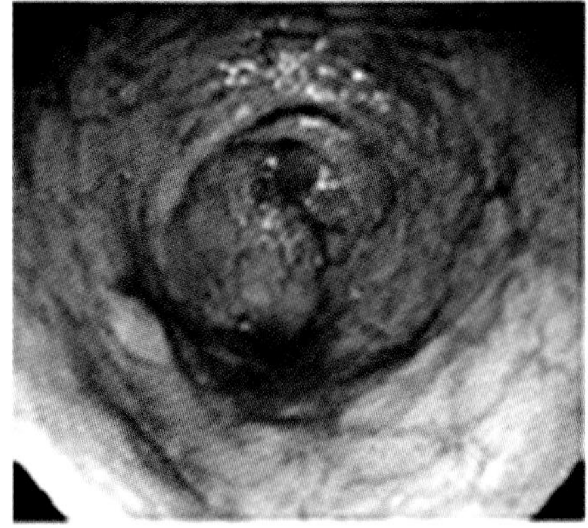

Fig. 25-6. Endoscopic demonstration of indigo carmine spraying of the distal antrum; note pooling within mucosal folds highlighting subtle topography. (With permission from Kodashima et al. Submucosal Dissection Using Flexknife. *J Clin Gastroenterol* 2006; 40(5).)

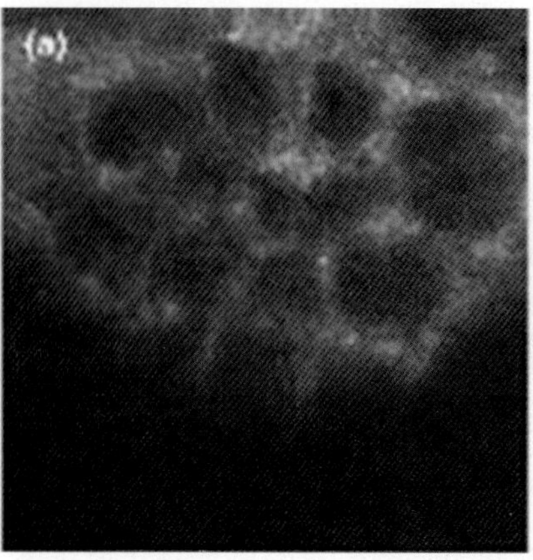

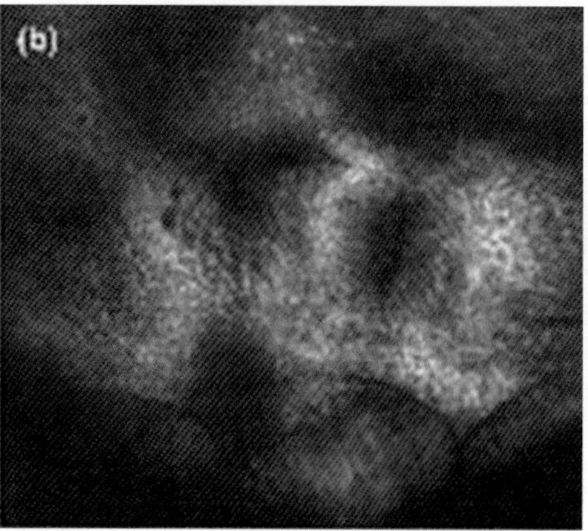

Fig. 25-7. Endoscopic confocal microscopic images of **(A)** normal gastric body mucosa compared with **(B)** intestinal metaplasia. (With permission from Evans et al. Endoscopic Confocal Microscopy. *Curr Opin Gastroenterol* 2005;21:578–584.)

changes in premalignant conditions or adenomatous changes while the green light penetrates deeper and offers subepithelial vascular visualization. This technology has recently become available with the latest generation of commercial endoscopes.

EMERGING DIAGNOSTIC MODALITIES

There are several innovations in the investigative phase aimed at improving the accuracy of endoscopic diagnoses (Raman spectroscopy probes, zoom endoscopy, optical coherence tomography, etc.). "Optical biopsy" refers to the concept of endoscopic histologic diagnosis without the use of any tissue biopsy or conventional histology. One such technique currently available but not yet clinically robust is endoscopic confocal microscopy (ECM). ECM utilizes either laser diode reflectance or fluorescence with an exogenous fluorophore to provide magnified views of cross-sectional epithelium in vivo nearly comparable to microscopic histology. Using ECM techniques, the diagnosis of *H. pylori* has been established in vivo, and there is ongoing work to determine if the technique can reliably make the diagnosis of proximal gastric intestinal metaplasia (Fig. 25-7).

Staging

The staging of gastric cancer relies on obtaining three parameters about a tumor: (1) the depth of invasion into or through the gastric wall, (2) the presence or absence of lymph node metastases, and (3) the presence or absence of distant metastases. In countries where it has become the standard of care, such as Japan and Korea, resection can be performed endoscopically for selected cases of early gastric adenocarcinoma (cancer confined to the mucosa or submucosa). The critical information required to determine if a given case of early gastric cancer (EGC) can be resected endoscopically with curative intent is whether (1) there are lymph node metastases and (2) the tumor has spread into or beyond the submucosa. Staging efforts are targeted at providing this information by endoscopic and histologic features as well as through an array of imaging modalities.

For EGC, the Japanese have developed a classification system based upon the endoscopic appearance of a lesion that is distinct from the Borrmann classification for more advanced lesions (Fig. 25-8). These different morphologies have been correlated with the risk of submucosal invasion and lymph node metastases. The excavated type is associated with a significantly greater chance of lymph node metastases compared with other morphologies. Because of this, curative endoscopic resection in Japan generally includes types I and II.

Poorly differentiated histology or larger diameter lesions portend a much greater risk of lymph node metastases compared with a more differentiated or intestinal type histology (4.2% vs. 0.4%). Therefore, EMR recommendations restrict curative endoscopic resection attempts to lesions ≤20 mm and of a differentiated histological type.

Imaging with endoscopic ultrasound is highly valuable in the staging of gastric cancer depth prior to any planned resection. Utilizing either an echoendoscope or an ultrasound microprobe deployed through the working channel of a conventional endoscope, the wall of the stomach can be visualized in five distinct layers (Fig. 25-9): (1) the mucosal fluid interface (hyperechoic), (2) the deeper mucosa, lamina propria, and muscularis mucosa (hypoechoic), (3) the submucosa (hyperechoic), (4) the muscularis propria (hypoechoic), and (5) the interface between serosa and surrounding tissues (hyperechoic). Using endoscopic ultrasound (EUS) images, the depth of tumor can be determined with an accuracy of greater than 80%. The depth of invasion, as determined by EUS, is perhaps the single most important determinant for endoscopic resectability (Fig. 25-10). EUS also assesses the presence of regional lymph node metastases, with an accuracy as high as 79% in some series.

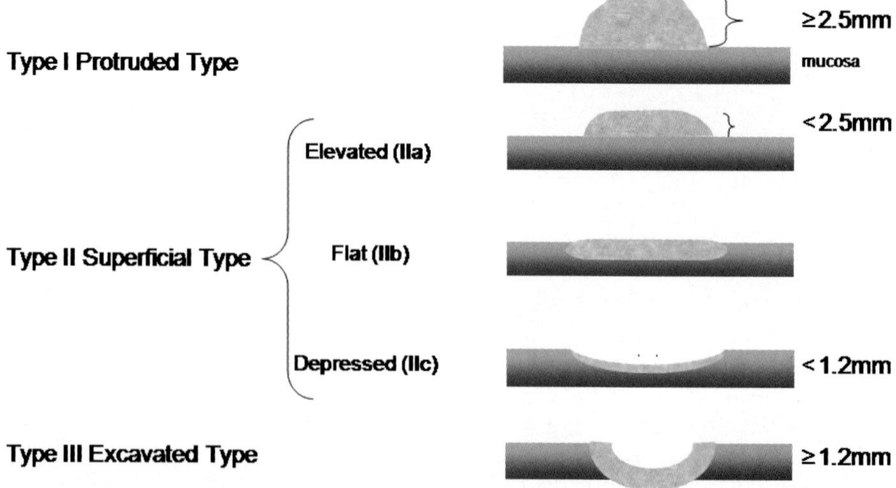

Fig. 25-8. Japanese and Paris Classification of superficial gastric cancer, by macroscopic appearance. Types I, IIa, and IIb are endoscopically resectable if <2 cm in diameter, as is IIc if <1 cm in diameter. These criteria serve to reduce the likelihood of a non-curative resection.

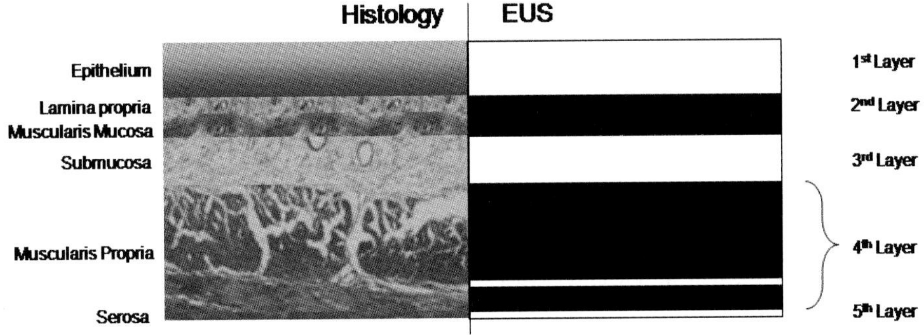

Fig. 25-9. Diagram of histologic layers of gastric wall and correlating endoscopic ultrasound (EUS) layers.

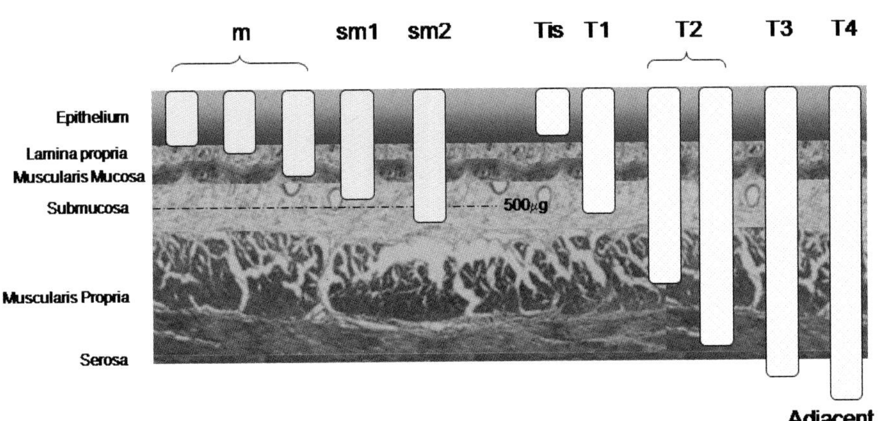

Fig. 25-10. (Left) The Japanese and Paris histologic classification of early gastric cancer by depth of invasion. Submucosal invasion of <500 μg (sm1) is associated with lymph node metastases 8.8% of the time compared with 23.7% rate of lymph node metastases when >500 μg invasion (sm2). These distinctions are missed within the Tis and T1 TMN designations (right).

Resection

Gastric lesions amenable to endoscopic treatment can undergo either ablation or resection. Endoscopic resection includes EMR as well as the more recently developed extension of EMR, endoscopic submucosal dissection (ESD). Additionally, an endoscopic stapled full-thickness gastric resection technique (FTGR) has been developed and used in a preliminary human clinical trial in Europe for the resection of early gastric cancer.

The current National Comprehensive Cancer Network (NCCN) guidelines for the treatment of early gastric cancer in the U.S. recommend that endoscopic resection take place within the context of a clinical trial at a center with extensive endoscopic experience. In countries such as Japan and Korea, however, the use of endoscopic resection has become the standard of care for selected cases of early gastric cancer.

EMR

Recommendations regarding EMR for curative resection from the Japanese Gastric Cancer Association restrict the procedure to early gastric cancers or highly dysplastic lesions that meet the following criteria: (1) non-ulcerated, (2) differentiated histology, (3) no submucosal tumor depth, and (4) a diameter ≤2 cm for elevated lesions (Type I or IIa) or a diameter ≤1 cm for depressed or flat lesions (Type IIb or IIc) without ulcer formation (Table 25-1). These guidelines minimize the chance of associated positive lymph nodes. The size restriction also reduces the need for piecemeal resections and the likelihood of leaving undetected positive margins.

After administration of an appropriate antibiotic prophylaxis, the first step in any EMR procedure for an EGC or highly dysplastic lesion is to proceed with conventional endoscopy. After visualizing the lesion, staining it with indigo carmine via a spray catheter will help to confirm the margin of the lesion. Cautery with a needleknife or the tip of a snare is used to delineate and mark out the margin of planned resection. The next step is infiltrating the submucosa beneath the lesion using a 4-mm 23- or 25-gauge needle through the endoscope. Numerous different solutions can be used to accomplish the injection, including normal saline, D20W, hypertonic saline, a dilute epinephrine solution (0.5 ml of 0.1% epinephrine in 100 ml of normal saline), and even hyaluronic acid or glycerine solutions. Indigo carmine or methylene blue, contrast stains used in chromoendoscopy, can be added to dye the submucosa blue upon injection as a visual marker to deter resection deeper than the submucosa. The choice of solution should be governed by the planned procedure. For longer procedures (for example, the piecemeal resection of a large lesion or a lesion in a difficult position such as the pyloric region or the cardia) hyaluronic acid or glycerine solutions provide a longer lift and require fewer reinjections. For shorter planned procedures, normal saline with or without diluted epinephrine may provide adequate duration of lift and is less costly.

To inject, the needle should be introduced into the submucosa beneath the lesion. In order to optimize continuous visualization, the injection should always begin at the distal margin of the lesion and move proximally. The exact amount of

TABLE 25-1. LESION CHARACTERISTICS RECOMMENDED FOR CURATIVE EMR

Japanese Gastric Cancer Association recommendations for curative EMR
Non-ulcerated
Differentiated histology
No submucosal tumor invasion
Diameter
≤2 cm for elevated lesions (I, IIa), or
≤1 cm for depressed or flat lesions without ulcer (IIb, IIc)

material injected depends on the size of the lesion and the solution used, but more than 20 ml will usually be required to provide the polypoid morphology necessary for successful snare application. The raised welt of mucosa upon successful injection, called the lifting sign, is an essential step in any EMR procedure as it both provides the pseudopolypoid shape necessary for snare application and also serves as an electrocautery buffer, reducing the likelihood of inadvertent perforation. If the lifting sign is absent, the injection may have been inappropriately placed (i.e., placed too deeply). More importantly, an absent lifting sign may signify a tumor more deeply invasive than previously appreciated, which would preclude the use of conventional EMR techniques.

Tada's original strip biopsy (Fig. 25-11A), also known as "inject and cut," consists of applying an endoscopic snare around the now polypoid lesion after injection. The resection is then carried out by strangulation coupled with electrocautery using a blended current. The resected lesion can then be extracted using either the snare itself or a biopsy forceps.

A modification of the original strip biopsy, termed the "inject, lift, and cut" technique, requires a dual-channeled endoscope (Fig. 25-11B). In this technique, the submucosal injection is again carried out as previously described. An endoscopic snare and a pair of grasping forceps are introduced, each through a different channel. The forceps are positioned through the open snare, with the snare tightened around the forceps. The forceps are then used to grasp the injected lesion. Following this, the snare is opened and the forceps are used to pull the lesion up through the snare. The snare is then tightened snugly around the lesion, with resection performed via strangulation and electrocautery applied with a blended current. The specimen can then be removed with either the snare or the forceps.

Another technique for EMR is called cap-assisted EMR, or EMR-C (Fig. 25-11C). After marking the lesion's margins and injecting it submucosally as previously described, a transparent cap is fitted to the end of a conventional single-channeled endoscope. A specially designed crescent-shaped snare is then prelooped along the inside rim of the cap (Fig. 25-12). After prelooping the snare in the cap, the target mucosa is suctioned fully inside the cap. The snare encircling the lesion is then closed and current applied. The resected lesion can be retrieved by gently aspirating it into the cap while removing the endoscope. There are several different caps

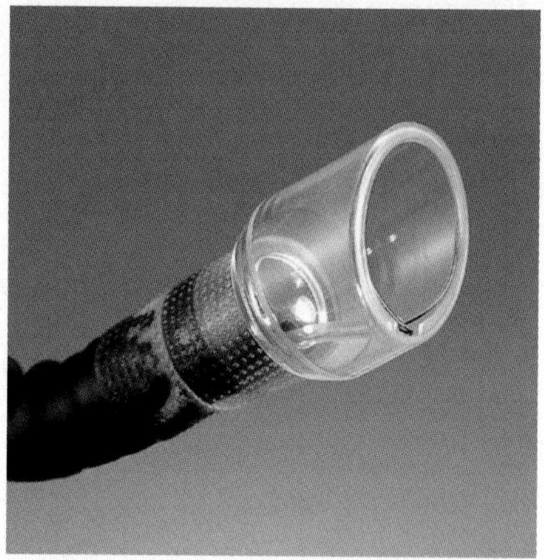

Fig. 25-12. A close-up picture of the EMR-C oblique cap taped to the end of a conventional single-channeled endoscope. Note the snare already prelooped along the rim of the cap. (Photograph courtesy of Olympus, Inc.)

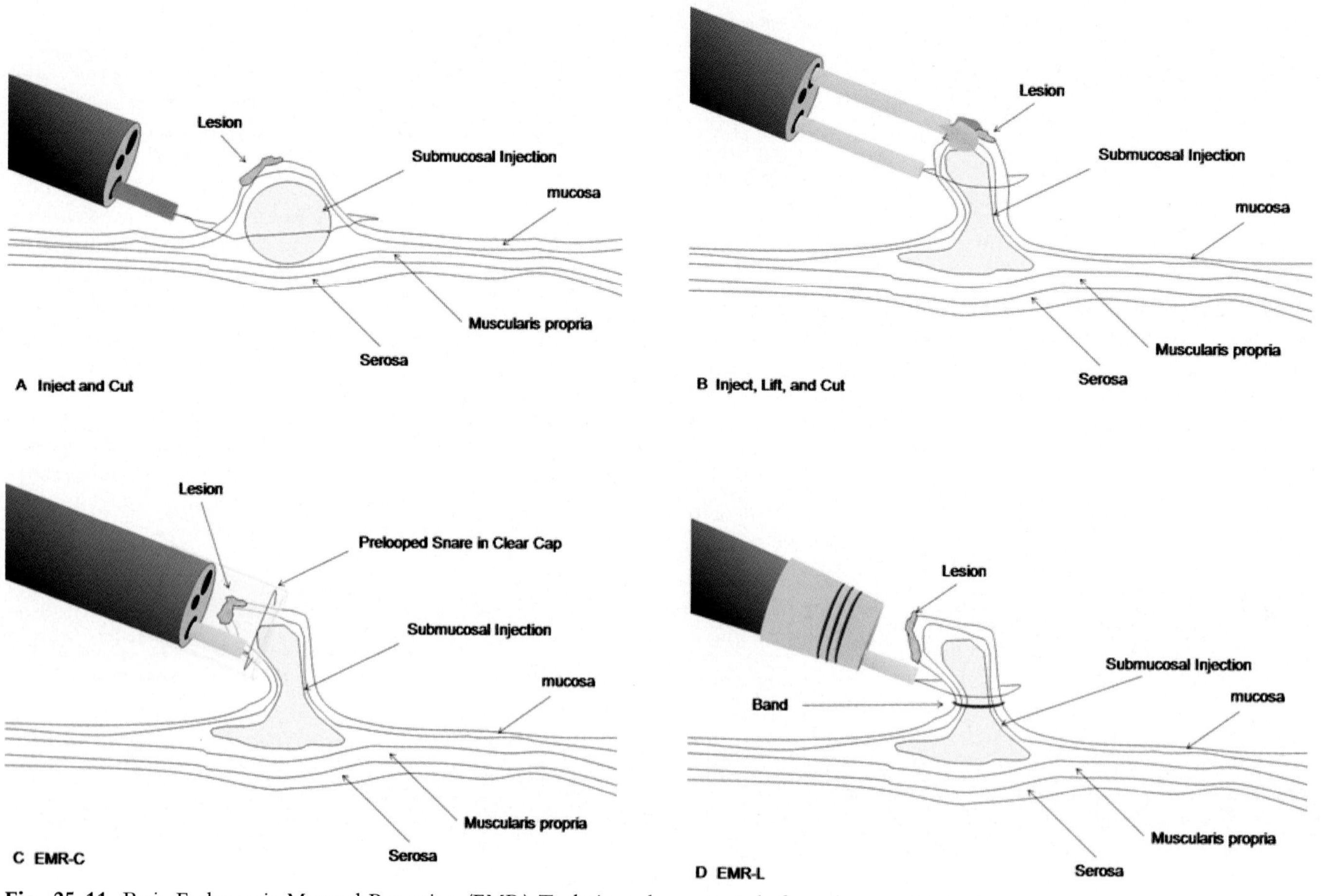

A Inject and Cut: Lesion; Submucosal Injection; mucosa; Muscularis propria; Serosa

B Inject, Lift, and Cut: Lesion; Submucosal Injection; mucosa; Muscularis propria; Serosa

C EMR-C: Lesion; Prelooped Snare in Clear Cap; Submucosal Injection; mucosa; Muscularis propria; Serosa

D EMR-L: Lesion; Band; Submucosal Injection; mucosa; Muscularis propria; Serosa

Fig. 25-11. Basic Endoscopic Mucosal Resection (EMR) Technique demonstrated after submucosal injection.

designed for this technique, with different caps providing different sizes as well as orientations (e.g., 0-degree caps, 30-degree oblique).

It is also possible to perform EMR with ligation, or EMR-L (Fig. 25-11D). This technique requires a single-channel endoscope and an esophageal variceal banding device. Using the banding device and endoscopic suction, the lesion is ligated with a variceal rubber band. EMR-L can be performed either with or without preceding submucosal injection. After the lesion is ligated to provide a polypoid shape, a standard snare is used with a blending current to transect the lesion either above or below the variceal band. The lesion can then be retrieved with biopsy forceps.

If one of these EMR techniques fails to fully resect the lesion, piecemeal resection can be used to complete the procedure, which usually requires repeating the full sequence of submucosal injection. Careful orientation of an EMR specimen immediately after resection is imperative for tumor margins, particularly in cases requiring multiple EMR applications.

If available, EUS may be employed during EMR to optimize the efficacy and safety of the procedure. Using a dual-channeled endoscope, an EUS microprobe can be used to visualize the extent of mucosal lift after submucosal injection and prior to the actual resection. Such visualization serves to ensure both appropriate placement of the submucosal injection as well as sufficient volume of injection to provide an adequate buffer layer between the mucosa and the muscularis propria. Once the lesion is strangulated within the snare, this same probe can sometimes confirm that tissue within the endoscopic snare does not include any of the deeper hypoechoic or black layers prior to electrocautery resection. This can minimize the chance of injury to the deeper muscularis propria tissues and lessen the likelihood of perforation during the procedure.

After an uncomplicated EMR procedure, patients are prescribed a mucosal protective agent (e.g., Maalox or sucralfate) along with oral antibiotics. Clear liquids are begun several hours after an EMR procedure with a soft, mechanical diet on the first postoperative day followed by a regular diet on the second postoperative day.

ESD

Endoscopic Submucosal Dissection or ESD is a new EMR technique that involves a freely drawn incision through the mucosa surrounding a lesion of interest and subsequently a careful dissection underneath the lesion within a submucosal plane. This is performed with an electrosurgical knife instead of the polypectomy snare used in conventional EMR techniques. This approach to resecting EGC allows en bloc resection of lesions much larger than the 2 cm upper limit recommended for conventional EMR. Using ESD, intramucosal non-ulcerated lesions of almost any size, ulcerated lesions less than or equal to 3 cm, and even small lesions with less than 500 micrometers of submucosal invasion can technically be resected. The long-term oncologic outcomes for these larger and deeper lesions with ESD are not yet well known.

To perform the procedure, margins of the lesion are again first confirmed using indigo carmine, as in conventional EMR. The line of planned incision is then delineated using cautery delivered by either a needleknife or an argon plasma coagulator (APC) to make discrete marks circumferentially every 2 mm apart. A 5-mm distance should be maintained between the edge of the tumor and the markings to preserve a histologically normal specimen margin and also reduce the potential for coagulation artifact to the tumor itself. A cautery mark applied separately from the proposed incision line designates "proximal" to assist in properly orienting the specimen after retrieval.

Injection is then performed starting distally as previously described with EMR, using a 4-mm 23- or 25-gauge needle. The injection should be beneath the previously marked line of incision as well as the lesion itself. After injection, an initial small mucosal incision is created, typically with needleknife electrocautery. Following this, a specific electrocautery knife is chosen, and the complete margin is incised circumferentially; typically this is started distally and carried proximally. A number of different electrocautery knives have been developed for ESD mucosal incision and subsequent submucosal dissection (Fig. 25-13, page 226). Maintaining an optimal endoscopic angle throughout the procedure is important so as to be able to accurately estimate the depth of mucosal incision and avoid perforation. In addition, superficial, incomplete mucosal incisions are associated with troublesome bleeding that may obscure the operative field; therefore, complete mucosal incisions should be performed on the first attempt. In areas such as the pylorus, ESD can be particularly challenging because of the complex, folded mucosal shape. In this region, circumferential submucosal injection can increase mucosal folding, which further obscures the lesion margin. This can be avoided by injecting and incising the distal margin of a prepyloric lesion prior to injecting and incising more proximally.

Following circumferential mucosal incision, an electrosurgical snare can separate the lesion from its submucosal attachments without formal submucosal dissection for smaller tumors and lesions. For larger lesions, an appropriate electrocautery knife is used to dissect the submucosal tissue off the deeper gastric wall tissues (Fig. 25-14, page 226). A number of different specially designed endoscopic caps or hoods can be used to facilitate this part of the procedure. These hoods help to maintain visualization of the submucosal plane of interest by spreading apart the overlying superficial mucosal tissue from the deeper gastric wall tissues as well as allowing the endoscope itself to provide some blunt dissection through the submucosal plane. Once the transection of the specimen is completed, the specimen is retrieved. Given a frequently larger en bloc specimen size associated with an ESD procedure compared with EMR, retrieval cannot always be accomplished with simple forceps. In such cases, specialized polyp retrieval devices such as the Roth Net (US Endoscopy; Mentor, OH) may be used.

After the resection is completed and the specimen is retrieved, sucralfate liquid (20 ml) is sprayed as a coating over the post-procedure ulcer base. The patient is observed afterwards and allowed a soft, mechanical diet on the first postoperative day. Similar to the post-EMR regimen described, oral mucosal protective agents (e.g., Maalox or sucralfate) along with oral antibiotics are administered. In many Japanese centers, the patient undergoes a repeat endoscopy one week after the procedure to ensure reasonable post-procedural ulcer healing. A repeat endoscopy is performed 2 months after the procedure to confirm adequate healing and evaluate for any local recurrence.

COMPLICATIONS

Complications from EMR and ESD procedures include bleeding and perforation. Much of the bleeding, particularly in EMR, resolves spontaneously. Protracted bleeding can be controlled with standard endoscopic techniques, generally with a combination of modalities such as injection and cautery.

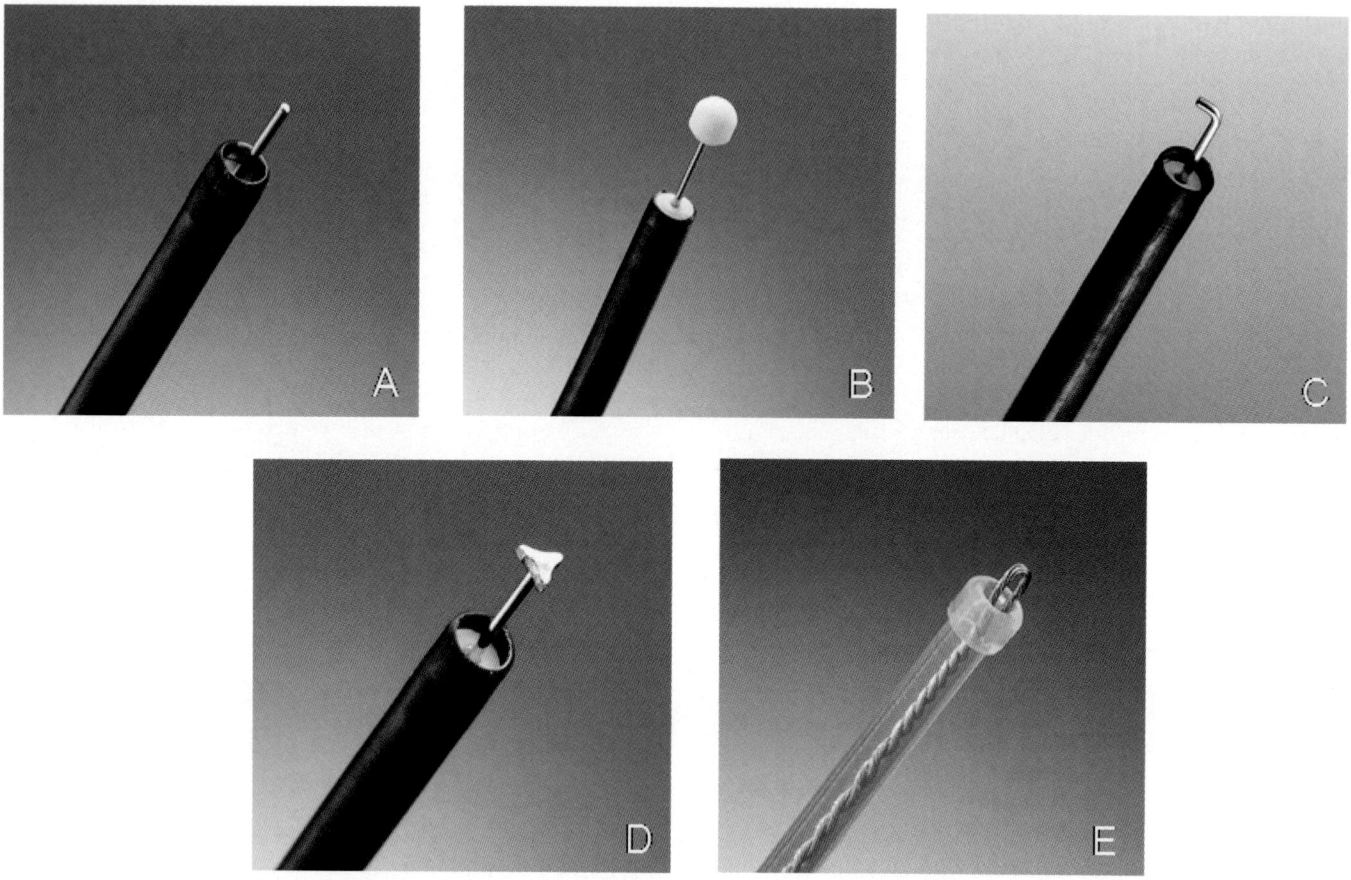

Fig. 25-13. Different electrosurgical knives available for endoscopic submucosal dissection: **A.** A needleknife. **B.** An insulated tip (IT) knife. **C.** A hook knife. **D.** A triangular tip (TT) knife. **E.** A flex knife. (Pictures courtesy of Olympus, Inc.)

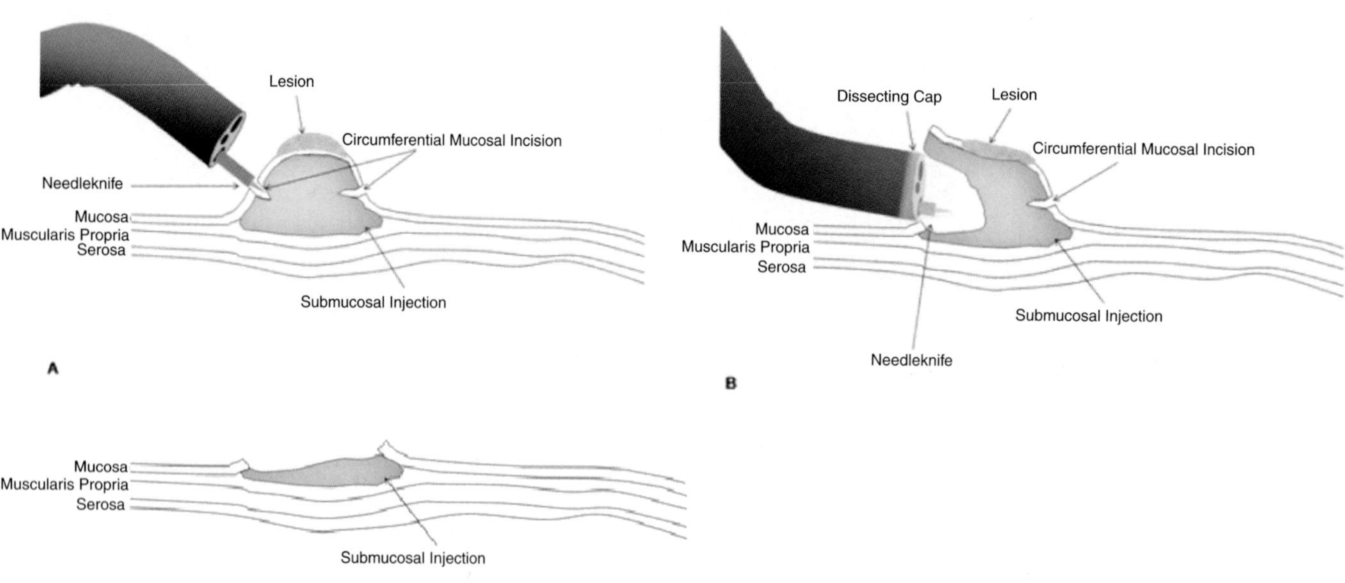

Fig. 25-14. A. A cross-sectional diagram demonstrating a circumferential mucosal incision made around the lesion. **B.** Using an electrosurgical knife and dissecting cap, the lesion is separated from the deeper gastric wall tissues. A surgically induced ulceration remains after resection.

Endoscopic clips can also be applied if necessary.

Perforation occurs in 1.2% of conventional EMR cases and 3.6% of ESD cases. In the majority of cases, the perforation is noted at the time of the procedure. While surgery remains the standard of care for iatrogenic gastric perforation, there are numerous case reports of treating iatrogenic perforations recognized at the time of mucosal resection nonoperatively. To do this the stomach is partially deflated to facilitate placement of endoscopic hemostatic clips, which coapt the edges of the perforation (Fig. 25-15). Irrigation is avoided until after satisfactory gastric closure. Upon closure, a transabdominally placed angiocatheter is used to evacuate the pneumoperitoneum as fully as possible. The patient is maintained without oral diet along with nasogastric tube decompression and intravenous antibiotics. Surgical repair has been reserved for large perforations not suited for endoscopic clip application or for endoclip closure that has clinically failed.

PATHOLOGY AND CURATIVE RESECTION

After completion of either EMR or ESD, specimens are carefully oriented on a plate before being fixed in 10% formalin. The size, shape, and gross margins of the specimen are recorded along with indication of the proximal resection margin. The specimen is serially sectioned every 2 mm, parallel to a line indicating the margin closest to the tumor on gross inspection. The specimen is histologically inspected for lymphatic or vascular invasion, depth of invasion (M, SM1, SM2), and vertical and lateral margin status. By conventions established in Japan, a lateral margin is considered negative if there is a greater than 1 mm distance between the edge of the tumor and the edge of the resection—this distance corresponds to approximately ten normal glands.

SURVEILLANCE

Cancer recurrences may be either metachronous cancers found upon surveillance (14% of patients at 5 years) or they may represent recurrences at the site of resection (5.6% of patients at 3 years). Because EMR and ESD are relatively new procedures, there is no well established optimal interval for surveillance endoscopy examinations. However, most endoscopists perform surveillance endoscopy at 1-year intervals following a curative resection. When mucosal resections are not curative (e.g., equivocal lateral margins) or margins cannot be evaluated properly, repeat examinations are pursued every 6 months for at least the first 3 years following a mucosal resection.

FTGR

Endoscopic full-thickness gastric resection (FTGR) has been developed using an electromechanically powered cutting stapler delivered via a flexible, steerable shaft. This technique has been described in one preliminary report to remove an EGC and a gastric carcinoid tumor in human subjects. The procedure involves the simultaneous side-by-side introduction of the endoscope and a flexible remote-controlled stapler device through the esophagus and into the stomach, using a temporarily placed overtube. The gastric wall containing the lesion of interest is then pulled by an endoscopic grasper into the opened jaws of the remote-controlled stapler (Fig. 25-16). The resection is completed with the firing of the stapler. The specimen is then removed through the esophagus using the endoscope.

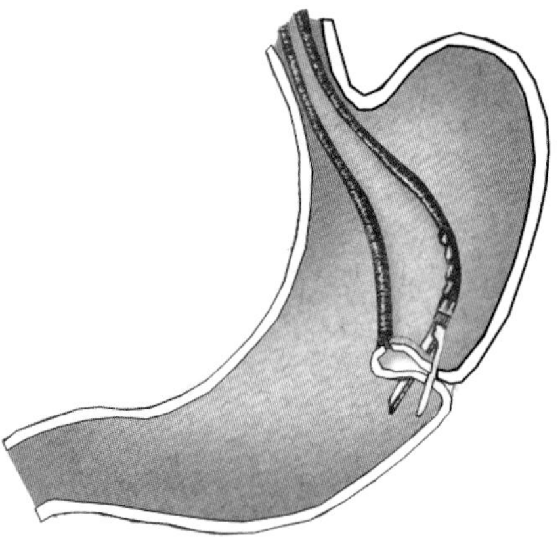

Fig. 25-16. A cross-sectional diagram of the full-thickness resection (FTR) technique for gastric lesions. Both endoscope and flexible cutting stapler instrument are introduced through the esophagus and into the stomach. A grasper is used through the scope to invaginate the full-thickness gastric wall of interest, pulling it into the jaws of the stapler, which are then fired to achieve a full thickness resection.

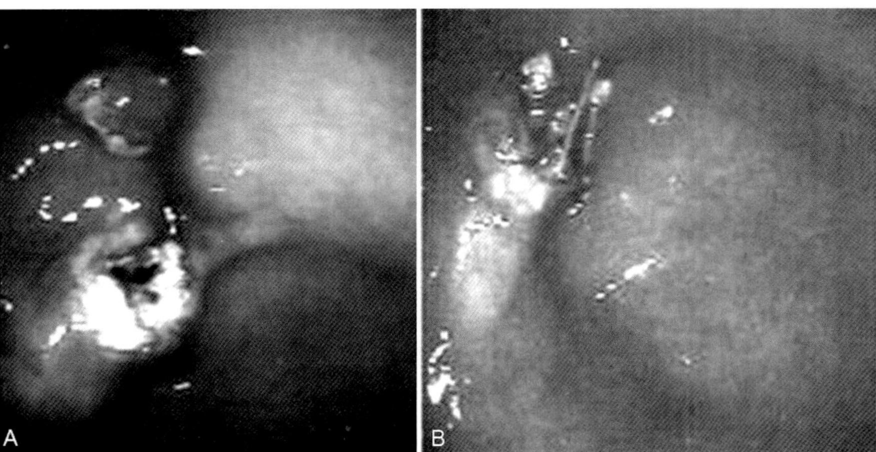

Fig. 25-15. A. Demonstration of a gastric perforation sustained during a mucosal resection. **B.** The perforation is treated with the application of two endoscopic endoclips. (With permission from Katsinelos et al. Endoclipping Gastric Perforation after Endoscopic Polypectomy. *Surg Laparosc Endosc Percutan Tech* 2004;14(5):279–281.)

Ablation

Ablation includes several different techniques: photodynamic therapy (PDT), laser therapy, and argon plasma coagulation (APC). At least one clear disadvantage of ablation over endoscopic resection techniques is the inability to pathologically examine tissue that is removed to determine margin status. Ablation therapy is therefore reserved for the treatment of early gastric cancer in patients deemed poor candidates for tumor resection or for the palliation of advanced gastric cancer causing bleeding or obstruction.

PDT

Photodynamic therapy (PDT) is based on the principle of applying laser light irradiation to activate a photodynamic agent selectively retained by the target tumor tissue. Upon applying laser energy, tumor cells are destroyed by the intracellular release of toxic singlet oxygen. To date, a number of different methods have been developed for PDT ablation

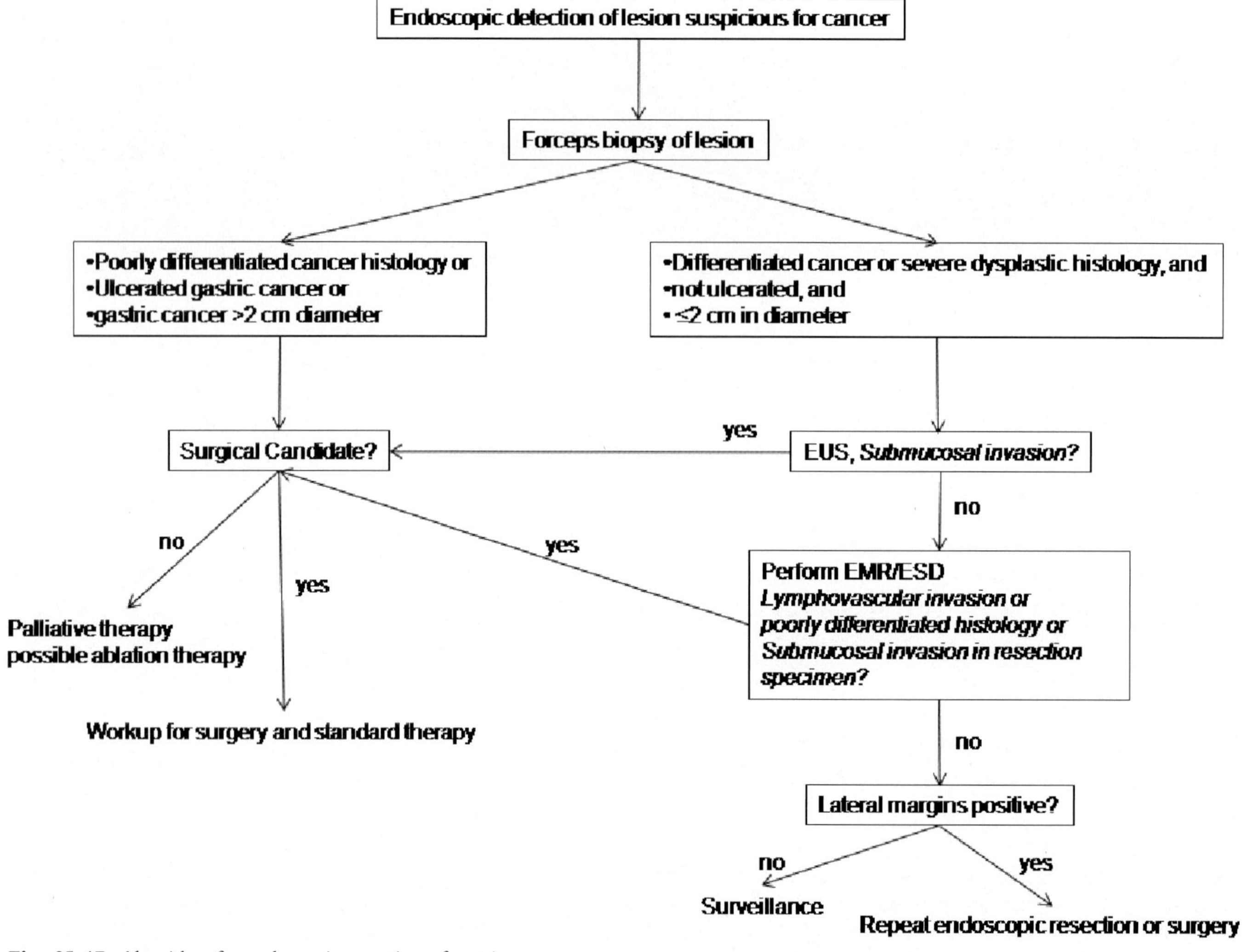

Fig. 25-17. Algorithm for endoscopic resection of gastric cancer.

of gastric neoplastic tissue. PDT treatments of EGC typically use either porfimer sodium (Photofrin) or mesotetrahydroxyphenylchlorin (mTHPC) as an intravenously delivered photosensitizer followed by the endoscopic treatment of the tumor tissue with red dye lasers. Complete treatment may require more than a single session of PDT therapy for complete ablation, depending on the size and extent of a given lesion. Several studies have had complete response rates greater than 80% for EGC with short-term follow-up. Laser ablation without a photosensitizer, typically using a neodymium-doped yttrium aluminum garnet (Nd:YAG) laser, has also been successfully used for the endoscopic palliation of obstruction or bleeding in advanced or unresectable cases of gastric cancer.

APC

Argon plasma coagulation (APC) is a form of tissue coagulation using high-frequency electrical current transmitted to target tissue by ionized argon gas that has been used endoscopically to treat EGC. The technique generally requires only a single session for smaller, flat lesions and several sessions for larger, more polypoid tumors. In one series of 40 patients with EGC not fit for surgery or EMR, APC achieved a complete remission rate of 90% at 52 months median follow-up and had a complication rate of 7.5%, including one perforation. In advanced cases, APC can also be used to palliate obstruction by debulking gastric tumors.

CONCLUSIONS

As endoscopic treatment of gastric lesions evolves and gains acceptance, it is important to realize that early lesions amenable to this technique are relatively uncommon in Western centers. Appropriate pretreatment staging and characterization of the lesion are as important as technical abilities for best outcomes (Fig. 25-17).

SUGGESTED READING

Akahoshi K, Kojima H, Fujimaru T, et al. Grasping forceps assisted endoscopic resection of large pedunculated GI polypoid lesions. *Gastrointest Endosc* 1999;50(1):95–98.

Chen CH, Yang CC, Yeh YH. Preoperative staging of gastric cancer by endoscopic ultrasound: the prognostic usefulness of ascites detected by endoscopic ultrasound. *J Clin Gastroenterol* 2002;35(4):321–327.

Ell C, Gossner L, May A, et al. Photodynamic ablation of early cancers of the stomach by means of mTHPC and laser irradiation: preliminary clinical experience. *Gut* 1998; 43(3):345–349.

Evans JA, Nishioka NS. Endoscopic confocal microscopy. *Curr Opin Gastroenterol* 2005; 21(5):578–584.

Fujii T, Iishi H, Tatsuta M, et al. Effectiveness of premedication with pronase for improving visibility during gastroendoscopy: a randomized controlled trial. *Gastrointest Endosc* 1998; 47(5):382–387.

Gotoda T, Yanagisawa A, Sasako M, et al. Incidence of lymph node metastasis from early gastric cancer: estimation with a large number of cases at two large centers. *Gastric Cancer* 2000;3(4):219–225.

J. A. NCCN Clinical Practice Guidelines in Oncology: *Gastric Cancer* 2006.

Japanese Gastric Cancer A. Japanese Classification of Gastric Carcinoma—2nd English Edition. *Gastric Cancer* 1998;1(1):10–24.

Kaehler G, Grobholz R, Langner C, et al. A new technique of endoscopic full-thickness resection using a flexible stapler. *Endoscopy* 2006;38(1):86–89.

Kapadia CR. Gastric atrophy, metaplasia, and dysplasia: a clinical perspective. [Review] [44 refs]. *J Clin Gastroenterol* 2003;36(5 Suppl): S29–36; discussion S61–62.

Kitamura T, Tanabe S, Koizumi W, et al. Argon plasma coagulation for early gastric cancer: technique and outcome. *Gastrointest Endosc* 2006;63(1):48–54.

Mimura S, Ito Y, Nagayo T, et al. Cooperative clinical trial of photodynamic therapy with photofrin II and excimer dye laser for early gastric cancer. *Lasers Surg Med* 1996;19(2): 168–172.

Nasu J, Doi T, Endo H, et al. Characteristics of metachronous multiple early gastric cancers after endoscopic mucosal resection. *Endoscopy* 2005;37(10):990–993.

Oberhuber G, Stolte M. Gastric polyps: an update of their pathology and biological significance. *Virchows Arch* 2000;437(6): 581–590.

Oda I, Saito D, Tada M, et al. A multicenter retrospective study of endoscopic resection for early gastric cancer. *Gastric Cancer* 2006; 9(4):262–270.

Rembacken B, Fujii T, Kondo H. The recognition and endoscopic treatment of early gastric and colonic cancer. *Best Pract Res Clin Gastroenterol* 2001;15(2):317–336.

Tada MMMTT, et al. The development of "strip-off" biopsy. [In Japanese]. *Gastroenterol Endosc* 1984;26(833).

Tada M, Tanaka Y, Matsuo N, et al. Mucosectomy for gastric cancer: current status in Japan. *J Gastroenterol Hepatol* 2000;15 Suppl:D98–102.

The role of endoscopy in the surveillance of premalignant conditions of the upper gastrointestinal tract. American Society for Gastrointestinal Endoscopy. *Gastrointest Endosc* 1998;48(6):663–668.

Update on the Paris classification of superficial neoplastic lesions in the digestive tract. *Endoscopy* 2005;37(6):570–578.

Waxman I, Saitoh Y. Clinical outcome of endoscopic mucosal resection for superficial GI lesions and the role of high-frequency US probe sonography in an American population. *Gastrointest Endosc* 2000;52(3):322–327.

COMMENTARY

Drs. White and Lin provide an overview of the use of endoscopy for the diagnosis, staging, and removal or ablation of neoplastic disorders of the stomach. Given the much higher prevalence of gastric cancer in Asia, much of the impetus for developing these endoscopic techniques has come from the Japanese experience. Unfortunately, most cases of gastric cancer diagnosed in the United States are advanced beyond the ability to perform endoscopic resection techniques and fall into the realm of surgical or palliative treatment. However, there are still many early lesions that can be approached endoscopically.

Similar to the endoscopic diagnosis of esophageal disease, several techniques can be used to enhance the detection rate of mucosal neoplastic lesions. These include chromoendoscopy and narrow band imaging, which are described herein. Endoscopic ultrasound, analogous to its utility for esophageal disease, plays a large role in the appropriate staging of neoplastic gastric lesions. Endoscopic mucosal resection techniques are clearly only indicated for superficial lesions, emphasizing the importance of accurate pretreatment staging. Endoscopic resection of superficial lesions has become much more sophisticated and robust in the recent past due to the increasing Japanese experience. The mucosa with overlying lesions can be resected, or the dissection can be carried into the submucosal plane. Experimental efforts are underway currently to allow full thickness resections; these efforts will certainly be enhanced by the recent push to develop tools applicable for natural orifice surgery.

NJS

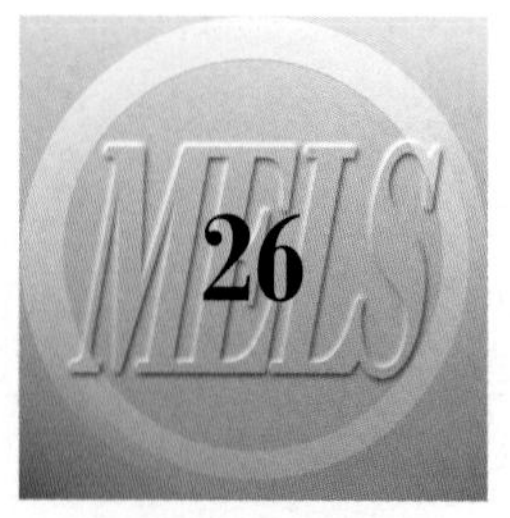

Resection of Nonadenomatous Gastric Tumors

DERON J. TESSIER AND BRENT D. MATTHEWS

INTRODUCTION

The evolution of gastric surgery has taken many steps since its beginnings, when Theodore Billroth performed the first successful gastrectomy in the 1880s. This includes numerous technical and mechanical advances such as the description and implementation of various types of anastomoses, the development of surgical staplers, and the use of nasoenteric sump tubes. One of the most important advances was the invention of the flexible endoscope and the skill sets necessary to perform diagnostic and therapeutic upper endoscopy. Medical progress has impacted gastric surgery as well; the advent of selective histamine-receptor blocker medications, proton pump inhibitors, and, subsequently, the description and treatment strategies for *Helicobacter pylori* have almost eliminated the previously common operations for peptic ulcer disease.

Technical innovations involving minimally invasive surgery have generated renewed interest in upper gastrointestinal surgery. There is little doubt that laparoscopy, with its resultant reduction in morbidity and recovery time, has been responsible for a dramatic growth in gastric surgery over the last decade. Patients who were previously palliated with medications or were observed for a variety of reasons now seek to have definitive therapies performed via minimally invasive techniques. Only a few areas in surgery have experienced the growth documented in the area of the lower esophagus and stomach. The number of antireflux operations such as Nissen fundoplication, paraesophageal hernia repair, esophageal myotomy for achalasia, and bariatric procedures for morbid obesity has grown exponentially since a near-systematic conversion to a laparoscopic approach. A growing number of patients are referred for minimally invasive gastric resection for localized nonadenomatous tumors, predominately gastrointestinal stromal tumors (GIST). Many of these spindle cell neoplasms previously had been managed by surveillance endoscopy. despite previously under appreciated malignant potential. The applicability of a minimally invasive approach to gastric resection is facilitated by the accessibility of the stomach both laparoscopically and endoscopically. The experience gained from laparoscopic antireflux surgery and the availability and reliability of laparoscopic staplers has led to widespread use of laparoscopy in the management of GISTs. Enabling technologies such as ultrasonic coagulating shears and bipolar vessel sealers and the fact that curative resection for many gastric tumors requires only negative margins without lymphadenectomy make GISTs excellent candidates for a minimally invasive procedure. With an expanding experience over the past decade, a relatively systematic approach to treatment has been developed. This chapter includes a description of nonadenomatous gastric tumors that require resection, their diagnostic and preoperative workup, and the minimally invasive operative approaches employed according to the location of the tumor within the stomach.

Gastrointestinal Stromal Tumors

CLINICAL PRESENTATION

While gastrointestinal stromal tumors (GISTs) are fairly rare, with an annual incidence in the United States of 1000 to 2500 cases per year, they still represent the most common nonadenomatous lesion requiring gastric resection. Patients with GISTs typically present between 50 and 70 years of age. Although a 2:1 male predominance of these tumors has been reported, recent data indicate that the incidence is evenly distributed between males and females. Approximately 80% of GISTs are located in the fundus or body of the stomach. On endoscopic and gross examination, GISTs are firm, distinct, and rounded or lobulated submucosal lesions (Fig. 26-1). When symptomatic, gastrointestinal bleeding and abdominal pain are the most common manifestations. Likewise dysphagia may occur for proximally located tumors near the gastroesophageal junction and lesions of the pylorus may cause symptoms of obstruction.

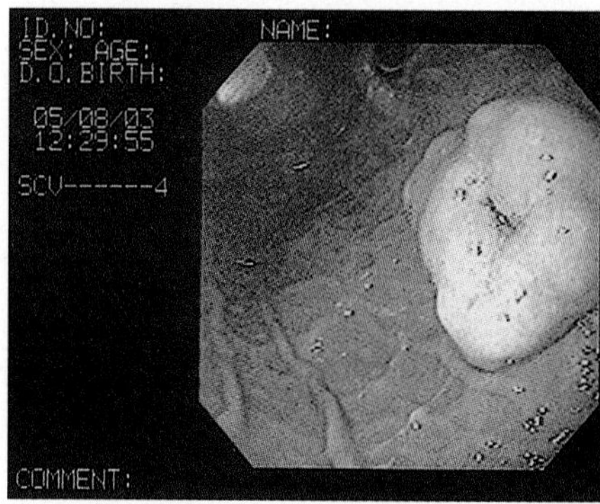

Fig. 26-1. A typical endoscopic view of a gastric gastrointestinal stroma tumor (GIST), located in the gastric fundus.

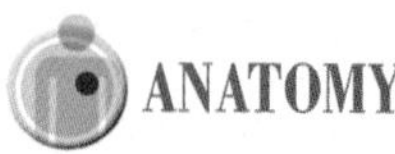

ANATOMY

The cellular origin of these tumors was previously recognized to be smooth muscle. Benign tumors were characterized as leiomyomas and malignant tumors as leiomyosarcomas. Identification of the interstitial cell of Cajal as the cell of origin of smooth muscle tumors led to the change in nomenclature to GIST. The interstitial cell of Cajal is a pacemaker cell of the gastrointestinal tract and is found within the myenteric plexus, submucosa, and muscularis propria. Immunohistochemistry established the derivation of GIST from the interstitial cell of Cajal by demonstrating the expression of cellular markers such as CD117, a marker of the c-kit gene product, and CD34, a human progenitor cell antigen.

Distant metastasis or local invasion may not present until many years after diagnosis of the primary tumor. A combination of prognostic factors (patient age, histologic grade, mitotic rate, tumor size, and DNA analysis) has been used to predict their biologic behavior and to determine a patient's eligibility for adjuvant treatment strategies. The most significant clinical predictors of tumor behavior are tumor size and mitotic activity. A tumor size greater than 5 cm and more than 5 mitoses/50 high-power fields are considered indicators of malignant potential. Other significant characteristics of malignancy include hemorrhage and/or necrosis of the tumor, mucosal invasion, and cellular atypia. Aneuploid DNA is associated with malignant GIST. Survival has been correlated with DNA content (P <0.001), and DNA ploidy is an independent predictor of survival. Nevertheless, GISTs with completely benign characteristics have recurred and/or metastasized. The only absolute signs of malignancy are metastasis and/or invasion into adjacent organs.

It is common that GISTs of the stomach are diagnosed incidentally in the course of an endoscopic evaluation for unrelated complaints. Because these tumors are submucosal, endoscopic biopsy will most often only demonstrate normal mucosa. Contrast upper gastrointestinal series can demonstrate a smooth-edged filling defect in the gastric lumen, but this modality lacks specificity and requires further diagnostic evaluation and/or confirmation. Endoscopic ultrasound (EUS) is perhaps the most valuable imaging technique for the evaluation of submucosal lesions in the upper gastrointestinal tract and for diagnosing GIST of the stomach. EUS morphology that is indicative of a gastric stromal tumor is a well-demarcated, hypoechoic mass that is contiguous with the fourth layer of the gastric wall (muscularis propria). The combined presence of two out of three EUS features (irregular extraluminal margins, cystic spaces, and lymph nodes with a malignant pattern) has a high positive predictive value for malignant or borderline GIST. While percutaneous fine-needle aspiration (FNA) biopsy of gastric stromal tumors should be avoided for fear of spilling tumor cells into the peritoneal cavity, transgastric biopsy utilizing EUS can give tissue for preoperative diagnosis. This is especially important in the setting of patients with potential metastatic disease to the liver, where transgastric FNA cytology can provide important diagnostic information for neoadjuvant treatment or enrollment in clinical trials. The yield for EUS-assisted biopsy is low, however. A recent review of 33 patients undergoing laparoscopic resection for GISTs at the Mayo Clinic found that preoperative EUS with biopsy was performed in 73% of patients; only 54% of this group had biopsy proven GIST by immunohistochemical staining and c-kit positivity. Computed tomography (CT) and magnetic resonance imaging (MRI) have value by allowing for a more comprehensive evaluation of the intraabdominal cavity to delineate the tumor's relationship to adjacent structures and to investigate for metastatic disease. Despite these advances in imaging and biopsy techniques, resection of these lesions is generally required from both a therapeutic and diagnostic standpoint.

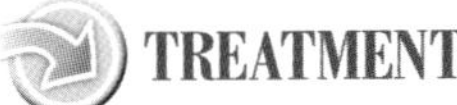

The treatment for GIST of the stomach is surgical resection. Whether via laparotomy, laparoscopy, or endoluminal resection (using a combination of flexible endoscopy and percutaneous transgastric laparoscopy), excision is the only currently available means of achieving long-term, disease-free survival. Two-centimeter margins were once presumed necessary for an oncologic resection and to provide the greatest opportunity for surgical cure. However, a study from the Memorial Sloan-Kettering Cancer Center revealed that tumor size and not negative microscopic surgical margins determines long-term survival. Currently, the goal is to obtain negative surgical margins, not an anatomical resection. Lymphatic spread of GIST is unusual; therefore, a lymph node dissection with the primary tumor is not part of the standard operative approach. Most of our patients are given the option of a minimally invasive approach for the resection of gastric stromal tumors. We have been able to demonstrate that a laparoscopic resection can obtain adequate margins, improve cosmesis, and offer an earlier return to normal activity and self-reliance compared to an open technique. The operative approach depends on tumor location. Most of the laparoscopic techniques are analogous to an open approach, although laparoscopic transgastric resection and endoscopically assisted endoluminal surgery are unique to minimally invasive surgery.

Pancreatic Rests and Adenomyomas

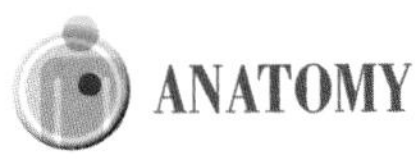

Ectopic pancreas, first described by Barbosa in 1946, is pancreatic tissue that lacks anatomic and vascular continuity with the pancreas. Ectopic pancreatic tissue is a rare condition with a reported incidence of 1% to 2% of autopsy specimens. The condition is thought to arise at the time of embryonal development, when tissue from the pancreas becomes implanted in the bowel wall and then is carried to its final location. "Rests" of pancreatic tissue have the microscopic appearance of pancreatic lobules with acini and ducts. Ectopic pancreatic tissue may be found anywhere along the alimentary tract, with the stomach and duodenum being the most common locations. Although most patients with gastric ectopic pancreatic tissue are asymptomatic, others present with nonspecific complaints or symptoms similar to peptic ulcer disease. The most common presenting symptoms are abdominal pain or epigastric discomfort, nausea and vomiting, and bleeding. Aberrant pancreatic tissue has the potential for neoplastic change. While the natural history of the tissue is difficult to determine, there are a few rare reports of islet cell tumors and ductal adenocarcinoma arising in ectopic pancreas.

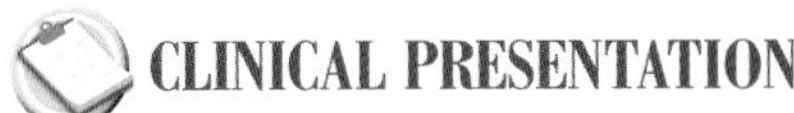

Gastric adenomyomas are rare, benign submucosal tumors of the antrum and pylorus. In general, the lesions are located within 4 cm of the pylorus. Histologically, they are characterized by ductal structures lined with cuboidal to columnar epithelium surrounded by smooth muscle bundles. Occasionally they are also incorporated within Brunner glands and heterotopic pancreas. Although obstruction and bleeding can occur with these lesions, there are no reported cases of malignancy. Most often adenomyomas are diagnosed incidentally and are asymptomatic.

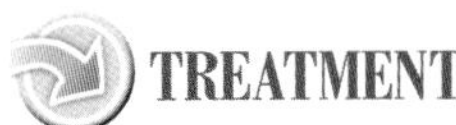

Diagnostic workup and operative strategies for pancreatic rests and adenomyomas are identical to that for GIST. These tumors are submucosal and typically presumed to be GISTs. Endoscopic biopsies are usually deferred due to their low diagnostic yield. As previously stated, EUS may be able to differentiate these submucosal tumors preoperatively due to certain subtle architectural differences. On EUS, aberrant pancreatic tissue tends to be located in the third or fourth layer of the gastric wall and to have an indistinct margin and a heterogeneous appearance (mainly hypoechoic). Nevertheless, the operative approach is ultimately similar. We have removed several pancreatic rests laparoscopically that were presumed to be GISTs until histologic evaluation confirmed their pathologic origin.

Carcinoids

CLINICAL PRESENTATION

Gastric carcinoid (neuroendocrine) tumors are rare and account for only 0.3% of all gastric neoplasms, although that number may actually underestimate their incidence. Approximately 9% of gastrointestinal carcinoids are found in the stomach. Carcinoids are typically divided into three main categories, classified on the basis of pathogenesis and histomorphologic characteristics. Types I and II gastric neuroendocrine tumors are highly susceptible to gastrin trophic stimulus. Hypergastrinemia, such as found in pernicious anemia (type I) or gastrin-producing neoplasms as in Zollinger-Ellison syndrome or multiple endocrine neoplasia I (type II), is believed to be responsible for the formation of these types of carcinoids. They are characteristically localized to the gastric body or fundus. Gastric neuroendocrine tumor types I and II are usually considered benign, with a low risk of malignancy. Invasion, uncommon in smaller tumors, occurs with increasing frequency in tumors larger than 2 cm. Type III gastric carcinoids are composed of poorly differentiated endocrine and exocrine cells, which grow sporadically, irrespective of gastrin hypersecretion. Most of these tumors show a low-to-high grade malignant transformation, and the majority have metastasized by the time of diagnosis. Indeed, only two-thirds of gastric carcinoids are localized at the time of discovery.

Most patients with small gastric carcinoids are asymptomatic, and tumors are discovered incidentally on upper endoscopy, although patients occasionally present with ulcer-like symptoms. The lesions appear as pink to yellow submucosal nodules that may project into the gastric lumen. Despite their submucosal location, these lesions usually can be diagnosed via endoscopic biopsy. In addition, gastric carcinoids often can be snared and removed in total.

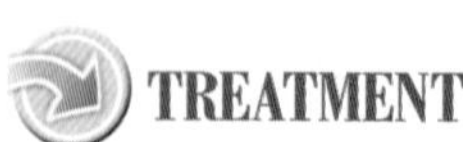

TREATMENT

Treatment of type I and type II tumors is simple excision. This can be performed by endoscopic polypectomy for negative margins or simple surgical excision via open surgery or laparoscopy. EUS can be used to delineate the depth of penetration of the carcinoid tumor and possibly to determine if it is resectable endoscopically. If a lesion has been endoscopically resected and subsequently is found to have a positive margin, we strongly recommend a laparoscopic resection within several days or a repeat gastroscopy with injection of India ink around the area of resection to mark the site for subsequent surgical resection. If time passes and the site is allowed to heal prior to the definitive resection, it may be impossible to identify the location of the tumor at surgery, even with the use of intraoperative flexible endoscopy. Invasion, which is uncommon in small tumors, occurs with increasing frequency as tumors grow larger than 2 cm. In lesions reaching this size, a more aggressive behavior of the tumor should be suspected. This would warrant a more extended gastric resection, as would be performed for a gastric carcinoma.

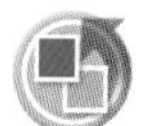

CONTRAINDICATIONS

There are few absolute contraindications to laparoscopy; most often surgeon experience and disease state dictate the relative feasibility and possible advantages of laparoscopic therapy. Several of these might include uncorrected coagulopathy, severe cardiopulmonary compromise, lack of experience with advanced minimally invasive techniques, and locally aggressive or advanced tumors that preclude safe handling or resection. Relative contraindications would include extensive previous surgery, peritonitis, or pancreatitis.

The ability to overcome purely technical obstacles in the application of laparoscopy has been pervasive throughout general surgery. Problems inherent in the laparoscopic approach to cancer surgery were suggested by early reports describing missed cancers, inadequate tumor margins, and the development of port-site metastasis. We believe that tumors of the stomach with limited metastatic potential (lack of lymph node metastasis) can be approached both safely and with the patient outcome advantages that have been seen in other operations that are performed using minimally invasive surgery techniques.

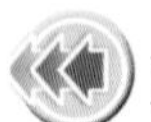

PREOPERATIVE PLANNING

Patient selection, including the diagnosis, location of the tumor, previous surgical history, and patient comorbidities, can play a key role in a surgeon's successful implementation of a minimally invasive procedure. The patient's overall medical condition should be assessed and cardiopulmonary comorbidities evaluated preoperatively, as conducted for any major operation. Patients should be able to tolerate general anesthesia and a potential laparotomy. Key points in a patient's history should include the type and extent of previous abdominal operations, confirmation of the patient's diagnosis (if possible), and a review/discussion of the diagnostic studies completed to date. A lengthy dialogue concerning the proposed operation, the options, risks, and possible outcomes should be included in the preoperative encounter.

In the more immediate period prior to surgery, the patient should be NPO (*non per os*, or nothing orally) for at least 8 hours. If gastric dysmotility is diagnosed preoperatively, one should consider maintaining a clear liquid diet for a full day preceding the operation in an effort to reduce the chance of having retained solid material within the stomach. An H_2 receptor blocker or proton pump inhibitor is often given preceding surgery. A broad-spectrum antibiotic is administered prior to the initial incision. Sequential compression devices are applied to the lower extremities to reduce the risk of deep venous thrombosis. After general anesthesia is established, a bladder catheter is placed and an orogastric tube is inserted. After the stomach has been aspirated, the orogastric tube is removed and the absence of other tubes in the esophagus is confirmed with the anesthesia team.

The set-up in the operating room is the same for most upper gastrointestinal surgeries. The patient is in a supine position with arms abducted on arm boards or tucked at the patient's sides. We use a split-leg table in nearly all circumstances, and the patient is secured to the bed with a beanbag and belt. This allows the surgeon to stand between the patient's legs and directly face the stomach. This also allows for assistants to stand on the patient's left and right sides very comfortably. Monitors are placed over the patient's shoulders bilaterally (Fig. 26-2). The typical size and locations of the ports are demonstrated in Figure 26-3. One assistant, on the right side, maintains the liver retractor via the right subcostal port and holds the camera. The assistant on the left uses the left lateral port for retraction. The assistant on the right side can be replaced by simply mounting a stationary liver retractor, in which case the assistant on the left takes over the duties as camera operator. The surgeon primarily uses the upper midline and left midabdominal ports. The port in the left lateral rectus sheath is the primary operative port

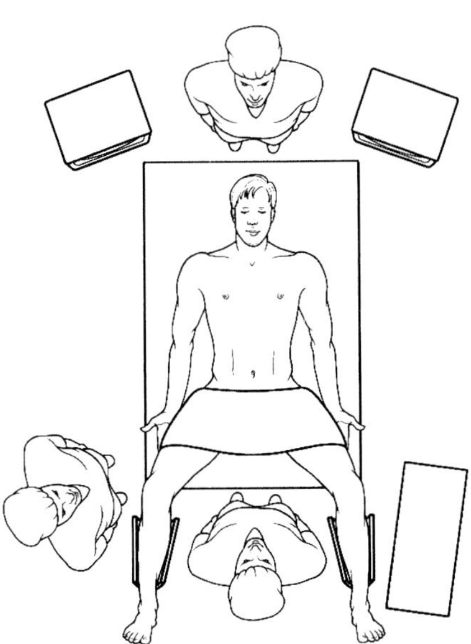

Fig. 26-2. A typical operating room setup for a laparoscopic gastric surgery.

through which an endoscopic linear stapler is introduced. However, any port can be replaced with a 12-mm sleeve to allow a different angle in which to transect the stomach. The first port placed is usually in the midline, one-quarter to one-third of the distance between the umbilicus and the xiphoid, and is used for the camera. This port is typically not placed at the umbilicus unless the lesion in question is located in the distal one-half of the stomach. An umbilical port tends to be somewhat low when the dissection is focused around the proximal stomach. The same can be stated for the other ports as well. When the lesion is in the distal portion of the stomach, all of the trocar positions can be moved slightly inferiorly to keep the ports from being directly over the operative site.

After insertion of the initial ports, the patient is placed in a steep reverse-Trendelenburg position. The orogastric tube and esophageal stethoscope are removed as soon as the stomach is noted to be decompressed. Stapling across a nasogastric tube is an embarrassing and troublesome event that most surgeons would like to avoid. Intraoperative endoscopy has become an integral part of most of our laparoscopic gastric resections. It is used to identify the exact location of small lesions, evaluate and plan the extent of resection margins, and examine and test the reconstruction or gastric closure. Troublesome overinsufflation of the small intestine with the loss of intraabdominal working space is uncommon. An experienced endoscopist and the judicious use of air insufflation are important. Occlusion of the duodenum with an atraumatic grasper also can reduce this problem. In all cases, our specimens are placed in a retrieval bag. We believe this technique may help prevent tumor spread within the abdomen and/or trocar sites and may decrease bacterial contamination of the wound.

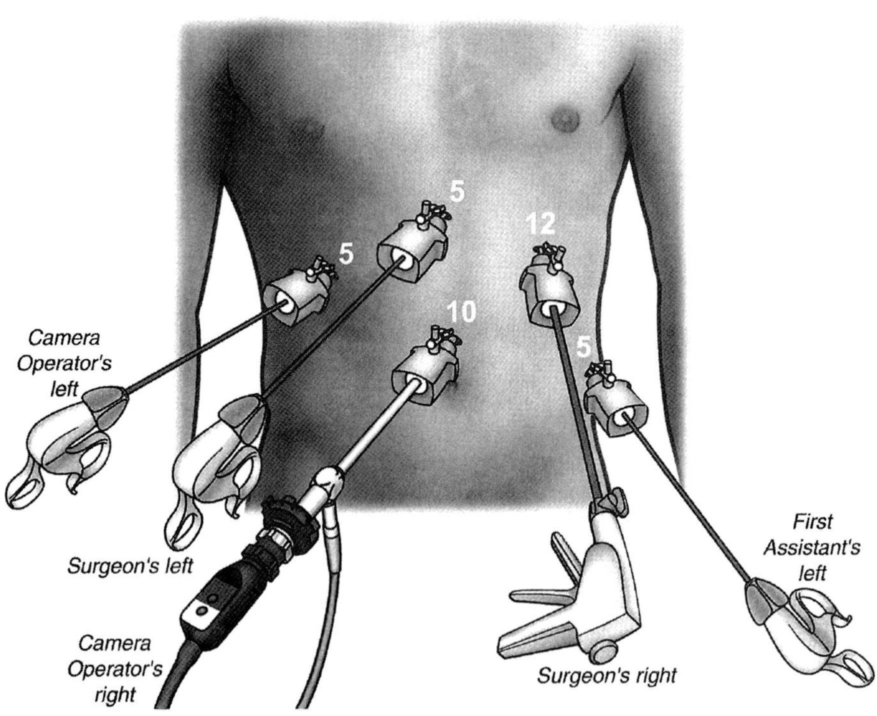

Fig. 26-3. Port placement and instruments for a gastric resection by laparoscopy. One 12-mm, one 10-mm, and three 5-mm ports are indicated.

Prior to the resection, a formal abdominal exploration is performed to rule out peritoneal spread or hepatic metastasis. The diaphragm, peritoneum, and surface of the liver are examined. Following a visual abdominal exploration, intraoperative ultrasound is performed for tumors with malignant potential. Intraoperative ultrasound provides distinctive anatomic detail of the liver for evaluation of metastatic deposits and provides real-time guidance for intraoperative biopsies of suspicious lesions. During a laparoscopic approach, intraoperative ultrasound also can provide anatomic details regarding the primary tumor's location, as well as adjacent vital (vascular) structures.

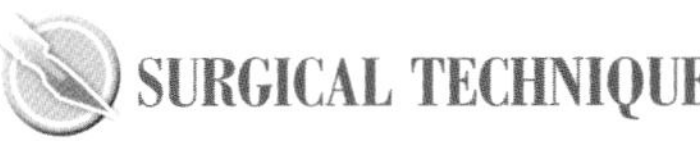

SURGICAL TECHNIQUE

Anterior Gastric Wall

Masses located on the anterior wall of the stomach are amenable to wedge resection using a linear endoscopic gastrointestinal anastomosis (GIA) stapler. If the tumor is extraluminal, it usually is visualized on initial inspection with the laparoscope. Those lesions that are intraluminal often are identified by a characteristic dimpling of the gastric serosal surface or by bimanual palpation of the stomach with laparoscopic instruments. As mentioned previously, intraluminal visualization by a flexible endoscope assists with tumor localization and may guide resection to ensure adequate margins and to safeguard against compromising the gastric inlet or outlet. After identifying the lesion, the short gastric vessels are ligated and divided as needed. Typically, this maneuver is performed with the assistant on the left retracting the omentum and gastrosplenic ligament laterally while the surgeon retracts the stomach medially and transects the vessels with ultrasonic coagulating shears.

Following this initial step, one must decide between one of two techniques to perform the gastric wedge resection. The simplest technique is to elevate the anterior gastric wall near the tumor with an atraumatic bowel grasper and simultaneously slide an endoscopic GIA stapler under the tumor (Fig. 26-4, page 234). An adequate margin of uninvolved, normal stomach is included with the tumor as the gastric wall is divided with the stapler. An alternative method to elevating the anterior gastric wall with bowel graspers is to place two seromuscular sutures on each side of

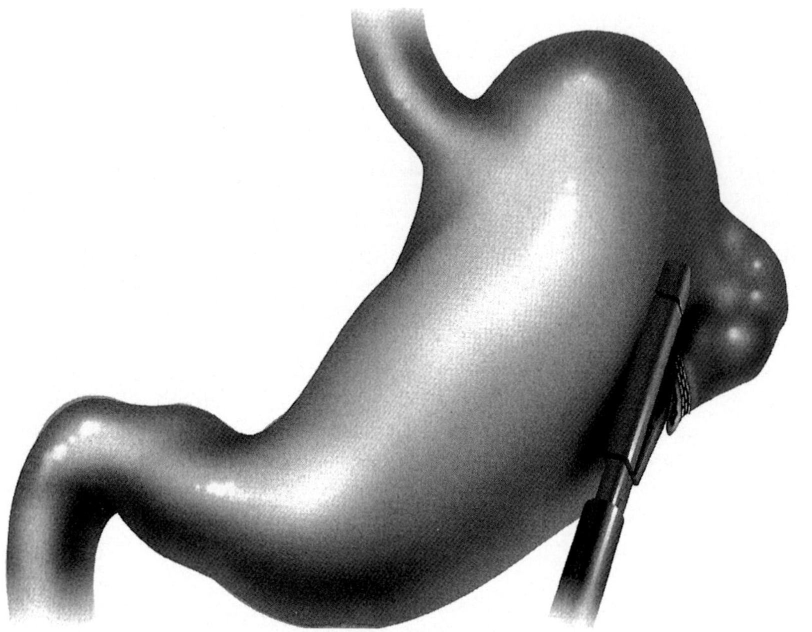

Fig. 26-4. A simple method of stapler resection of anterior gastric wall lesions.

the lesion approximately 1 to 2 cm beyond the lesion to ensure that the stitches do not penetrate or perforate the tumor. The sutures are elevated simultaneously and the stapler is placed just under the sutures to resect the tumor and a small margin of normal stomach.

Another technique is to circumferentially excise the gastric tumor and a surrounding margin of normal tissue using ultrasonic coagulating shears. This technique is simplified by insufflating the stomach with a flexible endoscope, allowing the site where the stomach will be opened to be determined by observing the tumor both endoscopically and via the laparoscope. Typically, the incision into the stomach is made 2 cm from the lesion to make certain that the tumor is not lacerated. This technique allows for a more precise excision of normal tissue at the margins of the tumor compared to the technique using an endoscopic GIA stapler. The gastrotomy can be closed by laparoscopic intracorporeal suturing or by placing two to four full-thickness traction sutures along the cut edge of the gastrotomy and using an endoscopic linear stapler to reapproximate ("close") the gastrotomy (Fig. 26-5).

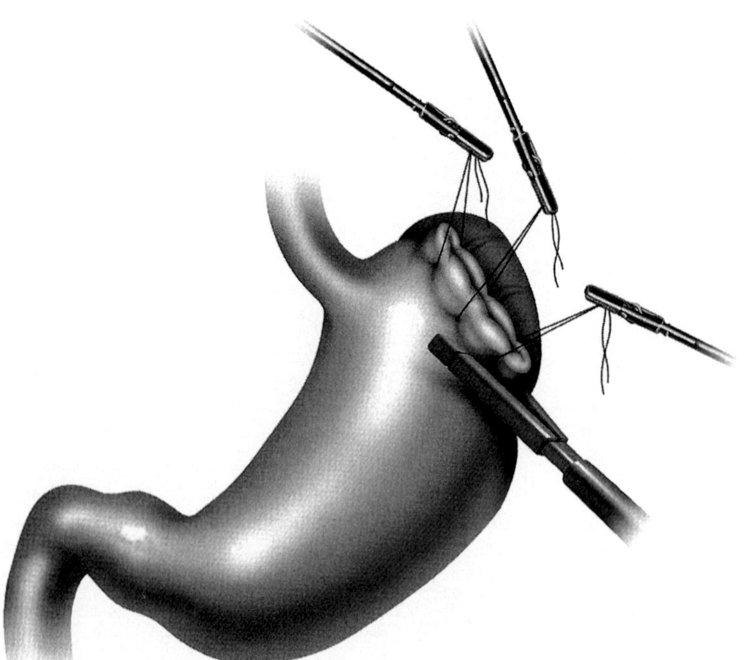

Fig. 26-5. An alternative for larger lesions is to excise the gastric wall and then close the defect with a stapler.

Posterior Gastric Wall

There are two techniques to approach posterior gastric wall masses. One method entails creating an anterior gastrotomy over the lesion after it is endoscopically localized. As described previously, the location of the gastrotomy is determined by visual cues from the gastroscope and laparoscope while simultaneously palpating the anterior gastric wall with laparoscopic graspers. Through the anterior gastrostomy, normal gastric tissue adjacent to the tumor is grasped with a laparoscopic bowel grasper (Fig. 26-6) or, alternatively, traction sutures can be placed on each side of the tumor, much as described for anterior gastric tumors. The tumor and a surrounding margin of normal stomach are elevated through the gastrotomy and resected by an endoscopic linear stapler. The staple line is examined for bleeding, and any bleeding points are oversewn. The anterior gastrotomy is closed as previously described.

An innovative technique for posterior gastric wall masses less than 3 to 4 cm in greatest diameter is percutaneous intragastric resection. Laparoscopic intragastric or "endoluminal" surgery involves the placement of balloon- or mushroom-tipped laparoscopic trocars (2 to 10 mm) percutaneously into the stomach (insufflated by a flexible endoscope), similar to the placement of a percutaneous endoscopic gastrostomy tube (Fig. 26-7). The pylorus may be occluded with a balloon-tipped nasogastric tube, but this is infrequently needed. An angled laparoscope, positioned through one of the percutaneous gastric trocars, is preferred for visualization of the operative field, but a flexible endoscope can be used in combination with two working trocars. A dilute epinephrine solution (1:100,000) is injected circumferentially around the tumor as a tumescent to aid in dissection of the submucosal plane surrounding the tumor and to limit bleeding. The lesion is enucleated from the submucosal–muscular junction using an electrocautery hook. The mucosal defect is left open to heal or can be closed with laparoscopic intragastric suturing. The tumor is placed in a retrieval

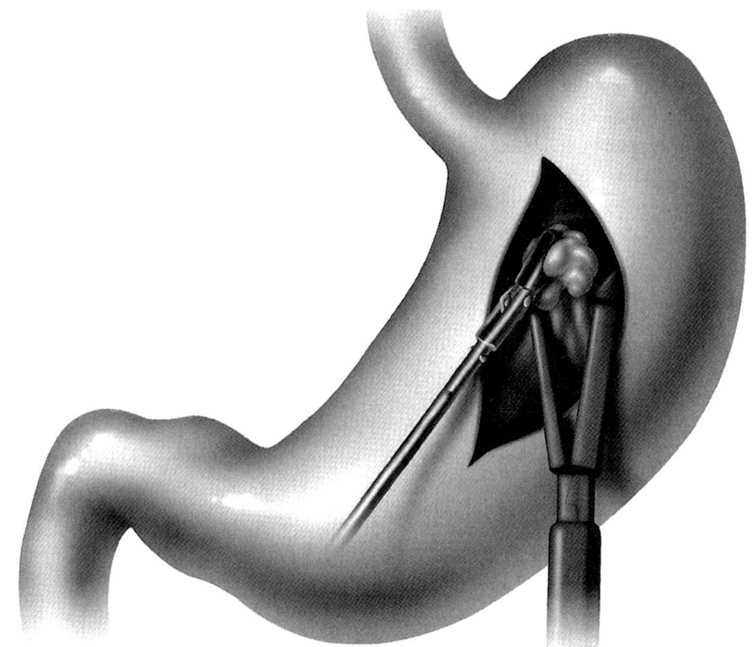

Fig. 26-6. Posterior gastric wall lesions are best accessed by an anterior gastrotomy.

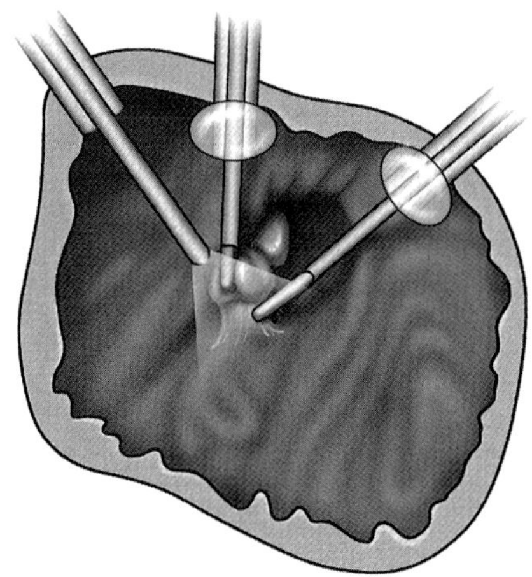

Fig. 26-7. Laparoscopic endoluminal resections are a good alternative for small lesions or ones in a difficult-to-access location.

bag and removed transorally with the flexible endoscope. Although some authors have described morcellating certain tumors and removing them piecemeal through one of the working trocars, appropriate staging of GIST may be limited.

Greater and Lesser Curvatures

Tumors of the greater and lesser curvatures are typically amenable to simple wedge resection with an endoscopic linear stapler. The trocar strategy is identical to that employed for the resection of anterior and posterior gastric wall masses. The greater omentum needs to be divided for greater curvature tumors, and the lesser omentum/gastrohepatic ligament divided for those tumors located on the lesser curve. Ultrasonic coagulating shears allow for a rapid, hemostatic division of the short gastric vessels on the greater curvature and branches of the left gastric artery and coronary vein on the lesser curvature. An important part of this technique is to rotate the greater or lesser curve of the stomach so that the tumor faces anteriorly. This allows the tumor to be removed as if it were an anterior approach. The tumor is resected using an endoscopic linear stapler and removed in an impermeable extraction bag.

Distal Stomach/Pylorus

Small tumors in the prepyloric region may be excised by wedge resection with an endoscopic linear stapler as previously described. Tumors near the pylorus, but not truly involving the pylorus, are approached using methods to achieve negative margins while not obstructing the pylorus. Posterior lesions that lie at least 1.5 to 2 cm from the pylorus and whose depth of penetration is limited to the mucosa or submucosa usually can be removed without compromising the pylorus. We have found EUS confirmation of the tumor's depth of penetration invaluable in planning our approach to pyloric masses. Our usual approach is through a horizontal, anterior gastrotomy, which can be effectively performed with the ultrasonic coagulating shears. The position of the gastrotomy is again localized with the aid of an endoscope, but the gastric opening is made no closer than 3 to 4 cm from the pylorus. Traction sutures are then placed proximally and distally within 1 cm or so of the tumor, and the tumor is pulled through the anterior gastrotomy out into the abdominal cavity. The mass can then be enucleated with an electrocautery hook or it can be elevated and removed with an endoscopic linear stapler. The enucleation site is closed with a running suture. If the tumor is to be enucleated, we frequently inject a dilute epinephrine solution (1:100,000) circumferentially around the tumor as described for the endoluminal technique. The horizontal, distal, anterior gastrotomy is closed vertically so as to not compromise the luminal diameter of the distal stomach. Two to four full-thickness traction sutures are used to approximate the gastric wall, and a thick-tissue GIA cartridge(s) is used to close the stomach. The endoscope, which is usually pulled back into the proximal stomach during the resection, is used to insufflate the stomach in order to evaluate the resection site and gastrostomy closure for bleeding, check the patency of the distal stomach, and to assess the integrity of the gastrostomy closure.

Large or full-thickness tumors in close proximity to the pylorus or those tumors causing gastric outlet obstruction often require a more formal resection (antrectomy and gastrojejunostomy) due to the high probability that a wedge resection will result in narrowing of the distal stomach, causing iatrogenic gastric outlet obstruction.

Gastroesophageal Junction

Masses in the proximity of the gastroesophageal (GE) junction can be managed similarly to tumors near the pylorus. The goals remain, if possible, to achieve an adequate surgical margin while maintaining the normal function of the lower esophageal sphincter mechanism. Lesions found more than 2 to 3 cm from the GE junction are approached according to their location, as an anterior, posterior, or greater/lesser curve mass, as previously described. Placement of a 40F or 44F bougie during the resection and closure prevents narrowing of the gastric inlet. The resection of a tumor at the GE junction is more difficult. If it is a mucosal or submucosal lesion, enucleation is a viable option and is one that we have used effectively on multiple occasions. As previously mentioned, EUS verification of the tumor's depth of penetration is invaluable

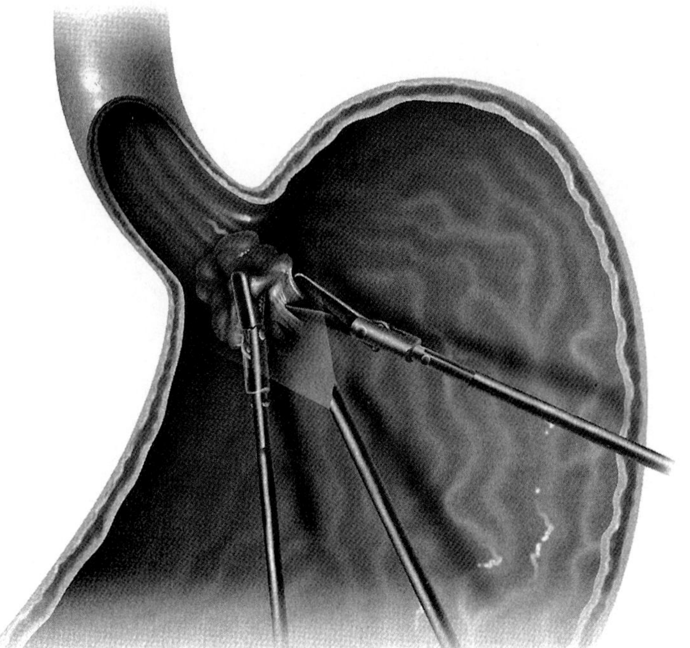

Fig. 26-8. Complex endoluminal procedures can involve a flexible endoscope as the camera and insufflator.

in determining the tactics of resection for these masses. Posterior lesions at the GE junction are easier to approach in this fashion because the instrument's insertion angle is naturally pointing toward the posterior GE junction.

In this technique, the vessels around the fundus and cardia of the stomach usually are not transected unless the lesion lies on the greater or lesser curvature. If the upper portion of the greater curve needs to be mobilized, the assistant on the left gently retracts the gastrosplenic ligament toward the lateral abdominal wall with a laparoscopic bowel grasper placed through the left lateral port. The surgeon uses the upper midline port to pull the stomach medially and inferiorly and the midright subcostal port to coagulate and transect the short gastric vessels using the ultrasonic coagulating shears. The anterior gastrotomy can be made linearly or horizontally, but one needs to remember that the gastrostomy closure must not constrict the upper stomach. Enucleation proceeds with an electrocautery hook after submucosal, peritumoral injection with dilute epinephrine. After removal of the lesion within an entrapment sac, we typically close the mucosa of the GE junction but have, on occasion, left it open to heal on its own. If the area is left open, the patient is treated prophylactically with a proton pump inhibitor for 6 weeks. In those patients on whom interval endoscopy was performed, there is essentially no residual scarring where the tumor was resected.

A novel technique we described for small GE junction stromal tumors (<4 cm) is a laparoscopic or minilaparoscopic intragastric resection. The technique can be performed in a manner similar to the endoluminal technique previously described. The minilaparoscopic, intragastric resection uses the flexible endoscope as the "camera" and insufflator (Fig. 26-8). Working ports are provided by two 2-mm, mushroom-tipped trocars placed percutaneously through the abdominal wall and into the distended stomach. We again perform a local injection with dilute epinephrine, but its instillation requires it to be performed via a 7-inch, 22-gauge spinal needle placed through one of the 2-mm ports or by injection needle though the endoscope. An electrocautery hook is used to enucleate the GE junction tumor, and the mass is removed transorally with the flexible endoscope.

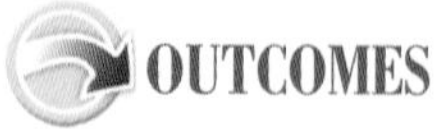

OUTCOMES

The effectiveness and reproducibility of laparoendoscopic techniques for the resection of GISTs of the stomach have been fairly well documented and are mostly positive. While numerous series have been published to date, there are only a few large single institution experiences to draw some conclusions from. In a recent series of 50 patients undergoing laparoscopic or laparoendoscopic resection, there was no morbidity or mortality. At a mean follow-up of 36 months 92% of patients were disease-free. In patients with recurrence, the tumor predominately reccurred in the liver, with one patient having diffuse intraperitoneal recurrent disease. There were no local recurrences. The authors found that disease progression was associated with increasing tumor size, tumor ulceration, tumor necrosis, and greater than 10 mitoses/50 high-power field. Patient sex, tumor location, resection margin status, and positive histochemical markers were not associated with adverse prognosis. In another experience of 38 laparoscopic resections compared to 22 open resections for gastric GISTs with a mean follow-up of 53 months, the authors concluded that disease-free survival was improved for tumors less than 5 cm regardless of operative approach. No conclusions can be made in regard to the appropriateness of laparoscopy for larger tumors from this study, as the authors resected all tumors larger than 5 cm using open or laparoscopic-assisted techniques.

We recently reviewed the Washington University Medical Center experience with 56 gastric GISTs in 55 patients with a mean age of 58.7 years. The tumors were located at the GE junction/cardia (12.5%), fundus (30.5%), body (29%), antrum (25%), or pylorus (4%). The most common presentation was an upper gastrointestinal bleed (46%). Laparoscopic partial gastrectomy (nonanatomical resection) was the most common procedure, performed in 80% of patients. Other procedures included antrectomy, esophagogastrectomy, and endoscopic-assisted transgastric resection. One patient required a conversion to an open procedure to control bleeding from the spleen. The mean tumor size was 3.8 cm ± 1.8, and negative surgical margins were obtained in all but one patient. There was an overall perioperative complication rate of 18%, with one case each of deep venous thrombosis, postoperative bleeding requiring reoperation, anastomotic stricture requiring dilation at 3 months, and incisional hernia at 12-month follow-up. There was one postoperative death (1.8%) secondary to respiratory failure. At a mean follow-up of 15 months, three (5.4%) patients had developed metastatic disease, each with high-risk tumors (>5 cm, >5 mitosis/high-power field).

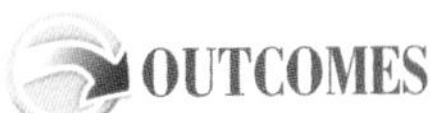

OUTCOMES

At this point, perioperative, immunologic, and/or oncologic advantages or disadvantages of the laparoscopic approach cannot be assessed pending results from prospective, randomized studies comparing minimally invasive techniques to conventional open techniques. When outcomes of patients undergoing an open or laparoscopic approach to resect gastric stromal tumors have been compared, a significant reduction in postoperative hospitalization, time to ambulation, return of bowel function, and resumption of oral intake has been seen in the laparoscopic group. Long-term follow-up has shown no difference in oncologic outcome.

In 2002 the Food and Drug Administration approved imatinib mesylate (STI-571, Gleevec) for patients with GISTs. Imatinib is a tyrosine kinase inhibitor that has been shown to provoke a substantial tumor response in patients with advanced or metastatic disease. The approval for the use of imatinib in patients with GISTs came after a study of 147 patients with unresectable disease found that 38% had a partial response with oral therapy. Subsequently, multiple other trials have demonstrated partial responses in patients with metastatic disease ranging from 55% to 80%. The dose, timing, and appropriate patients to receive imatinib and other tyrosine kinase inhibitors in development remains to be determined as data from numerous clinical trials become available.

CONCLUSION

The diagnosis and treatment of patients with GIST and other nonadenomatous tumors of the stomach has evolved over the past decade. Minimally invasive surgery affords a more patient-friendly means of resecting these masses, and newer adjuvant therapies are providing promise for potentially minimizing or controlling unresectable and/or metastatic disease. Nevertheless, clinical trials evaluating minimally invasive techniques, adjuvant treatments, and long-term follow-up are needed to more accurately predict the biologic behavior of gastric stromal tumor.

As technological advancements continue to allow the performance of more complex laparoscopic surgery in nearly all segments of the gastrointestinal tract, the ability to perform both palliative and curative gastric resections via a minimally invasive approach is increasingly possible. Combined with the utilization of preoperative and intraoperative flexible endoscopy, gastric lesions of nearly any size or histology can be localized, characterized, and resected using laparoscopic and/or intragastric techniques. We believe that continued emphasis upon minimally invasive foregut surgery will result in improved patient outcomes and expand the therapeutic options available to patients with both benign and malignant gastric tumors.

SUGGESTED READING

Brand B, Oesterhelweg L, Binmoeller KF, et al. Impact of endoscopic ultrasound for evaluation of submucosal lesions in gastrointestinal tract. *Dig Liver Dis* 2002;34:290–297.

Demetri GD, van Osterom AT, Garrett CR, et al. Efficacy and safety of sunitinib in patients with advanced gastrointestinal stromal tumour after failure of imatinib: a randomized controlled trial. *Lancet* 2006;368:1329–1338.

Gold JS, Dematteo RP. Combined surgical and molecular therapy: the gastrointestinal stomal tumor model. *Ann Surg* 2006;244:176–184.

Matthews BD, Walsh RM, Kercher KW, et al. Laparoscopic vs open resection of gastric stromal tumors. *Surg Endosc* 2002;16:803–807.

Novitsky YW, Kercher KW, Sing RF, et al. Long-term outcomes of laparoscopic resection of gastric gastrointestinal stromal tumors. *Ann Surg* 2006;243:736–747.

Rivera RE, Eagon JC, Soper NJ, et al. Experience with laparoscopic gastric resection. Results and outcomes for 37 cases. *Surg Endosc* 2005;19:1622–1627.

Schindl M, Kaserer K, Niederle B. Treatment of gastric neuroendocrine tumors. *Arch Surg* 2001;136:49–54.

Schnadig ID, Blanke CD. Gastrointestinal stromal tumors. Imatinib and beyond. *Curr Treat Options Oncol* 2006;7:426–437.

Walsh RM, Heniford BT. Laparoendoscopic treatment of gastric stromal tumors. *Semin Laparosc Surg* 2001;8:189–194.

COMMENTARY

Resection of nonadenomatous gastric tumors has undergone a partial transformation over the past 5 years. Increasingly we see a more liberal use of totally endoscopic approaches to resect these masses. Furthermore, the combined use of endoscopy and laparoscopy has become the routine rather than the exception when approaching such lesions. The advances seen with natural orifice transluminal endoscopic surgery (NOTES), as well as advances in endoluminal therapies, have led to a more aggressive utilization of minimally invasive techniques when approaching these tumors.

Many technological advances are still needed in the realm of closure of resected stomach and intestine with NOTES or submucosal endoscopic resections. One should approach full-thickness endoluminal resection of such a mass with extreme caution due to the limitations of our current closure instrumentation. It is anticipated that appropriate devices will be available to all during the life expectancy of this publication so that more aggressive endoluminal approaches to full-thickness resection of the stomach wall will find its place as a standard option in the armamentarium of gastrointestinal surgeon.

Drs. Tessier and Matthews present approaches to various types of tumors such as gastrointestinal stromal tumors (GISTs), carcinoid tumors, pancreatic rests, and adenomas. The primary focus of the authors' discussion is on the management of gastrointestinal stromal tumors and the evolution of the management of these masses. One should note that the minimally invasive approach to gastrointestinal stromal tumors is appropriate for smaller tumors. Some patients present with extremely large masses that are not amenable to a laparoscopic technique. My first gastrointestinal stromal tumor at my current university was 27 centimeters in diameter at the time of presentation, with invasion of four adjacent organs. Certainly, massive tumors such as these are to be approached with an open procedure and usually are managed with neoadjuvant therapies.

The techniques described by the authors are used by many, and the pearls offered are extremely helpful and

(continued)

demonstrate the broad experience of the senior author in this field. An additional technical point is that many of the tumors on the gastric wall can be suspended by sutures that are passed through the anterior abdominal wall. One can place a suture that is attached to a straight Keith needle directly through the anterior abdominal wall, continue it through the gastric wall proximal or distal to the mass, and then take the same needle back out through the anterior abdominal wall near the entry point. A second suture is placed on the opposite side of the mass and brought out through the abdominal wall in a like fashion. This allows one to suspend the mass with the sutures, much like a puppeteer, without the addition of one or two trocars. Once suspended, the mass can be resected through stapling, ultrasonic shears, or electrocautery.

WSE

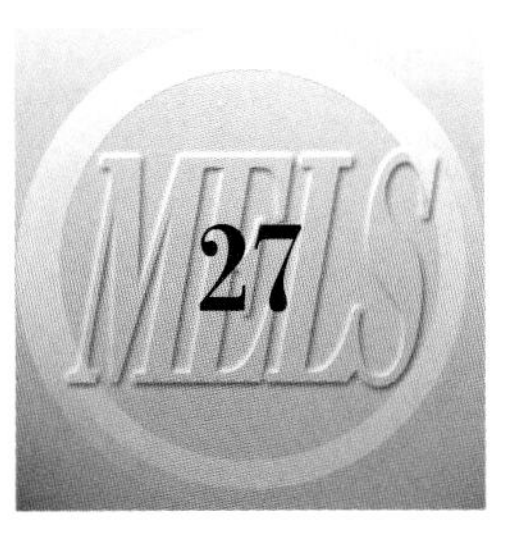

Laparoscopic Resection for Gastric Adenocarcinoma

WILLIAM W. HOPE, KENT W. KERCHER, AND B. TODD HENIFORD

INTRODUCTION

Gastric cancer is the second leading cause of cancer mortality worldwide. Although gastric cancer was the leading cause of cancer deaths in the United States in the 1930s, the incidence and mortality rate has fallen in the past several years. Gastric cancer now ranks as the fourteenth most common cancer in the U.S. In 2006, there were an estimated 22,280 new cases of gastric cancer and 11,430 deaths.

Surgery for gastric cancer began in 1881 when Theodore Billroth successfully resected an adenocarcinoma of the antrum with a distal gastrectomy. Although Billroth was not the first to attempt resection, he was the first surgeon whose patient survived the surgery. Unfortunately the patient died 4 months later from disseminated disease. Since the time of Billroth, there have been many technical and mechanical advances in the field of surgery that lend themselves to a minimally invasive approach for the management of gastric pathology. These advances include the description and implementation of various types of anastomoses, development of surgical staplers, use of nasoenteric sump tubes, and improved hemostatic coagulation devices. Perhaps the most important breakthrough was the invention of the flexible endoscope, which has not only improved diagnostic capabilities but also opened up a new frontier of therapeutic options that can be used on both benign and malignant gastric pathologies.

Since laparoscopic cholecystectomy was shown to have clear advantages over open surgery, new minimally invasive approaches have been applied to all areas of surgery. With the ability to approach the stomach both laparoscopically and endoscopically, gastric surgery is a perfect arena for minimally invasive techniques. Due to the growing volume of antireflux and obesity surgery, surgeons have gained the expertise needed to apply these approaches to other gastric pathologies. Kitano was the first to report a successful laparoscopic-assisted distal gastrectomy for early gastric cancer in 1994. Since that time, the number of laparoscopic resections for gastric cancer has increased dramatically as has the applicability of these techniques to various other gastric tumors, including gastrointestinal stromal tumors (GIST) and gastric carcinoids.

Currently, there are several controversies involving surgery for gastric cancer. The extent of lymph node dissection is an often debated topic and centers on the disparate results published in the Western and Asian literature. The use of laparoscopy for cancer has also been a subject of debate due to concerns regarding the oncologic adequacy of surgical resection and nodal sampling. Finally, new endoscopic techniques for resection of gastric tumors and sentinel lymph node evaluation are being evaluated, and this may change how gastric surgeries are performed.

In this chapter, we review the diagnosis, indications, and minimally invasive management strategies for patients with gastric cancer and discuss some of the current controversies.

Diagnostic Considerations

The majority of patients with gastric cancer in the U.S. present late in the course of their disease, in contrast to the Japan experience, where 50% of patients are diagnosed with early gastric cancers. The reasons for this discrepancy are primarily related to the aggressive endoscopic screening program employed by the Japanese. Patients with gastric cancer usually are asymptomatic; however, they may present with nonspecific complaints such as abdominal pain, weight loss, early satiety, nausea, reflux, and indigestion. Late findings include obstructing symptoms with intolerance to food and vomiting, steady pain, malnutrition, and anemia. Physical exam findings are typically varied; however, spread of gastric cancer can be manifested by enlarged lymph nodes in the supraclavicular fossa (Virchow's node), masses at the umbilicus (Sister Mary Joseph's nodule), pelvic floor (Blumer's shelf), or ovary (Krukenberg's tumor).

Upper endoscopy is critical for diagnosis and localization of the tumor. Endoscopic ultrasound (EUS) is also important to help differentiate the extension of the tumor and to establish a tumor (T) stage. Computed tomography (CT) scanning is of benefit to evaluate for liver and/or lymph node metastasis and to assess the local extent of disease. Laboratory investigations should include complete cell counts, a metabolic profile, liver chemistries, and tumor markers including carcinoembryonic antigen (CEA) and carbohydrate antigen (CA) 19-9.

STAGING

Two major classification systems have been developed for staging gastric cancer. The tumor, node, metastases (TNM) staging, developed by the American Joint Committee on Cancer (AJCC) and the International Union Against Cancer (UICC), is generally used in Western countries. The TNM staging system classifies lesions according to the depth that the primary tumor penetrates the gastric wall, the extent of lymph node involvement, and the presence or absence of distant metastases (Table 27-1, page 239). The Japanese staging system is an elaborate system that focuses on the anatomic involvement of specific (numbered) lymph node stations. Tumor staging is important not only for prognosis but also to assist with surgical decision making. EUS remains critical in the preoperative differentiation of gastric cancer extension as mucosal or submucosal or what is considered early gastric cancer. Although the diagnostic accuracy of EUS for the depth of cancer invasion can be greater than 80%, it often cannot precisely differentiate between mucosal and submucosal carcinomas.

The ultimate goal of staging is to direct therapy, both before and after surgery. Preoperatively, accurate staging may prevent futile attempts at surgical resection in patients with widely disseminated disease. In this regard, diagnostic or staging laparoscopy is an important modality in evaluating patients with gastric cancer. Staging laparoscopy has been proven to be a sensitive and specific test to accurately

TABLE 27-1. AMERICAN JOINT COMMITTEE ON CANCER (AJCC) STAGING SYSTEM FOR GASTRIC CANCER

Category	Criteria		
	Primary tumor (T)		
TX	Primary tumor cannot be assessed.		
T0	No evidence of primary tumor.		
Tis	Carcinoma in situ: intraepithelial tumor without invasion of the lamina propria.		
T1	Tumor invades lamina propria or submucosa.		
T2	Tumor invades muscularis propria or subserosa.		
T2a	Tumor invades muscularis propria.		
T2b	Tumor invades subserosa.		
T3	Tumor penetrates serosa (visceral peritoneum) without invasion of adjacent structures.		
T4	Tumor invades adjacent structures.		
	Regional lymph nodes (N)		
NX	Regional lymph node(s) cannot be assessed.		
N0	No regional lymph node metastasis.		
N1	Metastasis in 1 to 6 regional lymph nodes.		
N2	Metastasis in 7 to 15 regional lymph nodes.		
N3	Metastasis in more than 15 regional lymph nodes.		
	Distant metastasis (M)		
MX	Distant metastasis cannot be assessed.		
M0	No distant metastasis.		
M1	Distant metastasis.		
	Stage grouping		
Stage 0	Tis	N0	M0
Stage 1A	T1	N0	M0
Stage IB	T1	N1	M0
	T2a/b	N0	M0
Stage II	T1	N2	M0
	T2a/b	N1	M0
	T3	N0	M0
Stage IIIA	T2a/b	N2	M0
	T3	N1	M0
	T4	N0	M0
Stage IIIB	T3	N2	M0
Stage IV	T4	N1–3	M0
	T1–3	N3	M0
	Any T	Any N	M1

From *AJCC Cancer Staging Manual, 6th ed.* New York, Springer-Verlag, 2001.

stage patients and is encouraged before or at the time of a planned resection.

LYMPH NODE DISSECTION

Significant controversy persists regarding the appropriate extent of lymph node dissection required for gastric cancer. Some of the confusion stems from the different patient populations treated in the United States and Japan. As mentioned previously, 50% of patients in Japan are diagnosed with early gastric cancer, whereas fewer than 15% of patients in the United States are diagnosed at this early stage. Therefore, improved cure rates in the Japanese series may be related more to earlier stage at the time of surgical intervention than to aggressiveness of lymph node dissection.

While this topic can be confusing, a D1 lymphadenectomy refers to the removal of perigastric lymph nodes, which include the right and left pericardial, lesser and greater curvature, and the suprapyloric and infrapyloric nodes (Fig. 27-1). A D2 lymphadenectomy involves an extended lymphadenectomy and includes the nodes located along the vascular supply of the stomach: left gastric artery, common hepatic artery, celiac axis, the splenic hilum, splenic artery, hepatoduodenal ligament, root of the mesentery, middle colic artery, retropancreatic nodes, and paraaortic nodes (Fig. 27-2). In general a D1 lymphadenectomy is routinely practiced in the U.S., whereas a D2 lymphadenectomy is more commonly practiced in Japan. Japanese literature has demonstrated a survival benefit with a D2 dissection; however, this has not been duplicated by Western trials. Because Western trials have not demonstrated a survival benefit and have shown increased morbidity with a D2 compared to a D1 dissection, D1 lymphadenectomy continues to be practiced in most Western countries.

Laparoscopic Surgery for Gastric Cancer

Once a gastric cancer is diagnosed, surgical resection offers the best prognosis for long-term survival and the only chance for cure. Controversy regarding laparoscopic surgery for the management of malignant disease has centered on the adequacy of the oncologic resection. The main issues with regard to oncologic safety in laparoscopy are the ability to obtain an adequate negative margin, the equivalency of lymph node sampling, and the potential for local tumor dissemination. While many of the fears of laparoscopic surgery for cancer, such as port site metastasis and the detrimental effect of carbon dioxide, have been calmed by favorable long-term results in the laparoscopic treatment of other cancers such as colorectal, there remains little adequate long-term data with regard to laparoscopic gastric resection for cancer.

Various minimally invasive techniques ranging from endoscopic mucosal resection (EMR) to laparoscopic gastrectomy have been described for surgical treatment of gastric cancer and depend on the stage and location of the tumor. Early stage gastric cancers (those confined to the mucosa or submucosa) have traditionally been considered the best candidates for laparoscopic surgery. Minimally invasive techniques for removing early gastric cancer include EMR, laparoscopic wedge resection, and intragastric mucosal resection. There are three types of laparoscopic gastrectomy used to treat later stage gastric

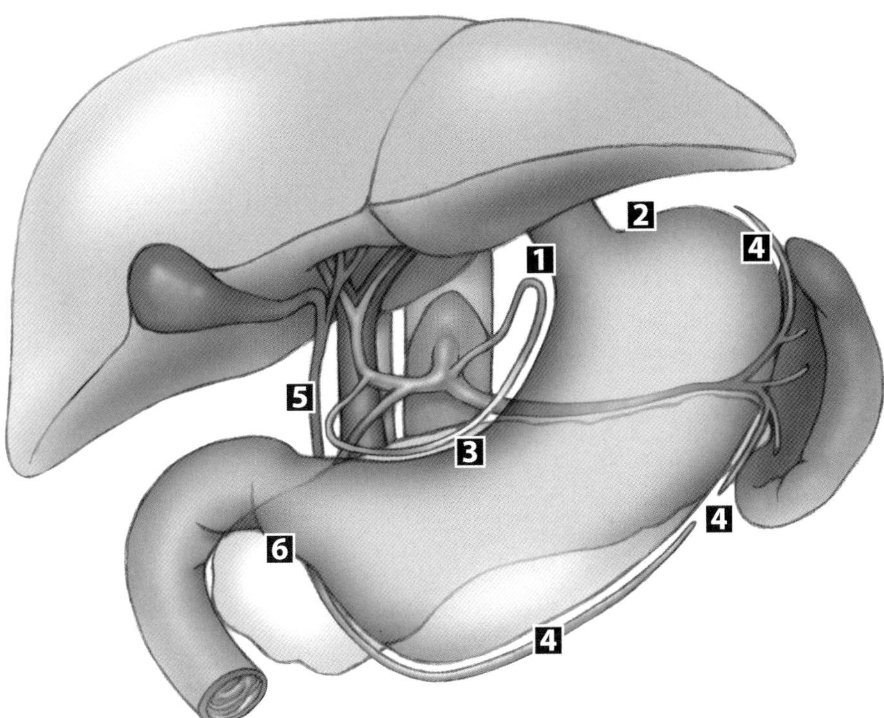

Fig. 27-1. D1 lymphadenectomy for gastric cancer. (Modified from: Roder JD, et al. *World J Surg* 1995;19:546–553; Fig. 1.)

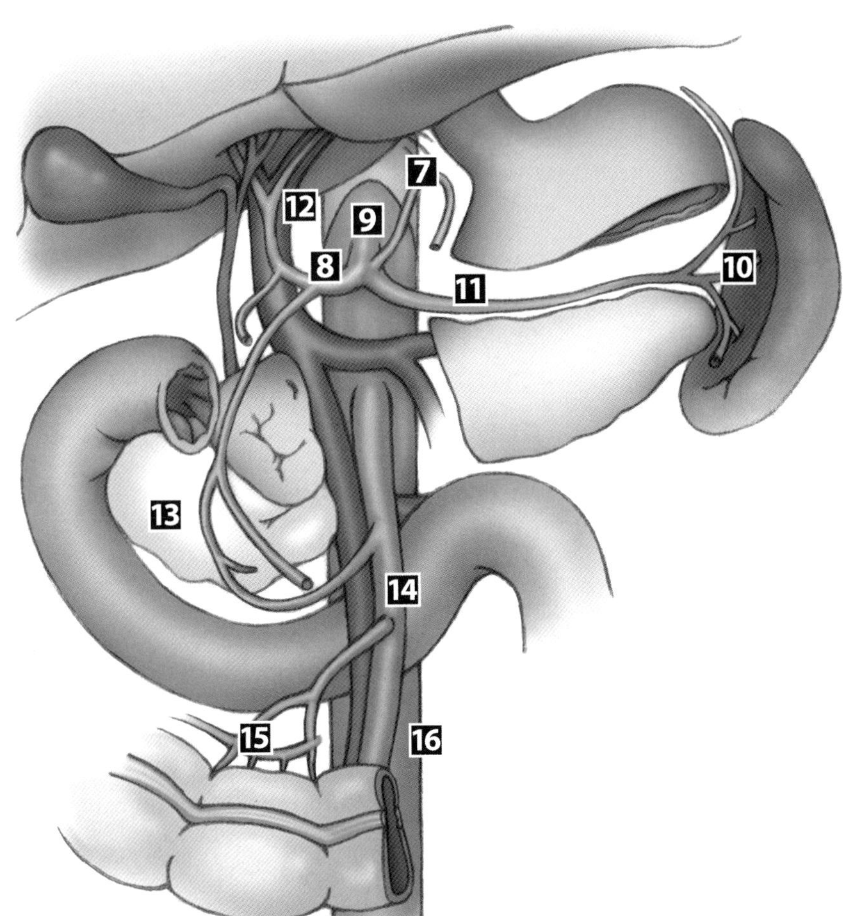

Fig. 27-2. D2 lymphadenectomy for gastric cancer. (Modified from: Roder JD, et al. *World J Surg* 1995;19:546–553, Fig. 1.)

cancer: the totally laparoscopic technique, the laparoscopic-assisted technique, and the hand-assisted technique. These techniques, including their indications and benefits, will be discussed later in the chapter.

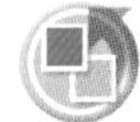

CONTRAINDICATIONS

There are few absolute contraindications to laparoscopy. A unique contraindication for patients with gastric cancer is the presence of metastatic disease, unless a staging laparoscopy or palliative procedure is planned. Uncorrected coagulopathy or inabilities to tolerate general anesthesia or a laparotomy remain absolute contraindications. Relative contraindications include extensive previous surgery, previous peritonitis, severe cardiopulmonary disease, and tumor size that would preclude its safe handling. Typically, the surgeon's experience and expertise with laparoscopy help to dictate which patients should be offered a laparoscopic approach. If unable to afford the patient similar surgical margins and lymph node resection with laparoscopic techniques, then open surgery should be contemplated.

PREOPERATIVE PLANNING

Patient selection, including the diagnosis, location of the tumor, previous surgical history, and patient comorbidities, can play a key role in the success of a minimally invasive procedure. The patient's overall medical condition as well as major cardiopulmonary conditions should be thoroughly assessed as for any major abdominal operation. In general, patients being considered for a laparoscopic procedure should be able to tolerate general anesthesia as well as laparotomy.

Key points in the patient's history include previous abdominal operations, confirmation of diagnosis and evaluation for metastatic disease, and a review of the diagnostic studies. A thorough discussion regarding the diagnosis, operation proposed, alternative treatment options, and risks and benefits should be included in the preoperative encounter.

Prior to surgery, the patient should be NPO (*non per os*, or nothing by mouth) for at least 8 hours, or longer in patients with signs and symptoms of gastric outlet obstruction. In these patients, preoperative nasogastric tube decompression may be required to decrease the risks of aspiration. An H2 receptor blocker or proton pump inhibitor is given prior to surgery along with a broad spectrum antibiotic prior to incision. Sequential compression devices are applied to the lower extremities to reduce the risk of deep vein thrombosis. After general anesthesia is established, a bladder catheter is placed, and an orogastric tube is inserted.

The operating room set-up is the same for most upper gastrointestinal surgeries. The patient is placed in a supine position with arms abducted on arm boards or tucked at the patient's sides. We use a split-leg table in nearly all circumstances, allowing the surgeon to stand between the patient's legs and to directly face the epigastrium. This also allows assistants to stand on the patient's left and right sides very comfortably. Video monitors are placed above the patient's shoulders bilaterally (Fig. 27-3). The typical size and location of trocars are demonstrated in Figure 27-4. The first port is usually placed in the midline, one-quarter to one-third of the distance between the umbilicus and the xiphoid, and is used for the camera. This port is typically not placed at the umbilicus unless the lesion in question is located in the distal half of the stomach, as an umbilical port tends to be somewhat low when the dissection is focused on the proximal stomach. When the lesion is in the distal portion of the stomach, all of the trocar positions can be moved slightly inferior to keep the ports from being directly over the operative site.

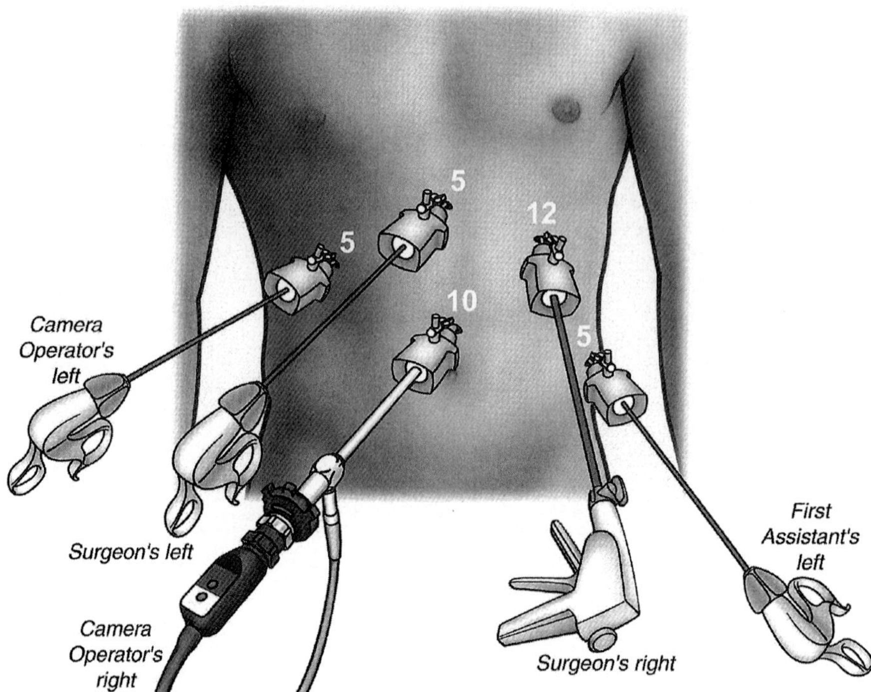

Fig. 27-4. Port placement and instruments for a gastric resection by laparoscopy.

After inserting the initial ports, the patient is placed in a steep reverse-Trendelenburg position. The initial oral gastric tube and esophageal stethoscope are removed as soon as the stomach is decompressed; stapling across a nasogastric tube is a troublesome event that all surgeons would like to avoid. Prior to surgical resection of the stomach, a formal abdominal exploration is performed to rule out peritoneal seeding or hepatic metastasis. The diaphragm, peritoneum, and surface of the liver are examined. Following a visual abdominal exploration, intraoperative ultrasound is performed for tumors with malignant potential. Intraoperative ultrasound provides distinctive anatomic detail of the liver for evaluation of metastatic deposits and provides real-time guidance for intraoperative biopsies of lesions suspected to be cancer. During a laparoscopic approach, intraoperative ultrasound also can provide anatomical details regarding the primary tumor's location, as well as adjacent vital (vascular) structures.

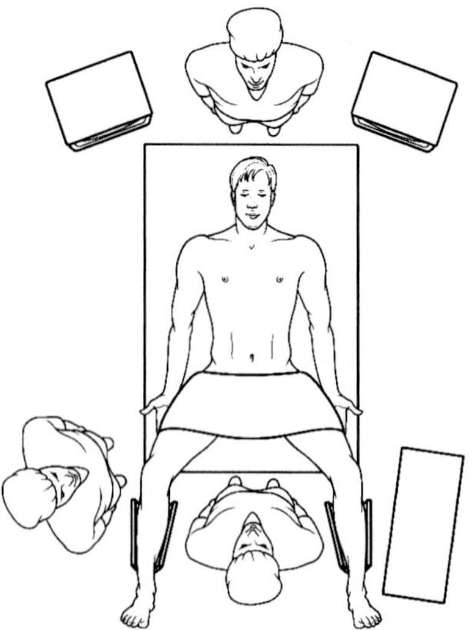

Fig. 27-3. Typical operating room setup for a laparoscopic gastric surgery.

Intraoperative endoscopy has become an integral part of most of our laparoscopic gastric resections. It is used to identify the exact location of small lesions, evaluate and plan the resection margins, and examine and test the reconstruction after gastric closure. The possibility of troublesome over-insufflation of the small intestine with the loss of working space is uncommon as long as the endoscopist performing the procedure uses judicious (limited) insufflation. Occlusion of the duodenum with an atraumatic grasper can also help avoid this complication.

During the procedure, one assistant, on the patient's right side, maintains the liver retractor via the right subcostal port and holds the camera. The assistant on the left uses the left lateral port for retraction. The assistant on the right side can be replaced by simply mounting a stationary liver retractor, in which case the assistant on the left takes over duties as camera operator. The surgeon primarily uses the upper midline and left midabdominal ports. The port lateral to the left rectus sheath is the primary operative port through which an endoscopic linear stapler is introduced. However, any port can be replaced with a 12-mm sleeve to allow a different angle from which to transect the stomach. In all cases, our specimens are placed in a retrieval bag prior to extraction. We believe that this technique may help prevent tumor spread within the abdomen and/or trocar sites, and may decrease bacterial contamination of the abdomen and port site.

Minimally Invasive Procedures for Early Gastric Cancer

Early gastric cancer is defined as cancer confined to the mucosa or submucosa, irrespective of lymph node involvement. There are three procedures for local resection of early gastric cancers: the laparoscopic wedge resection, the intragastric mucosal resection, and the endoscopic mucosal resection. Patient selection and preoperative evaluation of the tumor by endoscopic ultrasound are critical in the success of local resection for gastric cancer. Lymph node metastasis occurs in 2% to 5% of mucosal cancers and in 15% to 20% of submucosal cancers. The pathologic characteristics of early gastric cancer remain controversial; however, indications for local resection, proposed by Ogami et al., include a preoperatively diagnosed mucosal cancer, an elevated lesion less than 25 mm in diameter, or a depressed lesion less than 15 mm in diameter without ulcer formation.

LAPAROSCOPIC LOCAL RESECTIONS

The approach for laparoscopic local resection of early gastric cancer depends substantially upon the anatomic location of the tumor within the stomach. Laparoscopic wedge resection is applied to cancers involving the anterior wall, lesser curvature, or greater curvature of the stomach whereas intragastric mucosal resections are applied to cancers on the posterior wall of the stomach or near the cardia or pylorus. Those that are intraluminal can often be identified by the characteristic dimpling of the gastric serosal surface, by bimanual palpation of the stomach with laparoscopic instruments, or by localization with an endoscope. Flexible endoscopy remains a critical adjunct to localize the tumor, plan adequate surgical resection without compromising the lumen of the stomach, and test the anastomosis or gastric closure for integrity.

SURGICAL TECHNIQUE

After identifying the tumor, the short gastric vessels are ligated and divided as needed, typically with ultrasonic coagulation shears. There are three ways to perform the gastric wedge resection for tumors located on the anterior gastric wall. One is to elevate the tumor with an atraumatic grasper and to staple underneath the tumor using an endoscopic GIA stapler, making sure to include a margin of normal stomach (Fig. 27-5). The second technique involves placing two seromuscular sutures on either side of the lesion approximately 1 to 2 cm beyond the lesion so as not to penetrate or perforate the tumor. The sutures are then elevated and the tumor and normal adjacent stomach is resected using an endoscopic GIA stapler. Another technique is to circumferentially excise the tumor with a surrounding margin of normal tissue using the ultrasonic coagulation shears. This technique is simplified by insufflating the stomach with a flexible endoscope, allowing the site where the stomach will be opened to be determined by observing the tumor both endoscopically and by the laparoscope. Typically the incision is made 2 cm from the tumor to ensure adequate margin and to avoid inadvertently lacerating the tumor. The gastrotomy is closed using laparoscopic intracorporeal sutures or by placing traction sutures on the cut edge and using an endoscopic linear stapler to close the defect (Fig. 27-6).

Tumors on the posterior wall can be approached through an anterior gastrotomy. After the tumor has been appropriately localized endoscopically, an anterior

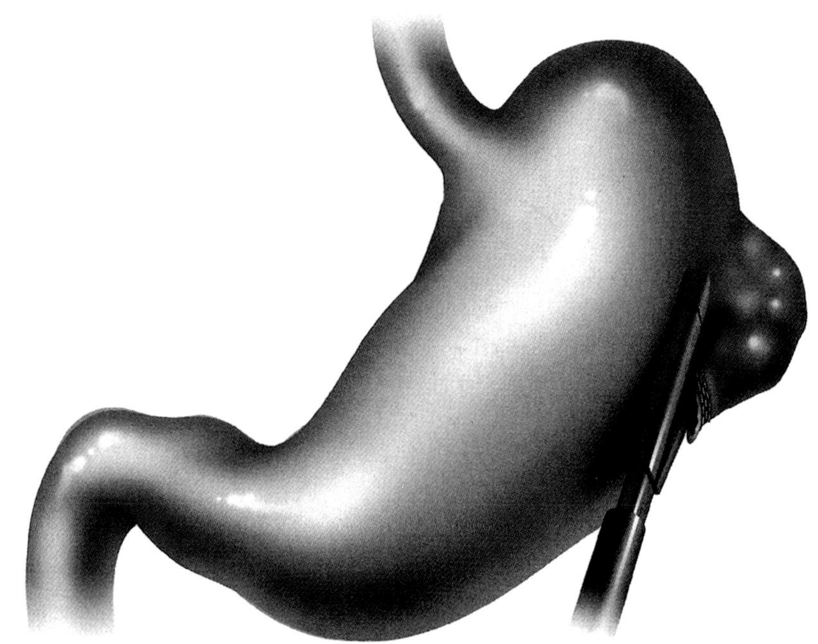

Fig. 27-5. A simple method of stapler resection for anterior gastric wall lesions.

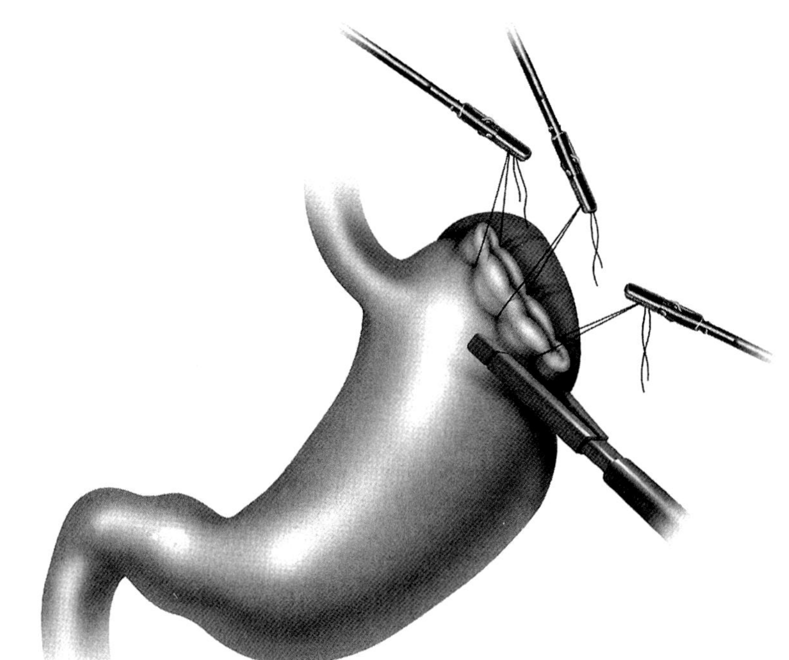

Fig. 27-6. An alternative for larger lesions is to excise the gastric wall and then close the defect with a stapler.

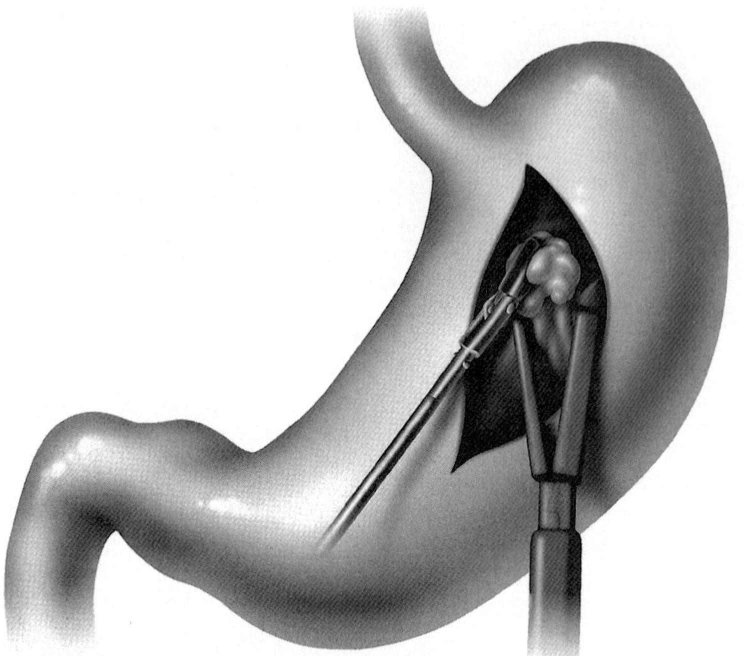

Fig. 27-7. Posterior gastric wall tumors are best accessed by an anterior gastrostomy over the lesion and then removal with an endoscopic stapler.

gastrotomy is made over the lesion. Through the gastrotomy the tumor with surrounding normal stomach can be elevated with atraumatic graspers or traction sutures and divided using endoscopic linear stapler, as described previously (Fig. 27-7). The anterior gastrotomy is then closed as previously described.

Tumors of the greater and lesser curvature are typically amenable to wedge resection with an endoscopic linear stapler. The greater omentum should be divided for greater curvature tumors and the lesser omentum divided for lesser curvature tumors. An important part of this technique is to rotate the lesser or greater curve of the stomach so the tumor faces anteriorly. Resection is then performed as if it were an anterior tumor.

Small tumors in the prepyloric region can be excised by wedge resection with an endoscopic linear stapler as previously described. Posterior lesions that lie at least 1.5 to 2 cm from the pylorus and are confined to the mucosa or submucosa can typically be removed without compromising the pylorus. EUS evaluation of depth of tumor invasion is critical when dealing with pyloric cancers. A horizontal gastrotomy is made with ultrasonic coagulation shears no closer than 3 to 4 cm from the pylorus. The tumor is then elevated with traction sutures and then either enucleated with hook electrocautery or excised with an endoscopic linear stapler. If the tumor is enucleated we typically inject a dilute epinephrine solution (1:100,000) circumferentially around the tumor to aid in the dissection. The enucleation site is closed with a running suture. The horizontal, distal anterior gastrotomy is then closed vertically so as not to narrow the gastric lumen. This is performed with traction sutures and a thick tissue (4.8 mm) GIA cartridge. Endoscopy is then used to test the anastomosis as well as check for patency of the lumen of the distal stomach.

INTRAGASTRIC MUCOSAL RESECTION

Intragastric mucosal resection or "endoluminal surgery" was first described by Ohashi in 1995 for local resection of gastric mucosa. This novel technique involves operating within the lumen of the stomach using laparoscopic instrumentation under endoscopic or laparoscopic guidance. This treatment modality is used to treat early gastric cancers that are not candidates for endoscopic mucosal resection because of tumor size or location. Intragastric mucosal resection is typically applied to cancers on the posterior wall of the stomach or near the cardia or pylorus.

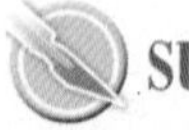

SURGICAL TECHNIQUE

The preoperative preparation is as previously described. The operation is begun by placing balloon or mushroom-tipped laparoscopic trocars (2 to 10 mm) percutaneously into the stomach (insufflated by a flexible endoscope), similar to the placement of a percutaneous endoscopic gastrostomy tube. The pylorus may be occluded with a balloon-tipped nasogastric tube, but this is infrequently needed. An angled laparoscope, positioned through one of the percutaneous gastric trocars, is preferred for visualizing the operative field, but a flexible endoscope can be used in combination with two working trocars. A dilute epinephrine solution (1:100,000) is injected circumferentially around the tumor as a tumescent to aid in dissection of the submucosal plane surrounding the tumor and to limit bleeding. Mucosal resection is then performed using forceps and the electrocautery hook (Fig. 27-8). The mucosal defect can be left open to heal or closed with laparoscopic intragastric suturing. The tumor is placed in a retrieval bag and removed transorally with a flexible endoscope, although morcellating the tumor and removing it through one of the gastric trocars has been described.

Tumors of the gastroesophageal (GE) junction are dealt with in a manner similar to those at the pylorus, with the goal being to obtain adequate surgical margins without compromising the gastric lumen. When the tumor is mucosal or submucosal, enucleation is a viable option. Figure 27-8 shows the technique for laparoscopic intragastric resection: 2-mm to 5-mm trocars and instruments are placed through the gastric wall with endoscopic insufflation of the stomach and diagnostic laparoscopy (like a percutaneous endoscopic gastrostomy, or PEG). Visualization and insufflation during resection is provided by the flexible endoscope. Enucleation is performed with an electrocautery hook, and the mucosal defect is closed with sutures. Port site gastrotomies are closed laparoscopically with interrupted sutures after completion of the resection and removal of the intragastric trocars.

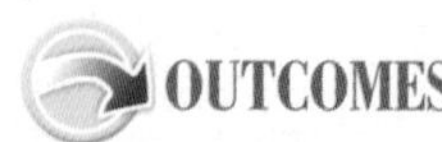

OUTCOMES

The few reports on the short- and long-term outcomes of laparoscopic local resection and intragastric mucosal resection there are come from the Japanese literature. Although the literature is limited, it appears that these techniques are safe and curative when the appropriate indications are used. Further evaluation pending outcomes of larger, prospective trials are needed to adequately assess these techniques.

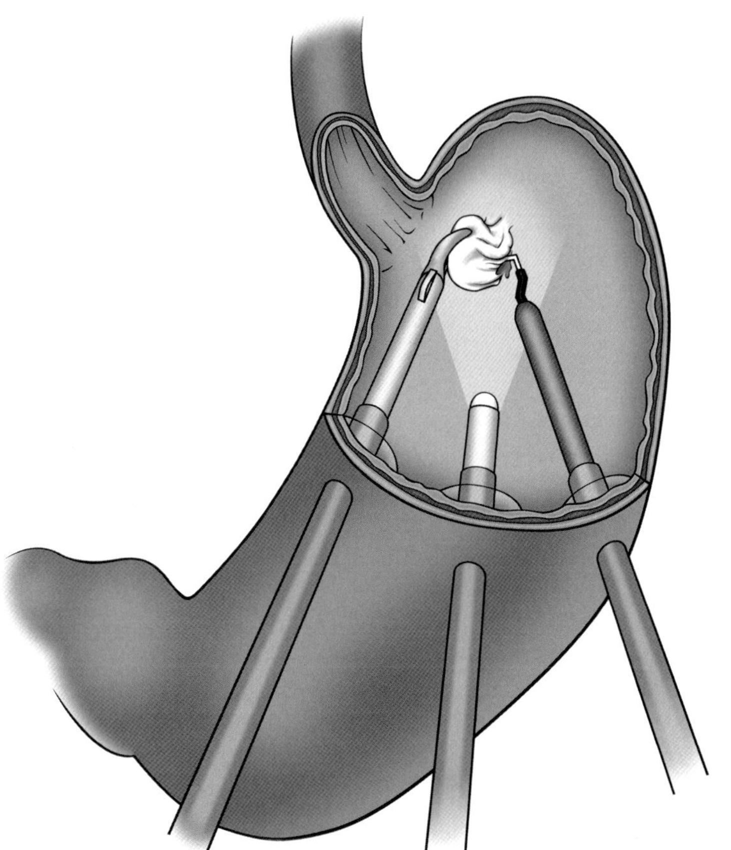

Fig. 27-8. Intragastric mucosal resection using laparoscopic graspers and the electrocautery hook.

Laparoscopic Gastrectomy for Gastric Cancer

Laparoscopic gastrectomy for gastric cancer remains controversial. However, if meticulous technique and the principles of oncologic surgery are maintained, many surgeons believe that survival statistics after laparoscopic surgery will equal those of open surgery.

There are three types of laparoscopic gastrectomy: the totally laparoscopic procedure, the laparoscopic-assisted procedure, and the hand-assisted laparoscopic procedure. Laparoscopic distal, proximal, and total gastrectomy are performed according to the location of the tumor and depth of invasion, as in open surgery. Laparoscopic partial gastrectomies, especially the laparoscopic-assisted distal gastrectomy, have been widely accepted in Japan for early gastric cancer with risk of lymph node involvement. Laparoscopic gastrectomies can be performed with perigastric lymph node dissection (D1) or extended lymph node dissection (D2) (Figs. 27-1 and 27-2).

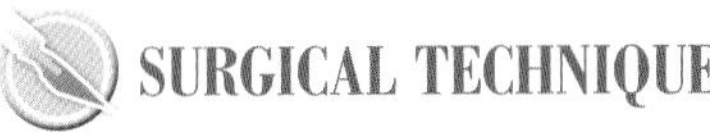

SURGICAL TECHNIQUE

Laparoscopic Total Gastrectomy

Patient and trocar positioning are similar to that described earlier, except 12-mm ports are used more liberally to allow for versatility in employing the endoscopic linear stapler from many different angles. The first step in the operation is to perform a general exploration for intraabdominal malignancy. Examination of the peritoneal surfaces, visual (laparoscopic and intraabdominal ultrasound) inspection, and manual (laparoscopic instrumentation) palpation of the liver and exploration of the lesser sac are critical when the resection is performed for curative intent. In approximately 25% of patients, laparoscopic exploration detects metastasis that precludes curative resection despite standard preoperative radiographic examinations indicating that the tumor appeared to be resectable.

The technique for a laparoscopic gastrectomy with D2 extended lymphadenectomy begins with coloepiploic detachment with omentectomy, followed by dissection of the gastrocolic ligament as far as the gastrosplenic ligament. These maneuvers can typically be accomplished with ultrasonic coagulating shears or bipolar vessel sealing devices. The left gastroepiploic vessels are then divided with laparoscopic clips.

Dissection is then carried out around the pylorus, where the right gastroepiploic vein is clipped flush with its trunk. The right gastroepiploic artery is clipped and cut at its origin from the gastroduodenal artery just above the pancreatic head. The pyloric vessels are then sectioned, the pylorus is freed, and infrapyloric tiers 4 and 6 lymph node basins are resected together. Lymphatic dissection of groups 1 (right paracardial), 3 (lesser curve), 5 (suprapyloric), and 12a (hepatoduodenal ligament) is then performed after incising of the lesser omentum and dissecting of the lesser curvature.

A 45-mm or 60-mm endoscopic stapler (3.5-mm staple load) is used to transect the duodenum. The duodenal staple line can be imbricated with 2-0 silk sutures for added security. Lymphadenectomy then continues with dissection of level 8 (common hepatic artery), 9 (celiac axis), and 11p (proximal splenic artery). The left gastric artery is then ligated with clips or an endoscopic stapler (2.0 to 2.5 mm) and the group 7 nodes (left gastric artery) are removed. Excision of the right paracardial nodes in the esophagogastric region (tier 1) is accomplished by lifting the gastric remnant.

The short gastric vessels, posterior lesser curve attachments, and phrenoesophageal ligament are divided using ultrasonic coagulating shears, and the distal esophagus is mobilized well into the mediastinum. The division of the phrenoesophageal ligament and the mediastinal dissection is facilitated by an assistant, who retracts the stomach in a caudal direction using a Penrose drain placed around the GE junction. The posterior dissection of the stomach and anterolateral dissection of the esophageal hiatus occur in a fairly bloodless plane and can be performed mostly with blunt techniques. The distal esophagus is mobilized by bluntly pushing the left and right crura away from the esophagus. The esophagus should be clearly visualized at all times, as esophageal injuries can occur with blind dissection. In general, any tubes in the esophagus (oro-/nasogastric, bougie, esophageal stethoscope, etc.) are

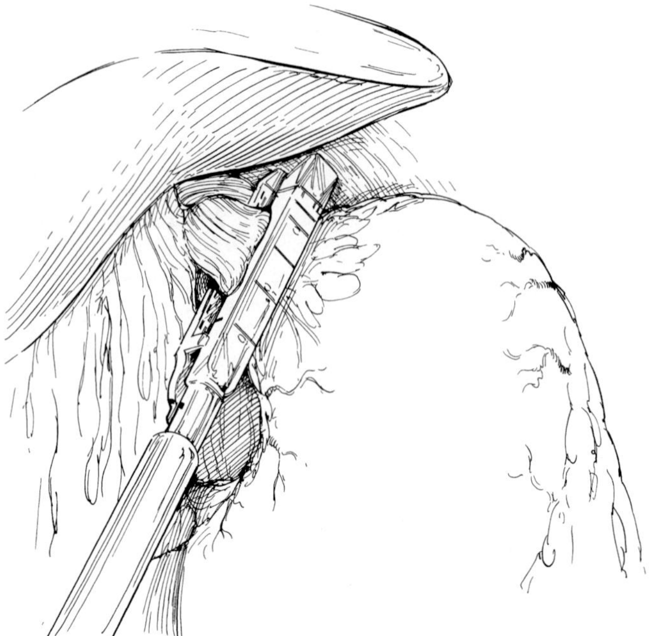

Fig. 27-9. After careful and complete mobilization, the esophagus is divided with a linear endoscopic stapler.

removed prior to initiating the hiatal dissection. These tubes can make the esophagus more rigid and difficult to manipulate safely. Posterior to the esophagus, segmental arteries from the aorta are divided with the ultrasonic coagulating shears. After the esophagus is mobilized, the anterior and posterior vagal trunks are identified and divided between clips.

Group 2 (left paracardial) lymph nodes are resected. The esophagus is transected with a linear stapler (Fig. 27-9), and the whole stomach is collected in an endobag and left in the peritoneal cavity.

The circular, flip-top EEA stapler (U.S. Surgical Corporation; Norwalk, CT) or endoscopic linear stapling device can be used to complete the esophagojejunostomy. This is similar to stapler techniques used to perform Roux-en-Y gastrojejunostomy for laparoscopic gastric bypass. Prior to performing an esophagojejunostomy, the ligament of Treitz is identified, and the proximal jejunum is divided approximately 30 to 45 cm distal to the ligament of Treitz with the endoscopic linear stapler. The biliary limb is subsequently anastomosed to the more distal jejunum, approximately 30 to 40 cm distal to the staple line on the Roux limb.

To complete a circular-stapled anastomosis, a flipped, 25-mm anvil is sutured to the distal end of a 16F orogastric tube that has been previously transected proximal to the sump air port (Fig. 27-10). The proximal end of the orogastric tube with the flipped anvil secured to the distal end is passed transorally and guided down the esophagus. A small enterotomy is made in the esophagus near the staple line, and the proximal end of the orogastric tube is gently pulled into the abdomen and out one of the trocar sites. As the tube is pulled through the enterotomy in the esophagus, the anvil is guided through the oropharynx by the anesthesiologist. After the anvil tip emerges from the esophagotomy, the orogastric tube is cut free of the anvil and removed. The circular stapler is placed through a 33-mm trocar or enlarged trocar site in the left upper quadrant and advanced into an enterotomy created along the staple line on the proximal Roux (jejunal) limb. The stapler is advanced antegrade through the Roux limb and the spike of the anvil is advanced through the antimesenteric border of the jejunum. The anvil protruding through the esophagotomy is united with the EEA stapler, and the stapler is tightened and fired. The enterotomy in the proximal Roux limb is closed with an endoscopic linear stapler. A completed gastrojejunostomy following a total gastrectomy is pictured in Figure 27-11.

To perform an esophagojejunostomy using an endoscopic linear stapler, enterotomies in the midpoint of the esophageal staple line and on the antimesenteric border of the Roux limb have to be made for the jaws of the stapler. One jaw of the endoscopic linear stapler is inserted into the enterotomy in the Roux limb, and the jejunum is brought up to the distal esophagus, where the second jaw of the endoscopic linear stapler is inserted into the enterotomy in the distal esophagus. Typically, one firing of the 4.5-cm stapler (3.5-mm cartridge) creates an adequate posterior anastomosis. The remaining anterior enterotomy is closed with laparoscopic, interrupted intracorporeally tied sutures. The anastomosis can be tested for patency and leaks by inserting a flexible endoscope and gently insufflating under a saline bath.

Slight enlargement of one of the 12-mm port sites is typically needed to remove the bag containing the stomach and lymph nodes. A drain can be placed in Morison's pouch near the duodenal stump. Port sites

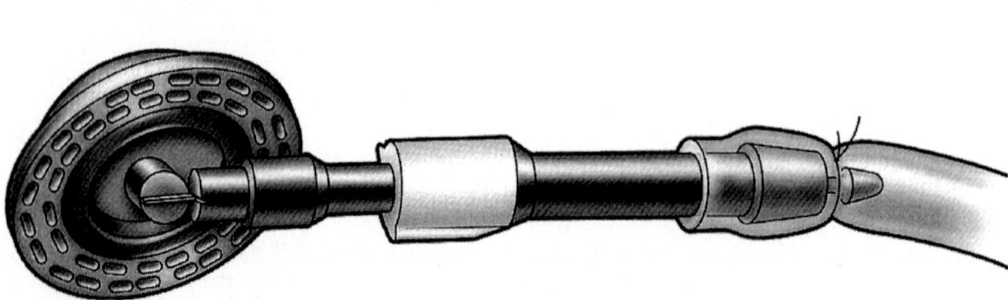

Fig. 27-10. A circular stapled esophagojejunal anastomosis requires alteration of the anvil of the stapler.

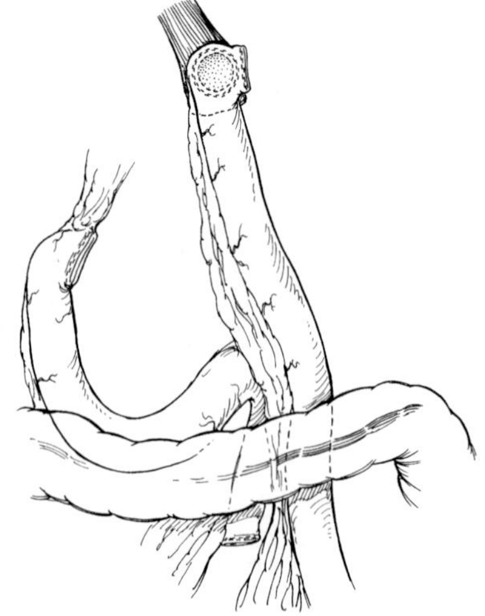

Fig. 27-11. Completed gastrojejunostomy following a total gastrectomy.

that are larger than 10 mm are then closed with a suture passer.

Alternative minimally invasive procedures have been described to facilitate the performance of laparoscopic total and subtotal gastrectomies. In the laparoscopic-assisted procedure, a 5-cm incision is made below the xiphoid after the stomach is mobilized laparoscopically. The duodenum and distal portion of the stomach are exteriorized through the minilaparotomy. Proximal gastric transaction and Roux-en-Y reconstruction is then performed through this incision. In the hand-assisted technique, an incision is made in the midline approximately 1 cm smaller than the surgeon's glove size. The procedure is carried out as described above with the use of a hand for retraction. Once mobilized, the specimen can be extracted through the hand port incision and the reconstruction completed in an "open" fashion though the hand-assist incision.

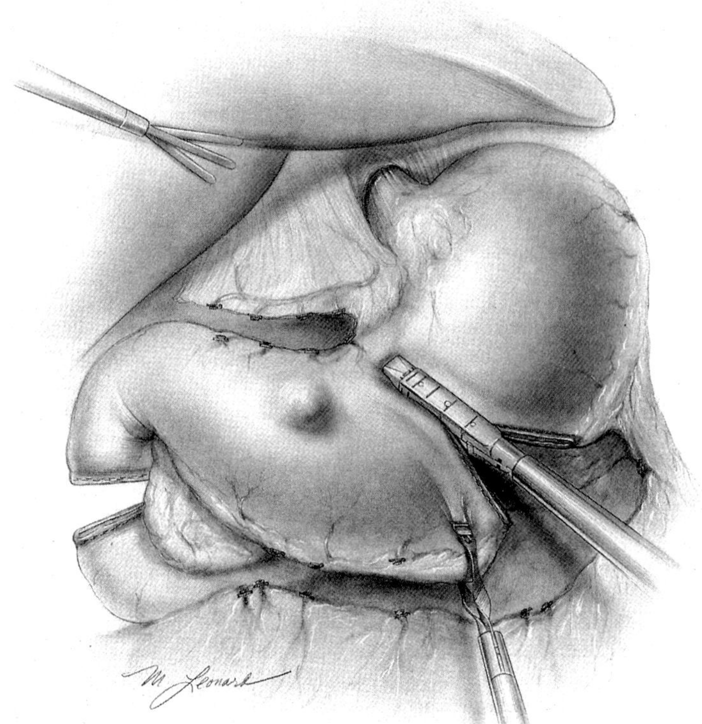

Fig. 27-12. Proximal gastric transection using a linear endoscopic stapler.

Laparoscopic Subtotal and Distal Gastrectomy

Laparoscopic subtotal and distal gastrectomies are performed using a similar technique to that described for total gastrectomy except for the mobilization of the fundus and abdominal esophagus. Proximal transection sites on the stomach are selected according to the location of the tumor. The proximal stomach is transected with a linear endoscopic stapler (Fig. 27-12). Three or four staple loads (3.5-mm or 4.8-mm cartridges) of a 45-mm or 60-mm stapler are usually required depending on the level of the stomach to be transected. In the more proximal stomach, we have found a 3.5-mm stapler works well and reduces bleeding. The more distal and thicker portions of the stomach may require a 4.8-mm staple cartridge.

Several techniques are used for reconstruction following a subtotal gastrectomy. We prefer a standard loop gastrojejunostomy or, when the gastric pouch is small, a Roux-en-Y gastrojejunostomy. This portion of the operation is initiated by taking the patient out of reverse-Trendelenburg position and maintaining him or her in a more neutral position. The omentum is rolled upward and over the colon, and colonic epiploica are grasped and pulled upward to expose the full undersurface of the transverse colon mesentery and to identify the ligament of Treitz. We measure approximately 20 to 35 cm distal to the ligament of Treitz and bring this portion of jejunum upward to the gastric remnant. When the intestine easily reaches the gastric remnant, an antecolic route is chosen. To facilitate the antecolic positioning of the jejunal limb, one can split the omentum in the midline in a caudal-cranial fashion using the ultrasonic coagulating shears. Otherwise, a small window can be made in the avascular area of the transverse mesocolon just above and lateral to the ligament of Treitz. The loop of the jejunum can be brought through the mesocolon easily in a retrocolic fashion. The anastomosis can be performed in an isoperistaltic or antiperistaltic manner. We typically choose an antiperistaltic anastomosis, which allows us to place a stapler from the cut edge of the stomach, angling slightly upward on the stomach and distally on the small intestine (Fig. 27-13). When possible, the anastomosis

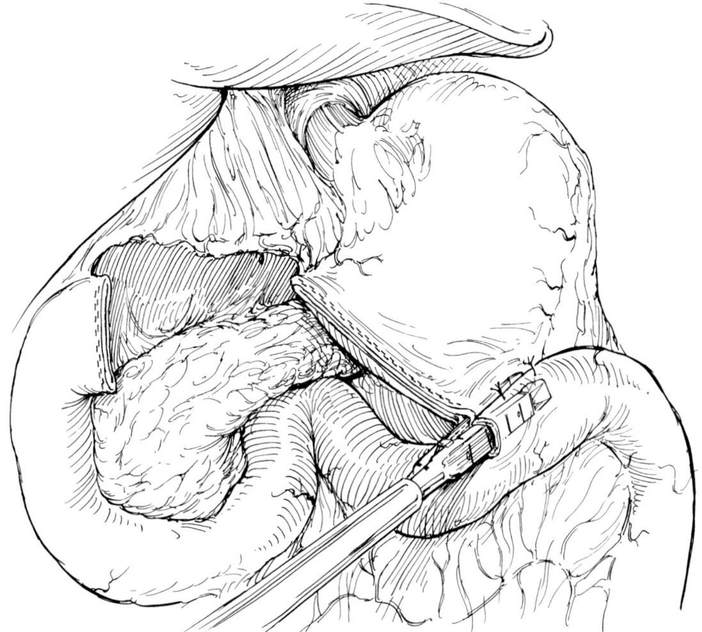

Fig. 27-13. Gastrojejunostomy created with an endoscopic linear stapler.

is performed on the dependant, posterior wall of the remaining stomach.

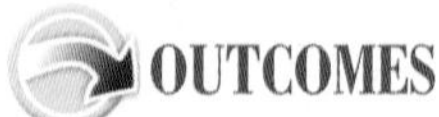

OUTCOMES

Results of laparoscopic-assisted distal gastrectomy have been investigated since 1995, including several case-control trials comparing it with open gastrectomy and a few randomized controlled studies with short-term outcomes. These studies have found advantages to the minimally invasive approach, including more rapid recovery, less pain, less blood loss, earlier return of gastrointestinal function, and shorter hospital stays. Laparoscopic gastrectomy, however, continues to require significantly longer operating times in most studies and is related to the learning curve of the surgical team. Japanese literature has shown very low morbidity and mortality rates with the laparoscopic-assisted distal gastrectomy, suggesting it to be a safe procedure. Comparative studies looking at surgical margins and number of lymph nodes evaluated have shown the laparoscopic-assisted distal gastrectomy to be equal to that of an open gastrectomy. Long-term outcome data are scarce for laparoscopic-assisted distal gastrectomy. In a series reported by Kitano et al., over 1000 patients underwent laparoscopic gastrectomy for early gastric cancer. They reported a 0.6% cancer recurrence rate at a median follow-up of 36 months with a 5-year disease-free survival rate of 99.8%, 98.7%, and 85.7% for stage IA, stage IB, and stage II disease, respectively. Recently, a prospective trial comparing laparoscopic and open partial and total gastrectomies showed improved postoperative recovery, shorter hospital stays, and improved cosmesis with no significant difference in number of lymph nodes dissected and no positive surgical margins. Randomized controlled trials to compare long-term survival are needed to further assess the efficacy of laparoscopic gastric resections for gastric cancer.

CONCLUSION

Minimally invasive approaches for the treatment of gastric cancer continue to evolve. Laparoscopic wedge resection, intragastric mucosal resection, and endoscopic mucosal resection have all been shown to be safe and effective for early gastric cancer without the risk for lymph node metastasis. With continued advances in endoscopic technology and skill, the use of laparoscopy for early gastric cancer may decline.

For early gastric cancer at risk for lymph node metastasis, laparoscopic gastrectomy with lymph node dissection is widely accepted and has potential advantages over open surgery, including earlier recovery and shorter postoperative stays.

For later stage cancers, laparoscopic partial and total gastrectomies with lymph node dissection are now being performed. Because of the steep learning curve and longer operating times associated with these procedures, alternative techniques such as hand-assisted laparoscopy and sentinel lymph node mapping are now being investigated. As technology and instrumentation evolve along with improved understanding of gastric cancer pathophysiology, minimally invasive procedures will have increasing roles in the treatment of gastric cancer.

SUGGESTED READING

Gotoda T, Yamamoto H, Soetikno RM. Endoscopic submucosal dissection of early gastric cancer. *J Gastroenterol* 2006;41:929–942.

Huscher CG, Mingoli A, Sgarzini G, et al. Laparoscopic versus open subtotal gastrectomy for distal gastric cancer: five-year results of a randomized prospective trial. *Ann Surg* 2005;241:232–237.

Kitano S, Shiraishi N. Minimally invasive surgery for gastric tumors. *Surg Clin North Am* 2005;85:151–164, xi.

Kitano S. Sjoraosjo N, Uyama I, et al. Japanese Laparoscopic Surgery Study Group. A multicenter study on oncologic outcome of laparoscopic gastrectomy for early cancer in Japan. *Ann Surg* 2007;245:68–72.

Noh SH, Hyung WJ, Cheong JH. Minimally invasive treatment for gastric cancer: approaches and selection process. *J Surg Oncol* 2005;90:188–193.

Oghami M, Otani Y, Furukawa T, et al. Curative laparoscopic surgery for early gastric cancer: eight years experience. *Nippon Geka Gakkai Zasshi* 2000;101:539–545.

Rosen MJ, Heniford BT. Endoluminal gastric surgery: the modern era of minimally invasive surgery. *Surg Clin North Am* 2005;85: 989–1007, vii.

Shiraishi N, Yasuda K, Kitano S. Laparoscopic gastrectomy with lymph node dissection for gastric cancer. *Gastric Cancer* 2006;9:167–176.

Uedo N, Iishi H, Tatsuta M, et al. Longterm outcomes after endoscopic mucosal resection for early gastric cancer. *Gastric Cancer* 2006; 9:88–92.

Ziqiang W, Feng Q, Zhimin C, et al. Comparison of laparoscopically assisted and open radical distal gastrectomy with extended lymphadenectomy for gastric cancer management. *Surg Endosc* 2006;20:1738–1743.

COMMENTARY

The Carolinas Medical Center authors have provided an update on the techniques and current status of laparoscopic resections for adenocarcinoma of the stomach. Although gastric cancer is relatively uncommon in the United States, the stomach is an organ that is eminently suitable to endoscopic and laparoscopic approaches. The endoscopic approaches to resecting mucosal tumors have been described elsewhere. The authors discuss staging and the locations of lymph nodes to be removed during a standard gastrectomy. They describe the technique for laparoscopic intragastric mucosal resection for tumors that are not candidates for endoscopic resection because of tumor size or location. These approaches require combined access techniques using a flexible endoscope as well as laparoscopic instruments passed into the lumen of the stomach.

Laparoscopic approaches to the stomach and gastric resection have been aided tremendously by the recent explosion in laparoscopic bariatric procedures. Surgeons who previously had minimal exposure to gastric surgery now feel comfortable approaching all parts of the stomach, using staplers for division and anastomosis, etc. Given the recent trials from Japan suggesting the oncologic equivalence of laparoscopic and open operations for gastric cancer, surgeons with experience in laparoscopic gastric operations should feel emboldened to perform laparoscopic gastrectomy for cancer. As long as they understand the lymph node basins and the techniques used to include the appropriate lymph nodes in the en bloc resection, patients with gastric adenocarcinoma will be well served. This chapter illustrates the techniques well and should allow a laparoscopic approach to many gastrectomies performed for malignancy.

NJS

C. Surgery for Morbid Obesity

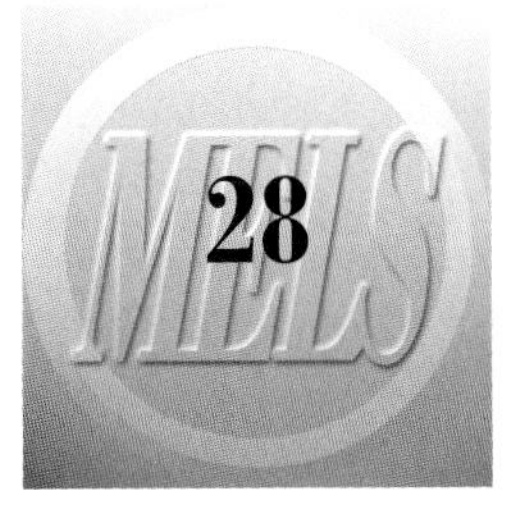

Restrictive Procedures for Morbid Obesity

TAGORE M. GRANDHI AND EMMA J. PATTERSON

INTRODUCTION

Obesity is a major health issue that is increasing in epidemic proportions and posing a difficult therapeutic challenge for clinicians in the United States, where it is currently the second leading cause of preventable death. According to the Centers for Disease Control, more than two-thirds of Americans are overweight and nearly one-third are obese. Furthermore, approximately 12 million Americans are considered morbidly obese, as defined by body mass index (BMI) greater than or equal to 40 kg/m^2. Obesity is associated with serious medical comorbidities (Table 28-1), and society pays a high cost for this condition in terms of health care dollars and obesity-related deaths. Conservative measures to achieve weight loss such as diet, exercise, and behavioral modifications have high failure rates in the setting of morbid obesity. A surgical approach may be required to prevent or treat the associated morbidities.

TABLE 28-1. WEIGHT-RELATED COMORBIDITIES

Diabetes type II
Hypertension
Dyslipidemia
Coronary artery disease
Congestive heart failure
Edema
Asthma
Sleep apnea
Obesity-hypoventilation syndrome
Arthritis
Osteoarthritis
Back pain
Degenerative joint disease
Nonalcoholic steatohepatitis (NASH)
Gastroesophageal reflux disease (GERD)
Gallstones
Menstrual irregularity/infertility
Polycystic ovary syndrome
Urinary stress incontinence
Depression
Venous thromboembolic disease
Cerebral vascular disease

Bariatric operations are either restrictive (limiting food intake), malabsorptive (limiting the amounts of nutrients absorbed), or a hybrid of the two. Laparoscopic adjustable gastric banding (LAGB), vertical banded gastroplasty (VBG), and sleeve gastrectomy (SG) are purely restrictive procedures. The jejunoileal bypass (JIB) and bilopancreatic diversion (BPD) with or without duodenal switch (BPD-DS) are malabsorptive procedures. The Roux en-Y gastric bypass (RYGB) is a hybrid procedure. The choice of operation is guided by multiple factors, including patient's age, the extent of his or her obesity, the presence of comorbid conditions, and the patient's and surgeon's preferences.

HISTORY

The word "bariatric" is derived from the Greek *baro,* meaning "weight," and the suffixes *iatr* ("treatment") and *ic* ("pertaining to"). Kremen et al. reported the first bariatric surgical procedure, the JIB, in 1954, bypassing a large segment of the nutrient-absorbing small bowel. In the late 1960 and early 1970s, JIB became popular. BPD, developed by Scopinaro in 1976, consists of a limited gastrectomy and long Roux-en-Y reconstruction with a short distal ileum common channel. In 1998 Hess developed a hybrid operation of a BPD with duodenal switch, which combines a greater curvature gastrectomy and a long Roux-en-Y duodenojejunostomy and theoretically allows reduction of the incidence of stomal ulcer and dumping syndrome.

In 1967 Mason and Ito developed the gastric bypass procedure. A partial gastrectomy with a loop gastroenterostomy was initially performed; later, gastric resection was replaced with gastric partition. Subsequent modifications include a small gastric pouch of 30 ml or less, transection of the stomach, narrow gastroenterostomy, and use of Roux-en-Y technique. Wittgrove et al. described laparoscopic Roux-en-Y gastric bypass (LRYGB) in 1994; today it is the most commonly performed bariatric surgical procedure in the U.S. In 1982 Mason developed the vertical banded gastroplasty by creating a 14-cm^3 vertical gastric pouch along the lesser curvature with a polypropylene mesh band around the lower end of the vertical pouch; a later modification was silastic band instead of mesh. In 1986, the first adjustable gastric band was created by Kuzmak, whose technique allowed for size adjustments to be done through an injection port placed subcutaneously. This lead to the introduction of LAGB in 1993, now the most frequently performed bariatric surgical procedure worldwide, outside the U.S.

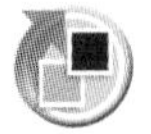

INDICATIONS

In 1991, the National Institute of Health Consensus Development Panel recommended criteria for patient selection for bariatric surgery. Patients whose BMI exceeds 40, or whose BMI is between 35 and 40 and have comorbid conditions of obesity such as cardiopulmonary problems, diabetes, or sleep apnea, may be considered for surgery if they have failed medical therapy. Patients should be selected carefully by a multidisciplinary team with medical, surgical, psychiatric, nutritional, and physical therapy expertise. In particular, patients need to have realistic weight loss expectations and to be motivated, well informed, and committed to long-term follow-up after surgery. The two most widely performed procedures today in the U.S. are RYGB and LAGB. Bilopancreatic diversion with or without duodenal switch, VBG, and sleeve gastrectomy are rarely performed.

PREOPERATIVE PLANNING

A multidisciplinary team sees patients preoperatively, over the 6- to 8-week period prior to surgery. During this time, all patients should attend an information session that educates patients about all aspects of surgery and provides an opportunity for patients to ask questions. Patients are evaluated by a multidisciplinary team that includes a nurse practitioner, psychologist, dietician, physical therapist, and surgeon. Due to co-morbidities, the patients often require extensive preoperative medical workup.

Investigations

Our routine laboratory tests for all patients include complete blood count (CBC), comprehensive metabolic panel (CMP), liver and thyroid function tests, hematinics (B-12, folate, iron levels), vitamin D levels, *H. pylori* antibody, and parathyroid assays. We do not routinely perform chest X-ray, esophageal manometry, or upper GI barium swallows, although some centers do. Patients with cardiac history are evaluated by a cardiologist, with necessary investigations including an echocardiogram (ECHO), myocardial perfusion scan, stress test, and coronary angiogram. Patients with anemia or significant reflux symptoms or those on long-term protein pump inhibitors (PPIs) will have esophago-gastro-duodenostomy (EGD) and, if necessary, a 24-hour pH test and esophageal manometry. All patients will have a sleep study; patients with moderate or severe sleep apnea will be recommended to have 2 to 3 weeks of nighttime continuous positive airway pressure (CPAP) or bi-level positive airway pressure (Bipap) therapy before surgery. Women beyond age 40 will be encouraged to have a mammogram, and all patients beyond 50 will be encouraged to have colonoscopy prior to surgery to screen for carcinomas.

SURGICAL TECHNIQUE

The various restrictive procedures are laparoscopic adjustable gastric band, sleeve gastrectomy, vertical banded gastroplasty, and laparoscopic Roux-en-Y gastric bypass. The gastric bypass is a hybrid procedure (restrictive and malabsorptive) and is described elsewhere in this textbook.

Vertical Banded Gastroplasty

The VBG involves creating a 14-cm^3 vertical gastric pouch along the lesser curvature with a polypropylene mesh band around the lower end of vertical gastric pouch, which acts as a stoma, preventing it from stretching. The use of a silastic band instead of mesh was later introduced. This procedure was largely replaced by the gastric bypass in the 1970s and 1980s and is now only performed in a few centers.

Sleeve Gastrectomy

This is a form of gastroplasty including subtotal gastric resection for creation of a long lesser curve based gastric conduit. This procedure evolved from two different procedures: it is part of the duodenal switch operation, but also closely mimics the Magenstrasse-Mill procedure popularized in the U.K. This can be a first-step procedure before gastric bypass or duodenal switch or a one-step restrictive procedure. The dissection begins on the greater curvature 2 to 3 cm from the duodenum. The gastroepiploic vessels and short gastric vessels must be coagulated and divided. The linear stapler-cutter device should be oriented so that the tip of the instrument should be oriented to the left of the visible endings of the lesser curvature vessels. A plastic tube (30 to 50F) should be inserted into the stomach. After five or six firings of the stapler, the greater curvature is detached completely from the stomach, which is removed in a retrieval bag. The dissection extends to the root at the left pillar of the hiatus. A methylene blue test is performed to test for staple-line leakage. The American Society of Metabolic and Bariatric Surgery recognizes that the performance of a sleeve gastrectomy may be an option for high-risk or super-super obese and that the concept of staged bariatric surgery may have value as a risk reduction strategy in high-risk patient populations.

Adjustable Gastric Banding

Patient Selection

With adjustable gastric banding using the LAP-BAND (Fig. 28-1), available from Allergen, Inc.; Irvine, CA, optimal patient selection enables the maximization of results most suited to the procedure and the avoidance of unsatisfactory outcomes for inappropriate candidates. A number of conditions are associated with a significantly lower percent excess weight loss (%EWL): increasing age and insulin resistance syndromes (hyperinsulinemia, type 2 diabetes, and polycystic ovary syndrome). There was also less weight loss if the SF-36 quality of life measure showed a poor physical activity score, high pain score, or poor general health score. In all of these conditions the effect was small and insufficient to preclude this approach to the treatment of obesity. The one positive predictor with greater weight loss is alcohol consumption of more than 10 standard drinks per week. The conditions that have no relation to weight loss after LAP-BAND placement are gender, presence of mental illness, comorbidities except those linked to insulin resistance, previous bariatric surgery, and sweet-eating behavior. Absolute contraindications to LAP-BAND include malignant hyperphagia (Prader-Willi syndrome). Relative contraindications include severe cardiovascular or pulmonary disease, severe portal hypertension, and an inability to comprehend and follow dietary changes.

Patient Positioning

The patients are admitted on the day of surgery. They are given preoperative intravenous antibiotics, usually a cephalosporin and subcutaneous chemoprophylaxis for thromboembolism, such as Lovenox. Thigh-high sequential compression devices are also applied prior to the procedure. The patient is placed supine in a reverse-Trendelenburg position with the legs together; no stirrups are used. Patients are secured to the table at the hips with wide tape and a Velcro strap; a foot-board or foot-stops are used. The surgeon stands on the patient's right side, with the monitors at the head of the bed and at either side (Fig. 28-2, page 252).

Trocar Placement

A 1.5-cm incision is made in the left subcostal region. Access into the abdomen is gained with a 12-mm direct-viewing trocar using a 0-degree laparoscope. The abdomen is insufflated to a pressure of 15 mmHg. The laparoscope is changed to 30-degree instrument, and the abdomen is explored to exclude any obvious bowel or vascular injury. The remaining trocars are placed under direct vision, as depicted in Figure 28-3, page 253. The ports include a 15-mm trocar in the right upper quadrant just to the right of the midline, 5-mm trocars in the right and left anterior axillary lines, and another 5-mm trocar placed in the subxiphoid region, which is removed and replaced with the Nathanson liver retractor (Cook Medical; Brisbane, Australia), which is used to elevate the left lobe of the liver off the gastroesophageal junction.

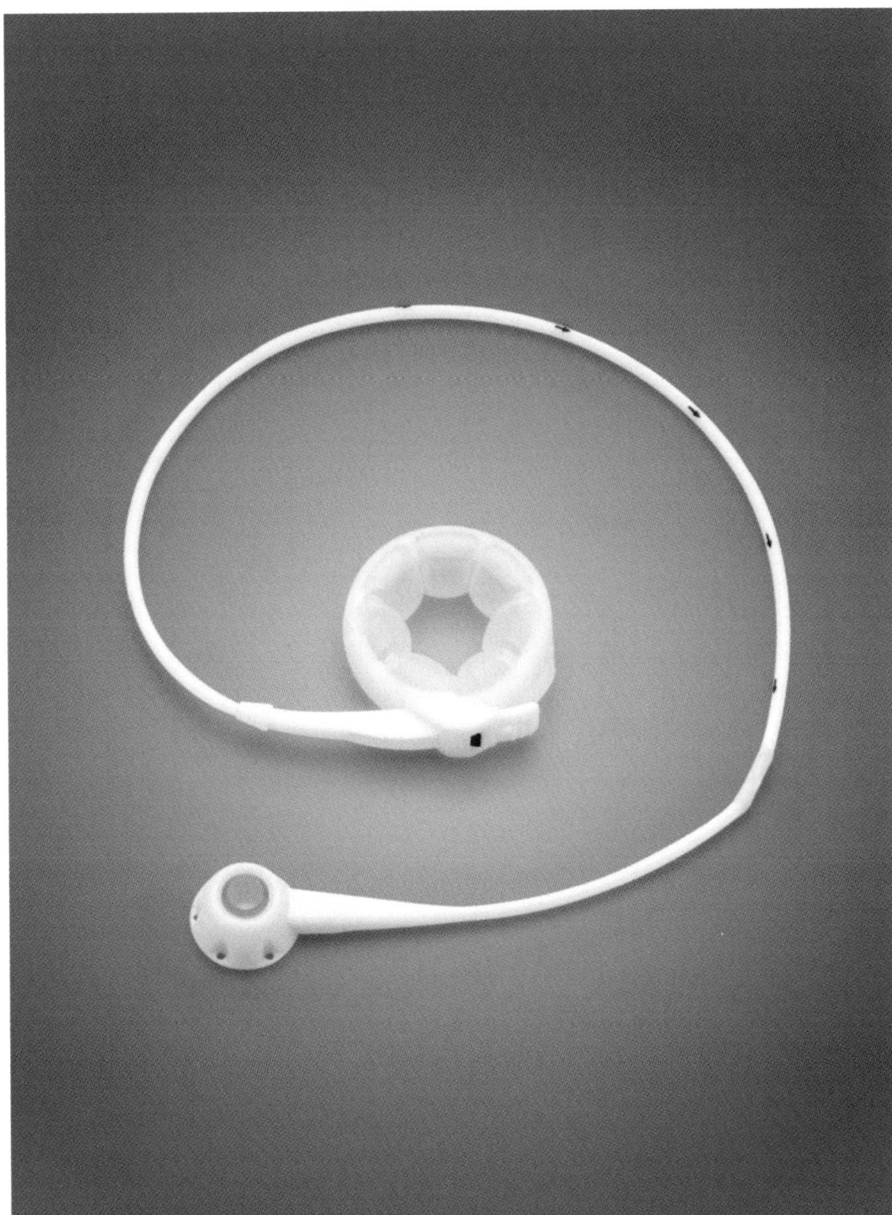

Fig. 28-1. A LAP-BAND device for gastric banding.

This is secured using a fixed device such as a Thompson retractor (Thompson Surgical Instruments, Inc; Traverse City, MI). The assisting surgeon and technician stand on the patient's left side.

Band Placement

The anesthesiologist decompresses the stomach with an orogastric suction tube. The assistant places a long atraumatic grasper through the left anterior axillary port, between the greater curvature of stomach and spleen. With this instrument, the omentum covering the angle of His is swept inferiorly, to place the fundus of the stomach on a stretch without directly holding it. With the camera in the left upper quadrant, this sweeping retraction of omentum is a key step in providing an unparalleled view of the angle of His.

The surgeon places another long, atraumatic grasper through the right lateral port and a diathermy spatula through the 15-mm port. The gastroesophageal fat pad is held with the grasper and pulled superiorly and to the right to expose the angle of His (Fig. 28-4, page 254). The peritoneum lateral to the angle of His is incised, and the fundus of stomach is freed from the left crus of the diaphragm using a combination of electrocautery and blunt dissection. This dissection is cephalad to the first short gastric vessel. The anterior fat pad is removed using coagulation cautery (Fig. 28-5, page 254).

Theoretically it is very important to dissect out the diaphragmatic crura, both anteriorly and posteriorly, and repair any defect around the gastroesophageal junction (Figs. 28-6 and 28-7, page 255). This helps prevent pouch dilatation, band slip, and heartburn. The hiatus hernia is repaired prior to band placement, as failure to do this results in a high chance of band slippage. The 30-degree laparoscope is rotated to view the lesser omentum, and the clear space in the gastrohepatic omentum is opened using electrocautery. The caudate lobe is seen through the clear space of gastrohepatic ligament. If an aberrant left hepatic artery is encountered, an attempt should be made to preserve it, but sometimes the dissection is otherwise impossible; in these cases the vessel should be double clipped on both sides and divided. The right crus is seen inferiomedial to the caudate lobe of the liver, curving to the right and disappearing in the retroperitoneal fat. It is very important to identify the inferior vena cava, which runs to the right of and parallel to the right crus. In the presence of large amounts of intraabdominal fat, the vena cava can be mistaken for the right crus. The peritoneum just medial to the base of the right crus is incised with electrocautery. This should be at the level of the start of the lesser curve of stomach.

An atraumatic grasper inserted through the right lateral port is gently passed through the incised peritoneum medial to the right crus in a flat trajectory behind the esophagus to emerge at the previously dissected area of angle of His, creating a retrogastric tunnel. Virtually no force should be used during this maneuver, and the grasper travels only a short distance: 3 to 4 cm at most. Any resistance met should be dealt with caution; the grasper should be withdrawn and the step repeated. The inferolateral placement of the 5-mm port (in the right anterior axillary line) gives a flat approach of the instrument behind the cardia of the stomach free of any torque or force. It is important to stay directly on the top of right and left crura to prevent injury to the posterior gastric wall or vagus nerve. The adjustable gastric band is primed on the back table with normal saline and inserted into the abdomen through the 15-mm port. The end of the tubing of the band is brought up to the retrogastric grasper and pulled through, encircling the stomach (Fig. 28-8, page 256). Due to the minimal dissection, it is necessary to release a few peritoneal attachments medial to the right crus in order to allow the shoulder of the band to be pulled completely around the stomach. The tubing is passed into the

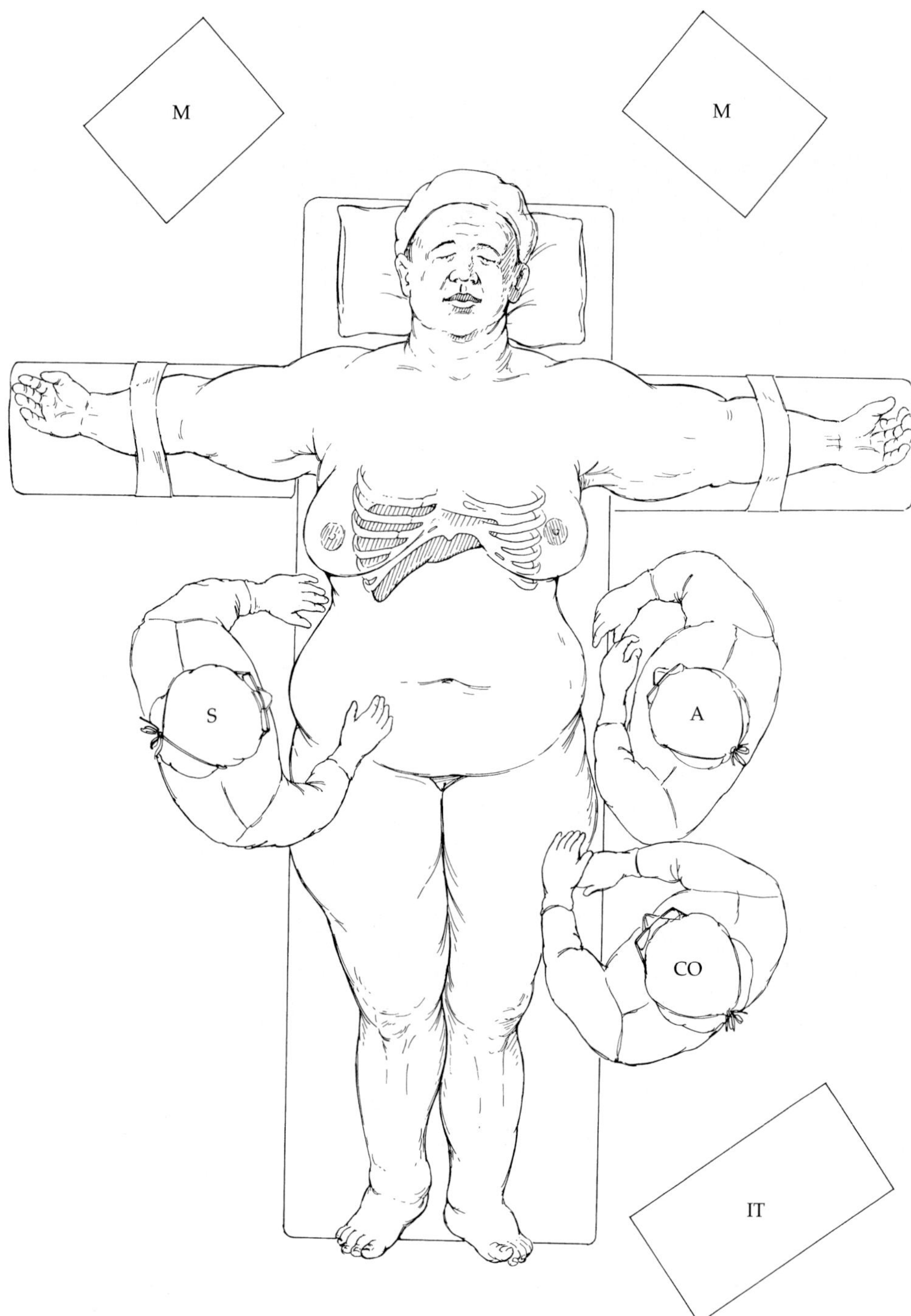

Fig. 28-2. Patient positioning and setup for laparoscopic adjustable gastric banding (LAGB). A, assistant; CO, camera operator; IT, instrument table; M, monitor; S, surgeon.

opening in the buckle and pulled through (Fig. 28-9, page 256). Closure of the band is performed by simultaneous left and right traction, with the grasper in the left hand holding the buckle and the right one grasping the tubing near the buckle (Fig. 28-10, page 257).

The laparoscope is transferred into the 15-mm port in order to use the ports on either side for suturing. An anterior fundoplication is performed, with two to three interrupted or running gastrogastric sutures using a permanent suture such as 2-0 Ethibond (Ethicon Inc; Somerville, NJ) from the fundus to the gastric pouch above the band. The first suture should approximate the highest part of the greater curvature to the "bare area" of the stomach created by excision of the fat pad (Fig. 28-11, page 257). A 5-mm instrument should pass freely between the band and stomach. If it does not, the band is likely to be constricting, and fatty tissue between the band and stomach should be removed. The function of the gastrogastric sutures is to prevent herniation of the stomach upward through the band. It is important to avoid tension and also to avoid bringing the stomach over the buckle of the band, to prevent erosion. We place a 2-0 Ethibond

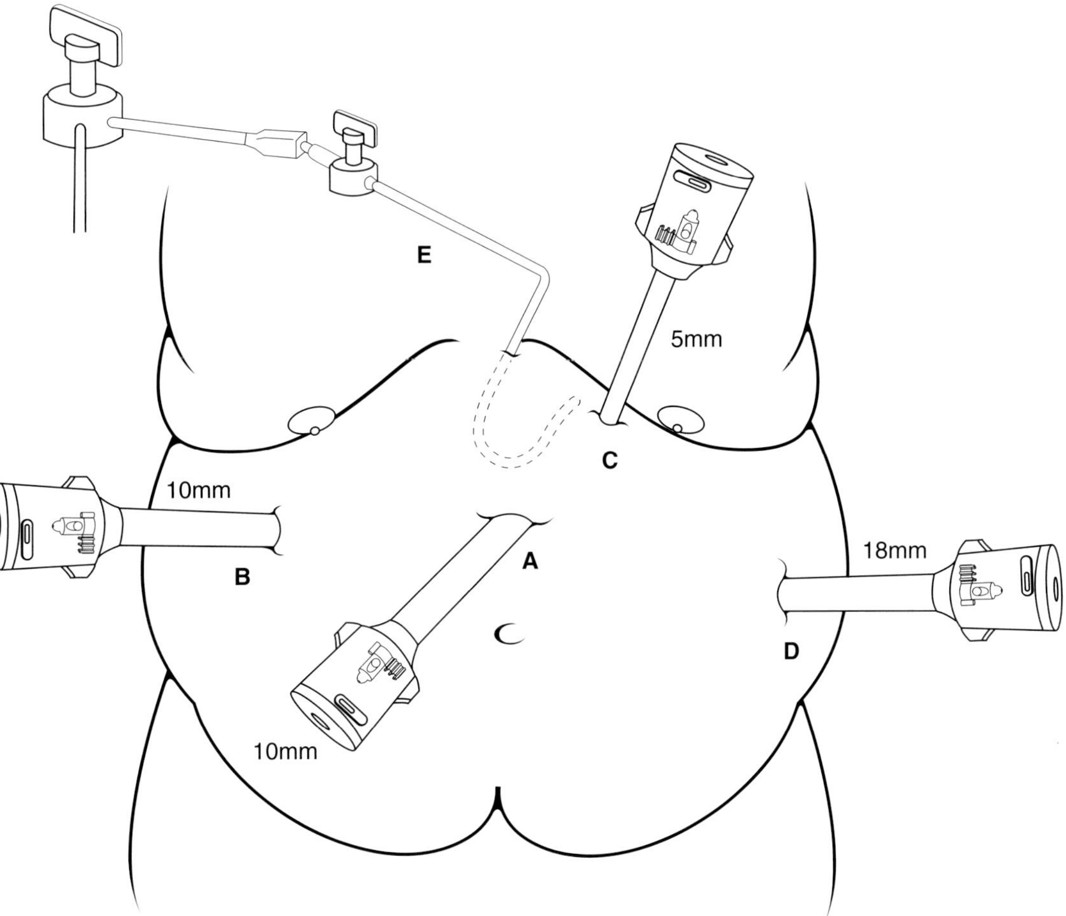

Fig. 28-3. Trocar positioning. **Port A:** 12-mm trocar for abdominal access and camera placement. **Port B:** 15-mm trocar in right upper quadrant for band insertion and surgeon's right hand. **Port C:** Nathanson liver retractor. **Port D:** 5-mm trocar in right anterior axillary line below falciform ligament to avoid instrument trauma to liver edge; used for surgeon's left hand. **Port E:** 5-mm trocar in left anterior axillary line and assistant's port.

suture to imbricate the greater curvature to the lesser curvature of the stomach below the band (Fig. 28-12, page 258), also known as a Patterson stitch. We feel this reduces the chance of band slippage. Once suturing is performed, the liver retractor is removed and the camera is transferred to left upper quadrant port. The tubing of the band and the excised fat pad are grasped and brought out through the 15-mm trocar site. With this, the laparoscopic part of the procedure is complete: the abdomen is desufflated and the trocars removed.

Reservoir Port Placement

The 15-mm port site incision in the right upper quadrant is extended by 2 cm laterally and the dissection carried down to the anterior rectus sheath, which is incised exposing the muscle. Four 1-0 Ethibond sutures are placed in four quadrants of the anterior rectus fascia (Fig. 28-13, page 258). Narrow Deavor retractors help in retracting the fat and exposing the fascia. The port is attached to the tubing and the redundant tubing is placed back into the abdomen. The port is then secured to the anterior rectus fascia by passing the Ethibond sutures through the four holes of the access port and then tying them (Fig. 28-14, page 259). The fascia of Scarpa is reapproximated using 3-0 vicryl sutures. All skin incisions are reapproximated using 4-0 monocryl in a subcuticular fashion. The port should be placed at a site that is easily accessible for adjustment and that will not create pressure on the band by clothing.

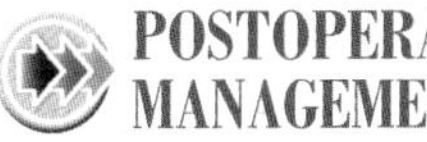

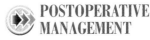

POSTOPERATIVE MANAGEMENT

An upper gastrointestinal radiograph using gastrografin contrast is performed to exclude gastric perforation, malposition, and obstruction (Fig. 28-15, page 259). The patient is advised to stay on a liquid diet for 2 weeks, followed by a pureed diet for 2 weeks, before advancing to normal food. This is important to allow proper healing and scarring of the band in the appropriate position without undue stress caused by vomiting solid food. In most cases, the procedure can be performed on an outpatient basis. Postoperative follow-up should be at 1 month by the dietician and the surgeon in order to evaluate the need for band adjustment.

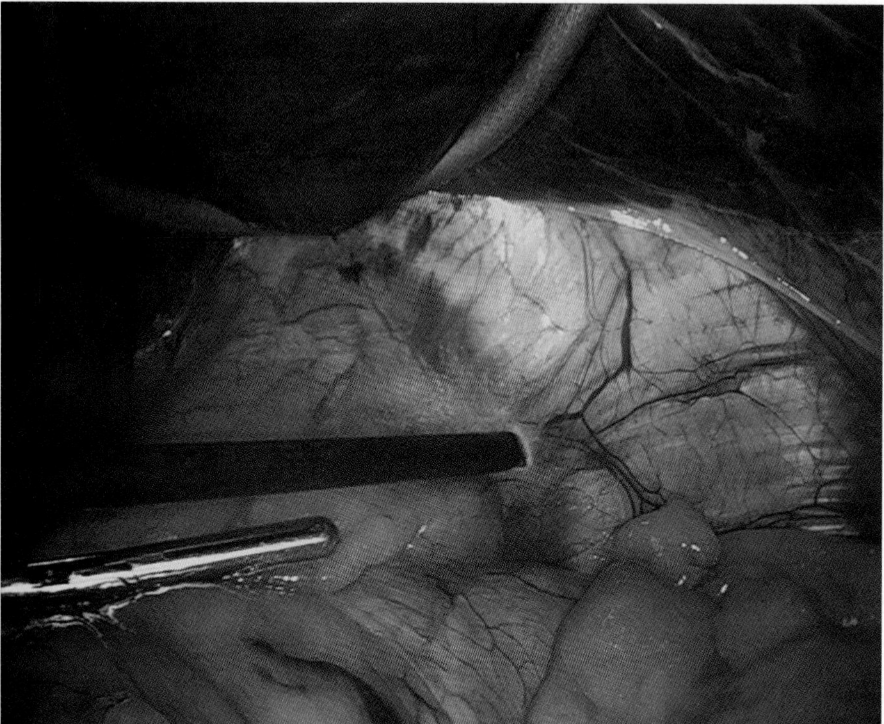

Fig. 28-4. A dissection of the peritoneum along the angle of His releases the gastric fundus, creating an exit site from the retrogastric dissection.

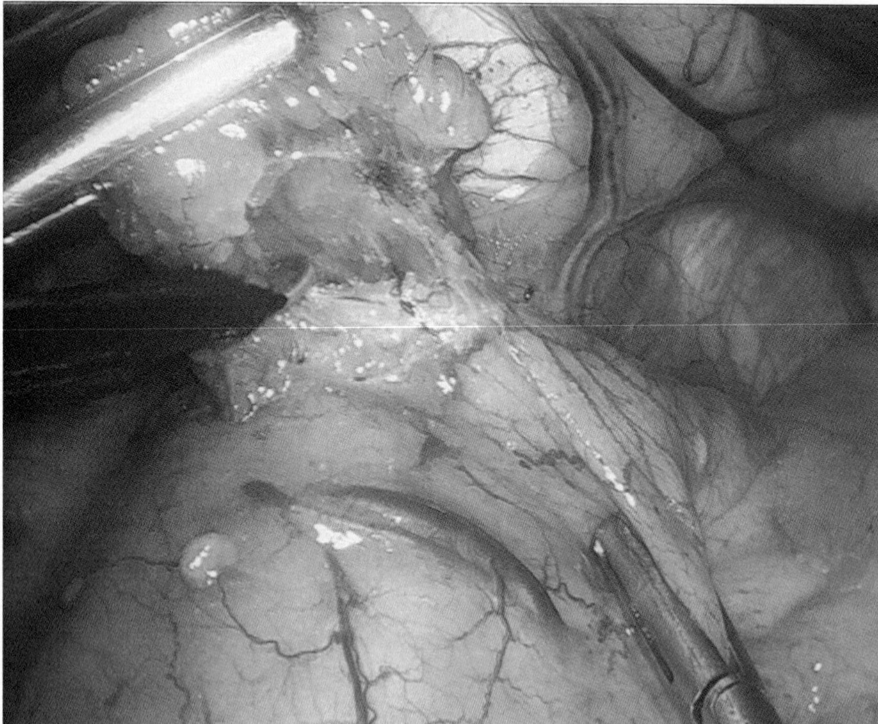

Fig. 28-5. Excision of the anterior fat fad.

Band Adjustments

The need for adjustment depends on several factors: persistent hunger, lack of satiety, lack of adequate weight loss, and lack of restriction. Adjustments can be performed by blind percutaneous technique in the office or under fluoroscopic guidance. A 20-22 gauge non-coring Huber needle is used to access the port. It is important to use non-coring needle to prevent port damage and leakage from the system. Saline should be easily injected and withdrawn to confirm the appropriate position within the port.

Blind percutaneous adjustments offer the advantage of being quick, easy, and inexpensive. Patients usually require five to six adjustments before achieving an adequate-sized stoma. Patients are advised to drink water before leaving office to make sure the band is not too tight. Following adjustment, patients are instructed to remain on a liquid diet for 2 days and a soft diet for 2 days and to slowly advance to regular food. While fluoroscopic adjustments, which involve X-ray exposure for the patient, are more time-consuming and expensive, the advantages may be fewer adjustments in the first year and the ability to monitor for complications such as band slippage or pouch or esophageal dilatation.

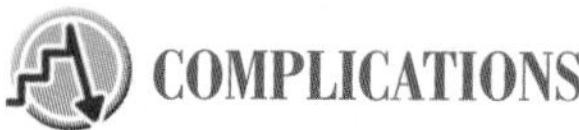

COMPLICATIONS

Laparoscopic adjustable gastric banding is a relatively safe operation. Nonetheless it is associated with complications (Table 28-2),

TABLE 28-2. COMPLICATIONS OF THE LAPAROSCOPIC ADJUSTABLE GASTRIC BAND (LAGB)

General complications
Deep venous thrombosis
Pulmonary embolism
Pneumonia
Myocardial infarction
Early complications
Gastric perforation
Wound infection
Access port infection
Delayed emptying of the pouch
Acute stomal obstruction
Misplacement of band
Pouch esophageal reflux
Late complications
Band slippage or gastric prolapse
Gastric necrosis
Pouch dilatation
Band erosion
Esophageal dilatation
Chronic nausea and vomiting
Gastroesophageal reflux (GERD)
Access port or tubing leakage
Migration or inversion of port
Tubing disconnection/kinkage

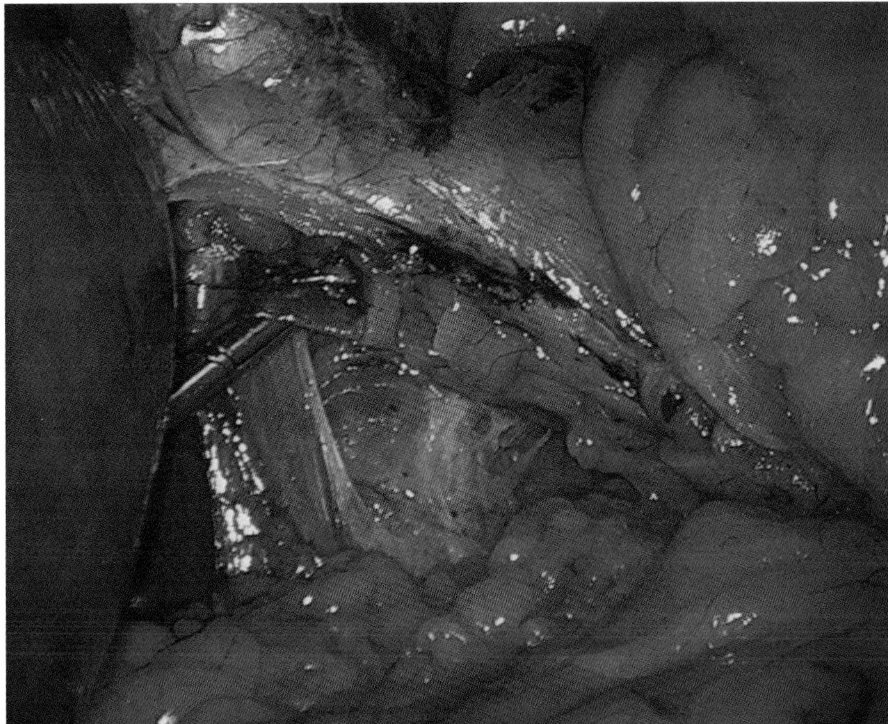

Fig. 28-6. Posterior dissection showing a crural defect.

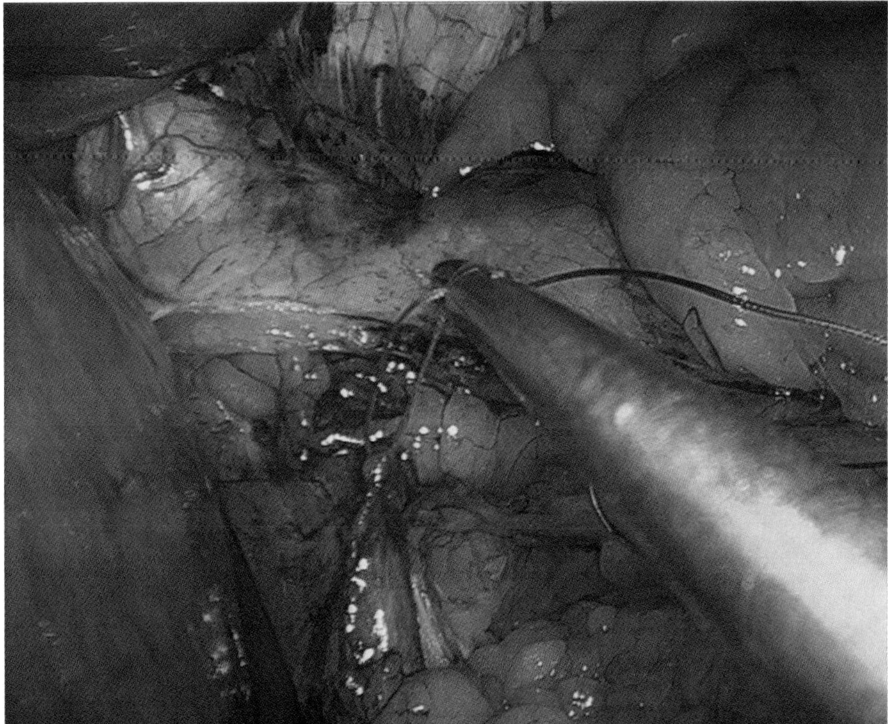

Fig. 28-7. Suture closure of a crural defect.

which can be divided into two groups: early and late. Early complications include gastric perforation, wound infection, access port infection, delayed emptying of the proximal pouch and short-term obstruction, and general complications of any major operation, including deep vein thrombosis, pulmonary embolism, pneumonia, cardiac arrhythmia, and myocardial infarction. Late complications are more common with bands and include band slippage or gastric prolapse, pouch dilatation, band erosion, esophageal dilatation, chronic nausea and vomiting, gastroesophageal reflux, and access port or tubing leakage.

Gastric Perforation

Gastric perforation during LAP-BAND placement is rare, ocurring in less than 0.5% of patients. This complication has been associated with the perigastric technique in which dissection along the stomach was performed (historically) and is very rare with the pars flaccida dissection technique, in which dissection is performed along the left crus of the diaphragm. On rare occasions this complication is caused by nasogastric tube placement. Postoperative upper gastrointestinal series (UGI) X-rays can be helpful in detecting unrecognized perforation and should be indicated early in a surgeon's experience with banding or if there are any technical difficulties with the dissection. Immediate repair of gastric perforation and band explantation is indicated. *Acute stomal obstruction* may occur in 1.4% of patients and resolves spontaneously with conservative treatment. This complication has decreased significantly with the development of larger-circumference and lower-pressure bands. *Misplacement* of the band is normally caused by the surgeon's lack of experience. The band may be placed in the perigastric fat or in the lower part of the stomach, the latter causing severe gastric outlet obstruction.

Gastric Pouch Dilatation

Gastric pouch dilatation is the most common late complication of LAGB, occurring in up to 5% to 25% of cases. This complication can be detected by radiology before clinical symptoms appear; therefore many surgeons perform routine annual screening upper GI X-rays of these patients. Pouch dilatations are of three types: acute concentric pouch dilatation, chronic concentric pouch dilatation, and eccentric pouch dilatation. *Acute concentric pouch dilatation* is due to an overly tight stoma and as a result of overinflation of the gastric band or edema following food or pill obstruction and vomiting. Concentric pouch dilatation presents as acute dysphagia, vomiting, or heartburn. Prompt decompression is the best treatment in the early stages. *Chronic concentric dilatation* may be due to chronic overeating, band overinflation, or a missed hiatal hernia. If left untreated, chronic concentric dilatation may progress to eccentric pouch dilatation or band slip. The first line of therapy

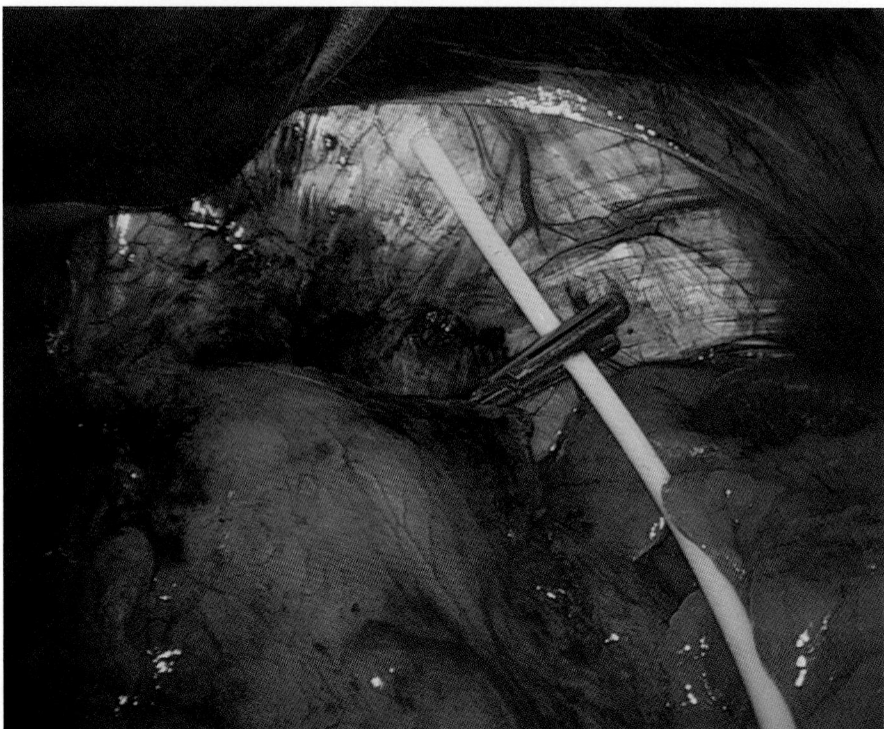

Fig. 28-8. The retrogastric tunnel is created anterior to the crura. Dissection is started along the right crus. The end of the tubing of the band is brought up to the retrogastric grasper and pulled through, encircling the stomach.

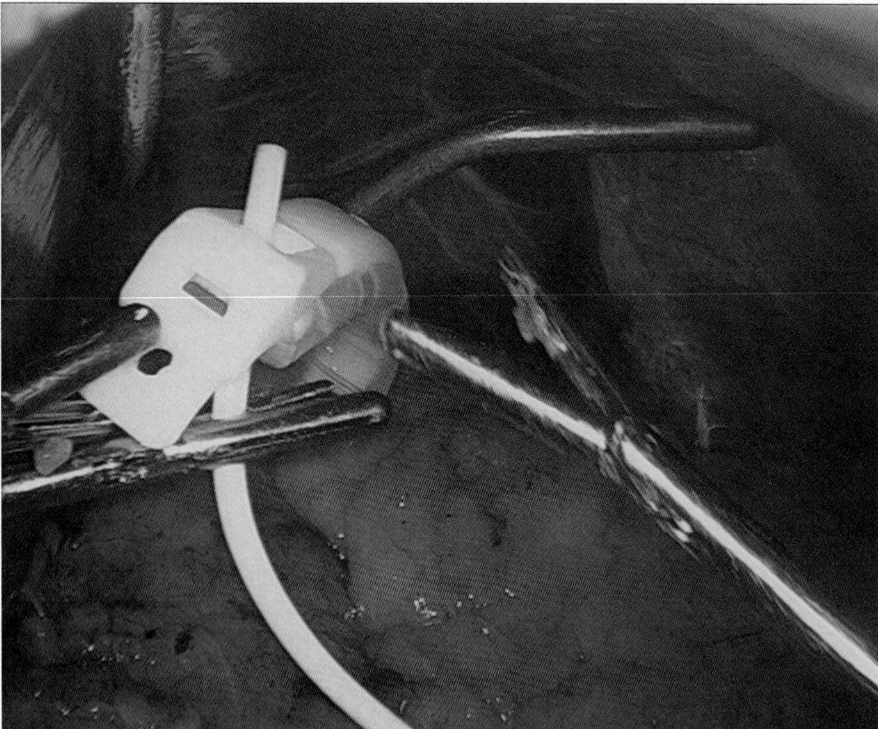

Fig. 28-9. The tubing is passed through the opening in the buckle.

includes removing some fluid and nutritional counseling. However, if the patient cannot experience restriction without gastrointestinal reflux disease (GERD), then a surgical revision is required, replacing the band to higher location and repairing of the hiatal hernia if one exists. *Eccentric pouch dilatation* is due to slippage of the band. With the pars flaccida technique, almost all slips are anterior, as the lesser sac should not be entered. Posterior slips were common with the historical perigastric technique.

Gastric Prolapse

Gastric prolapse, previously known as slippage, comprises herniation of the stomach up through the band in the cephalad direction, resulting in an enlarged gastric pouch and a partial or complete gastric occlusion. Patients may be asymptomatic in 20% of cases or present with nausea, vomiting, an inability to eat or drink, and reflux. Abdominal pain is a rare presentation of gastric prolapse and may represent gastric ischemia, a surgical emergency. Slippage may also present with weight gain due to increased capacity of food in the gastric pouch. Band slippage can manifest immediately during the early postoperative phase or as a late complication a few months later. Gastric prolapse can occur anteriorly or posteriorly. This complication occurs most commonly with the perigastric technique. With the change in technique to the pars flaccida approach, the incidence of prolapse has reduced markedly from 25% to 4%. *Posterior prolapse* is characterized by the posterior part of the fundus moving up through the band, resulting in the creation of a large posterior gastric pouch. The band is lower and anterior and its orientation is changed clockwise. *Anterior prolapse* occurs when the anterior part of the stomach prolapses through the band to create a large anterior gastric pouch. The band changes its position to a counterclockwise position and becomes more horizontally oriented. Overeating with overfilling of the gastric pouch, overinflation of the gastric band at the time of adjustments, and excessive vomiting are risk factors for band slippage. Posterior or anterior pouch dilatation leads to excessive stomach tissue inside the ring and obstruction between the upper stomach and lower stomach. The incidence of gastric prolapse has decreased due to refinements in surgical technique, such as reduction in the size of the gastric pouch to less than 15 ml (virtual pouch), placement of gastrogastric sutures, and a high positioning of the posterior aspect of the band, in close proximity to the gastroesophageal junction.

Initial management should include a UGI X-ray to confirm the diagnosis, complete deflation of the band system, and intravenous hydration. A flat plate X-ray of the abdomen is a useful screening test for slippage, as it will show the downward tilt of the band toward the left lower quadrant

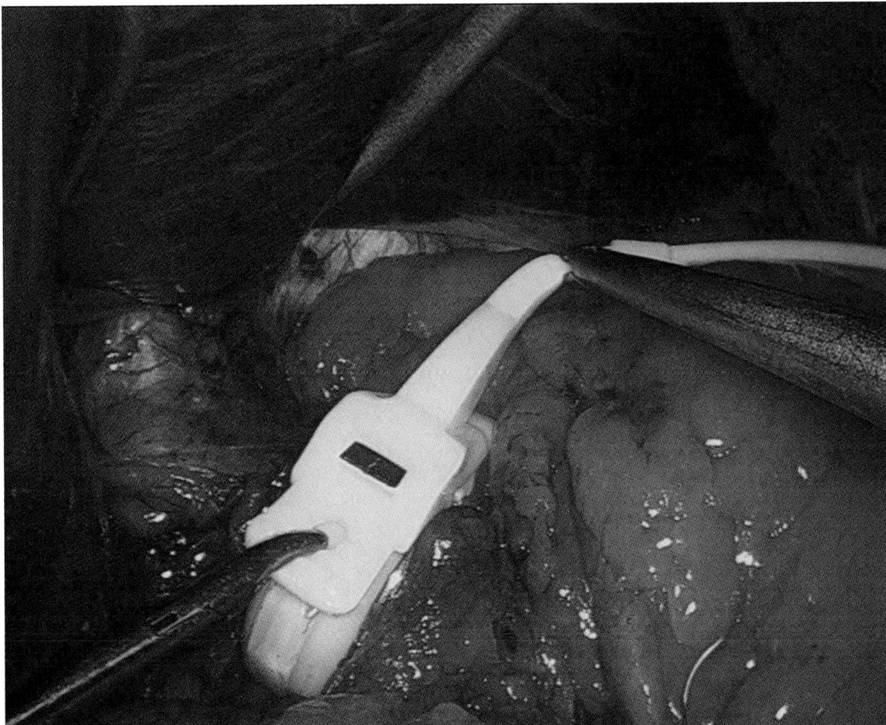

Fig. 28-10. Laparoscopic adjustable band closure.

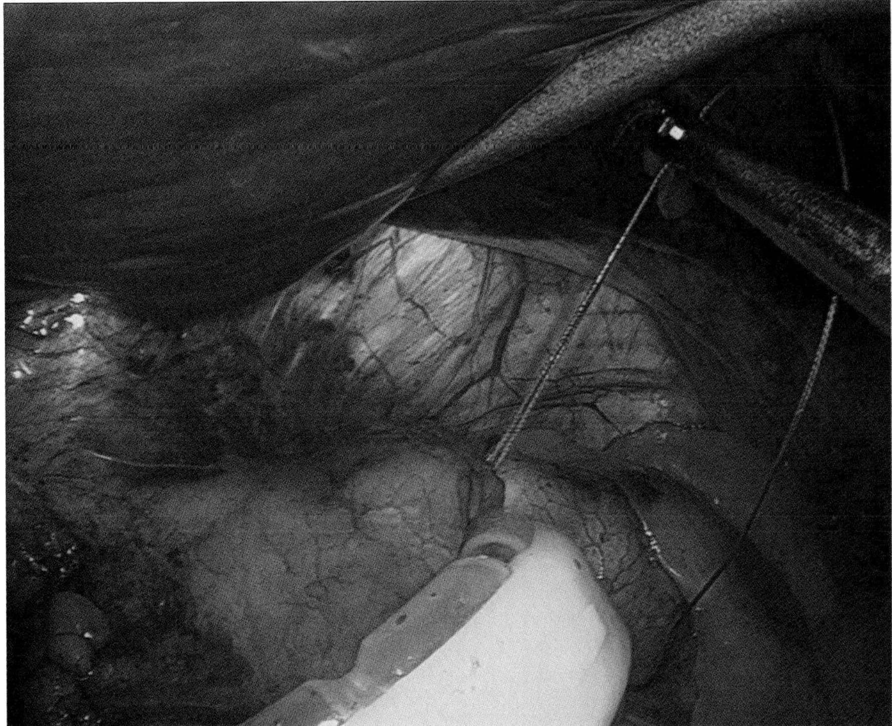

Fig. 28-11. Gastrogastric suture placement. The first suture should be high up on the greater curvature near the spleen.

instead of its proper position, pointing toward the left shoulder (Fig. 28-16, page 260). True prolapse, in contrast to gastric pouch dilatation, does not respond to conservative measures. The options of treatment are (1) repositioning of the band, (2) removal and replacement of the band, and (3) removal of the band without replacement.

Band Erosion

Band erosion is a situation in which a part of the band has eroded through the full-thickness gastric wall and migrated into the lumen. Band erosion is a rare and usually late complication, occurring in 1% to 3% of cases. The clinical presentation varies and involves either regain of weight or late infection at the access port site. Generally, the band is totally expelled into the gastric lumen. The band is transported by peristalsis in an aboral direction, but the progression is halted by the anchoring tube connected to the access port. Contact with hydrochloric acid turns the silicone brown. This rare complication may be related to ischemia due to a band that is too tight, a band that is infected from some other intraabdominal process (such as perforated appendicitis), intraoperative damage to the outer gastric wall (such as wrapping the stomach over the buckle of the band), and, some suggest, the use of nonsteroidal anti-inflammatory medicines that may increase the risk of erosion. Erosion has either an acute or chronic presentation. In band erosion, the band abrades constantly and slowly against the lumen and is eventually engulfed by the stomach. Many patients are asymptomatic and present only with a nonfunctioning band and loss of restriction to food. In many cases the first indication of possible erosion is a late infection at the access port site. The connecting tube provides drainage of gastric content to the port site, which causes the infection. Erosion should be ruled out at the first sign of late port site infection. Injuries to the gastric wall should be avoided by meticulous, gentle, and careful operative dissection. Another consideration during surgery is placing all the gastric-to-gastric sutures to left side of rather than over the locking mechanism (buckle). Placing them over the locking mechanism causes pressure necrosis to the fundus that covers it, and the band can erode into the wrap. In these situations, the patient may still have good weight loss, and erosion may only be detected by routine endoscopy. Band erosion is diagnosed by the intraluminal position of the band with contrast outlining both the inside and outside of the band, appearing as a intraluminal filling defect. Computed tomography (CT) may show extraluminal gas, peritoneal fluid, or abscess along the gastric wall or near the access port. At endoscopy there are three stages of band migration. In stage 1 a small part of the band is visible through a hole in the

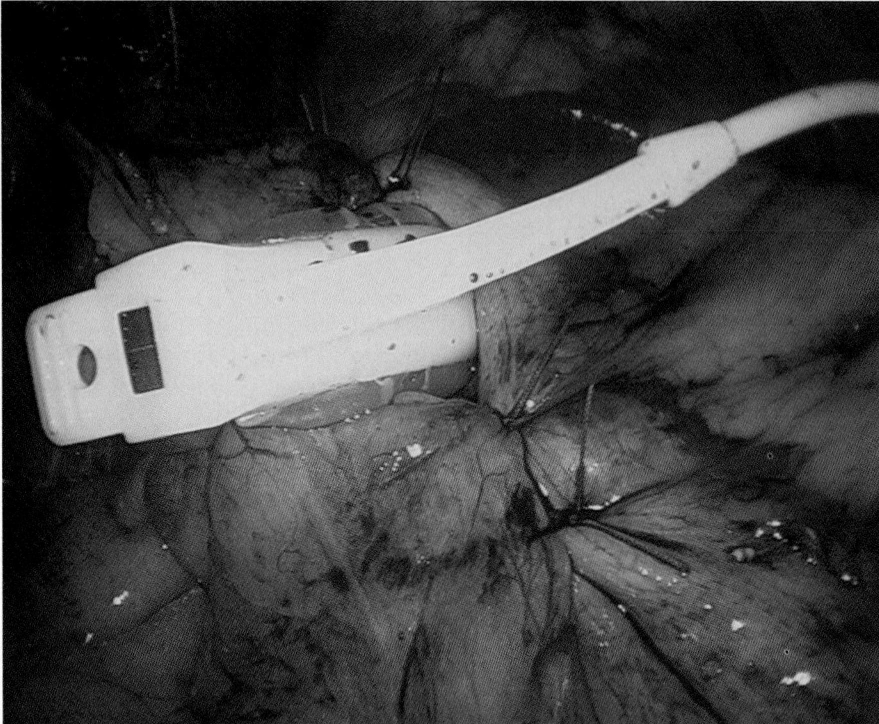

Fig. 28-12. Final band position showing the crural repair anteriorly, the gastrogastric suture, and the Patterson stitches (inferior to the band).

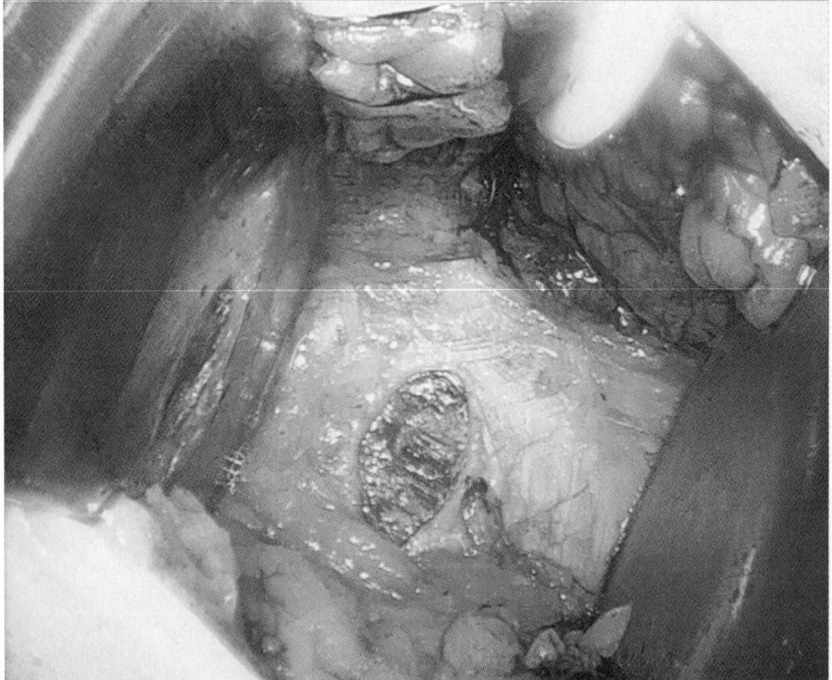

Fig. 28-13. Dissection showing the anterior rectus sheath, which is incised, exposing the rectus muscle.

mucosa; in stage 2 there is partial migration, with more than half of the band in the gastric lumen; in stage 3 there is complete migration of the band. Treatment involves removal of the band, repair of stomach wall, and later replacement of the band or conversion to a different procedure. Some advocate removal of the band with an endoscope if there has been partial or total migration.

GERD

The presence of a hiatal hernia in the morbidly obese patient dictates simultaneous crural repair prior to band placement. The diaphragmatic hiatus should be dissected anteriorly and posteriorly. All hiatal defects should be aggressively sought out and approximated with permanent sutures. Reflux occurring postoperatively is due to four major reasons:

1. Gastric prolapse
2. Gastric pouch dilatation due to band overinflation or edema
3. Esophageal dysmotility
4. The presence of an unrecognized hiatal hernia

Symptoms are treated with antacids and PPIs. Definitive treatment depends upon the diagnosis. A UGI X-ray will show the rate of esophageal emptying, band position, stoma size, and gastric pouch size. The most common cause of GERD after band placement is overinflation of band, which is treated with the simple removal of a small amount of fluid. Gastric prolapse and esophageal dysmotility are treated surgically.

Complications with Connecting Tubing and Access Port

Complications may include infection related to indwelling foreign bodies, leakage of saline from any part of the system with resultant band deflation, and migration or inversion of the port preventing band adjustments. These complications most often occur late and usually require surgical repair. Leakage of saline may occur at the level of the band, the connector tube, or at the access port. Leakage is suspected when filling and insufficient deflating volumes of the banding system combined with loss of eating restriction are observed. While nuclear medicines studies may be helpful in diagnosing a leak in the system, another reasonable option is just to replace the port, as this is where the leak occurs in most of the cases. The site of leak can be localized with 99m TC albumin, which shows a decrease in the count in the defective part with accumulation of nuclear tracer adjacent to it. Tubing disconnection and fluid leakage can be fixed by exploratory laparoscopy, retrieval of tubing, mobilization of the access port, and reconnection of the tubing with

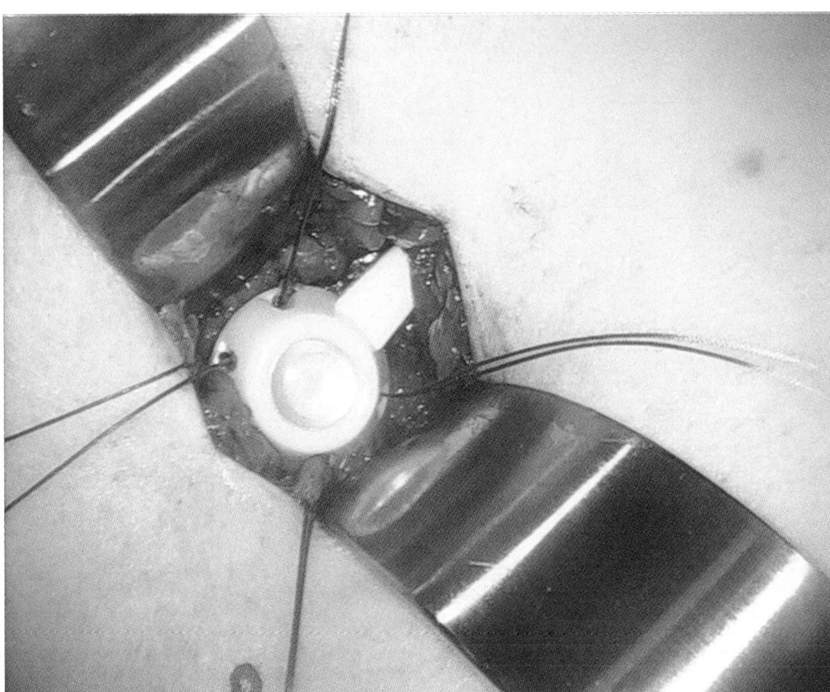

Fig. 28-14. Final port position.

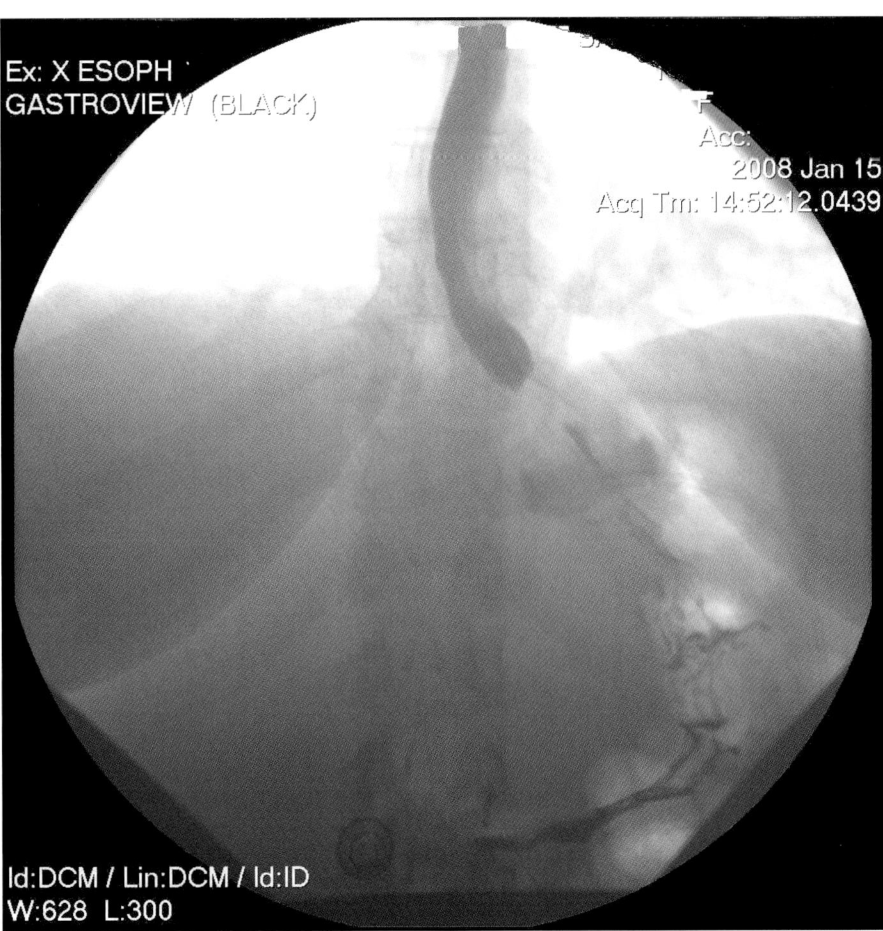

Fig. 28-15. A gastrografin swallow with an easy flow of contrast through the band and an absence of extravasation.

a new access port. If fluid leakage is suspected to be due to a chronic loss of restriction, the band and port should be completely replaced. Port migration can be managed with local wound exploration and port fixation. The injectable port should be sutured to the anterior rectus sheath to prevent port migration. If sutures fail, the port may migrate, become inverted, or rotate.

In refractory cases of port site infection, the port may need to be removed. Strict asepsis while accessing the port is therefore necessary. Other reported problems related to the connecting tubing include intraabdominal abscess, disconnection of tubing with migration into the small bowel, erosion of tubing into bowel as a consequence of wound infection with enterocutaneous fistula, and intracolonic penetration of the tubing.

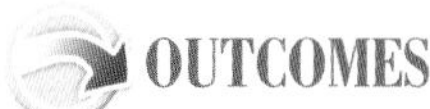

OUTCOMES

Inflatable bands have been placed in Europe and Australia since the first LAP-BAND was placed by Mitiku Belachew in Huy, Belgium in 1993. The LAP-BAND received FDA approval and was introduced in the U.S. in 2001. Weight loss after LAGB is gradual and steady for up to 3 years, after which a steady plateau of 51% to 56% EWL is maintained out to 5 years. Average weight losses at years 1, 2, 3, 5, and 6 are 44.7%, 54.9%, 57.5%, 53%, and 57% respectively. O'Brien and Dixon have reported a fall in BMI from 46 to 30 kg/m^2 and 54% EWL at 6 years. Weiner et al. have 8-year data on 984 patients showing 57% EWL. Fielding and Duncambe reported 2,110 bands, with an average 5% EWL at 6 years. A combined series from Europe of 5,827 patients who had an average BMI of 46 showed a decrease to an average of 31 at 5 years. Steffen et al. prospectively followed 824 patients after LAGB for 5 years and found that 83% achieved and maintained greater than 50% EWL.

Changes in Comorbidities

The most important outcomes from LAGB have been marked improvements in health and quality of life (QOL). Weight loss causes resolution or remission of diabetes in two-thirds of patients and improved blood glucose control for the remainder. These changes are related to the dual effects of improvement in insulin sensitivity and pancreatic beta cell function. Hypertension is strongly driven by obesity; there is evidence

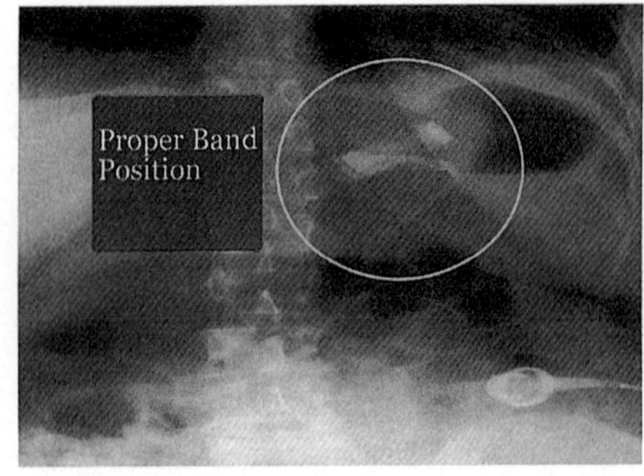

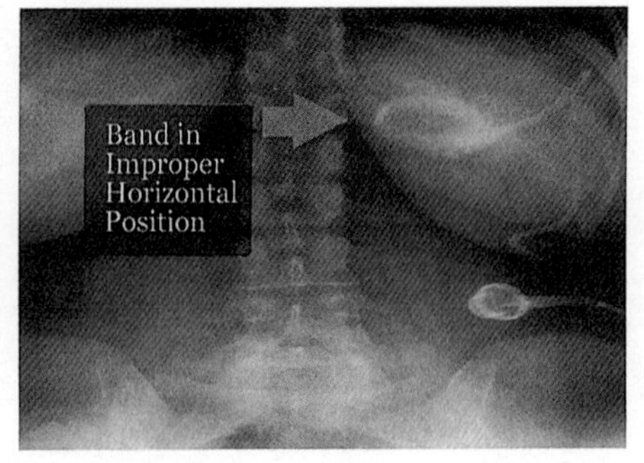

Fig. 28-16. Abdominal film with **(A)** proper band placement and **(B)** improper horizontal position secondary to band slippage.

of a reduction in both systolic and diastolic blood pressure following band placement. LAGB causes favorable changes in the levels of fasting triglycerides, HDL-C, and the total cholesterol:HDL-C ratio. Major improvement in asthma following LAGB is attributed to improved respiratory mechanics and possibly a reduction in gastroesophageal reflux. Gastric banding is also an effective treatment for gastroesophageal reflux. However, low band placement or failure to recognize and repair a hiatus hernia at the time of placement may exacerbate or induce gastroesophageal reflux, and prolapse and overtightening of the band may cause reflux symptoms. Major improvements in sleep quality and a reduction of excessive daytime sleepiness, snoring, nocturnal choking, and observed obstructive sleep apnea have been reported with weight loss following band surgery. Central obesity is associated with ovulatory dysfunction and infertility. Weight loss following LAGB reduces active testosterone and usually restores normal ovulation and fertility. Gestational diabetes and hypertension are also improved. LAGB also provides a dramatic and sustained improvement in QOL, self-evaluation of appearance, and depression.

CONCLUSION

Since its introduction in 1993, laparoscopic adjustable gastric banding has been the subject of many studies and evolution. The continuous progress in surgical technique and the increasing experience of surgeons have decreased the rates of many complications. LAGB is a safe and effective means of weight loss in the morbidly obese patient. A successful procedure requires a team approach consisting of the surgeon, dietician, physical therapist, and psychologist. Band adjustment strategies are critical to weight loss success, as is patient compliance with dietary restrictions and physical activity. The real appeal of LAGB is mainly in its safety profile for the patient and the ease of performance from a technical standpoint, making it an achievable laparoscopic treatment option even for high-risk patients. Resolution of obesity-related comorbidities parallels weight loss after LAGB. There are a number of published series with patients with 5 or more years of follow-up. An excess weight loss (EWL) of 50% to 60% in LAGB patients is comparable to gastric bypass. The lower mortality and morbidity of the procedure, the ease of placement, adjustability, and reversibility of the band, and the successful weight loss that results will likely continue to increase popularity and placement of the LAGB.

SUGGESTED READING

Carucci LR, Turnar MA, Szucs RA. Adjustable laparoscopic gastric banding for morbid obesity: Imaging assessment and complications. *Radiol Clin N Am* 2007;45:261–274.

Dixon JB, O'Brien PE. Selecting the optimal patient for LAP-BAND placement. *Am J Surg* 2002;184:17s–20s.

Dixon JB, O'Brien PE. Changes in comorbidities and improvements in quality of life after LAP-BAND placement. *Am J Surg* 2002;184: 51s–54s.

Fielding GA, Allen JW. A step-by-step guide to placement of the LAP-BAND adjustable gastric banding system. *Am J Surg* 2002;184: 26s–30s.

Fielding GA, Ren CJ. Laparoscopic adjustable gastric band. *Surg Clin N Am* 2005;85: 129–140.

Mehanna MJ, Birjawi G, Moukaddam HA, et al. Complications of adjustable gastric banding, a radiological pictorial review. *AJR* 2006;186: 522–534.

O'Brien PE, Dixon JB. Laparoscopic adjustable gastric banding in the treatment of morbid obesity. *Arch Surg* 2003;138:376–382.

Piorkowski J, Ellner S, Mavanur A, et al. Preventing port site inversion in laparoscopic adjustable gastric banding. *Surg Obes Relat Dis* 2007;3(2):159–162.

Provost DA. Laparoscopic adjustable gastric banding: an attractive option. *Surg Clin N Am* 2005;85:789–805.

Ren CJ, Fielding GA. Laparoscopic adjustable gastric banding *Current Surgery* 2003;60:30–33.

Roy-Choudhury S, Nelson W, El Cast J, et al. Technical aspects and complications of laparoscopic banding for morbid obesity—a radiologic perspective *Clin Radiol* 2004;59(3): 224–236.

Salameh JR. Baritric surgery: Past and present *Am J Med Sc* 2006;331(4):194–200.

Spivak H, Faveretti F. Avoiding postoperative complications with the LAP-BAND system *Am J Surg* 2002;184:31s–37s.

COMMENTARY

Restrictive procedures for morbid obesity have a standard place in our armamentarium of the bariatric surgeon. Thousands of patients have benefited from the performance of laparoscopic restrictive bariatric operations. Proponents of restrictive procedures claim enhanced technical ease, lower morbidity, and comparable weight loss to laparoscopic Roux-en-Y gastric bypass. Proponents of the Roux-en-Y gastric bypass claim that despite the increased technical difficulties and potential for increased morbidity, patients with the combined restrictive and malabsorptive procedures experience increased resolution of their associated metabolic problems and, in some series, greater sustained weight loss. Despite one's position in these debates, it is obvious that many patients respond extremely well to restrictive procedures for morbid obesity.

The approach to restrictive procedures for morbid obesity is undergoing significant change. Broad acceptance of this procedure in the U.S. lagged behind acceptance in Europe and Australia. Competitive bands are currently being developed and several are expected to be released within the coming months to years. Additionally, innovative totally endoscopic approaches are being tested. These endoluminal procedures have a very reasonable chance of obtaining and maintaining a place in the armamentarium of those who treat obesity.

The authors of this chapter have described the evolution of these procedures as well as significant technical tips. Appropriately, they have discussed in detail potential complications and methods for avoiding such complications. One cannot overemphasize the importance of a team approach to treating patients with morbid obesity. The role of the dietician and the bariatrician is significant, and one who approaches the surgical management of morbid obesity as purely a technical procedure is likely to have poor long-term outcomes. The appropriate preoperative preparation of these patients, proper technical execution of the operation, and long-term follow-up and management provides the patient with the best chance of an optimal outcome.

WSE

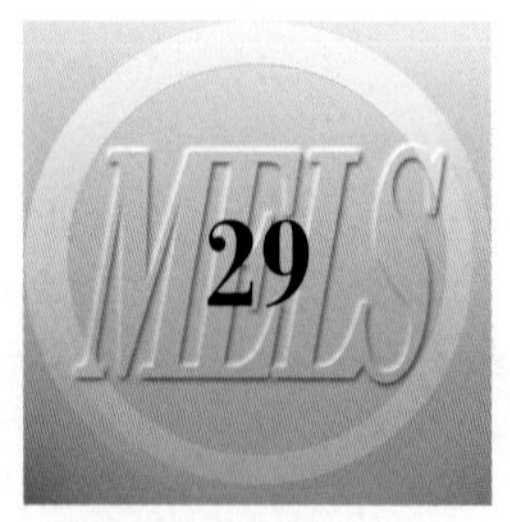

Laparoscopic Roux-en-Y Gastric Bypass

DANIEL B. LESLIE, TODD A. KELLOGG, AND SAYEED IKRAMUDDIN

INTRODUCTION

Gastric bypass is the most commonly performed bariatric procedure in the United States. Though the term "gold standard" is perhaps overreaching, this operation represents the benchmark by which all other bariatric procedures are currently compared. The standard gastric bypass performed today is an isolated Roux-en-Y gastric bypass (RYGB), meaning that the stomach is completely divided. A small gastric pouch approximately 15 to 30 cc in size is constructed and connected to a Roux limb. The Roux limb is made typically 75 to 150 cm in length and is in turn connected to the biliopancreatic limb. The procedure is performed in either an antecolic or retrocolic configuration. The procedure can be performed through a midline incision but the majority of procedures performed today use the laparoscopic approach. The operation has established itself over the last two decades as a durable operation with excellent outcomes when performed both open and laparoscopically. The incidence of mortality is extremely low. This chapter will summarize the history of the gastric bypass, the current techniques used to perform it, and outcomes of the RYGB in terms of weight loss, the resolution of comorbid illness, and complications.

Background

The RYGB as it is currently performed is the product of both years of technical modifications of the original gastric bypass and the technical limitations of laparoscopic instrumentation. Edward Mason at the University of Iowa originally described the gastric bypass operation for the treatment of morbid obesity in 1967. In his original description, a 90% gastric bypass was created with a horizontal gastric pouch and a loop gastrojejunostomy to bypass the distal stomach. The stomach was divided and sutured closed. The next iteration involved cross-stapling the stomach without dividing it in order to reduce gastrointestinal anastomotic leaks and decrease some of the morbidity associated with the original operation. Alkaline bile reflux led to long-term complications with many of these operations, a problem eventually overcome with conversion of the loop gastrojejunostomy to a Roux-en-Y intestinal reconstruction. The undivided bypass had a significant rate of failure due to staple line breakdown and the subsequent development of gastrogastric fistulae. Though attempts were made to decrease the incidence of staple line breakdown by increasing the number of staple lines, ultimately this problem was solved by actual division of the stomach to create an isolated gastric pouch.

It bears emphasis that the gastric bypass, like adjustable banding and the biliopancreatic diversion/duodenal switch, is only a *tool* for the treatment of obesity. All such procedures for obesity can be overcome by the consumption of highly refined carbohydrate snacks. In order to compensate for failure or inadequate initial weight loss, many technical modifications of the traditional gastric bypass procedure have been performed. These have included banding of the stoma or the pouch with either a prosthetic or an autologous material and lengthening of the Roux limb.

The first recorded laparoscopic RYGB was performed by Wittgrove et al. in 1994. They reported a circular-stapled gastrojejunostomy with a retrogastric, retrocolic RYGB. In their original series they did not report closure of any of the potential mesenteric defects. There are other approaches to this operation, including a linear-stapled technique for the gastrojejunal anastomosis with the Roux limb being passed in either a retrocolic-antegastric or antecolic-antegastric path. There are many described ways to complete the gastrojejunostomy. A totally hand-sewn procedure has been described using a suturing device, the da Vinci robot (Intuitive Surgical, Inc; Sunnyvale, CA), or conventional laparoscopic techniques. Most surgeons prefer either the linear or circular stapling technique as it requires less facility with laparoscopic suturing.

Regardless of the approach, it is important that surgeons master one technique for the operation and at least be familiar with other techniques, should technical complications during surgery require flexibility. A mastery of intracorporeal suturing is also necessary.

It is beyond the scope of this chapter to discuss the open approach to RYGB, but it is important to emphasize that a firm understanding of exposure techniques in morbidly obese patients using the open approach is a fundamental component of bariatric surgery. Without this knowledge and experience, converting a patient from a laparoscopic approach to an open approach would be less safe.

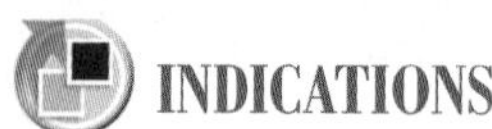

INDICATIONS

The National Institutes of Health has published indications criteria for all bariatric surgery. Patients should have a body mass index greater than or equal to 40 kg/m^2. Patients with a BMI less than 40 kg/m^2 may undergo surgery if they have significant comorbid illness such as diabetes mellitus, hypertension, or obstructive sleep apnea. In our experience, it is preferred that all patients demonstrate 6 months of dietary and lifestyle modification under the guidance of their primary care physician or in our bariatric practice. All patients are seen for a minimum of 3 months prior to undergoing obesity surgery; during this period they have a routine psychological evaluation. Though the utility of this evaluation in predicting weight loss is not clear, assessments can be made about a patient's level of intelligence and whether he or she understands the complications of the procedure and that surgery is only a tool, the presence of any untreated psychiatric disorder, and the adequacy of the patient's support system.

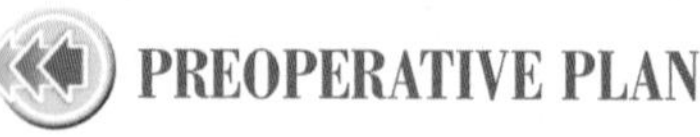

PREOPERATIVE PLANNING

Patient Evaluation

The evaluation and management of patients preoperatively must be comprehensive and can be lengthy. It is important that patients understand that surgery is a very powerful tool for the management

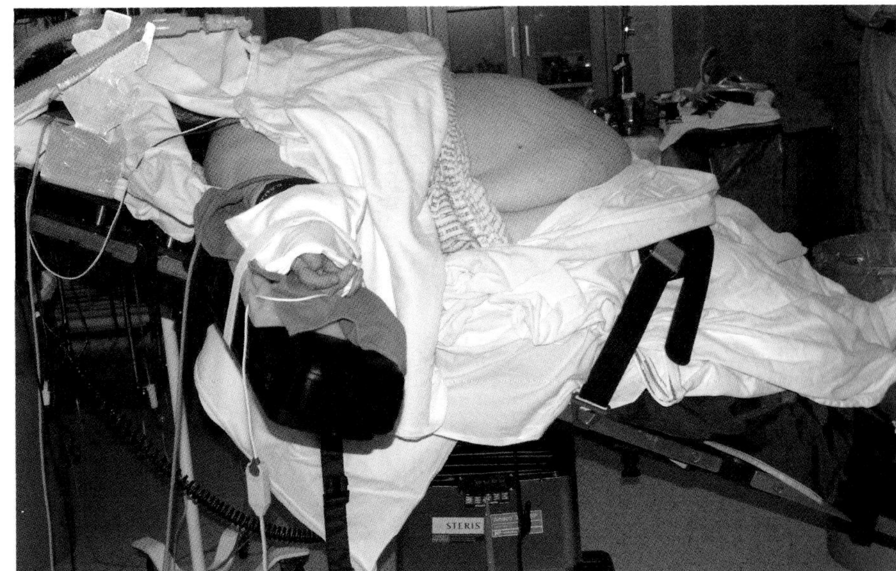

Fig. 29-1. Steep reverse-Trendelenburg is necessary for optimal visualization during the operation.

of morbid obesity. The patient will have the best result after surgery when the procedure is used in the correct context of exercise and lifestyle modification, which should be instituted preoperatively. Along those lines, it's important to focus on all aspects of health care before operating. For example, patients are required to stop smoking, and referral to a smoking cessation program is offered if needed.

The workup begins by obtaining a letter from the primary care physician detailing weight loss attempts the patient has made under their care during the previous year and all attempts at weight loss, including counseling, the use of medications, and other interventions that may have been used. In addition, the number of years the patient has been severely or morbidly obese is documented. Patients with central obesity and those who are massively obese are required to lose some weight preoperatively. Even for those patients who are not massively obese, a 5- to 10-pound weight loss is encouraged, as this solidifies the patient's commitment to the procedure and discourages the "last supper" syndrome. For patients with a history of snoring or central obesity, a sleep study is obtained preoperatively to assess for apneic episodes and continuous positive airway pressure (CPAP) therapy is started if obstructive sleep apnea is diagnosed. Appropriate instruction in the use of CPAP is necessary as its use can induce swallowing of air with subsequent dangerous dilatation of the gastric remnant. Abdominal distention can also further compromise respirations. Preoperative sleep apnea is a risk factor for anesthesia and postoperative complications, so protection of the airway in these patients is paramount.

An echocardiogram should be obtained on any patient who has a history of fenfluramine and phentermine (Fen-Phen) use for 6 months or if the patient is unsure of the duration and it appears to have been greater than 3 months. For those patients with type 2 diabetes above the age of 45, a cardiology consultation is requested. Otherwise, cardiology consultation is obtained for any patient older than 50 with risk factors such as dyslipidemia, a history of smoking, or a history of hypertension. Thrombophlebitis and deep venous thrombosis (DVT) can be significant problems in the morbidly obese patient. Hematology consultation is obtained for any patient with history of a blood clot without a known etiology, such as being on oral contraceptives or during pregnancy. For those patients with severe pulmonary hypertension, a temporary inferior vena caval filter is placed prior to surgery as the pulmonary reserve in the event of a pulmonary embolism would be very low. For patients with limited exercise reserve or for those who are wheelchair-bound, physical medicine and rehabilitation consults are obtained. The physiatrist's expertise in determining a patient's functional status and limitations is crucial for planning an exercise regimen for these patients, as is the physiatrist's ability to put such an assessment in the context of existing medical problems, such as autoimmune disease, severe degenerative joint disease, and neuromuscular disorders such as multiple sclerosis or spinal stenosis. Once again, surgery is just a tool; for those patients without the capacity to exercise, the outcome of surgery will not be as favorable.

All patients are screened for anemia preoperatively. Serum ferritin level and other measures of iron stores such as a total iron binding capacity and iron level are evaluated. In many cases iron saturation is low, which may be a hallmark of obesity as an inflammatory disorder with decreased utilization. This is treated preoperatively as repletion of iron postoperatively can be even more difficult after bypass of the duodenum. In addition, vitamin B12 levels and folate levels should be checked preoperatively.

Operating Room Setup and Equipment

A specialized heavy-duty operating table that can hold up to 1000 pounds and provide 45 degrees of reverse-Trendelenburg position is used (Fig. 29-1). The table should also have the ability to have extenders for both length and width, and footboards should be available to prevent patient movement during table tilts. Air-filled hover mats are especially useful for moving patients safely to and from the operating table and preventing injuries to the operating room teams. Extra-long instruments, including toothed and atraumatic graspers, ultrasonic scissors, endoscopic staplers, liver retractors, and suction aspirators, should be available.

Preoperative Preparation

On the morning of surgery, subcutaneous low molecular weight heparin and a broad spectrum intravenous antibiotic are administered, and sequential compression devices are placed as a DVT prophylaxis. Patients are placed supine on the operating table, and a pillow is placed below the knees to bend them. The feet are secured on gel pads, with a towel placed above the feet and taped to the base of the footboard. A security strap is placed at the knees. A transurethral bladder catheter is placed. Both arms are left abducted and secured on a board with adequate padding.

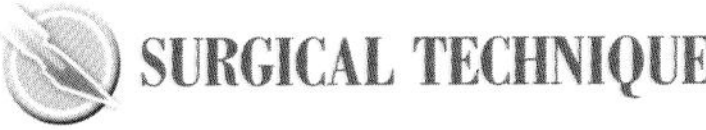

SURGICAL TECHNIQUE

We perform a laparoscopic RYGB using an antecolic, antegastric Roux limb and a gastrojejunostomy performed with a linear stapler, the enterotomy of which is oversewn in two layers over a 30F stent, typically using a 30F endoscope. A stapled jejunojejunostomy is performed 150 cm distal to the gastrojejunostomy on the Roux limb, and the biliopancreatic limb is 100 cm.

The technique of laparoscopic gastric bypass has undergone many revisions over the past 10 years and continues to be modified. The following technique offers a number of technical advantages gained with increasing experience on the part of the authors. First, we will describe an antecolic antegastric procedure in which the greater omentum is not divided. Second, the mesentery between the distal biliopancreatic limb and the Roux limb of jejunum is not typically divided with ultrasonic shears or a stapler, meaning the size of this defect is smaller. Third, in the rare event that a loop of jejunum does not reach to the gastric pouch in a tension-free manner, the Penrose drain can be moved slightly downstream since the bowel has not been divided yet. This maneuver allows one to isolate a more mobile loop of bowel in order to perform a tension-free gastrojejunostomy and avoid the retrocolic pathway, which is associated with a higher risk of internal herniation. Fourth, by immediately placing a back row between the gastric pouch and the Roux limb, there are more points of fixation for the small bowel, which makes measuring the Roux limb technically less challenging. Finally, since the distal biliopancreatic limb is located further into the left upper quadrant, the angle used for construction of the jejunojejunostomy is more ergonomic for suturing.

Limitations of the described approach arise when a very thickened small bowel or very short mesentery is found, in which case it is preferable to pass the Roux limb in the retrocolic, retrogastric pathway.

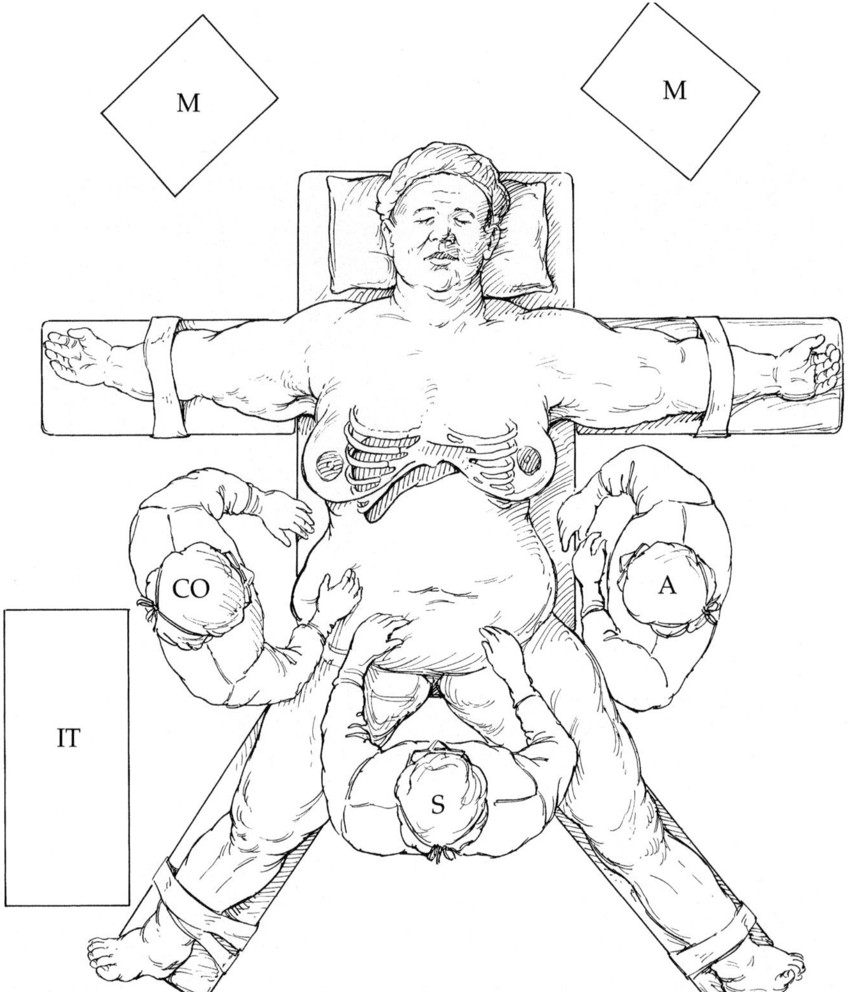

Fig. 29-2. Room setup and surgeon position for gastric bypass. A, assistant; CO, camera operator; IT, instrument table; M, monitor; S, surgeon.

Operating Room Setup and Port Placement

We use a six-port technique. The surgeon stands on the patient's right and the assistant on the left. The camera is usually held on the left side by the assistant (Fig. 29-2). A mixture of 0.5% Marcaine and 1% lidocaine is instilled at each trocar site prior to port placement. A 150-mm Veress needle (Ethicon Endo-Surgery, Inc.; Cincinnati, OH) is placed in a subcostal location in the left upper quadrant in the midclavicular line and used to establish pneumoperitoneum. A Hasson access technique is used at an appropriate location for patients with previous left upper quadrant abdominal surgery, large ventral hernia repair with mesh, or a history of a bowel obstruction.

The abdomen is insufflated with carbon dioxide to a maximum pressure of 15 mmHg, and a total of six ports are placed (Fig. 29-3). All trocars are non-bladed to reduce the rate of herniation. A 5-mm non-bladed trocar is inserted at the Veress needle site. Next, using a 5-mm laparoscope through the first port for visualization, a 12-mm trocar is placed 15 to 20 cm below the xiphoid process to the left of midline, and the camera is used from this port. A 45-degree laparoscope is used to perform the procedure, allowing great ease in navigating around complex angles.

The patient is then positioned in steep reverse-Trendelenburg. Another left lateral 5-mm port is placed inferiorly and just subcostal on the left side, more lateral to the first trocar site. Two working ports are then placed for the surgeon: a 5-mm port at the right subcostal site and a 12-mm port just 10 cm away, roughly at the same level as that of the camera port. One 5-mm right lateral port is placed for the liver retractor (Fig. 29-3). An angulating triangular liver retractor is positioned and held in place with a side clamp for the table (Genzyme Corp.; Cambridge, MA).

Gastric Pouch Creation

We begin the operation by using scissors to take down adhesions at the angle of His and to separate the left crus from gastric cardia and fundus (Fig. 29-4). The hepatogastric ligament is then incised with an ultrasonic shears, and the lesser sac is entered (Fig. 29-5, page 266). In most

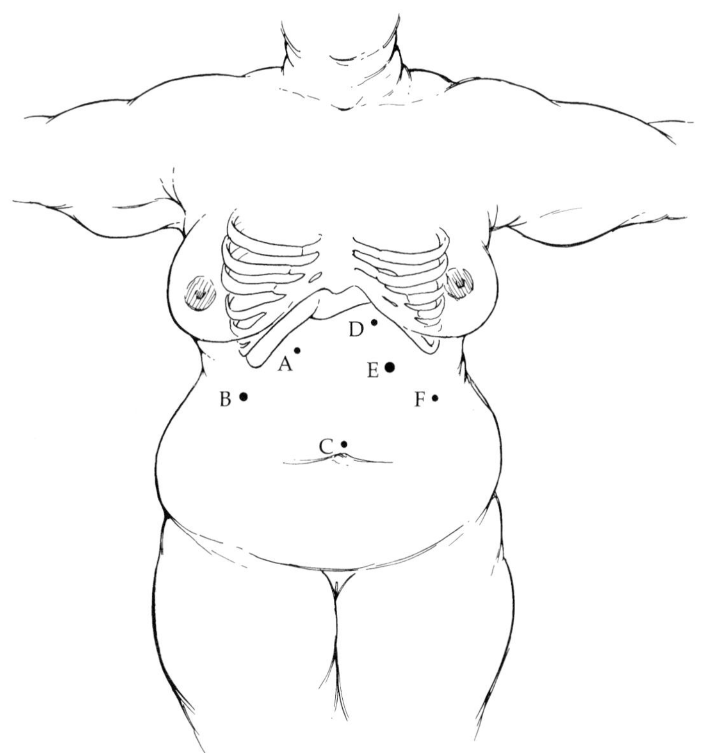

Fig. 29-3. Port configuration with six-port technique.

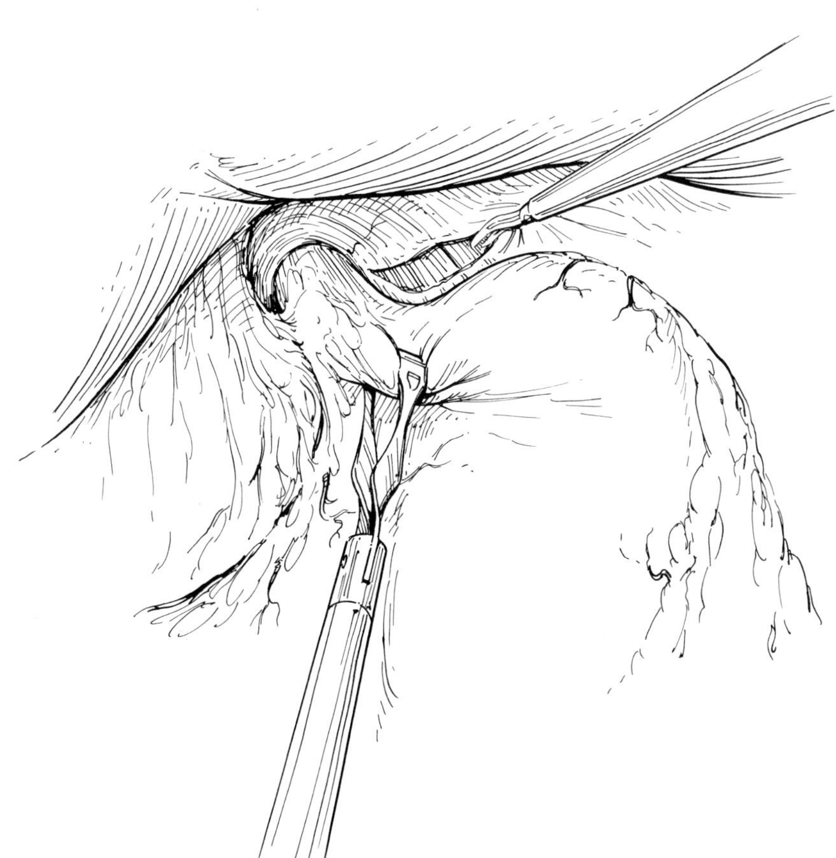

Fig. 29-4. The peritoneal attachments at the angle of His are sharply divided.

cases, the lesser sac is free of adhesions, but in patients with a history of pancreatitis or gallbladder disease there may be significant adhesions, and a combination of sharp and blunt dissection may be necessary to visualize the retrogastric tunnel. Care is taken to avoid injury to the splenic vessels, the pancreas, or the posterior wall of the stomach.

Formation of the gastric pouch is begun immediately below the left gastric artery, which courses toward the stomach about 3 cm down from the gastroesophageal junction on the lesser curve. A roticulating 60-mm blue load triple linear stapler with GORE SEAM-GUARD Bioabsorbable Staple Line Reinforcement (W. L. Gore & Assoicates; Flagstaff, AZ) is used to divide the lesser curvature neurovascular bundle (Fig. 29-6, page 266).

Division with additional blue loads on the stapler is carried up to the angle of His, the goal being a very small, narrow gastric pouch, approximately 15 to 30 cc in size, with complete fundic transection (Fig. 29-7, page 267). The ultrasonic shears are used to dissect any posterior gastric adhesions free, with care taken to avoid injury to the left gastric artery, which can be found medially on the pouch.

The Gastrojejunostomy

This next phase of the operation combines construction of the gastrojejunostomy with jejunojejunostomy preparation. The patient is brought into supine position. The colonic mesentery is elevated just above the ligament of Treitz to clearly identify the proximal jejunum and to create a space for bowel limb measurement. The jejunum is marched 100 cm distally, and the proximal bowel is rotated one-half turn clockwise and moved to the patient's left side. At 100 cm, the bowel is elevated with graspers, and a Maryland dissector is passed through the mesentery just adjacent to the small bowel and used to pass a Penrose drain to encircle the loop of jejunum. The future distal biliopancreatic limb is now to the patient's anatomic left, and the proximal Roux limb is to the patient's right of the Penrose drain. The operating table is moved back to steep reverse-Trendelenburg position, and the drain is used as a handle to pass the loop of jejunum in antecolic, antegastric position to a point adjacent to the small gastric pouch. The greater omentum is not divided to

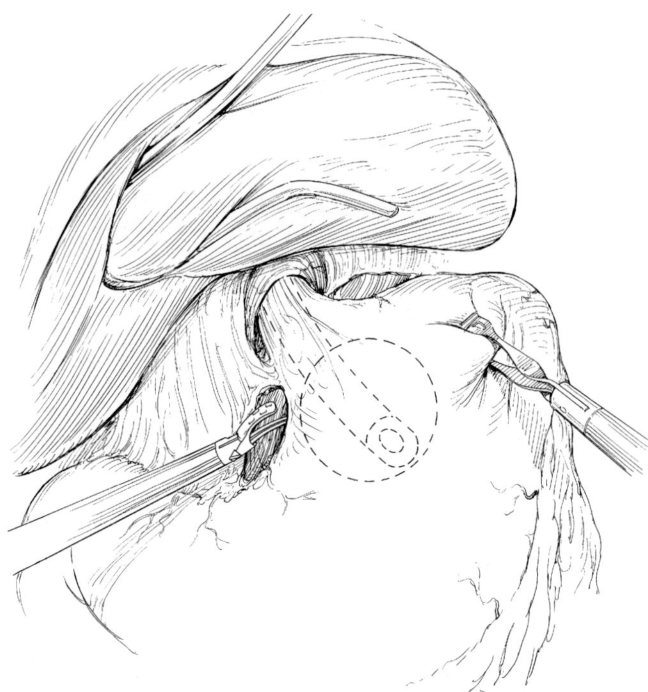

Fig. 29-5. The hepatogastric ligament is divided with a harmonic scalpel. Care is taken to avoid a replaced or accessory left hepatic artery.

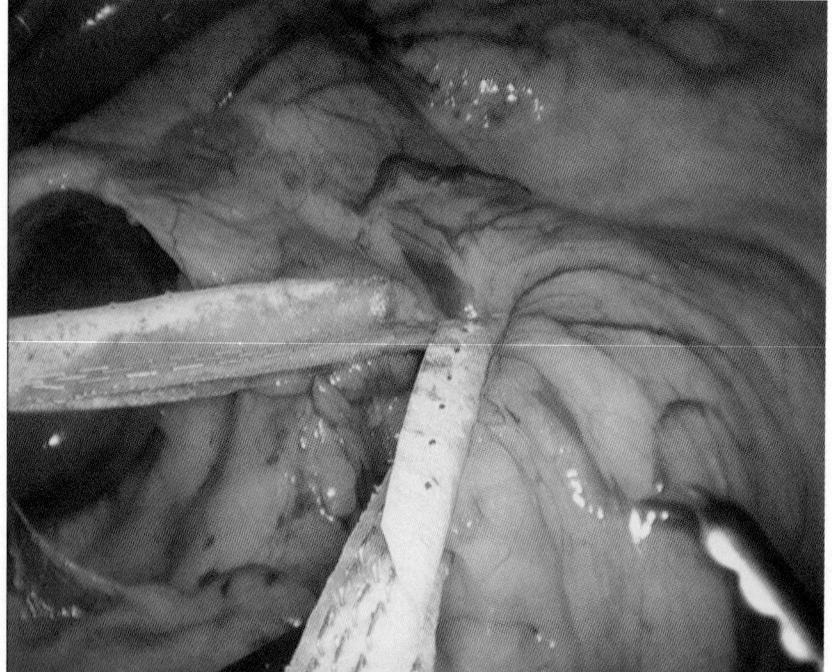

Fig. 29-6. The lesser curvature has been divided to the stomach using a SEAM-GUARD-reinforced triple linear stapling device.

accomplish this maneuver (Fig. 29-8, page 268).

With the Penrose drain still in place to take off traction, a non-absorbable 2-0 suture is used to run a back wall suture between the gastric pouch and the loop of small bowel on the patient's right. With this jejunal loop secured to the gastric pouch, the operation may readily proceed to construction of the jejunojejunostomy, as described later, or may follow with completion of the gastrojejunostomy as follows.

A roticulating, 60-mm white load stapler is used to divide the small bowel, maintaining what is to the patient's left as the biliopancreatic limb and what is to the right as the Roux limb. The Penrose drain is removed from the abdomen, and the distal biliopancreatic is reflected inferiorly using gentle traction to elongate the mesenteric defect slightly by about 1 to 2 cm. Note that this mesenteric defect has not been formally divided with staplers or with the ultrasonic shears.

Enterotomies are made on the gastric pouch and on the Roux limb with the harmonic scalpel, and a blue load stapler is inserted to 2 cm and fired (Fig. 29-9, page 269). In the process, the back row stitch is directed toward the left upper quadrant to facilitate the stapling angle.

A 3-0 absorbable suture is then used to sew the residual enterotomies of the anastomosis, beginning at the right corner and the left corner of the anastomosis, and the two sutures brought together in the middle without tying. This can be either an interrupted or running suture line. Absorbable suture is chosen to decrease the incidence of marginal ulcer, which may be associated with permanent suture. A 30F gastroscope is passed through the anastomosis into the Roux limb, and the suture is tied. A second layer of 2-0 non-absorbable suture is placed anteriorly to complete a two-layer anastomosis (Fig. 29-10, page 270). The patient is moved to a supine position; with a bowel clamp on the Roux limb, the anastomosis is tested using saline immersion to inspect for any evidence of bubbling or leakage. Small holes can be oversewn if necessary.

The Jejunojejunostomy

The Roux limb is run 150 cm and sutured to the distal biliopancreatic limb at this location. Small enterotomies are made on each limb with the ultrasonic shears, and a non-roticulating, 60-mm white load stapler is inserted into the lumen of each bowel and fired to create the jejunojejunostomy (Fig. 29-11, page 270). A single stitch is then placed to secure the heel of the anastomosis.

The midpoint of the enterotomy defect is approximated with a single suture; using graspers on the proximal Roux limb corner and on the distal biliopancreatic limb corner, the entire enterotomy is rotated between 100 and 180 degrees counterclockwise

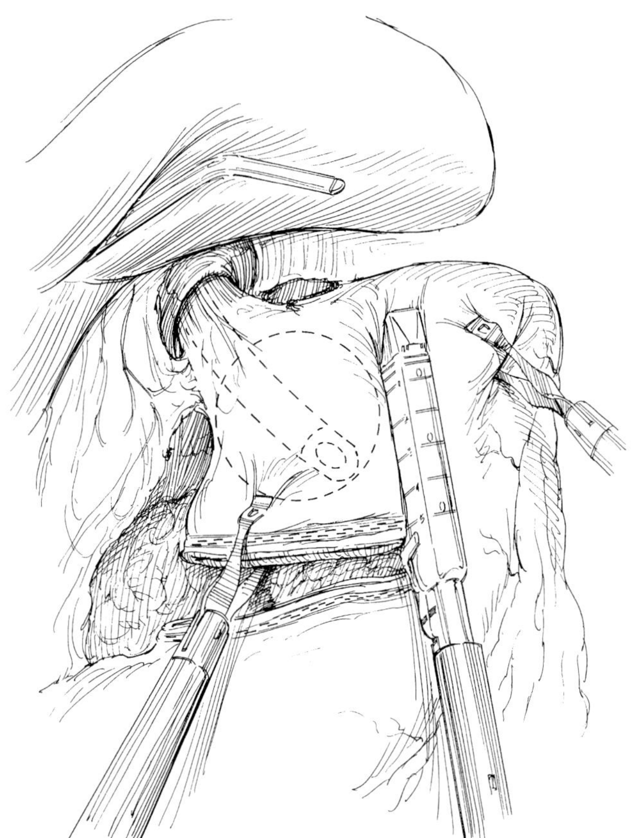

Fig. 29-7. A fully roticulated 60-mm blue load is directed toward the angle of His to complete the construction of the gastric pouch. The 15- to 30-cc gastric pouch is completely separated from the gastric remnant.

and moved into the left upper quadrant. A second non-roticulating, 60-mm white load stapler is used to close the enterotomy. An anti-torsion stitch is placed between the two limbs of the bowel, and mesenteric defect sutures (Fig. 29-12, page 271) are run toward the root of the mesentery to completely close the small bowel mesenteric defect. The biologic glue TISSEEL (Baxter Healthcare Corp.; Deerfield, IL) is applied to each anastomosis, hemostasis is assured, and the operation is complete. The liver retractor and all ports are removed under direct visualization where possible, and all skin incisions are stapled with sterile dressings applied.

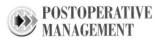

POSTOPERATIVE MANAGEMENT

A typical stay in the hospital is 2 days following laparoscopic RYGB. Some bariatric practices that have identified patients who have a lower risk profile and are therefore able to be discharged after a 23-hour hospital stay. If the practice profile is more slanted toward high-risk patients, then the hospital stay is longer.

Patients remain nil per os and receive intravenous fluids until a postoperative upper gastrointestinal (GI) study is obtained on the day after surgery. Pain control is intravenous hydromorphone via patient-controlled analgesia pump and intravenous ketorolac. After a negative upper GI study, clear liquids and oral pain medications are started. All patients see a dietician while in the hospital. The patient will be discharged when he or she is tolerating oral liquids and medications and ambulating well, which usually occurs on postoperative day two. Skin staples are removed and replaced with steristrips on the day of discharge.

In order to avoid constipation, patients are typically started on a stool softener such as docusate and asked to increase water and fiber in their diet. Patients are asked to crush their medications and sent home with clear liquids only. Medications are carefully reviewed; diabetic medications are typically reduced dramatically prior to discharge. Patients discharged home with antihypertensive or diuretic medications are instructed to carefully monitor symptoms of orthostasis because the need for such medication is frequently reduced dramatically in the post-RYGB setting. Ursodiol is given to patients who still have a gallbladder in order to prevent gallstone formation during the period of rapid weight loss.

The postoperative visits typically occur at 1 week, 1 month, 3 months, 6 months, 9 months, and 1 year. The patients are then seen every 6 months up until year five and annually thereafter. Multivitamins, supplemental iron, calcium, and vitamin B12 are recommended in an outpatient setting one week after surgery. Patients are asked to start a pureed diet beginning one week after surgery. Laboratory testing is obtained at 3 months and again at 1 year after surgery. Patient follow-up is extremely important because of long-term risks of vitamin deficiencies, though very few bariatric programs are successful in achieving high rates of follow-up.

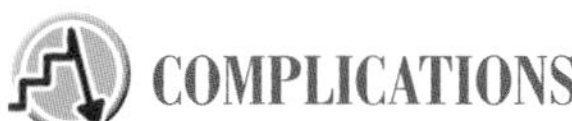

COMPLICATIONS

The mortality of the gastric bypass performed in most major series is quite low, ranging from 0.3% to 3.3%. This stands apart from series that look at short-term outcome data using coding, which suggests short-term (within 30 days of surgery) mortality may potentially be higher in these patients.

Postoperative complications are unusual but can be devastating or even lethal if not immediately recognized and acted on. The most dreaded complication of a gastric bypass is a gastrointestinal leak. This may occur from the gastric pouch, the gastrojejunal anastomosis, the bypassed stomach, or from the jejunojejunostomy. Most leaks occur either at the level of the gastric pouch or around the gastrojejunostomy; taken together, both are referred to as an anastomotic leak. The incidence of leak was as high as 5% in early series, but now has dropped markedly in most published series. Leakage can be a potentially difficult problem, and all patients must be counseled regarding the possibility prior to operation. The approach for any patient who demonstrates a leak is to operate promptly, rather than attempt nonoperative management. The patient is immediately re-explored laparoscopically under controlled conditions and a saline immersion test is performed to identify the anastomotic leak site. With a 30F

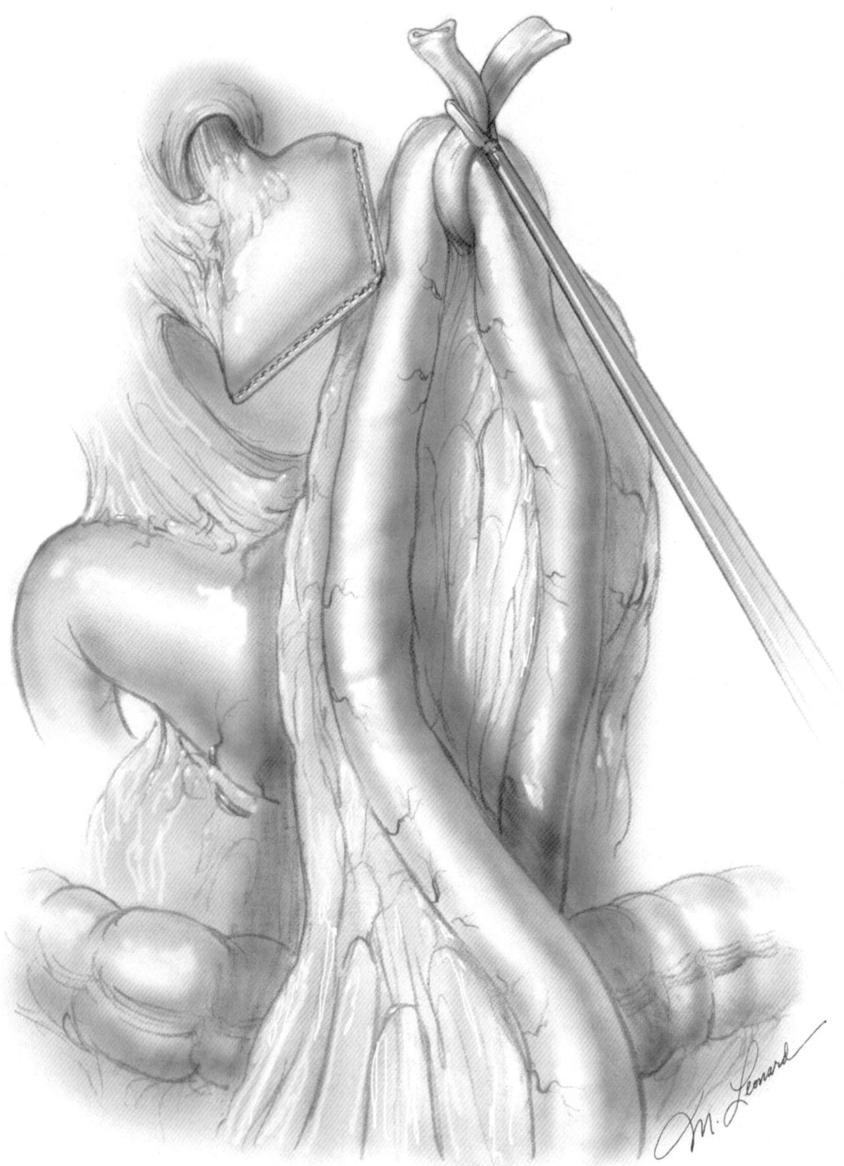

Fig. 29-8. This loop of jejunum has been secured with a Penrose drain 100 cm past the ligament of Treitz. A 180-degree clockwise turn has been introduced; the future Roux limb is to the left of the Penrose drain and biliopancreatic limb is to the right on the photograph. The Penrose drain is used to pull the jejunum to the left upper quadrant adjacent to the gastric remnant.

endoscope in place, the leak site is oversewn and the area is drained widely. If it appears that the anastomosis is very significantly compromised, a gastrostomy tube is placed in the gastric remnant. Although quite uncomfortable, this is a very safe and useful way to feed the patient postoperatively.

Bleeding is infrequent, with about 1 in 200 patients requiring a reoperative exploration for bleeding. The incidence of stricture following surgery varies markedly from center to center and may be as high as 10%. One of the difficulties in interpretation of this is the definition of what a stricture may be. Oftentimes this is based solely on clinical data. Some surgeons may do this based on clinical symptoms of nausea or vomiting, prompting the use of upper endoscopy. Regardless, strictures are relatively easy to treat and respond very well to outpatient balloon dilatation. Our approach is to perform upper endoscopy as early as 21 days after surgery, at which time this can be accomplished quite safely. A balloon can be directly passed through the stricture site and inflated using a 36F balloon inflated to 6 atmospheres pressure for 5 minutes. This usually results in prompt resolution of the stricture, and the patient is able to go home that day.

Management of internal hernias postoperatively is a complex problem as they can be difficult to identify. Internal hernias after RYGB can occur at one of three different sites: (1) the Petersen defect, which is underneath the mesentery of the Roux limb, (2) the retrocolic defect, which can be present in the case of a retrocolic gastrojejunal anastomosis, and (3) the jejunojejunostomy mesenteric defect, which is between the distal biliopancreatic limb and the side of the Roux limb. In early series of laparoscopic RYGB, these defects were not routinely closed, which led to marked morbidity including bowel ischemia and infarction in the event of internal herniation. More recent techniques have focused attention on trying to eliminate these sites of herniation, including using the antecolic pathway for gastrojejunal anastomosis, sewing the jejunojejunostomy mesenteric defect closed, and orienting the Roux limb toward the right at the gastrojejunostomy. Even with this, there is still a risk for posterior Petersen-type hernias. There should be a high degree of suspicion for a patient who has had a brisk weight loss approximately 8 months or more after RYGB who complains of episodes of crampy abdominal pain, especially if the gallbladder has already been removed and there is no history of marginal ulcer. Neither CT scan nor upper GI is effective in identifying this problem, and the best treatment is an elective diagnostic laparoscopy. Patients with acute crampy abdominal pain associated with tachycardia, peritonitis, leukocytosis, or fever should be operated on immediately. This typically can be done laparoscopically, reducing and occasionally resecting the small bowel and repairing the defect.

Nutritional deficiencies following the gastric bypass can be significant problems. Pre-existing nutritional defects should be identified and corrected before bariatric surgery. The incidence of iron deficiency and anemia in female candidates for bariatric surgery is 14% to 20%. Bypass can exacerbate the problem as the duodenum is a primary site of iron absorption. Iron, ferritin, hemoglobin, and mean corpuscular volume (MCV) levels should be checked preoperatively and again

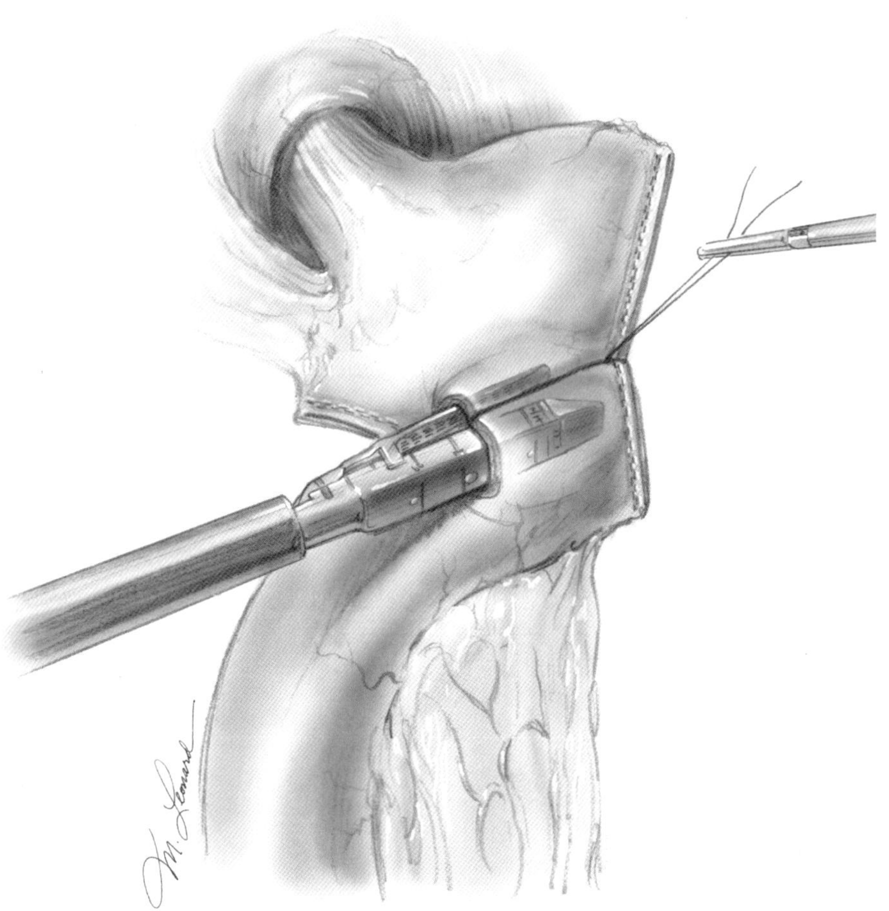

Fig. 29-9. Enterotomies have been made on the gastric pouch and jejunum, and traction is held on the back row stitch toward the left upper quadrant to facilitate stapling of the inner portion of the gastrojejunostomy.

several weeks following surgery. Oral replacement is appropriate, though we occasionally use an intravenous iron infusion prior to surgery. In addition, patients are encouraged to take vitamin B12 via oral, sublingual, or parenteral route starting before surgery. Particular care must be taken for patients who are contemplating pregnancy. For these patients, iron, folate and other B-vitamin levels are closely monitored. Homocysteine levels are also evaluated as they may be a reliable indicator of B-vitamin precursors. Nutritional complications are rare in patients who take vitamin supplements. When they do occur it is usually in patients with persistent vomiting. Particular care should be taken hydrating such patients, as dilution may worsen their deficiencies.

Another problematic complication is marginal ulcer. The incidence of marginal ulcer is around 10% after surgery in spite of a nearly ubiquitous use of over-the-counter proton pump inhibitors and histamine 2 (H2) blockers. In the majority of cases, marginal ulcer is related to the use of non-steroidal anti-inflammatory drugs (NSAIDS), smoking, and alcohol consumption. The use of NSAIDs and smoking are strongly discouraged postoperatively. Marginal ulcers have been known to perforate when they occur on the jejunal side.

A common problem following the gastric bypass is constipation. This may be due to a reduced fluid or fiber intake. Constipation may also be related to hormonal changes following the gastric bypass. Enteroglucagon, or GLP-1, is a hormone produced by the intestinal L cells in the proximal colon and the terminal ileum. The L-cell product of GLP-1 is responsible for slowing motility of the gastrointestinal track, impairing gluconeogenesis, blocking pancreatic glucagon secretion, and improving insulin sensitivity. Increased levels of this hormone following bypass contribute significantly to constipation in these patients. Patients should be cautioned to avoid constipation and placed on a thorough bowel regimen, avoiding laxatives if possible.

Excessive flatulence can also be a significant complaint, but this can be ameliorated in most patients by keeping a careful food log and avoiding foods that cause gas.

OUTCOMES

The laparoscopic RYGB has fared very favorably compared to the open technique in terms of percent excess weight loss (%EWL) as well as complications. The hospital stay for open gastric bypass is approximately 4 to 6 days, compared to 1 to 2.5 days following laparoscopic RYGB. Though the initial incidence of mortality and gastrointestinal leak rate appeared to be higher with laparoscopic gastric bypass compared to the open literature, in many larger series this does not appear to be borne out. One area in which there is a major difference is in the incidence of wound-related complications. The incidence of hernias following open RYGB ranges from 14% to 20%, but is markedly lower following laparoscopic bypass.

Percent excess weight loss for the laparoscopic RYGB is reported to be 50% to 80% in 5 years in most major series.

Resolution of comorbid illness is quite profound following RYGB. In many series, a complete resolution of type 2 diabetes is seen in 80% or more of the cases, and partial resolution is seen in most of the remaining patients. The best outcomes are seen with those with the least severe type 2 diabetes and shortest duration of the disease.

Hypertension is also commonly improved. The Swedish Obesity Study has demonstrated that both diabetes and hypertension have been markedly improved after gastric bypass, although after 10 years, the impact on hypertension does tend to be significantly diminished. A recent outcomes study by Christou et al. described the effect of gastric bypass on mortality and improvement of comorbid illnesses. In a group of 1035 bariatric surgical patients, 81% of whom underwent RYGB, the nonsurgical mortality rate was 0.68% compared with 6.17% in 5746 matched control patients who did not undergo surgical weight loss. This is a 5.5% absolute and 89% relative risk reduction for death after weight loss surgery.

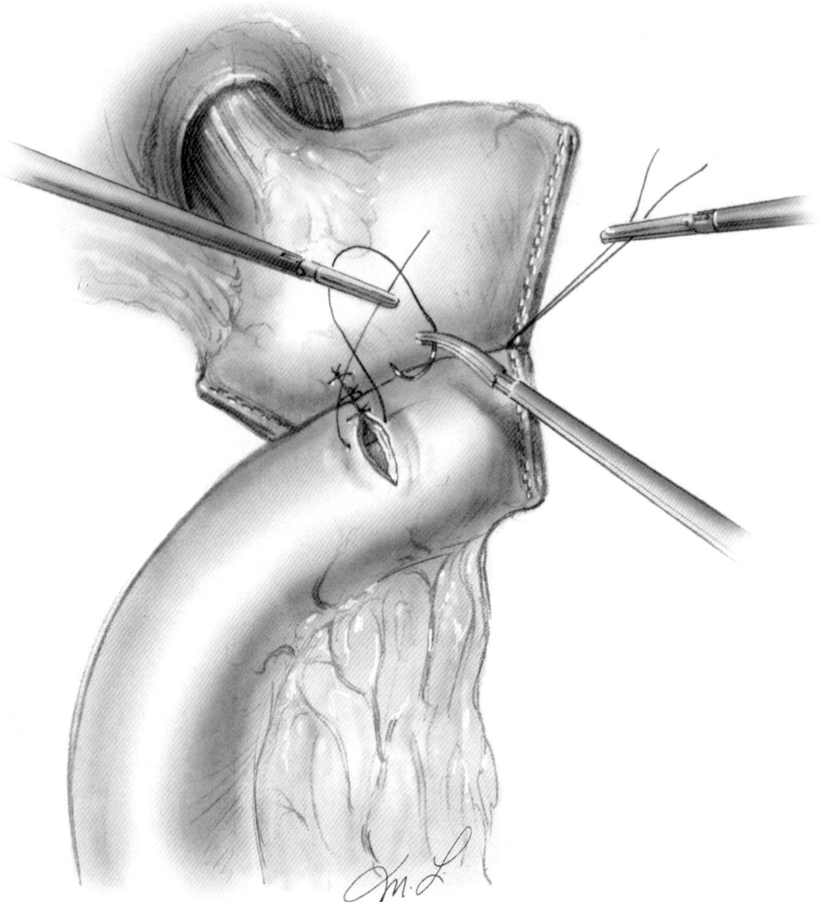

Fig. 29-10. The enterotomies are closed in a two-layer suture fashion.

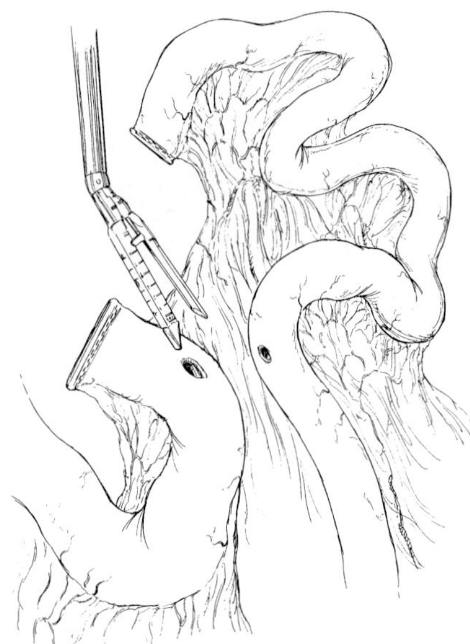

Fig. 29-11. A white load on the triple linear stapling device is inserted into the enterotomy defect on the distal biliopancreatic limb on the left of the figure and on the Roux limb on the right to create the jejunojejunostomy.

SUMMARY

Minimally invasive surgery has revolutionized the practice of bariatric surgery to date, and the field is likely to change further as new technologies emerge. The laparoscopic Roux-en-Y gastric bypass is the current gold standard procedure that will serve as a benchmark for all other approaches. Outcomes improve with experience. Surgery is a tool and must be used in the context of a multidisciplinary program.

SUGGESTED READING

Christou NV, Sampalis JS, Liberman M, et al. Surgery decreases long-term mortality, morbidity, and health care use in morbidly obese patients. *Ann Surg* 2004;240:416–423; discussion 423–424.

Higa KD, Boone KB, Ho T. Complications of the laparoscopic Roux-en-Y gastric bypass: 1,040 patients—what have we learned? *Obes Surg* 2000;10:509–513.

NIH conference. Gastrointestinal surgery for severe obesity. Consensus Development

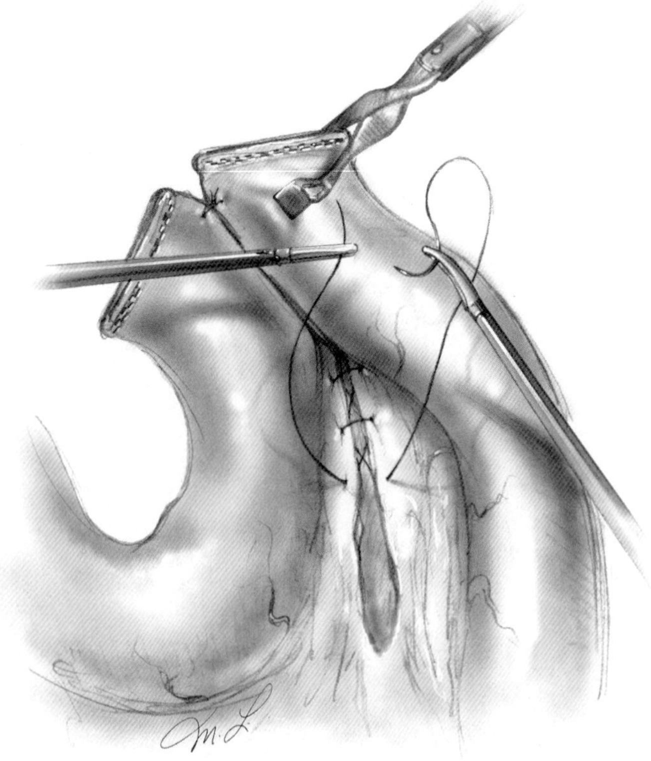

Fig. 29-12. An anti-obstruction stitch is placed between the Roux limb and the distal biliopancreatic limb; this is continued toward the root of the mesentery to close the mesenteric defect.

Conference Panel. *Ann Intern Med* 1991; 115:956–961.
Pories WJ, Swanson MS, MacDonald KG, et al. Who would have thought it? An operation proves to be the most effective therapy for adult-onset diabetes mellitus. *Ann Surg* 1995;222:339–350; discussion 350–352.
Schauer PR, Burguera B, Ikramuddin S, et al. Effect of laparoscopic Roux-en-Y gastric bypass on type 2 diabetes mellitus. *Ann Surg* 2003;238:467–484; discussion 84–85.
Schauer PR, Ikramuddin S, Gourash WF. Laparoscopic Roux-en-Y gastric bypass: a case report at one-year follow-up. *J Laparoendosc Adv Surg Tech A* 1999;9:101–106.
Schneider BE, Villegas L, Blackburn GL, et al. Laparoscopic gastric bypass surgery: outcomes. *J Laparoendosc Adv Surg Tech A* 2003; 13:247–255.
Wittgrove AC, Clark GW, Tremblay LJ. Laparoscopic gastric bypass, Roux-en-Y: preliminary report of five cases. *Obes Surg* 1994;4:353–357.

COMMENTARY

Laparoscopy truly brought bariatric surgery "out of the closet," where it had been since the 1970s. Until recently surgeons practicing bariatric surgery were both rare and quiet; morbid obesity was a socially shameful condition, and bariatric surgery was stung by some disastrous outcomes with early iterations. By the time the Roux-en-Y bypass was refined and popularized it seemed that it was too late. Two developments in the early- and mid-1990s served to change that: The first is a phenomenal epidemic of morbid obesity worldwide, with a growing awareness by society of the cost and morbidity of the condition. It is certainly no longer possible to hide these people away when they comprise 30% to 40% of the population and cost health systems hundreds of millions of dollars each year. The second development was the application of laparoscopy to the procedure. This introduced the concept of bariatric surgery to a new generation of surgeons—a generation raised on the concept of leveraging minimally invasive access to introducing new techniques into programs and practices—for academic or entrepreneurial benefit. Both factors have led to a tremendous growth in the practice of bariatrics; more patients are requesting this less morbid procedure and more surgeons and hospitals are performing it. On the whole this growth has been a good thing, making the surgery available to a larger number of patients, stimulating investment in technology and basic science research, facilitating outcomes research, and creating a career path for young surgeons. There have also been downsides to this rapid adoption, such as ill-prepared individuals launching practices without adequate training or preparation and institutions launching programs without establishing all of the support systems described by Drs. Leslie, Kellogg, and Ikramuddin. In some cases, this has led to patient harm, bad perceptions of the practice of bariatrics, and a restriction of insurance coverage.

This chapter illustrates another benefit of the increased volume and distribution of bariatric surgery—it allows surgeons to rapidly explore innovations and refinements in traditional techniques. These innovations can be anything from slight alterations in traditional technique that decrease complications or increase efficiency to a major rethinking of the surgery itself, as we are seeing with descriptions of endoluminal approaches. Such innovation seldom occurred in earlier days, when there were few practitioners and each person jealously clung to the exact methods of his or her mentor with almost superstitious fervor. The authors describe several elegant time-saving and complication-preventing "tricks" used in their method of laparoscopic gastric bypass, which certainly justifies their inclusion in a "mastery of surgery" textbook. Surgeons interested in bariatric surgery would do well both to closely study the small details of this operative description and to observe the spirit of innovation that stimulated their discovery.

LLS

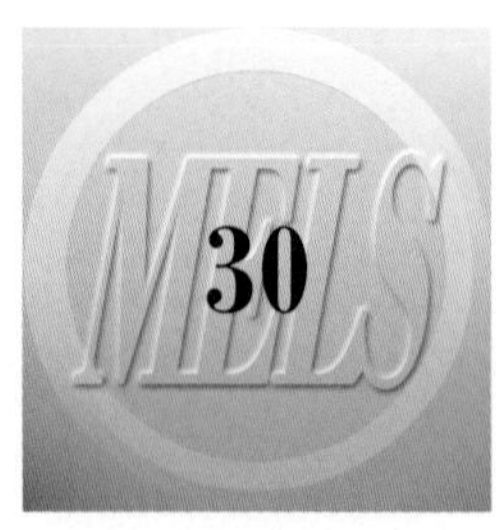

30 Laparoscopic Duodenal Switch and Sleeve Gastrectomy

VIVEK N. PRACHAND

INTRODUCTION

There has been a growing recognition on the part of the public and the medical profession that (1) obesity is an epidemic chronic disease affecting nearly every organ system; (2) behavioral and pharmacologic attempts at achieving significant and sustained weight loss are generally ineffective, particularly in the case of severe obesity; and (3) the development of laparoscopic techniques for bariatric procedures have made them relatively safe and effective. As a consequence, the number of individuals in the U.S. receiving bariatric operations increased nine-fold, from 13,000 to over 121,000, between 1998 and 2004. Roux-en-Y gastric bypass (RYGB) and laparoscopic adjustable gastric banding (LAGB) comprise over 90% of these operations. There has been a growing interest, however, in biliopancreatic diversion (BPD) with duodenal switch (DS), particularly in regard to the surgical treatment of superobese patients (body mass index, or BMI $\geq$50 kg/m^2). This interest is based on the finding in two recent meta-analyses suggesting that weight loss following BPD or DS may be superior to RYGB or LAGB, as well as the recognition of inadequate weight loss following RYGB or LAGB in superobese patients. The latter observation is of particular concern given that the prevalence of superobesity has increased nearly five-fold over the past 15 years.

Biliopancreatic diversion with duodenal switch is a hybrid operation described by Hess in 1988 and first performed laparoscopically by Gagner in 1999. It combines the DeMeester duodenal switch, initially developed for the treatment and prevention of bile reflux following gastric resection, with the Scopinaro biliopancreatic diversion, first performed in 1976, and offers another option for the treatment of severe obesity. In contrast to the 15 to 30 cc gastric pouch created during RYGB, the restrictive component of DS is provided by a vertical or "sleeve" gastrectomy that results in resection of approximately 80% of the gastric reservoir and parietal cell mass while leaving the antrum and pylorus anatomically and functionally intact (Fig. 30-1). The distal end of the 150 to 200 cc DS "pouch" consists of a short segment of postpyloric duodenum, which is hypothesized to provide improved calcium and iron absorption and to decrease the risk of stomal ulceration. The malabsorptive component of the procedure is provided by a distal Roux-en-Y reconstruction, with limb lengths measured in a retrograde fashion from the ileocecal junction (rather than antegrade from the ligament of Treitz, as in RYGB) and the distal anastomosis fashioned 50 to 100 cm proximal to the ileocecal junction. As with RYGB, the presence of antegrade flow of biliopancreatic secretions is thought to preclude the "blind loop syndrome" seen with the earlier, and more malabsorptive, jejunoileal bypass with sequelae including arthropathy and liver failure. By limiting the admixture of biliopancreatic secretions and ingested food to a relatively short "common channel" (CC), there is reduced absorption of macro- and micronutrients, with fat and starch malabsorption particularly marked. The relative contributions of restriction and malabsorption to

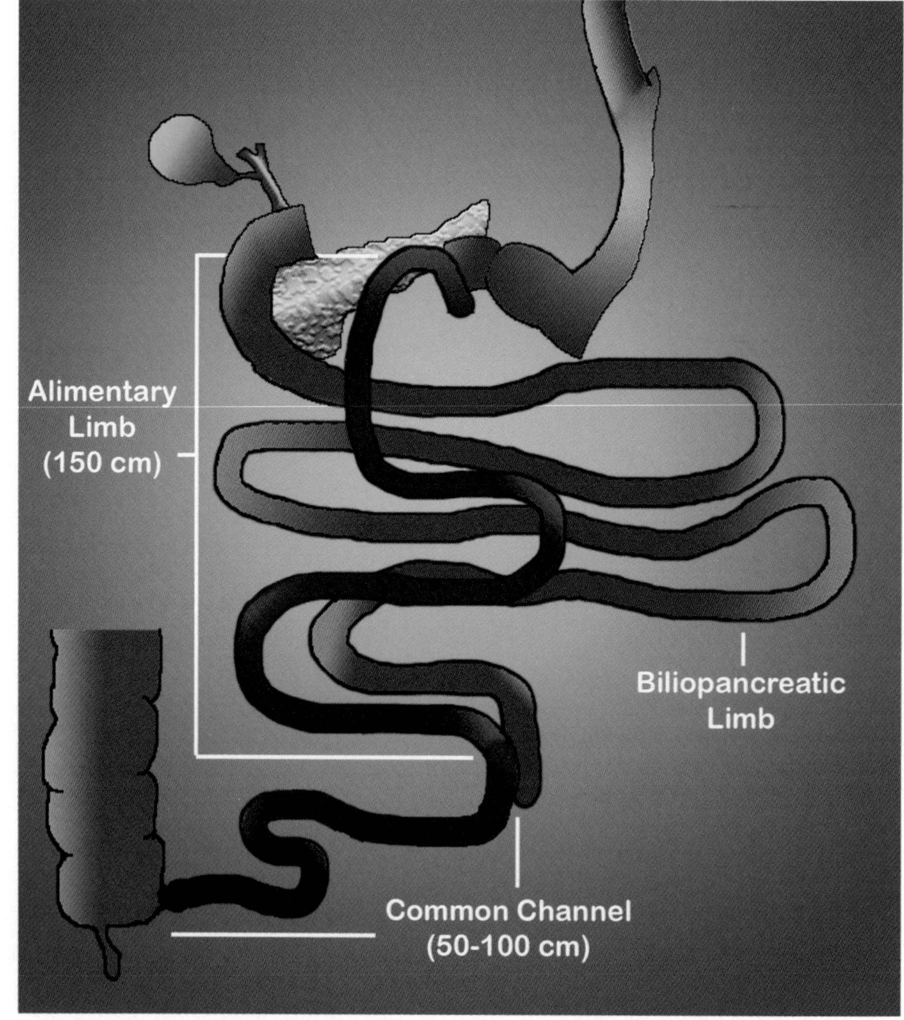

Fig. 30-1. Duodenal switch anatomy.

weight loss and maintenance of weight loss following DS are not well characterized.

While it is our practice to use the fixed limb lengths (150-cm alimentary limb, 100-cm common channel) to perform the Roux-en-Y reconstruction, there is considerable disagreement amongst surgeons in this regard. Hess and others describe using an alimentary limb that is 40% of the entire small bowel length with a common channel that is 10% of the small bowel length, both rounded to the nearest 25-cm increment with a maximum common channel length of 100 cm. We have chosen a fixed limb length approach to allow improved standardization, and have chosen the common channel length of 100 cm, erring on the side of potentially inadequate weight loss in an effort to reduce the likelihood of excessive malabsorption.

Another area of significant contention is the method used for bowel measurement, given that the degree of bowel stretch (moderate vs. unstretched) and the anesthetic technique used (general ± epidural) can substantially influence the measurements obtained. Our approach has been to use moderate stretch, using the known measurements of the bowel graspers to visually gauge 10-cm increments. While other authors describe the routine use of premeasured umbilical tapes or rulers, ultimately it is the consistency of the application of the technique that is of greater importance than the actual technique utilized. After all, the measurement of bowel length is a rough approximation of the luminal surface area, which is dependent on the epithelial microstructure (and as such cannot be practically measured) to a far greater degree than the length of the bowel itself.

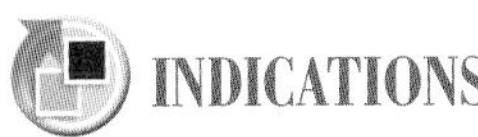

INDICATIONS

The perceived increased perioperative and nutritional risks of DS as well as the greater technical complexity of the procedure, particularly when performed laparoscopically, have limited its widespread adaptation. All patients undergoing DS should be appropriate candidates for bariatric surgery based on current National Institute of Health (NIH) criteria: severe obesity (BMI ≥40 kg/m^2 or 35 to 40 kg/m^2 with significant obesity-related comorbidities); history of multiple previous nonsurgical weight loss attempts; adequate comprehension and support; and absence of active substance abuse or poorly controlled psychological disorders. In our experience, however, we generally limit our recommendation for DS to superobese patients (BMI ≥50kg/m^2), as it is this group of patients for whom the potential benefit of a higher likelihood of successful weight loss may justify the greater potential of developing nutritional deficiencies. While it can be reasonable to perform DS on non-superobese patients, it is particularly important that the lack of demonstrably advantageous weight loss or comorbidity improvement in this patient group as well as the risks of excessive weight loss, macro- and micronutrient deficiencies, and steatorrhea be substantially discussed as part of the informed consent.

Given the higher morbidity and mortality rates seen in several series following DS in super-superobese patients (BMI ≥60 kg/m^2), Gagner has proposed a two-stage approach as a safer alternative to DS in this patient group. The approach, which has demonstrated substantial reduction in complication rates as compared to a historical cohort, consists of laparoscopic sleeve gastrectomy followed by interval duodenoileostomy and ileoileostomy 6 to 12 months later. While we have used this planned two-staged approach in the setting of extreme superobesity (BMI ≥70 kg/m^2), quite often the intraabdominal findings favor a reasonably expeditious completion of the entire procedure, particularly in female patients. Conversely, we have had instances when intraoperative findings such as massive hepatomegaly or an excessively thick, noncompliant abdominal wall precluded effective laparoscopic completion of the entire DS. In these cases, rather than convert to an open procedure with its attendant increased risk of wound complications and potentially challenging visualization, we stopped the procedure after completion of the sleeve gastrectomy. As such, we feel that sound intraoperative surgical judgment, rather than absolute BMI criteria, should determine whether a staged approach is used, and that this possibility be discussed with the patient at the time of informed consent.

CONTRAINDICATIONS

Prior to incorporating laparoscopic DS into their bariatric practice, the surgeon should have experience in all aspects of the perioperative management of bariatric surgical patients, have progressed well beyond the technical learning curve associated with laparoscopic RYGB, and have a multidisciplinary team available that includes advanced nutritional expertise and a commitment to achieve at least a 75% long-term follow-up. Contraindications to laparoscopic DS are similar to those of laparoscopic RYGB. Medical contraindications include the inability to safely tolerate general anesthesia, non-correctable coagulopathy, massive abdominal wall hernia, preexisting potentially malabsorptive disorders such as inflammatory bowel disease or celiac sprue, diarrhea-predominant irritable bowel syndrome, or active malignancy with reduced life expectancy. Psychosocial contraindications include poor nutritional knowledge, inadequate support, inability or unwillingness to maintain postoperative follow-up, and active alcohol or drug abuse. Additionally, we do not offer bariatric surgery to smokers, given the increased perioperative pulmonary, wound-healing, and anastomotic risks associated with cigarette use. Mandatory smoking cessation provides an opportunity to assess the patient's motivation and ability to institute a significant lifestyle change similar in magnitude to that required following surgery. Finally, it is important to assess the patient's willingness and ability to purchase postoperative vitamin supplements, as these are not always covered by the insurer.

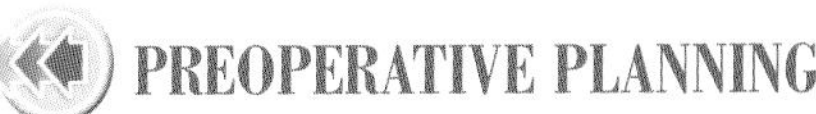

PREOPERATIVE PLANNING

All patients undergo a multidisciplinary evaluation by the surgeon, dietician, and a psychologist. In performing a complete history and physical examination, it is particularly important that the surgeon carefully assess the patient for the presence of obesity-related comorbidities, as these are often unsuspected by primary care providers in this relatively young, functional patient cohort. Specifically, diabetes and lipid panel screening are obtained if not performed within the past 12 months, and the surgeon should have a high index of suspicion for obstructive sleep apnea and a low threshold for recommending polysomnography. When identified, comorbidities should be well controlled prior to surgery so as to reduce their associated perioperative risks, despite the high likelihood that most comorbidities will substantially improve or resolve following surgery. Screening colonoscopy should be performed if not already done in patients greater than age 50, and women should be up-to-date with pelvic examinations, Pap smears, and mammography as appropriate for their age and medical history.

Patient education is a critical component of both the evaluation and the informed consent process. In an information session prior to evaluation, patients are informed regarding the rationale for bariatric surgery and the various surgical interventions available, including their relative advantages, disadvantages, and risks. The recommendation of a specific procedure is provided by the surgeon at the time of individual evaluation, based on the severity of obesity, nature of obesity-related comorbidities, and patient preference. A full day of education and preparation is scheduled 2 to 3 weeks prior to surgery, during which patients return to the clinic for an updated history and physical, nutrition education, and nursing education regarding postoperative expectations, as well as an initiation of the postoperative vitamin regimen. A detailed information session thoroughly describing surgical risks, complications, outcomes, and follow-up is held, with mandatory concomitant attendance by the patient's identified support person.

Consultation in the anesthesia clinic is scheduled on this day as well. In addition to laboratory testing ordered by the anesthesiologist, nutritional parameters (complete blood count, complete metabolic profile, iron studies, B12, zinc, selenium, PT/INR, and vitamins A, E, and D) are obtained. Preoperative deficiencies are surprisingly frequent, and repletion is initiated when they are identified. Additionally, patients who are at exceptionally high risk of thromboembolism (BMI ≥60 kg/m^2, history of previous deep vein thrombosis (DVT) or pulmonary embolism (PE), chronic venous insufficiency, age greater than 55 years, non-ambulatory patients, hypercoagulability) are referred to a vascular surgeon for evaluation for perioperative placement of a retrievable inferior vena cava (IVC) filter. The device is usually inserted after anesthesia induction immediately prior to DS, except in cases where a two-staged DS is being contemplated (BMI ≥70 kg/m^2). These massive patients are at increased risk of pressure-related neuropraxias and gluteal rhabdomyolysis with prolonged anesthetic immobilization. As such, in this setting the device is placed a few days earlier so as to provide the bariatric surgeon with additional continuous anesthetic time to be used to potentially perform a single-staged DS based on intraoperative findings and surgical judgment.

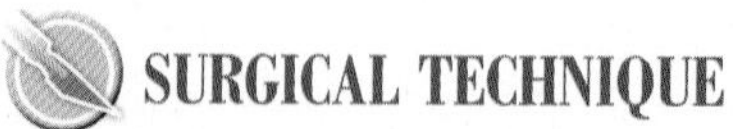

SURGICAL TECHNIQUE

A clear liquid diet is initiated the day prior to surgery. We routinely use a mechanical bowel prep (phospho-soda) to facilitate laparoscopic visualization via small bowel and colon decompression. In addition to bathing, patients are instructed to use 2% chlorhexidine gluconate wipes the night before and the morning of surgery. If the patient uses a continuous positive airway pressure (CPAP) or bi-level positive airway pressure (BiPAP) device, they are instructed to bring their mask and machine for the hospital stay. A second-generation intravenous antibiotic is given prior to skin incision.

Patient Positioning and Port Placement

While several groups have described the use of the "French" position with the patient supine and legs abducted, our preference is for the supine position with upper extremities placed out on arm boards. Padded belts are used across the hips and lower extremities for added security during table manipulation. In general, ports are placed slightly lower than those for gastric bypass to optimize duodenal mobilization and proximal anastomosis. The operating surgeon stands on the patient's right side during gastric mobilization and duodenal transection and moves to the patient's left side for the remaining portions of the procedure.

Initial peritoneal access is gained under direct visualization using an optical trocar just to the left of midline approximately 17 cm below the xiphoid. After obtaining pneumoperitoneum and confirming safe abdominal entry, a 5-mm port is placed in the right anterior axillary line 2 cm below the costal margin for placement of a liver retractor (Diamond-Flex triangular retractor; Snowden-Pencer; Atlanta, GA), which elevates the left liver, exposing the anterior stomach, and is secured using a self-retaining holder. We find this to be preferable to the use of the Nathanson liver retractor (Cook Medical; Bloomington, IN) in the subxiphoid position, as it facilitates retractor repositioning as different gastroduodenal exposures are needed. The remaining four ports are positioned as shown in Figure 30-2A. Of particular importance is the triangulated positioning of the operating ports and camera for optimal creation of the duodenoileostomy (Fig. 30-2C) and bowel measurement, ileal transection, and ileoileostomy (Fig. 30-2D). Dilating ports are used throughout except for the 15-mm bladed trocar placed just to the right of the falciform ligament, which allows the use of thick-tissue stapler during sleeve gastrectomy and facilitates the retrieval of the

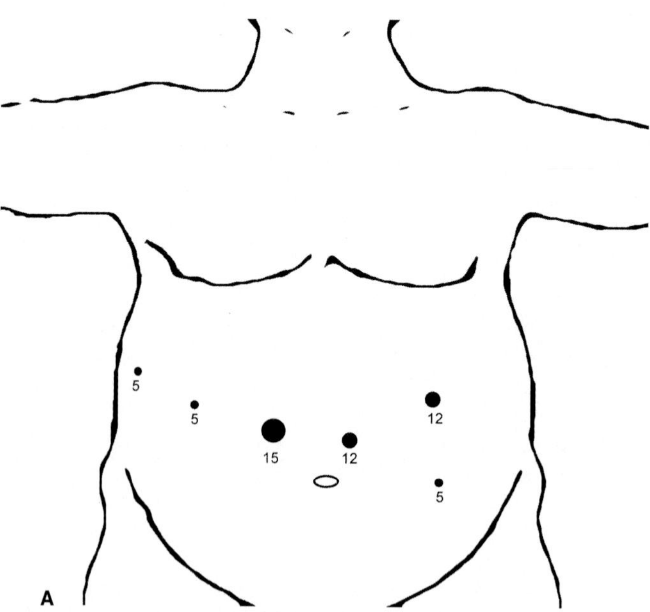

Fig. 30-2. Port placement for laparoscopic duodenal switch. **A.** Trocar postioning and sizes. **B.** Sleeve gastrectomy/duodenal transection. The surgeon stands on the patient's right side and the assistant on the left. **C.** Duodenoileostomy. The table is slightly rotated towards the surgeon standing on the left side. Additional lifts for the surgeon are often necessary to improve suturing ergonomics. **D.** Bowel measurement and ileoileostomy.

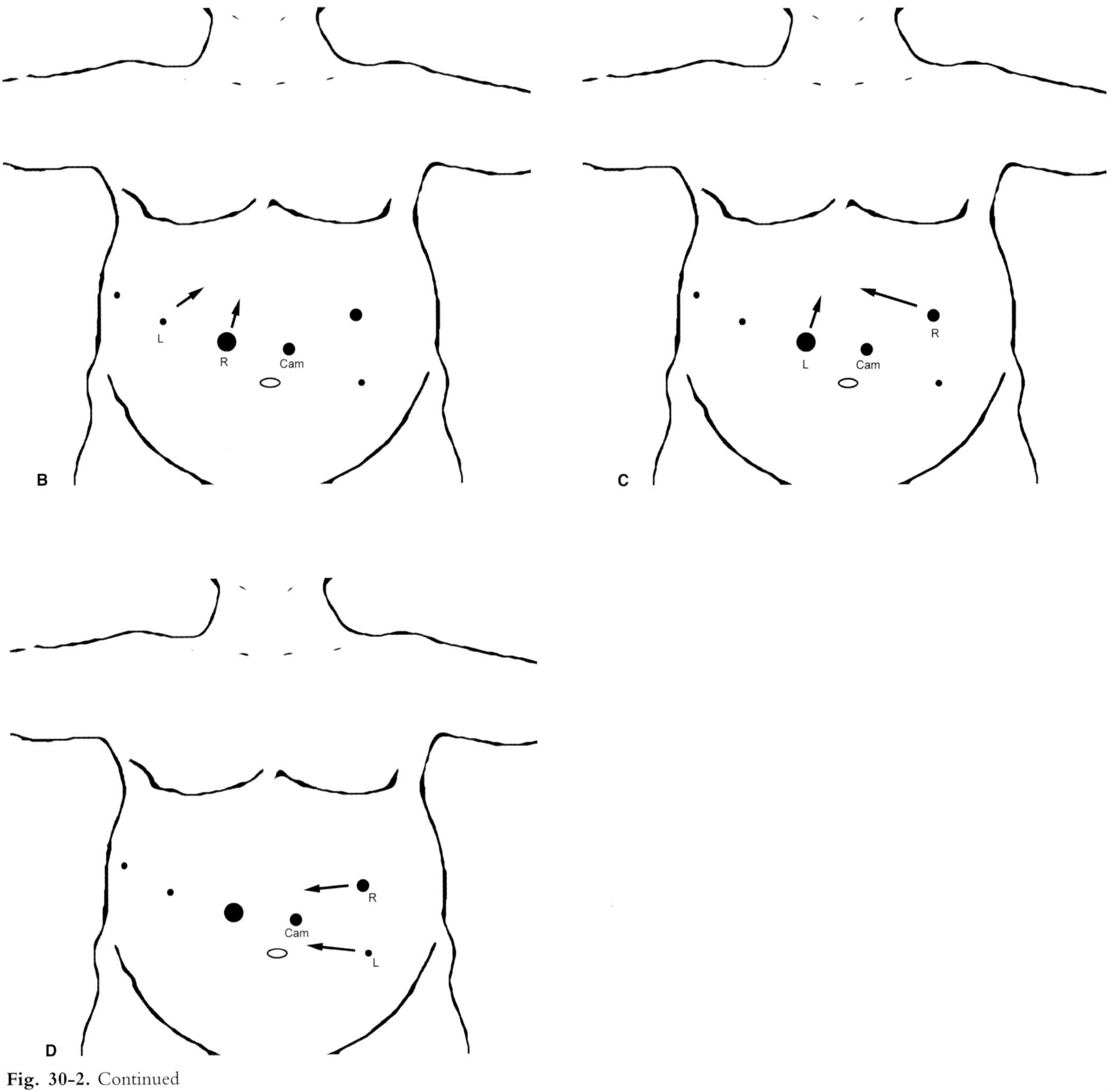

Fig. 30-2. Continued

resected stomach without extensive additional fascial dilation. While it is useful to have extra-long ports available, particularly for the 5-mm left lateral port site, they are not generally necessary. A 5- or 10-mm 45-degree laparoscope is used for the entirety of the operation after initial abdominal access. If the falciform ligament is particularly bulky and obscures the proximal duodenum, a "falciform sling" is created using a heavy suture passed via an epigastric counter-incision and a fascial closure device on either side of the most redundant portion of the falciform.

Sleeve Gastrectomy

With the surgeon standing on the patient's right side (Fig. 30-2B), a 2-0 braided polyester seromuscular stitch is used to mark the pylorus anteriorly, creating a readily visible landmark during both gastric and duodenal mobilization. This stitch can be particularly helpful when a two-stage procedure is performed, as adhesions encountered at the second stage may obscure ready visual identification of the pylorus. The entire greater curve is mobilized from the antrum 5 to 6 cm proximal to the pylorus to the left crus, including division of all posterior gastropancreatic adhesions, using ultrasonic coagulating shears or bipolar device. If the device cannot safely reach the cephalad aspect of the mobilization, it is our preference to place an additional 5-mm subxiphoid port rather than open an extra-long dissecting device. A 60F bougie is then passed transorally and oriented along the lesser curve. This is facilitated by retracting the greater curve anteriorly, allowing gravity to move the bougie to the desired position (Fig. 30-3, page 276).

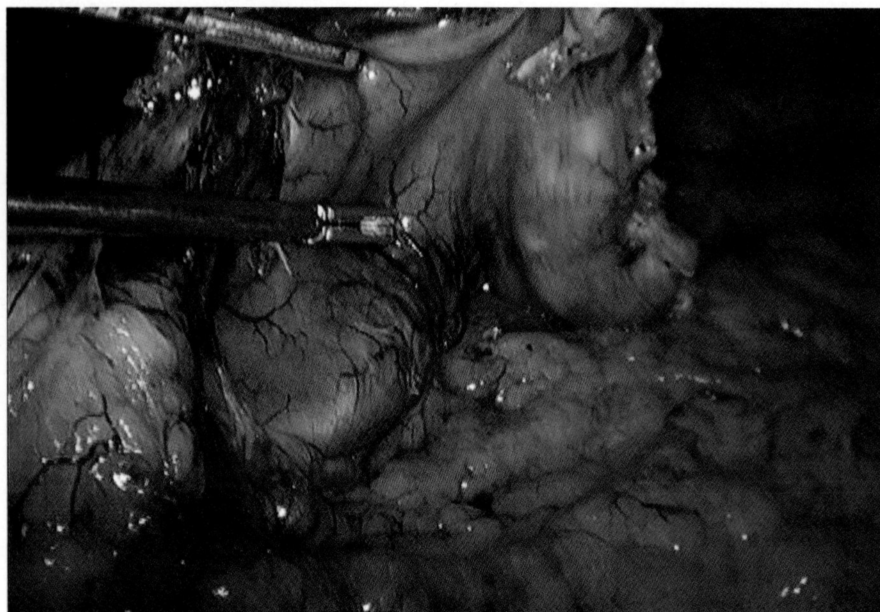

Fig. 30-3. Bougie positioning. Gravity is used to position the bougie along the lesser curvature by retracting the greater curvature anteriorly.

With the bougie in place, six to nine firings of a thick-tissue linear 60-4.8 (green) stapler with bioabsorbable buttressing material are used to perform the resection. In some cases, marked thickness of the distal antrum may preclude the use of buttressing material. Care is taken to keep the staple lines within the same horizontal plane so as to avoid "corkscrewing" of the sleeve, which can result in a functional obstruction that is not easily amenable to endoscopic dilation. We do not tightly oppose the stapler to the bougie as some authors suggest. Proximal gastric division takes place near the angle of His to avoid leaving any significant fundus, which can dilate substantially over time, resulting in an hourglass shape of the gastric sleeve and partial gastric outlet obstruction (Fig. 30-4). Similarly, care must be taken to avoid excessive angulation of the staple line near the incisura. Following resection, the gastrectomy specimen is placed in the left upper quadrant for retrieval near the completion of the operation to avoid compromise of the pneumoperitoneum and port displacement following fascial dilation.

At this point of the operation, if there has been any physiologic compromise of the patient, or the surgeon judges the technical feasibility of the remaining malabsorptive portion of the operation to be questionable, the specimen can be retrieved and the procedure terminated. A return to the operating room takes place after a 100- to 150-pound weight loss plateau is reached, usually between 9 and 15 months after surgery. As previously mentioned, this possibility should be discussed with the patient preoperatively, and if the staged approach was unplanned, the rationale needs to be carefully documented.

Sleeve gastrectomy alone as a primary bariatric operation has been gaining in popularity amongst both bariatric surgeons and patients, with early weight loss results approaching those seen with adjustable gastric banding and even gastric bypass. The technique is similar to that described above, though a smaller bougie (34 to 46F) is typically used. There is a perceived advantage in the avoidance of significant malabsorption and its attendant risk of long-term malnutrition, as well as the technical expertise required and risks entailed during creation of duodenoileal anastomosis. It is important to note, however, that many (if not the majority) of the leaks following DS occur high along the sleeve staple line, often near the angle of His, as opposed to either enteroenteral anastomosis. Furthermore, long-term weight loss efficacy (beyond four years) has not been established with sleeve gastrectomy alone, and substantial sleeve dilation has been anecdotally described.

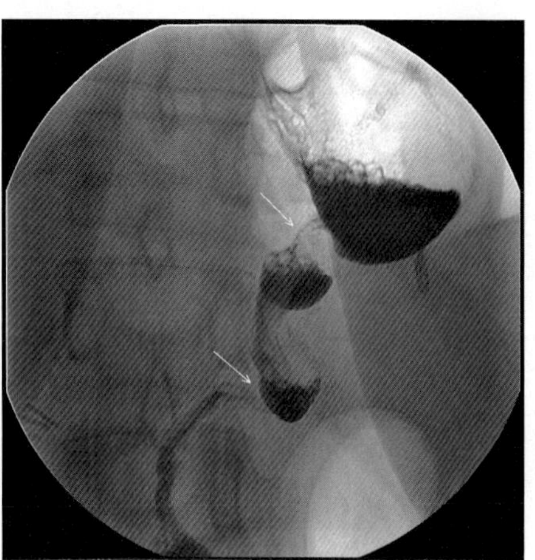

Fig. 30-4. "Hourglass" sleeve gastrectomy.

Duodenal Transection

The assistant on the patient's left side retracts the antrum laterally to linearize the first portion of the duodenum. Monopolar hook electrocautery is used first to incise the peritoneum along the inferior aspect of the duodenum to the head of the pancreas, then along the superior margin to the junction of D1 and D2. A formal Kocher maneuver is not usually required for adequate D1 mobilization. Careful circumferential retroduodenal dissection just proximal to the duodenal fusion with the head of the pancreas is performed. This generally takes place 3 to 5 cm distal to the pylorus and usually requires the division of one or two vessels traveling from the pancreas to the duodenum using ultrasonic coagulating shears. The duodenum is then transected using a roticulating linear 60-3.5 (blue) stapler with bioabsorbable buttressing material placed only on the anvil side, with the non-buttressed cartridge passed beneath the duodenum anterior to the pancreas. In addition to providing mechanical reinforcement and reducing bleeding from the staple line, the buttressing material straightens the duodenal cuff staple line, facilitating subsequent creation of the duodenoileostomy. We do not routinely oversew the duodenal stump staple line. Passing the blunt and relatively thick stapler cartridge beneath the duodenum requires creation of a larger retroduodenal window but reduces the risk of injury to the pancreas and duodenum, and omission of the buttressing material on the cartridge side reduces the resistance of its passage through the retroduodenal window. After careful inspection of the staple lines, a seromuscular 2-0 braided polyester suture is placed near the inferior corner of the duodenal cuff staple line, with its tail cut 3 to 4 cm in length to facilitate the proximal anastomosis described below.

Creation of Alimentary (ROUX) Limb

The greater omentum is retracted cephalad, and a sagittal slit is created in the omentum beginning at the edge of the right transverse colon to facilitate antecolic passage of the alimentary limb to the duodenal cuff. The surgeon moves to the patient's left side and, using atraumatic bowel graspers, identifies the ileocecal junction. The ileum is measured 100 cm in a retrograde fashion, whereupon two antimesenteric seromuscular marking stitches are placed. By convention, we cut the distal suture short and leave the proximal suture long to maintain proper bowel orientation. From this point, the ileum is measured an additional 150 cm proximally. Care is taken to place the measured ileum along the ascending colon to avoid twisting of the mesentery. The transection point is selected within a few centimeters from this site so as to optimize the mobility of the alimentary limb, and the bowel and its mesentery divided with a linear 60-2.5 (white) stapler with bioabsorbable buttressing material in the surgeon's right hand while the distal pancreaticobiliary limb is held in the surgeon's left hand. Without letting go with the left hand, a 2-0 seromuscular marking stitch is placed in the antimesenteric corner of the distal biliopancreatic limb to obviate confusion with the alimentary limb. The latter is then brought cephalad in an antecolic fashion to the postpyloric duodenal cuff through the previously fashioned omental slit with its mesentery facing to the patient's left side. In the rare instance (2% to 3%) of excessive tension with this configuration, the alimentary limb is passed in a retrocolic fashion through a mesocolic window created to the right of the middle colic vessels.

Duodenoileostomy

A variety of anastomotic techniques for creation of the duodenoileostomy have been described, including circular-stapled, linear-stapled, and hand-sutured. Early in our experience, we used the circular-stapled approach as described by Gagner. We occasionally encountered difficulties passing both the 25- and 21-mm EEA anvils through the pylorus, however, and while this difficulty could be overcome by placement of the anvil directly in the duodenal cuff, at times the lumen of the alimentary limb would not easily accommodate even the 21-mm EEA device. We then used a linear-stapled technique with hand-sutured closure of the common enterotomy, similar to that used for gastrojejunostomy by several authors during gastric bypass, but were dissatisfied with the anastomotic diameter consistently obtained. Since mid-2004, we have been using a two-layer hand-sutured technique with negligible leak and stricture rates.

The surgeon remains on the patient's left side, but moves his left hand from the 5-mm left lateral port to the 15-mm right medial port, with the camera remaining between his hands in the initial 12-mm port (Fig. 30-2C). The table is tilted toward the surgeon, who may use additional lifts as necessary to provide an appropriate ergonomic suturing position with elbows in and shoulders relaxed. The assistant stands on the patient's right side and uses a grasper via the 5-mm right upper lateral port to follow the suture and maintain tension.

The posterior outer layer of the anastomosis is created by approximating the staple line of the duodenal cuff to the antimesenteric border of the proximal alimentary limb in a running manner, using a 20-cm length of 2-0 braided polyester suture on an SH needle beginning at the cephalad corner and tied to the traction stitch placed following duodenal transection. Enterotomies are made in the anterior wall along the entire length of this posterior row to maximize the anastomotic diameter using ultrasonic coagulating shears. The inner layer is started at the midpoint of the enterotomies using two separate 25-cm 2-0 polyglycolic acid sutures on an SH needle using full-thickness continuous suturing posteriorly (Fig. 30-5) transitioned to a running Connell stitch at the corners and tied together at the midpoint of the anterior inner layer. The outer anterior layer is then performed in a running Lembert fashion, again using a 20-cm length of 2-0 braided polyester and also tied to the inferior duodenal cuff traction stitch.

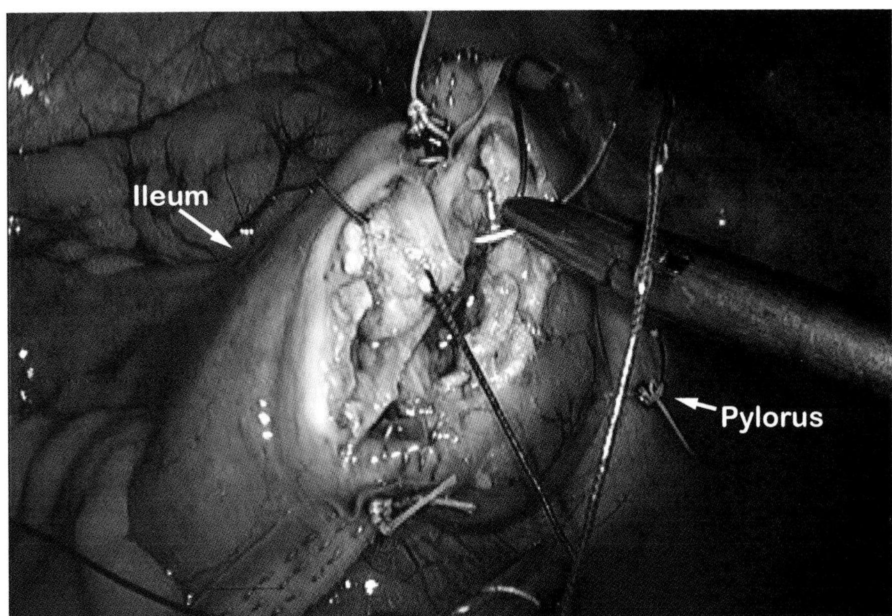

Fig. 30-5. Duodenoileostomy. The inner layer is performed with a 25-cm length of 2-0 polyglycolic acid suture on an SH needle.

Ileoileostomy

The patient is rotated back to the midline, and the surgeon moves his left hand back to the 5-mm left lateral port. The alimentary limb is followed distal to the duodenoileostomy, tucking it along the medial aspect of the ascending colon, until the two marking stitches previously placed 100 cm proximal to the ileocecal valve are encountered. The distal end of the pancreaticobiliary limb, which is readily identified in the foreground by its marking stitch when the alimentary limb is tucked laterally, is approximated to the alimentary limb at this level using interrupted 2-0 braided polyester Lembert sutures. When properly oriented, the edge of the pancreaticobiliary limb mesentery faces the left upper quadrant and forms a "V" with the edge of the mesentery of the alimentary limb. Small enterotomies just large enough to accommodate the linear stapler are created in the antimesenteric border of either limb of intestine through which the jaws of the EndoGIA 60-2.5

(white) stapler are introduced. After the stapler is deployed, we routinely hand-suture, rather than staple, the resulting common enterotomy using a single layer running Connell stitch with 2-0 braided polyester, as there is substantial risk of narrowing the anastomosis with stapled closure given the relatively small caliber of the ileum at this level. Two Brolin seromuscular antiobstruction stitches are placed just proximal and distal to the linear staple line.

Closure of Hernia Defects

The mesenteric defect of the ileoileostomy is closed in a running fashion using 2-0 braided polyester suture. Optimal management of the Petersen hernia defect remains controversial, however, with some authors recommending complete closure, including seromuscular incorporation of the transverse colon, while others recommend leaving the defect widely open with the assumption that a wider defect reduces the risk of incarceration. We have generally used the latter approach unless the Roux limb was passed retrocolic, in which case the defect is closed by approximating the mesenteric staple line to the transverse mesocolon, or if additional division of the ileal mesentery was necessary to provide adequate alimentary limb mobilization without undue tension. Regardless of the approach taken, the surgeon needs to have a high index of suspicion for internal hernia as the etiology of abdominal pain in all postbariatric patients with a Roux-en-Y reconstruction, as the radiographic evaluation of internal hernia is relatively insensitive, and internal hernia defects may reopen years after the initial operation.

The fascia of the 15-mm port site is slightly dilated and a large specimen retrieval bag is introduced, into which the resected stomach is placed. By keeping a small corner of the proximal or distal gastric staple line just outside the cinched bag, the resected stomach can usually be removed without extending the skin or fascial incision. Three or four 0-polyglycolic acid ties are passed using the fascial closure device for eventual port site closure, and the 15-mm port reinserted.

Anastomotic Testing

After confirming adequate hemostasis, a laparoscopic bowel clamp is passed via the left upper lateral 12-mm port site and used to occlude the alimentary limb 30 cm distal to the duodenoileostomy. The gastric sleeve, antrum, and duodenoileostomy are submerged in saline irrigation, and upper GI endoscopy is performed using medium-flow endoscopic insufflation to test the integrity of the gastric sleeve staple line as well as the proximal anastomosis. If air bubbles are seen, Lembert sutures are placed until these are eliminated. The endoscope and bowel clamp are removed, and a 19 Blake drain placed via the right upper quadrant 5-mm port site oriented near the duodenoileostomy and extending along the gastric staple line into the left upper quadrant.

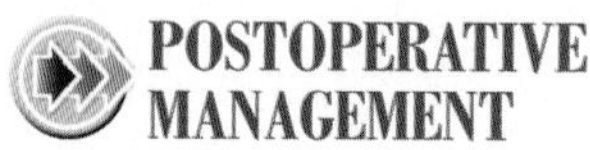

POSTOPERATIVE MANAGEMENT

Patients are extubated in the operating room and admitted to an intermediate care unit with telemetry and continuous pulse oximetry after discharge from the recovery room. Patient-controlled intravenous narcotic analgesia (without a continuous basal infusion dose) is used for pain control, with ketorolac added if renal function is normal. Ambulation and low-carbohydrate clear liquids are initiated on the morning of postoperative day 1, and enoxaparin 40 to 100 mg SQ bid is initiated and titrated to a near-therapeutic level, where it is continued for 2 to 3 weeks after discharge. If an IVC filter was placed, DVT prophylaxis is continued until device removal 4 to 6 weeks after surgery. The diet is advanced to pureed food on postoperative day 2. Discharge usually takes place between postoperative days 2 and 4, after demonstration of diet tolerance and return of bowel function. We do not obtain a routine postoperative upper GI contrast study. Pureed diet is maintained for 2 weeks, followed by soft diet for a month and regular diet thereafter with a goal of 80 to 90 g of protein/day. Regular vitamin supplements (multivitamin, B-complex, calcium citrate with vitamin D, vitamin A, and vitamin D) are started 2 weeks postoperatively. A proton pump inhibitor is used for the first month, and ursodeoxycholic acid is used for the first 6 months after surgery if the gallbladder is still present.

Patients are seen by the surgeon and bariatric dietician at all postoperative appointments. These include 1.5 weeks postoperative for drain removal, 2.5 weeks postoperative for diet advancement, and subsequent appointments at 1, 3, and 6 months, and then yearly. Nutritional parameters are rechecked at the 3-month, 6-month, and yearly visit, with supplementation adjusted accordingly.

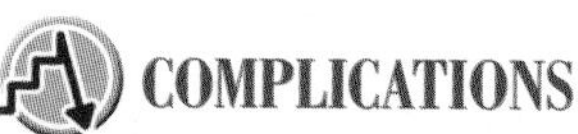

COMPLICATIONS

Laparoscopic DS is a substantially more complex procedure than RYGB and generally requires 60 to 90 minutes greater operative time with conversion rates ranging from 2% to 10%. Not surprisingly, in much of the bariatric surgical literature the perioperative complication rate of DS appears to be higher than that following RYGB, with 30-day mortality and complication rates following DS ranging from 0.9% to 8% and 15% to 38%, respectively. It is important to note, however, that the patient population in most DS series is generally heavier than in RYGB series, and usually includes a preponderance of superobese (BMI $\geq$50 kg/m^2) or super-superobese (BMI $\geq$60 kg/m^2) patients. Furthermore, in the few studies in which a direct comparison between DS and RYGB was performed, there is generally not a substantial difference in either the frequency or nature of complications, though the length of hospital stay is slightly longer with DS.

Leaks may occur at any staple line or anastomosis despite provocative intraoperative endoscopic or hydrostatic testing, and while the duodenoileostomy may appear to be the site at highest risk, in our experience (and that of other DS surgeons), the proximal gastric staple line (near the angle of His) is the most common site of leak (1% to 3%) following DS. Because radiographic-guided percutaneous drainage of this region is usually difficult, we routinely place a closed suction drain near the proximal anastomosis extending along the sleeve staple line to the left upper quadrant, as small, contained or well-drained leaks in can generally be managed nonoperatively (provided the patient is clinically stable) with antibiotics, NPO (*non per os*, or nothing by mouth), drainage, and total parenteral nutrition (TPN). Clinical instability or failure to respond to nonoperative therapy should prompt surgical intervention. In such a setting, in addition to attempting to repair the leak and placing one or more additional drain(s) adjacent to the repair, postoperative nutritional management is simplified by the insertion of a feeding jejunostomy tube in the proximal biliopancreatic limb 30 to 40 cm distal to the ligament of Treitz. Once the leak has resolved clinically and radiographically, which may require several weeks, diet is resumed and gradually advanced.

Pulmonary complications are best prevented by aggressive pulmonary toilet, incentive spirometry, early ambulation, and use of the patient's own positive airway pressure appliance if applicable. Other early complications include bleeding (4% to 5%), DVT and PE (0.5%), wound complications (1% with laparoscopy), splenectomy, and urinary tract infection. It is important to emphasize appropriate fluid intake at the time of discharge, as dehydration is the most common reason for postoperative ER visits and admissions.

The surgeon should maintain a high index of suspicion for internal hernia as the etiology of persistent recurrent abdominal pain, because the classic nausea and vomiting symptoms seen in bowel obstruction are often absent. Elevated bilirubin or transaminases may indicate biliopancreatic limb obstruction, and suggestive CT findings include spiralization of small bowel mesenteric vessels (Fig. 30-6) and duodenojejeunal dilation (Fig. 30-7). The threshold for operative reexploration should be low and can usually be performed laparoscopically in the absence of severe systemic compromise. The surgeon stands on the patient's left side and, using the previous three left-sided port incisions, begins systematic exploration at the ileocecal junction, following the alimentary limb first to the ileoileostomy, where the potential mesenteric defect is inspected, then proximally to the duodenoileostomy. If a Petersen hernia is present, this maneuver will clearly demonstrate the presence or absence of herniating bowel (usually the pancreaticobiliary limb), which can be reduced and the defect repaired. The alimentary limb is then followed distally from the duodenoileostomy to the ileoileostomy. The distal biliopancreatic limb is then identified and followed proximally to the ligament of Treitz. This systematic approach allows the surgeon to visualize all defects and maintain the proper orientation of the small bowel and its mesentery.

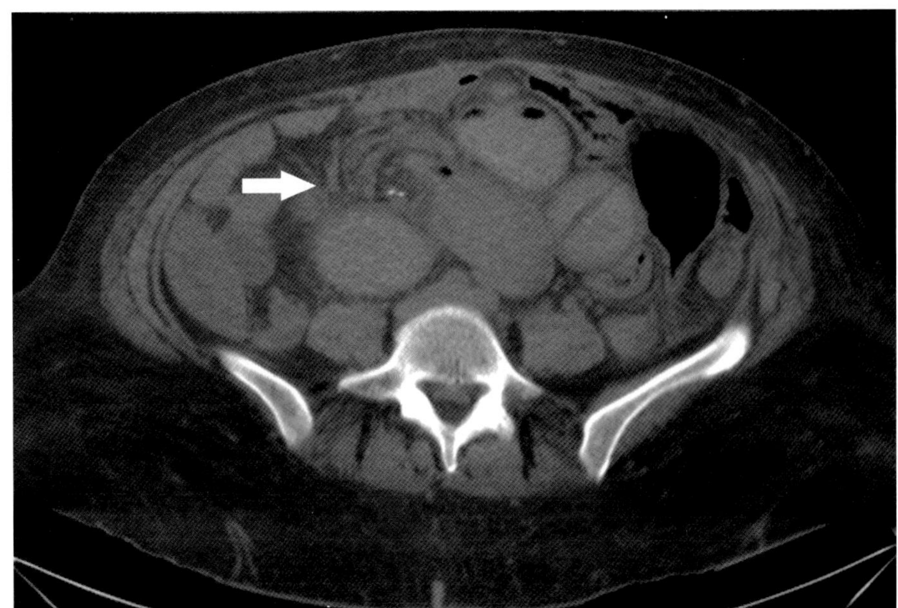

Fig. 30-6. Internal hernia. The arrow demonstrates spiralization of the mesenteric vessels. At exploration, the bioliopancratic limb was found to be herniating through the Petersen defect.

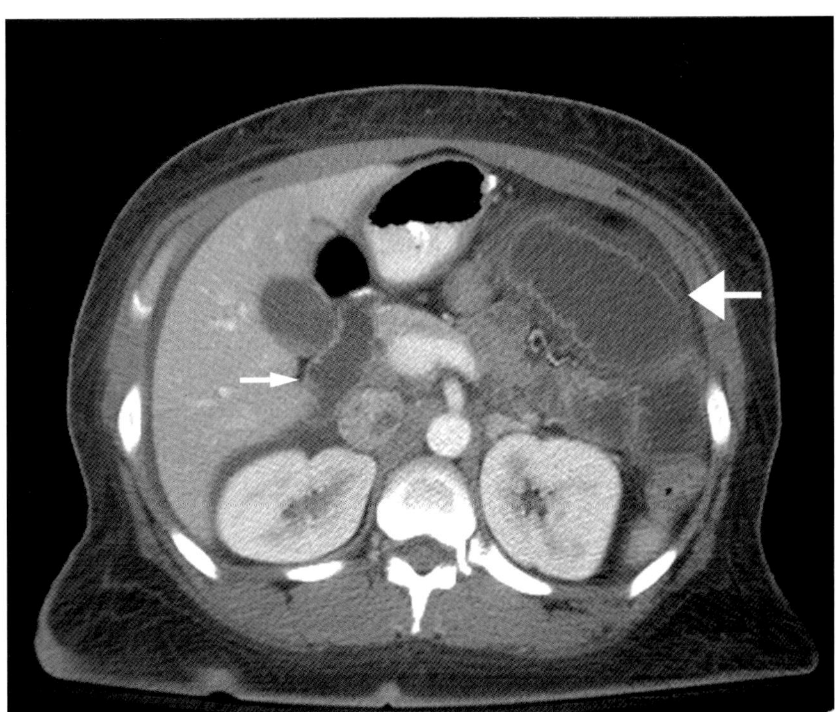

Fig. 30-7. Biliopancreatic limb obstruction. A dilated pancreaticobiliary limb (large arrowhead) and duodenal stump (small arrow) are readily apparent.

Nutritional Deficiencies

The development of the serious complications seen following the now-discredited jejunoileal bypass (JIB), including severe arthropathy and liver failure, has made many bariatric surgeons hesitant to offer procedures that utilize malabsorption as a significant mechanism of action given the lack of demonstrable advantage over restrictive procedures (RYGB and adjustable banding). While the severe complications of JIB are attributed to bacterial overgrowth and blind loop syndrome in the long segment of bypassed jejunoileum (and thus should be obviated by the Roux-en-Y reconstruction of the DS), significant nutritional deficiencies can still develop due to both the restrictive and malabsorptive components of the procedure.

Protein deficiency, manifested by a serum albumin level <3.6 g/dl, occurs in up to 25% of patients in the first 6 months following surgery and is persistent in 5% of patients 2 years after surgery. Reduced protein intake (<80 to 90 g protein/d) and obligate daily GI protein loss of up to 30 g (normal is 6 g), rather than malabsorption per se, appears to play the major role: Scopinaro has shown that 70% of ingested protein is absorbed following BPD with a 50-cm common channel. Moderate hypoalbuminemia (3.0 to 3.6 g/dl) is treated with protein supplements, dietary counseling, and close follow-up. Patients with severe hypoalbuminemia (<3.0 g/dl) may require hospitalization for albumin infusion with aggressive diuresis and parenteral nutritional support, as severe protein deficiency itself may impair intestinal absorption and liver function. Refeeding syndrome has been observed in these patients.

Despite regular vitamin supplementation, a high incidence of significant micronutrient deficiencies (30% to 60%) has been described following DS in some series, particularly with regards to certain fat-soluble vitamins (A, D, and K), calcium, zinc, and iron. Although it seems counterintuitive, severely obese patients may have significant preoperative micronutrient deficiencies including iron (25% to 40%), zinc (30% to 40%), selenium (40% to 60%), vitamin B12 (5% to 10%), thiamine (5% to 30%), vitamin A (10% to 15%), and vitamin D (20% to 70%). Contributing factors include poor diet quality, obesity-related inflammatory state, and biologic nutrient non-availability due to sequestration in adipose tissue. Routine identification and treatment of these macro- and micronutrient deficiencies preoperatively may help to prevent postoperative nutritional complications.

While the surgeon may not have control over the prevalence of deficiencies preoperatively, the choice of limb-length measurements used during DS likely impacts the degree of both protein and fat malabsorption. Scopinaro demonstrated a 28% fat absorption rate with a 50-cm common channel, and in studies that describe a high incidence of post-DS vitamin deficiencies, the common channel was between 50 and 75 cm. While there are no data comparing common channel length and incidence of deficiencies, several series report improvement in deficiencies when the common channel and alimentary limb are lengthened. Accordingly, we have chosen to routinely use a 100-cm common channel length in an effort to reduce their incidence.

Daily lifelong vitamin supplementation is an absolute requirement following DS and should be strongly emphasized prior to surgery. Patients should be made aware that supplements may not be covered by insurance and may cost \$20 to \$40/month. There is no evidence-based consensus regarding optimal supplementation: our protocol includes (1) multivitamin with iron; (2) calcium citrate (carbonate is not well-absorbed) with added vitamin D (1000 to 1200 mg + 800 U/d) in two doses; (3) a B-complex vitamin (without additional herbal products); (4) vitamin A (dry) 10,000 IU daily; and (5) vitamin D (dry) 10,000 IU daily in two divided doses. Gel-based and enteric coated vitamins should be avoided.

The importance of compliance with follow-up appointments and routine laboratory nutritional testing cannot be overemphasized. Indeed, difficulty maintaining adequate follow-up is another reason to proceed with caution when offering DS to patients. Documented efforts should be made to contact patients who miss appointments by phone or mail (certified if necessary). If the insurance policy no longer allows the patient to be seen by the surgeon, arrangements should be made for the primary care physician to obtain the necessary tests with adjustment of supplementation performed accordingly.

Given the current absence of evidence-based guidelines for repletion of vitamin deficiencies, it is important that bariatric programs develop protocols for vitamin repletion when deficiencies are encountered. While most deficiencies may be correctable with aggressive oral repletion, at times intravenous or intramuscular injections are necessary. Response to repletion should be followed at 1- to 3-month intervals, depending on the severity of the defect, with adjustments made accordingly.

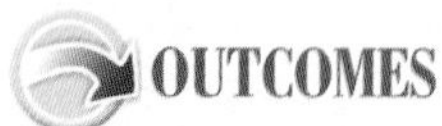

OUTCOMES

A recent meta-analysis by Buchwald et al. suggests that the percentage of excess weight lost (% EBWL) following DS may be superior to that seen with RYGB (70.1% vs. 61.2%). Direct comparative data between the two procedures, however, remains limited to single-institution cohort studies, and when the comparison includes both severely obese and superobese patients, advantageous weight loss for DS has not been demonstrated. Furthermore, because relatively few DS patients have been recruited to participate in the ongoing NIH-funded multi-center Longitudinal Assessment of Bariatric Surgery study, the question of the comparative efficacy between DS and RYGB for severe obesity will remain unresolved for the near future. Nonetheless, we have recently reviewed the weight loss outcomes in a cohort of 350 consecutive superobese patients undergoing DS (n = 198) or RYGB (n = 152) and demonstrated statistically significant differences in absolute weight loss, % EBWL, change in BMI, and likelihood of achieving >50% EBWL, all of which favored DS.

The available comparative data regarding comorbidity improvement and resolution is even more scant than that comparing weight loss, and is primarily limited to the aforementioned meta-analysis. While these data suggest a possible advantage for DS regarding diabetes, dyslipidemia, hypertension, and obstructive sleep apnea, in the absence of additional corroborating evidence, at this time these differences should not be used in the process of procedure selection.

A number of patients seek DS because they are under the impression that the reduced restriction (in comparison to RYGB) affords them the opportunity to eat "normal-sized" meals yet still lose weight. Similarly, some surgeons share this impression and refuse to offer DS because they do not want to be an "accomplice" to "cheating" of this nature. In our experience, however, the average meal size one year post-DS is 25% to 50% of the size of a typical pre-DS meal, which is very similar to that seen following RYGB.

There is a widespread perception that because of its malabsorptive component, frequent passage of malodorous stools (6 to 8 BMs/day) and flatus is a universal occurrence following DS. To a large extent, however, post-DS bowel habits can be influenced by the quantity of ingested fats and starches. On average, 6 months following DS, patients average 2 to 4 BMs/day, with two or three typically occurring within the 2 two hours after waking with another one or two in the late afternoon or evening. Interestingly, we have not always seen a robust correlation between stool frequency and magnitude of weight loss. Indeed, it may be that other poorly-understood mechanisms play significant roles, such as increased energy expenditure associated with intestinal adaptation, alterations in gut flora, or reabsorption of digestive secretions in the biliopancreatic limb.

REVISIONAL SURGERY

Inadequate weight loss is rare following DS and is generally amenable to dietary counseling and increased physical activity. We do not have any experience performing revisions that result in a reduction in the length of the common channel, and there is little description of this procedure in the literature. Rather than increasing the degree of malabsorption, some authors advocate increasing the extent of restriction by "re-sleeving" the gastric sleeve if it has dilated over time. Experience using this approach is limited to case reports,

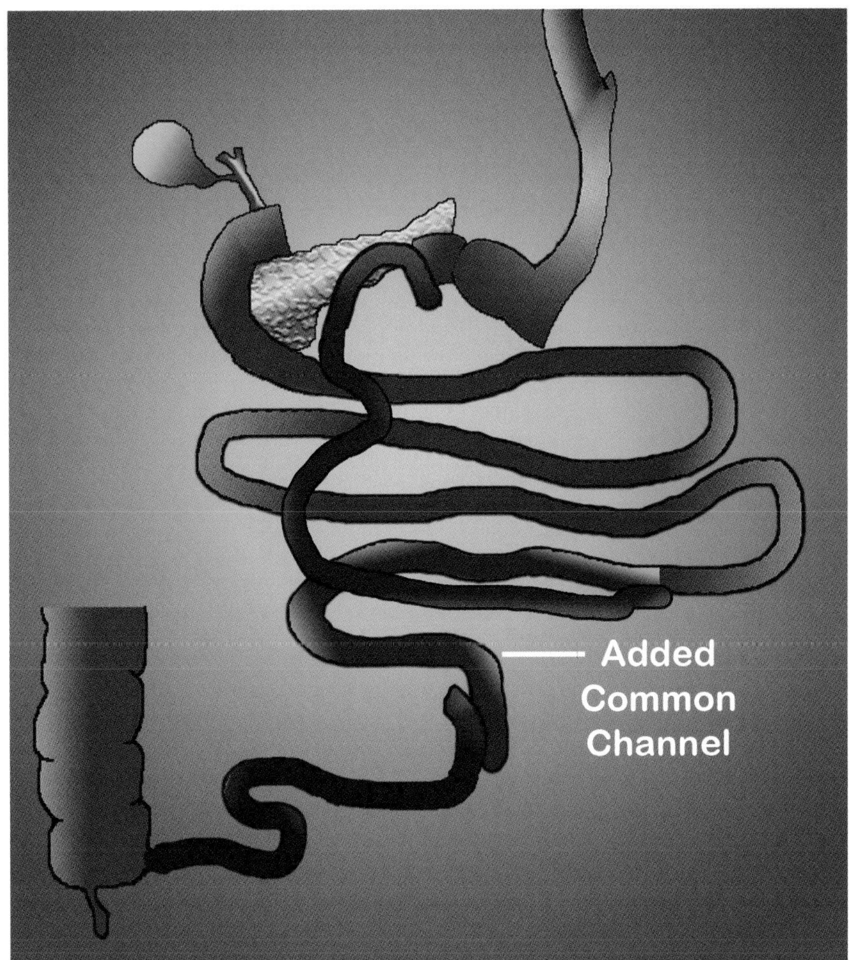

Fig. 30-8. Duodenal switch revision. Division of the alimentary limb proximal to the ileoilcostomy and performing a new anastomosis proximally along the biliopancreatic limb adds length to the common channel. Near-total reversal of malabsorption is obtained by creating the anastomosis just distal to the ligament of Treitz.

however, and an increased rate of gastric staple line complications might be anticipated in this setting.

Non-correctable nutritional deficiencies, excessive weight loss, severe alterations in bowel habits, and inability to remain compliant with post-op dietary and supplement requirements are the major indications for DS revision, which is required in 1% to 6% of all patients following DS. In DS revision, the alimentary limb is divided just proximal to the ileoileostomy. The proximal transected alimentary limb is then re-anastomosed to the biliopancreatic limb a variable distance, ranging from 100 cm proximal to the original ileoileostomy (Fig. 30-8) to a site along the proximal jejunum just distal to the ligament of Treitz. Performing the revision in this manner lengthens both the alimentary limb and the common channel, and in the latter example results in a near-complete reversal of malabsorption. The extent of the revision is based on the clinical scenario and the surgeon's judgment, and patients should be instructed that some degree of weight regain and return or exacerbation of comorbidities can occur. Laparoscopic DS revision is generally straightforward and uses the identical approach to that described earlier for the evaluation of internal hernia. A systematic approach is crucial so as to avoid any ambiguity in intestinal limb identification.

Finally, there may be a role for DS as a salvage procedure for failed restrictive procedures. While conversion to DS following adjustable gastric banding is quite straightforward, conversion to DS (laparoscopically or open) following vertical banded gastroplasty (VBG) and RYGB is exceptionally difficult, with complication rates that are generally three to five times greater than that following primary bariatric surgery. In essence, normal GI anatomy must be restored prior to proceeding with DS. If the patient has had a previous VBG, however, a Scopinaro BPD, rather than DS, might be preferable so as to avoid the dense subhepatic adhesions inevitably encountered from the prior gastroplasty and the previous vertical staple line. Regardless of the reconstructive approach taken, in these cases we almost always place a feeding jejunostomy catheter in the biliopancreatic limb 30 to 40 cm distal to the ligament of Treitz to provide enteral nutrition while the proximal staple lines and anastomoses have the opportunity to heal.

SUGGESTED READING

Anthone GJ, Lord RV, DeMeester TR, et al. The duodenal switch operation for the treatment of morbid obesity. *Ann Surg* 2003;238:618–628.

Biron S, Hould FS, Lebel S, et al. Twenty years of biliopancreatic diversion: what is the goal of the surgery? *Obes Surg* 2004;14:160–164.

Buchwald H, Avidor Y, Braunwald E, et al. Bariatric surgery: A systematic review and meta-analysis. *JAMA* October 13, 2004;292:1724–1737.

DeMeester TR, Fuchs KH, Ball CS, et al. Experimental and clinical results with proximal end-to-end duodenojejunostomy for pathologic duodenogastric reflux. *Ann Surg* 1987;206:414–426.

Deveney CW, MacCabee D, Marlink K, et al. Roux-en-Y divided gastric bypass results in the same weight loss as duodenal switch for morbid obesity. *Am J Surg* 2004;187:655–659.

Hess DS, Hess DW, Oakley, RS. The Biliopancreatic diversion with the duodenal switch: results beyond 10 years. *Obesity Surg* 2005;15:408–416.

Marceau P, Hould FS, Simard S, et al. Biliopancreatic diversion with duodenal switch. *World J Surg* 1998;22(9):947–954.

Prachand VN, DaVee RT, Alverdy JC. Duodenal switch provides superior weight loss in the super-obese (BMI ≥50 kg/m^2) compared with gastric bypass. *Ann Surg* 2006;244(4):611–619.

Ren CJ, Patterson E, Gagner M. Early results of laparoscopic biliopancreatic diversion with duodenal switch: a case series of 40 consecutive patients. *Obesity Surg* 2000;10:514–523.

Scopinaro N, Gianetta E, Adami GF, et al. Biliopancreatic diversion for obesity at eighteen years. *Surgery* 1996;119:261–268.

Slater GH, Ren CJ, Siegel N, et al. Serum fat-soluble vitamin deficiency and abnormal calcium metabolism after malabsorptive bariatric surgery. *J Gastrointest Surg* 2004;8:48–55.

Strain GW, Gagner M, Inabnet WB, et al. Comparison of effects of gastric bypass and biliopancreatic diversion with duodenal switch on weight loss and body composition 1–2 years after surgery. *SOARD* 2007;3:31–36.

Sturm R. Increases in morbid obesity in the USA: 2000–2005. *Public Health* 2007, in press.

COMMENTARY

Dr. Prachand, in this detailed and well-illustrated chapter, describes the laparoscopic duodenal switch (DS) procedure performed for the treatment of severe obesity. Although the majority of patients will either undergo a laparoscopic adjustable band procedure or Roux-en-Y gastric bypass, there is great interest in using the duodenal switch procedure in those with super obesity. The indications, contraindications, and preoperative management of the bariatric patient are described in detail. Of note, preoperative nutritional deficiencies should be identified and corrected prior to operation. Although not mentioned by the author, many bariatric surgeons now advocate a "liver shrinking" low calorie-high protein diet for several weeks preoperatively to facilitate exposure of the proximal stomach. The DS procedure is described in meticulous detail, including the precise use of the surgeon's left and right hands, the changing of positions at the table, and maintaining triangulation of the operative field.

The use of a staged procedure is also discussed. In some individuals, an initial sleeve gastrectomy is performed, and the remainder of the operation is delayed until significant weight loss has occurred. This has led some surgeons to advocate a sleeve gastrectomy by itself for weight loss. However, there are no long-term studies that assess whether weight loss can be maintained, given the natural proclivity of the stomach to dilate over time. The complete duodenal switch operation is technically challenging, and there is a higher incidence of complications than that for either laparoscopic banding or gastric bypass. This approach should probably be used only by surgeons with an extensive experience in bariatric surgery, including having performed a large number of gastric bypasses. Hopefully, prospective randomized trials comparing the duodenal switch to other more commonly performed bariatric procedures will allow an adequate comparison of these approaches to the morbidly obese patient.

NJS

Diseases of the Liver and Biliary Tract

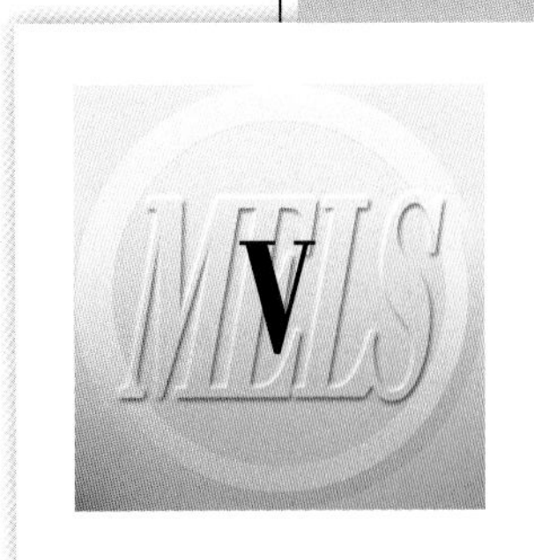

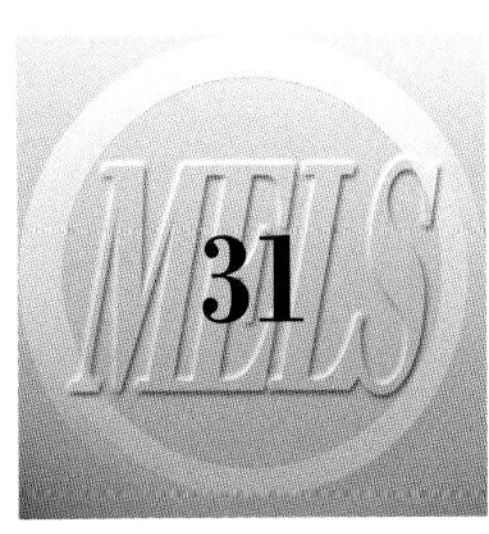

Endoscopy of Bile and Pancreatic Ducts

GARY C. VITALE, IGOR GOUSSEV, AND BRIAN R. DAVIS

INTRODUCTION

Since the advent of minimally invasive therapy, simple endoscopic pancreaticobiliary procedures such as sphincterotomy, stone removal, stent decompression, cyst drainage, and biopsy have become a primary treatment in the overall management of many different patient populations. Endoscopic procedures avoid skin incisions and typically require only minimal sedation and a short postprocedure recovery interval. These favorable aspects of interventional endoscopy make it preferred over operative approaches. The efficacy and safety of many interventional endoscopic procedures are highly dependent on the skill and experience of the endoscopist, necessitating skilled training in these areas of treatment. Advances in imaging modalities such as computed tomography (CT), magnetic resonance imaging (MRI), preoperative magnetic resonance cholangiography, and even positron emission tomography have yielded highly accurate diagnostic results, thus relegating endoscopic retrograde cannulation of biliary and pancreatic duct, or endoscopic retrograde cholangiopancreatography (ERCP), to an interventional treatment modality role. The evolution of minimally invasive procedures currently is such that there will be an ever-expanding role of endoscopy and ERCP in the primary treatment of many diseases previously treated with more invasive surgery.

TOOLS AND SETUP

Endoscopic retrograde cholangiopancreatography is usually performed in a dedicated endoscopy suite under fluoroscopy. The suite should have a dedicated fluoroscopy table that is also capable of film or digital radiography. A side-viewing, double-chambered duodenoscope is required for visualization of the ampulla. Multiple varieties of cannulation catheters are required to address the ampulla, including ball-tipped, needle-tipped, sphincterotomes, and needleknife catheters. Hydrophilic guidewires are also used to obtain access to the ampulla and ducts.

The endoscopy team consists of the surgeon, a catheter nurse, and a sedation nurse. Ergonomic room setup requires the need for both the endoscopist and catheter nurse to visualize the fluoroscopy and endoscopy monitors simultaneously. The optimal placement of the two video monitors is directly opposite the endoscopist and the catheter nurse. If an X-ray technician is used, he or she is positioned to the left of the endoscopist or, in modern suites, seated at a distant console. The sedation nurse stands at the head of the bed with placement of the physiologic monitors (electrocardiogram, O_2 saturation, blood pressure) to his or her right, also in view of the endoscopist.

PATIENT FACTORS

Patient position and preparation is prone with the head turned to the right and the right shoulder slightly elevated. The right hip is flexed as well as the right knee. Extension of the neck degrades optimal scope positioning and ampullary lineup, so the patient's neck should generally be flexed. The properly sedated patient does not require an anesthetic spray of the posterior pharynx, but this is necessary in instances where sedation will be used sparingly. We use a midazolam- and meperidine-based sedation.

There are different factors, such as external pelvic fixation, an unstable chest cage due to fractures, cervical spine immobilization, etc., that make it impractical or impossible to place the patient in a prone position or to turn his or her head to the right. Alternative positions such as dorsal decubitus and left lateral have been proposed and performed by experienced endoscopists. These positions create a difficult angle for cannulation and instrumentalization of the common bile duct and pancreatic duct. Prior to sphincterotomy, a coagulation profile should be documented and anticoagulation therapy suspended. Pacemakers and automatic defibrillators may need to be adjusted.

Antibiotics may be indicated (obstructive jaundice, cholangitis, infected pancreatic pseudocyst, etc.) prior to the procedure. Attention should be directed to providing good gram-negative coverage to treat the most likely pathogens in cholangitis, such as *Escherichia coli* (*E. coli*) and *Klebsiella pneumoniae*. General anesthesia should be considered for patients with a known allergy to meperidine, midazolam, or morphine or an unsuccessful sedation in the past.

OPERATOR ENDOSCOPIST FACTORS

The success of ERCP depends on the skill of the endoscopist and catheter nurse as well as the experience of the sedation nurse. These three function as a team. The endoscopist should contact other specialists when undertaking emergent ERCP so that other drainage procedures can be accomplished if the ERCP is unsuccessful. Most endoscopists who perform ERCP have over 100 cases of experience, as recommended by the American Society for Gastrointestinal Endoscopy.

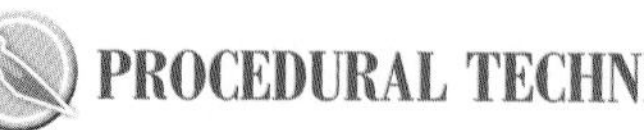

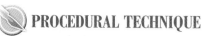

PROCEDURAL TECHNIQUE

The side-viewing endoscope is not passed under direct vision but rather relies on guidance from the endoscopist's finger and the patient's intact swallow response. The scope is guided through a bite block and into the posterior oropharynx. The left index finger of the endoscopist guides the scope tip caudally to just above the larynx (usually 15 to 20 cm at the incisors). The neck is flexed slightly. The patient is verbally prompted to swallow. Upon elevation of the larynx, the surgeon gently feeds the endoscope down the upper esophagus. If there is resistance, the scope has most likely deviated into a lateral pyriform recess. Forcing the scope in this blind pouch can result in a pharyngeal tear or perforation.

Once past the upper esophageal sphincter, the side-viewing endoscope is passed gently into the stomach. Advancing the slightly flexed tip along the greater curvature, the pylorus is seen after passing the incisura. The pylorus is placed at the 6 o'clock position, and the scope is advanced through the pylorus. The up/down and right/left dials are turned to their maximal clockwise direction and locked in place. The lumen should be in view before the scope is reduced into the second portion of the duodenum while torquing the scope shaft to the right. The scope is then withdrawn, causing a paradoxical forward movement by reducing the gastric loop that was developed on scope insertion. The reduced position is called the "short" position, where the scope handle should face the catheter nurse. In the "long" position, the scope is not reduced into position; the greater curvature loop is maintained while advancing more length until the ampulla is visualized. In this position, the scope handle faces away from the catheter nurse (180 degrees, toward the patient's feet). The short position is better for major papilla procedures. The long position is typically only used for those minor papilla procedures where the short position proves suboptimal.

The method of scope placement and optimal position will vary depending on the anatomy. The natural relationship of the gastroesophageal (GE) junction to the gastric outlet is variable from nearly 180 degrees (straight stomach) to the two structures being located side by side (J-stomach). Also, pathological conditions that produce a mass effect, such as pancreatitis, peptic ulcer disease, and malignancies, may necessitate additional techniques to obtain optimal scope positioning. In cases of choledochoduodenostomy access, the anastomosis is encountered up and to the right in the proximal duodenum. In Billroth II and post-Whipple patients, the afferent limb is intubated and the scope is advanced retrograde to the ampulla or bilioenteric anastamosis. Fluoroscopy is very useful in these patients to achieve final position.

ACCESS AND INTERVENTIONS

Cannulation of the pancreatic duct and biliary tree are the rate-limiting factors for interventional ERCP. An atraumatic and accurate cannulation technique will provide the best results with the least complications. The endoscopist should have an appreciation for the anatomy of the ampullary region, as well as knowing when to cease futile attempts at cannulation. After one or two unsuccessful attempts at wireless catheterization, we have a very low threshold to employing wire-sounding techniques using a hydrophilic floppy-tipped wire. In difficult cases, wire sounding is less traumatic and seems to have a higher success rate than wireless catheterization. Also, this avoids the situation of biliary contrast injection without deep cannulation, which, when followed by unsuccessful attempts at cannulation/decompression, may increase the risk of cholangitis following ERCP (Fig. 31-1).

Cannulation with a sphincterotome and guidewire is used initially in cases where an endoscopic sphincterotomy (ES) is likely. ES over a wire helps maintain correct scope alignment and facilitates atraumatic instrument exchange with extraction balloon catheters, stents, and balloon dilators, etc. (Fig. 31-2).

The cutting wire is positioned between 11 and 1 o'clock. Pure cutting current is used to decrease pancreatic orifice inflammation and post-ERCP pancreatitis. There are multiple types of sphincterotomes, including special Billroth II catheters, and there are multiple forms of energy sources.

Biliary ES should precede ES of the pancreatic outlet if needed and is done with the same technique and instrumentation. Minor papilla ES also is achieved using the same principles. However, deep cannulation of the minor papilla can be facilitated in the long position, with a small hydrophilic wire through a catheter tip cannula. The smaller-diameter diagnostic ERCP scope is better suited for this, because the larger therapeutic ERCP scope can be cumbersome in the long position.

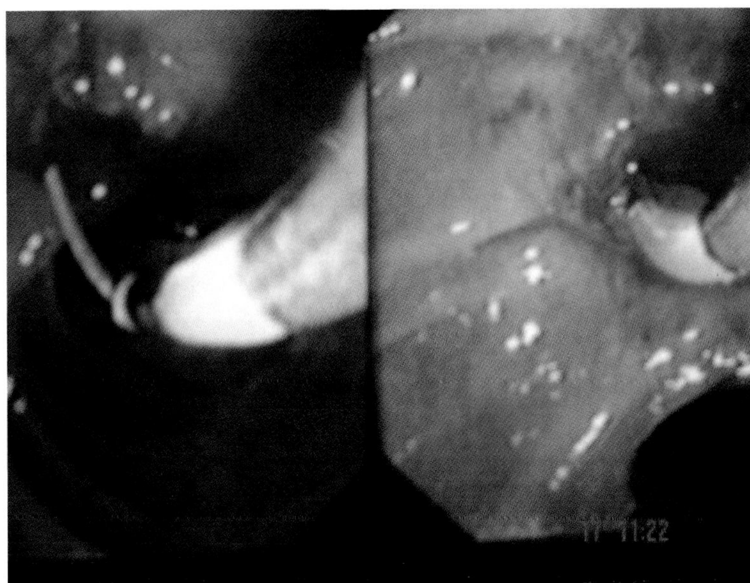

Fig. 31-1. Endoscopic view of cannulation attempt with guidewire sounding.

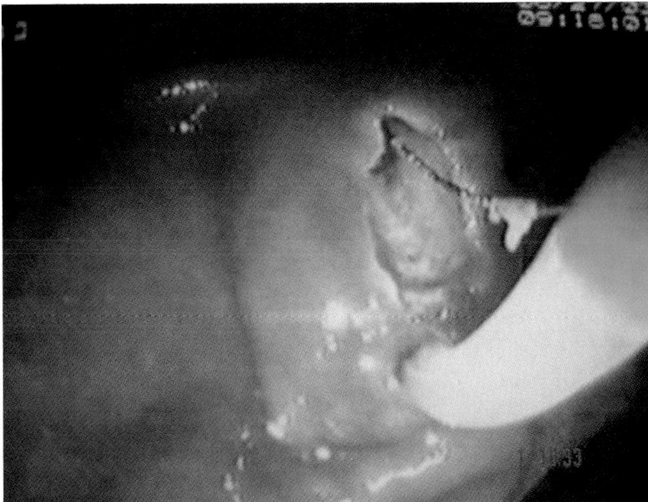

Fig. 31-2. Endoscopic view showing picture of sphincterotome.

A precut sphincterotomy (PCS) is used when access to the ampulla is refractory to standard techniques and there is a solid indication for interventional ERCP. One technique is an infundibulotomy with a needleknife, where the initial incision is centered over the bulge in the distal common bile duct (CBD), incising the infundibulum of mucosa and submucosa over the transduodenal bile duct and progressing inferiorly. After the duct lumen is accessed, a standard sphincterotome is used to complete ES. The other technique of PCS uses a precut needle catheter, begins the PCS at the orifice, and extends the incision proximally.

The percutaneous transhepatic cholangiography (PTC) rendezvous technique is another maneuver to deal with a difficult ampulla. This is especially useful when an ES is indicated, but retrograde access has been unsuccessful. A 450-cm ERCP wire is placed via PTC through the ampulla and into the duodenum. The wire is brought out of the ERCP scope with a snare, and a sphincterotome is placed over the wire for an ES. Large-caliber dilators or stents can be placed endoscopically, and the PTC access can be kept small (limiting intrahepatic trauma and bleeding) and completely removed. A strictly PTC approach is efficacious but may require multiple procedures or a safety catheter to convert the PTC drain to an internal stent. Current biliary metallic PTC stent kits are as small as 7F, and the access site catheter can be pulled after a few days. Extraction of stones should begin at the bile duct bifurcation, and stones should be dragged distally. The ampullary region is susceptible to trauma if the outlet is significantly smaller than the stone. In these cases, mechanical lithotripsy may be helpful. Wire extraction baskets are available in a variety of configurations and can even serve to break up soft stones without the need for a large caliber lithotripter.

We treat strictures with specifically designed high-pressure balloons available in 4-, 6-, 8-, and 10-mm sizes after complete inflation at 12 atmospheres. Contrast within the balloon can be used to delineate the morphology of the stenosis treated in real time. Stent-deployment systems are available in kits, usually as over-the-wire delivery systems, sometimes involving tapered stent introducers for larger end prostheses (10- and 11.5F stents). Daughter scopes, laser lithotriptors, and a variety of other equipment are now widely available.

Abdominal Pain of Unknown Etiology

In the evaluation of abdominal pain of unknown etiology, ERCP has a limited role as it bears infrequent but potentially serious complications. Even when patients describe typical pancreatic or biliary pain, the yield of ERCP is going to be very low in the absence of abnormal laboratory studies or other diagnostic imaging. With the recent advances in magnetic resonance cholangiopancreatography (MRCP) technology, it has become a noninvasive alternative that is comparable to ERCP in accuracy in a wide array of pancreatobiliary problems.

Choledocholithiasis

The role of ERCP in the management of choledocholithiasis with advances in MRCP, CT, and endoscopic ultrasound (EUS) is mainly interventional. There is still no consensus on the optimal management of choledocholithiasis, particularly in patients who undergo cholecystectomy. Local expertise in a given institution is critical to the decision making for the treatment of common bile duct (CBD) stones. A given unit may have varying experience with ERCP, laparoscopic transcystic CBD exploration, and laparoscopic transcholedochal exploration. Familiarity and availability of stone fracture techniques such as electrohydraulic lithotripsy and pulsed-dye laser lithotripsy also may influence the treatment strategy. As a result, there is not one single gold standard for bile duct stone removal. Each patient's condition must be evaluated and treated according to institutional strengths.

Patients presenting with signs and symptoms of biliary stones may be stratified into three groups based on their age, clinical exam, laboratory data, and initial diagnostic imaging results. Patients younger than 60 years of age with normal liver enzyme levels, normal bilirubin, no history of pancreatitis or large gallstones, and normal calibre bile ducts by transabdominal ultrasound are considered to have a slight risk (2%) of harboring a CBD stone. Patients younger than 60 years of age with a history of pancreatitis or jaundice, elevated preoperative bilirubin and alkaline phosphatase (ALP) with multiple small gallstones detected by transabdominal ultrasound are considered to be an intermediate risk (30% to 50%) of harboring a CBD stone. Patients older than 60 years of age with the clinical and biochemical picture described above or patients presenting with a clinical picture of jaundice or cholangitis and evidence of a CBD stone or CBD dilatation by transabdominal ultrasound are considered at high risk (50%) of harboring a CBD stone.

For patients in a low risk group with cholelithiasis and no evidence of malignancy, the management of choice is laparoscopic cholecystectomy. Intraoperative cholangiogram in this group can be carried out routinely or selectively depending on surgeon's preference. For patients in the intermediate risk group, laparoscopic cholecystectomy with an intraoperative cholangiogram (IOC) is the gold standard. However, even in the high-risk group, stones will be discovered in only 30% of cases. An alternative to IOC is laparoscopic ultrasound (LUS) where available. Several studies have shown that LUS has higher specificity and sensitivity than IOC, while shortening the intraoperative time, preventing radiation exposure, and being more cost-effective. The problem with the preoperative ERCP is that even in the high-risk group the study will be negative in 70% to 80% of cases. However, there are relative indications for preoperative ERCP, which will be discussed later in this chapter.

Stones that are discovered intraoperatively may be dealt with by using a single-stage approach, a dual-stage approach, or observation. In a single-stage approach stones discovered by IOC or LUS are extracted without leaving the operating room. In several recent randomized control trials (RCT) reinforced by meta-analysis, it was shown that laparoscopic CBD exploration was comparable to ERCP in stone removal rates with a shorter hospital stay. The technique and further discussion on laparoscopic CBD exploration can be found elsewhere in this book. In cases of failure to clear the CBD laparoscopically and an unreliable postoperative ERCP in a given institution, open CBD exploration remains a viable alternative. Intraoperative passage of a guidewire through the cystic duct in order to facilitate postoperative ERCP has been described. In a limited number of centers intraoperative or postprocedure ERCP under the same general anesthetic has been described. This avoids a choledochotomy or duodenotomy with an advantage of creating a sphincterotomy, although an antegrade laparoscopic sphincterotomy has been described. Very few centers have this capability, and this option is rarely used. That is why we see little reason to pursue this approach. The dual-stage approach involves either a preoperative ERCP with no obligation for an IOC if the duct is clear or, more commonly, a postoperative ERCP after a positive IOC and failed or unavailable laparoscopic CBD exploration, provided that ERCP success rates are high in a given institution. The University of Louisville experience demonstrates a 90% or greater stone extraction rate at ERCP (Fig. 31-3).

There are specific relative indications for preoperative ERCP. Typically, if the efficacy of local ERCP is questionable, surgeons seek a preoperative ERCP. If preoperative ERCP is unsuccessful, then the patient will not leave the operating room until the duct is cleared, because a postoperative ERCP cannot be relied upon for that patient. If liver enzymes are high or increasing, it may be best to consider an ERCP before the operation as it may indicate an impacted stone, which could be more difficult to remove laparoscopically (Fig. 31-4).

Pancreatic head enlargement, which can be seen in both malignant and benign processes, warrants further investigation before cholecystectomy. ERCP with an EUS with or without a fine needle aspiration (FNA) could be carried out if PET/MRCP scans are not available. The positron emission tomography (PET) scan is a noninvasive, sensitive modality and should be used liberally. If pancreatic cancer is diagnosed after it is symptomatic, then it is unlikely that a curative resection will be successful. The possibility of occult malignancy should be raised for elderly patients with obstructive jaundice. Even minor elevations of liver function tests, particularly without definite stones in the gallbladder, should be cause for investigation. The ampulla is difficult to assess at the time of operation, and it is best evaluated before operation with ERCP. Early identification of an ampullary tumor can lead to definitive surgical treatment with curative intent.

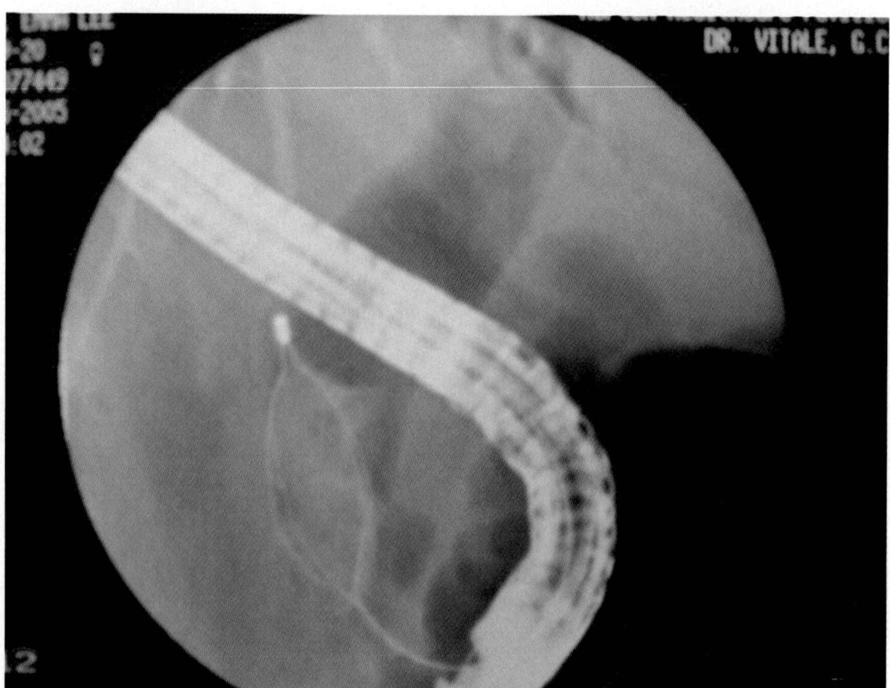

Fig. 31-3. Radiographic view of a stone extraction with basket.

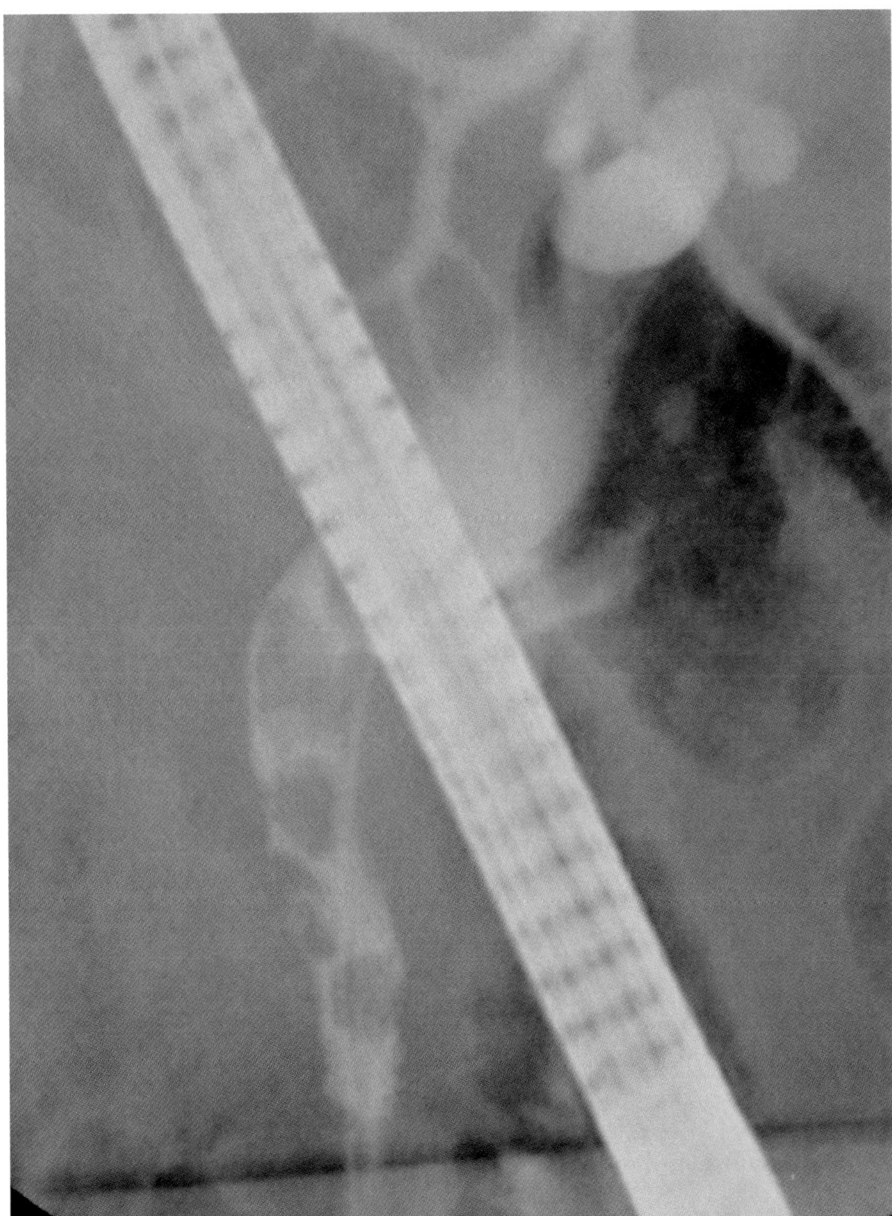

Fig. 31-4. Cholangiography showing a common bile duct stone and guidewire previous to the performance of a sphincterotomy.

Patients who are known to be alcoholic or patients with a known or suspected chronic pancreatitis history with enzyme changes should have preoperative evaluations to rule out distal CBD strictures caused by pancreatitis. These patients should undergo preoperative sphincterotomy and stent placement to reduce intrabiliary hypertension and possible post-cholecystectomy biliary leaks (stump blowout).

Worsening gallstone pancreatitis is a definite indicator for preoperative ERCP. In a recent meta-analysis, it was shown that early ERCP and sphincterotomy may decrease the severity and morbidity and mortality rates that are associated with pancreatitis. The presence of cholangitis in the setting of gallstone pancreatitis requires urgent ERCP. Preoperative treatment of cholangitis reduces complications when compared with a direct operative approach.

A documented history of cirrhosis or ascites in the presence of gallstones should prompt preoperative ERCP evaluation. In these cases, the elevation of liver enzymes may be due to hepatocellular dysfunction rather than choledocholithiasis. If gallstones are present, however, portal hypertension may make intraoperative dissection of the porta hepatis more difficult and hazardous; therefore endoscopic stone extraction may be preferable (Fig. 31-5, page 288).

The presence of intrahepatic stones that have been documented by ultrasonography or by CT is a relative indication for endoscopic clearance, as laparoscopic clearance might be difficult and operative management is likely to result in choledochotomy, which should only be performed if significant CBD dilatation is present. ERCP in this setting also offers the advantage of sphincterotomy, which would allow stones and fragments to pass.

The presence of very large stones in the CBD may be a relative contraindication to a laparoscopic approach. Large stones can be fractured and removed endoscopically in most cases. In patients with a very large, inflamed gallbladder with elevations of the liver enzymes and suspected choledocholithiasis, a preoperative ERCP and stone extraction may be advisable as attempting an IOC is problematic because of cystic duct obstruction, inflammation, foreshortening, and necrosis.

ERCP with ES alone could be used in frail and debilitated patients with a limited life span who are discovered to have CBD stones. In institutions where the success rate of ERCP is high, outside of aforementioned circumstances, ERCP is generally not requested preoperatively, because a preoperative ERCP is negative in 70% to 80% of cases. Although the risk of ERCP is low in experienced hands (1% to 3%), only those patients who have the greatest potential benefit should be exposed to these risks.

Postoperative ERCP for a CBD stone that is confirmed by IOC and not cleared by laparoscopic or open techniques requires aggressive ERCP techniques to gain access to the biliary tree. In these cases, we do not leave the ERCP suite until all efforts to access the biliary tree are exhausted. This includes higher-risk procedures such as PCS. We prefer to perform ERCP outside the operating room, in a dedicated ERCP suite at a time separate from the day of cholecystectomy. Other variations of dual-stage treatment include the adjunctive use of plastic stents that are placed antegrade by the laparoscopic surgeon to "bridge" the patient to a second-stage ERCP. If a preoperative ERCP is performed, we do not proceed with a same-day cholecystectomy, because endoscopic insufflation can render laparoscopy difficult.

The observation group is limited to asymptomatic patients with CBD stones that measure less than 3 to 4 mm. Intervention is delayed unless symptoms develop, which happens in only 30% of

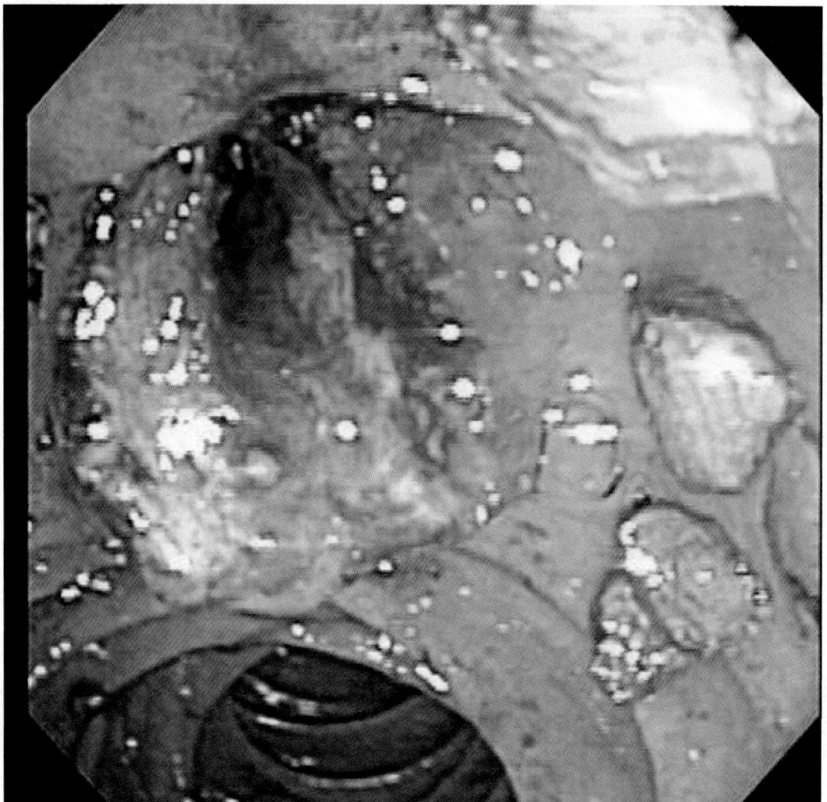

Fig. 31-5. Endoscopic view of common bile duct stone that passed into the duodenum after a sphincterotomy.

the cases. This approach is not recommended in the setting of gallstone pancreatitis or where a common channel is noted on an IOC.

Endoscopic Management of Bile Duct Injuries

Although rare, iatrogenic bile duct injuries still remain a formidable complication, with significant morbidity and occasionally mortality. The rate of bile duct injury, after an initial surge during the early 1990s, is 1 in 500 to 1000 patients. ERCP is a very valuable tool in diagnosis and treatment of bile duct injuries. Recently, MRCP emerged as a valuable diagnostic tool. The treatment and outcome of biliary injuries vary considerably and are dependent on the type of injury, its location, and the time of its diagnosis.

CLASSIFICATION OF BILE DUCT INJURY

The anatomic classification of Bismuth has been adopted widely for the classification of biliary tract injuries. In the Bismuth classification (Table 31-1), five stricture types are recognized that reflect the location with respect to the confluence of the hepatic duct (types I-IV) or the involvement of an aberrant right sectoral hepatic duct with or without a concomitant hepatic duct stricture (type V).

This classification was later further broadened by Strasberg et al. Injuries are classified as type A to type E. Type A injuries are bile leaks from minor ducts that are still in continuity with the CBD. Type B injuries involve occlusion of part of the biliary tree. Type C injuries occur when the duct is transected without ligation. Type D injuries are lateral to an extrahepatic bile duct, which is similar to a type A injury in that the extrahepatic biliary tree remains in continuity but is classified separately to underscore the greater severity and potential need for major reconstruction. Type E injuries are biliary strictures and are further subdivided into 5 categories, E_1 to E_5, which are based on the Bismuth classification.

Patients with iatrogenic injuries generally present either early with bile leaks or later with strictures. Patients with bile leaks after cholecystectomy (type A, C, and D) generally are seen within the first week after operation; however, some injuries may not be apparent for several weeks, and very few injuries are diagnosed intraoperatively. Most patients experience abdominal pain that is coupled with fever or other signs of sepsis. Biliary ascites without overt signs of sepsis may develop in a few of these patients. A small number of patients have none of these signs and symptoms but have rather nonspecific complaints of weakness, fatigue, or anorexia. Elevated alkaline phosphatase levels are characteristic. Some patients may have mild hyperbilirubinemia; markedly elevated serum bilirubin levels (>3 mg/dL) are uncommon. The initial diagnostic procedures of choice are ERCP, MRCP, PTC, and hepatobiliary iminodiacetic acid (HIDA) scanning. ERCP is the most definitive procedure and can be used to treat many injuries; therefore, this is the procedure of choice in most cases in which the suspicion of injury is high. If the suspicion of injury is low, a MRCP or HIDA scan may allow the identification of the injury earlier than would be possible if one awaited clinical symptoms. PTC is useful in cases of complete obstruction or in cases in which part of the bile duct has been excised. In these cases, ERCP will not opacify the most proximal ducts, and

TABLE 31-1. BISMUTH CLASSIFICATION OF BILIARY STRICTURE

Type	Description
Type I	A low common hepatic duct stricture. Hepatic duct stump greater than 2 cm.
Type II	A proximal common hepatic duct stricture. Hepatic duct stump less than 2 cm.
Type III	A hilar stricture with no residual common hepatic duct. Hepatic duct confluence intact.
Type IV	Destruction of hepatic duct confluence. Right and left hepatic ducts separated.
Type V	Involvement of aberrant right sectoral hepatic duct alone or with concomitant stricture of the common hepatic duct.

PTC is necessary to better delineate the entire anatomy before definitive therapy is undertaken. Recently, MRCP has been evaluated for diagnosis of bile duct injuries and appeared to have specificity and sensitivity similar to ERCP (Fig. 31-6).

Cases of minor bile leaks from cystic duct stump and ducts of Luschka and some focal major bile leaks without loss of tissue may be managed endoscopically by ERCP with ES, stone clearance, and stent placement with good success rate. If a biloma becomes infected, it can be managed by percutaneous drainage or by returning to the operating room. The loss of bile duct tissue or complete transection of the bile duct requires operative management with bilioenteric anastomosis.

Benign postoperative biliary strictures can often be managed by endoscopically placed stents. Polyethylene stents (10F) are inserted for a 6- to 12-month period. Balloon dilatation or dilatation with progressively larger wire-guided axial dilators is performed initially and at 3- to 4-month intervals. The main disadvantage of endoscopic management is that it requires a series of ERCPs. Our approach is to stent these lesions over a year's time, which requires an initial stent placement and about two exchanges (temporary stents last about 4 months before becoming occluded). Each exchange is accompanied by an assessment of stricture morphology and optional dilatation. If patients fail this course of minimally invasive outpatient ERCP therapy, then operative options are still available. For lesions that are longer than 1 to 2 cm, ERCP therapy is less likely to succeed. However, it appears to do no harm to attempt a course of stenting, and most patients and surgeons prefer this. The University of Louisville experience demonstrates an 83% success rate in the endoscopic treatment of benign bile duct strictures after laparoscopic cholecystectomy.

Traditionally, bile duct strictures have been treated surgically with a Roux-en-Y hepaticojejunostomy. The advantages of endoscopic management are the avoidance of general anesthesia as well as a bilioenteric anastamosis. The long-term course after a bilioenteric anastamosis has many potential complications, including cholangitis, strictures, and a shortened life expectancy.

ERCP plays an important role in diagnosing and treating bile duct injuries. In our experience for lesions after laparoscopic cholecystectomy, cannulation and opacification of the duct have been successfully achieved in 95% of the patients. When interventional ERCP was chosen as the primary treatment, sphincterotomy and stenting were achieved in 83% of the patients.

TRAUMATIC BILIARY INJURIES

ERCP has an important role in the diagnosis and management of traumatic biliary injuries in both the adult and pediatric population. In several recent studies, endoscopic biliary decompression with ES and stenting have been shown to be effective in managing a wide variety of biliary injuries. Most biliary fistulas were amenable to endoscopic management. The results of treatment of traumatic biliary duct injuries were similar to iatrogenic bile duct injuries.

Hemobilia should be approached with angiography. The rare case of bilhemia—extreme jaundice from a biliary-venous intrahepatic fistula (major liver trauma)—is best managed endoscopically. ERCP is successful in these patients even in the presence of problems such as open abdomens and pelvic fractures. However, some patients require an alternate position (supine) for the procedure.

ENDOSCOPIC TREATMENT OF MALIGNANT BILE DUCT STRICTURES

Obstruction of the biliary tree can result from a variety of malignant tumors. The two most common entities are pancreatic adenocarcinoma and cholangiocarcinoma. In rare cases obstruction can be caused by metastatic spread of other cancers or periportal metastatic lymphadenopathy. ERCP plays an important role in diagnosis and management of these cancers. The University of Louisville experience demonstrates stenting in 77% of patients that present with malignant strictures and a 97% success rate in treating those strictures.

Cholangiocarcinoma

ERCP has an established role in the diagnosis of cholangiocarcinoma (CC). The cholangiographic appearance is essentially diagnostic with brushings for cytology, forceps biopsy, and cytological analysis of the bile being a useful adjunct in centers where pathologists are experienced with this malignancy. ERCP, CT angiography, and newly emerging MRI/MRCP are used in staging and planning of surgery.

The treatment of CC depends on timing of presentation, localization, and spread of the tumor. The mainstay of treatment for CC remains surgery when the tumor is deemed to be resectable. Unfortunately, only one-third of patients present with potentially resectable tumors, with a 5-year survival rate after resection of only 10% to 20%. In the other two-thirds, palliation is the main goal. Surgical palliation was believed to be the best method of palliation, but it had a high

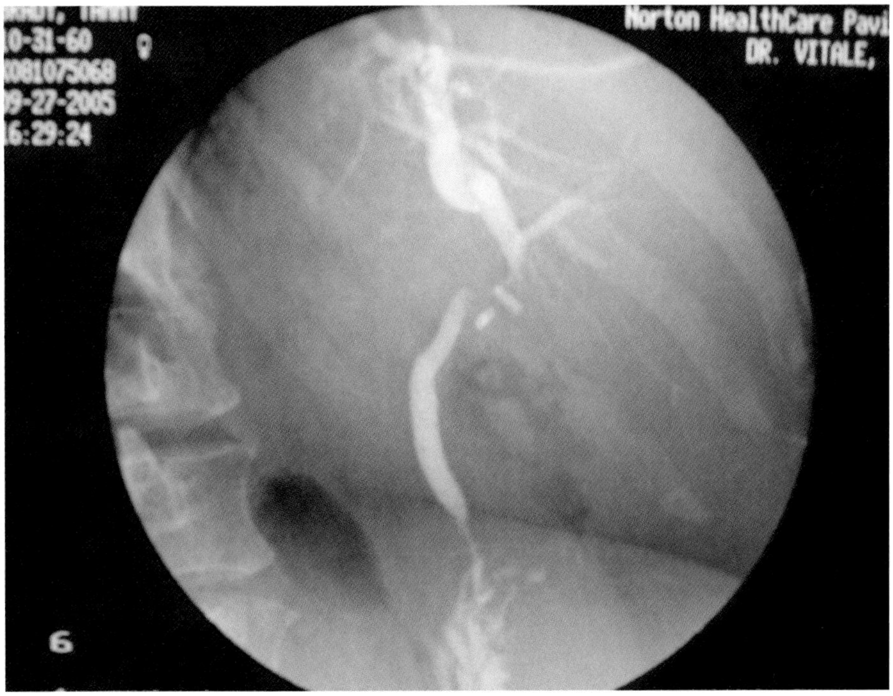

Fig. 31-6. Cholangiography showing a common bile duct ligation after a laparoscopic cholecystectomy.

morbidity and long hospital stays and bore up to 20% mortality in some series. A big operation with high risk is obviously acceptable in potentially curable patients, but for terminally ill patients this needlessly degrades what little time the patient has left. Multiple RCTs completed in recent years showed that endoscopic palliation with stent placement was superior to surgery, with 50% less morbidity and nearly zero mortality. An effective palliation was achieved in 75% to 80% of proximal tumors (Klatskin tumor) and over 90% in distal tumors. For the endoscopic approach, there was no mortality related to the procedure; 41% of the patients reached 12-month survival (one as long as 84 months) after initial stenting. Endoscopic treatment with stenting relieves jaundice and can provide long-term palliation comparable to the surgical approach (Fig. 31-7).

The average survival of patients with unresectable tumors ranges from 4 to 12 months, and this leads to a controversy over whether to use metallic or plastic stents. Plastic stents rarely last past 3 to 4 months secondary to the growth of a biofilm, which eventually leads to stent occlusion. If the patient is alive at this stage, a stent exchange would be required. A metallic stent lasts 3 to 4 times longer than a plastic stent, and the majority of patients will die with their first stent in situ. If a metallic stent is left in situ beyond 2 years, it could lead to serious complications of stent erosion and bleeding. A recent meta-analysis of 24 randomized controlled trials containing 2436 patients confirmed the superiority of endoscopic management to surgical management and also showed that metallic self-expandable stents were superior to plastic stents in patients surviving longer than 4 months, with longer patency and fewer procedures needed per patient to keep the bile ducts open. Cost-effectiveness was limited in patients surviving less than 4 months. Therefore, in a patient with a questionable long-term survival, it would be reasonable to initially place a plastic stent with a scheduled stent exchange. At that next procedure, a metallic stent may be placed, depending on the patient's overall health.

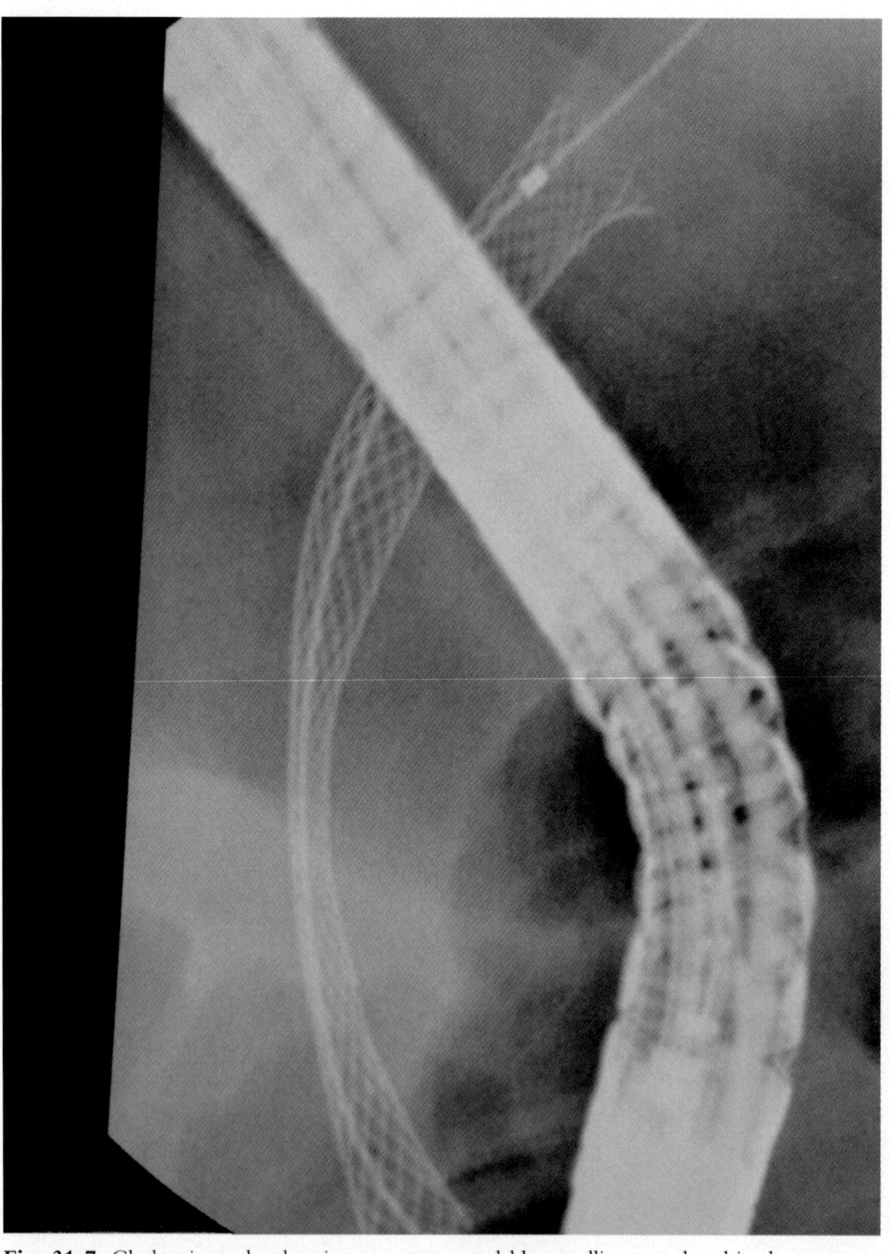

Fig. 31-7. Cholangiography showing an auto-expandable metallic stent placed in the common bile duct for palliation in a patient with cholangiocarcinoma.

Recently, photodynamic therapy (PDT) has emerged as a novel method in managing unresectable CC. In several nonrandomized trials as well as in one RCT, it was shown that PDT and stenting versus stenting alone improved median survival up to 21 months in one series. Interestingly, PDT and stenting had the same median survival as surgery. More RCTs are needed in this area, but this therapy shows some promise.

Pancreatic Adenocarcinoma

As in cholangiocarcinoma, ERCP has a role in the diagnosis and management of pancreatic carcinoma. In patients with pancreatic cancer, ERCP has a sensitivity between 90% and 97% in the detection of tumors and a false-positive and a false-negative result in 4% and 7% of cases, respectively. Classic signs of ductal adenocarcinoma on ERCP include irregular stenosis of the duct, or a "double duct" sign. These are not specific for cancer and may be seen in certain inflammatory lesions, including pancreatitis. Several other diagnostic modalities such as pancreatic protocol CT scan, MRI/MRCP, PET scan, and EUS with FNA are valuable adjuncts in diagnosing pancreatic cancer. ERCP biopsies are most sensitive with a forceps biopsy; however, this requires an accessible tumor and an ES. Endoscopic FNA, brushings, and fluid aspirations for cytology are less sensitive. EUS-guided FNA also is useful, but limited in availability.

The mainstay of pancreatic cancer treatment is surgery. As with CC, the majority of patients with pancreatic cancer presents late in the course, with unresectable disease at the time of diagnosis. Palliative intervention is directed primarily at the relief of obstructive jaundice, pain, nausea, and vomiting because of duodenal obstruction. Endoscopic palliation consists mainly of biliary stenting to relieve obstructive jaundice that results from cancer of the pancreatic head. The success rate for the insertion of stents into the bile duct exceeds 90%. After stenting is performed, jaundice is relieved in more than 85% of patients, thereby improving the quality of life in 70% of those patients who underwent stenting. Recent reports from the MD Anderson Cancer Center (University of Texas; Houston, TX) and several other institutions showed that duodenal obstruction can also be managed endoscopically when applicable with good results and less morbidity and mortality than surgical bypass. These reports are retrospective reviews that need to be validated by RCTs, but this approach shows some promise.

Pancreatitis

ACUTE PANCREATITIS

The role of ERCP in managing acute pancreatitis is limited to severe or worsening gallstone pancreatitis. The mainstay of controversy was confounding cholangitis, which is an independent indication for ERCP. A recent meta-analysis of 3 RCTs containing 511 patients showed that early ERCP with or without ES reduces the odds of complications. This meta-analysis controlled for this confounding effect of cholangitis. These patients can be a challenge for the endoscopist. The anatomic changes of significant pancreatitis can make even intubation of the duodenum difficult, and suboptimal ampullary line-up is frequent. Ampullary changes from stone passage and pancreatitis can make cannulation difficult. A sphincterotome and guidewire are used initially. If the CBD is refractory to cannulation but the pancreatic duct (PD) is not, there is a low threshold for placement of a PD stent. This is done to straighten the often sigmoid-shaped orientation of the swollen ampullary biliary passage in patients with long common channels. Also, a PD stent can provide postprocedure decompression and decreases the likelihood and severity of any procedure-related pancreatitis. A PD stent placed for these indications can be removed days to weeks following discharge from the hospital.

CHRONIC PANCREATITIS

Chronic pancreatitis is a most difficult clinical problem for the physician and the patient. There is a well-known association with alcohol, and occurrence and progression years after exposure and abstinence is notorious. The exact pathophysiologic features of this disease are still ill-defined. Chronic pancreatitis is most likely the result of a heterogeneous compilation of diverse, but occult, causative factors that share a chronic inflammatory effect on the pancreas as their end result.

The initial evaluation of chronic pancreatitis patients should focus primarily on the identification of any possible etiological agent. Recurrent bouts of preventable subacute pancreatitis can result in fibrosis and scarring, with an anatomic predisposition toward a persistent course of chronic pancreatitis. Therefore, it is important to identify and limit the exposure of potentially causative agents as soon as possible. This is sometimes omitted by referring physicians (i.e., stopping alcohol consumption and evaluating lipids, calcium, prescription medications, etc.). The diagnosis of chronic pancreatitis is confirmed with objective evidence of the disease, by CT, MRI, US, ERCP, or (rarely) pancreatic biopsy. Of all the modalities available besides biopsy, EUS is the most sensitive. When EUS was compared with CT, ERCP, and abdominal US in the evaluation of 81 patients with chronic pancreatitis, it was found that EUS had a sensitivity of 88% (abdominal US, 58%; ERCP, 74%; CT, 75%); specificity was 100% for ERCP and EUS, 95% for CT, and 75% for abdominal US.

The primary treatment issue in chronic pancreatitis is typically pain control. It is worthwhile to consider an anatomic evaluation to identify treatable conditions whenever there is a significant worsening of pain. This entails a CT or ultrasound scan to identify treatable cystic complications and an ERCP or MRCP for ductal obstructive problems. The treatment of anatomic lesions can improve the patient's pain significantly if the lesion is symptomatic. However, in these patients, this often can only be proved with a trial of lesion-directed treatment (i.e., cyst drainage, stone removal, or ductal stenting).

A PD stricture theoretically may produce an outlet obstruction of the pancreatic excretory flow. Ductal hypertension has been associated with pain in these patients and may play a limited role in the progression of the disease process. Dominant PD strictures in these patients respond well to dilatation and stenting, with a 74% success rate. Surgery should be reserved as a late-stage intervention. The morbidity that is associated with endoscopic treatment (e.g., stents, dilatation, sphincterotomy) is less than for an operation. The results of an endoscopic approach may provide the patient with significant relief and avoid an operation. The University of Louisville experience demonstrates that 83% of patients experienced a decreased pain level after pancreatic stenting. Endoscopic interventions may provide short-term pain relief, but with progression of the disease they will become less beneficial and eventually unsuccessful.. In these cases, the delay in operative therapy is useful for guiding surgery (Fig. 31-8, page 292).

If the patient notes a significant improvement with endoscopic drainage of the pancreatic ductal system, a surgical drainage procedure should give similar results. More importantly, in cases in which stenting does not benefit the patient, a resection should be pursued no matter how large the pancreatic ducts have become (Fig. 31-9, page 292).

Endoscopic treatment for postoperative recurrences of symptoms is less likely to be useful compared with interventions that are performed before operation, unless there is a surgical complication (such as an anastomotic stricture). In summary, endoscopic treatment of pancreatic ductal strictures in chronic pancreatitis may guide surgery and even avoid operation in some cases. Pancreatic lithiasis occurs in a few patients with chronic pancreatitis. Endoscopy with or without lithotripsy is useful in clearing the pancreatic duct of stones. Relief of pain should follow the removal of symptomatic obstructing PD stones or protein plugs. However, the removal of stones is thought to have little impact in the overall course of the disease (Fig. 31-10, page 293).

Patients with pancreas divisum who have symptoms may present with acute recurrent pancreatitis, chronic pancreatitis, or a chronic pain syndrome. Endoscopic drainage of the minor papilla with sphincterotomy and stent placement is beneficial for patients who present with acute recurrent pancreatitis or chronic pain. Long-term results demonstrate that up to 80% of patients have a reduction of symptoms, with an estimated 25% recurrence rate at

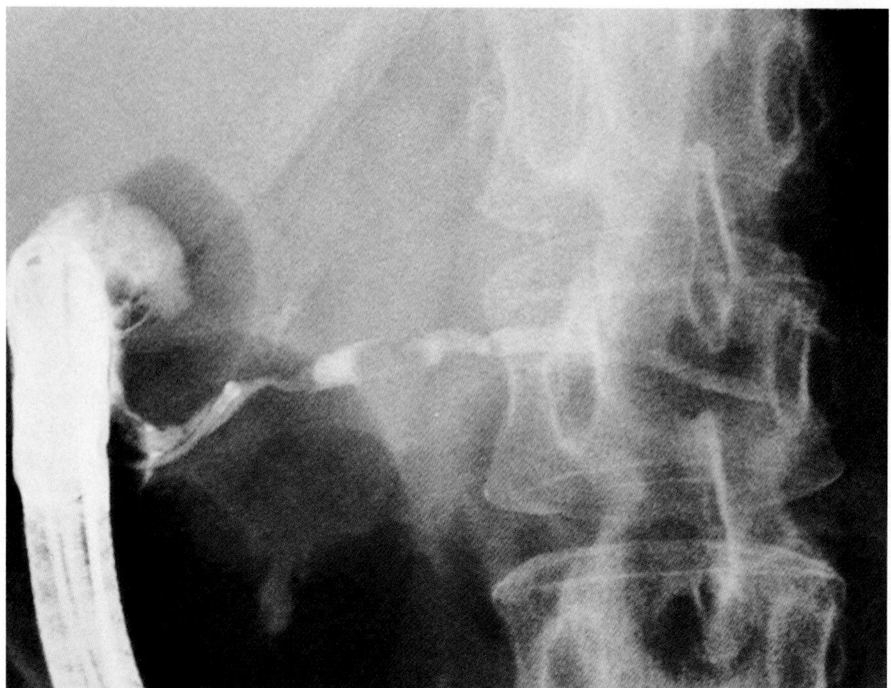

Fig. 31-8. Pancreatography and guidewire placement in a patient with chronic pancreatitis and a pancreatic duct orifice stricture.

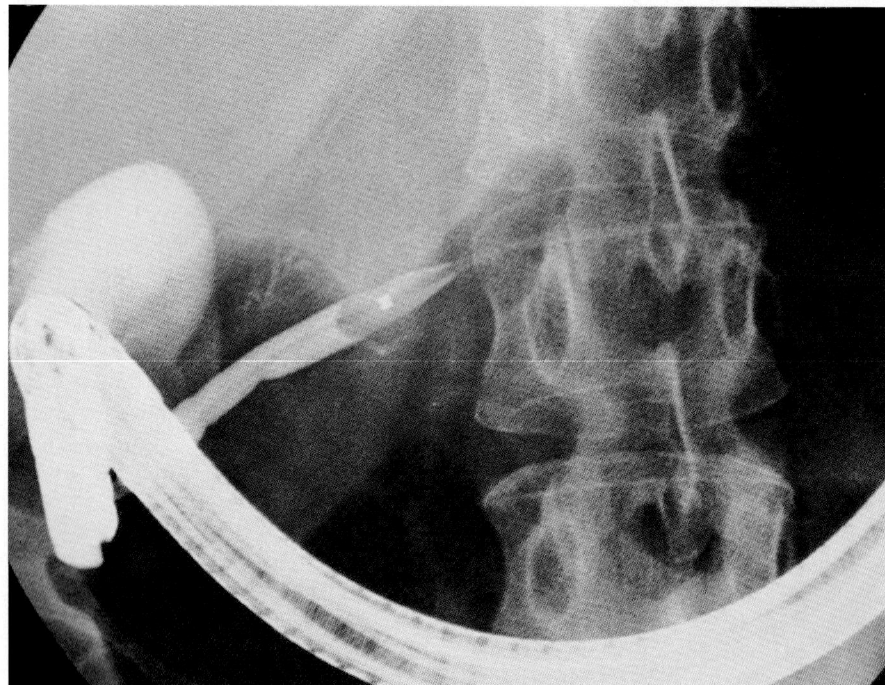

Fig. 31-9. Guidewire balloon dilatation of the strictured area of the pancreatic duct.

50 months. In chronic disease, drainage of the minor papilla is effective in only 25% to 50% of the patients, and most authors recommend surgical resection for those patients.

Pancreatic duct disruption may result from acute or chronic pancreatitis, pancreatic surgery, pancreatic malignancy, or trauma. Persistent PD disruption may lead to pancreatic ascites, fluid collection, or fistula formation. Surgical options include internal or external drainage of fluid collections or partial pancreatectomy or pancreaticojejunostomy. Radiologic percutaneous drainage of fluid collections is another option, with resolution in 42% to 90% of patients. Transpapillary PD stents have been successful in relieving pancreatic ascites, resolving localized fluid collections, and closing both internal and external fistulae in communication with the PD. The bridging position of the stent has been correlated with the outcome, and a 60% success rate in the resolution of the disruption has been reported with this technique. Ductal changes have been seen after stenting but have not been correlated with the clinical outcome.

The options available for endoscopic intervention in the management of pancreatic pseudocysts are numerous. However, it is important to remember that 20% of cystic lesions of the pancreas are neoplastic and endoscopic drainage is contraindicated. Caution should be given in cases where the cyst wall is thick (>1 cm), there is a lack of cyst to gut wall adherence, loculations occur, or the diagnosis is uncertain. We employ endoscopic management of pseudocysts liberally, but only in the appropriate clinical context.

ERCP is used to assess the pancreatic duct for communication with the cyst. If there is no communication, then the cyst is treated with endoscopic cyst enterostomy. The anatomy of the cyst as it impinges on either the stomach or the duodenum dictates which location is chosen: either cyst gastrostomy or a cyst duodenostomy. We do not routinely use EUS, but correlate the endoscopic findings with preprocedure CT scans. In some cases however, EUS is valuable. There are numerous variations in technique of endoscopic cystenterostomy, as well as types and sizes of stents and length of stenting intervals in the literature. The important factors are the characteristics of the pseudocyst: presence of acute or chronic pancreatitis, size, thickness of the wall, chronicity, degree of symptomatology, location, associated pancreatic parenchymal and/or ductal pathology, and the possibility of a cystic neoplasm. The small numbers of pseudocysts preclude construction of controlled studies to determine their optimal management. What clinical data are available are uncontrolled for the characteristics of the pseudocysts as well as the techniques used to treat them. Our success rate has been 83%, which is comparable to that reported by other investigators. Of course, in cases where drainage procedures (endoscopic, laparoscopic, or open) fail, the possibility of a misdiagnosis (cystic neoplasm) can arise (Fig. 31-11).

A series by the surgical endoscopy unit at the University of Louisville reported a

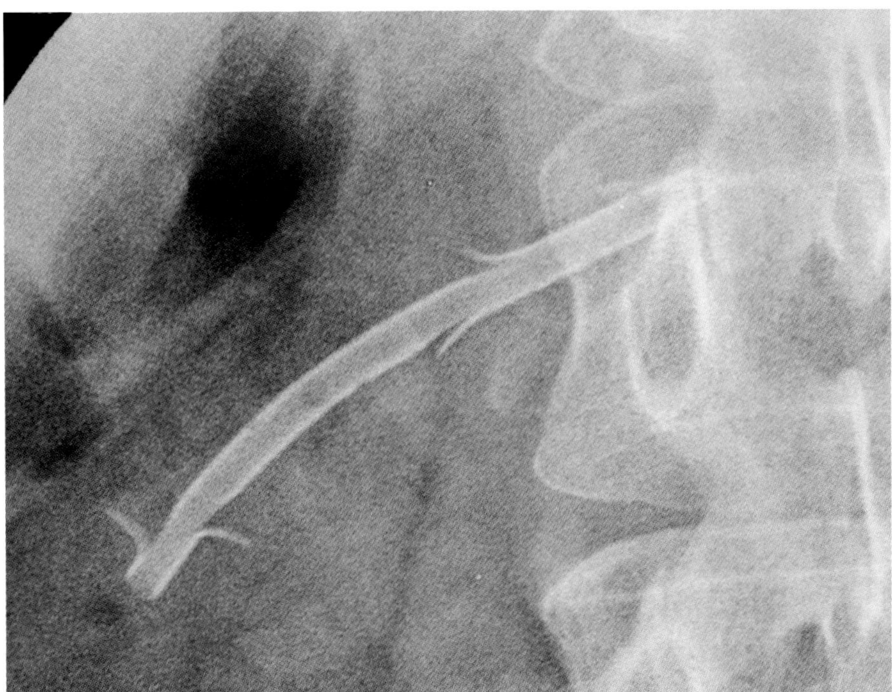

Fig. 31-10. Stent placed in the pancreatic duct beyond the stricture.

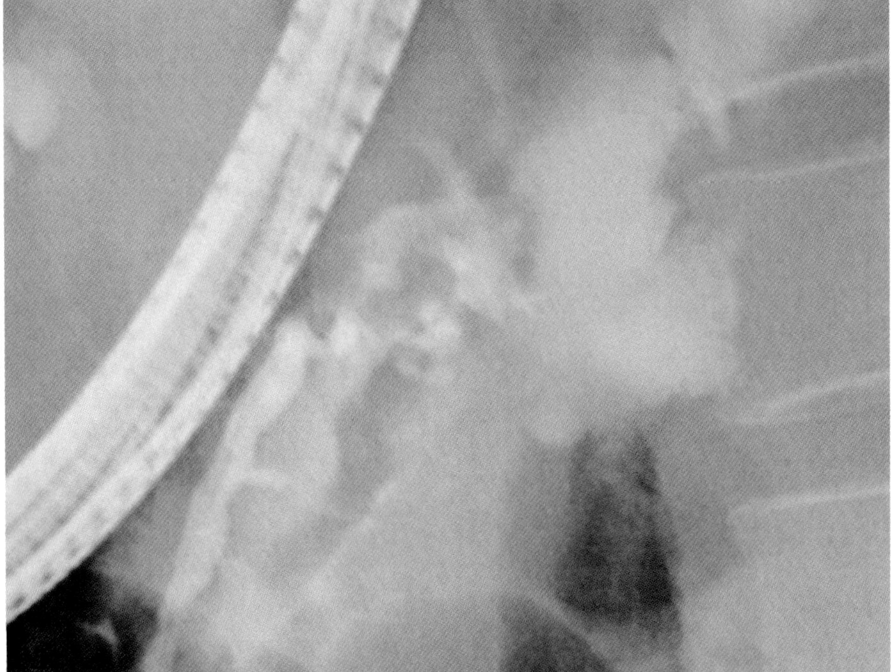

Fig. 31-11. Pancreatography of a patient with a pancreatic duct disruption at the tail level with pseudocyst formation.

83% success rate in draining pancreatic pseudocysts endoscopically. The average size of the pseudocysts was 8.5 cm in diameter; the mean follow-up was 34 months. Twenty-five cyst gastrostomies, 11 cystduodenostomies, and 20 transpapillary drainages were performed. Misdiagnosis of a cystic neoplasm was found in two patients, and pancreatitis postprocedure was the most common complication. No patient required blood transfusion or surgical management. There was no mortality related to the procedure. In our experience, endoscopic drainage should be considered in patients with symptomatic pseudocysts when the anatomic configuration is favorable (Fig. 31-12, page 294).

Endoscopic management in these complex patients is clearly valuable and should be used as part of a multidisciplinary approach. There should be no argument regarding whether endoscopic management is better or worse than surgery. It clearly adds to the armamentarium of treatment options available and, if used efficaciously, will benefit a significant number of these patients (Fig. 31-13, page 294).

Chronic pain treatment is best handled with a multidisciplinary approach. The early involvement of a pain service to treat the high analgesic requirements of these patients is recommended. The use of oral and transdermal narcotics should only be pursued in those patients with a firm diagnosis. Typically, narcotic use does become an issue with these patients and will sometimes confound the clinical picture. Once these patients are taking narcotics on a regular basis, they become socioeconomically handicapped. Furthermore, it seems that the gastrointestinal hypomotility that is induced from long-term narcotic usage may even worsen the abdominal complaints of these patients.

Peripheral nerve treatments can decrease the need for narcotics and hence limit the problems that are associated with chronic narcotic use, such as gastrointestinal dysmotility and addiction. Celiac ganglion injections (percutaneous or EUS-guided) and splanchnic nerve ablation are the primary modalities used for interventional pain therapy. Pancreatic pain can be improved in 80% of patients with the use of a celiac ganglion block, with an expected duration of approximately 6 months in patients with cancer. Unfortunately, the results do not appear as good for benign disease. Thoracoscopic splanchnicectomy seems to have better results than ganglion blocks in the treatment of benign disease. This is probably due to the difference in specificity of the two different modalities in the interruption of nerve stimulation. Surgical division of a nerve is more specific than an indirect paraganglionic injection. We preferentially use thoracoscopic splanchnicectomy liberally with good results. Approximately 83% of patients experience some benefit. The reduction in narcotic usage is the primary goal of this approach.

When symptoms become refractory to all the measures that have been mentioned

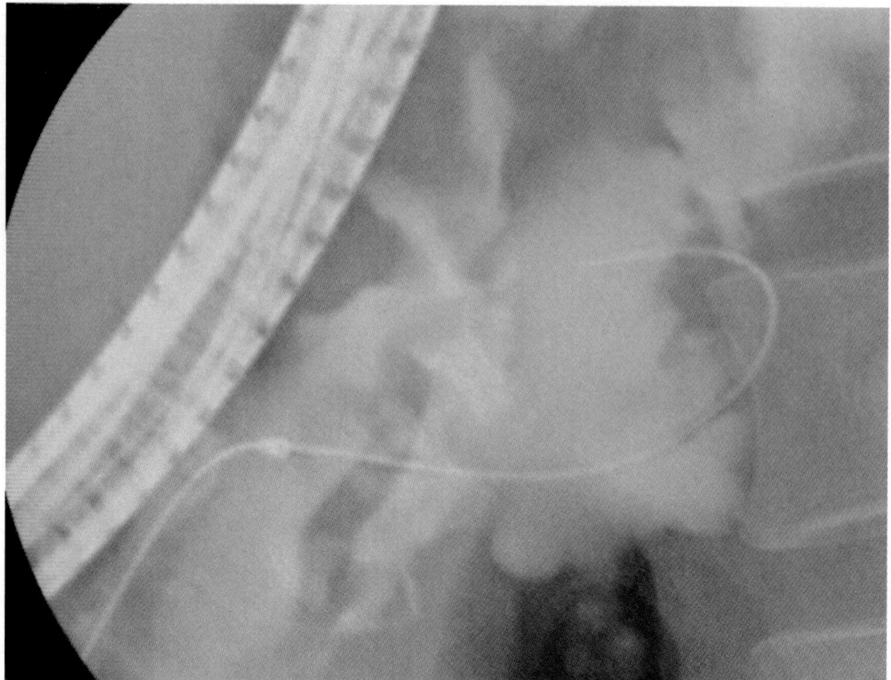

Fig. 31-12. Sequence of guidewire placement in the pancreatic duct up to the level of disruption.

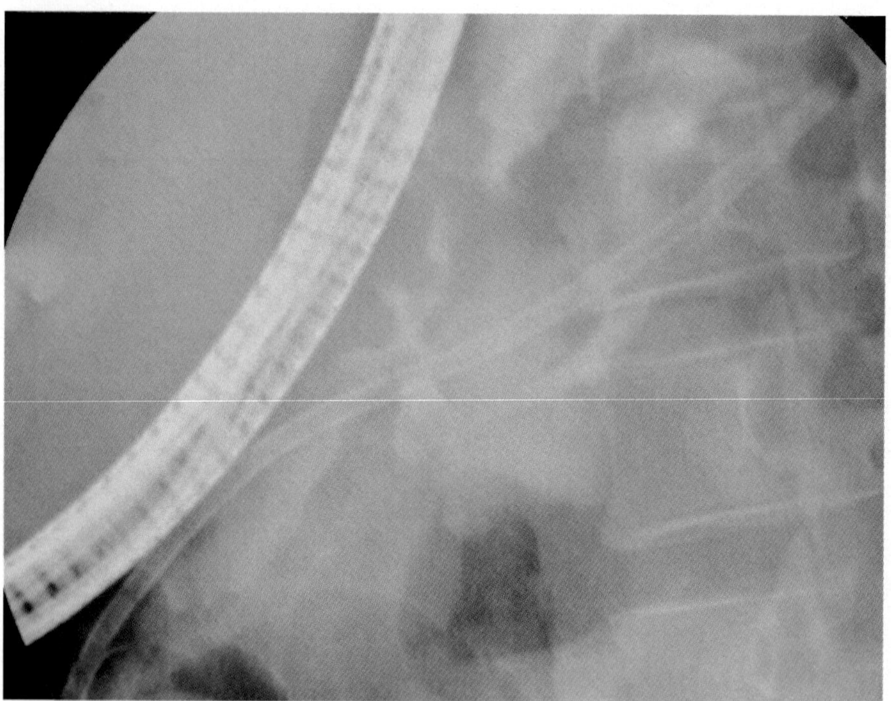

Fig. 31-13. Pancreatic stent placement to the level of pancreatic duct disruption.

here, operation should be considered. The results of surgery tend to mirror the results of nonoperative therapy in that a significant number of patients will have recurrence of pain in the late postoperative period. For this reason, operation should be used only after less invasive therapies have been exhausted. The operative approach is tailored to the anatomic manifestations of the disease. Typically, large duct disease is treated with a parenchymal-sparing pancreaticojejunostomy (a drainage procedure), unless preoperative stent decompression demonstrates little relief of pain. Patients with small duct disease are preferentially treated with pancreatic resection. Some patients will have an eccentric distribution to their chronic inflammatory changes, and the operation is tailored accordingly. There are many different variations of resections and drainage procedures, and the complications are generally proportional to the complexity of the procedures. No one operation has been proved to be superior. Overall, when selected properly, patients experience a significant benefit with operation in 70% to 90% of cases.

Alcohol is the leading cause of pancreatitis in North America. It is important to understand that chronic pancreatitis is managed chronically. It is not treated with an expectation for cure because there is no medical or surgical cure for this condition. Management tools vary from simple oral analgesics and pancreatic enzymes to endoscopic interventions and major surgical procedures. However, PD strictures, stones, and pseudocysts are amenable to endoscopic dilatation, stenting, stone extraction, and drainage no matter what the underlying cause of the pancreatitis.

Chronic Pancreatitis and Distal Bile Duct Stenosis

The intrapancreatic portion of CBD is susceptible to compression secondary to a cicatrical process. In the workup, it is imperative to exclude malignancy as it may be affecting up to one-third of these patients. ERCP with or without biopsy, high-definition CT scan, PET scan, MRCP, and EUS with or without biopsy are very useful in ruling out malignancy. Until recently, surgical decompression with choledochoduodenostomy or choledochojejunostomy was the preferred option in patients in whom malignancy had been ruled out. The endoscopic management of cholestatic complications of chronic pancreatitis is now evolving, with a potential permanent shift away from operative decompression. Multiple studies have shown that ERCP with biliary stent placement effectively resolves jaundice and cholangitis, though it has no effect on chronic pain. Because of the problems with stent occlusion inherent with plastic stents, long-term treatment entails repeat ERCPs and stent exchanges three to four times a year, whereas a biliodigestive bypass is more permanent. The development of microbial-resistant plastic stents and dual-layer stents (with longer patency rates) may change this balance. Metallic stents rarely are considered for benign disease, even in the high-risk surgical patient (Fig. 31-14). The University of Louisville experience demonstrates that 80% of

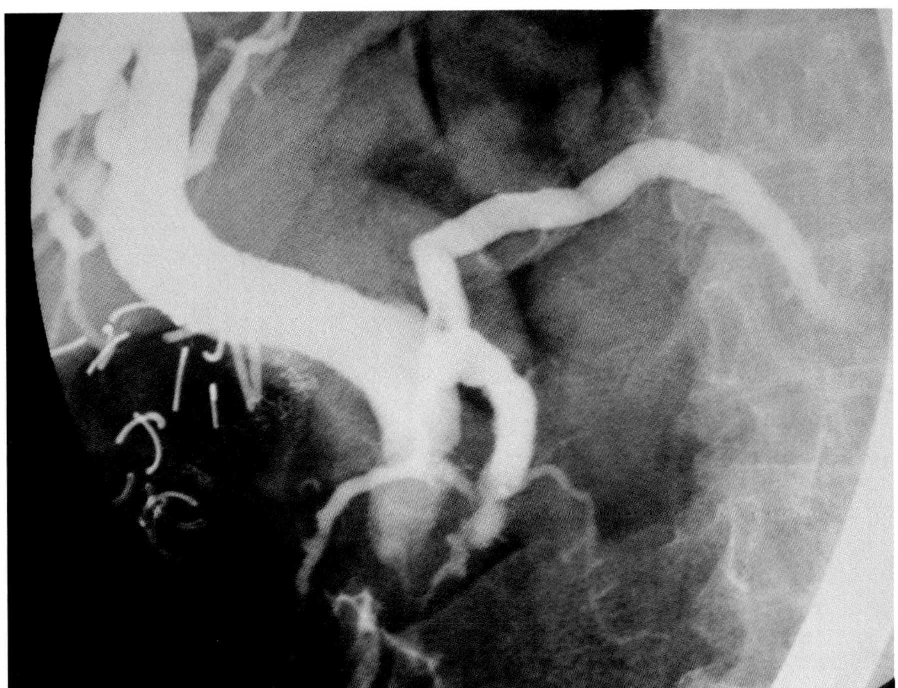

Fig. 31-14. Cholangiopancreatography of a patient with chronic pancreatitis and a distal common bile duct stricture with dilated distal duct and stones, showing a strictured intrapancreatic portion of the common bile duct.

strictures from chronic pancreatitis will respond and dilate after a year-long course of stenting.

Ampullary Dysfunction

The ampullary region is the point of exodus of the biliary and main pancreatic excretory systems. Distal outflow obstruction is usually due to an intraluminal lithiasis but can also be caused by extrinsic compression caused by periampullary tumors, choledochoceles, or inflammation. An intrinsic obstruction of the ampullary sphincter, in the absence of these lesions, may be due to scarring from previous episodes of stone passage, known as ampullary stenosis (AS), or a failure to decrease tone at the physiologically appropriate time (sphincter of Oddi dysfunction). This functional ampullary stenosis may manifest as a clinical syndrome with symptoms of either biliary or pancreatic disease. Ampullary stenosis is uncommon and essentially a diagnosis of exclusion. Symptoms should not be attributed to ampullary stenosis until other conditions have been excluded, including malignancy.

Biliary ampullary stenosis is typically diagnosed by ERCP in the evaluation of patients with persistent or recurrent biliary colic after cholecystectomy. ERCP is pursued in these patients because one-third of the patients will have stones; a malignancy is found in up to 8% of patients, and ampullary stenosis is present in approximately 10% of patients. These patients respond well to duct clearance and ES. Without objective findings on ERCP, a clinical diagnosis of sphincter of Oddi dysfunction is based on the triad of (1) elevated liver functions tests, (2) a dilated CBD, and (3) delayed contrast drainage at ERCP. The presence of this triad in a patient with biliary colic predicts an excellent response (90% to 95%) to endoscopic sphincterotomy, the standard method of sphincter ablation. Patients without this triad of findings sometime undergo sphincter of Oddi manometry. Manometry offers an objective measurement of sphincteric function to identify which patients have a disorder of the ampulla that may improve with sphincter ablation. Manometry-proven stenosis responds well (80% to 85%) to sphincter ablation. Normal manometry predicts a 60% response, but placebo yields a 40% to 50% response. This suggests that a tight sphincter is perhaps just one component of a multifactorial, somewhat nebulous disorder. Therefore, an overlap of symptoms with irritable bowel syndrome (IBS) should be explored, as well as potential contributing psychosocial factors.

A dysfunctional ampulla appears to be central in the symptoms of another subset of patients: those with recurrent biliary colic after lithotripsy. In these patients, 68% have recurrent symptoms without stones. Acalculous post-lithotripsy patients with recurrent symptoms treated with ES, even without manometry, have good results.

The ampulla, being the point of exodus of both the biliary and pancreatic secretions, may also be the origin of more complex symptoms. Two-thirds of patients with sphincter of Oddi dysfunction will have abnormal pancreatic sphincter manometry. A hyperactive pancreatic sphincter can produce pancreatic pain and/or pancreatitis. Similar to endoscopic sphincterotomy in patients with biliary colic, selective pancreatic sphincterotomy is beneficial to patients with pancreatitis and documented abnormal pancreatic sphincter manometry. We treat post-sphincterotomy stenosis with balloon dilatation and stenting only when there is no more sphincter muscle to divide. The risk of postprocedure pancreatitis is lessened with placement of prophylactic PD stents. Each endoscopic procedure is also used to rule out periampullary tumors by biopsying any suspicious lesions.

Ampullary Tumors

Ampullary tumors can be either associated with familial adenomatous polyposis (FAP) (20% to 30%), or more commonly occur sporadically (70% to 80%). They present with vague abdominal pain, liver enzyme elevation, jaundice, and pancreatitis or more rarely with bleeding or duodenal obstruction. Rare combinations of bleeding ampullary tumors obstructing the CBD present with melenic stools deprived of bile, resulting in so-called silver stools (which are in fact dark grey).

Because of the different malignant potential of sporadic and FAP-associated tumors they will be considered separately. The sporadic group of tumors includes adenomas distal variants of biliary papillomatosis, ampullary hamartomas, adenomyoma, stromal tumors, inflammatory pseudotumors, heterotopias and carcinomas. Ampullary adenomas can be either a more tubular or more papillary type. Malignant transformation of benign lesions into carcinoma have been documented, and papillary adenomas are thought to mimic the colonic adenoma-to-carcinoma sequence. This tumor affects both sexes equally and is uncommon before the age of 50 years. Carcinoma is an uncommon neoplasm that accounts for approximately 6% of all periampullary tumors, with an incidence of approximately 5.7 cases per million per year. Although rare, neoplasms of the ampullary region are now being diagnosed more frequently. Ampullary tumors are usually evaluated using a side-viewing duodenoscope with biopsies taken to evaluate histologic characteristics of the tumor. Reliance on endoscopic features alone is insufficient for the discrimination of benign and malignant neoplasms. In the setting of a papillary mass, distal pancreatic or CBD strictures are predictive of invasive cancer. EUS has been used to augment ERCP and conventional imaging techniques in the staging of carcinoma of the major duodenal papilla. However, EUS cannot reliably distinguish benign from malignant lesions, and peripapillary inflammation further distorts the findings. Intraductal US may be promising in the evaluation of depth of penetration of certain tumors (Fig. 31-15).

Management of these neoplasms depends on histologic characteristics. Pancreaticoduodenectomy is the procedure of choice, with transduodenal ampullectomy performed at some centers for frank carcinoma and high-grade dysplasia. Less invasive alternatives are being sought increasingly for the definitive treatment of benign papillary adenomas. Endoscopic resection has been reported more frequently in the last few years. The problem with endoscopic management is a high recurrence rate; 10% to 30% on average with some series reporting 90% to 100%. The recurrence is generally managed by re-resection with good results. However, endoscopic management is not without complications, with pancreatitis being the most common (up to 20%), followed by bleeding (5% to 15%), cholangitis (5%), and in one series perforation. Deaths from this technique have been reported. Considering the high recurrence and complication rates, endoscopic management is usually reserved for elderly, high-risk patients. Careful endoscopic surveillance is needed for resected ampullary tumors.

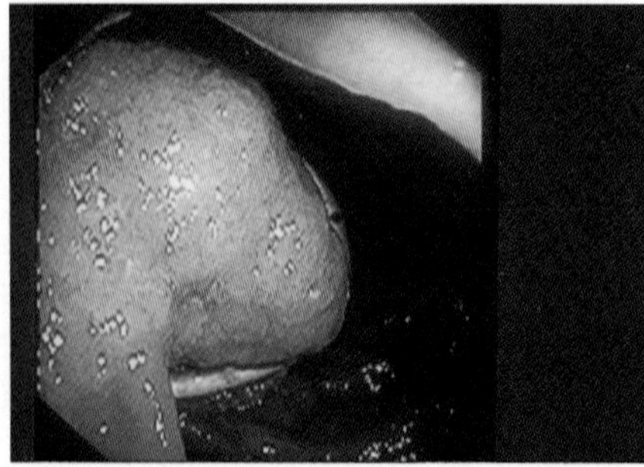

Fig. 31-15. Endoscopic view of an ampullary tumor protruding into the duodenal lumen.

Ampullary Tumors in Familial Adenomatous Polyposis

Familial Adenomatous Polyposis (FAP) is an autosomal dominant disease that is characterized by the development of multiple adenomas of the gastrointestinal tract. The treatment of colorectal polyps with total abdominal colectomy is more or less standardized. Periampullary and duodenal adenomas are reported to be present in up to 80% of FAP patients in most studies from Western countries. Next to the colon, the duodenum and the periampullary areas are the most common sites for neoplasms to develop. Tumors in these areas occur in approximately 4% of patients and are the most common cause of cancer death in this population. The risk of cancer in the duodenum and periampullary region in FAP patients is 100-fold greater than in the general population. The adenoma-carcinoma sequence is assumed to occur in the duodenum. In a retrospective study of 559 patients, the sequence of adenoma-carcinoma has been confirmed with a high percentage of patients with the histologic diagnosis of "parts of an adenoma," where other regions of the tumor already contain a carcinoma. Recently, a large prospective five-nation study set the cumulative incidence rate of duodenal cancer at 4.5% by the age of 57 years. The median age of duodenal cancer development was 52 years (range of 26 to 58 years). Therefore, proper screening and surveillance (preferably with ERCP side-viewing scopes) and biopsy are extremely important in achieving long-term survival for these patients.

The Spigelman criteria can be useful in managing these patients. This system is a four-stage scoring system that is based on the number (1 to 4, 5 to 20, >20), size in millimeters (1 to 4, 5 to 10, >10), histologic features (tubular, tubulovillous, villous), and degree of dysplasia (mild, moderate, severe) of duodenal polyps. It is widely believed that patients with the risk of periampullary carcinoma are presumed to be those with Spigelman stage IV disease. Surveillance recommendations are to perform duodenoscopy every 2 to 3 years in low-risk groups (I and II) with more frequent follow-up for duodenoscopies with biopsies (every 6 months) for groups III and IV.

It was previously thought that duodenal adenomas were static lesions, but recently several investigators have shown that duodenal polyposis may progress. A prospective study from the U.S. followed 114 FAP patients for 51 months and found progression of polyps in size (26%), number (32%), and histology (11%). A study from Finland involving 98 FAP patients, reported worsening polyposis in 73% of 71 FAP patients followed for 11 years, with a median interval for progression by one stage occurring in 4 to 11 years. Another group from France reported a stage change in 60% of patients with an average time of evolution by one stage occurring in 4 years. The risk of malignancy correlates with Spigelman's stage with stage II having 2.3%, III having 2.4%, and IV having a 36% risk of duodenal cancer.

In a recent study from the University of Louisville, 54 patients with FAP were followed for 10 years. Twenty patients developed duodenal adenomas and 13 underwent excision of the neoplasm. Seven patients had their neoplasm removed endoscopically with four recurrences, and six underwent pancreaticoduodenectomy. This study demonstrated (1) that duodenal adenomas are common in FAP, and endoscopic surveillance should be initiated at the time of diagnosis of FAP, (2) local resection has a high recurrence rate, and (3) although pancreaticoduodenectomy is the procedure of choice in this population, it may adversely affect bowel habits in ileal pouch patients. ERCP is a very useful surveillance tool in a setting of FAP, but the threshold for traditional operative treatment and a definitive cancer resection should not be diminished.

Primary Sclerosing Cholangitis

Primary sclerosing cholangitis (PSC) is a disease of unclear etiology that typically affects young men and is associated strongly with ulcerative colitis. Interestingly, the surgical treatment of ulcerative colitis has no positive effect on the course of the hepatobiliary disease, and patients with both ulcerative colitis and PSC are more likely to harbor a colonic neoplasm. PSC should be in the differential diagnosis of all patients with chronic cholestasis.

ERCP is the diagnostic test of choice. Although liver biopsies are frequently inconclusive, they aid in ruling out other causes of chronic cholestatic states. The classic cholangiographic beaded appearance with an irregular distribution of multifocal strictures is reflective of the pathophysiologic process. This is characterized histologically by biliary periductal fibrosis with associated obliterating luminal fibrous cores and secondary cholangiectasis (prestenosis dilatation). MRCP has been evaluated in the diagnosis of PSC with some promise. The magnetic resonance characteristics of PSC changes are hepatic peripheral wedges of high T2 signal with segmental biliary dilatation. This is most likely due to localized changes in tissue perfusion that are associated with the multifocal biliary ductal inflammation. The gross appearance of the liver at laparoscopy and open surgery includes multifocal surface depressions in advanced cases, with whitish-yellowish hues and a leopard-skin appearance.

Cholangiocytes do not regenerate as hepatocytes do, so damaged bile ducts never return to normal. At present, there is no cure. Experimental medical treatments within randomized controlled clinical trials that use immune modulators, cupretics, choleretics, and/or anti-fibrogenics offer the most promise. If an effective medical therapy is found, its application to patients in the asymptomatic stage of the disease will be the best strategy. This approach will rely on earlier detection by screening patients who are at risk (ulcerative colitis) with the use of a genetic assay and/or some form of cholangiography (MRCP or ERCP). For now, clinical decision making is based on a rational long-term treatment plan for the disease condition. Current treatment is aimed at relieving biliary obstruction, which may in turn delay the progression of secondary cirrhosis. In the patient who does not have cirrhosis, the achievement of biliary drainage can be accomplished with endoscopic techniques (80% success rate), percutaneous techniques, or surgical bilioenteric anastomosis. Once cirrhosis develops, the best outcomes are achieved with orthotopic liver transplantation. Although with orthotopic liver transplantation there is a 20% recurrence rate at 5 years, endoscopic therapy of postsurgical and transplant biliary anastomotic strictures is effective in 70% to 90% of cases (Fig. 31-16).

Treatment of patients with PSC is also driven by the looming possibility of cholangiocarcinoma, which is the most common cause of death in this population, developing in 10% to 30% of patients with PSC. Therefore, when dealing with a dominant stricture in a patient with PSC, obtaining negative cytologic brushings and carcinoembryonic antigen and CA 19-9 levels on a regular basis is wise when nonresective therapy is pursued. Alcohol consumption has been associated with an increased risk of cholangiocarcinoma in patients with PSC; therefore, alcohol avoidance should be discussed with these patients. Ursodeoxycholic acid is used prophylactically and may limit intrahepatic stone formation, which occurs in up to 10% of patients. The endoscopist should be aware that a hypercoagulable state can be present in up to 40% of these patients.

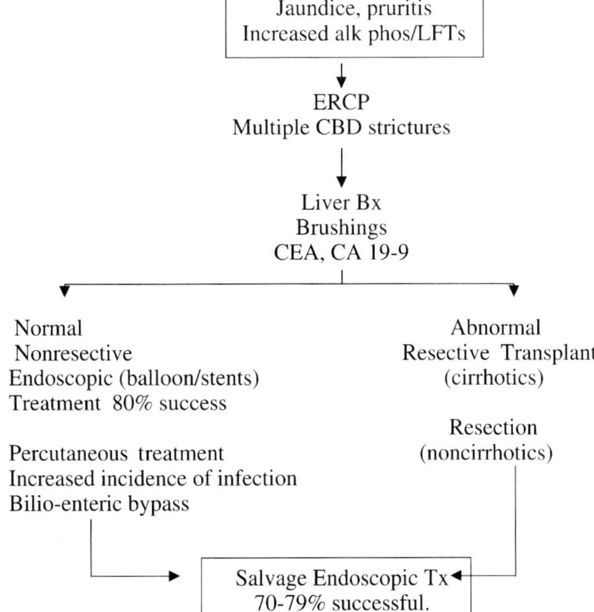

Fig. 31-16. Clinical options in management of primary sclerosing cholangitis (PSC).

CHOLEDOCHAL CYSTS

The cause of choledochal cysts is not fully understood. There is a definite congenital type, in addition to an acquired type, which is suggested by a delayed clinical presentation. There are five different anatomic variants, depending on the location of the cystic changes (Longmire/Alonso-Lej classification, types I to V). The treatment for patients with choledochal cysts is dependent on the cyst anatomy or type, age, and symptoms. All symptomatic patients are treated. Currently, resectional surgery is the first choice of therapy, unless the anatomic location introduces surgical risks out of proportion to patient benefit (Fig. 31-17, page 298).

The treatment of biliary cysts in general is surgical because of the association with malignancy. The frequency of cholangiocarcinoma developing in a biliary cyst is 10%. This risk increases with age and is more often associated with Alonso-Lej types I and IV and Caroli disease. Malignancy should be suspected strongly in patients with symptoms of cholangitis, weight loss, or anemia. Lithiasis is associated with malignancy, and the radiologic appearance is similar. Carcinoma arising in biliary epithelium distant from the cyst has been described, even after excision, but the actual incidence is unclear. Nonetheless, this possibility and the potential for biliary cirrhosis and cancer require lifelong follow-up and monitoring (Fig. 31-18, page 298).

Endoscopic cholangiography defines the anatomic type of cyst for surgical planning and allows cytologic brushings and biliary carcinoembryonic antigen levels to identify any occult malignancy. Excluding a malignancy is not necessary for symptomatic patients with favorable anatomic features and few surgical risk factors, but it is useful in asymptomatic, high operative risk patients or in cases with complex anatomic features. In these circumstances, patients may be better served with careful observation or limited endoscopic treatment. Cholangitis is best treated with a period of endoscopic stent decompression and antibiotics before any surgical approach. Complete cyst excision is the treatment of choice, when anatomically possible.

Cyst excision is most readily accomplished in patients with type II cysts. Dissection of the type II cyst is followed with diverticulectomy and closure of the stump with an absorbable suture. If a significant circumference of the CBD is

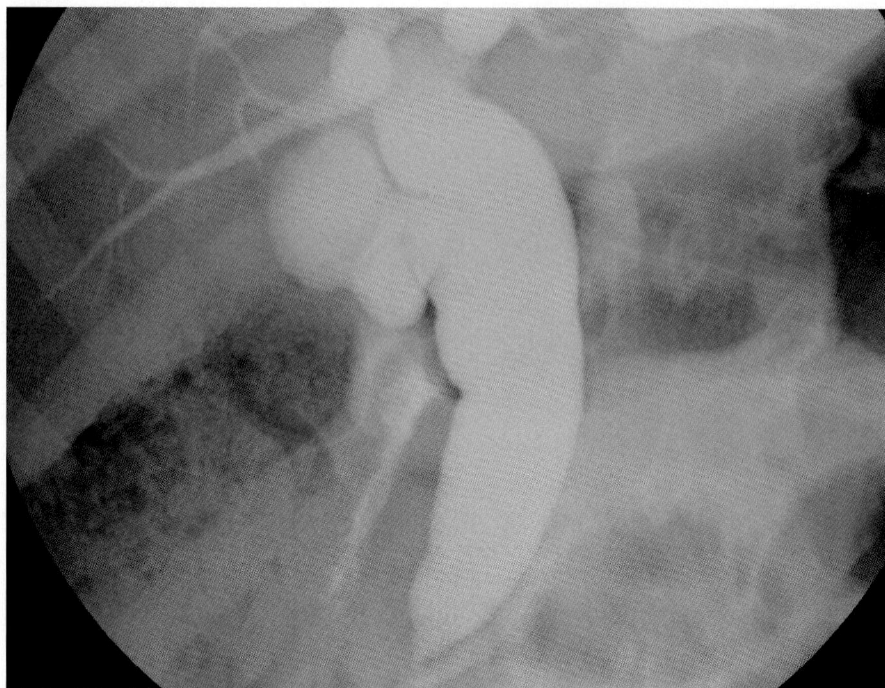

Fig. 31-17. Cholangiogram of a patient with a fusiform type I choledochal cyst.

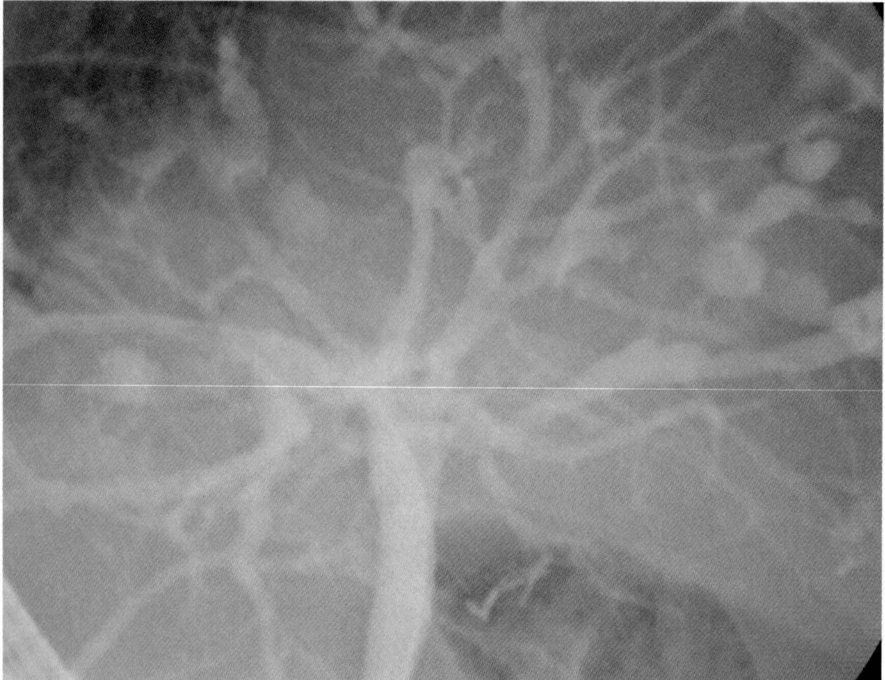

Fig. 31-18. Cholangiogram of a patient with multiple intrahepatic cysts (type V).

involved (usually in wider diverticular necks), a T-tube or bilioenteric bypass can be used. Type I cysts are treated with excision that avoids extensive mural dissection into the posterior pancreatic head, although as much biliary mucosa as possible should be removed because this is the tissue with malignant potential. Compared with patients with other types of choledochoceles, those patients with Alonso-Lej type III have been treated differently over the past 30 years. Nonresectional therapies (such as cyst-duodenostomy, extended sphincteroplasties, and endoscopic extended sphincterotomies) have been used with very good success rates for the relief of symptoms. Choledochoceles are rare, and the malignant potential is unclear. Malignancy has been reported in type III choledochoceles, but in only a few case reports. In cases of Caroli disease (type V) that are limited to a region of the liver, a partial hepatectomy is curative. Orthotopic liver transplantation is used for patients with pan-hepatic Caroli disease. Otherwise, the treatment of these patients is dictated by episodes of cholangitis, symptomatic strictures, and stones. The use of percutaneous techniques that are combined with endoscopic intervention limits the necessity to perform limited open surgical drainage procedures that may complicate an eventual liver transplantation.

Surgical therapy has an overall reported complication rate of up to 20% (which includes anastomotic leaks, wound infections, pancreatitis) and a mortality rate of 3%. Up to one-third of patients have a recurrence of symptoms. These patients should be evaluated carefully with repeat ERCP, cytologic sampling, and cancer surveillance. If present, postoperative strictures should be treated with a trial of dilatation and stenting, if malignancy is not suspected.

SUGGESTED READING

Chapman WC, Abecassis M, Jarnigan W, et al. Bile duct injuries 12 years after the introduction of laparoscopic cholecystectomy. *J Gastrointest Surg* 2003;7:412–416.

Harrell DJ, Vitale GC, Larson GM. Selective role for endoscopic retrograde Pancreatography in abdominal trauma. *Surg Endosc* 1998;12: 400–404.

Reed DN, Vitale GC. Interventional endoscopic retrograde cholangiopancreatography and endoscopic surgery. *Surg Clin North Am* 2000;80:1171–1201.

Spigelman AD, Williams CB, Talbot IC, et al. Upper gastrointestinal cancer in patients with familial adenomatous polyposis. *Lancet* 1989; 2:783–785.

Vitale GC, Cothron E, Vitale A, et al. Role of pancreatic duct stenting in the treatment of chronic pancreatitis. *Surg Endosc* 2004;18: 1431–1434.

Vitale GC, George M, McIntyre K, et al. Endoscopic management of benign and malignant biliary strictures. *Am J Surg* 1996; 171:553–557.

Vitale GC, Larson GM, George M, et al. Management of malignant biliary stricture with self-expanding metallic stent. *Surg Endosc* 1996;10:970–973.

Vitale GC, Larson GM, Wieman TJ, et al. The use of ERCP in the management of common bile duct stones in patients undergoing laparoscopic cholecystectomy. *Surg Endosc* 1993;7:9–11.

Vitale GC, Rangnekar NJ, Hewlett SC. Advanced interventional endoscopy. *Curr Probl Surg* 2002;39:26–32.

Vitale GC, Stephens G, Wieman TJ, et al. Use of endoscopic retrograde cholangiopancreatography in the management of biliary complications after laparoscopic cholecystectomy. *Surgery* 1993;114:806–814.

COMMENTARY

Drs. Vitale, Goussev, and Davis have provided a new chapter in this textbook covering endoscopy and its surgical applications in the pancreatobiliary system. This group of experienced surgical endoscopists details the indications and techniques for successfully performing ERCP. ERCP may be helpful to treat common bile duct stones discovered before, during, or after laparoscopic cholecystectomy. In some very elderly patients or those with significant comorbidities, an ERCP with sphincterotomy and stone removal for choledocholithiasis may be the only treatment necessary, even with an intact gallbladder containing stones. Endoscopic techniques, too, have assumed a prominent role in the treatment of postoperative bile duct strictures. This treatment modality is usually limited to those patients who do not have an excisional injury but a stenosis that is relatively short. This discussion of the endoscopic management of bile duct injuries extends that presented by Dr. Strasberg in Chapter 34.

The authors go on to clearly delineate the use of endoscopy in patients with acute and chronic pancreatitis as well as tumors and inflammatory conditions of the biliary and pancreatic ducts. Over the last 30 years ERCP has assumed a prominent role in the diagnosis and management of diseases and disorders of the pancreatobiliary tree. The presence of expert biliary endoscopists within a medical center allows the laparoscopic surgeon to be more aggressive in his or her treatment options. For instance, in a center where endoscopic expertise is lacking, the surgeon performing a cholecystectomy should probably never leave the operating room without definitively treating common bile duct stones. The surgeon and surgical endoscopist must work closely together in deciding the appropriate treatment algorithm for any specific patient, based upon the characteristics of the problem and the combined expertise of the two disciplines.

NJS

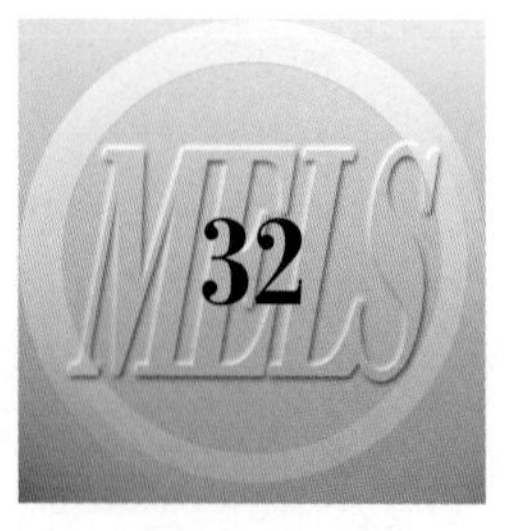

Laparoscopic Cholecystectomy

GERALD M. FRIED, LORENZO E. FERRI, AND KATHERINE E. HSU

INTRODUCTION

Gallstones are an extremely common condition, arising in approximately 10% to 20% of the adult population, and as such pose an important public health problem. Since the days of Carl Langenbuch, it has been recognized that the treatment for symptomatic gallstones is removal of the gallbladder, not because it contains stones, but because it causes them. For over 100 years the technique of cholecystectomy evolved little and required a generous abdominal incision to provide sufficient light and exposure to perform the operation safely. In the late 1980s, with the advent of improved optics and video laparoscopy, the technique of laparoscopic cholecystectomy was introduced and widely adopted by practicing general surgeons. By the time of the National Institutes of Health (NIH) consensus development conference on gallstones and laparoscopic cholecystectomy in 1992, the laparoscopic approach to cholecystectomy had become the standard of care. Overall, over 90% of cholecystectomies are now done using the minimally invasive approach.

Since its introduction, the laparoscopic cholecystectomy procedure has evolved progressively due to improvements in optics and instrumentation. Miniaturization of instruments and thus trocar sites has continued. It is now possible to perform a straightforward elective laparoscopic cholecystectomy using one 10- or 12-mm port and two or three ports as small as 2 to 3.5 mm. It is our current practice to use one 12-mm port at the umbilicus and three other 5-mm ports. We have found that 5-mm instruments are durable and versatile and a 5-mm laparoscope provides a bright and high-quality image. There seems to be little further advantage in decreasing port size below 5 mm.

The early experience with laparoscopic cholecystectomy was associated with an increased risk for common bile duct injuries. With advances in education and improved instrumentation, this risk has been decreased. In the hands of properly trained surgeons, laparoscopic cholecystectomy can be safely performed in the majority of patients.

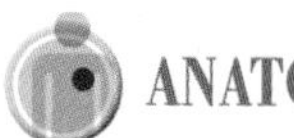

ANATOMY

Surgeons operating on the biliary tract are aware that this region is prone to anatomic anomalies. Surgeons should be cognizant of the main anatomic variations and constantly look for them when operating on the biliary tract. Interpretation of the anatomy is made more difficult in laparoscopic surgery because of a fixed angle of view and monocular optics that make depth perception more difficult. This can be helped with the use of an angled (30-degree) laparoscope that allows viewing from different angles.

Hepatocystic Triangle and Triangle of Calot

The hepatocystic triangle is the space bordered by the inferior edge of the liver, the gallbladder, and the cystic duct. The cystic artery passes through this space. Careful dissection of this area is crucial to safe performance of laparoscopic cholecystectomy. The triangle of Calot is the space bordered by the cystic duct, the cystic artery, and the gallbladder. Dissection of this space is necessary to ensure that there is no tubular structure entering the putative cystic duct between the point of planned clip placement and the gallbladder. The cystic duct should be dissected and clearly visualized circumferentially where it joins the neck of the gallbladder. It is important to obtain the "critical view of safety," first described by Strasberg et al., to ensure that common bile/hepatic duct injury does not occur. In this technique, the tissues of the hepatocystic triangle are completely dissected such that only two structures are entering the gallbladder, which is otherwise still attached to the upper liver bed. The base of the liver bed is exposed through both the hepatocystic and Calot triangles. If this view is achieved, the two structures must be the cystic duct and artery. It is neither advisable nor necessary to perform added dissection for the purpose of exposing the common bile duct (Fig. 32-1). Once this is confirmed, the cystic duct can be safely clipped and divided.

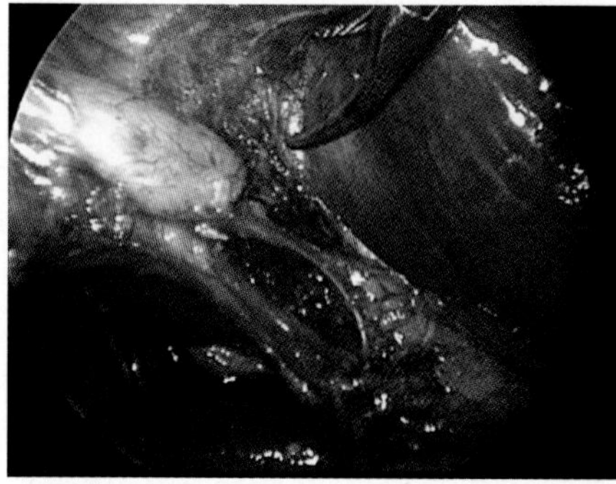

Fig. 32-1. The "critical view of safety" is obtained when the triangle of Calot is dissected such that only two structures are present and the base of the liver can be viewed through the triangle of Calot when viewing it from the anterior position.

Arterial Anatomy

The cystic artery usually arises from the right hepatic artery and divides into anterior and posterior branches near the gallbladder. If dissection of the triangle of Calot is carried out close to the gallbladder wall, anterior and posterior branches may have to be ligated and divided separately. The posterior branch of the cystic artery should be looked for in every case; failure to do so may lead to troublesome bleeding. A useful anatomic marker for the cystic artery is the cystic duct lymph node, which usually lies over the artery.

The right hepatic artery can loop very close to the gallbladder and, in the presence of acute cholecystitis or in patients with a chronically inflamed contracted gallbladder, the right hepatic artery can be easily mistaken for the cystic artery. Also, 15% of the population may have an aberrant right hepatic artery (RHA) originating from the superior mesenteric artery. In this situation the RHA may course across the Triangle of Calot. Therefore, any dissected arterial structure should clearly be seen going to the gallbladder before it can be presumed to be the cystic artery.

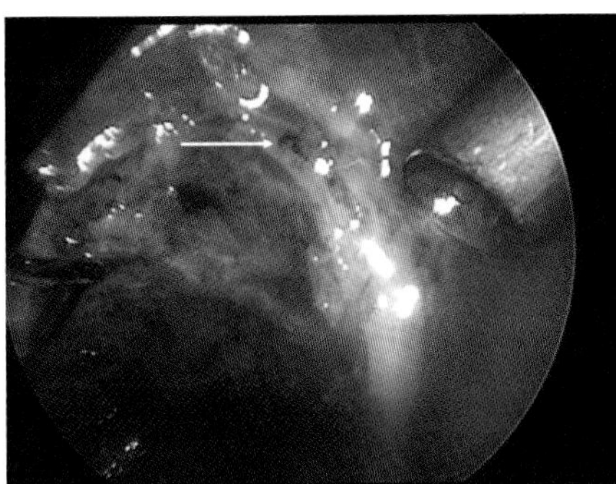

Fig. 32-2. Duct of Luschka (arrow) draining bile from the liver bed after gallbladder removal.

Biliary Duct System

The cystic duct joins the common hepatic duct to form the common bile duct. The point of insertion of the cystic duct is variable and can be low near the duodenum and frequently on the medial side of the bile duct. During laparoscopic surgery, it is important to put traction on the neck of the gallbladder *perpendicular* to the bile duct in order to best differentiate the cystic duct from the common duct. If traction is applied superiorly and medially, the cystic duct will align with the common duct and the common duct can be easily mistaken for the cystic duct and be injured. Infrequently, the cystic duct may enter the right hepatic duct or a segmental ductal branch. For this reason, careful dissection must be performed before clipping or dividing any structure in the hepatocystic triangle.

Accessory bile ducts (of Luschka) have been described between the gallbladder and the liver (Fig. 32-2). Although these have been blamed for postoperative bile leaks, it is more likely that these leaks arise from injury to small bile ducts in the liver parenchyma coursing just deep to the liver capsule as a result of dissection in the incorrect plane.

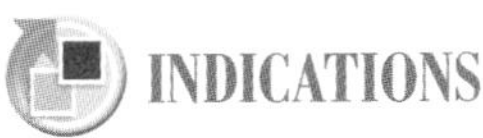

INDICATIONS

Gallstones are very prevalent, yet the majority of these stones are not symptomatic. The natural history of asymptomatic gallstones does not mandate elective cholecystectomy in every patient, because the risk of an asymptomatic patient becoming symptomatic is estimated at only 1% to 2% per year. Thus, the confirmed presence of *symptomatic* gallstones, with or without complications, remains the primary indication for cholecystectomy. The classic presentation of uncomplicated gallstones includes a spectrum of symptoms under the umbrella term of "biliary colic": intermittent right upper quadrant or epigastric pain or severe pressure, which may radiate to the back or tip of the right scapula, associated with nausea and vomiting, and diaphoresis. The development of complications of gallstones, including acute cholecystitis, jaundice, and pancreatitis, is an indication for urgent cholecystectomy. Patients with biliary colic should be scheduled for an elective cholecystectomy, because once gallstones become symptomatic, the risk for recurrent attacks or complications rises dramatically.

Lessons learned from the open cholecystectomy era in patients with acute cholecystitis are applicable to laparoscopic cholecystectomy. Patients who present with up to 72 hours of severe pain should undergo urgent laparoscopic cholecystectomy. In the presence of acute cholecystitis, the rate of conversion from laparoscopy to laparotomy is higher than for patients with simple biliary colic and is estimated to be as high as 10% to 12%. Patients with symptoms of acute cholecystitis longer than 72 hours by the time of presentation present an even more difficult problem for the surgeon. These patients are likely to have a significant degree of dense and very vascular inflammatory adhesions with loss of normal tissue planes. Conversion rates from laparoscopic to open procedures have been quoted as high as 20% to 29%. An option for their management may be a trial of conservative therapy, including fasting and intravenous antibiotics. If these patients respond rapidly to this treatment, they can be discharged from hospital and readmitted for an interval cholecystectomy in approximately 6 to 8 weeks.

In acute biliary pancreatitis, laparoscopic cholecystectomy should be performed on the same admission once the signs and symptoms of pancreatic inflammation have resolved. Delay in the removal of the gallbladder after an episode of pancreatitis puts the patient at significant risk for recurrent attacks of pancreatitis or gallstone complications. Up to 20% of patients will have a recurrent attack of acute pancreatitis within 30 days of a first attack if a cholecystectomy is not performed. Bile duct imaging is indicated in all patients with biliary pancreatitis. Options include intraoperative cholangiography (our preferred approach), intraoperative ultrasonography, or preoperative magnetic resonance cholangiography. Since the prevalence of bile duct stones in these patients at one week or longer after an acute attack is in the range of 15%, diagnostic ERCP is not recommended unless there is high suspicion of bile duct stones (e.g., jaundice, dilated duct, or visible common duct stones on ultrasound).

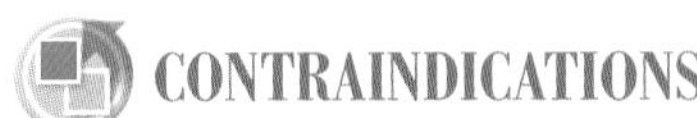

CONTRAINDICATIONS

As experience has been gained with laparoscopic cholecystectomy, the number of contraindications has progressively diminished. Absolute contraindications to laparoscopic cholecystectomy include suspicion of gallbladder cancer, inability to identify relevant anatomical structures, and uncontrolled bleeding disorders.

Almost all of the traditional relative contraindications may be addressed by an experienced and prudent minimally invasive surgeon. Special consideration should be given to patients with previous abdominal surgery, pregnancy, and cirrhosis.

Previous Abdominal Surgery

Although early series demonstrated that previous abdominal surgery with accompanying risk of adhesions was a predictor of conversion, it is clear that laparoscopic cholecystectomy may be performed safely on most of these patients. Certainly, previous lower abdominal operations add little difficulty in performing cholecystectomy, as long as the initial trocar can be placed safely. Patients with previous upper abdominal operations, especially in the right upper quadrant, present much more difficulty in gaining access to the area of the gallbladder. Despite this, a trial of the laparoscopic approach is warranted in these patients. It is important to note that not all patients with previous operations have adhesions to the anterior abdominal wall and, conversely, the absence of prior surgery does not necessarily predict the absence of adhesions. To diminish the risk of intraperitoneal injury in patients with prior surgery, we routinely use the open Hasson technique for placement of the initial trocar. Many other surgeons advocate the use of the Veress needle and percutaneous insertion of the initial trocar in these patients, choosing an insertion site remote from the abdominal wall scars.

Pregnancy

Any operative intervention during pregnancy must be carefully considered. Fetal loss due to spontaneous abortion or developmental abnormalities are risks with any surgery during the first trimester. Surgery during the third trimester may precipitate premature labor. The enlarged uterus late in pregnancy may require alteration in trocar placement and patient positioning when surgery cannot be avoided.

In the early days of laparoscopic surgery, there was concern expressed over its safety in pregnancy with respect to both the patient and the fetus. Pneumoperitoneum was thought to cause diminished uterine blood flow, increased fetal acidosis, and general fetal distress; however, these risks appear to be overstated. Although it is generally accepted that elective cholecystectomy for biliary colic should be delayed until after birth, these risks must be measured against the risk of ongoing inflammation in a patient with acute cholecystitis. When laparoscopic cholecystectomy must be performed during pregnancy, it is most safely done in the second trimester. The patient should be rotated to the left to move the uterus off the inferior vena cava and away from the operative field, and CO_2 pneumoperitoneum should be administered at the lowest pressure required to provide exposure.

Cirrhosis

Patients with cirrhosis and portal hypertension are at increased risk for any surgical procedure, including laparoscopic cholecystectomy. Optimal preoperative preparation is mandatory, including replacement of clotting factors. Intravenous vasopressin also may be useful to decrease intraoperative bleeding in selected patients with portal hypertension. Trocar placement must be performed with particular care, avoiding large collateral vessels in the abdominal wall. Bleeding from the liver bed can be quite profuse during dissection of the gallbladder, but can be minimized by remaining within the correct tissue plane. Electrocautery and innovative energy sources, such as bipolar welding devices and the ultrasonic shears, are helpful to diminish bleeding from the raw liver surfaces. When bleeding develops, direct compression with an adrenaline-soaked sponge placed through the 12-mm trocar is helpful, and local agents to promote coagulation should be available (oxidized cellulose, fibrin glue, etc.). Properly prepared, compensated cirrhotics can undergo laparoscopic cholecystectomy with risk comparable to open cholecystectomy.

PREOPERATIVE PLANNING

A detailed history can facilitate operative planning and decrease the risk of perioperative morbidity. Eliciting a history of reduced cardiopulmonary reserve may identify patients who will not tolerate CO_2 pneumoperitoneum. A careful history is the best way to diagnose patients with occult bleeding diatheses. A history of jaundice or pancreatitis should alert the surgeon to an elevated risk of choledocholithiasis.

Preoperative investigations should include biochemical analysis of liver function and ultrasound imaging of the gallbladder and biliary tree. Significant abnormalities in either of these tests may prompt further investigations. The primary goals of these preoperative investigations are to confirm the presence of gallstones and to determine if the patient is likely to have common bile duct stones. By identifying patients with choledocholithiasis preoperatively, the surgeon may plan to clear these stones either preoperatively by endoscopic means or at the time of surgery by laparoscopic or open techniques.

A selective approach to cholangiography and biliary tree clearance preoperatively benefits those at highest risk and limits the potential complications of these additional invasive procedures in those at low risk for common bile duct stones. Patients with clinical jaundice, ultrasonographic evidence of a dilated common bile duct, or visible common duct stones are considered at high risk for choledocholithiasis. Our practice with these patients is to perform endoscopic sphincterotomy and duct clearance, followed in 24 hours by laparoscopic cholecystectomy. A history of pancreatitis, multiple small stones on ultrasonography, and mild elevations of serum direct bilirubin or alkaline phosphatase represent moderate risk factors. With these patients, we do either intraoperative fluoroscopic cholangiography or preoperative magnetic resonance cholangiography (MRCP). Patients with large solitary gallstones, normal biliary tree on ultrasonography, and a normal biochemical liver profile are considered to be at low risk for common duct stones; we do not do routine cholangiography in these patients. Other authors recommend routine cholangiography in all patients. There is no high-level evidence to help decide between these two approaches.

Prophylactic Antibiotics

The rate of surgical site infections in uncomplicated cholecystectomy is 1% to 4%. Despite numerous prospective trials, a definitive benefit of routine antibiotic prophylaxis in uncomplicated elective gallstone disease has not been established. Accordingly, we do not recommend routine antibiotic prophylaxis. Rather, a selective approach is used. Patients at high risk for having bacterial contamination of their bile are given a single dose of a second-generation cephalosporin 15 to 30 minutes before the incision. These patients include those with acute cholecystitis, prior biliary tree instrumentation, choledocholithiasis, or who are older than 70 years of age. Patients who are immunosuppressed and those with prosthetic devices also should receive preoperative antibiotics. In the absence of a prospective trial to validate these criteria, the surgeon needs to individualize the use of antibiotic prophylaxis in his or her practice.

Prophylaxis against Deep Vein Thrombosis

The increased intraabdominal pressure due to pneumoperitoneum, reverse-Trendelenburg position, and systemic vasodilatation associated with general anesthesia in laparoscopic cholecystectomy may confer a theoretical increased risk for the development of deep vein thrombosis (DVT). Despite scientific studies that demonstrate diminished venous outflow in femoral veins of patients undergoing laparoscopic procedures, implying stasis, no study to date has demonstrated a decrease in DVT with pharmacologic prophylaxis (unfractionated or low molecular weight heparin). Given the low rate of DVT in this patient population (1% to 3%), an appropriately powered study designed to show a benefit of prophylaxis would require a vast number of patients. In the absence of convincing evidence in the literature, we recommend DVT prophylaxis in laparoscopic cholecystectomy (heparin and/or pneumatic compression devices) according to the guidelines for open procedures: previous DVT, cancer, obesity, exogenous estrogens, projected operating time >2 hours, and age >40 years.

SURGICAL TECHNIQUE

Step 1: Patient Positioning

The patient is placed in the supine position with the right arm tucked by the side and the left arm free for access by the anesthesia team. The operating surgeon stands to the patient's left, the camera operator to the surgeon's left, and the assistant on the patient's right. The primary video monitor is placed on the patient's right at the level of the shoulder, to give an unobstructed view for the surgeon and camera assistant. A second monitor, if available, is placed to the surgeon's right to allow the assistant to comfortably view the procedure. We routinely use a radiolucent operating table to facilitate operative cholangiography. An electric table is preferred because patient positioning is used to facilitate exposure.

Step 2: Introduction of Initial Trocar and Generation of Pneumoperitoneum

The insertion of the first trocar not only allows for the development of pneumoperitoneum, but also allows for the safe insertion of additional operative trocars under direct vision with the laparoscope.

In patients without previous surgery near the umbilicus, the 12-mm trocar is first placed through a 10- to 15-mm transverse or vertical incision through or adjacent to the umbilicus. This location may be altered in certain circumstances, such as obesity, previous abdominal surgery, or pregnancy. The benefits of this location include its central position in the abdomen, the cosmetic benefit, and the lack of subcutaneous fat beneath the umbilicus, making access to the fascia easy even in obese individuals. The base of the umbilical raphe is grasped with a Kocher forceps, allowing the surgeon to bring the linea alba up to the wound. At this point, either the percutaneous or open routes may be used to initiate pneumoperitoneum.

Our preference is the open approach using a blunt-tipped Hasson cannula. We make a 12-mm transverse incision through the linea alba and peritoneum and insert the trocar under direct vision. Intraperitoneal positioning is confirmed by insertion of a blunt instrument or the surgeon's finger. Stay sutures are placed on either side of the fascial incision to not only aid in fixing the Hasson cannula to the fascia and preventing an air leak, but also to close the eventual defect at the conclusion of the procedure. We find this open approach is very quick and virtually eliminates the risk of major vascular injury. Although this complication is rare, it is catastrophic, and repeatedly reported with the percutaneous insertion of a sharp trocar, even in experienced hands.

The percutaneous approach uses a Veress needle, which is passed through the fascia into the peritoneal cavity, aiming for the midline in the direction of the sacral hollow. Lateral deviation increases the risk of puncturing the iliac vessels. Proper intraperitoneal positioning can be verified by first aspirating and then allowing saline to pass through the needle by gravity alone. The gas tubing is connected to electronic insufflator tubing and insufflation begun. Good flow and low pressure provides further evidence of proper placement of the trocar.

Carbon dioxide traditionally has been used for the generation of pneumoperitoneum in laparoscopic surgery. This gas is highly soluble and does not support combustion, yet may result in significant systemic absorption and acidemia in prolonged cases. In the majority of patients this is well tolerated and can be minimized by increasing the ventilation, eliminating CO_2 in the expired gas. However, patients with underlying severe respiratory or cardiac disease may not tolerate the CO_2 load. Alternative gases are available, such as nitrous oxide, and can be used in selective cases.

Intraabdominal pressure should be individualized for each case. The surgeon should aim for the minimal pressure required to provide an adequate working space, keeping in mind the potential deleterious consequences of sustained elevated intraabdominal pressures. High intraabdominal pressure may mimic abdominal compartment syndrome with diminished venous return due to compression of the inferior vena cava and elevated airway pressure due to forces exerted on the diaphragm. We usually start with 12 mmHg and adjust accordingly, avoiding pressures above 15 mmHg. An open line of communication between the surgical and anesthesia teams is of paramount importance in all laparoscopic cases; the pressure may need to be adjusted up to obtain adequate working space, or down to limit the deleterious physiologic effects of the pneumoperitoneum.

Step 3: Placement of Accessory Trocars

After pneumoperitoneum is achieved, the laparoscope is placed through the umbilical trocar to confirm adequate operating space and aid in the insertion of the accessory operating trocars under direct vision. We always use an angled laparoscope (30 degrees) for laparoscopic cholecystectomy. An angled scope can provide angles of view that cannot be obtained with a 0-degree scope, and this greatly adds to the safety of the operation. In most circumstances, a total of four trocars is optimal to perform a cholecystectomy. At times a fifth trocar may be required to aid in retraction of redundant transverse colon or bulky omentum. There is minimal risk to using an additional 5-mm trocar, and there should be no reluctance to use one if it can help in the exposure during a difficult case.

It is important to note that the location of the three accessory trocars should not be rigidly standardized. The surgeon should place these trocars according to the intraabdominal anatomy. Thus stated, however, most surgeons place a 5-mm port, through which a grasping forceps is placed on the fundus of the gallbladder, in the right anterior axillary line, approximately halfway between the costal margin and the anterior superior iliac spine. A second accessory port is placed high in the epigastrium, immediately to the right of the falciform ligament. This trocar may be 5 or 10 mm. This trocar will need to accommodate a clip applier and (during extraction of the gallbladder) a laparoscope, so the trocar size will depend on whether a 5- or 10-mm clip applier and scope are being used. It is our usual practice to use a 5-mm 30-degree scope and a 5-mm reusable clip applier (with locking nylon clips); we therefore use three 5-mm trocars for our accessory ports. The final accessory port of 5 mm is placed according to surgeon preference either just below the liver edge in the right midclavicular line (Fig. 32-3A, page 304) or, alternatively, in the midline adjacent to the falciform ligament in the midepigastrium, at the same horizontal level as the gallbladder (Fig. 32-3B, page 304). The exact choice of trocar location will depend not only on the patient's anatomy but also the technique used by the surgeon. We prefer the surgeon to use two hands, holding the gallbladder neck in one hand while operating with the other hand. The right midclavicular line port placement may be better suited to right-handed dissection, while the midepigastric placement is better suited for left-handed dissection.

Step 4: Adhesiolysis and Exposing the Cystic Duct and Artery

Adhesions obscuring the right upper quadrant due to previous surgery or inflammation may require division prior to

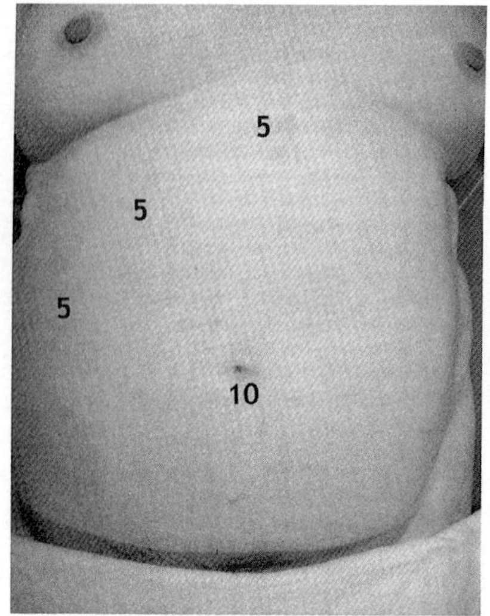

A

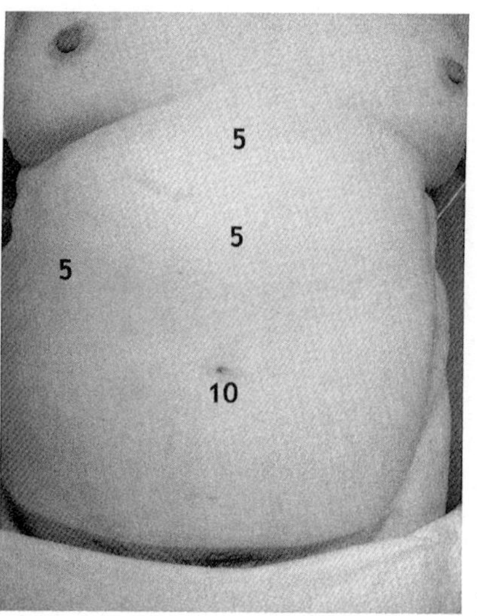

B

Fig. 32-3. Two options demonstrating possible port placement, depending on the surgeon's preference. **A.** Midclavicular right subcostal, for a right-handed dissection. **B.** Midline epigastric, for a left-handed dissection.

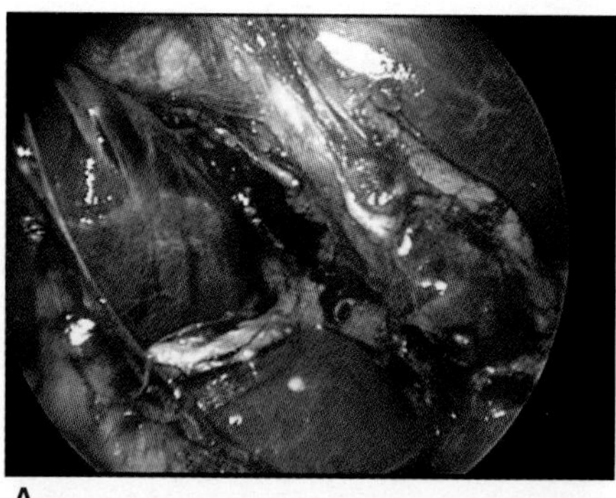

A

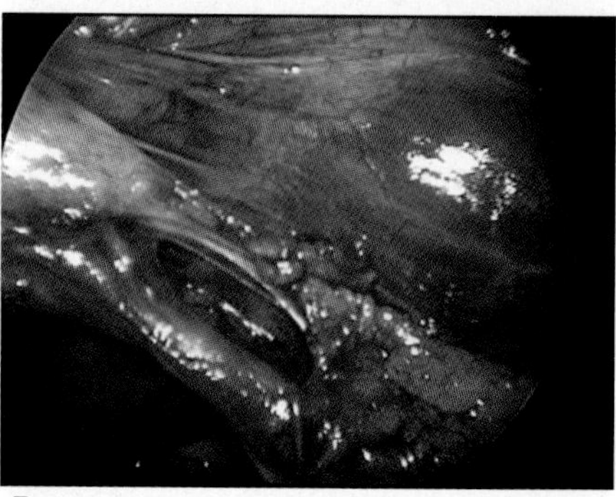

B

Fig. 32-4. Retraction of Hartmann pouch. **A.** Improper retraction superoanteriorly causes the cystic and common hepatic ducts to come into alignment. This may lead to major duct injury, as the common hepatic/common bile ducts (CHD/CBD) are misidentified as the cystic duct. **B.** Proper retraction inferolaterally separates the cystic duct from the CHD/CBD and opens the triangle of Calot.

commencing the dissection of the gallbladder. The plane between the anterior abdominal wall and the omentum is usually avascular. Adhesiolysis should be sharp, and electrocautery should be employed sparingly if at all to minimize the risk of thermal injury to adjacent bowel. The surgeon should be able to develop an avascular plane between the adhesions and the gallbladder wall by gently grasping the adhesions at their insertion.

Adequate exposure of the hepatocystic triangle is of paramount importance and is required prior to proceeding with a laparoscopic cholecystectomy. By tilting the patient in reverse-Trendelenburg position and to the left, gravity is used to expose the gallbladder as it retracts the colon, duodenum, omentum, and stomach. If necessary, gastric decompression may be achieved by an orogastric tube passed by the anesthetist.

Once freed from adhesions, the fundus of the gallbladder is grasped by the assistant through the most lateral trocar, applying retraction superiorly and to the right. If the gallbladder is distended and tense due to acute cholecystitis or hydrops, it is helpful to aspirate the gallbladder with a 14-gauge needle passed percutaneously prior to grasping the fundus. This retraction effectively rotates the liver and exposes the gallbladder body and the Hartmann pouch. With this maneuver alone the hepatocystic triangle is very narrow, causing the cystic and common hepatic ducts to be in parallel alignment (Fig. 32-4A). This parallel alignment may lead to inadvertent injury to the common hepatic duct as it is erroneously identified as the cystic duct. In order to open the triangle of Calot, the surgeon grasps the Hartmann pouch and retracts it caudally and to the right. By opening the hepatocystic triangle, the cystic–common hepatic duct angle widens, separating these two structures and thereby permitting safe dissection (Fig. 32-4B). Using a curved dissector through the main operating trocar, the peritoneal layer overlying the gallbladder–cystic duct junction is circumferentially peeled away, starting posteriorly. The neck of the gallbladder is dissected away from its attachments to the liver and the junction of the gallbladder; the cystic duct can now be seen clearly from all directions. The surgeon should alternate between inferolateral and superomedial retraction of the Hartmann pouch to view the three-dimensional anatomy of the hepatocystic triangle.

Step 5: Dissection and Division of Cystic Duct and Artery

With the overlying peritoneum stripped, dissection should start close to the gallbladder until the gallbladder–cystic duct junction is completely dissected and encircled, to limit the risk of confusing the right hepatic, common hepatic, or common bile duct for the cystic duct. Electrocautery is used with extreme caution during this stage, to avoid electrical injury to the biliary ducts. We retract the Hartmann pouch and cystic duct inferolaterally and, while looking with the angled laparoscope from anteriorly to posteriorly, we make certain that we can see the liver through this space, ensuring that no hepatic ducts are entering the structure we have interpreted as the cystic duct. No structure is clipped or divided until this "critical view of safety" is achieved where only two structures are clearly entering into the gallbladder and the base of the liver can be visualized through the dissected triangle of Calot (Fig. 32-1). Only by achieving this critical view can a surgeon be certain that the two structures are indeed the cystic artery and duct. Once identified, the cystic duct is dissected only to allow the safe placement of two or three clips. Further dissection down to the cystic duct–common duct junction is not only unnecessary, but also may increase the risk of injury to these structures. Although the long-term effect of a long cystic duct remnant is unknown, the relationship to postcholecystectomy syndrome is probably overstated. Once the cystic duct is dissected free, the cystic duct should be milked toward the gallbladder so that any stones present will be pushed into the gallbladder. If indicated, a cholangiogram is done at this time (this will be discussed later) or, alternatively, after dissection and division of the cystic artery.

The artery is located cephalad to the duct and usually runs parallel to it. The cystic artery usually is anatomically related posterior to the cystic duct node, which serves as a useful landmark for this structure. When dissection is carried out very close to the gallbladder, the cystic artery may have already divided into multiple small ramifications; occasionally, a major cystic artery may not be identified. Care should be taken to ensure that the artery identified is actually entering the gallbladder. The right hepatic artery can course very close to the gallbladder and can be easily mistaken for the cystic artery. In addition, a posterior branch of the cystic artery may be encountered and should be sought in all cases to avoid troublesome bleeding. Once fully dissected, the cystic duct and artery are controlled with clips and divided.

Inflammation from current or previous episodes of cholecystitis may make the cystic duct difficult to control using regular clips. Other options to occlude the cystic duct may need to be employed if the cystic duct is significantly thickened, wide, or shortened. Standard clips may not be large enough to completely occlude a wide duct; therefore multiple clips, extra- or intracorporeal ligation of the duct (Fig. 32-5), the use of an endoloop, or, rarely, an endoscopic stapling device may be required. The application of multiple clips involves an initial clip occluding as much of the duct as possible, followed by a partial cut of the duct with the laparoscopic scissors. The remaining unoccluded duct is then clipped at the apex of incision. The use of an endoloop has been well described for the management of wide cystic ducts, but requires division of the duct prior to ligation, risking retraction of the cystic duct. Our preference is to encircle the duct with a ligature and to secure this with either an intracorporeal or extracorporeal tie while the duct is in continuity.

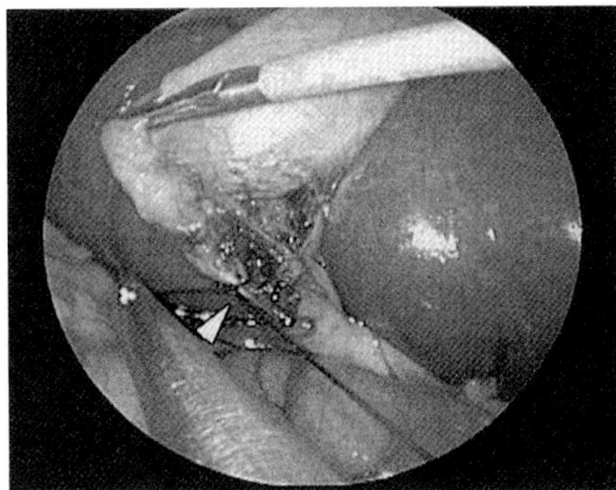

Fig. 32-5. Controlling a difficult cystic duct with extracorporeal ligation (arrow).

Step 6: Intraoperative Cholangiogram

The routine use of intraoperative cholangiography is controversial. Proponents cite the relatively high rate (10%) of choledocholithiasis in all patients undergoing cholecystectomy, the need to define the exact biliary anatomy, and the need to be comfortable with the technique in cases when the indication is certain. Opponents argue that there are no objective data to demonstrate that the routine use of cholangiography in low-risk patients diminishes complications due to biliary injury or choledocholithiasis. Despite this controversy, pre- or intraoperative findings may warrant an intraoperative cholangiogram. After identification and dissection of the cystic duct, a clip is placed at the gallbladder–cystic duct junction and a small partial cut is made in the anterolateral wall of the cystic duct. A saline-flushed 4- or 5F catheter is then passed into the resulting hole by one of two methods: specially designed cholangiogram (Olsen) forceps can be used through a right subcostal port, or a catheter can be introduced percutaneously through a 14-gauge intravenous catheter. The cholangiogram catheter is advanced into the cystic duct and secured with a clip or the clamp. Radiopaque instruments should be moved away from the operative field and the C-arm positioned. Water-soluble contrast is injected slowly under fluoroscopic guidance. Video fluoroscopy provides a dynamic image of the contrast filling the biliary tree and is superior to static films. However, if fluoroscopy is not available, at least two static films are taken for a cholangiogram. The first film is taken after 5 ml of contrast diluted with equal parts of saline is injected. The contrast is diluted in this case as the cholangiogram is not taken while filling the bile ducts with contrast, and full strength contrast may overshadow any filling defects when looking at one static film. The first film should document contrast freely flowing through the common bile duct into the duodenum. A further 10 to 15 ml of contrast are injected, and the second film taken. This film should show the common hepatic duct, bifurcation, and minor duct anatomy. It is imperative to visualize the entire biliary tree from the intrahepatic ducts to the duodenum. Once the cholangiogram is completed, hard copy films are printed or digital images saved, and the cholangiogram catheter is removed. Two clips are placed on the distal cystic duct prior to completely dividing the duct. Stones identified by cholangiogram may be managed intraoperatively by laparoscopic techniques or postoperatively by ERCP (endoscopic retrograde cholangiopancreatography) (described in Chapter 31). An alternative means to identify stones in the bile duct is laparoscopic ultrasound. This is a rapid and accurate technique. It avoids the radiation exposure of cholangiography, but it does not provide as detailed anatomic information of the biliary tree.

Step 7: Dissection of the Gallbladder from the Liver Bed

With the cystic duct and artery secured and divided, the gallbladder is then dissected from the liver bed. Dissection is facilitated by placing the areolar tissue attaching the gallbladder to the liver bed under tension with appropriately directed traction and countertraction. This is achieved by alternating retraction of the neck of the gallbladder from an inferolateral to superomedial position (Fig. 32-6). The tissue placed under tension is then easily divided with the use of monopolar electrocautery. Throughout the operation, monopolar cautery settings are placed at the lowest level to provide hemostasis, usually 25 watts. The plane between the gallbladder and liver is usually quite avascular; bleeding usually signifies that the surgeon has deviated from the plane and has violated the integrity of the liver. If encountered, bleeding can be controlled by electrocautery in the vast majority of cases.

If the surgeon deviates from the avascular plane in the other direction, the result is the perforation of the gallbladder, often with spillage of both bile and stones.

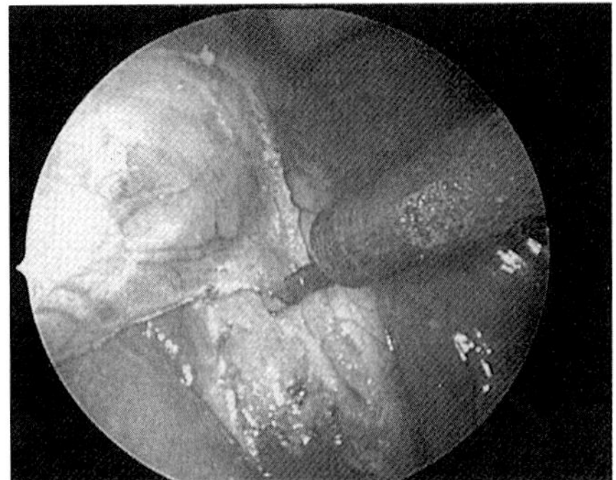

Fig. 32-6. Inferolateral retraction of gallbladder for dissection off the liver bed; note the avascular plane under appropriate tension.

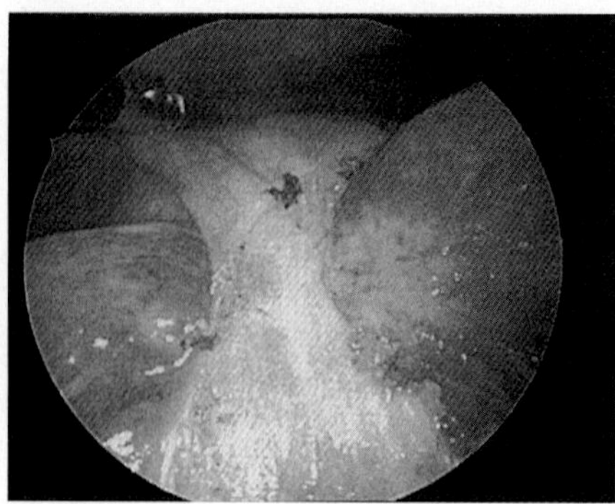

Fig. 32-7. A final narrow bridge of peritoneum attaching the gallbladder to the liver bed.

To limit contamination and the continued spillage of stones, the hole can be controlled in several ways. The surgeon can grasp the wall adjacent to the hole and the gallbladder can be retracted from that point for the remainder of the procedure, or the hole can be closed with a suture ligature or an endoloop. Dissection continues until the gallbladder fundus is attached by a thin strip of peritoneum (Fig. 32-7). Using the gallbladder as a handle to maintain exposure, the areas of dissection are carefully examined for bleeding or bile leak, with particular attention paid to the clipped cystic duct and artery stumps. The surgeon may wish to irrigate the area at this time; however, routine irrigation is not necessary in the absence of bile spillage. If stones are spilled into the abdominal cavity, every effort should be made to retrieve the stones as these can lead to future abdominal wall and intraabdominal abscesses. After hemostasis is assured, the final attachment to the gallbladder is divided, and the gallbladder is placed above the right lobe of the liver without removing the grasping forceps.

Step 8: Extraction of the Gallbladder

The laparoscope is repositioned in the epigastric port and a heavy grasping forceps is introduced through the umbilical port to grasp the neck of the gallbladder. Under direct vision, the gallbladder is extracted via the umbilical trocar insertion site. The fascia and skin incisions may need to be enlarged in order to retrieve the gallbladder; however, simple stretching with a Kelly forceps usually suffices. If perforation of the gallbladder occurred during the procedure, the gallbladder should be placed in a sterile bag prior to extraction to limit bile contamination of the abdomen and wound, as well as stone spillage. Every attempt should be made to collect and remove spilled stones. This may be achieved by placing them in the sterile bag with the excised gallbladder. Alternatively, an effective means to remove small- and medium-sized spilled stones is the use of a 10-mm suction–irrigation probe or suctioning small stones through a 28F chest tube placed through a 10 to 12 mm trocar. If the security of the cystic duct closure is in doubt, or the common bile duct was explored, a closed suction drain is left in the right subhepatic space and exteriorized through the right lateral trocar site.

Following extraction of the gallbladder, the pneumoperitoneum is recreated and the trocars are removed under direct vision to ensure that there is no bleeding from the trocar sites. The fascia at the umbilicus and at any trocar site larger than 5 mm should be closed to prevent hernia formation.

CONVERSION TO LAPAROTOMY

It is important to keep in mind that the primary goal of laparoscopic cholecystectomy is the *safe* removal of the gallbladder; therefore, conversion to open laparotomy should not be deemed a failure. Conversion to laparotomy may be required to definitively identify surgical anatomy or to address intraoperative complications such as bleeding or biliary or bowel injury. Ideally, conversion should be carried out before complications arise. Conversion also may be required when the procedure is technically not feasible due to inability to grasp a necrotic gallbladder and retract it appropriately to open the hepatocystic triangle.

Conversion rates of 5% overall and 20% for acute cholecystitis generally have been reported in the literature. The ability to better predict the probability of conversion preoperatively allows both the surgeon and the patient to adequately prepare for the procedure. Patients deemed to have a high risk of conversion preoperatively might not be the best candidates for outpatient cholecystectomy. Factors determined to be predictive of conversion include acute cholecystitis (present or past), male gender, age >65 years, and gallbladder wall thickening >3 mm as determined by ultrasound. Other factors with less predictive value include morbid obesity, previous upper abdominal surgery, and severe pancreatitis.

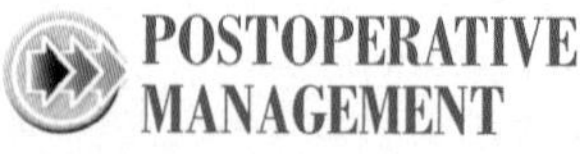

POSTOPERATIVE MANAGEMENT

Most patients may be managed in an ambulatory surgery setting and discharged several hours after surgery. Routine postoperative investigations or antibiotics are unnecessary, and patients are allowed regular diet if they are not experiencing nausea. Oral analgesics are usually sufficient for control of pain after laparoscopic cholecystectomy. We find that incisional injection of bupivacaine, the use of nonsteroidal antiinflammatory drugs (NSAIDs) administered as a suppository or intramuscularly at completion of the procedure, and minimizing the use of narcotics are helpful in minimizing postoperative pain, nausea, and vomiting. Other adjuncts include the use of a single intravenous injection of dexamethasone. Persistent pain that requires prolonged parenteral opioids should alert the surgeon of possible complications and may mandate further investigations or admission to the hospital. Discharged ambulatory patients are advised to be cognizant of signs of potential complications, such as increasing abdominal pain, fever, unremitting nausea, and jaundice. Follow-up in the office or clinic is set at around 2 weeks. If no problems arise, no further follow-up is required.

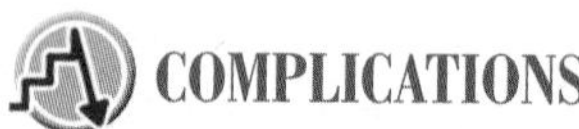

COMPLICATIONS

The blind percutaneous approach to establish pneumoperitoneum may cause intraperitoneal injury with either the Veress needle or trocar. Puncture of bowel by the Veress needle does not necessarily require treatment in the absence of leakage of bowel contents. However, the site of injury should be marked and rechecked at the completion of the procedure. More significant bowel injury by the Veress needle and some trocar injuries to bowel can be exteriorized through an enlarged umbilical incision and repaired securely prior to proceeding with the laparoscopic cholecystectomy. Another option is to suture a small laceration laparoscopically. In all cases the bowel should be carefully inspected for the possibility of a through and through injury. A more severe trocar injury to the bowel, mesentery, or vascular structures mandates prompt laparotomy for repair.

Bleeding can arise at several points in the procedure. Trocar insertion may impale a blood vessel. This can result in laceration but subsequent tamponade of abdominal wall vessels; therefore, bleeding may only be noted after the trocar is removed at the conclusion of the case. This point underlines the importance of visualizing the insertion sites at the end of the procedure. Injury to abdominal wall vessels can be controlled with a figure-of-eight stitch placed under direct vision, either with a straight needle or suture passer. Alternatively, a Foley catheter can be passed through the trocar insertion site and a 30-ml balloon inflated and pulled under tension to tamponade the vessel for 4 to 6 hours.

Bleeding from the liver bed can be controlled with electrocautery in most cases. If this does not work, options include direct pressure with an adrenaline-soaked sponge, packing with oxidized cellulose or similar hemostatic agent, or the use of fibrin sealant. Bleeding arising from the porta hepatis requires a more careful approach. Indiscriminate clipping or electrocautery in this area is likely to cause injury to the bile duct or hepatic vasculature. Arterial bleeding is usually due to loss of control of the cystic artery or its posterior branch. Irrigation and suction, through an additional trocar if necessary, should be used liberally to identify the source of bleeding. If the bleeding site is clearly identified, a curved dissector can be used to grasp the vessel so that it can be carefully clipped. Brisk bleeding in this area that cannot rapidly be controlled laparoscopically should prompt immediate conversion.

Bile leaks occur in approximately 1% of laparoscopic cholecystectomy cases and most often are noted only after the patient has been discharged from hospital. Symptoms typically arise 4 to 10 days after the procedure and include increasing abdominal pain, fever, and abdominal distension. Ultrasound examination demonstrating a significant fluid collection should prompt an hydroxyl iminodiacetic acid (HIDA) radionuclide scan to confirm a suspected ongoing leak. Once a bile leak is confirmed, it is usually drained percutaneously and the biliary anatomy defined with cholangiography (MRCP or ERCP). The cystic duct is the most common source of bile leaks after laparoscopic cholecystectomy. Most can be managed by percutaneous drainage and endoscopic sphincterotomy with temporary stenting. Rarely is reoperative management required for a bile leak from the cystic duct.

Major bile duct injuries may be unrecognized at the time of surgery and can present several days after the procedure with abdominal pain, fever, or jaundice. The best chance to repair major biliary injuries is the first chance, and success is the highest when this is undertaken by an experienced biliary surgeon. If referral to another institution is required, external drainage should be performed and the patient transferred for definitive management.

SUGGESTED READING

Adamsen S, Hansen OH, Funch-Jensen P, et al. Bile duct injury during laparoscopic cholecystectomy: a prospective nationwide series. *J Am Coll Surg* 1997;184:571–578.

Al-Fozan H, Tulandi T. Safety and risks of laparoscopy in pregnancy. *Curr Opin Obstet Gynecol* 2002;14:375–379.

Barkun AN, Barkun JS, Fried GM, et al. Useful predictors of bile duct stones in patients undergoing laparoscopic cholecystectomy. McGill Gallstone Treatment Group. *Ann Surg* 1994;220:32–39.

Barkun AN, Rezieg M, Mehta SN, et al. Postcholecystectomy biliary leaks in the laparoscopic era: risk factors, presentation, and management. McGill Gallstone Treatment Group. *Gastrointest Endosc* 1997;45:277–282.

Fried GM, Barkun JS, Sigman HH, et al. Factors determining conversion to laparotomy in patients undergoing laparoscopic cholecystectomy. *Am J Surg* 1994;167:35–39.

Gracie WA, Ransohoff DF. The natural history of silent gallstones: the innocent gallstone is not a myth. *N Engl J Med* 1982;307:798–800.

Lo CM, Liu CL, Fan ST, et al. Prospective randomized study of early versus delayed laparoscopic cholecystectomy for acute cholecystitis. *Ann Surg* 1998;227(4):461–466.

National Institutes of Health Consensus Development Conference Statement. Gallstones and laparoscopic cholecystectomy. September 14–16, 1992. *J Laparoendosc Surg* 1993;3:77–90.

Poggio JL, Rowland CM, Gores GJ, et al. A comparison of laparoscopic and open cholecystectomy in patients with compensated cirrhosis and symptomatic gallstone disease. *Surgery* 2000;127:405–411.

Sigman HH, Fried GM, Garzon J, et al. Risks of blind versus open approach to celiotomy for laparoscopic surgery. *Surg Laparosc Endosc* 1993;3:296–299.

Society of American Gastrointestinal Endoscopic Surgeons (SAGES). Guidelines for laparoscopic surgery during pregnancy. *Surg Endosc* 1998;12:189–190.

Strasberg SM. Avoidance of biliary injury during laparoscopic cholecystectomy. *J Hepatobiliary Pancreat Surg* 2002;9(5):543–547.

COMMENTARY

Drs. Fried, Ferri, and Hsu have described their practical approach to the performance of laparoscopic cholecystectomy. All surgeons performing cholecystectomy should be aware of the fact that "normal" biliary ductal anatomy is seen in less than 50% of patients. The Achilles' heel of laparoscopic cholecystectomy remains bile duct injury. The authors have illustrated their technique for safe performance of laparoscopic cholecystectomy; when combined Dr. Strasberg's discussion in Chapter 34 on the prevention of bile duct injuries, the reader should understand techniques that will minimize the likelihood of bile duct injury.

Few absolute contraindications exist for laparoscopic cholecystectomy, but a number of conditions render the operation more difficult. Acute cholecystitis is one of these conditions. Within the first few days of onset of the acute inflammation, the dissection may be simplified by the presence of edema in the tissue planes. Over the next few days, however, these planes become obscured by hypervascular tissue, and the conversion rate increases. This has led to talk of a "golden period" lasting for up to 72 hours after initiation of pain with acute cholecystitis. My approach to the management of patients who present late in the course of acute cholecystitis is to assess whether the patient can safely undergo *open* cholecystectomy. In a young, otherwise healthy patient, we will generally proceed with an attempted laparoscopic cholecystectomy with the knowledge that the rate of conversion will be higher (even if the conversion occurs after the patient has cooled off and returns to the operating room in 8 weeks). In those patients who would not tolerate an open cholecystectomy well and in those with an acute comorbidity, we try to delay the operation for 8 to 10 weeks, when the subacute inflammation has evolved to chronic inflammation. This may require the placement of a percutaneous cholecystotomy tube for resolution of the acute symptoms and signs.

Other adjunctive techniques for laparoscopic cholecystectomy bear mentioning. In the cirrhotic, most gallstones

(continued)

can simply be observed, as the incidence of gallstones is high, and there are many other causes for right upper quadrant pain in this subset of patients. However, when a cholecystectomy is truly deemed necessary in the presence of portal hypertension, it may be safer to leave the back wall of the gallbladder attached to the gallbladder bed and simply remove the anterior two-thirds of the gallbladder and its contents, a so-called subtotal cholecystectomy. In the patient in whom the hepatocystic triangle is very difficult to dissect due to acute or chronic inflammation, several strategies may help the surgeon. One is to perform an early laparoscopic ultrasound to assess the location of the common bile duct and its junction with the cystic duct to be able to judge where a safe dissection can be initiated. The second is to perform a "top down" cholecystectomy, as was championed by many individuals in the era of open cholecystectomy. This is somewhat more difficult to perform, as the plane between the peritoneum of the gallbladder fundus and its serosa must be entered and dissected to be able to maintain superior traction on the liver. However, having entered this plane, the gallbladder may be dissected safely down to its neck. If it is still impossible to dissect out the cystic duct, the gallbladder can be amputated at this location, the stones removed, and the neck of the gallbladder occluded with sutures or staples. Any exposed mucosa left in situ should be cauterized to prevent mucus formation postoperatively.

Although it is likely that "cystic duct syndrome" has been exaggerated in the past, I am convinced that leaving longer cystic duct stumps may lead to retained stones within these ducts that can either pass into the common duct or present later as a "mini gallbladder," causing symptoms. Prior to clipping the cystic duct I advocate incising it near its proximal end as though one were to perform a cholangiogram. A blunt grasper is then used to exert pressure on the lateral aspect of the porta hepatis and to sweep proximally toward the cystic duct and assess whether there is free flow of bile from the cystic ductotomy. The dissected segment of cystic duct is then "milked" by compressing it with a grasper back toward the opening in the cystic duct to both feel for stones and to remove them should they be present. Only after this maneuver has been performed will I put clips on the distal cystic duct. If a surgeon encounters a cystic duct that is too large to be occluded by a medium-to-large clip, this should be a warning sign that in fact this structure is not the cystic duct but a misidentified common bile duct. Additional dissection, intraoperative ultrasound, or intraoperative cholangiography may be necessary to resolve this issue.

The issue of routine versus selective investigation of the common bile duct during cholecystectomy is more of a religion than a science. A few recent large, population-based studies have suggested that routine cholangiography does decrease the overall risk of common bile duct injury. Many large clinical series exist, however, that demonstrate the safety of cholecystectomy without routine cholangiography. Still others advocate routine intraoperative ultrasonography. I believe the hallmark of a safe cholecystectomy is a meticulous dissection technique, not rushing the dissection, and never assuming that a tubular structure near the neck of the gallbladder is the cystic duct or artery without having completely dissected them in continuity.

NJS

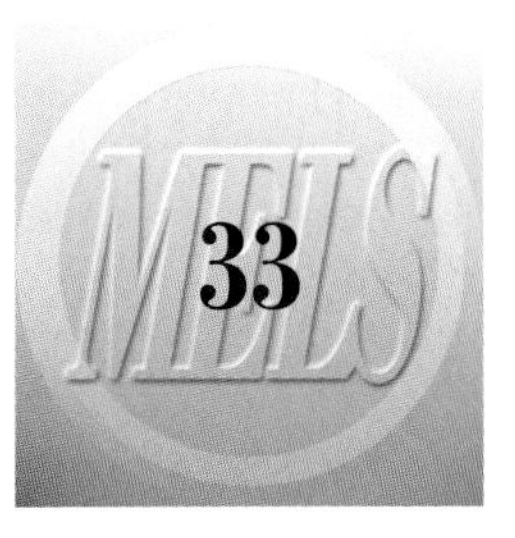

Surgery of the Extrahepatic Bile Ducts

ASOK DORAISWAMY AND EDWARD H. PHILLIPS

INTRODUCTION

For hundreds of years, the nonoperative management of patients with common bile duct (CBD) stones was not only standard practice but also the lone option. Because most calculi pass spontaneously, benign neglect was often successful. However, some untreated patients develop biliary enteric fistulae or die of sepsis or hepatic failure. The early surgical treatment of biliary disease involved the creation of external or internal biliary fistulae in an attempt to copy nature's cure. It wasn't until 1867, when John S. Bobbs performed the first cholecystostomy in Indianapolis, that attempts were made to manage CBD stones by either forcing them back into the gallbladder via the cystic duct or by fragmenting them in the CBD using external pressure, facilitating spontaneous passage. With the introduction of ether, anesthesia, and longer, safer surgery, cholecystectomy became possible, opening a whole new but controversial and complicated world for the surgeon. A few years later, in 1889, Robert Abbe, in the United States, and J. Knowlsey Thorton, in the United Kingdom presented their experiences with direct incision of the CBD to remove calculi, forever changing the treatment of patients with CBD stone disease. In 1899, Halsted performed the first choledochoduodenostomy and cautioned that every biliary operation should be an exploratory one, with the type of procedure dictated by the operative findings.

Even with this revolutionary approach to biliary disease, operative morbidity was high, and decisions were based on subjective clinical experience. It was not until 1931, when Mirizzi introduced intraoperative cholangiography, that the mortality of CBD surgery was decreased. Prior to intraoperative cholangiography, a negative CBD exploration occurred in as many as 50% of patients explored. This incidence was reduced to 6% when guided by cholangiography. In addition, the incidence of retained CBD calculi decreased from 25% to 11%. A more selective approach to CBD exploration substantially contributed to the decrease in morbidity and mortality. Reoperation carried a 30% morbidity rate and a 5% mortality rate. The next advance in operative biliary surgery was the introduction of choledochoscopy, with the first choledochoscope consisting of a metal funnel with a mirror and light, and the advent of the flexible scope in 1963. Unfortunately, choledochoscopy was not widely accepted until the late 1970s. Choledochoscopy further reduced the incidence of retained calculi to 3%. The most important advance in the management of CBD stones occurred in 1974, with the introduction of endoscopic retrograde cholangiopancreatography (ERCP) with endoscopic sphincterotomy (ES). Patients with cholangitis have subsequently been shown to have improved outcomes if they had ES preoperatively rather than an open CBD exploration.

Trials of the preoperative clearance of CBD stones prior to open cholecystectomy versus open CBD exploration alone were reported by Neoptolemos et al. in 1990 and 1992, Heinerman, Ponchon, and Stiegmann and colleagues in 1989, and Stain and coworkers in 1991. All but Stain et al. showed reduced hospitalization with the one-step procedure; none showed a decrease in morbidity or mortality with preoperative ES. In fact, Stain showed an increase in morbidity when preoperative ES was added to cholecystectomy, compared with cholecystectomy and open CBD exploration. The study by Heinerman and associates was the only one to show a reduction in morbidity in patients undergoing ES compared with open CBD exploration, but 74% of patients having open CBD exploration had undergone concomitant transduodenal sphincterotomy. Consequently, preoperative ES for patients suspected of harboring CBD stones did not become common practice until the introduction of laparoscopic cholecystectomy.

Laparoscopic Common Bile Duct Exploration

The treatment of CBD stones prior to laparoscopic cholecystectomy was fairly straightforward: patients underwent cholecystectomy, and, if stones were suspected, cholangiography was performed. If stones were found, a CBD exploration via choledochotomy was performed. However, the advent of laparoscopic cholecystectomy brought with it an aversion to convert to "open" surgery, which initially was the only surgical option for removing CBD stones. Consequently, preoperative ERCP became the standard for patients suspected of having choledocholithiasis, while postoperative ES was reserved for patients whose CBD stones were found either intraoperatively or postoperatively. One of the problems with a protocol of preoperative ES is that it is difficult to predict which patients have choledocholithiasis. If strict criteria are used, many patients with CBD stones will be missed, while if liberal indications are used, the majority of preoperative endoscopic retrograde cholangiography (ERC) examinations will be negative. In fact, all series utilizing preoperative ERC have a 40% to 70% negative rate for CBD stones. This is consistent with the negative CBD exploration rate in the era prior to intraoperative cholangiography. Another problem with a preoperative ES protocol is the cost of the study. A single negative ERC costs approximately $3000. This would pay for more than 15 intraoperative cholangiograms. In addition, the long-term effects of sphincterotomy in young patients with a normal-diameter CBD is unknown, but strictures and cancer induction are a concern.

Now that surgeons are more experienced with laparoscopic cholecystectomy and intraoperative cholangiography, less reliance should be placed on preoperative ERCP. Surgeons should learn the various techniques of laparoscopic CBD exploration to treat patients with CBD calculi in one session and to avoid potential complications of ES. Transcystic duct exploration with balloon dilation of the cystic duct, fluoroscopic wire-basket retrieval of calculi, flexible choledochoscopy, and laparoscopic choledochotomy are all accepted techniques. Intraoperative ES, either antegrade or retrograde, and ampullary balloon dilation have also been used, but are rarely necessary.

CLINICAL PRESENTATION

Patients undergoing laparoscopic cholecystectomy routinely have preoperative ultrasound examination of the liver, gallbladder, CBD, and pancreas. Careful analysis of the ultrasound can provide important information and may indicate the need for further studies (i.e., ERCP). Liver function tests are also important to evaluate preoperatively. About two-thirds of patients with CBD stones have elevated liver function tests, but only one-third of patients with elevated liver function tests will have CBD stones (Table 33-1). A serum amylase level should be obtained in patients with abdominal or back pain and tenderness. A baseline amylase level can be helpful when ERC or CBD exploration is anticipated. Nuclear biliary studies are rarely helpful in the diagnosis of choledocholithiasis. Magnetic resonance imaging (MRI) has recently been shown to be an excellent method of visualizing the CBD, even the intrapancreatic portion, and is gaining popularity now that the laparoscopic approach to CBD stones has proven to be safe and cost-effective.

The clinical presentation of choledocholithiasis can be subtle. An attack can include epigastric pain that tightens around the waist and radiates to the back, shoulder, or neck. It may be associated with nausea, vomiting, darkening of the urine, and lightening of the color of the stool. Fever and rigors can occur. Often, it is difficult to differentiate between acute cholecystitis with empyema of the gallbladder with or without choledocholithiasis and cholangitis. In our experience, 18% of patients with acute cholecystitis have choledocholithiasis at the time of surgery.

TRANSCYSTIC DUCT TECHNIQUE

The transcystic duct technique offers an excellent approach to CBD stones, while avoiding a choledochotomy and the difficulty of suture repair of the CBD. Most transcystic duct techniques of CBD exploration involve dilation of the cystic duct with balloon dilators (preferred) or sequential graduated bougies. Biliary flexible endoscopy is our primary approach to the CBD regardless of entrance site. Nevertheless, balloon trolling of the CBD, fluoroscopy-guided wire-basket stone retrieval, ampullary balloon dilation with lavage, and transcystic endoscopy-assisted sphincterotomy are all techniques that can be employed laparoscopically via the cystic duct without the need for dilation.

Flexible biliary endoscopy with wire-basket retrieval of calculi is our preferred technique. It appears to be the safest technique because the endoscope, wire-basket manipulations, and stone capture are performed under direct vision without manipulating the ampulla. This technique is feasible in 80% to 90% of patients. One limitation is that the endoscope cannot be passed into the proximal CBD in 90% of patients. Multiple stones, small, fragile cystic ducts, and stones proximal to the cystic duct–CBD junction must usually be dealt with by choledochotomy, ES, or ampullary balloon dilation. Larger stones (greater than 8 mm) should be dealt with via a choledochotomy but can be removed with the transcystic technique if the stones can be fragmented with a pulsed dye laser or electrohydraulic lithotripsy. These more difficult situations occur in about 10% of cases of choledocholithiasis in the U.S.

TABLE 33-1. INCIDENCE OF SPECIFIC LIVER FUNCTION TEST ABNORMALITIES AND PREDICTION OF COMMON BILE DUCT STONES (n = 727)

Abnormality	n	%	CBD stones	%
ALP	35	5	12	34
SGOT/PT	32	4	5	16
ALP + SGOT/PT	31	4	13	42
ALP + SGOT/PT + bilirubin	22	3	12	55
Bilirubin	19	3	4	21
Bilirubin + SGOT/PT	13	2	5	38

CBD, common bile duct; ALP, alkaline phosphatase; PT, prothrombin time; SGOT, serum glutamic oxaloacetic transaminase, or aspartate transaminase.

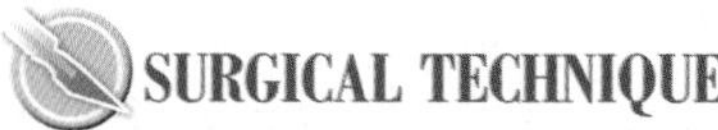

SURGICAL TECHNIQUE

The patient is positioned on the operating room table in the supine position similar to laparoscopic cholecystectomy. Because any patient can have unsuspected CBD stones, trocar location is critical. The most medial subcostal 5-mm trocar should always be placed in as lateral a position and as close to the costal margin as possible. This facilitates insertion of the scissors for incising the cystic duct and introducing the cholangiogram catheter. It eventually provides the best angle of approach for the flexible choledochoscope (Fig. 33-1). If needed, the placement of an additional 5-mm trocar to retract the duodenum and expose the CBD is recommended.

After dissecting the cystic duct and the cystic artery, a clip is placed as high as possible on the gallbladder at the junction of the gallbladder and the cystic duct. A cholangiocatheter, or a 4F end-hole ureteral catheter, is inserted in the cystic duct and secured in place with a clip or cholangiocatheter clamp (Fig. 33-2), and cinefluoroscopic cholangiography is performed. Although the procedure can be performed solely with static films, we recommend digital fluoroscopy. Considerable time is saved during the cholangiogram, and this equipment greatly improves accuracy and facilitates insertion of the guidewires, catheters, and other instruments during CBD exploration.

If it is difficult to intubate the cystic duct and a better intubation angle is needed, an additional 5-mm trocar should be inserted. This can be used for direct insertion or for a special endoscope grasper to gently guide the endoscope into the cystic duct (Fig. 33-3, page 312). When stones are seen on intraoperative cholangiography, the number, size, and location should be noted, as well as their relationship to the entrance of the cystic duct and CBD. The anatomic pattern is studied with particular attention to the entrance of the cystic duct to the CBD (Fig. 33-4, page 312). We recommend against using a dye solution greater than 50% to avoid obscuring CBD stones, if present.

After review of the intraoperative cholangiogram, a strategy for the treatment of choledocholithiasis should take into account the number of stones and their location. If the location of the stones and the patient's condition permit, the cystic duct should be dissected bluntly down close to its junction with the CBD. It is often necessary to make an incision in the larger portion of the

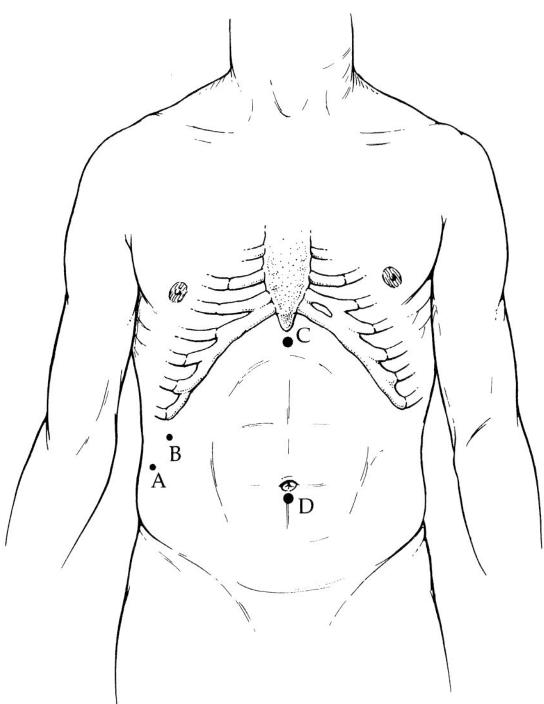

Fig. 33-1. Trocar sites and instrumentation ports for laparoscopic transcystic common bile duct explorations. **A.** Large-claw gallbladder grasper. **B.** Scissors, cholangiocatheter, guidewire/balloon dilator, choledochoscope. **C.** Hook coagulator, grasper. **D.** Video camera.

cystic duct closer to the CBD so that less cystic duct requires dilation. The location of the incision should allow an adequate length of cystic duct stump for closure with a suture loop at the end of the procedure. A no. 5 balloon dilating catheter, which has a balloon that is 4 cm long and 6 mm in outer diameter, is preloaded with a 0.35-inch, 150-cm long hydrophilic guidewire (see Fig. 33-3). The assemblage is inserted via a 5-mm reducer sleeve in the trocar in the right anterior axillary line just under the costal margin.

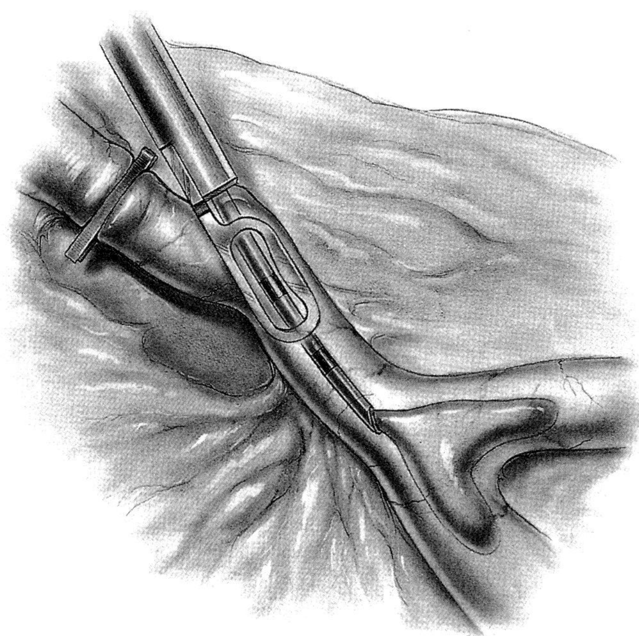

Fig. 33-2. Cholangiographic clamp used to insert and secure a cholangiocatheter in the cystic duct for intraoperative cholangiogram.

When one is learning the technique, it is best to obtain X-ray or fluoroscopic confirmation of the guidewire location before advancing the balloon dilating catheter or sequential bougies over the guidewire (Fig. 33-5, page 312). Two-thirds of the balloon should be inserted. The balloon is then slowly inflated with a LeVeen syringe attached to a pressure gauge. The balloon and cystic duct are observed laparoscopically while an assistant or nurse slowly inflates the balloon as the pressures are read aloud. The balloon should be inflated to the insufflation pressure recommended by the manufacturer (usually 12 atm) and held there for 3 minutes (Fig. 33-6, page 313). If the cystic duct begins to tear, inflation should stop for 1 minute before further inflation is attempted. With patience, most cystic ducts can be dilated to 7 mm, but they should never be dilated larger than the inner diameter of the CBD. When a small CBD is being explored, care must be taken to choose the proper diameter-dilating balloon based on the intraoperative cholangiogram. The cystic duct must be dilated to the size of the largest CBD stone so that the stone entrapped in the wire-basket does not become impacted on removal. Stones larger than 9 mm must usually be fragmented with a pulsed dye laser or electrohydraulic lithotripsy, or removed via choledochotomy. After the cystic duct is dilated, the balloon catheter is deflated and withdrawn.

The endoscope can be inserted over a 150-cm guidewire, inserted freehand, or gently guided with an atraumatic grasper. The working channel of some endoscopes is eccentric to their cross section, making insertion over the guidewire difficult. The endoscope should have bidirectional deflection and a working channel of at least 1.2 mm; an outer diameter of 2.7 to 3.2 mm is ideal. Smaller scopes compromise the working channel, and larger scopes are more difficult to pass. A camera is attached to the endoscope with the image projected on a monitor with an audiovisual mixer (picture in picture) or projected on its own monitor. It is best and most convenient to set up a mobile cart with a monitor, light source, camera box, video recorder, endoscope, wire baskets, balloon dilating catheters, and other instruments needed for a laparoscopic CBD exploration. This cart can function as an emergency laparoscopic cart and/or a backup cart for other laparoscopic procedures. Having all the required instruments in one place decreases frustration and delays when CBD calculi are encountered.

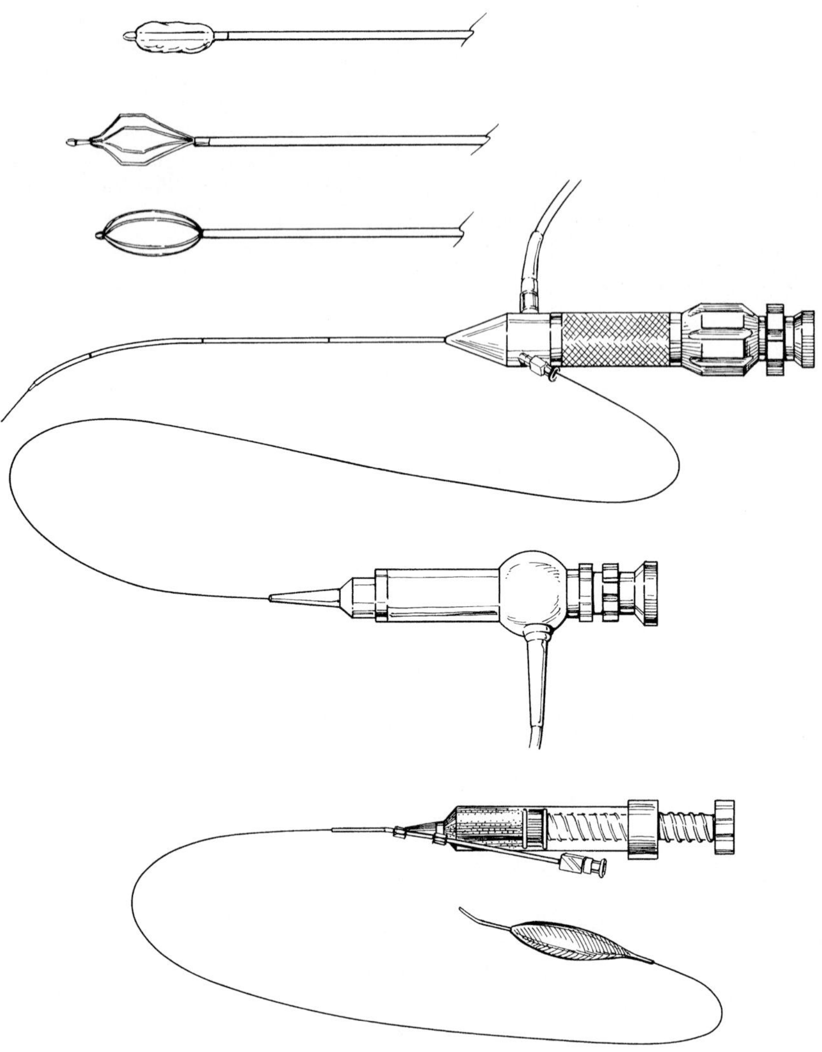

Fig. 33-3. Choledochoscope and instruments used to facilitate laparoscopic common bile duct explorations.

Once the endoscope is in the cystic duct, irrigation with warm saline should be initiated. The temperature of the irrigant must be monitored, as hypothermia can occur from instillation of cold fluid. The operating surgeon manipulates the scope, inserting and torquing with the left hand while deflecting the endoscope with the right hand or the deflecting lever. Once the stone is seen, irrigation is turned off or decreased. The stones closest to the scope should always be entrapped first and none should be bypassed, as they may be irrigated up into the liver. A straight no. 4 wire basket (2.4F) is preferable. The closed basket should be advanced beyond the stone, opened, and then pulled back to entrap it (Fig. 33-7). The basket should be gently closed around the stone and pulled up lightly against the end of the endoscope so that they can be withdrawn together (Fig. 33-8, page 314). This process is repeated until all stones are removed. A completion cholangiogram is essential. At this point, a decision regarding cystic duct tube drainage may be made. Elderly or immunosuppressed patients with cholangitis should have a latex (not silicone) tube placed for postoperative decompression of the biliary system. In patients who are likely to be harboring a retained stone, a tube should be placed for postoperative cholangiography and percutaneous tube tract stone extraction, if necessary. If the pre-exploration intraoperative cholangiogram shows a different number of CBD stones than those found on endoscopy, a tube should be placed. The cystic duct

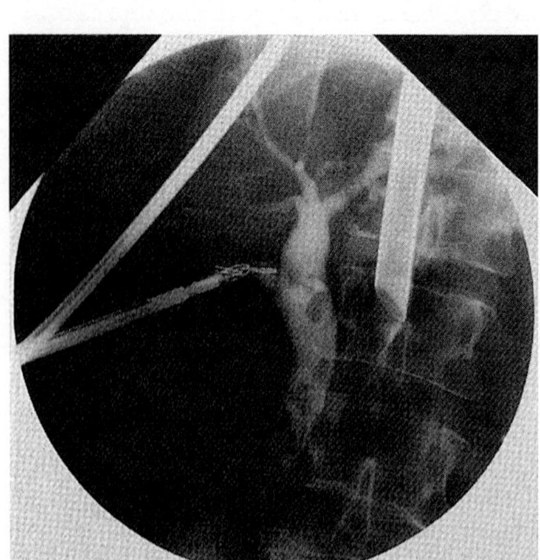

Fig. 33-4. Operative cholangiogram shows multiple common bile duct stones in a dilated duct and their relationship to the cystic duct.

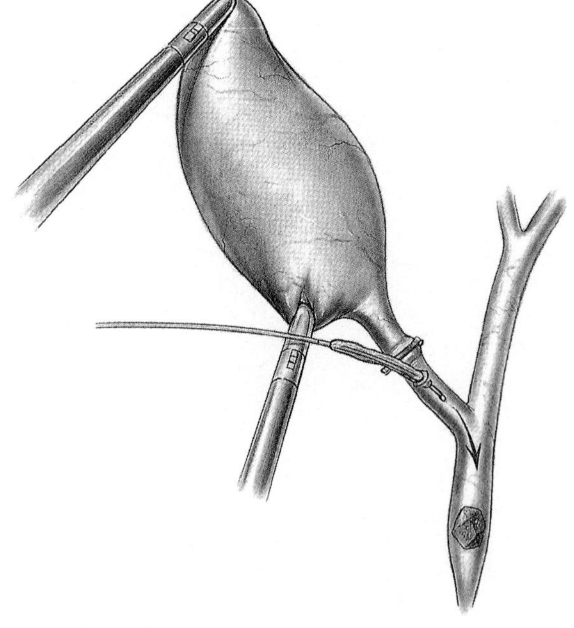

Fig. 33-5. Positioning of a guidewire in preparation for advancing a balloon dilating catheter for cystic duct dilation.

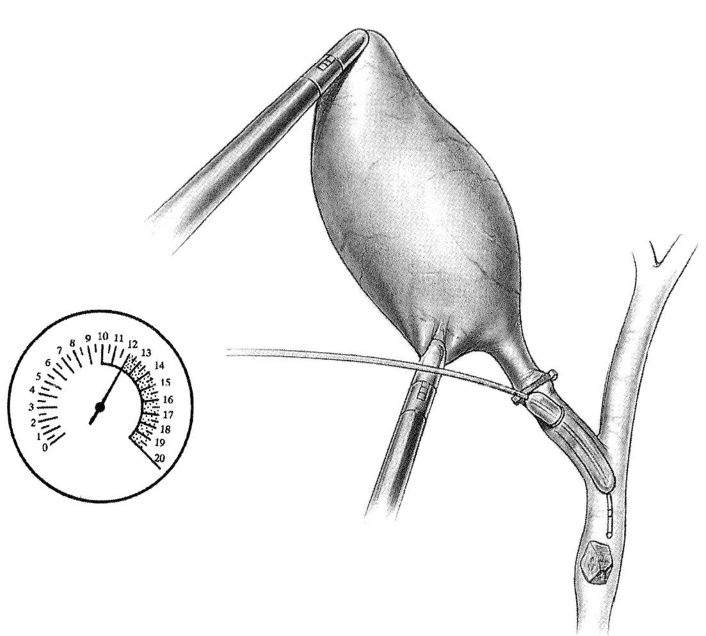

Fig. 33-6. Balloon catheter attached to LeVeen syringe during cystic duct dilation.

stump must be closed with a loop ligature as clips may slip off the thinned duct.

If the cystic duct cannot be dilated sufficiently to allow insertion of an endoscope or the cystic duct becomes transected, there are three other transcystic duct techniques that may be employed. Intraoperative fluoroscopy is crucial for these maneuvers:

1. One mg of glucagon is administered intravenously, 3 minutes are allowed to pass, and the CBD is forcibly lavaged to flush the stones through the ampulla into the duodenum. This may work with stones 2 mm or smaller and is usually tried before cystic duct dilation.
2. Fluoroscopic wire-basket stone retrieval requires special spiral wire baskets with flexible leaders to avoid injuring the CBD (Fig. 33-9, page 314). The basket is placed in the CBD via the cystic duct and advanced with fluoroscopic guidance into the distal CBD and opened. A 25% Hypaque solution is injected through the wire-basket catheter. The basket is then pulled back until the stone is captured. The advantage of not having to dilate the cystic duct is offset by the problem of extracting the wire basket with the captured stone through the nondilated cystic duct. In our experience, this technique is not as successful as other transcystic duct techniques and can lead to an impacted basket and stone that would require choledochotomy for removal. Nevertheless, it can be an easy and successful technique in selected patients, namely those patients with relatively few CBD calculi that are close to the inner diameter of the cystic duct.
3. Biliary balloon catheter stone retrieval is useful, especially in cases with a dilated cystic duct. A biliary balloon catheter can be passed blindly or under fluoroscopic control via the cystic duct into the distal CBD or the duodenum. The balloon is gently inflated, and the catheter is then withdrawn, modulating the pressure on the balloon. This is often successful via choledochotomy but, when used via the cystic duct, has the potential to pull the stone into the common hepatic duct, out of reach of an endoscope.

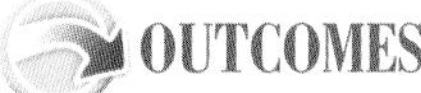

OUTCOMES

To analyze long-term clinical outcome and patient satisfaction following transcystic common bile duct exploration with biliary endoscopy, a prospective cohort study of unselected patients found to have common bile duct stones during laparoscopic cholecystectomy between October 1989 and April 1998 was conducted. Laparoscopic transcystic bile duct exploration (LTCBDE) with choledochoscopy was performed in all 217 patients. A mailed survey assessed symptoms, outcome, and satisfaction; 116 (54%) surveys were returned. Mean follow-up was 60 months. Six patients (4%) had LTCBDE fail and, in four patients (3%), ERC was performed. No patient had late recognition of retained stones or a bile duct stricture. The majority (95%) of patients were satisfied or mostly satisfied with LTCBDE.

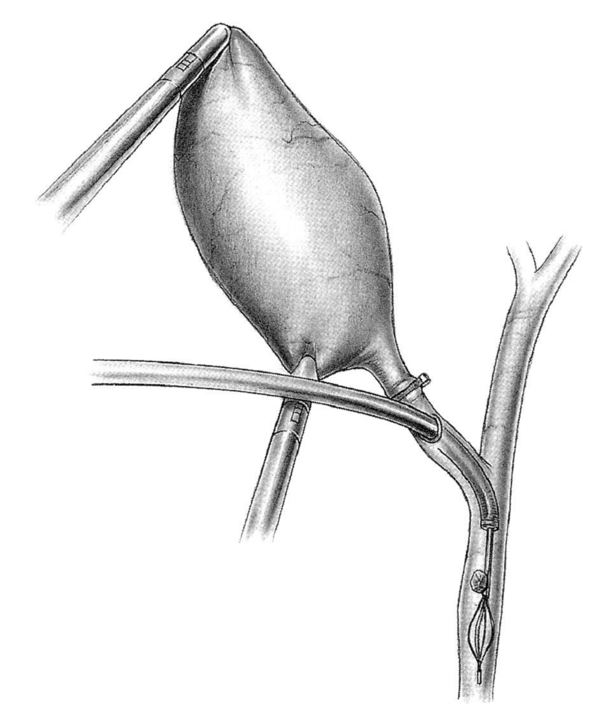

Fig. 33-7. Advancement of a wire basket through the choledochoscope for stone entrapment.

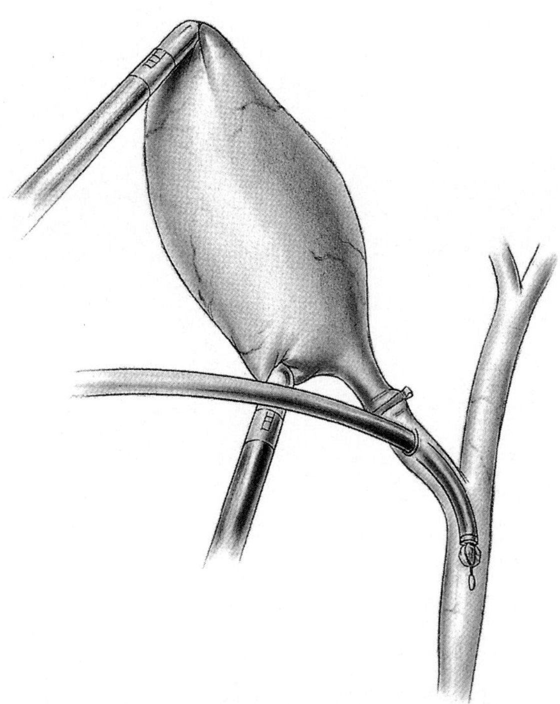

Fig. 33-8. A choledochoscopic view of a basket capturing a common bile duct stone.

Other reported studies have shown that both the laparoscopic transcystic and choledochotomy routes of common duct exploration have a high rate of duct clearance with low morbidity and mortality (Tables 33-2 and 33-3).

TRANSCYSTIC AMPULLARY BALLOON DILATION

In an effort to enhance our ability to lavage small stones and debris from the CBD when an endoscope cannot be inserted into a small, fragile cystic duct, we apply the laparoscopic technique of balloon dilation of the sphincter of Oddi (SO) via the cystic duct. Although our series is small, initial results indicate that this technique is a useful adjunct to laparoscopic CBD exploration techniques. However, it should be used when the only alternative is ES.

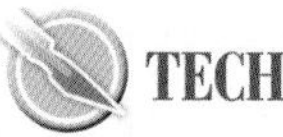

TECHNIQUE

When CBD stones and/or debris discovered at fluorocholangiography during laparoscopic cholecystectomy are less than 4 mm in diameter and cannot be extracted by endoscopic wire basket or lavage, laparoscopic transcystic balloon dilation of the SO can be performed. A 6-mm balloon-dilating catheter (no. 5 Phantom) is inserted via the right subcostal trocar over a floppy-tipped 0.035-inch hydrophilic guidewire (Fig. 33-10). The wire is advanced through the incision into the cystic duct and gently passed under fluoroscopic control into the CBD and then the duodenum. The balloon catheter is advanced over the guidewire, through the cystic duct, into the CBD, and then through the SO. Radiopaque markers on the balloon catheter identify its position spanning the SO. Repeated in-and-out manipulations through the SO should be avoided. Using a LeVeen syringe, the balloon is slowly dilated under fluoroscopic view with 50% Hypaque to the diameter of the largest stone in the CBD; it should never be dilated larger than the inner diameter of the CBD. After 3 minutes (using a pressure not greater than 12 atm), the balloon is deflated. Forceful irrigation into the cystic duct is then performed with warm saline solution, and completion cholangiogram is obtained (Fig. 33-11, page 316). The cystic duct is then ligated with an endoloop, and a drain is placed in the Morison pouch. Placement of a cystic duct tube should be considered in cases in which percutaneous access or follow-up cholangiography may be required.

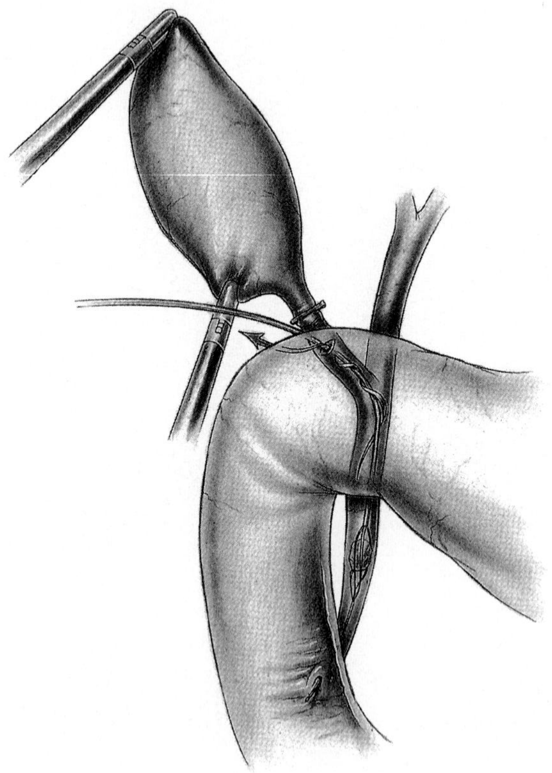

Fig. 33-9. Fluoroscopic transcystic basket retrieval of a common bile duct stone.

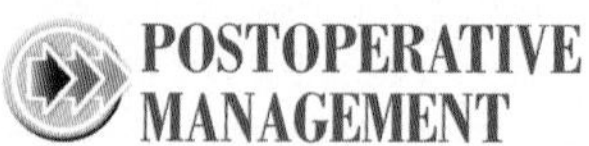

POSTOPERATIVE MANAGEMENT

Postoperatively, patients are observed for sepsis, bleeding, pancreatitis, or bile leak, complications that will usually occur within the first 24 hours. Routine postoperative laboratory tests should include a hematocrit, liver function, and serum amylase.

TABLE 33-2. LAPAROSCOPIC COMMON BILE DUCT EXPLORATION EXPERIENCE

Surgeon	Year	Total class	Transcystic route	%	Choledochotomy route	%	Total successful clearance	%	Mortality
DePaula	1994	119	107	90	12	10	108	91	1
Dion	1994	59	18	31	41	69	52	88	0
Ferzli	1994	24	13	54	11	46	24	100	0
Franklin	1995	113	2	1.8	111	98	112	99	1
Petelin	1995	173	154	89	19	11	168	97	1
Phillips	1995	162	145	90	17	10	150	93	1

TABLE 33-3. LAPAROSCOPIC COMMON BILE DUCT EXPLORATION COMPARISON OF LONG-TERM OUTCOMES

	TCD (%)	OTOMY (%)	Morbidity (%)	Mortality (%)	Retained stones (%)
Dorman	21	79	NR	NR	2
Berthou	51	49	9	0.9	3
Martin	58	42	7	0.3	NR
Keeling	66	34	5	0	NR
Phillips	92	8	6	0.3	5

TC, transcystic route; OTOMY, choledochotomy route; NR, not reported.

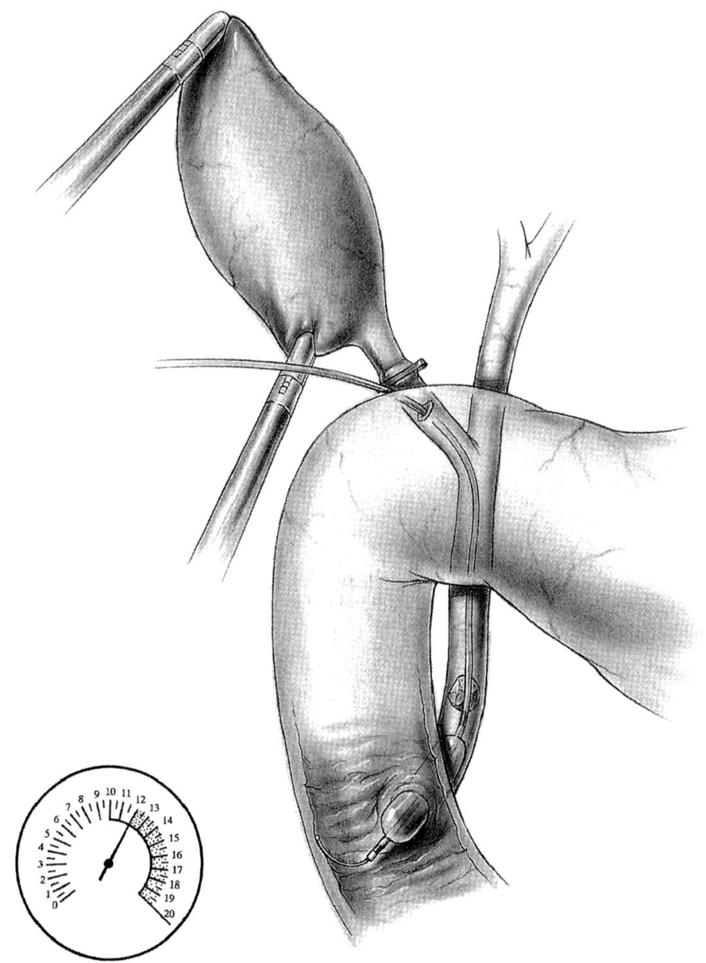

Fig. 33-10. Laparoscopic transcystic ampullary balloon dilation of the papilla.

If there is a question of bile leak, an ultrasound examination is the best first test; occasionally, a hydroxy iminodiacetic acid (HIDA) scan is helpful. An ERCP is sometimes needed not only to diagnose a leak but also to place a transampullary stent in association with percutaneous drainage. Reoperation will rarely be necessary.

Patients who have had a transcystic duct approach can be separated into two groups: those with suspected CBD stones, and those with unsuspected CBD stones. Patients whose stones were preoperatively suspected are discharged on average 3.6 days postoperatively. Patients with unsuspected stones are discharged on average 1.7 days postoperatively. Both groups tend to return to work and regular activities on average 10 days after surgery.

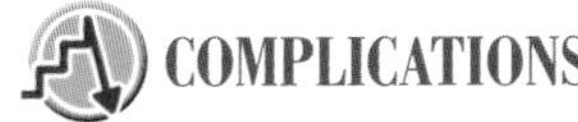

COMPLICATIONS

Complications with the transcystic duct stone extraction technique include perforation of the cystic or extrahepatic bile duct, cystic duct stump leak, pancreatitis, persistent cholangitis due to high intraductal pressures with lack of CBD decompression, delayed strictures due to mechanical injury or thermal injury from lithotripsy, and retained stones. All these complications can be minimized by careful attention to detail and proper patient selection. Patients with stones greater than 8 mm, multiple stones, or stones proximal to the cystic duct insertion are better served by choledochotomy.

Surgical judgment is the key in selecting the proper approach to treat a patient's common duct stones and minimizing complications. Knowledge of the outcomes of the different treatments can improve one's judgment. A prospective multicenter study

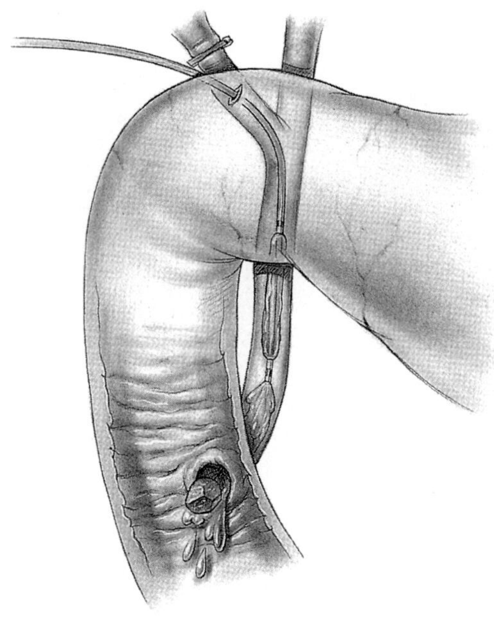

Fig. 33-11. Laparoscopic transcystic flushing of common bile duct after ampullary dilation.

of ES in 2347 patients showed procedure-related morbidity was 9.8%, procedure-related mortality was 0.5%, and total mortality was 2.3%. Surgical results should be compared and therapeutic recommendations should consider these morbidity figures. Myocardial infarction was the leading cause of postoperative mortality. Aspiration pneumonia occurred in 2% of the patients and was the cause of death in one (see Table 33-2).

Morgenstern and Wong performed a review of 1200 cholecystectomies on the teaching service at our own hospital just prior to the introduction of LC. They analyzed 220 patients who underwent open CBDE and found that patients under age 60 had no mortality while patients over 60 had 4.3% mortality. On the other hand, only two LTCBDE procedure-related complications (2%) were reported, and there was no mortality in patients under 65 years of age and one death in 256 LTCBDEs. There were no cases of delayed stricture and a 90% satisfaction rate.

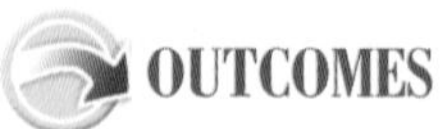

OUTCOMES

Any manipulation of the ampulla of Vater can produce hyperamylasemia and/or clinical pancreatitis. In our experience, 17 (85%) of 20 patients had successful laparoscopic transcystic balloon dilation of the SO with clearance of stones from the CBD. Hyperamylasemia occurred in 15% of patients, and clinical mild pancreatitis occurred in three patients. Although this procedure appears to have a lower rate of clinical pancreatitis than endoscopic retrograde methods of SO dilation, surgeons should take this risk into consideration when applying this technique.

LAPAROSCOPIC CHOLEDOCHOTOMY

Laparoscopic choledochotomy is an excellent approach in patients with a dilated CBD (greater than 8 mm), calculi 1 cm or larger, multiple calculi, or stones located in the proximal ducts, or in those who require lithotripsy for impacted calculi. It is contraindicated in small ducts because of the risk of stricture. The advantages of choledochotomy are that calculi can easily be irrigated out of the CBD and an endoscope can be inserted up into the intrahepatic ducts. Common bile duct explorations, especially for solitary large stones, can be performed without a choledochoscope by milking the CBD stone into the choledochotomy. However, this technique cannot be relied on to accurately locate and/or remove all stones on a consistent basis. Therefore, we recommend use of a 10.5F (3.3-mm) choledochoscope that can be flexed in two directions with a 1.2-mm working channel that can accommodate larger and less delicate wire baskets. Another advantage of this technique is that a T-tube, which can decompress the duct and provide access for cholangiography and retrieval of calculi, can be used. The disadvantages of choledochotomy are that a T-tube is required and considerable laparoscopic suturing skill is needed to close the choledochotomy. Laparoscopic choledochotomy should not be performed without first performing an intraoperative cholangiogram. After completing the cholangiogram and ascertaining the exact location and number of CBD stones, a choledochotomy can be made at the point most desirable for extraction of the stones.

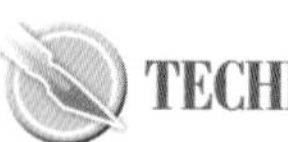

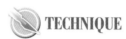

TECHNIQUE

The procedure is performed before the gallbladder is removed so that the gallbladder can be used to elevate the liver and apply tension to the cystic duct (Fig. 33-12). The anterior wall of the CBD is bluntly dissected. Occasionally, it is necessary to aspirate bile to confirm the CBD. Intraoperative ultrasound is an additional method that can be used to identify the CBD and locate stones. The choledochotomy is placed in the anterior aspect of the CBD, preferably below the junction of the cystic duct into the CBD. This placement results in less chance of compromise to the lumen during closure of the choledochotomy. Two stay sutures should be placed in the CBD and its anterior wall should be tented before an incision is made with microscissors (Fig. 33-13). The choledochotomy should be made only as long as the circumference of the largest calculus to minimize the suturing required for closure. The stay sutures on the edge of the choledochotomy may need to be crossed alongside the endoscope so that the irrigation can distend the CBD.

The most efficient technique is to insert a choledochoscope into the CBD and irrigate with warm saline solution. The choledochoscope should be oriented so that flexion is in a vertical manner, as this assists in its passage through the choledochotomy. The CBD should be entered at a right angle, and the scope turned after entering the CBD. A biliary balloon catheter, wire basket, or both can be used to remove calculi in most patients (Fig. 33-14, page 318). Occasionally, a three-pronged grasper or biliary lithotripsy is necessary to remove an impacted calculus.

Pulsed-dye laser energy is the safest technique of lithotripsy, but electrohydraulic lithotripsy can be used safely if it is performed carefully under direct vision.

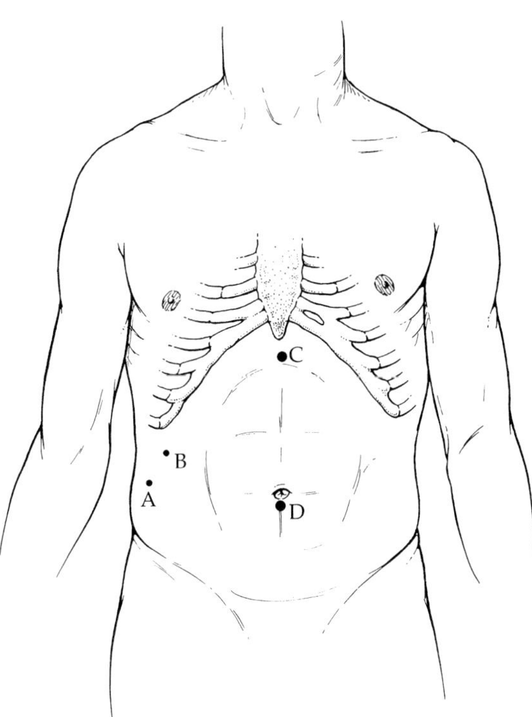

Fig. 33-12. Trocar sites and instrumentation for the laparoscopic choledochotomy. **A.** Large-claw gallbladder grasper. **B.** Latex T-tube, scissors, grasper, cholangiocatheter, needle holder. **C.** Hook coagulator, grasper, flexible scope, scissors, needle holder. **D.** Video camera.

After the CBD is cleared, a decision must be made regarding the need for a drainage procedure. This can be accomplished laparoscopically by performing a choledochoduodenostomy, Roux-en-Y choledochojejunostomy, or postoperative- or intraoperative-facilitated ES. When a drainage procedure is not needed, a latex T-tube must be inserted entirely intracorporeally to avoid carbon dioxide loss and to permit easier manipulation of the tube. We frequently use a 10F to 14F T-tube that has been tailored with a long and short end. The entire T-tube is brought into the abdominal cavity, and the long tail is allowed to extend over the top of the liver. The long end of the cut T-tube is introduced into the distal aspect of the CBD and the short end into the proximal end (Fig. 33-15, page 318). After the T-tube is well situated in the CBD, a pre-tied loop, which is very advantageous for the first suture, is placed immediately below the neck of the T-tube as it is being pushed cephalad (Fig. 33-16, page 319). This traps the T-tube and minimizes the chance of subsequent dislodgement. The next suture should be placed in the most proximal end of the choledochotomy and two sutures lifted to facilitate closure of the choledochotomy. Our preference is to close the choledochotomy with interrupted sutures of VICRYL (Ethicon; Somerville, NJ) lubricated with mineral oil. The long end of the T-tube is brought through the abdominal wall, and completion cholangiography is performed. Care must be taken to ensure a watertight seal, or as close as one as possible, without causing ischemia to this segment of the duct. It is better to have a small leak than to have an ischemic duct.

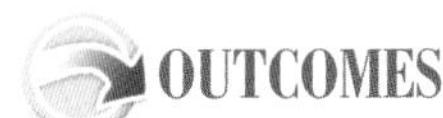

OUTCOMES

Results with this technique have been excellent (see Table 33-2). Franklin et al. performed 111 procedures, with one retained calculus. Morbidity was 5% and mortality 1%. Surgeons who perform transcystic CBD exploration as the first technique in the treatment of CBD calculi perform laparoscopic choledochotomy only in the most challenging cases of choledocholithiasis (10%). This explains why the incidence of complications associated with laparoscopic choledochotomy (11% to 17%) and retained calculi (8% to 22%) is higher for these procedures than with laparoscopic transcystic or even open CBD exploration as the primary method of calculi removal. Biliary drainage procedures should be performed in many of these difficult situations to reduce the incidence of retained calculi. Endoscopic sphincterotomy or choledochoduodenostomy can be performed laparoscopically; however, because drainage procedures are needed in only 1% of all patients undergoing laparoscopic cholecystectomy, converting these operations to open procedures seems appropriate, except in the hands of experienced laparoscopic surgical teams.

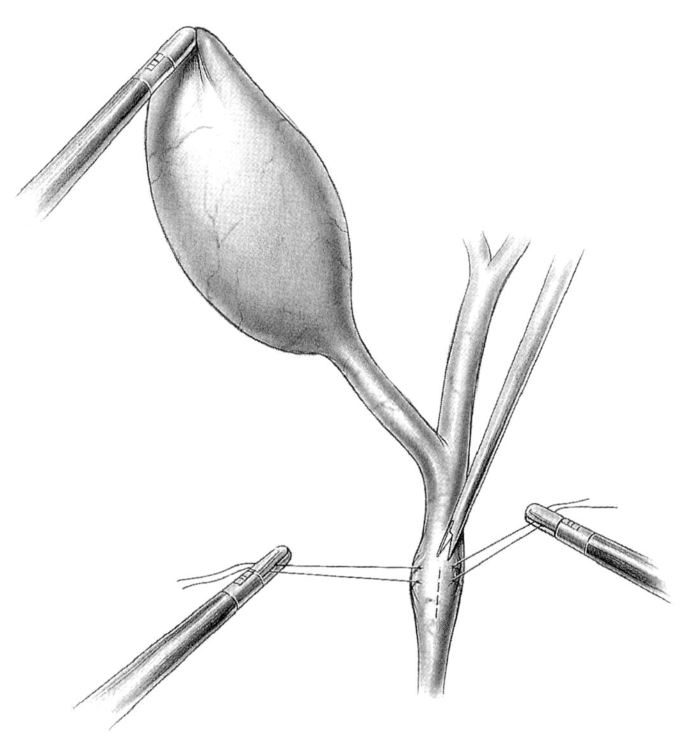

Fig. 33-13. Laparoscopic choledochotomy after the placement of stay sutures.

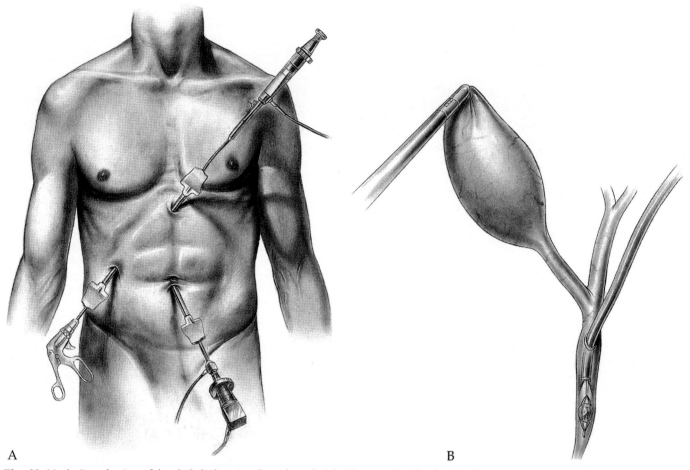

Fig. 33-14. A. Introduction of the choledochoscope through a subxiphoid trocar. **B.** The choledochoscope is inserted through the choledochotomy into the CBD. A wire basket is then used to capture and remove calculi.

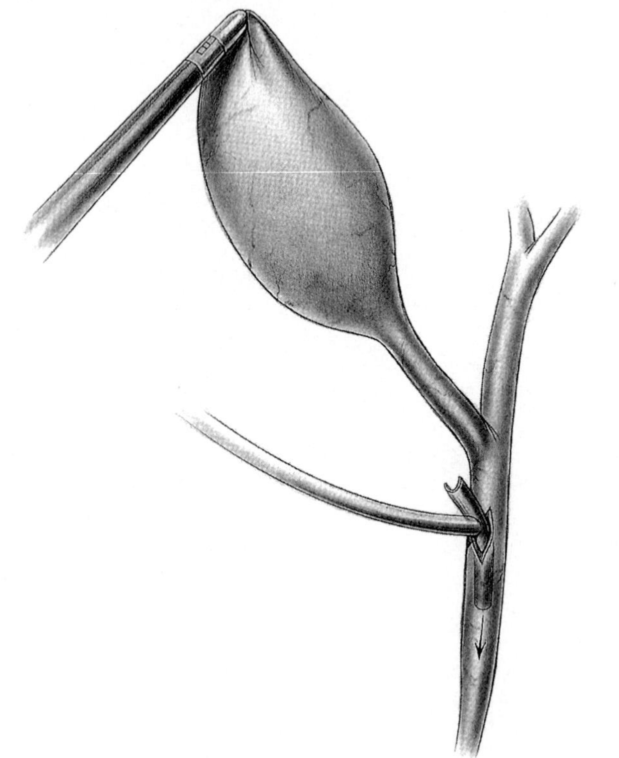

Fig. 33-15. A T-tube placed via choledochotomy after stone removal. The T-tube will be brought out through a subcostal trocar site.

Laparoscopic Antegrade Transcystic Sphincterotomy

In 1993, DePaula et al. described a technique that combined methods of laparoscopic CBD exploration and ES. According to their report, this procedure is indicated for any patient with multiple CBD stones, a CBD measuring greater than 20 mm, ampullary dyskinesia, or any evidence of impaired CBD emptying. Most surgeons who perform this procedure do it for patients with complex choledocholithiasis in whom transcystic CBD exploration and laparoscopic choledochotomy have failed to clear the CBD, which should be less than 3% of patients.

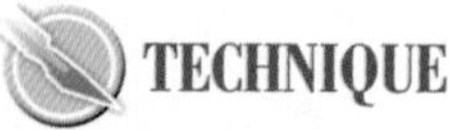

TECHNIQUE

A cart should be available that contains a side-viewing duodenoscope, a selection of endoscopic sphincterotomes, guidewires,

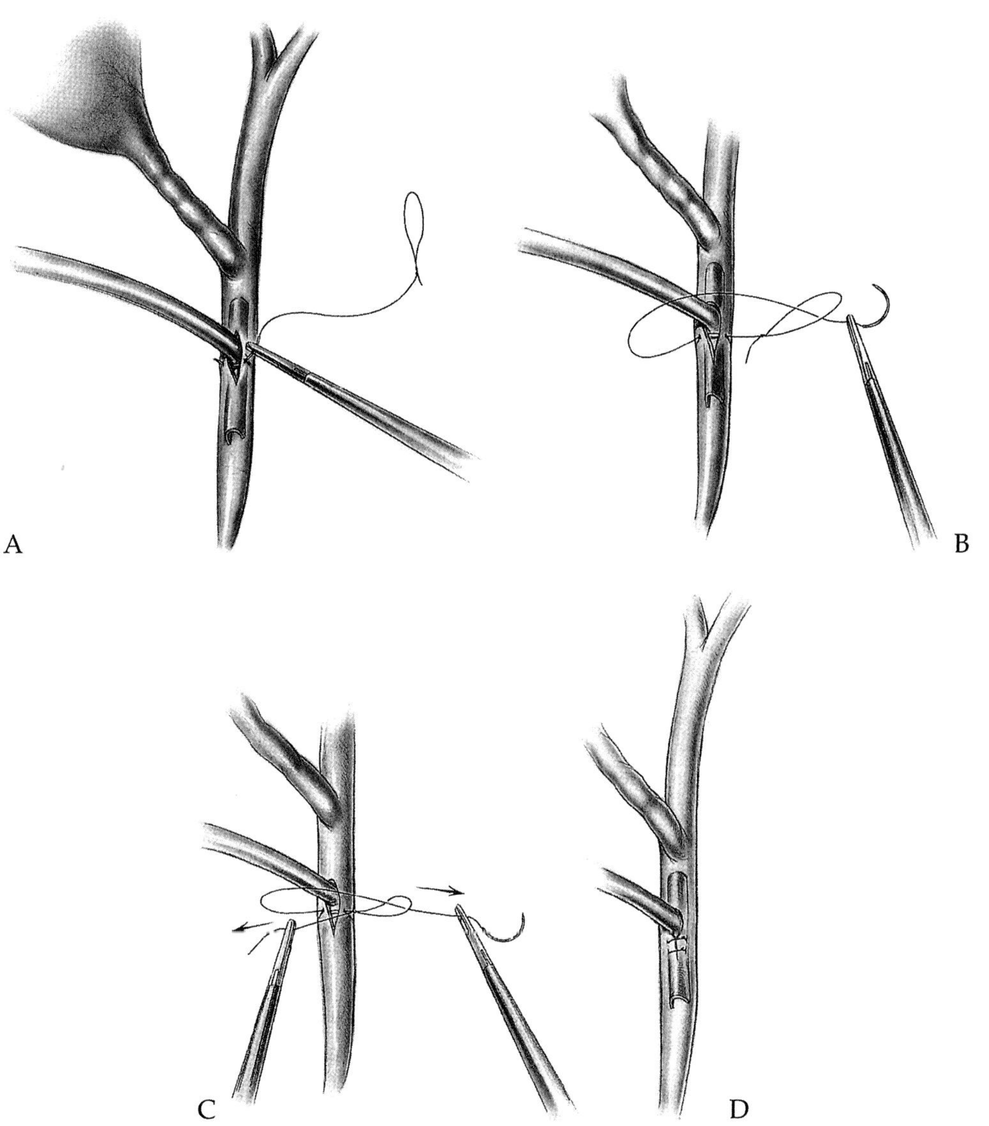

Fig. 33-16. A to **D**. The T-tube being sutured in place.

and a cautery cable compatible with the sphincterotomes. Antegrade sphincterotomy is usually performed after an attempt has been made at laparoscopic CBD exploration. The transcystic or choledochotomy access to the CBD can be used for performing antegrade sphincterotomy (Fig. 33-17, page 320). The first step is to pass the sphincterotome directly into the distal CBD and across the ampulla (Fig. 33-18, page 320). Different types of endoscopic sphincterotomes are commercially available, including a 30-mm short-nose sphincterotome or a Classen-Demling sphincterotome, which was originally designed for intubating the ampulla following a Billroth II gastrectomy. The sphincterotome is introduced via the right upper quadrant port. A grasping forceps is inserted through the subxiphoid sheath and then used to guide the sphincterotome into the lumen of the cystic duct or through the choledochotomy. While the sphincterotome is being manipulated into the biliary tree, a second member of the surgical team passes a side-viewing video duodenoscope through the mouth and into the duodenum. Glucagon, 0.5 to 1.0 mg, is then administered intravenously to minimize duodenal peristalsis. The duodenoscope is positioned across from the ampulla (Fig. 33-19, page 321). As the sphincterotome passes through the ampulla, it is visualized. The surgeon withdraws and manipulates it, usually by twisting it, until the cutting wire is bowed at the 12 o'clock position (Fig. 33-20, page 321). Cautery is applied until the sphincter and overlying mucosa are divided up to the first transverse fold of the duodenum. An outpouring of bile and/or stones usually signifies a successful sphincterotomy. The CBD is then flushed copiously with saline to wash out any remaining stones or debris. The choledochoscope can then be reinserted to explore the CBD, flush the duct, and push stones out through the widened ampulla. If one or more stones are impacted in the distal CBD or ampulla, it may be difficult to pass the sphincterotome antegrade into the duodenum. In these cases, one can advance the choledochoscope as far distally as possible, maneuver a smaller guidewire through the working channel across the ampulla, and then follow the previously mentioned steps. If the sphincterotomy is successful, insertion of a T-tube

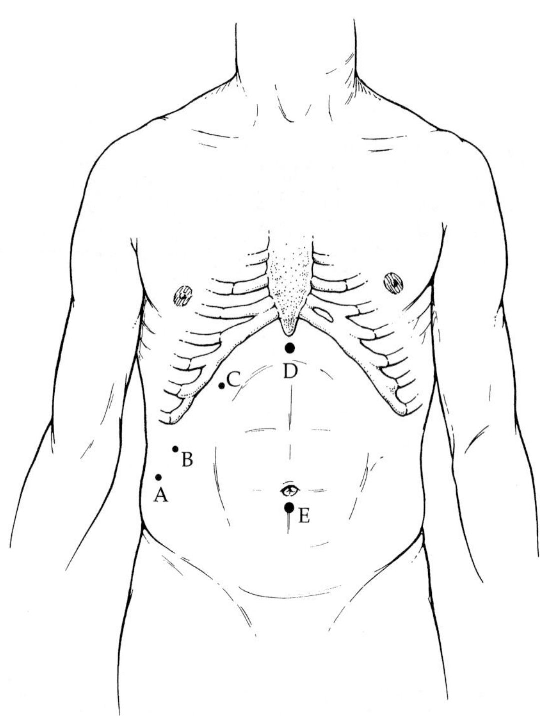

Fig. 33-17. Trocar sites and instrumentation for the laparoscopic antegrade transcystic sphincterotomy. A fifth cannula (5-mm) can be inserted in the right upper quadrant for introduction of the choledochoscope, sphincterotome, and so on. **A.** Gallbladder grasper. **B.** Grasper, cholangiocatheter. **C.** Flexible scope, cautery cable, side-viewing duodenoscope. **D.** Clip applicator, scissors, cautery hook, grasper. **E.** Video camera.

for postoperative biliary decompression is not necessary. Often, a small amount of bleeding is visualized from the sphincterotomy site but it usually stops, although it occasionally requires injection of epinephrine or coagulation.

Laparoscopic antegrade sphincterotomy has a number of advantages over conventional methods of ES. First, the sphincterotome is passed quickly through the bile ducts and across the ampulla. DePaula and associates reported a mean time of 17 minutes to perform this procedure, and Zucker was able to complete antegrade sphincterotomy in just over 25 minutes (excluding time spent at attempted CBD exploration). Inadvertent cannulation of the pancreatic duct is also eliminated and other complications associated with ERCP should be dramatically reduced, such as the creation of false passages, perforation of the CBD or duodenum, and the so-called "trapped basket" or "sphincterotome." In addition, patients expect complete management of all their biliary tract problems in one sitting, which this provides. However, antegrade sphincterotomy does have its disadvantages: operative and anesthesia time are prolonged and the procedure does require additional equipment and experience in upper gastrointestinal endoscopy. Despite these disadvantages, laparoscopic antegrade sphincterotomy may have an increasingly important role in the surgical management of complex choledocholithiasis.

CONCLUSION

Laparoscopic cholecystectomy has become the primary treatment for symptomatic cholelithiasis. Concomitant CBD stones are present in 10% to 15% of patients, and several approaches to the management of these stones have been described. Laparoscopic transcystic CBDE will be applicable in 80% to 90% of cases, and laparoscopic choledochotomy in most of the others. Laparoscopic transcystic CBDE with choledochoscopy and stone extraction should be the primary technique because it is safe, efficient, and the most cost-effective for managing CBD stones in one session. If unsuccessful, it still allows other laparoscopic approaches, open choledochotomy, or postoperative ES.

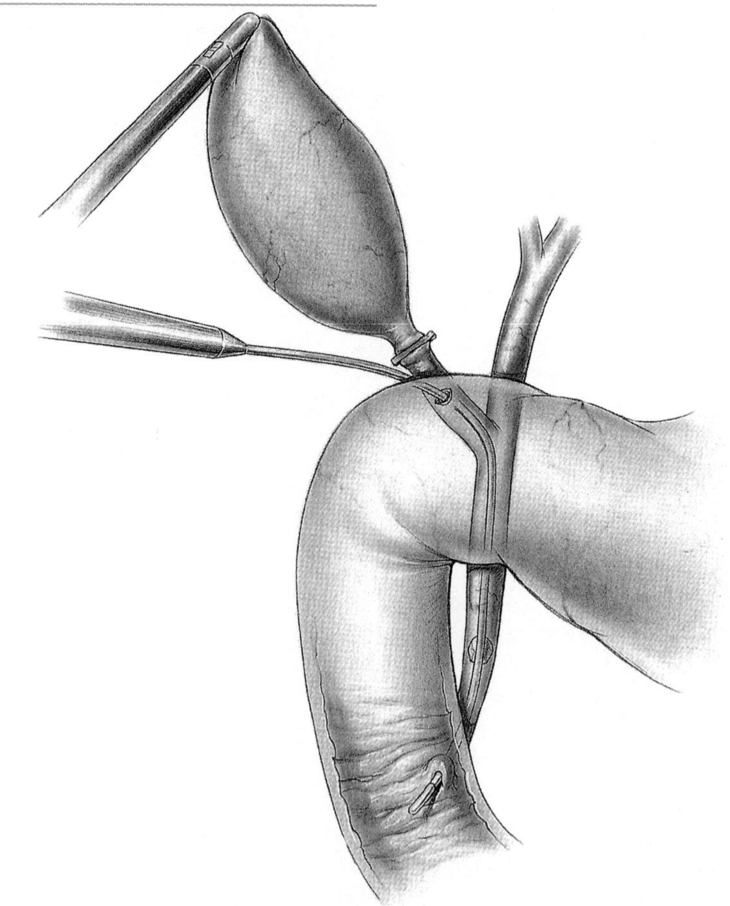

Fig. 33-18. An endoscopic sphincterotome is inserted using a suture introducer to minimize gas leakage.

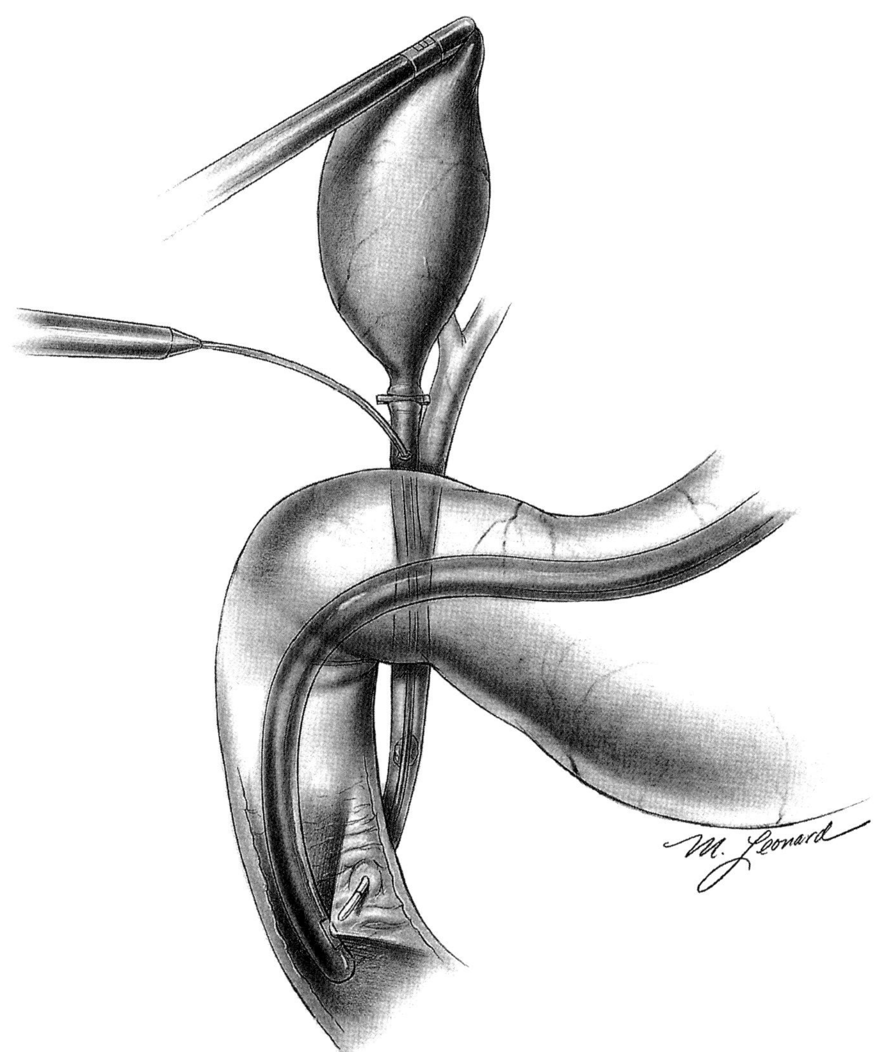

Fig. 33-19. The side-viewing duodenoscope is positioned directly opposite the ampulla so that the sphincterotome may be guided into proper position under direct vision.

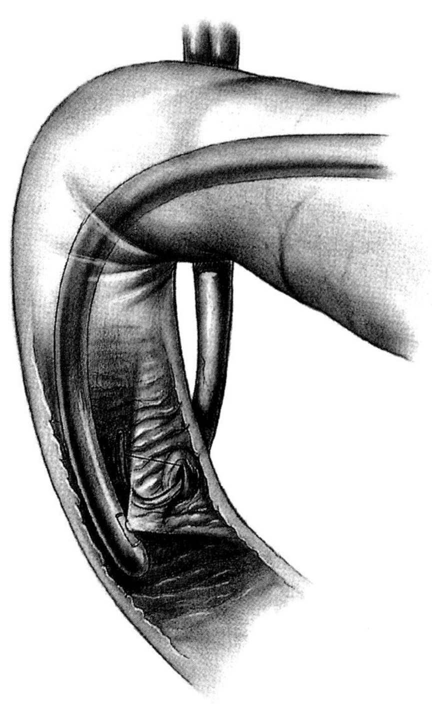

Fig. 33-20. The sphincterotome is bowed, exposing the cutting wire, which is maneuvered until it is at the 12 o'clock position.

Laparoscopic Biliary Bypass

The two traditional treatment options for patients with noncalculous biliary obstruction are laparotomy with biliary bypass and endoscopic stenting. Open biliary bypass is a durable method of restoring bile flow, with only 15% of patients experiencing recurrent jaundice over their remaining life span. Endoscopic stenting, on the other hand, is complicated by occlusion in 50% of patients by 1 year despite the development of covered Wallstents (Schneider Stent Inc.; Minneapolis, MI) The drawback of palliative open bypass is the substantial associated morbidity (20% to 60%), mortality (15% to 30%), and length of hospital stay (14 to 21 days) in debilitated patients with advanced cancer. Open bypass is the treatment of choice in patients with benign obstructive conditions who have an extended life expectancy and can safely tolerate a general anesthetic.

Patients with a malignant non-resectable obstruction are more often managed with endoscopic stents, avoiding a surgery and prolonged recovery that can consume a significant portion of their limited life span. Van den Bosch has recommended that patients expected to live more than 6 months should undergo surgical bypass. This recommendation was based on a review of 148 pancreatic cancer patients palliated with either endoprostheses or surgical biliary bypass. The late morbidity was 60% in patients who lived longer than 6 months in the endoprostheses group, compared to only 5% in the surgery group.

Laparoscopic biliary bypass is an ideal palliative procedure as it combines the durability of an open bypass while approximating the minimally invasive nature of endoscopic stenting. Although first performed over 15 years ago, there are very few reports of laparoscopic biliary bypass in the literature. Laparoscopic biliary bypass requires advanced suturing skill and precision because of fixed suturing angles and unforgiving tissue that if mishandled leads to ischemia, stricture, or bile leak. Some of these limitations may be overcome in the future by anastomotic devices or the use of robotics, which provide improved range of motion and the filtering of hand tremor, allowing for more precise suturing. The technical advantages of performing biliary bypass laparoscopically are improved lighting and magnification of the operative field, while the disadvantages are lack of tactile sensation and only visual clues for depth of field discrimination. However, in experienced hands laparoscopic biliary bypass can be performed safely and has the same durability as the open operation while allowing for rapid recovery and shorter hospitalization. In addition, laparoscopy is often used as a part of staging for pancreatic cancer. In patients found to have unresectable disease on laparoscopy, palliative biliary and or gastric bypass can be performed at the same setting. As of yet, there are no prospective randomized trials comparing open surgical bypass, laparoscopic bypass, and endoscopic stenting.

PROCEDURE SELECTION

The three described laparoscopic biliary bypass procedures include: cholecystojejunostomy (CJ), choledochoduodenostomy (CDD), and choledocho/hepaticojejunostomy (CDJ). The choice of procedure depends on several factors, including the presence of the gallbladder, patency of the cystic duct, location of the tumor relative to the cystic duct-bile duct junction, size of the bile duct, prior surgical history, and, most importantly, the skill and experience of the laparoscopist. A previous cholecystectomy obviously precludes a cholecystojejunostomy and even makes choledochoduodenostomy and choledochojejunostomy more difficult as the gallbladder cannot be used for retraction. A small and contracted gallbladder suggests that either the cystic duct is not patent or that chronic cholecystitis has led to a fibrotic gallbladder wall. Whichever the cause, a cholecystojejunostomy in this setting is bound to fail. On the other hand, the presence of a Courvoisier gallbladder is indicative of a patent cystic duct and likely a good outcome with cholecystojejunostomy. Still, a CDJ is preferable as it has longer-term patency compared with CJ. The degree of obstruction and the diameter of the CBD are important considerations as well; a bile duct of at least 1.5 cm improves the feasibility of a CDD or CDJ.

A well-established contraindication for performing CJ is presence of tumor within 1 cm of the hepatocystic duct junction. With tumor in such close proximity there is a high likelihood of growth and subsequent obstruction. Tarnasky performed a retrospective study of ERCP in patients with malignant biliary obstruction to assess what percentage would be candidates for cholecystojejunostomy based on established anatomic criteria. One hundred out of 218 patients who underwent ERCP were excluded based on either prior biliary surgery (e.g., cholecystectomy) or the presence of a hilar tumor. Over half of the remaining patients had non-patent hepatocystic junctions, leaving just 50 of the original 218. Of these patients, 28 had tumors less than 1 cm from the hepatocystic junction, leaving just 22 of the initial 218 patients as candidates for CJ. This demonstrates the importance of preoperative or intraoperative cholangiography to assess for patency of the hepatocystic junction and to measure the distance between the tumor or stricture and the hepatocystic junction prior to performing CJ.

In order to further evaluate which type of bypass (cholecystoenterostomy and choledochoenterostomy) would lead to better palliation, Urbach retrospectively examined 1919 patients palliated with biliary bypass for pancreatic cancer. Of the 945 patients who underwent gallbladder bypass at 1, 2, and 5 years, 7.5%, 17.4%, and 26% had additional biliary interventions as compared to 2.9%, 11%, and 13% of those who were treated with bile duct bypass. These data supported previous studies that suggest the bile duct provides more durable palliation with less chance of reintervention. Although an anastomosis to the bile duct is more durable than one to the gallbladder, cholecystojejunostomy is still more commonly used as a palliative procedure. It can be performed laparoscopically with relative ease compared with hepaticojejunostomy because a circular or linear endoscopic stapler can be used and exposure is easier to obtain. Some argue that its lower long-term patency rate is justified because of its ease of performance and safety profile, especially given a population with a median life expectancy of 8 months. When it obstructs, an endostent can be placed; the patient's life expectancy at that point is short and repeated stent placements are less likely.

Choledochoduodenostomy has traditionally been used for benign disease because of the fear that anatomic proximity to a malignant tumor would risk encroachment on the anastomosis. However, there have been recent challenges to this traditional thinking. Di Fronzo retrospectively reviewed 79 consecutive patients presenting with malignant biliary obstruction, 71 of whom underwent choledochoduodenostomy for palliation. The other eight underwent hepaticojejunostomy because of tumor encroachment on the proximal bile duct or the inability to adequately mobilize the duodenum. None of these 71 patients developed recurrent biliary obstruction, which supports choledochoduodenostomy as a reasonable approach to palliate malignant biliary obstruction.

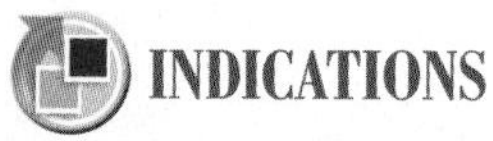

INDICATIONS

A patient being considered for laparoscopic biliary bypass requires a systematic workup beginning with an assessment of nutritional state and performance status. The patient's ability to tolerate an invasive procedure will play a role in selection of the location of the bypass (gallbladder vs. bile duct) or whether the patient is even a candidate for bypass.

Regardless of whether the bypass is being performed for benign disease or palliation of malignancy, a detailed knowledge of the biliary anatomy preoperatively is essential to avoid surprises and misadventures at the time of laparoscopy. An ultrasound, MRCP, PTC, or ERCP is useful to identify the location of the obstruction, confirm the presence of stones, and measure the diameter of the bile duct. An obstruction high in the biliary tree is not amenable to a laparoscopic approach and in many cases, open biliary bypass. A bile duct of at least 1.5 cm diameter makes the laparoscopic approach more feasible, although it is still possible to perform a bypass in a smaller diameter duct. If a CJ is to be performed, the strictured portion of the bile duct should be at least 1 cm away from the hepatocystic junction. Finally, the patient's surgical history must be taken into account as the laparoscopic approach is made much more difficult in the setting of prior surgeries, such as cholecystectomy and right hemicolectomy, which may have caused scarring in the area of the portahepatis.

LAPAROSCOPIC CHOLECYSTOJEJUNOSTOMY

Cholecystojejunostomy can be performed more simply compared to CDD and CDJ. There is minimal dissection required to expose the area for anastomosis, whereas CDD and CDJ require careful dissection of the porta hepatis. In addition, CJ can be performed with a triple staple technique, avoiding the need for suturing.

The first successful laparoscopic cholecystojejunostomy was performed in 1992. Shimi reported four cases of palliative CJ for advanced pancreatic cancer. All four patients were discharged within ten days and required minimal postoperative analgesics. The initial CJ was performed

TABLE 33-4. REPORTED CASES OF LAPAROSCOPIC CHOLECYSTOJEJUNOSTOMY

Author/Year	Number of cases	Operating time* in minutes	Mortality	Morbidity	Inpatient stay in days
Shimi/1992	4	90	1	0	10
Fletcher/1992	1	NR	0	0	4
Rhodes/1995	7	75	1**	0	4 (3 to 33)
Raj/1997	2	45 to 60	0	0	2
Casaccia/1999	2	127***	0	0	4.5
Chekan/1999	3[a]	NR	0	0	9.25
Kuriansky/2000	12[a]	89	3	1	6.4
O'Rourke/2004	1	44	0	1[b]	5

NR, not reported.
*Median operating time
**Stroke (included in the series are seven patients with biliary bypass alone, five patients with gastrojejunostomy alone, and three patients who had double bypass; it was not specified which group the patient with the stroke belonged to)
***Time for both biliary and gastric bypass
[a]All cases were both cholecystojejunostomy and gastrojejunostomy
[b]Death occurred 8 months post-op unrelated to surgery

using an intracorporeal linear cutting stapler with the common defect closed by suturing. These initial reports were followed by several single-institution series showing quick recovery and low morbidity (see Table 33-4).

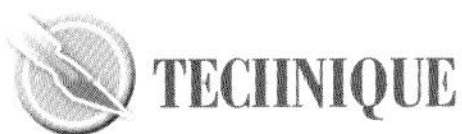

TECHNIQUE

The patient can be placed either supine, with the surgeon on the patient's right side, or in lithotomy, with the surgeon standing between the patient's legs. Four or more ports are required; a 10-mm infraumbilical port for a 30-degree telescope, a 12-mm port for the stapling device laterally under the right costal margin, and two 5-mm working ports (one inferior to the 12-mm port and the other in the left upper quadrant) to assist with tissue retraction.

The first step in the procedure is to assess the status of the gallbladder. A contracted gallbladder is indicative of either a non-patent cystic duct or chronic cholecystitis, both of which are contraindications to CJ. The preoperative cholangiogram must show both a patent cystic duct as well as at least a 1 cm distance between the cystic duct entrance into the common duct and the strictured area of the bile duct or tumor.

Several authors have described using a Roux-en-Y jejunal limb to create the biliary bypass. Although creating a Roux limb increases the complexity of the procedure and even the potential for complications, there are several advantages. The Roux limb has added length to decrease tension, and there are fewer septic complications as food is less likely to reflux into the bile duct.

Another method of performing the CJ is to create a side-to-side antecolic anastomosis with a jejunal loop 40 cm distal to the Treitz ligament. Two stay sutures are used to approximate and suspend the jejunum and gallbladder together. The harmonic scalpel (Ethicon Endo-Surgery, Cincinnati, OH) is then used to create an enterotomy and cholecystotomy. The stapler contains a 3.5-mm cartridge and is inserted through the right lateral 12-mm port; the jaws are inserted into both the gallbladder and jejunum and fired (Fig. 33-21, page 324). The resultant defect can be closed with either a running absorbable suture in two layers or with a second load of the stapler.

LAPAROSCOPIC CHOLEDOCHODUODENOSTOMY

Choledochoduodenostomy (CDD) is an excellent choice for patients with benign biliary obstruction. When performed in the setting of pancreatic malignancy, there is concern of late duodenal obstruction. Unlike the cholecystojejunostomy, which is very amenable to a purely stapled anastomosis, a completely stapled technique for CDD is much more challenging. Although a stapled technique for CDD has not been described in the literature, it can be performed by inserting a circular stapler through the stomach and into the duodenum while sewing the anvil to the dilated common bile duct. CDD is less technically challenging in that CDJ as the anastomosis involves only one suture line and does not require creation of a Roux limb or jejunal loop. Another advantage of CDD over CDJ includes endoscopic access to the biliary tree and more physiologic bile drainage.

The most common indications for CDD are benign diseases such as impacted stones with failed ERCP, retained stones, ampullary or distal common duct stricture from chronic pancreatitis, recurrent cholangitis, and recurrent choledocholithiasis, etc. There is controversy regarding the use of choledochoduodenostomy for palliation of malignant obstruction due to a fear of the tumor causing distal duodenal obstruction. Birkenfeld performed side-to-side choledochoduodenostomy in 46 patients with malignant periampullary tumors, and none had invasion of the stoma causing recurrent obstruction. In another study of palliative operations for pancreatic cancer performed at the Cleveland Clinic over 5 years, patients who underwent choledochoduodenostomy were found to have a lower rate of biliary sepsis than those patients undergoing choledochojejunostomy. Despite these and other similar studies showing the effectiveness of CDD in palliating malignant obstruction, the majority of the laparoscopic CDDs reported have been for benign disease.

There is some debate about whether a side-to-side or end-to-side CDD is the preferred technique of anastomosis. Most favor a side-to-side anastomosis, arguing that the distal bile duct blood supply is poor and performing an end-to-side anastomosis risks ischemia and recurrent stenosis. Those in favor of an end-to-side anastomosis argue the "sump syndrome" can occur with a side-to-side anastomosis as a result of stones or debris collecting in the nonfunctional distal bile duct with bacterial overgrowth manifesting clinically as pain or even sepsis. The reported incidence of the sump syndrome is between 0.14% and 3.3%. The anastomosis should be at least 1.5 cm to avoid postoperative stenosis and allow food and other debris to easily pass in and out of the stoma. Given the lack of prospective studies showing clear advantage of one method over the other, the side-to-side anastomosis is used much more often, as it is more amenable to the laparoscopic approach requiring a limited anterior bile

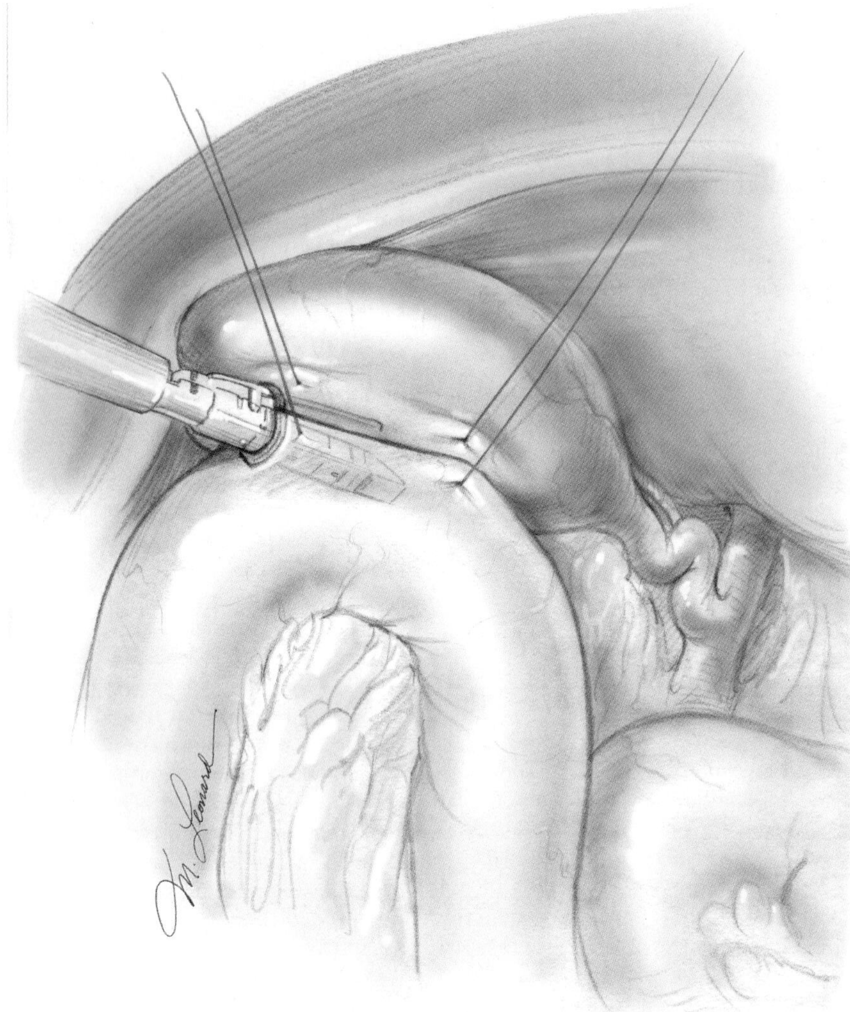

Fig. 33-21. Stapled side-to-side cholecystojejunostomy.

duct dissection. To date there is 1 case report in the literature of a laparoscopic end-to-side choledochoduodenostomy, with all other reported cases performed in a side-to-side fashion.

Franklin performed the first laparoscopic CDD in 1991 for benign recurrent bile duct obstruction. This was followed by several other case series that reported very low morbidity and short hospital stay (Table 33-5). Long-term follow-up after laparoscopic CDD is too sparse to accurately compare timing of re-strictures with open CDD, where two-thirds occur within 2 years and 90% occur within 7 years.

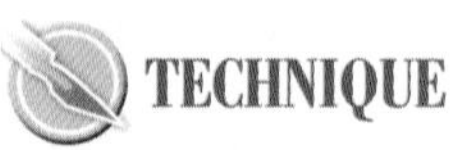

TECHNIQUE

The port placement for CDD is similar to that used for a laparoscopic cholecystectomy. A 10-mm port is placed at the umbilicus with 5-mm ports placed at the subxiphoid region, right upper abdomen, right lower abdomen, and an additional port in the left upper quadrant, which along with the subxiphoid port allows for suturing of the anastomosis. A 30-degree 10-mm scope is used through the umbilical port.

The first step in performing the anastomosis is dissection of the anterior surface of the bile duct. If necessary the identity of the CBD can be confirmed by aspirating bile. A longitudinal choledochotomy is made in the suprapancreatic part of the common duct using microscissors. The incision should be between at least 1.5 cm and up to 2 cm if possible. If stones are present they can be removed by a variety of techniques described earlier in this chapter, including the use of lithotripsy, stone forceps, saline flushing, or flexible endoscopic extraction with balloon catheter or wire basket through the working channel of the endoscope. Choledochoscopy should then be used to confirm clearance of the bile duct.

A generous Kocher maneuver should be performed to bring the duodenum in close proximity to the CBD without tension. A longitudinal duodenostomy is then created, which is perpendicular to choledochotomy to allow the anastomosis to be naturally tented open (Fig. 33-22). The size of the duodenostomy should match the size of the choledochotomy. An initial seromuscular stay suture can be placed at the distal aspect of choledochotomy and attached to the midportion of the inferior aspect of the duodenostomy; this will facilitate proper alignment prior to creating the single-layer mucosa-to-mucosa anastomosis. The posterior row of sutures should be placed in an interrupted fashion using an absorbable material such 3.0 VICRYL (Fig. 33-23, page 326). Once the posterior row is

TABLE 33-5. REPORTED CASES OF LAPAROSCOPIC CHOLEDOCHODUODENOSTOMY

Author/Year	N	Benign disease %	Operating time*	Morbidity	Mortality	Inpatient stay (mean days)
Rhodes/1996	2	100	180	0	0	4
Tinoco/1999	25	76	115	0	1	4.2
Gurbuz/1999	2	100	NR	0	0	8
Jeyapalan/2002	6	100	222	0	1	6
Tang/2003	12	100	137	1	0	7.5
O'Rourke/2004	3	100	330	0	0	4
Bhandarkar/2005	1	100	NR	0	0	5

NR, not reported.
*Median operation time in minutes

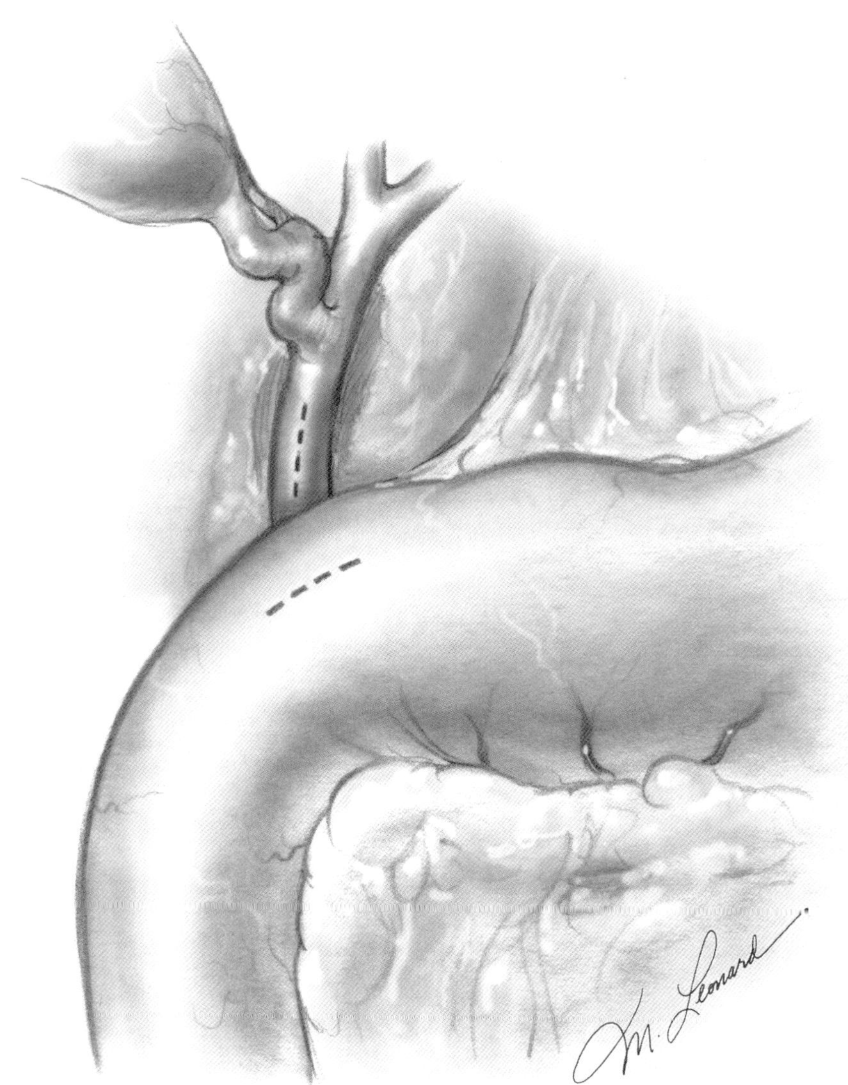

Fig. 33-22. Perpendicular longitudinal incisions in common bile duct and duodenum.

finished, the anterior row of sutures can be completed in a running fashion with the last stitch being tied at the medial aspect of the anastomosis. Three more seromuscular stay sutures can be placed at the corners to assure tension-free fixation.

LAPAROSCOPIC HEPATICOJEJUNOSTOMY AND RESECTION OF CHOLEDOCHAL CYST

Laparoscopic hepaticojejunostomy (HJ) requires an extensive dissection to expose the proximal bile duct or hepatic duct close to the hilar plate. In addition, creation of the Roux jejunal limb adds to the complexity of this operation and makes it the most difficult of the three laparoscopic biliary bypass procedures. Despite the difficult technical nature of HJ, favorable results were reported as early as 1992, when Phillips performed a laparoscopic excision of a choledochal cyst with Roux-en-Y hepaticojejunostomy reconstruction (Table 33-6, page 326). The main advantages of the hepaticojejunostomy are an improved patency and fewer septic complications compared with either CJ or CD. In a meta-analysis of 600 patients who underwent open biliary bypass, 93 of 400 patients (23%) developed recurrent jaundice after CJ, compared to 14 out of 200 (7%) after HJ.

The vast majority of the reported cases of laparoscopic HJ have been for either benign stricture or as the reconstruction after excision of a choledochal cyst (Table 33-6). Few cases have been reported as palliation for malignant obstruction because there is often a more simple method of decompression. On the other extreme, patients with choledochal cysts are usually diagnosed during infancy and childhood, with the rare case presenting later in life as recurrent cholangitis, choledocholithiais, and/or cholelithiasis. These patients must be treated by complete cyst excision with hepaticojejunostomy in order to avoid malignant degeneration.

Nearly all reported cases of laparoscopic choledochal cyst excision come from either China or Japan, where the incidence of choledochal cyst is as high as 1 in 1000 compared to the U.S., where the incidence is estimated at 1 in 100,000 to 150,000. Li has the largest current series of laparoscopic choledochal cyst excision with hepaticojejunostomy comprised of 35 patients aged 3 months to 9 years. There was just one immediate postoperative bile leak that stopped spontaneously; the other 34 patients were free of postoperative complications, with a mean of 1.5 years of follow-up.

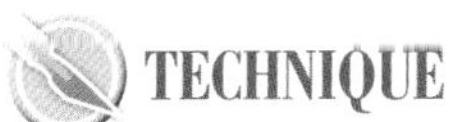

TECHNIQUE

The surgeon is positioned to the left of the patient, who is placed supine. Five ports are used: a 10-mm supraumbilical port for a 10-mm, 30-degree scope, a 10-mm epigastric port for the surgeon's right hand, a 10-mm port in the left mid upper abdomen for suturing, a 5-mm right subcostal port for the surgeon's left hand, and a second more lateral 5-mm right subcostal port for liver retraction.

In cases of choledochal cyst, the gallbladder is retracted cephalad to expose the dilated bile duct, which is carefully dissected posteriorly along the portal vein. Once circumferential dissection is achieved, an umbilical tape can be passed around the duct to aid in retraction. The duct is dissected toward the duodenum until a narrow normal portion of CBD is reached. The bile duct is then divided at this point using either a stapling device or with shears after placement of an endoloop. The divided end is used for retraction and the rest of the cyst is dissected up to normal hepatic duct, where it is subsequently divided (Fig. 33-24, page 327). The gallbladder is then removed en bloc with the cyst. In cases of malignant or benign obstruction the bile duct is prepared in a similar fashion, with

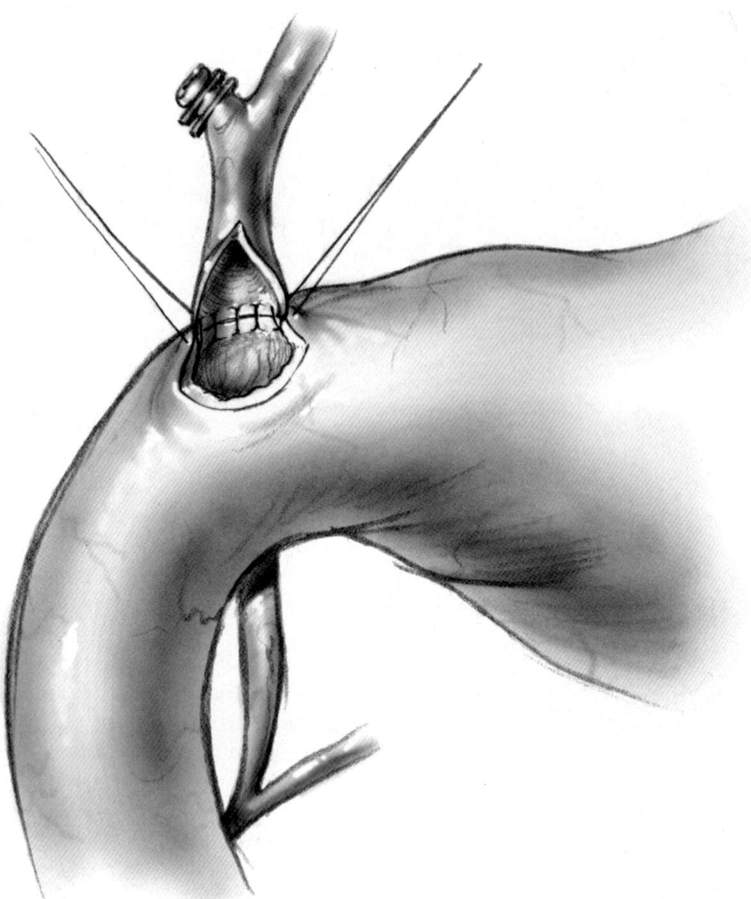

Fig. 33-23. Posterior row of interrupted sutures in a choledochoduodenostomy.

upward traction on the gallbladder to expose the bile duct. Circumferential dissection is not necessary as a side-to-side anastomosis can be performed.

Tanaka suggested leaving a small cuff of proximal cyst to facilitate the laparoscopic anastomosis. However, Todani reported that insufficient excision of the terminal portion of the choledochal cyst accounted for malignant degeneration in four out of 12 patients who underwent reoperation after cyst excision. Therefore, complete excision of the choledochal cyst is recommended to avoid future malignant degeneration.

Once the bile duct has been prepared, the Roux limb is created by dividing the small bowel 30 cm distal to the Treitz ligament with an endo-GIA stapler (white load). The mesentery is divided in a similar fashion until the Roux limb will easily reach the port hepatis in an antecolic fashion without tension. A triple-staple technique is completed to create a side-to-side jejunojejunostomy. A small enterotomy is created on the antimesenteric border of the jejunum. Stay sutures are placed at either end of the bile duct and bowel (Fig. 33-25). Leaving one end untied facilitates visualization, and the anastomosis is performed using a running suture on the posterior aspect of the jejunum and an interrupted layer to complete the anterior aspect of the end-to-side anastomosis.

TABLE 33-6. REPORTED CASES OF LAPAROSCOPIC ROUX-EN-Y CHOLEDOCHO-HEPATICOJEJUNOSTOMY

Author/Year	N	Indication	OR time	Morbidity	Mortality	Inpatient stay (days)
Phillips/1992	1	Cyst	120	0	0	7
Farello/1995	1	Cyst	NR	0	0	7
Shimura/1998	1	Cyst	NR	0	0	11
Rothlin/1999	3	Malignant	129*	1	0	9*
Machado/2000	1	Malignant	NR	0	0	6
Tanaka/2001	5	Cyst	616	1	0	25
Han/2003	6	Benign	358	1	0	NR
Ali/2003	1	Malignant	210	0	0	4
Li/2004	35	Cyst	260	1	0	4.5
O'Rourke/2004	2	1 Cyst, 1 Benign	501	1	0	3.5
Ure/2005	9	Cyst	289	2	0	5
Ure/2005	1	Cyst	270	1	0	4
Choweby/2005	9	6 Cyst, 3 Benign	297	2	0	5.1

OR, operating room; NR, not reported.
*Includes data from a series of gastroenterostomy (7) and diagnostic laparoscopy (3)

CONCLUSIONS

Laparoscopic biliary reconstruction is a feasible option for those with appropriate laparoscopic skills and experience with hepatobiliary surgery. The choice of operation must be made on an individual basis, taking into account both comorbidities and the underlying disease process. Although the results reported to date are very encouraging, long-term follow-up is lacking to compare patency rates of laparoscopic versus open bypass procedures. Until larger long-term studies are available, these operations should be approached with caution and a low threshold for conversion to open surgical technique.

SUGGESTED READING

Chekan EG, Clark L, Wu J, et al. Laparoscopic biliary and enteric bypass. *Semin Surg Oncol* 1999;16:313–320.

Cotton PB, Lehman G, Vennes J, et al. Endoscopic sphincterotomy complications and their management: an attempt at consensus. *Gastrointest Endosc* 1991;37:383–393.

Date RS, Siriwardena AK. Current status of laparoscopic biliary bypass in the management of non-resectable peri-ampullary cancer. *Pancreatology* 2005;5:325–329.

Franklin ME Jr, Pharand D, Rosenthal D. Laparoscopic common bile duct exploration. *Surg Laparosc Endosc* 1994;4:119–124.

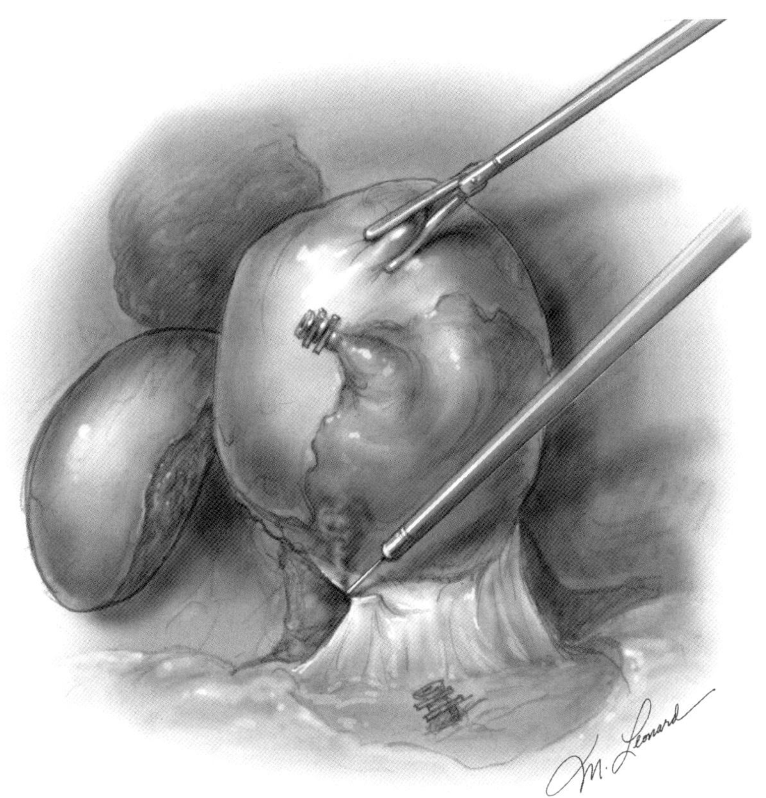

Fig. 33-24. Excision of a choledochal cyst.

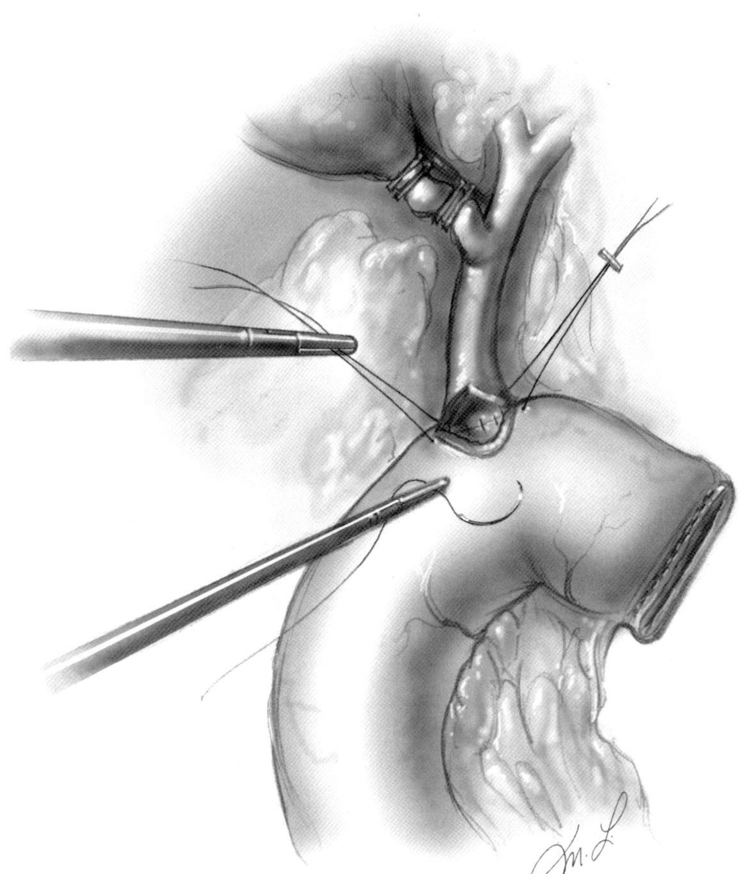

Fig. 33-25. Choledochojejunostomy.

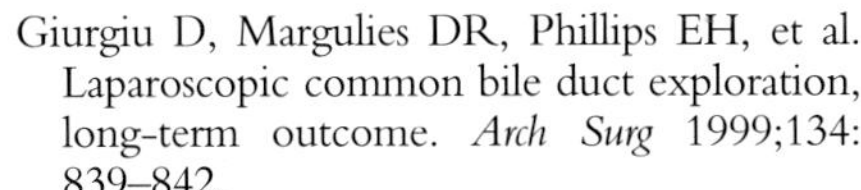

Giurgiu D, Margulies DR, Phillips EH, et al. Laparoscopic common bile duct exploration, long-term outcome. *Arch Surg* 1999;134: 839–842.

O'Rourke RW, Lee NN, Chen J, et al. Laparoscopic biliary reconstruction. *Am Jour Surg* 2004;187:621–624.

Phillips EH, Carroll BJ, Pearlstein AR, et al. Laparoscopic choledochoscopy and extraction of common bile duct stones. *World J Surg* 1993;17:22–28.

Phillips EH, Liberman M, Carroll BJ, et al. Bile duct stones in the laparoscopic era: is preoperative sphincterotomy necessary? *Arch Surg* 1995;130:880–886.

Phillips EH. Controversies in the management of common duct calculi. *Surg Clin North Am* 1994;74:931–951.

Schreurs WH, Juttmann JR, Stuifbergen WN, et al. Management of common bile duct stones: selective endoscopic retrograde cholangiography and endoscopic sphincterotomy: short- and long-term results. *Surg Endosc* 2002;16:1068–1072.

Scott-Conner CEH. Laparoscopic biliary bypass for inoperable pancreatic cancer. *Semin in Lap Surg* 1998;5:185–188.

Urbach DR, Bell CM, Swanstrom LL. Cohort study of surgical bypass to the gallbladder or bile duct for the palliation of jaundice due to pancreatic cancer. *Ann Surg* 2002; 237(1):86–93.

COMMENTARY

This comprehensive chapter on laparoscopic procedures involving the extrahepatic bile ducts is written by one of the first surgeons to perform the laparoscopic removal of common bile duct stones. Many surgeons performing laparoscopic cholecystectomy have abdicated the management of common bile stone to the gastroenterologist. This places the patient at risk from a second procedure and the unknown long-term effects of the sphincterotomy itself. Preoperative ERCP is often unnecessary, and if common bile duct stones discovered intraoperatively are left for postoperative ERCP, the possibility of failure of this second procedure exists. For surgeons opting for this latter option, it is probably beneficial to leave a transcystic cholangiocatheter in place postoperatively; this catheter allows for subsequent cholangiography (to assess whether the stones have passed spontaneously) and duct decompression in the early postoperative period, and will enable placement of a guidewire into the duodenum to assure successful cannulation of the bile duct.

One key to facilitate laparoscopic management of bile duct stones is to have all of the required equipment kept in a single location in the operating room supply area. When common bile duct stones are discovered (which inevitably occurs after regular hours or on weekends), the equipment is easily organized, even by operating room personnel who may not be familiar with its use. In general, the transcystic duct approach is applicable in the majority of the patients seen in most practices: relatively few, small, and distally located stones. For those stones that are large, multiple, located proximally, or associated with a very distal or tortuous insertion of the cystic duct, a choledochectomy should be used, assuming the common bile duct is adequately dilated. With the transcystic approach, the patient can usually be managed perioperatively, similar to those undergoing cholecystectomy alone. To successfully perform choledochotomy, the surgeon must be proficient at laparoscopic suturing. Certainly, those who perform laparoscopic cholecystectomies on a regular basis should familiarize themselves with the techniques for laparoscopic management of common duct stones, as they are present in 5% to 15% of patients undergoing elective cholecystectomy.

The section dealing with laparoscopic bypass operations describes various techniques available for palliation of malignant obstruction of the bile duct and the use of laparoscopy for excision of choledochal cysts. The majority of U.S. surgeons do not deal with choledochal cysts. However, malignant obstruction of the bile ducts is relatively common and should be amenable to laparoscopic treatment. Especially in those centers where laparoscopy is used as a staging procedure for patients with pancreatic cancer, the discovery of unresectable disease should lead the surgeon to consider one of the biliary bypasses described in this chapter. If a choledochojejunostomy is entertained as a possibility and preoperative cholangiography has not been undertaken, a transcystic cholangiogram should be performed to assess the distance between the cystic duct insertion and the proximal extent of the obstructing lesion. Surgical bypass often affords longer-term palliation for this group with unresectable disease, and the laparoscopic approach minimizes morbidity and duration of hospitalization. Surgeons should not be too quick to assign the palliation of biliary obstruction to the endoscopist for placement of endoscopic stents.

NJS

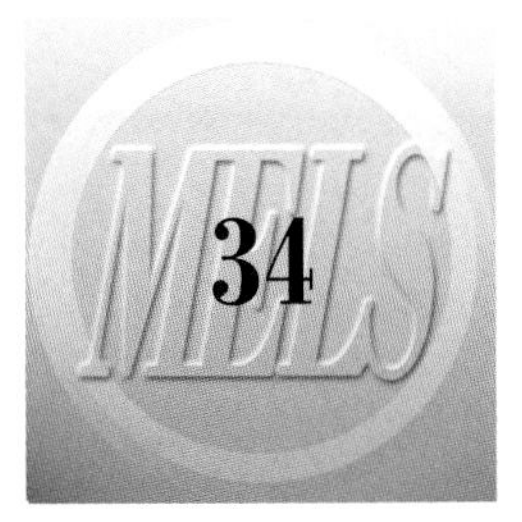

Bile Duct Injury

STEVEN M. STRASBERG

INTRODUCTION

Biliary injury is the most severe common complication of cholecystectomy. It is always morbid, increases cost, and often leads to litigation. Injury may occur during laparoscopic cholecystectomy, planned open cholecystectomy, or after conversion from laparoscopic to open cholecystectomy. Injury rates have decreased from the levels encountered in the early 1990s. However, injury rates are probably still higher than those in the era of open cholecystectomy, although accurate data are unavailable. The causes of injury are increasingly better understood, and improvements in strategies for preventing injury have occurred. When injury occurs, a high rate of permanent cure is possible using advanced techniques of reconstruction in specialized centers.

Terminology

The *prevailing anatomic pattern* is the most common anatomical pattern and it may be present almost always or in less than in 50% of patients depending on the structure. In actuality it is very uncommon for the prevailing pattern to be present in less than 50% of persons even when discussing the biliary tree. *Anomalies* are variations from the prevailing pattern. Anomalies may be common or rare. There may be anomalies of position, number, or size of structures. *Aberrancy* refers to abnormal position of a structure. An *accessory* structure is one that is in addition to the normal prevailing pattern and whose function can be deleted without loss of overall function of the organ. The term *replaced* is used synonymously with aberrant when referring to aberrant arteries to the liver. Because anomalies of bile ducts and vascular structures the porta are frequently present, it has been said that there is no "normal" pattern of anatomy in this area of the body. This is incorrect; the prevailing anatomic pattern is the "normal" pattern in the sense that it is the most common pattern.

Classification of Biliary Injuries

The Bismuth classification, which is actually a classification of benign biliary strictures, as opposed to biliary injuries, was the standard means of classifying biliary injuries in the era of open cholecystectomy. It classified strictures into five types based mainly on the upper level of injury. This classification became somewhat less useful with the introduction of laparoscopic cholecystectomy, as some of the most common injuries encountered were not strictures. We introduced a classification that includes the injuries seen with increased frequency after the advent of laparoscopic cholecystectomy but still retains important features of the Bismuth classification (Fig. 34-1, page 330).

Type A: Bile leak from a minor duct retaining continuity with the common bile duct (Fig. 34-2, page 330). These leaks are usually caused by a failure to adequately occlude the cystic duct or by inadvertent entry into a small bile duct in the liver bed. Type A biliary injuries are the least serious, because major ducts are not involved. However, even these injuries can be morbid. They are usually lateral injuries to the biliary tree. Therefore, decreasing intrabiliary pressure by endoscopic sphincterotomy usually resolves the problem.

Types B and C. Creation of a discontinuity of part of the biliary tree with occlusion (Type B) or intraperitoneal leak (Type C). These are end injuries that isolate a part of the biliary tree. They usually result from damage to an aberrant right hepatic duct, but a completely occluded or transected normally positioned right hepatic duct would also fit here. About 2% of patients have an aberrant low-lying right hepatic duct that usually drains one or two segments of the right hemiliver. Sometimes the cystic duct joins the aberrant duct, which then continues to join the main ductal system. This variation contributes to the likelihood of injury because the appearance of the confluence of the aberrant duct with the common hepatic duct is virtually identical to that of the confluence of a cystic duct with the hepatic duct. When the injury is a ductal occlusion, it is designated as Type B. When it is a transection without occlusion it is Type C. Generally, occlusions are injuries of lesser severity. The liver upstream from the occlusion usually undergoes asymptomatic atrophy. If symptoms such as cholangitis do occur they are often delayed for years. Transections without occlusion (Type C) result in local intraperitoneal bile collections or bilious ascites with peritonitis. In the Bismuth classification isolated aberrant right ductal strictures were lumped with other Type V strictures. Not only are these injuries much more common in the laparoscopic era but they are almost always transections. As the management and prognosis of B and C injuries are so different, they were given separate categories in our classification.

Type D: Lateral injury to major bile ducts. Type D injuries are partial (< 50%) transections of major bile ducts, usually lacerations of the common duct. When the transection involves more than 50% of the circumference of the duct, the injury should be considered an E type. Like the Type A variant, they are lateral injuries and will usually resolve after decompression by endoscopic sphincterotomy. If discovered at the time of surgery they may be repaired with sutures and the placement of a T-tube. Such injuries have the potential to be much more serious, particularly if thermal in origin or associated with devascularization of the bile duct. Then they may progress to a circumferential, or Type E, injury.

Type E: Circumferential injury of major bile ducts (Bismuth class I to V). These are circumferential injuries of major bile ducts, as described by Bismuth. Subclassification into Types E1 to E4 is based on the level of injury, while the E5 is a combination of common hepatic duct and aberrant right duct injury. Type E injuries separate the hepatic parenchyma from the lower biliary tract, due to stenosis, simple occlusion, or

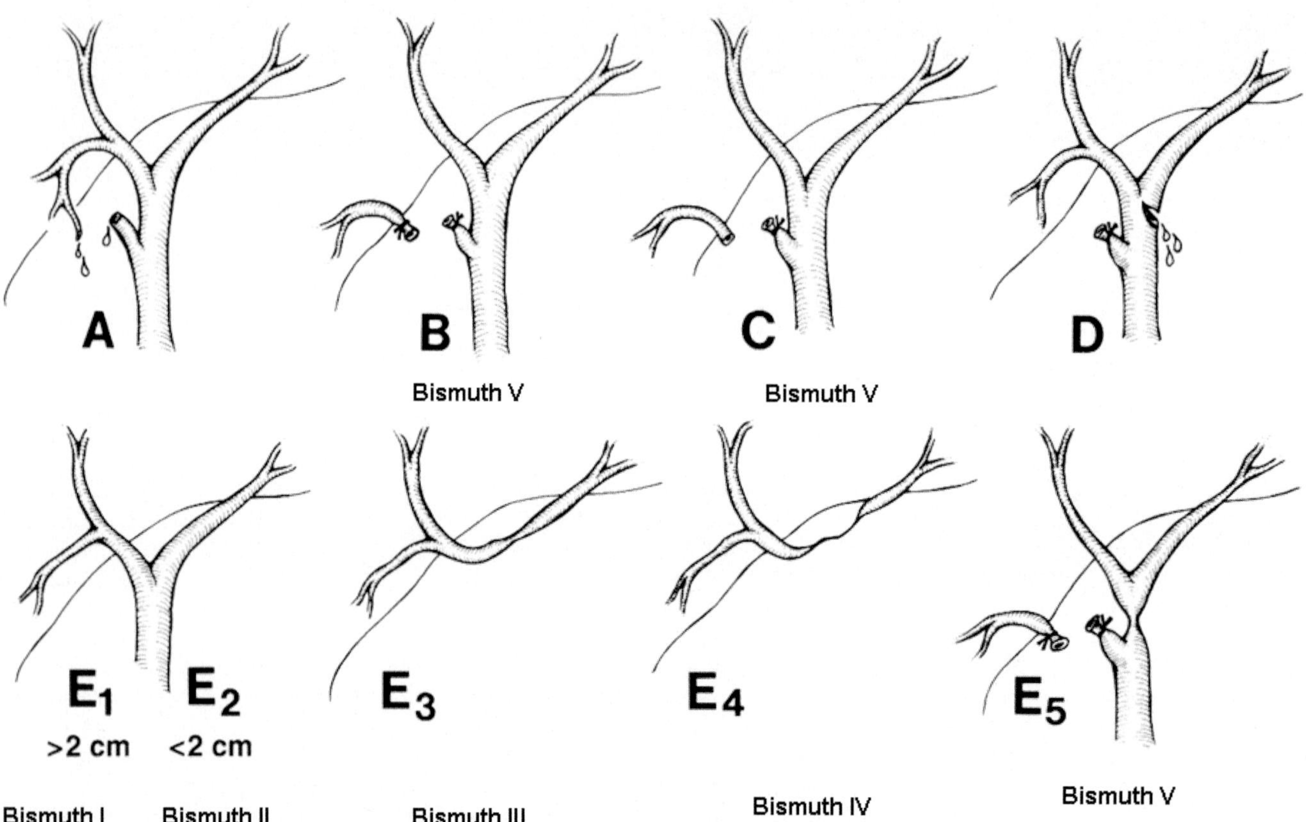

Fig. 34-1. A classification of laparoscopic injuries to the biliary tract. Type A injuries originate from small bile ducts that are entered in the liver bed or from the cystic duct. Type B and C injuries almost always involve aberrant right hepatic ducts. The notations >2 cm and <2 cm in Type E1 and Type E2 indicate the length of common hepatic duct remaining. The corresponding Bismuth classification numbers are given when possible. Note that Types A and D do not exist in the Bismuth classification, which is a classification of bile duct strictures rather than injuries. Likewise types B and C correspond to Bismuth type V, although in that classification they would be a stenosis rather than a transection with or without occlusion.

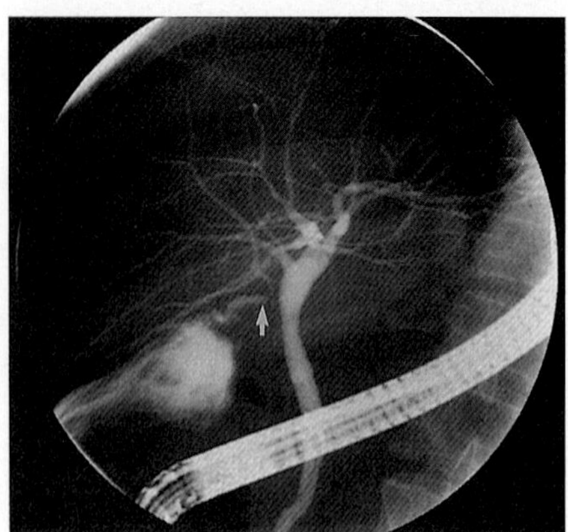

Fig. 34-2. A postoperative ERCP in a patient who developed a biloma. Note that the injury is to a small tributary of a hepatic duct. (By permission of the *Journal of the American College of Surgeons*.)

transection, sometimes accompanied by resection of bile ducts. As noted above, the Bismuth classification is of bile duct stenoses. However, our classification is of all bile duct injuries; therefore to classify the injury correctly it must be stated whether the injury is a partial occlusion (stenosis) or complete occlusion, whether the duct has been transected, and whether and how much bile duct has been excised, for example: "E3, 2-cm duct length excised, transection without proximal occlusion, distal occlusion present." For purposes of repair, the upper limit of injury is the key variable and is given in the E type itself.

Vascular injuries may accompany biliary injuries. They occur more commonly with higher biliary injuries. Vascular injuries are associated with a greater tendency for restricture of bile duct repairs, but this seems to be true only when bile ducts associated with vascular injuries are not repaired after an interval in expert centers using the Hepp-Couinaud approach but rather repaired more immediately in community hospitals. There is a tendency to higher rates of mortality when an associated vascular injury has occurred. Arterial injuries may involve the proper hepatic artery, the right hepatic artery, and replaced right hepatic arteries coming off the superior mesenteric artery. Portal vein transection and traumatic thrombosis have also been reported. The vascular component may become the predominant feature of the injury with necrosis of the intrahepatic biliary system (similar to that seen with hepatic artery thromboses after liver transplantation) or even hepatic infarction. Infarction of the intrahepatic biliary tree requires transplantation, while hepatic infarction may lead to the need for hepatic resection or transplantation. Portal vein thrombosis may lead to cavernous transformation of the portal vein. This increases the difficulty of later repairs and may itself lead to bile duct compression. The worst vascular injuries we have been referred have occurred after conversion from laparoscopic cholecystectomy to open cholecystectomy in patients with severe inflammation and in whom the "top-down" technique was used after conversion.

Pathogenesis of Bile Duct Injuries

Determining the cause of a biliary injury is often difficult. Usually the only record of the injury is an operative note. There is no mandated standard for operative notes, and they vary greatly in detail and explanatory value. Sometimes when the injury is recognized intraoperatively, the pathogenesis of the injury is clear. In many cases, especially when the injury is unrecognized intraoperatively or when the note is lacking in detail, the mechanism of injury is indeterminable. Furthermore, two readers of a particular note may come to different conclusions regarding the mechanism, depending on their views regarding the general mechanisms of injury. For instance, although it is agreed that visual deception is an important pathogenetic mechanism in biliary injury, some (such as this author) stress that the deceptions are highly dependent on the techniques adopted in cholecystectomy for ductal identification, whereas others have emphasized psychological factors associated with human error as the root cause.

PATIENT-RELATED FACTORS

Inflammation

Cholecystectomies are usually performed on pathological gallbladders; inflammation is almost always present, but severe inflammation increases the risk of biliary injury, and unusual grades of inflammation may make cholecystectomy very difficult.

Acute Cholecystitis

The incidence of biliary injury is higher when laparoscopic cholecystectomy is performed during acute cholecystitis than it is for elective indications. Acute inflammation causes thickening of tissues, increases their friability and vascularity, and promotes adhesions. These factors obscure normal anatomical relationships (Fig. 34-3A) and increase the difficulty of exposure and dissection. An important consequence is that the inflammatory mass may effectively obliterate the triangle of Calot (Fig. 34-3B). When using certain techniques, this tends to result in the visual deception that the inflammatory mass that in fact consists of the gallbladder, the cystic duct, and the common hepatic duct is the gallbladder alone and that the common bile duct is the cystic duct. Severe inflammation is more likely to be encountered when the time between the onset of symptoms and surgery for acute cholecystitis is greater than 72 hours, when there is a palpable inflammatory mass, or if the white blood cell count is greater than 18,000 cells/cu mm.

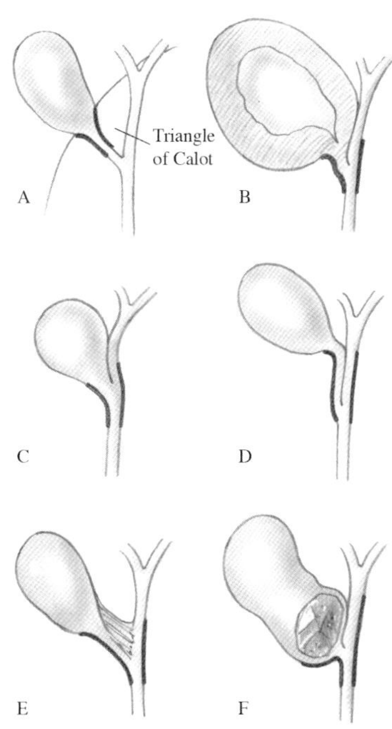

Fig. 34-3. Conditions that predispose to the deception that the common bile duct is the cystic duct, especially when the infundibular technique is used. **A.** Condition of minimal inflammation in which the triangle of Calot is open and the funnel shape of the junction between the gallbladder and cystic duct (heavy line) is readily apparent. The infundibular technique is effective under these conditions. Conditions that may give a misleading funnel shape (heavy lines) because of obliteration or concealment of triangle of Calot (in these cases the common bile duct is being dissected as it appears to be the cystic duct widening into the gallbladder). **B.** Severe acute cholecystitis. **C.** Severe chronic inflammation. **D.** Parallel cystic duct insertion. **E.** Congenital bands. **F.** A large impacted stone.

Severe Chronic Inflammation with Dense Scarring

Numerous bouts of cholecystitis may result in severe fibrosis of the gallbladder and surrounding tissue. The gallbladder may become shrunken down to a structure no more than one centimeter in length and width. In these cases fibrotic retraction may bind the gallbladder to the common hepatic duct and right hepatic artery, effectively obliterating the triangle of Calot (Fig. 34-3C). Such inflammation may make dissection very difficult and contribute to visual deception when certain techniques are used. In extreme cases the inflammation may affect the whole porta hepatis.

Congenital Abnormalities

A number of congenital abnormalities increase the risk of biliary injuries. The most important of these anomalies are aberrant right hepatic ducts and parallel insertion of the cystic duct into the common bile duct.

Aberrant Right Hepatic Ducts

A low-lying aberrant right hepatic duct, present in about 2% of patients, is a well recognized risk factor for biliary injury. These ducts may lie in or close to the triangle of Calot and are in danger of injury during dissection. The most perilous situation occurs when the cystic duct actually unites with the low-lying aberrant right duct, which then continues to a confluence with the common hepatic duct. The appearance of the junction of the aberrant duct with the hepatic duct may be identical that of the normal confluence of the cystic duct with the common hepatic duct, and consequently there is great potential for injury. These injuries are underreported as occlusion of an aberrant duct may be asymptomatic and thus unrecognized. Aberrant right hepatic duct injuries are more common in laparoscopic than open cholecystectomy.

Parallel Union Cystic Duct

The parallel union cystic duct (Fig. 34-3D) occurs in about 20% of individuals. It was a well described risk factor for biliary injury in the era of open cholecystectomy and continues to be a risk factor today. It may effectively contract the triangle of Calot and cause the deception that the common bile duct is the cystic duct.

Aberrant Position of Cystic Duct Termination

The cystic duct may insert into the biliary tree at any point from the right hepatic duct to the termination of the common bile duct. Insertion into the right hepatic duct is very uncommon but exposes this duct to injury.

Congenital Adhesions Between the Gallbladder and Common Hepatic Duct

Such adhesions are prominent in some individuals; they obscure the triangle of Calot and may fix the common hepatic duct to the side of the gallbladder. In some cases the Hartmann pouch may actually lie over and to the left of the common bile and common hepatic ducts (Fig. 34-3E).

Abnormal Diameter or Length of Bile Ducts

There is considerable variation of bile duct size from person to person. Duct size differs depending on whether internal or external diameters are measured. The internal diameter of the cystic duct is normally 2 to 3 mm, which would make the external diameter about 3 to 5 mm. The normal supraduodenal common bile duct external diameter duct ranges from 4 to 13 mm, but the normal internal diameter measured by ultrasound is considered to be 3 to 8 mm, with wall thickness accounting for the difference. In rare cases duct size may be less than these norms, which exposes the ducts to injury especially when certain techniques of ductal identification are used. Cystic duct length is highly variable. A congenitally absent cystic duct is rare. An absent cystic duct is usually due to effacement of the cystic duct by a stone and is generally accompanied by severe inflammation.

Intrahepatic Gallbladder

An intrahepatic gallbladder is difficult to grasp and indirectly contributes to injury by making it difficult to expose the cystic duct.

Hepatic Duct Uniting with or Lying in Proximity to the Gallbladder

A duct of Luschka is an accessory duct that runs between an intrahepatic duct and the gallbladder. It penetrates the cystic plate in its course between the two structures. It usually is 1 mm or less in diameter. An injury to a duct of Luschka is difficult to recognize as the duct is tiny, and hepatic bile is dilute and often straw-colored as opposed to gallbladder bile, which is normally dark green. Ducts of Luschka are uncommon but not rare. In about 10% of individuals, a right hepatic duct measuring 2 to 3 mm in diameter lies immediately deep to the cystic plate. In this location it is in danger of injury if the cystic plate is penetrated when dissecting the gallbladder off the plate (gallbladder bed). Injuries to such ducts and ducts of Luschka produce Type A injuries. A major hepatic duct that enters directly into the gallbladder would be in great danger of injury during dissection of the gallbladder off the cystic plate. The incidence of such ducts is unknown other than they must be extremely rare. To the author's knowledge they have not been described in anatomical dissections. Their presence is most likely due to erosion of a stone into a major bile duct, causing a fistula between the gallbladder and the bile duct.

Other Patient-Related Factors

Large Impacted Gallstones

These are not infrequently mentioned in operative notes of cholecystectomies in which biliary injuries have occurred. They tend to impair retraction and hide the cystic duct (Fig. 34-3F). As noted they may efface the cystic duct, thus shortening or obliterating it, and in severe cases cause common bile duct compression or erosion with severe pericholecystic inflammation (Mirizzi syndrome).

Obesity and Body Habitus

Obesity, a risk factor for cholelithiasis, is common in patients having a cholecystectomy. Morbid obesity and large body size in general contribute to difficulty in operative exposure. The same is true of skeletal deformities. These may be contributing factors to biliary injury.

PROCEDURE-RELATED FACTORS

These are problems related to concepts or technique of procedure itself.

Misidentification—A Concept Problem

Secure identification is an issue in many areas of surgery ranging from patient, limb, and organ identification to identification of ureters, proximal jejunum, and bile ducts. Each has been misidentified. There are two main types of bile duct misidentification: misidentification of the common bile duct as the cystic duct (Figs. 34-4A to C) and misidentification of an aberrant right hepatic duct as the cystic duct (Figs. 34-4D to F). In the former type, misidentification results in the clipping and cutting of the common bile duct. If the injury is unrecognized the biliary tree will be divided again at a higher level in order to complete the cholecystectomy (Figs. 34-4A and B). This type of injury has been called the "classical injury." The type of injury produced may be E1 to E4 and depends upon the level of the second transection. Higher levels of transection may result from traction on the gallbladder pulling the hepatic ducts down into the field where they are divided. This second transection of the biliary tree is often not recognized. If bile is seen, the surgeon may think he or she has only made a hole in the gallbladder. In operative notes of such procedures it is not unusual to find references to a "second cystic duct" or an "accessory cystic duct," which really is the common hepatic duct or higher level biliary ducts. These injuries either result in bile duct obstruction or bile leak, depending upon whether the biliary tree is clipped and cut or only cut. Injury is often associated with laceration or clipping of the right hepatic artery. This may cause brisk bleeding that leads to conversion and diagnosis of biliary injury or can simply result in unrecognized occlusion of the artery, the surgeon believing that he or she has occluded a large cystic artery. Arterial occlusion may aggravate the biliary injury due to ischemia of the remnant bile duct.

The second type of misidentification leads to injury of an aberrant right hepatic duct (B and C injuries). The section of the aberrant right hepatic duct, between entry of cystic duct and junction with the common hepatic, is mistaken to be the cystic duct (Figs. 34-4D to F). The misidentified section is clipped and usually cut. To remove the gallbladder the aberrant duct must be cut again at a higher level.

Techniques and Their Relationship to Misidentification

The key to understanding why misidentification occurs rests with examining the rationale for identification of the cystic structures during cholecystectomy. There are five techniques in general use: the "infundibular technique," cholangiography, dissection of the cystic duct to the confluence with the common hepatic duct and the common bile duct, the "critical view of safety" technique, and the "top-down" technique. Previously we have classified the "top-down" method as a variant of one of the other methods, but in reality it has a different logic and should be discussed separately.

Infundibular Technique

This technique depends on the display of the funnel-shaped junction (infundibulum) of the lower end of the gallbladder

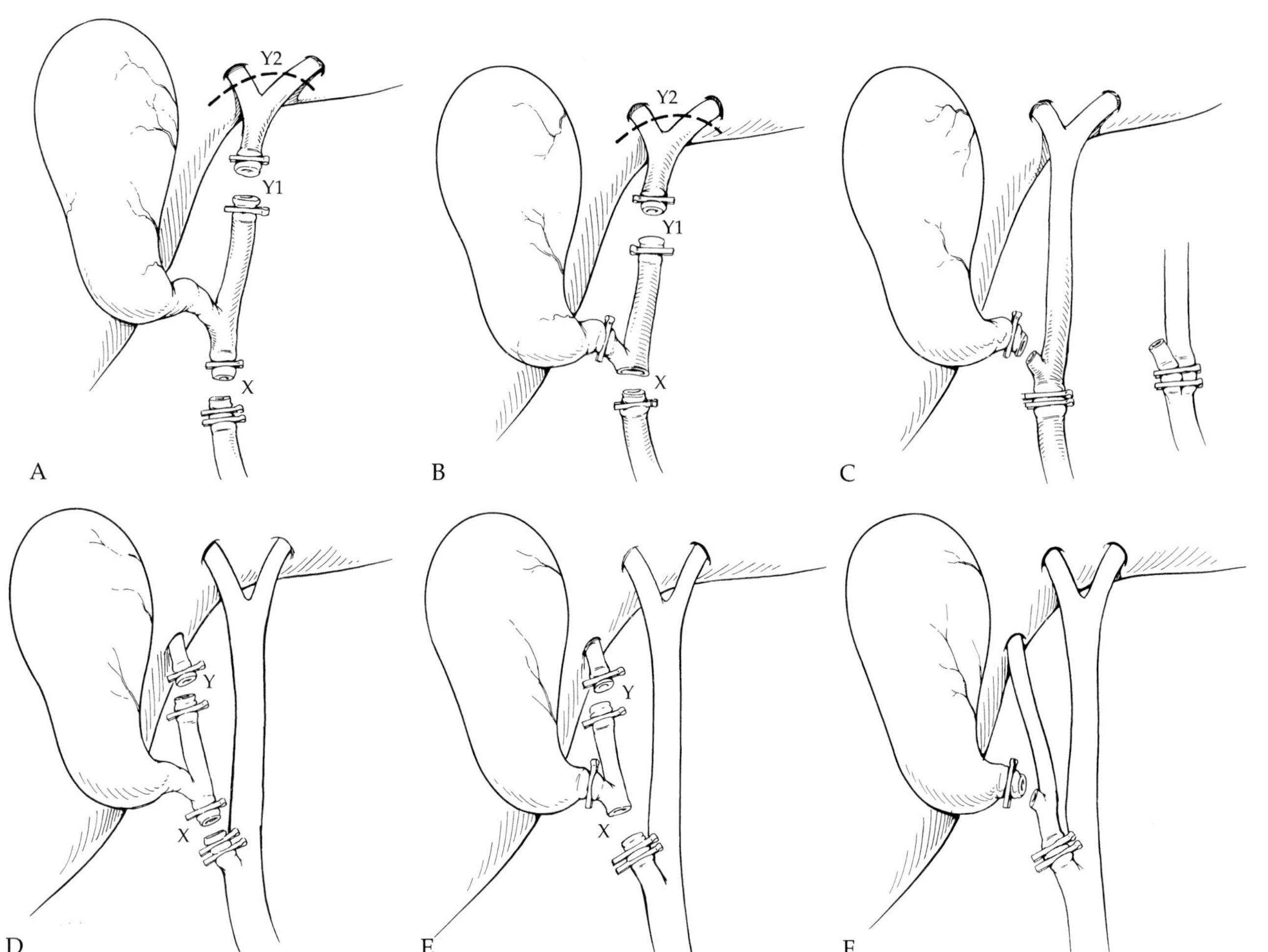

Fig. 34-4. Patterns of biliary injury due to misidentification. **A.** The "classical" type E injury in which the common duct is divided between clips at point x. The ductal system is later divided again to remove the gallbladder either at point Y1, producing E1 or E2 injuries, or at point Y2, producing E3 or E4 injuries. **B.** Variant of Type E injury which leads to bile leakage into the operative field and thereby an increased chance of recognition before the entire injury evolves. **C.** Variant of Type E injury leading to clipping but not excision of the duct. This injury also causes intraoperative bile leakage, except when cystic and common bile ducts are both occluded, as shown in the inset. **D, E,** and **F** represent variants of injury to aberrant right hepatic duct, producing Type B or Type C injuries. The injuries shown in D, E, and F correspond to the injuries shown in A, B, and C, but affect the aberrant right duct. (By permission of the *Journal of the American College of Surgeons.*)

with the cystic duct for identification of the cystic duct (Fig. 34-3, page 331). In the infundibular method the surgeon is instructed to follow the putative cystic duct up to the gallbladder or the gallbladder down to the cystic duct, at which point, *after circumferential dissection* of these structures, the funnel is displayed. It is this flaring or widening that was believed to give conclusive identification of the infundibulo-cystic junction and therefore safe identification of the cystic duct. It should be noted that the infundibular technique calls for circumferential or three-dimensional display of the funnel. Seeing the funnel in two dimensions, that is, simply clearing one surface of the funnel, is inadequate. However, we have collected numerous operative notes of biliary injuries in which the surgeon described following what was thought to be the cystic duct (actually the circumferentially dissected common bile duct) to a point that it seemed to flare into the gallbladder. In retrospect the mistaken "flare" occurred when the common bile duct was followed up to an inflammatory mass within which the cystic duct was hidden ("hidden cystic duct" syndrome). This visual deception is most likely to occur when one or more factors described above are present: severe acute or chronic inflammation, a large stone in the Hartmann pouch, adhesive bands, intrahepatic gallbladder, short cystic duct, etc. These make retraction and display of the real cystic duct difficult. Also, misidentification may lead to injury of the bile duct without division or clipping, as extensive dissection may cause devascularization, particularly if ductal arteries thought to be the cystic artery or its branches, are divided. This type of injury may present later as a stricture.

Intraoperative Cholangiography (IOC)

A large well-controlled study from Australia that proved that IOC reduces the incidence of biliary injury was subsequently confirmed in studies from the U.S. Other studies suggest that the severity of biliary injury is reduced by IOC. Operative cholangiography is best at

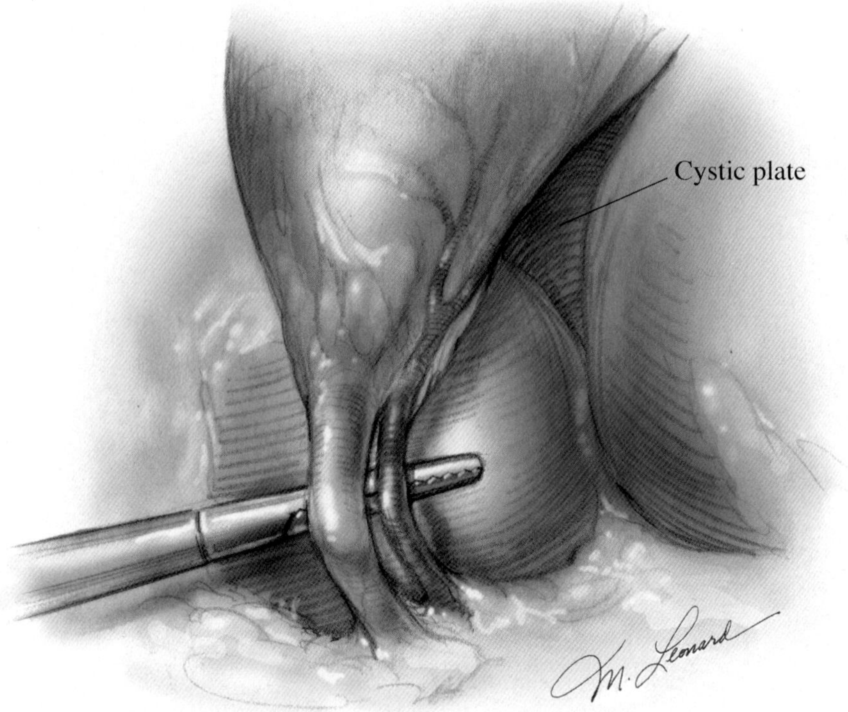

Fig. 34-5. The "critical view of safety." The triangle of Calot is dissected free of all tissue except for cystic duct and artery, and the base of the liver bed is exposed. When this view is achieved, the two structures entering the gallbladder can only be the cystic duct and artery. It is not necessary to see the common bile duct. (By permission of the *Journal of the American College of Surgeons.*)

detecting misidentification of the common bile duct as the cystic duct and will prevent excisional injuries of bile ducts, if the cholangiogram is correctly interpreted. Unfortunately, operative cholangiograms are sometime misinterpreted. The most common misinterpretation is the failure to recognize that when only the lower part of the biliary tree is seen, the common bile duct rather than the cystic duct has been incised and cannulated. IOC is not effective at detecting aberrant right ducts, which unite with the cystic duct before joining the common duct. The aberrant duct appears to be the cystic duct visually and on cholangiograms, especially as some non-aberrant right-sided ducts usually fill during the procedure (Fig. 34-6). Because it is not unusual to obtain only partial filling of the right hepatic ducts by IOC, this is taken as a normal pattern. Another drawback is that an incisional injury of the common bile duct, made in order to perform IOC, may not be innocuous. However, the benefits of IOC in ductal identification far outweigh its disadvantages.

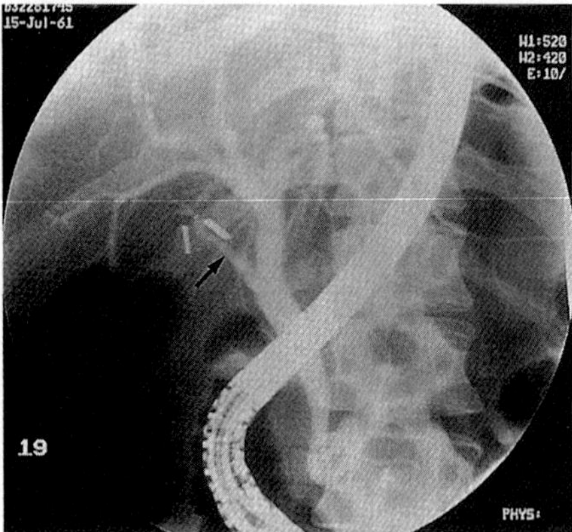

Fig. 34-6. Postoperative ERCP in a patient with an aberrant right hepatic duct (arrow). Note that the intrahepatic biliary system appears normal. Clips indicate the position of the cystic duct and artery. Note how the point of union of the aberrant duct with the common hepatic duct looks like a cystic duct-common duct junction. Mistakenly doing a cholangiogram through the aberrant duct rather than identifying it by dissection would have led to a ductal injury that would have been difficult to repair because of the small size of the aberrant duct. (By permission of the *Journal of the American College of Surgeons.*)

Dissection of the Cystic Duct to the Confluence with the Common Hepatic Duct/Common Bile Duct

This was a common and usually safe technique in performance of open cholecystectomy. There is reason to believe that its use during laparoscopic cholecystectomy has been associated with an increase in lateral injuries to the common hepatic duct (Type D), which have become much more common. Possibly this is due to poorer visibility as one dissects laparoscopically in the coronal plane approaching the common bile duct. Undoubtedly the injury is more prone to occur when this technique is used in patients with a parallel union cystic duct. This technique is not in widespread use judging from surgeon audience responses.

The "Critical View of Safety" Technique

Introduced in 1992 and modified in 1995, this technique recommends clearing the triangle of Calot of fat and fibrous tissue and taking the gallbladder off the lowest part of its attachment to the gallbladder bed (cystic plate). Only two structures will be connected to the lower end of the gallbladder once this is done. Raising the gallbladder off the lower part of the cystic plate is an important step, equivalent in the open technique to taking the gallbladder off the gallbladder bed. No attempt is made to expose the common bile duct or common hepatic duct. A picture of the critical view is shown in Figure 34-5. This view provides a convincing demonstration that the two structures entering the gallbladder are the cystic duct and artery. Note the resemblance between the critical view technique and the technique of identification in open cholecystectomy in which the cystic duct and artery were putatively identified and the gallbladder then taken off the liver bed (i.e., the gallbladder was pedunculated on its cystic structures). The latter is not done before occlusion of the cystic structures during laparoscopic cholecystectomy because of the tendency of the gallbladder to rotate after it is fully removed from the liver bed and because removal from the liver bed is eased by prior division of the cystic structures.

"Top-Down" Cholecystectomy

In this technique the cholecystectomy is started at the fundus, taking the gallbladder off the gallbladder bed prior to any dissection or identification of structures in the triangle of Calot. This is a technique favored by a number of authors. The "top-down" method seeks to pedunculate the gallbladder on the cystic artery and cystic duct, thus making secure identification. While it may be an effective technique of identification in most instances, our experience is that it may lead to serious biliary and vascular injuries in the presence of severe inflammation. The injuries are technical injuries rather than injuries of misidentification because they occur in the course of dissection before a structure is recognized. The problem is that the surgeon dissecting from above may "see" the inflammatory mass containing the gallbladder and critical vessels and bile ducts as the gallbladder alone and lacerate or divide one or more of these structures (Fig. 34-7). In fact, the worst bilo-vascular injuries that have been referred to us have occurred in this way, often after conversion to open cholecystectomy. Note that the critical view technique has no conceptual connection to the top-down technique of cholecystectomy, the key difference being that the critical view technique calls for the dissection to start in the triangle of Calot, and identification of cystic structures is complete before the fundus of the gallbladder is mobilized. Similarly the top-down technique is not the same as taking the gallbladder off the cystic plate starting at the fundus, after the cystic structures have been putatively identified and taped. That is a standard safe method of open cholecystectomy as noted previously.

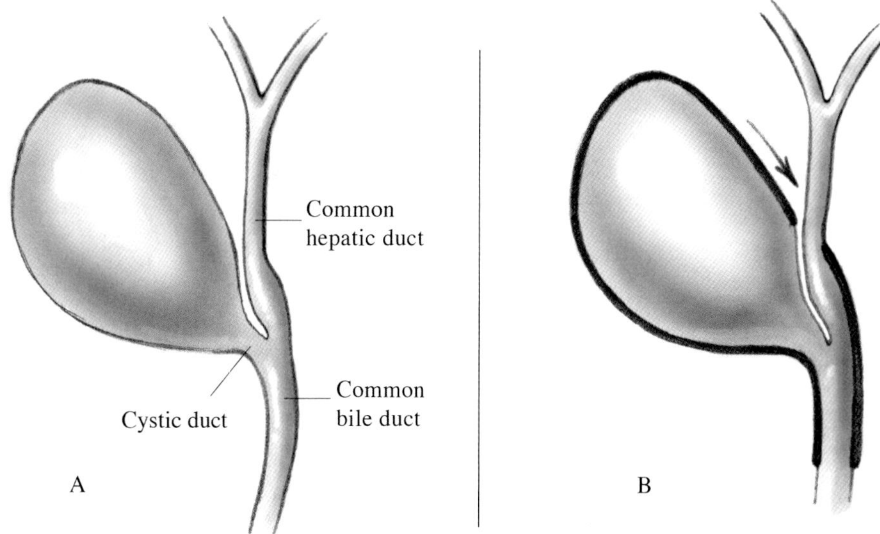

Fig. 34-7. The cause of bile duct injury in "top-down" cholecystectomy in the face of severe inflammation with obliteration of the triangle of Calot, which draws the side of the common hepatic duct to the side of the gallbladder. **A.** Real anatomical situation. **B.** Apparent anatomical situation is shown by heavy line. The surgeon sees the anatomy bounded by the heavy line as the gallbladder and the cystic duct, and as the gallbladder is excised top-down (arrow) the common hepatic duct is transected. Vascular injuries are also common with this mechanism of injury.

In addition, it has been recognized since the earliest days of laparoscopic cholecystectomy that the direction of traction of the gallbladder may contribute to the mistaken conclusion that the common bile duct is the cystic duct, and that this may lead to the misidentification injury. When the Hartmann pouch is pulled superiorly rather than laterally, the cystic and common bile ducts appear to be a single continuous structure (Fig. 34-8).

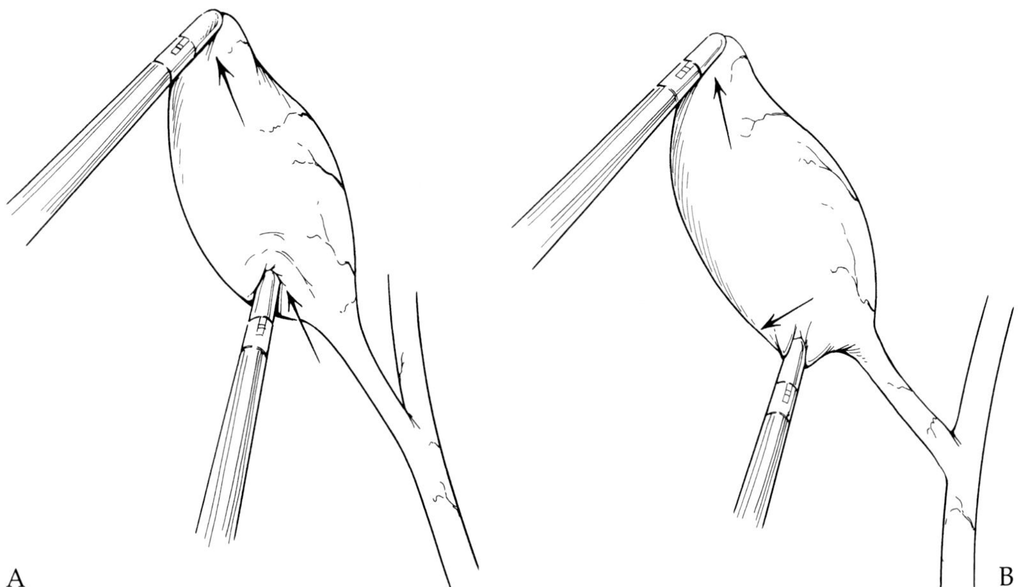

Fig. 34-8. The effect of the direction of traction on the appearance of the bile ducts. **A.** Both graspers pulling superiorly bring the common and cystic ducts into alignment, giving the appearance of a single duct. **B.** When the grasper on the Hartmann pouch is pulling laterally to the right, the cystic and common ducts appear as separate structures and the common bile duct is less likely to be mistaken for the cystic duct and injured. (From *Surgery of the Liver and Biliary Tract 2/E*;CD-ROM. Eds. LH Blumgart and Y Fong. Churchill Livingston.)

Technical Problems

Injury to a Bile Duct in the Course of Dissection

Bile ducts may be injured in the course of dissection much in the same way that an enterotomy occurs in the course of dissecting adhesions. Inflammation, aberrant anatomy, small duct size, and large body habitus contribute to the likelihood of this occurrence. As noted above this mechanism of injury has been responsible for severe injuries when the top-down method of cholecystectomy has been used. However, it may occur in the course of dissection irrespective of the method of identification. One variant of this type of injury is damage to a bile duct deep to the gallbladder bed when freeing the gallbladder from its attachment to the liver. This occurs most often when inflammation obscures or obliterates the plane between the gallbladder and the cystic plate or when visibility is hampered as in the case of an intrahepatic gallbladder. As noted above, about 10% of patients have a sizable hepatic duct that lies immediately deep to the cystic plate and is therefore prone to injury.

Failure to Obtain Secure Closure of the Cystic Duct

The cystic duct is normally occluded with metallic clips. These are not as reliable as ligatures or suture ligatures, which were the standard methods of cystic duct closure during open cholecystectomy. When the duct is thick, rigid, or wide, clips may fail. Thus, their use should usually be avoided under these circumstances. Retained common duct stones may contribute to clip failure by raising bile duct pressure. Clips may also cross or "scissor" during application, resulting in poor closure or be loosened by subsequent dissection.

Thermal Injuries

Thermal injuries (Fig. 34-9) are more likely to occur in the presence of severe inflammation, because hemorrhage is more common when dissecting in the face of acute inflammation, and higher power settings may be used to control hemorrhage. The result of application of diathermy to bile ducts is thermal necrosis. These injuries are often not recognized at surgery and usually result in bile duct stenosis rather than loss of continuity. Division of adhesions with cautery may lead to bowel or bile duct injury if the adhesion is connected to these structures by a narrow isthmus along which all the electrical energy must pass. The reader is referred to earlier chapters in this text that discuss dangers and avoidance of thermal injury in laparoscopic surgery.

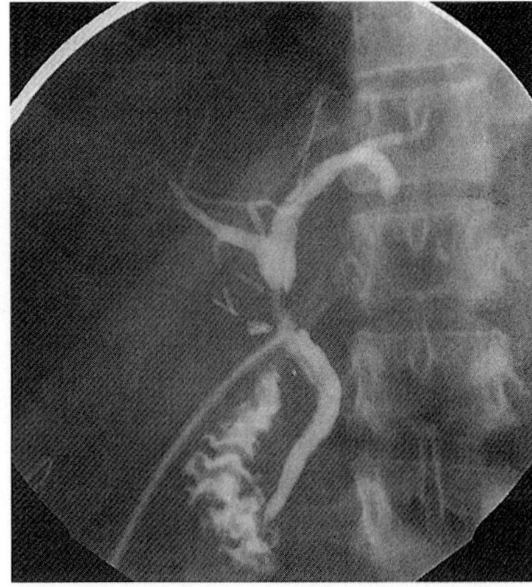

Fig. 34-9. T-tube cholangiogram in a patient 2 months after a thermal injury. The common hepatic duct (arrow) appears shrink-wrapped over the T-tube. At the time of reconstruction the common hepatic duct was replaced by scar. (By permission of the *Journal of the American College of Surgeons.*)

Tenting Injuries

The junction of the common bile duct and hepatic bile ducts may be occluded when clipping the cystic duct and pulling up forcefully on the gallbladder at the same time. This is a very uncommon laparoscopic injury, perhaps due to the magnification afforded by laparoscopy.

SURGEON- OR HOSPITAL-RELATED FACTORS

Learning Curve Effect

Inexperience with laparoscopic cholecystectomy was a well documented cause of bile duct injuries in the 1990s. The likelihood of biliary injury was much greater during the early experience of a surgeon than subsequently. Cholecystectomy during an attack of acute cholecystitis is a more difficult and less commonly performed operation than elective cholecystectomy. It is possible that inexperience in the procedure during acute cholecystitis is still contributing to injury. Possibly residents do not obtain sufficient training with this procedure prior to entering practice.

Another area of increasing concern is the lack of experience with open cholecystectomy, especially difficult open cholecystectomy. Recently we have observed a sharp increase in injuries that occurred after conversion to open cholecystectomy. Many of these injuries have been severe, involving major vascular structures as well as bile ducts, and have occurred in the hands of surgeons who have performed hundreds of laparoscopic cholecystectomies. In most residency programs today almost all open cholecystectomies are performed on normal gallbladders as part of another procedure, such as a liver resection or pancreatoduodenectomy. The experience gained in this way may not be sufficient for the surgeon to become adept at open cholecystectomy when the gallbladder is inflamed. The lack of experience with difficult open cholecystectomy may also be due in part to the almost universal acceptance of laparoscopic cholecystectomy by patients. We have previously documented that 15% to 20% of patients refused elective open cholecystectomy, whereas almost no patient refuses laparoscopic cholecystectomy. Therefore, the trend is to have fewer opportunities to treat patients who have put off treatment until they have had multiple attacks of pain and have more severely inflamed gallbladders.

The Psychology of Human Error

First Hugh and then Way et al. have emphasized certain traits of human behavior described by Reason that cause or contribute to biliary injury. Some of the key points made in their analysis are that surgery is a complex task, that visual disorientation will occur occasionally under such complex conditions, and that persistence in error due to the deadly mind-set error is a common human failing. The mind-set error is the tendency to interpret information incorrectly after one has first made a decision. For instance if one were to be convinced that the common bile duct was the cystic duct one would tend to interpret the right hepatic artery as being the cystic artery even if *in retrospect* good judgment would have questioned its identity based on a factor such as size or position. The point of departure of the author with this view is that visual disorientation is more likely to occur with certain methods of procedure and can be greatly diminished with the use of routine cholangiography or the critical view technique of identification.

Equipment-Related Injury

Laparoscopic equipment must be regularly maintained. Focal loss of insulation on cautery instruments can result in arcing and thermal injuries to bile ducts or bowel.

Avoidance of Biliary Injuries

Biliary injuries are best avoided by understanding the mechanism of injuries and adopting methods that circumvent these mechanisms. Biliary injuries cannot be completely eliminated. They may occur in the hands of highly skilled surgeons when operative conditions are difficult.

GENERAL

Only surgeons trained and proctored in laparoscopic cholecystectomy should perform the procedure. Because laparoscopic cholecystectomy for acute cholecystitis is more difficult and associated with a higher incidence of biliary injury, it should not be attempted until experience is gained. Special note should be taken of conditions that make surgery during acute cholecystitis particularly difficult and consideration given to percutaneous cholecystostomy as a temporizing measure. When inflammation is severe and mandates conversion to the open procedure, it may be unusually difficult, especially for the surgeon inexperienced in difficult open cholecystectomy. Cholecystostomy or partial cholecystectomy with occlusion of the cystic duct using a purse-string suture placed from the interior of the gallbladder as described by Bornman are excellent options under these conditions if structures cannot be displayed in the triangle of Calot. Cholelithiasis is a benign disease that in many cases is cured simply by stone extraction. Cholecystectomy at a later time may be necessary but local conditions will often be improved. Therefore, the surgeon should hesitate before entering a zone of danger during this procedure. Nonetheless, the decision to proceed is one of surgical judgment and depends upon local factors and experience. If factors associated with increased difficulty can be anticipated, then securing additional assistance in the operating room is helpful.

Misidentification Injuries

Although still in widespread use the author believes that the infundibular technique *ought to be discarded* as a sole means of ductal identification. It is an error trap in that it works well in most circumstances and seems to be very reliable, but it is actually prone to fail under particular circumstances, which are occasionally present in patients requiring cholecystectomy. Under these conditions the surgeon may carry out the technique correctly and will have achieved positive or "conclusive" (meaning convincing in this case) identification by the tenets of the technique (i.e., a funnel will be circumferentially displayed), yet the common bile duct will be mistaken for the cystic duct. Similarly, dissection of the cystic duct down to the union with the major bile ducts ought to be discouraged as a routine method of ductal identification for the reasons stated above. The author favors identification of biliary anatomy using the "critical view of safety" technique, because this method is good at identifying the cystic duct even when aberrant ducts are present. If this method is not used, the routine use of cholangiography is recommended.

Technical Problems

Injury to a Bile Duct in the Course of Dissection

Avoidance depends on the principles of careful dissection and experience, as well as recognition of circumstances in which the potential hazard in continued dissection may outweigh the benefit of completing a cholecystectomy as outlined above. Also the author recommends not using the "top-down" technique in the face of severe inflammation in either open or laparoscopic surgery. To prevent injuring an intrahepatic duct just deep to the cystic plate, one must attempt not to dissect deep to the plate when elevating the gallbladder off its bed. Use of the spatula dissector combined with irrigation to keep the field clear of blood may help. Cautery scissors are also useful, but there is no substitute for patience, gentle technique, and experience in this dissection.

Failure to Obtain Secure Closure of the Cystic Duct

Tips of clips should be noted to project beyond the cystic duct and to be free of any extraneous material. Clips should not be manipulated in the subsequent dissection. Preformed ligature loops should be used for closure of the cystic duct if the cystic duct is thick, rigid, or wide. Two loops should be applied on the side of the cystic duct to be retained. The application of additional clips is not advisable and may, in fact, lead to tenting injury. Locking clips and laparoscopic staplers may also be used provided that there is enough length on the cystic duct for their application.

Thermal Injuries

Cautery should be used with great care in the porta hepatis. The surgeon must be sure that low cautery settings are used, that only small 1 to 2 mm pieces of tissue are divided at one time, and that the coagulating surfaces of instruments are not contacting adjacent tissues. Low cautery settings are essential, characteristically 30 watts or less. Higher settings may lead to arcing of current to ducts. The cystic duct should not be divided by diathermy as this can lead to thermal necrosis of the cystic duct stump or adjacent bile duct. Attempting to stop hemorrhage by *blind* application of cautery, clamps, or clips is very unwise. Brisk bleeding requires conversion. Adhesions should be divided sharply or with minimum application of power. Active electrode monitoring may be helpful in avoiding this type of injury but is currently not in wide use.

Tenting Injuries

This sort of injury is avoided by not lifting the gallbladder forcefully when applying clips to the cystic duct. It is recommended that the surgeon sees that a length of cystic duct will remain below the clip closest to the common bile duct end of the cystic duct before applying that clip.

PRESENTATION AND INVESTIGATION

About one-third of the more serious injuries are diagnosed during surgery. Most of the rest are identified in the first 30 days after surgery, but a few may appear years after laparoscopic cholecystectomy. Intraoperative diagnosis may be made by cholangiography, by observation of bile in the field, or more rarely by seeing the lacerated or divided duct. Sometimes the diagnosis is made after conversion for bleeding or inability to proceed in a difficult dissection.

Postoperative presentations are influenced by the type of injury and whether a drain has been left. The commonest presentations are pain and sepsis with or without jaundice, jaundice without other symptoms, or biliary fistula. Some patients present only with distension and malaise. The latter is usually due to bile ascites. It is a particularly insidious presentation as it may lead to delay in diagnosis

Pain/Sepsis

CT scan is performed first to identify fluid collections, which may then be aspirated to determine if they are bilious. Usually a drain is placed in the biloma, and an ERCP follows. MRI with Magnetic

Resonance cholangiography (MRC) has the potential to replace CT scan plus ERCP with a single study. However MRC does not detect collapsed ducts well and is more likely to be useful when there is obstruction of the biliary tree than perforation with free drainage of bile into the peritoneal cavity. Many patients presenting with pain/sepsis without jaundice have Type A or D injuries, and definitive treatment is possible at the time of endoscopy.

Jaundice

Jaundice is usually indicative of the more severe Type E injuries. If jaundice is the only symptom, duct occlusion alone, for example by clips, is most likely. Conversely, transections are often accompanied by pain and sepsis due to accumulation of bile in the peritoneal cavity; this is especially true if the injury is several days old. In either case ERCP is the first-line investigation. The duct may be found to be partially or completely occluded, with clips often seen at the point at which the dye column stops (Fig. 34-10), or transected, with loss of continuity to the upper biliary tract. If the ducts are only partially occluded, the entire extent of injury may be diagnosed by ERCP. Next, a CT scan is performed. *In patients with complete occlusion of the bile duct(s)* the bile ducts will be dilated and no biloma will be seen. Percutaneous transhepatic cholangiography (PTC) is performed next to delineate the proximal ducts and to provide external drainage of bile. *In patients with transection of bile duct without occlusion* the ducts will be decompressed and a biloma or bile ascites is usually present. Our approach for such patients is to drain the biloma and wait for several weeks to perform the PTC. During this time the biloma cavity will contract around the drain. Then retrograde injection through the drain will display the biliary tree. This facilitates PTC when ducts are decompressed. This technique of displaying the ducts from below to facilitate PTC is not feasible until the biloma cavity has contracted.

Bile Fistula

The first-line investigation is a fistulogram. Subsequent management depends upon anatomical findings.

Other Symptoms

Occasionally patients with bile ascites may complain only of vague symptoms such as malaise, constipation, or distension.

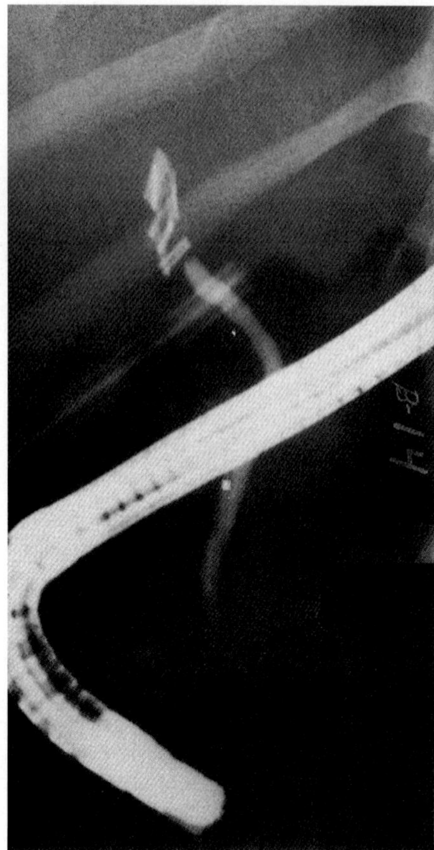

Fig. 34-10. Postoperative ERCP in a patient who was noted to have bile in the operative field at the time of surgery. The surgeon placed a drain in the right upper quadrant and referred the patient for further management. Note the complete occlusion of the bile duct and the position of clips at the top of the column of dye. (From *Surgery of the Liver and Biliary Tract 2E* CD-ROM. Eds. LH Blumgart and Y Fong. Churchill Livingston.)

This is because hepatic bile is relatively nonirritating. Hematobilia due to an arterial pseudoaneurysm is a rare but very dangerous presentation.

All patients with biliary injuries other than Type A injuries should be considered to potentially have a concomitant vascular injury. As previously noted injury to the right hepatic artery is the most common vascular injury, but any vessel in the porta hepatis may be injured. Therefore it is becoming common to routinely perform an investigation to evaluate the hepatic arteries and portal vein as part of the investigation of these injuries. Usually this is done by MRI or CT scan, and arteriography is reserved for cases in which the results of these investigations are unclear. Some have advocated MRI as the best first investigation of a biliary injury because it can show bile ducts, blood vessels, and fluid collections in a single investigation. There is theoretical merit in this argument, but in our experience MRI often lacks the detail required to make detailed plans regarding reconstruction.

Management of Biliary Injuries

MANAGEMENT OF INJURIES RECOGNIZED DURING THE INITIAL OPERATION

There is little written about the conduct of a laparoscopic cholecystectomy once a biliary injury is suspected. The following is based on the author's experience with referred biliary injuries. It is also predicated on highly suggestive evidence that repair of difficult biliary injuries often fail when performed by surgical teams infrequently engaged in upper biliary tree surgery.

Intraoperative recognition of biliary injury is usually an indication for conversion. The following two guidelines are suggested when laparotomy is undertaken for suspected injury: (1) repair should be attempted only if the techniques of dissection or reconstruction required for repair are commonly used by the operating team, and (2) the injury should not be worsened by dissection solely for the purpose of making an exact diagnosis. When appropriate expertise is not available, closed suction drains should be placed in the right upper quadrant laparoscopically and the patient referred.

Type A injuries, recognized at the time of surgery, are repaired by suture of the cystic duct and drainage. If the anatomy has been clearly demonstrated through dissection or cholangiography, laparoscopic repair by ligature loop or suture is sometimes possible. Type D injuries are repaired by closure of the defect using fine absorbable sutures over a T-tube and placement of a closed suction drain, in the vicinity of the repair. This usually requires conversion to an open procedure. Nonabsorbable sutures are contraindicated as they form a nidus for stone formation. The T-tube should exit through a separate incision in the duct, if possible. Avulsion of the cystic duct, a variant of Type D injury, may be similarly managed. When the Type D injury is thermal in origin or when the injury involves more than 50% of the circumference of the duct, the preferred treatment is Roux-en-Y hepaticojejunostomy, applying the principles of anastomosis given below. Type E injuries recognized intraoperatively should be repaired by hepaticojejunostomy. Choledochocholedochotomy should be avoided because of considerations of blood supply and tension. Choledochoduodenostomy has the theoretical disadvantage of tension on the anastomosis, as does a loop hepaticojejunostomy.

MANAGEMENT OF BILIARY INJURIES DIAGNOSED POSTOPERATIVELY

The approach depends on type of injury, type of initial management and its result, and time elapsed since the initial operation or repair.

Type A Injuries

The treatment is endoscopic sphincterotomy with placement of a stent or a nasobiliary catheter. Intraperitoneal bile collections may require percutaneous drainage. Operative repair is rarely needed.

Type B Injuries

Type B injuries may remain asymptomatic or present after many years with right upper quadrant discomfort, attacks of pain, or cholangitis. Symptomatic patients require hepaticojejunostomy or hepatic resection if biliary-enteric anastomosis is not possible. In asymptomatic patients, treatment is not recommended when the volume of liver affected is small or if the injury was remote and the isolated portion has atrophied. When the injury is recent and the section of liver is large (such as the whole right liver), repair is empirically recommended.

Type C Injuries

Type C injuries require drainage of the bile collections and biliary-enteric anastomosis, hepatic resection, or ligation of the duct. If the duct is tiny (<1 mm), then resection of the affected segment(s) or ligation is preferable because attempts to repair such ducts may result in strictures. Insertion of a transhepatic catheter prior to duct reconstruction is a useful aid. It also may be used to control bile drainage and to drain the subhepatic bile collection preoperatively.

Type D Injuries

Treatment by endoscopic sphincterotomy and stent is the treatment of choice in the postoperative period. When operation is required, the technique of repair is the same as when the problem is discovered at time of initial surgery unless the injury is thermal, in which case hepaticojejunostomy is probably the better choice.

Type E injuries

The best chance for lasting repair is the initial repair. Strictures and sometimes clip occlusions may be treated initially by dilation and stents placed by ERCP. In our experience nonsurgical therapy is most likely to be successful when the strictures are mild, appear months to years after surgery, or are of short length. Lillimoe reported 64% success rate with interventional techniques. The failures tended to occur when E3 or E4 lesions were treated, when a fistula was present, or when a stricture occurred shortly after a hepaticojejunostomy had been done. Nonsurgical therapy is most likely to be successful in cases in which operative repair is rather easy and nonsurgical treatment often requires multiple endoscopic procedures. The age and health of the patient as well as the likelihood of good long-term outcome should be considered when choosing therapy for a stricture. Operation is required for failure of stent therapy and when there is ductal discontinuity.

TIMING OF SURGERY

Factors favoring immediate repair are early referral, stable patient, lack of right upper quadrant bile collections, and simpler injuries that can be rapidly diagnosed and are unlikely to involve vascular injury. Many patients are referred between 1 to 6 weeks after the primary operation, when local inflammation may be expected to be great. In these patients percutaneous tubes are inserted to relieve obstruction from affected segments, to drain subhepatic collections, and to control sepsis. Repair is performed when inflammation has settled, usually about 3 months after the last operation. This delayed approach is sometimes used even when the patient is referred within the first week, especially in complex injuries and those in which either a thermal etiology or concomitant ischemic injury is suspected. Immediate repair may also be undertaken when the injury is diagnosed months after surgery, for instance after failure of stenting of a stenosis or the late failure of a biliary-enteric anastomosis.

PREOPERATIVE PLANNING

The complete extent of an injury must be diagnosed preoperatively; failure to do so may result in exclusion of bile ducts from the repair. The percutaneous transhepatic tubes placed to assure biliary drainage from all liver segments also serve as guides

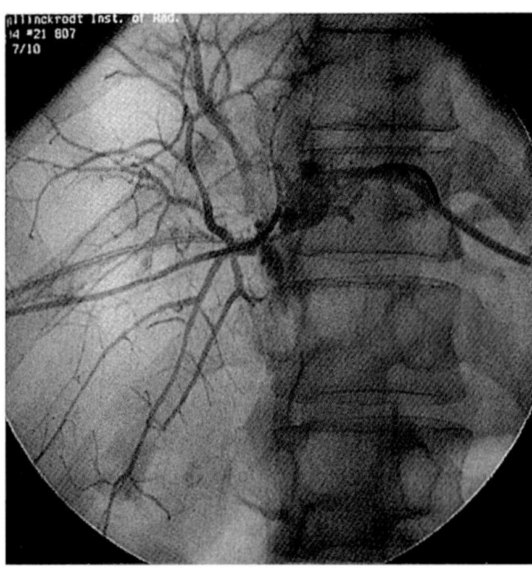

Fig. 34-11. An E4 injury in which there were three separately transected ducts: the left hepatic duct, the right anterior duct, and the posterior duct. Preoperative placement of percutaneous transhepatic tubes facilitated identification of anatomy at surgery. (From *Surgery of the Liver and Biliary Tract* 2E CD-ROM. Eds LH Blumgart and Y Fong. Churchill Livingston.)

to the position of the injured ducts at surgery (Fig. 34-11). Our policy is to perform conciliation between CT and PTC studies to be sure that all ducts in the liver are accounted for.

The guiding principles for repair are that the anastomosis must be tension-free, with good blood supply, mucosa-to-mucosa contact, and of adequate calibre. Most experts in this field recommend hepaticojejunostomy in preference to either choledochocholedochotomy or choledochoduodenostomy, as a tension-free anastomosis is always possible with hepaticojejunostomy. Whenever possible, we prefer to construct side-to-side anastomoses to avoid dissection behind bile ducts, which may affect their blood supply. Often the anastomosis is done to the extrahepatic portion of the left hepatic duct after it is lowered by dividing the hepatic plate (the Hepp-Couinaud approach). This approach is particularly suitable for injuries at or just below the bifurcation (Types E2 and E3). Right ducts do not lend themselves to this approach as well, as they have a short extrahepatic length. Sometimes the end of the right duct is used. We have described an approach to isolated right hepatic duct injuries (Fig. 34-12, page 340). Dissection of the left duct provides a guide to the coronal plane in which the intrahepatic right hepatic ducts will be found, and these may be exposed by removing liver tissue. Exposure is also facilitated by dividing the bridge of tissue between segments 3 and 4,

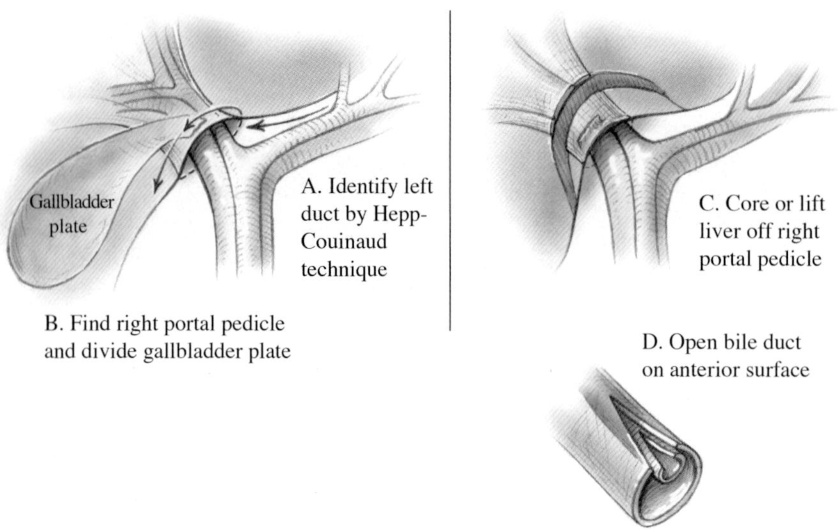
Gallbladder plate
A. Identify left duct by Hepp-Couinaud technique
B. Find right portal pedicle and divide gallbladder plate
C. Core or lift liver off right portal pedicle
D. Open bile duct on anterior surface

Fig. 34-12. A technique for identifying isolated right ducts. **A.** Step 1: Finding and dividing cystic plate to expose right pedicle. **B.** Step 2: Elevating liver off right portal pedicle, identifying, and incising right duct.

by fully opening the gallbladder fossa, which often collapses with adherence of its walls. If these maneuvers are not sufficient, resecting part of segment 4b and/or 5 will open the upper porta hepatis as described by Mercado.

The use of anastomotic stents is controversial. There is no evidence that they are helpful if a large calibre mucosa-to-mucosa anastomosis has been achieved. We use them when very small ducts have been anastomosed. In cases in which a primary repair has failed, it is not always necessary to perform a fresh hepaticojejunostomy. Stenting can sometimes be successful if the strictures are short. Readers interested in a more detailed discussion of the subject are referred to the author's chapter in the companion text *Mastery of Surgery*.

Occasionally biliary reconstruction is not possible or advisable. When ductal reconstruction to a part of the liver is impossible, then resection should be performed. Occasionally failure of reconstruction leads to secondary biliary cirrhosis and end-stage liver failure, at which point liver transplantation is required. In almost all examples of this outcome, high reconstructions have been attempted by surgeons lacking experience in these difficult procedures or there has been a combined biliary/vascular injury. Treatment of failed repairs with metallic stents gives very poor results in the long term, with 50% of treated patient suffering from repeated cholangitis. Re-repair at specialist centers is far more successful than metallic stenting.

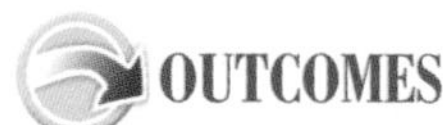

OUTCOMES

Most surgical series of biliary reconstruction cite very good short-term results. However, it is well established from older literature describing ductal injury during open cholecystectomy that there is a progressive re-stenosis rate. Two-thirds of recurrences are diagnosed in the first 2 years after repair, but re-stenosis has been described after 10 years. The re-stenosis rate varies from 5% to 28%. There is a recent indication that the results in the laparoscopic era may not be as good as these rates, perhaps because of increased severity of injury.

Comparison among surgical series is not easily done because of lack of standard reporting and the effect of differences in the severity of injuries treated in different series. Injuries above the bifurcation involving several bile ducts have a worse prognosis than injuries of the common hepatic duct, and the proportion of severe injuries in a series will affect outcome. Reporting of treatment failure is not uniform. Length of follow-up is another obvious variable affecting outcome and is not uniform among series. Several authors have reported that both quality of life and life span are adversely affected by a biliary injury.

SUGGESTED READING

Callery, MP. Avoiding biliary injury during laparoscopic cholecystectomy: technical considerations. *Surg Endosc* 2006;20:1654–1658.

Connor, S. Garden, OJ. Bile duct injury in the era of laparoscopic cholecystectomy. *Brit J Surg* 2006;93:158–168.

Fletcher DR, Hobbs MS, Tan P, et al. Complications of cholecystectomy: risks of the laparoscopic approach and protective effects of operative cholangiography: a population-based study. *Ann Surg* 1999;229(4):449–457.

Strasberg SM, Eagon CJ, Drebin JA. The "hidden cystic duct" syndrome and the infundibular technique of laparoscopic cholecystectomy—the danger of the false infundibulum. *J Am Coll Surg* 2000;191:6617.

Strasberg SM, Hertl M, Soper NJ. An analysis of the problem of biliary injury during laparoscopic cholecystectomy. *J Am Coll Surg* 1995; 180:101–125.

Strasberg. Reconstruction of the Bile Duct: Anatomic Principles and Surgical Techniques. In: *Mastery of Surgery 5th Edition*. Josef E. Fischer, Ed.

COMMENTARY

Dr. Strasberg describes the primary causes of bile duct injury during laparoscopic cholecystectomy, classifies those injuries, discusses methods to diminish the occurrence of such injuries, and details the means by which these injuries should be repaired. Bile duct injury is the Achilles' heel of laparoscopic cholecystectomy. The incidence of such injuries appears to be three to five times greater than that during open cholecystectomy, with the incidence only decreasing slightly over the last decade. The main message of this chapter is not how to treat biliary injuries, but how to prevent them. I consider this chapter to be a "must read" for all surgeons who perform laparoscopic cholecystectomy.

Several limitations of the laparoscopic technique must be overcome to minimize ductal injuries. First, as exposure of the porta hepatis is gained by cephalad retraction applied to the gallbladder, there is a natural tendency to pull the gallbladder vertically and align the cystic duct with the common bile duct, thereby giving the mistaken impression that the common bile duct is a continuation of the cystic duct. This optical illusion is likely the primary cause of most major bile duct injuries and can be minimized by lateral traction on the neck of the gallbladder, thereby exaggerating the angle between the cystic duct and the common bile duct. Second, two-dimensional visualization renders spatial discrimination difficult; the surgeon must therefore view the anatomy from all sides by moving the infundibulum back and forth and assessing its appearance from both the dorsal and ventral aspects of the hepatocystic triangle. The use of an angled laparoscope, which allows multiple viewing angles of the operative field, also enhances the surgeon's ability to determine the three-dimensional relationships of the regional anatomy. Third, monopolar electrocautery generally is used to obtain hemostasis and to dissect the gallbladder from its bed. When used injudiciously, cautery can injure the common bile duct and thus should only be used at a low wattage in short bursts. Alternatively, too deep a plane of dissection in the gallbladder bed may occur, unroofing peripheral bile ducts and leading to postoperative bile leakage that may be ascribed to the so-called ducts of Luschka. Fourth, the cystic duct usually is occluded by clips that may have been improperly applied or that control the duct inadequately; surgeons must be prepared to ligate the duct, usually with an endoloop, in the presence of a large friable cystic duct.

Cholangiography has been hailed by some authors as the primary means to prevent biliary injuries. However, misidentification of ducts prior to inserting the cholangiocatheter can result in injury, and bile duct injuries have been known to occur following cholangiography. Several large-scale population studies have demonstrated that routine application of cholangiography likely does decrease the global incidence of bile duct injury. It is most likely true that performance of cholangiography with correct interpretation of the resulting films may limit the extent of bile duct injury if the common bile duct has been misidentified for the cystic duct. It is therefore wise to obtain cholangiograms liberally and certainly to perform them if there is any doubt of the anatomy. However, the primary means of preventing bile duct injuries, in my view, is meticulous dissection of the neck of the gallbladder and attaining the "critical view of safety," in every case.

The laparoscopic surgeon also must have a "game plan" in mind should a laparoscopic bile duct injury occur. The acute management of these patients largely depends on the experience of the surgeon in performing complex biliary procedures. Except for minor injuries (Types A and D), most such injuries should probably be referred to centers with large experience in proximal biliary operations. If a surgeon is not experienced in these procedures, the best management plan is probably to place an active drainage catheter in the right upper quadrant and immediately transfer the patient to a tertiary care center.

Using the principles outlined by Dr. Strasberg for preventing bile duct injury, laparoscopic cholecystectomy should be able to be performed safely in virtually all patients. This should allow the operation to maintain its true position as a major advance in the treatment of cholelithiasis.

NJS

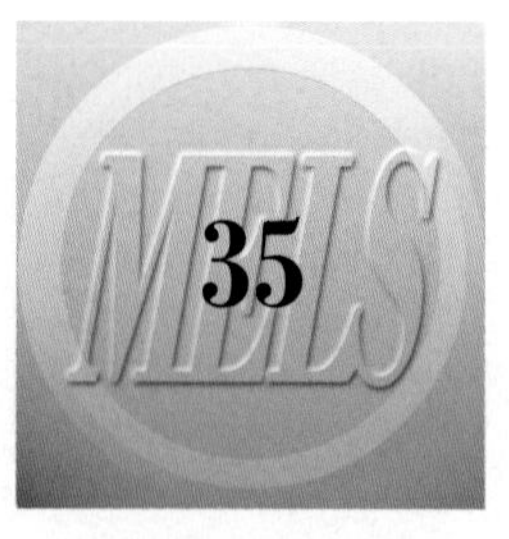

Nonresective Treatment of Liver Tumors

PAUL D. HANSEN AND DONALD BLAIR

INTRODUCTION

There is a wide variety of both benign and malignant tumors that develop in the liver. The most common benign tumors—hemangiomas, focal nodular hyperplasia (FNH), adenomas, and cysts—are generally asymptomatic. Identification of these asymptomatic hepatic lesions is increasing as the use of diagnostic imaging becomes more common in Western countries. While asymptomatic benign tumors rarely require any form of surgical management, they may require intervention if they begin to enlarge over time or become symptomatic. Potential treatments include endovascular techniques, local ablative techniques, or resection using minimally invasive or open surgical techniques. The goal of intervention is eliminating the symptom or halting growth using the least invasive procedure possible.

Malignant lesions are common in the liver. Metastatic breast, lung, and nonhepatic gastrointestinal cancers are the most common tumors; primary hepatic malignancies make up less than 10% of malignant tumors identified at autopsy. The treatment for malignant liver lesions depends on the specifics of the cancer and the presenting scenario. While the underlying goal is cure, this is seldom possible. In fact, less than 20% of patients who present to a surgeon with a primary or secondary hepatic malignancy will be candidates for curative surgical intervention.

Historically, open surgical resection offered the only hope of cure. Open resections, however, have a well-described and significant morbidity (30% to 50%) and mortality (0% to 10%) profile. Nonresectional interventions for the management of liver tumors are not a new concept but have been less common due to limitations in the technology. There has been a sharp upturn in the emphasis on utilizing less invasive techniques during the last decade, in part due to the introduction of laparoscopy into mainstream surgery. The clear and absolute benefit of using less invasive techniques has caught the attention of patient and surgeon alike.

A number of ablative techniques has been introduced over the years. One of the first described was ethanol injection. Injection of a small volume of ethanol was shown to generate long-term survival in patients with selected tumors such as small hepatocellular cancers, thus verifying the concept. Subsequently, technologies using thermal energy such as cryotherapy or radiofrequency ablation (RFA) were developed. The ultimate ability of an ablation to deliver a curative treatment in other tumor types is currently unknown and a topic of much debate.

Palliation can also be a goal of liver tumor treatment. Tumor debulking, for instance, may be quite helpful in patients with hormone-producing neuroendocrine tumors. Some patients will develop an acute worsening of their liver function with hepatocellular carcinoma (HCC) progression in the setting of cirrhosis. Tumor debulking with chemoembolization or yttrium^{90} infusions may allow liver function to return to baseline and the patient to be palliated for several months.

Each of the techniques and technologies discussed below has its strengths and weaknesses. There are nuances to every particular clinical situation, which may suggest a patient is better treated with one method rather than another. Additionally, factors such as local clinical expertise may play a role in treatment selection. An algorithm of nonresectional methods of treating the most common liver tumors is also provided.

Nonresectional Technologies

ENDOVASCULAR TECHNIQUES

Endovascular techniques are typically utilized to treat unresectable cancers, but they also have a role in managing some forms of benign disease. They may be used as the sole treatment or as a means of down-staging before a planned surgical intervention. Endovascular techniques are typically performed via the hepatic artery. The key to the technique is the fact that the normal liver parenchyma receives the majority of its blood supply from the portal vein, whereas liver malignancies derive nearly all their blood supply from the hepatic artery. Therefore, therapeutic agents delivered via the hepatic artery concentrate within the tumors and spare much of the normal parenchyma.

The therapeutic agent instilled is designed to have a tumoricidal effect only at the concentration achieved within the tumor. The lower concentration obtained within the normal liver parenchyma is minimally toxic to normal hepatocytes. The delivery points for these therapies have evolved from an earlier whole-liver approach to a lobar approach and then more recently, to a segmental and if possible a sub-segmental approach. This latter approach has been particularly important in hepatocellular carcinoma, where the patients typically have underlying liver disease. By delivering the therapeutic agent in a highly selective fashion, the amount of normal parenchyma exposed to the toxic agent is reduced.

The earliest form of embolization was bland embolization. This entails installation of particles or gel film to achieve flow stasis within the target vessel, resulting in tissue ischemia and infarction of the tumor. Its effect however, is limited by the recruitment of blood flow from the portal vein. Chemoembolization involves coupling an embolic agent with a chemotherapeutic agent. This technique has several theoretical mechanisms of action. The direct delivery of the chemotherapy to the tumor allows for increased concentration of chemotherapy in the target tissue. The ischemia induced by the embolic agent allows for prolonged contact between the chemotherapy and the tumor. The ischemia also induces a failure of transmembrane pumps within the tumor cells, causing decreased washout of chemotherapy and greater absorption of the chemotherapy.

Hepatic arterial infusion of yttrium^{90} is another therapeutic option. External beam radiation to the liver is not an option, as the maximum tolerable whole liver radiation dose is about 30 Gy and the required therapeutic dose to treat liver tumors is around 120 Gy. Yttrium^{90} infusion involves a focused transarterial delivery of microspheres impregnated with yttrium^{90} to hepatic tumors. Yttrium^{90} is a beta-emitter that deposits 90% of its energy within a 5.3-mm radius of the microsphere. While the total dose delivered may be equivalent to a 120-Gy whole-liver dose, it is focused within the tumor or the involved segments of the liver. This induces a tumoricidal effect, with minimal injury to the surrounding normal parenchyma.

The logistical setup for yttrium^{90} infusion is considerably more involved than chemoembolization, which has limited its widespread utilization. But the results are comparable to chemoembolization and yttrium^{90} infusion seems to be much better tolerated. Specifically, symptoms of fever, pain, and nausea and vomiting, which are common side effects of a chemoembolization, are seen much less frequently. And because yttrium^{90} infusion does not rely on an embolic effect, the arteries feeding the tumor are often preserved, allowing for the possibility of repeat therapy via the same hepatic artery (Fig. 35-1).

One of the newest technologies being investigated is the arterial infusion of drug-eluting beads (DEB). The beads used in this technique are embedded with high concentrations of chemotherapeutic agents. These agents are slowly released into the surrounding tissue after embolization. Early studies evaluating treatment by chemoembolization versus DEB have shown that there is a significant increase in drug concentration within the target tumor and decrease in systemic concentrations of the chemotherapeutic agents following therapy with DEB, leading to a greater local tumor effect with fewer side effects.

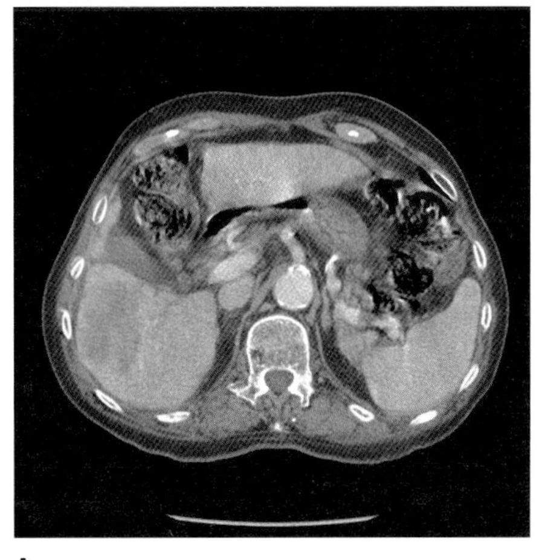

A

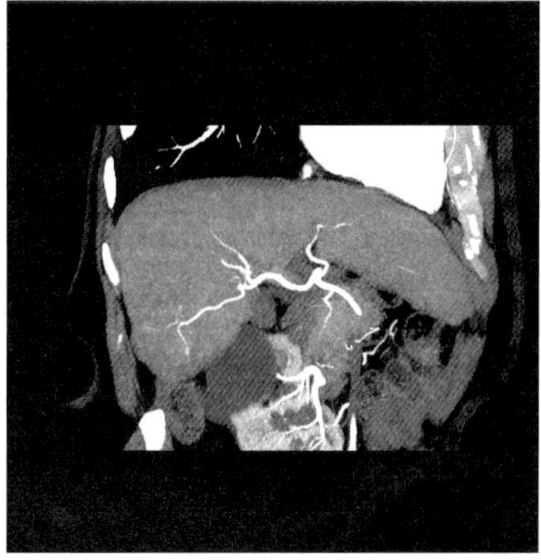

B

C

Fig. 35-1. Planning images for chemoembolization or yttrium^{90} treatment of an HCC. **A.** CT image of right-lobe HCC. **B.** CT angiogram demonstrating vascular supply of the HCC. **C.** Selective angiography of the HCC prior to the chemoembolization or yttrium^{90} infusion. HCC, hepatocellular carcinoma; CT, computed tomography.

Hepatic Arterial Infusion Pumps

Like other endovascular techniques, hepatic arterial infusion (HAI) pumps also work on the premise that malignancies derive the majority of their blood supply from the hepatic artery, while the normal hepatic parenchyma derives its supply from the portal vein. The principal agent infused via HAI pump is Floxuridine (FUDR), which is metabolized by the liver and results in a first-pass effect. The FUDR not absorbed by the tumor is metabolized by the liver, with only a small amount passing through to the systemic circulation. This allows the administration of a high concentration of drug to the hepatic artery with little in the way of systemic side effects.

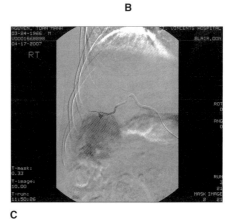

The hepatic arterial infusion of FUDR has been utilized since the 1980s, primarily for the treatment of isolated colorectal liver metastases. While most authors agree that this treatment reduces local hepatic progression of disease, it produces a limited increase in overall long-term survival. Additionally, there are a number of management issues and surgical complications that may arise, reducing the overall benefit to quality of life. Finally, several new systemic chemotherapeutic agents have come into use over the last few years that appear to induce similar rates of hepatic progression-free survival when compared to HAI. We currently utilize HAI when other forms of therapy have been exhausted and there is isolated progression of liver metastases.

ABLATION TECHNOLOGIES

The primary goal of any liver-directed tumor treatment is the eradication of 100% of the tumor cells. Any technology that can reliably achieve this end result might be considered an option for definitive treatment. There are several such technologies available today, most of which rely on chemical or thermal ablation of tissue. The advantages of these treatments are their repeatability, their general tolerability by the patient, and the possibility of local application with little destruction of surrounding tissue.

Ethanol Ablation

Injection of 95% ethanol into tumors was first described by Sugiura et al. in 1983: the injection of 0.5 cc of absolute ethanol could destroy 1 cc^3 of tissue. Ethanol is infiltrated throughout the target tissue and kills by inducing cytoplasmic dehydration, coagulative necrosis, and microvascular thrombosis. Injection of the tumor with ethanol can be performed percutaneously under ultrasound or computed tomography (CT) guidance or during open or laparoscopic surgical procedures with ultrasound guidance. The volume injected should be roughly similar to the volume of the tumor (spherical volume = $4/3\ \pi r^3$). Injection of small volumes is well tolerated, whereas the injection of volumes greater than 50 cc may be associated with hypotension and alcohol intoxication. Most authors suggest follow-up after ethanol injection with imaging looking for persistent viable tissue. Injections may be repeated as necessary to achieve complete ablation.

Successful tumor ablation depends on the diffuse infiltration of the ethanol throughout the tumor. While this may be possible in softer, more vascular tumors such as hepatocellular cancer and neuroendocrine tumors, it is not generally possible in harder, less vascular tumors such as metastatic adenocarcinoma. Tumor size is also a reliable predictor of treatment success. Tumors larger than 3 cm require large-volume infusions. Achieving the perfect distribution of ethanol, which would result in a 100% tumor cell kill, is more difficult and less reliable in larger tumors. Reinfusion, as many as six to eight times, may be necessary to achieve a successful treatment (Fig. 35-2).

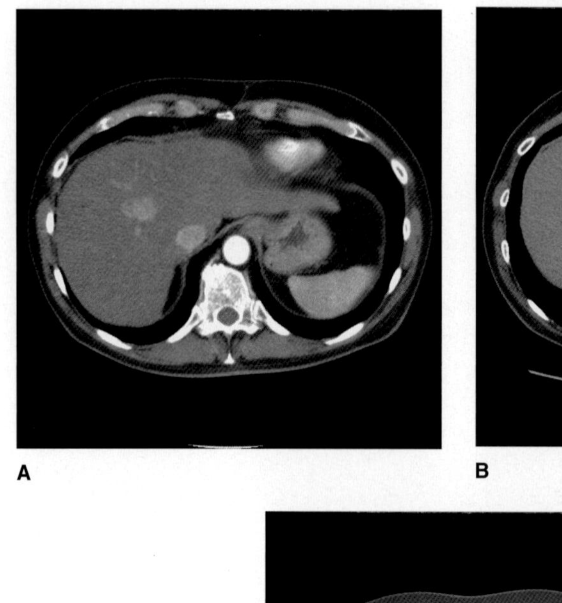
A

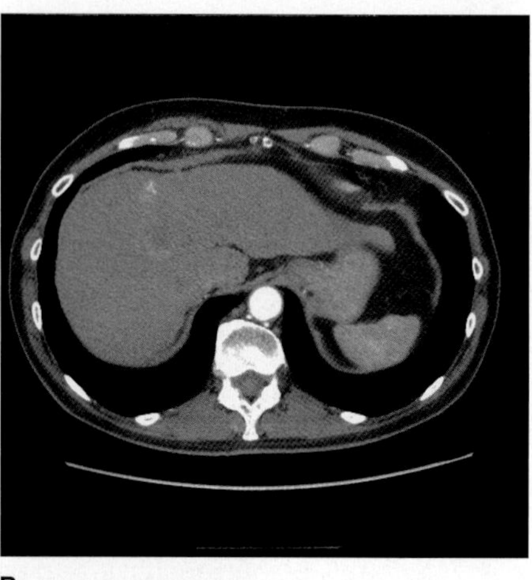
B

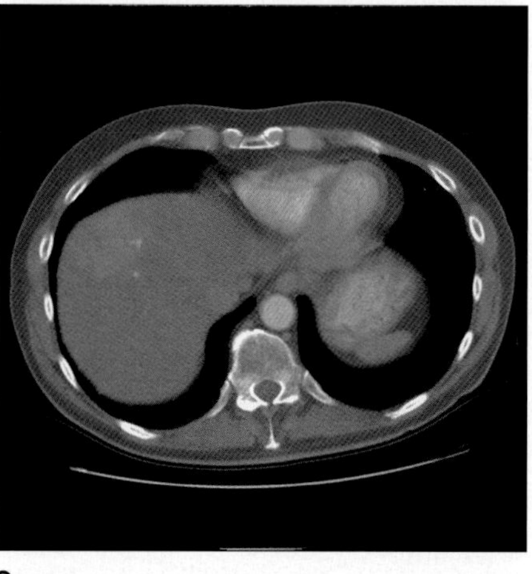
C

Fig. 35-2. Ethanol injection of an HCC. **A.** CT scan showing a hypervascular HCC. **B.** After the first laparoscopically guided injection of ethanol, a small posterior rim of viable hypervascular tissue remains. **C.** After a second injection of ethanol, the lesion is completely hypovascular. HCC, hepatocellular carcinoma; CT, computed tomography.

Radiofrequency Ablation

The radiofrequency ablation (RFA) of tissues has been utilized since the 1950s. Initial applications were for skin or bladder lesions, using a paddle to achieve a surface ablation. In the early 1990s, redesign of needle antennae and evaluation of bipolar techniques by McGann et al. led to technology capable of destroying much larger volumes of tissue.

Radiofrequency ablation uses electrical energy, with an alternating current at around 454,000 Hz. Ions within the surrounding tissue flip-flop their orientation with each change of current direction; this rapid ionic movement within the tissue results in frictional heating. Thorough heating of the target tissue depends on generation of an even and strong current density. If the tissue near the probe heats too quickly, dessication occurs, impedance rises, and no further or erratic tissue ablation occurs. Ablation technologies have overcome this problem by infusing saline into the surrounding tissues, cooling the probe tip with circulating saline, or integrating local tissue impedance into the control algorithm that drives the electrical generator. During the last few years, a series of technological redesigns has led to ablation devices and protocols that are far more reliable than the earlier models and destroy even larger volumes of tissue.

Factors that limit the ability of RFA to effectively destroy a target tumor include tumor size and composition, the tumor's relationship to surrounding vasculature, and the risk to surrounding vital structures. Co-opting a basic tenet of surgical resection, it is felt that successful tumor ablation requires destruction not only of the visible tumor but also a 1-cm margin of normal surrounding tissue. Thus, the destruction of a 3-cm tumor requires the creation of a 5-cm ablation lesion. It is widely reported in the literature that local ablation failure rates increase when the target tumor is larger than 3 cm and increase sharply with tumors larger than 4 cm.

Tumor type also plays an important role in ablation success. It was initially thought that hypervascular lesions would prove more difficult to ablate due to the cooling effect of the blood flow. In our experience, in fact, hypervascular tumors are generally easier to ablate. This is likely due to their higher ion content. Lower fluid content tumors, such as nonhepatic gastrointestinal metastases, have a lower ion content and tend to heat much more slowly.

Hypervascularity is a different issue from a tumor being adjacent to a large blood vessel. Blood vessels greater than 3 mm in diameter may not thrombose during RFA. The persistent blood flow will act to cool surrounding tissue and protect cells from thermal damage. If a tumor wraps around such a vessel, the vessel will act as a thermal shield. Tumor cells behind the vessel will not be exposed to lethal temperatures, and the treatment will fail locally.

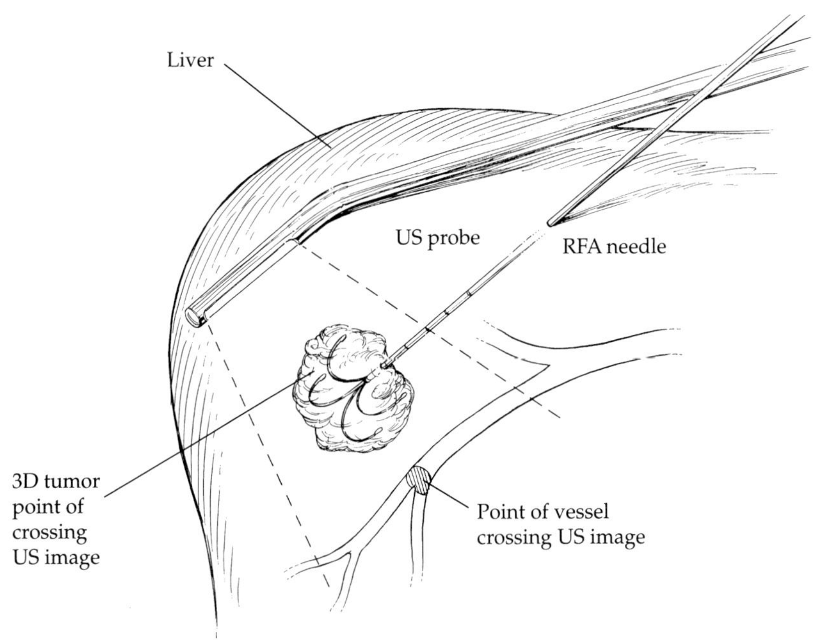

Fig. 35-3. Laparoscopic RFA requires facility with laparoscopic ultrasound (US). RFA, radiofrequency ablation.

Because heat causes indiscriminate damage, great care must be taken to avoid injury to surrounding vital structures. The major concern for injury within the liver is the central biliary system (Fig. 35-3). While most patients will tolerate ablation of segmental bile ducts, destruction of the main left or right duct or the hepatic or common bile duct may result in an obstructive biloma. These bilomas become infected and, depending on the degree of injury, may require percutaneous drainage or endobiliary stenting. Ablation of a lesion within 2 cm of a central bile duct, especially a large lesion requiring an aggressive ablation, should be considered high risk.

While we use a percutaneous application in selected cases (Fig. 35-4), we prefer the laparoscopic approach for most cases. Laparoscopic staging with peritoneoscopy and intraoperative ultrasound will find extrahepatic disease or additional intrahepatic disease in up to one-half of potential candidates, thus precluding RFA as an acceptable treatment option. Laparoscopic techniques to isolate and protect surrounding structures allow a more thorough and aggressive ablation. And finally, accuracy of probe placement within the tumor is highest with direct application of the ultrasound probe to the surface of the liver.

A drawback to laparoscopic RFA is that most surgeons have a limited familiarity with ultrasound. Successful tumor treatment depends on accurate ultrasound-guided RFA probe placement; even a few millimeters of error can result in local treatment failure. The final extent of tissue injury is not well seen on ultrasound imaging. Once an ablation is underway, steam formation and nitrogen outgassing increase the echogenicity of the ablation zone and preclude further meaningful ultrasound imaging. We believe this is the source of treatment failures when repositioning of the probe after the initial ablation is required.

Like other ablative technologies, RFA tends to destroy less of the surrounding functional hepatic tissue than a liver resection. This allows treatment of bilobar tumors and treatment in patients with advanced cirrhosis. Hepatic preservation also allows RFA to be used repeatedly for tumor recurrences.

Cryotherapy Ablation

Cryotherapy uses extreme cold as a means of thermal tissue destruction. Rapid freezing of tissue to −170° C followed by rapid thawing causes tissue death in several ways, dependant on how cold the ice ball gets and how rapidly temperature changes occur. Ice crystals will form within cells and expand to rupture cell walls. The redistribution of water and solutes within the intra- and extracellular spaces causes cellular dehydration. Dehydration causes pH shifts that denature proteins and degrade cell walls. Microvascular thrombosis occurs due to disruption of the endothelium and leads to the deposition of platelet thrombi. Injured tissue is even more susceptible to injury; thus, repeat freeze–thaw cycles are increasingly lethal.

Cryoablation was more frequently used to treat surgically unresectable tumors in the 1980s and 1990s. It has largely fallen out of favor, in deference to RFA. The complication rate associated with cryoablation was essentially the same as that seen with open resection in many reports. Massive hemorrhage during surgery

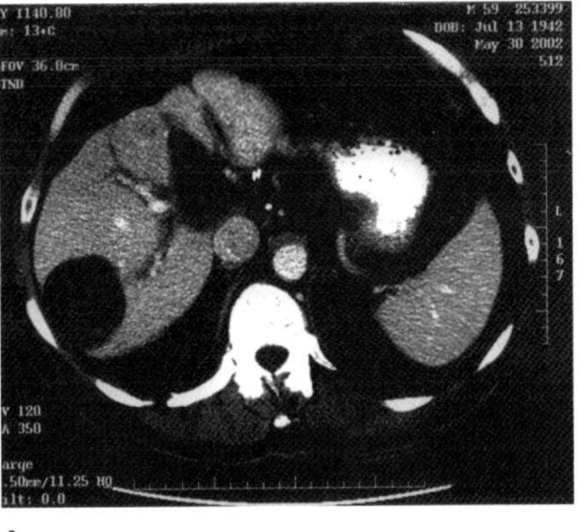

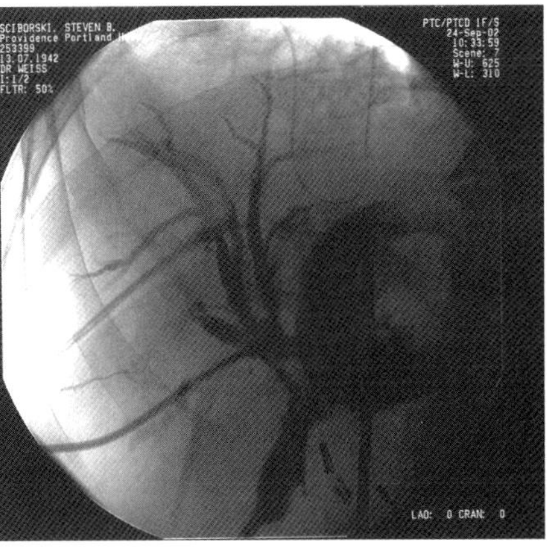

Fig. 35-4. RFA of caudate lobe colorectal metastasis led to the destruction of the left and common hepatic duct and an infected biloma. **A.** Post-RFA CT image of two colorectal liver metastases. **B.** Percutaneous transhepatic cholangiogram demonstrating the biloma obstructing the left and common hepatic ducts. RFA, radiofrequency ablation; CT, computed tomography.

in up to 5% of patients was often due to vascular injuries from the large cryoprobes or freeze fracture injuries across blood vessels. Postoperative bile leaks were also common. Finally, nearly 20% of postoperative mortality was caused by a poorly understood multi-organ system failure marked by a consumptive coagulopathy.

The principal advantage of cryotherapy is that the ice balls are clearly visible on ultrasound imaging. The treating physicians can more definitively understand the margins of their ablation and thus the tissue destroyed.

Microwave and Laser Ablation

Microwave and laser technologies hold much promise for hepatic tumor ablation. Both energy sources are used to heat surrounding tissues to temperatures above 100° C. Tissue heating is typically more rapid than RFA. The primary limitation has been the inability to create lesions of adequate size. These problems are likely to be overcome in the next few years.

Liver Tumors and Treatment Options

BENIGN LIVER TUMORS

The majority of lesions identified in the liver are benign and asymptomatic; this is especially true in an era where diagnostic imaging has become so readily available. Abdominal ultrasounds, CT scans, and magnetic resonance imaging scans (MRIs) are frequently obtained for vague abdominal symptoms or minor trauma. Hepatic hemangiomas, hepatic adenomas, FNHs, and benign liver cysts occur in up to 5% of the general population. Determining what an incidentally identified lesion is or determining whether the lesion may be the source of a symptom can be a vexing problem.

Hemangiomas

Hemangiomas are found at autopsy in up to 20% of liver specimens. Most are classified as capillary hemangiomas and are of no clinical significance. Cavernous hemangiomas are ectatic vascular malformations, not true neoplastic lesions. They are thought to be congenital, with 40% being multifocal. Lesions greater than 5 cm in diameter are classified as giant cavernous hemangiomas. They tend to be well circumscribed with a thin fibrous capsule.

The vast majority of hemangiomas are asymptomatic and do not require intervention or even follow-up. Occasionally, these lesions may cause pain due to thrombosis and inflammation or capsular stretch of the liver. Persistent growth can cause pain, biliary obstruction, or a cardiac steal phenomenon. Giant cavernous hemangiomas warrant follow-up imaging to identify persistent growth. A pattern of growth rather than absolute size may justify intervention. The risk of spontaneous rupture of hemangiomas is small—as of 1996, there were fewer than 50 cases of spontaneous rupture identified in the worldwide literature by Scribano et al.—and is not an indication for intervention. Finally, Kasabach-Merritt syndrome is a very rare indication for treatment in which patients with hemangiomata develop thrombocytopenia and a consumptive coagulopathy.

The principal treatment for symptomatic or growing hemangiomas has been resection. In selected circumstances, liver transplantation may be required. Nonresective treatments such as ablation, embolization, and focal radiation are generally not indicated. Ablation has a limited role because the size of the majority of symptomatic lesions (>6 cm) is prohibitive. Additionally, most large lesions are located near central hepatic structures, which are susceptible to an ablation injury.

A number of embolic techniques has been described in the literature. Factors that limit successful ablation include multiple sites of vascular inflow, erratic flow within the tumor, and high shunt fractions through the tumor. Still, several small studies have suggested embolization can be performed safely and may result in symptom reduction. These techniques have a limited ability to reduce the size of the hemangiomas and complications have been reported.

Our current policy is to restrict treatment to clearly symptomatic patients. In the rare circumstance of bleeding from a hemangioma, poor surgical candidates may be stabilized using endovascular techniques. The majority of patients will benefit from a definitive surgical resection or, less likely, RFA. Non-bleeding but symptomatic lesions smaller than 5 cm located more than 2 cm from the central bile ducts may be treated with RFA. Larger or central lesions are treated with laparoscopic or open liver resections. Embolic techniques are reserved for poor operative candidates.

Focal Nodular Hyperplasia

Focal nodular hyperplasia (FNH) is a benign, tumor-like structure of the liver. They are the second most common benign lesion of the liver after hemangiomas and they occur in both men and women of all ages. Histologically FNHs are composed of cords of hepatocytes, separated by fibrous septae. The structures have no portal or hepatic veins, but do have scattered biliary epithelium. They are characterized radiographically by the presence of a stellate central scar, absent in 15% of cases, and are predominantly solitary lesions, although up to 20% may be multifocal.

The etiology of FNH remains unclear. Oral contraceptives have been implicated, but these lesions occur in men, and up to half of the women with FNH have no history of taking oral contraceptives. The natural history of FNH is one of a benign course. Most stay dormant and some regress, but up to 10% may enlarge over time. The vast majority of FNH are asymptomatic; when patients with FNH do present with symptoms, other sources need to be excluded.

If a patient presents with symptoms and an FNH and no other source is identified by history or imaging, treatment may be considered. If the patient has been on oral contraceptives, these are stopped. Angioembolization has been shown to improve symptoms and induce regression in some tumors. RFA is an acceptable alternative in small peripheral lesions. Larger central lesions, which do not respond to angioembolization, may require surgical resection.

Simple Hepatic Cysts

Simple hepatic cysts are a very common incidental finding. Up to 5% of the general population has one or more. Fifty percent of patients have solitary cysts, while the rest may have a range from two to more than 20. Simple hepatic cysts are thought to be congenital ductal malformations and to have a cuboidal epithelium with a serous fluid-filled cavity. As cysts enlarge, they crowd out the normal hepatic parenchyma. Apparent septations in the cysts may be hepatic pedicles that cannot be pushed aside and are slung across the cyst cavity as it enlarges and crowds out the hepatic parenchyma. Simple hepatic cysts are benign and require intervention only when clearly symptomatic.

Simple cysts need to be differentiated from the much less common cystadenoma. The cystadenoma will typically have multiple locules with areas of polypoid or papillary projections. Although the lining is a single layer of cuboidal or columnar cells, cystadenomas typically stain positive for mucin. Cystadenomas have a malignant potential and should be resected.

Patients with true polycystic liver disease have a distinct disease process different from simple hepatic cysts. Patients with polycystic liver disease do occasionally require surgical debulking, but this is a progressive disease and the preservation of functional hepatic tissue is a priority. Few of these patients eventually require liver transplantation. Nonresective techniques, such as aspiration and ethanol injection, are used only in the rare situation where a dominant cyst is felt to be causing the bulk of the symptoms.

The vast majority of simple cysts are asymptomatic. Attributing symptoms to the presence of simple hepatic cysts should be undertaken with some caution. Our approach is to rule out other possible causes of the symptoms. If no cause is identified, a trial of percutaneous aspiration is performed to determine if the symptoms improve. If the symptoms improve, the patient is brought back when the cyst and symptoms recur. A percutaneous drain is placed and the cyst is drained. Contrast is injected to exclude communication with the bile ducts. A sclerosing agent is then injected, retained for 1 hour, and then removed.

There have been several small case reports and one prospective trial showing good objective and symptomatic improvement from percutaneous sclerotherapy as described above. The prospective trial demonstrated cyst volumes reductions from an average of 309 mL to 21.5 mL and that all patients experienced relief of their symptoms. If the cyst recurs, the next step is laparoscopic fenestration.

Hepatic Adenoma

Hepatic adenomas are primarily tumors of young, otherwise healthy women. There is a strong association with long-term oral contraceptive usage. There have been case-control studies demonstrating a direct correlation between increased dosage and increased length of utilization and the frequency of developing adenomas. While adenomas may be multiple in as many as 30% of patients, adenomatosis, defined as more than ten adenomas, appears to be a separate clinical entity from isolated adenomas.

Fifty percent of adenomas are symptomatic at presentation to a surgeon. Right upper quadrant pain is the most common symptom, but mass effect, nausea, and hemorrhage may also occur. The risk of malignant transformation of adenomas is thought to be 3% to 4% per year and 10% to 15% overall. The rate of malignant conversion is thought to be higher in tumors larger than 6 cm.

Currently, the management of adenomas depends on symptoms, size, and the history of contraceptive use. Patients taking oral contraceptives should stop if possible. Lesions less than 6 cm may be observed with serial scans for involution and/or resolution of symptoms. Persistent symptoms or continued growth require intervention. Some authors believe that persistence of the adenoma of any size is an indication for intervention. The literature more commonly supports intervention in any adenoma larger than 6 cm.

Treatment options for adenoma include bland arterial embolization, chemical embolization, thermal ablation, or resection. Embolization is the preferred method of initial treatment in acute hemorrhage. Embolization has proven effective in controlling symptoms in many patients, but typically does not result in complete involution. Both chemical and thermal ablation are effective methods of tumor destruction in lesions less than 4 cm in size. We have used RFA in selected peripheral adenomas up to 8 cm in size. Larger lesions almost invariably lay adjacent to central hepatic structures and are therefore difficult to treat with RFA and curative intent without jeopardizing the central biliary tree. The treatment of choice for larger lesions is currently resection—either laparoscopic or open.

PRIMARY LIVER CANCERS

Hepatocellular Carcinoma

Hepatocellular carcinoma (HCC) is one of the most common causes of cancer death worldwide. This is largely due to the relationship between viral hepatitis, cirrhosis, and the development of HCC. All patients with cirrhosis are at risk for the development of HCC and should be screened with an alpha fetoprotein (AFP) test and ultrasound every 6 to 12 months. Identification of a suspicious mass may require a biopsy. If a mass is more than 2 cm in size and has a classic HCC vascular pattern using two imaging modalities, or a classic HCC vascular pattern on one imaging modality and an elevated AFP, no biopsy is required.

When deciding on the treatment of confirmed or suspected HCC, a number of issues must be considered. First is whether there is extrahepatic disease. In the presence of extrahepatic disease, systemic treatment with surafenib may be beneficial but local approaches to the liver disease are generally unwarranted. Arguments for palliative endovascular tumor treatments have been made in selected cases where the extrahepatic tumor burden is small and the primary demise is expected to be from hepatic tumor progression.

The second issue is whether the HCC developed in a normal liver or in the setting of cirrhosis. In a patient without cirrhosis, surgical resection is the only treatment shown to generate long-term survival. Nonresective treatments may play a role in patients who are not candidates for major surgical intervention. In patients with cirrhosis, the most definitive treatment option is liver transplant. The Milan criteria for liver transplant require that the patient have no more than three tumors less than 3 cm in size or a single tumor less than 5 cm. Patients who are transplant candidates may benefit from bridging treatments such as chemoembolization, yttrium^{90} infusion, or RFA to prevent tumor progression while they are on the transplant waiting list.

The third issue in selecting the best treatment option is in determining the patient's general health and functional hepatic reserve. Patients with a history of hepatic encephalopathy, poorly controlled ascites, or significant portal hypertension do not tolerate liver interventions well. Ablative and endovascular treatments may be indicated because they tend to destroy or injure less of the residual functional hepatic tissue.

Nonresective treatment of HCC includes endovascular therapies and ablation. Because infusional treatments are not currently considered curative, we prefer RFA or ethanol injections when possible. For lesions less than 3 cm in size and more than 2 cm away from the central bile ducts, we start with RFA. If the lesion is within 2 cm of the central bile duct, we use ethanol injection. For lesions greater than 3 cm, we start with either chemoembolization or yttrium^{90} arterial infusions. If the lesions downsize, we may follow up with an RFA or ethanol injection (Fig. 35-5, page 348).

SECONDARY LIVER CANCERS

The liver is one of the most common sites in the body for the development of metastatic lesions. The prognosis for patients at this stage of disease is generally quite poor. Of patients with a gastrointestinal primary

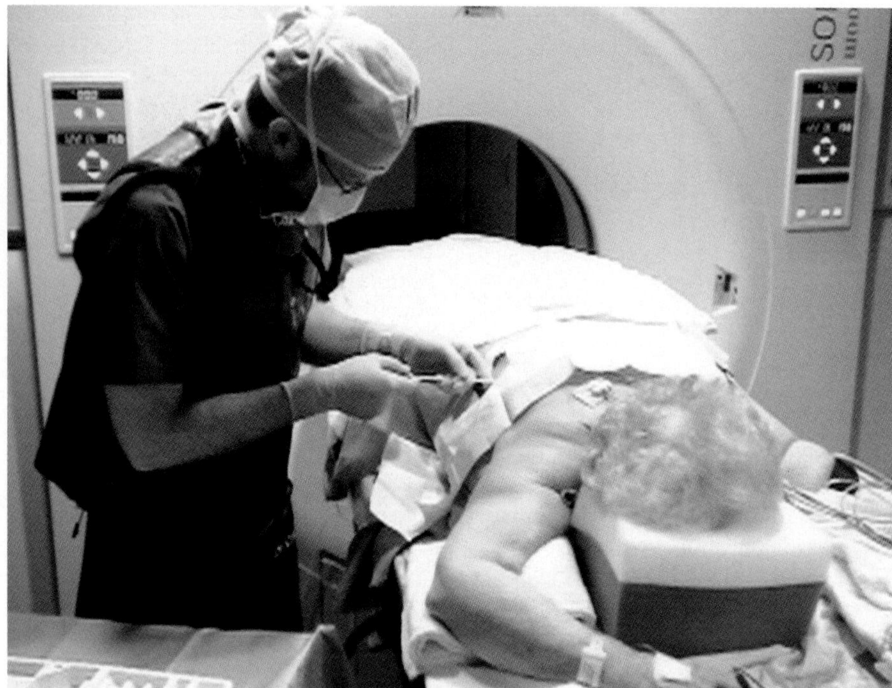

Fig. 35-5. CT-guided RFA with the patient in the prone position and under general anesthesia. CT, computed tomography; RFA, radiofrequency ablation.

tumor, only those with colorectal liver metastases are considered curable. Rarely a patient with a non-colorectal gastrointestinal primary cancer will develop limited liver metastases, which are slowly progressive, with the liver the only site of tumor progression. This is also seen occasionally with non-gastrointestinal primaries such as sarcomas or breast cancer. In these situations, liver-directed treatments may be beneficial. Because the expected prognosis remains poor, minimally invasive treatments may be preferable.

Metastatic Colorectal Cancer

Up to 60% of patients diagnosed with metastatic colorectal cancer will develop liver metastases. Although there have been dramatic breakthroughs in chemotherapeutic treatment options, liver resection was until recently the only treatment option proven to generate long-term survivorship. Ablative therapies may have several potential advantages over resection, but they must have proven efficacy before they obtain widespread acceptance. Liver-directed infusional therapies also have a role in down-staging treatable lesions or in palliating incurable disease.

As the gold standard for the treatment of isolated colorectal liver metastases, surgical resection is reported to generate 5-year survivors in 21% to 58% of patients. This is a highly select group of patients who are in good enough general health to tolerate a major surgical intervention. Their functional liver reserve must be greater than 20% following the resection. They must also have a tumor burden that allows resection while leaving viable remnant segments intact. Not infrequently, resection of even a small liver metastasis (<2 cm) will require resection of more than 60% of hepatic volume to achieve a curative result. Overall, less than 30% of patients with isolated colorectal liver metastases are candidates for surgical resection.

The rate of perioperative morbidity associated with surgical resection is up to 40% and includes pain, bleeding, bile leaks, and infectious complications. Open resections are typically followed by a week in the hospital and 8 weeks of postoperative recovery. Perioperative mortality in high-volume programs is reported to be 1% to 4%. While these results have improved remarkably over the last 20 years, there is clearly room for further improvement.

The primary option for nonresective, extirpative treatment of colorectal liver metastases is currently radiofrequency ablation. Ethanol injection does not work well in these harder tumors. Cryotherapy is an effective method of destroying tumors, but is associated with a complication profile similar to that of liver resection.

Radiofrequency ablation is a minimally invasive tumor-directed treatment, meaning tumors can be targeted individually, leaving remnant liver tissue largely unaffected. This allows the destruction of bilobar tumors or tumors that are disparately placed, either precluding a resection or requiring a large-volume resection. Additionally, RFA may also be utilized in conjunction with resection or it may be used repeatedly if the tumor recurs or sequentially if there is an overwhelming tumor burden that would preclude treatment of all tumors in a single setting.

Being able to use minimally invasive RFA allows treatment in many patients who would not tolerate an open hepatectomy. A highly select group of patients with small tumors away from adjacent viscera or liver capsule can be treated under sedation in a CT- or ultrasound-guided procedure. Most patients require very deep sedation or a general anesthesia.

While the overall magnitude of the laparoscopic approach is similar to a percutaneous one, the procedure offers several advantages. Laparoscopic peritoneoscopy will identify peritoneal implants or small-volume metastases on the surface of the liver that are too small to be seen via preoperative CT or PET. Laparoscopy allows the surgeon to evaluate the liver for unsuspected disease such as cirrhosis. Intraoperative ultrasound is the most accurate imaging for identifying small hepatic lesions or portal adenopathy.

The laparoscopic approach typically requires two 10-mm ports: one for the camera and one for the ultrasound device. Additional ports may be required for adhesiolysis. The morbidity profile of these procedures includes pain, bleeding, bile leak, and bile duct injury. Perioperative morbidity and mortality rates are less than 10% and 0.1%, respectively (see Fig. 35-6).

Limitations in the use of RFA include the inability to reliably destroy tumors larger than 3 to 4 cm in diameter. In our experience, tumors less than 3 cm in diameter and more than 2 cm away from the central biliary system can be destroyed with less than a 5% treatment failure rate. If tumors are close to the central bile duct, ablations are less aggressive and prone to fail. Similarly, tumors greater than 3 cm must be burned more and more aggressively as the risk of treatment failure increases. Using the technology available in 2008, we rarely attempt to ablate tumors larger than 4 cm unless there are no options. We will consider trying to down-size these tumors with systemic or regional chemotherapy or yttrium^{90} infusions prior to ablative techniques.

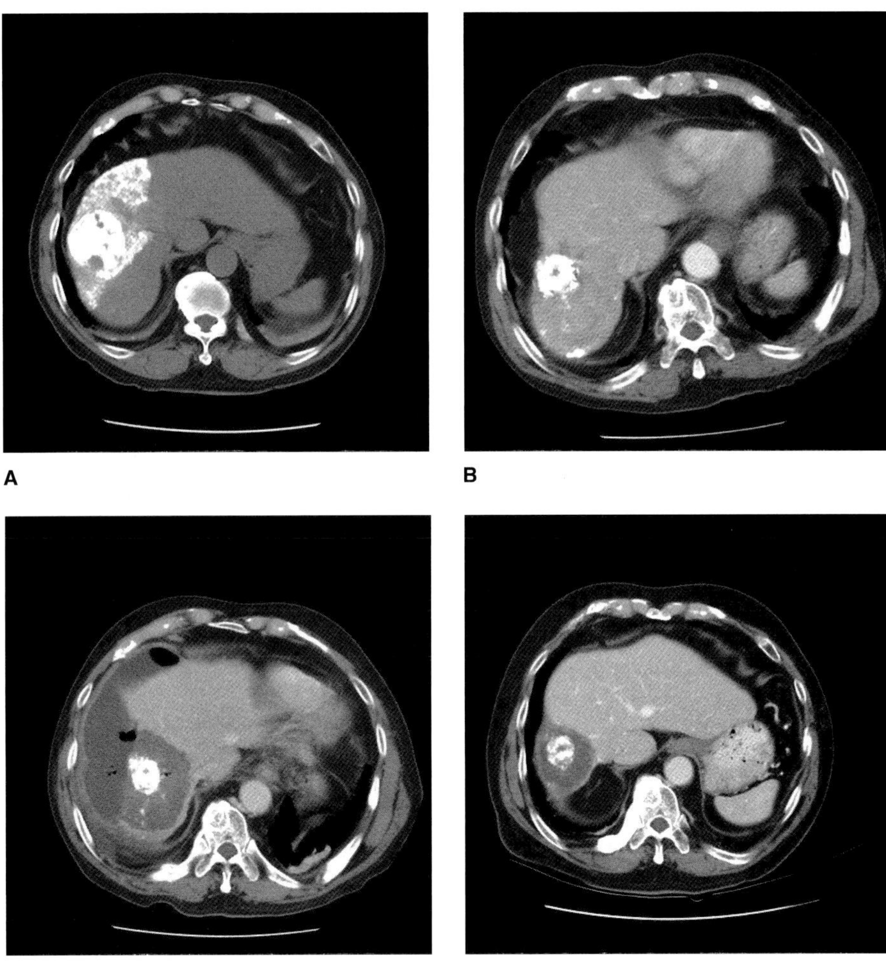

Fig. 35-6. An HCC treated by three courses of TACE and followed up by RFA. **A.** HCC lesion 1 week after TACE. **B.** Following three TACE procedures. **C.** 1 week after RFA. **D.** 2 years after RFA. HCC, hepatocellular carcinoma; TACE, Transcatheter arterial chemoembolization; RFA, radiofrequency ablation; HCC, hepatocellular carcinoma.

There remains significant controversy regarding the appropriate use of RFA in colorectal liver metastases. There are currently no randomized, controlled trials that directly demonstrate RFA as being equal to liver resection in producing long-term survivals. There are, however, several trials that have demonstrated 5-year survival rates between 18% and 25% in patients considered unresectable and where the majority had failed preablation chemotherapy.

In our 10-year experience with RFA of colorectal liver metastases, we have shown a 5-year survival rate of 25%. These findings occur in a group of patients where more than 80% had previously failed chemotherapy. We believe our results will continue to improve for two reasons. First, four iterations of progressively better ablation machines were used during this 10-year period. The first machines generated only 50 watts and the needle deployment was only 3 cm. The current machines generate up to 250 watts and have a needle deployment up to 7 cm. The second reason is our clinical experience. Patient selection and surgeon expertise play critical roles in determining outcome. This is especially true in terms of using of intraoperative ultrasound for staging, treatment planning, needle placement, and determination of a complete ablation. In our experience, the learning curve for laparoscopic RFA may be more than 30 cases.

For patients who present with initially unresectable or unablatable disease, down-staging should be considered. Newer chemotherapeutic agents have been shown to be effective in converting 10% to 15% of patients from unresectable to resectable. The 5-year survivorship following such conversion has been reported at 15%. While similar data is not yet available for ablative treatments, it is likely that the effect will be similar.

Infusional methods of down-sizing colorectal tumors include HAI of FUDR and yttrium^{90}. Bland embolization and chemoembolization have been shown to be ineffective. HAI with FUDR will induce tumor regression in up to 60% of chemonaive patients and in up to 40% of patients who have failed fluorouracil (5FU)-based regimens. The response rates for patients having failed oxaliplatin- or irinotecan-based regimens are unknown.

Data regarding down-sizing with yttrium^{90} is also limited. While approximately 30% to 40% of colorectal liver metastases decrease in size after yttrium^{9} treatment, much of the yttrium^{90} effect is achieved via devascularization and tumor fibrosis. These tumors become rubbery and subsequent RFA probe deployment can be difficult.

In summary, while surgical resection remains the mainstay of treatment for isolated colorectal liver metastases, it is likely that RFA will play an increasing role. Currently RFA is used in patients who are unresectable due to tumor location or because they are not candidates for a major surgical procedure. We believe that as experience and technology progress, ablation may become the treatment of choice.

Metastatic Neuroendocrine Cancer

The treatment of hepatic neuroendocrine metastases has different goals than the treatment of metastatic adenocarcinoma. Neuroendocrine tumors in general are more slowly progressive than other hepatic malignancies. Mean survival times of patients with metastatic neuroendocrine tumors have been reported between 3 and 8 years. Once metastatic to the liver, however, neuroendocrine tumors are incurable. There is debate about whether to treat asymptomatic patients. Hormonally active or symptomatic patients, however, will typically benefit from an aggressive approach to debulking.

Debulking tumors can be done in a number of ways. In the uncommon situation in which a patient has only a few identifiable tumors, surgical resection or RFA may be appropriate. In the more typical scenario, in which patients have innumerable small tumors, infusional treatment with bland embolization, yttrium^{90} infusion, or chemoembolization may be preferred.

Both symptomatic control and objective response can be obtained using these techniques. Symptomatic responses are seen in 82% to 96% of patients treated with infusional therapy, whereas objective responses range from 52% to 83%. Five-year survival ranges from 60% to 65%. It should be noted that carcinoid tumors have better objective responses and survival rates as compared with pancreatic islet cell carcinoma.

SUMMARY

Between 1950 and 1990, the tenets of safe and effective management of liver tumors by open liver surgery were developed. Open resection was, for practical purposes, the only curative option available and patient-friendly palliative options were limited. The introduction of minimally invasive surgical techniques into the mainstream of surgery during the 1990s opened the door to a number of innovative treatment options. Minimally invasive resections, as well as numerous ablative and endovascular techniques, are currently under development or are being evaluated. The rate at which new technologies are being introduced is currently growing faster than our ability to adequately evaluate their potential role in the treatment armamentarium for liver tumors.

The potential for such treatment options is undeniable. Due to the prevalence of liver tumors, the limit a patient's general health or liver capacity places on the possibility of performing curative resective treatments, and the general value of minimally invasive approaches, interest in these technologies will continue to increase. The primary challenge to practicing physicians will be in appropriately selecting treatments based on a thorough understanding of the available data and its careful application to a patient's clinical scenario.

SUGGESTED READING

Amerst FF, McElrath-Garza A, Ahmad A, et al. Long-term survival after radiofrequency ablation of complex unresectable liver tumors. *Arch Surg* 2006;381–388.

Bharat A, Brown DB, Crippin JS, et al. Pre-liver transplantation locoregional adjuvant therapy for hepatocellular carcinoma as a strategy to improve longterm survival. *J Am Coll Surg* 2006;203(4):411–420.

Blumgart LH, Fong Y, eds. *Surgery of the Liver and Biliary Tract*. 3rd ed. New York: W. B. Saunders Company Ltd, 2000.

Boige V, Malka D, Elias D, et al. Hepatic arterial infusion of oxaliplatin and intravenous LV5FU2 in unresectable liver metastases from colorectal cancer after systemic chemotherapy failure. *Ann Surg Oncol* 2008;15(1):219–226.

Carr BI. Hepatic arterial yttrium^{90} glass microspheres (theraspheres) for unresectable hepatocellular cancer: interim safety and survival data on 65 patients. *Liver Transpl* 2004;10(2): S107–S110.

Hong K, Georgiades CS, Gerschwind JF. Technology insight: image guided therapies for hepatocellular carcinoma—intra-arterial and ablative techniques. *Nat Clin Pract Oncol* 2006;3(6):315–324.

Khatri VP, Chee KG, Petrelli NJ. Modern multimodality approach to hepatic colorectal metastases: solutions and controversies. *Ann Surg Oncol* 2007;16(1):71–83.

Koffron AJ, Auffenberg G, Kung R, et al. Evaluation of 300 minimally invasive liver resections at a single institution: less is more. *Ann Surg* 2007;246(3):385–392.

Llovet JM, Real MI, Montana X, et al. Arterial embolization or chemoembolization versus symptomatic treatment in patients with unresectable hepatocellular carcinoma: a randomized controlled trial. *The Lancet* 2002;359: 1734–1738.

Lo CM, Ngan H, Tso WK, et al. Randomized controlled trial of transarterial lipiodol chemoembolization for unresectable hepatocellular carcinoma. *Hepatology* 2002;35: 1164–1171.

Rhee TK, Lewandowski RJ, Liu DM, et al. 90Y Radioembolization for metastatic neuroendocrine liver tumors: preliminary results from a multi-institutional experience. *Ann Surg* 2008;247(6); in press.

COMMENTARY

The authors make a compelling case for the role of ablative therapies in the management of nonresectable liver tumors. They identify the various types of tumors frequently encountered by the surgeon and describe the varied approaches to the management of these tumors, appropriately commenting upon the evolution of available technology over the past decade. Only a short time ago, ablative techniques were limited by the needle array and power generated during radiofrequency ablation. Today, much stronger devices are available with wider arrays, and as a result the ability to more effectively manage tumors has progressed. This rapid evolution of technology makes it quite difficult to compare current outcomes with those described only a few years ago under the same heading of radiofrequency ablation.

Currently, ablative techniques have not eliminated the need for hepatic resection or the chemotherapeutic management of diseases. In certain cases, ablative techniques may stand alone as the sole approach to a disease process. Far more commonly, however, multi-modal therapy is employed for nonresectable hepatic lesions. The authors have emphasized the ability to effectively treat smaller hepatic masses while preserving a greater percentage of normal hepatic parenchyma when using ablative techniques. Additionally, the authors have emphasized careful selection of patients to minimize complications such as bile duct injury and bile leaks. The surgeon's learning curve also plays a significant role in the outcomes. Experience depends upon far more than one's technical expertise with laparoscopy; the surgeon must also be knowledgeable regarding the various types of tumors and treatment options when dealing with hepatic disease. Additionally, expertise with the use of intraoperative ultrasound greatly impacts outcomes.

The field of ablative therapies for hepatic masses currently holds an important place in the armamentarium of treating these diseases. It is anticipated that the role of percutaneous and laparoscopic ablations will increase within the next decade as technologies, therapeutic agents, and knowledge improve.

WSE

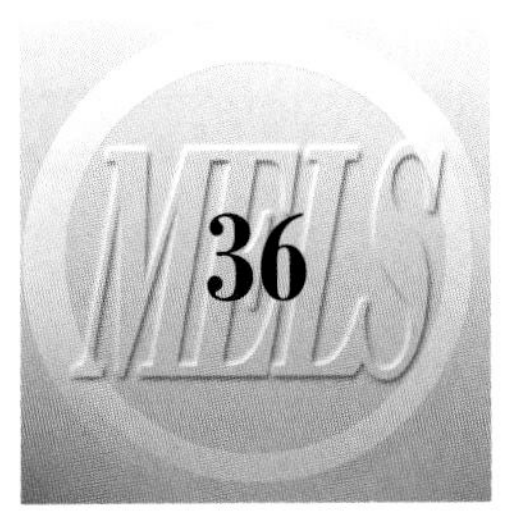

Liver Resection

ANDREW A. GUMBS AND BRICE GAYET

INTRODUCTION

Laparoscopic resection of peripheral hepatic segments has become increasingly common in the surgical treatment of both benign and malignant tumors. Although many centers have begun using the hand-assisted technique for minor hepatic resections and fenestration procedures, we prefer totally laparoscopic techniques for all procedures including major hepatic resections. Currently, the minimally invasive approach to major hepatectomies (three or more Couinaud segments) is only being performed in a few highly specialized centers. This is principally because of unsupported concerns of gas embolism or possible difficulty in controlling major hemorrhage via the laparoscopic approach. Further misconceptions include the lack of ability to obtain adequate resection margins for hepatic malignancies using minimally invasive techniques. At our institution we have successfully performed 62 major totally laparoscopic hepatectomies: 48 right (segments V-VII), 8 left (segments II-IV +/- I), 4 extended right (segments IV-VIII), 1 extended left (segments I-V and VIII) and 1 central (segments IV-V and VIII), as well as other trisegmentectomies and over 150 minor hepatectomies, consisting of bisegmentectomies, segmentectomies, and wedge resections (Table 36-1).

This chapter will discuss pertinent issues regarding preoperative patient selection, necessary equipment, trocar placement, intraoperative monitoring, and the steps necessary to perform major and minor hepatic resections of the liver using totally laparoscopic techniques. Laparoscopic radiofrequency, cryoablation, and the laparoscopic placement of hepatic arterial infusion pumps for the treatment of unresectable liver tumors are covered in other chapters of the text; therefore, none of the technical aspects of these procedures will be discussed in this chapter.

TABLE 36-1. LIST OF MAJOR TOTALLY LAPAROSCOPIC HEPATECTOMIES

Right (segments V to VII):	48
Left (segments II to IV +/- I):	8
Extended right (segments IV to VIII):	4
Extended left (segments I to V and VIII):	1
Central (segments IV to V and VIII):	1

INDICATIONS

The same indications exist for surgery for benign tumors of the liver whether it is done open or laparoscopically. Asymptomatic hemangiomas and patients with the diagnosis of focal nodular hyperplasia (FNH) are observed. When symptomatic, hemangiomas can be embolized via angiography or resected. The same is true for symptomatic patients with FNH. Hepatic adenomas always require resection due to the increased risk of carcinogenesis.

Small asymptomatic simple cysts are typically observed, and symptomatic (painful) cysts should be percutaneously aspirated as a diagnostic test. If there is no bile or evidence of infection on aspiration they are ablated by injecting the cavity with alcohol. If surgery is indicated, the cyst is laparoscopically excised or unroofed, and the bile leak is located and closed. The defect is filled with omentum, and a cholecystectomy is considered to rule out future confusion with right upper quadrant pain. If the bile leak cannot be located easily, a catheter can be inserted in the cystic duct to inject either methylene blue or air as a localization test. Because of pain issues, laparoscopic approaches to symptomatic cysts are well advised.

By definition, complex cysts have a solid component and represent a small but definite risk of malignancy. Because of this, complex hepatic cysts require resection so that a full histologic examination can be performed. Patients from areas of high risk should have hydatid cysts serology done, particularly if calcified septated liver cysts are present. If these tests are positive and surgery is indicated, the same principles of avoiding dissemination in the open technique exist for the laparoscopic one. Finally, even though polycystic liver disease can be particularly difficult to deal with and may involve prolonged surgery, we still prefer to approach this disease laparoscopically when surgery is indicated. Laparoscopy will minimize intraabdominal adhesions, which is an important advantage as these patients often require multiple interventions.

Although there is no randomized controlled prospective trial that proves that surgical resection is superior to ablative procedures for malignancies, we favor a laparoscopic resection whenever possible for primary and secondary hepatic tumors. As with open surgery, an estimated 25% of the normal liver must remain for adequate hepatic reserve postoperatively. In patients with hepatic steatosis or heptic complications after chemotherapy, 30% to 40% of the liver should de preserved postoperatively. In patients with fibrotic livers, at least 40% of the liver should be maintained. In our view, starting with laparoscopy is always indicated and may be especially useful in patients with primary and secondary liver cancers, because evidence of unresectability is not always apparent in preoperative imaging.

According to the EASL 2000 Barcelona Conference on diagnostic criteria of hepatocellular carcinoma (HCC), all lesions smaller than 2 cm require either histologic or cytologic confirmation. However, nodules that are hypervascular during the arterial phase of helical computed tomography (CT) scan, are larger than 2 cm, and either have a confirmatory radiological study with the same finding (via MRI or Doppler ultrasound) or an α-fetoprotein level greater than 400, are considered de facto HCC and do not require biopsy prior to surgery. Patients with nodules smaller than 2 cm that cannot be biopsied percutaneously and that are Child-Pugh class A should also undergo laparoscopic resection. All patients with the diagnosis of HCC undergo a full metastatic workup with clinical assessment of lymph node status and radiological examination with both thoracoabdominal CT and MRI of the liver, due to the superiority of MRI in identifying hepatic lesions. Brain and bone scans are only obtained in symptomatic patients.

According to the current Milan Criteria, surgery is indicated for patients with tumors less than 5 cm or when there are fewer than four nodules that are no greater than 3 cm in greatest diameter in the absence of thrombosis of a lobar branch or trunk of the portal system. We have extended these criteria and will laparoscopically resect larger HCC tumors (>8 cm) in a way that will still leave the patient with adequate hepatic reserve, using embolization if needed. All patients with HCC should discuss the possibility of a liver transplant service with appropriate personnel. Laparoscopic resection may be indicated prior to transplantation for patients who will have to wait for prolonged periods of time for an organ, because the decreased adhesion formation may make the subsequent transplantation easier. Radiofrequency ablation, chemotherapy, and chemoembolization are reserved for unresectable patients.

In the Western world, metastases secondary to colorectal cancer are the most common indication for hepatic surgery. Assessment of resectability of the hepatic metastases and a rigorous search for other evidence of metastatic disease is paramount. In addition to clinical and laboratory examinations, all patients must have thoracic and abdominopelvic CT scans with intravenous contrast and a positron emission test (PET) scan. Fong et al. developed a Clinical Risk Score that helps predict the presence of occult intrahepatic or extrahepatic disease, which may contraindicate surgery. The five factors that make up this Clinical Risk Score include the presence of more than one liver tumor, positive node status of the primary tumor, a disease-free interval of less than 1 year, the presence of liver tumor greater than 5 cm, and a carcinoembryonic antigen (CEA) level greater than 200 ng/mL. In patients with more than two of these factors, occult disease rendering patients unresectable will be found in up to 42% of the patients. As with HCC, the routine use of laparoscopy and laparoscopic ultrasound in the management of liver metastases can spare these patients, in particular, from unnecessary laparotomy. Notably, ideal resection margins are at least 1 cm, but 0.5 cm margins are acceptable.

When hepatic metastases from rectal cancer are diagnosed synchronously we perform the hepatic resection first and then proceed to resection of the primary tumor at the same operation. Removal of the hepatic disease is prioritized because of the increased risk of infection or fistula formation after rectal surgery. Such a complication can cause prolonged delay in the initiation of chemotherapy. In some patients with complex hepatic metastases, we may even opt to perform the liver surgery first and the rectal surgery at a second setting. Colon cancers have a much lower incidence of leaks or fistulae and are resected before the hepatectomy. If liver metastases are discovered during the colon surgery, we perform the colon resection and removal of any small metastases laparoscopically; for patients with larger metastases, the laparoscopic hepatic metastasectomy is deferred for 1 to 3 months. Laparoscopy is particularly useful in patients requiring a second operation due to the decrease in adhesions. When celiac and/or portal lymph nodes are found to be positive intraoperatively, resection is still performed if no more than a left or right hepatectomy will be required.

When resection for cure is not possible in one setting due to the extent of intrahepatic tumor, surgery for cure is still attempted when total resection can be obtained within two operations. In disease that will result in less than the necessary liver remnant, the ipsilateral branch of the portal vein that is to be resected can be embolized preoperatively to allow for hypertrophy of the contralateral lobe. In these patients, surgery must be performed within 30 to 45 days to limit the risk of disease spreading into the contralateral lobe of the liver. If patients also present with resectable pulmonary metastases, we prefer hepatic metastasectomy prior to lung resection.

In patients found to have unresectable disease, chemotherapy is given, and patients are re-evaluated after no more than three cycles. The use of laparoscopic radiofrequency ablation, embolization, and hepatic intraarterial chemotherapy can further increase the candidate pool for curative resection but must be assessed on a case-by-case basis. Postoperative chemotherapy should be discussed with all patients after hepatic metastasectomy. As a rule, however, we opt for surgery alone for patients who present with metachronous disease in the liver.

CONTRAINDICATIONS

Contraindications to major laparoscopic hepatic resections include the usual contraindications to laparoscopy; mainly anesthesia risk factors, such as an American Society of Anesthesiologists (ASA) score of 4 or more. Contraindications specific to the pneumoperitoneum include closed angle glaucoma, intracranial hypertension and diffuse bullous emphysema. Contraindications specific to liver surgery include a need for complex vascular or biliary reconstruction. Previous surgery, including previous open hepatectomy, may make the dissection more difficult but is only a relative contraindication for a laparoscopic approach.

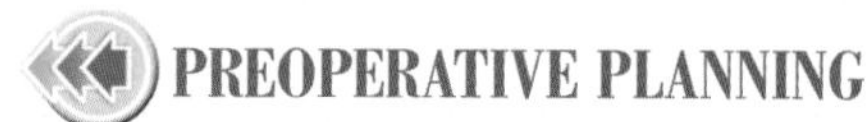

PREOPERATIVE PLANNING

Lesions should be assessed preoperatively with CT scan, MRI, ultrasound, PET scan, or a combination of these. For lesions close to large vascular or biliary structures, three-dimensional reconstruction should be obtained (Fig. 36-1). Lesions whose resectability is uncertain based on preoperative imaging should be re-evaluated with intraoperative laparoscopic ultrasound. Ultimately, the decision to proceed with minimally invasive hepatectomy is the same as for an open resection, and both depend on operator ability.

Equipment

Equipment for the laparoscopic hepatectomy includes high-definition video cameras and monitors controlled by a voice-controlled robotic holder (AESOP 3000; Intuitive Surgical Inc.; Sunnyvale, CA), an atraumatic liver retractor with a self-retaining table-mounted holder, and standard laparoscopic instruments such as dissectors and atraumatic graspers. A bipolar cautery forceps is critical to safely performing the dissection through the hepatic parenchyma to allow for identification of the major vascular branches of the portal and hepatic veins. An ultrasonic coagulating shears is particularly useful for the division of the hepatic parenchyma. A flexible laparoscopic ultrasound probe with color-flow Doppler capability is used to confirm the presence of the lesion, to note its proximity to major vascular structures, and to identify other lesions. Once the large vessels are identified and skeletonized, laparoscopic linear staplers are used to transect the principal branches. A full laparotomy tray and a hand port are placed in every operating room to be on hand should urgent conversion become necessary.

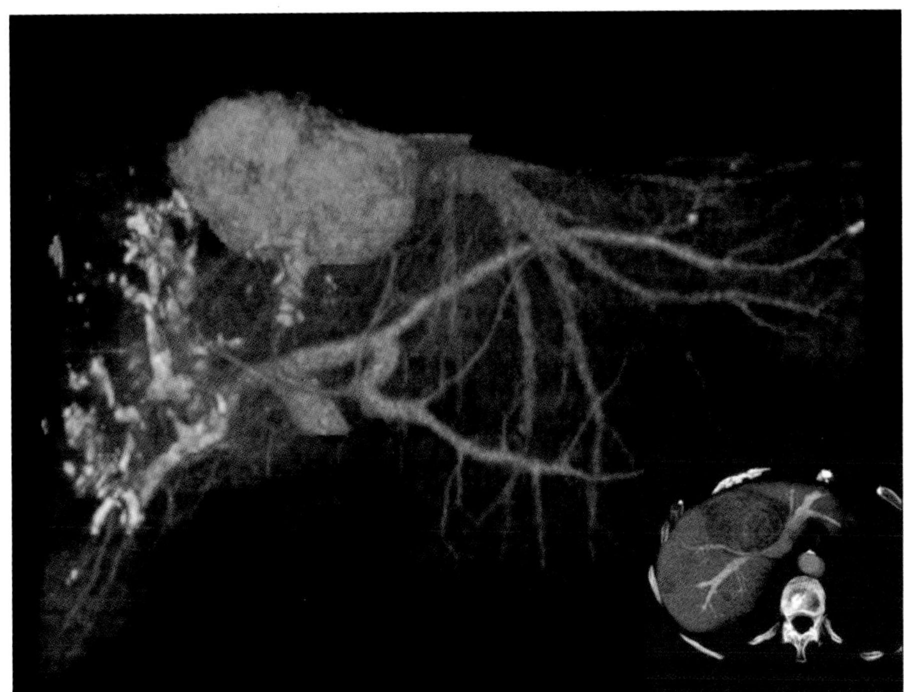

Fig. 36-1. Three-dimensional vascular reconstruction showing tumor (in light blue) in segment VIII. Because the tumor was next to the middle vein and the left lobe was particularly small on preoperative computed tomography (CT) scan (please see picture in picture), the patient underwent right portal vein branch embolization 3 weeks prior to surgery. Note the white enhancement in the right side of the liver where the embolization was done and the marked hypertrophy of the left hepatic lobe.

Patient Positioning and Room Set Up

Patients are placed in the supine position on the operating table. All patients receive deep venous thrombotic prophylaxis preoperatively with subcutaneous heparin. An orogastric tube is place to decompress the stomach and removed at the end of the procedure. A central venous line is placed for central venous pressure (CVP) monitoring preoperatively and continued postoperatively in patients with a history of congestive heart failure. Intraoperatively, the pneumoperitoneum affects the transducer, during which time CVP is better assessed visually or with a laparoscopic ultrasound. The ideal CVP is when the inferior vena cava (IVC) appears half full and fluctuates with the movements of the heart and ventilator.

Proper patient position is critical to the successful performance of the procedure. The arms are tucked at the patient's sides, and the operating table is placed in slight reverse-Trendelenburg. The legs are spread apart and bent at the knees to just under 90 degrees (a "French" or "low lithotomy" position) to ensure maximal freedom of motion of the laparoscopic instruments. The upper body of the patient is strapped down to prevent sliding during the procedure. The self-retaining table-mounted liver retractor is placed on the patient's right side (Fig. 36-2). For lesions in the right liver, the right upper abdomen is elevated with padding. The robotically-controlled camera holder is placed on the left side of the operating room table. The operating surgeon stands between the patient's legs, the surgical assistant stands on the patient's left side, and the surgical technician stands on the right (Fig. 36-3, page 354).

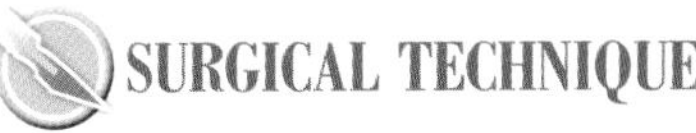

SURGICAL TECHNIQUE

Trocar Placement

Pneumoperitoneum to a pressure of 10 to 12 mmHg is obtained with the Veress needle. In the absence of previous abdominal surgery, the first trocar (10 mm) is placed approximately 7 cm below the right costal margin, between the midclavicular line and midline. In the case of surgery for a possible malignancy, the abdomen is inspected for evidence of obvious carcinomatosis or additional lesions not visualized preoperatively. Four additional ports are placed under direct visualization. A 12-mm port is placed along the midclavicular line 1 to 2 fingerbreadths below the costal margin, to be used for the laparoscopic ultrasound and vascular staplers.

If resectability is determined, two 5-mm ports are placed to the left and right of the camera port. These ports should be placed to ensure optimal ergonomics for the surgeon, as these procedures can take 4 to 6 hours to perform. Another 5-mm

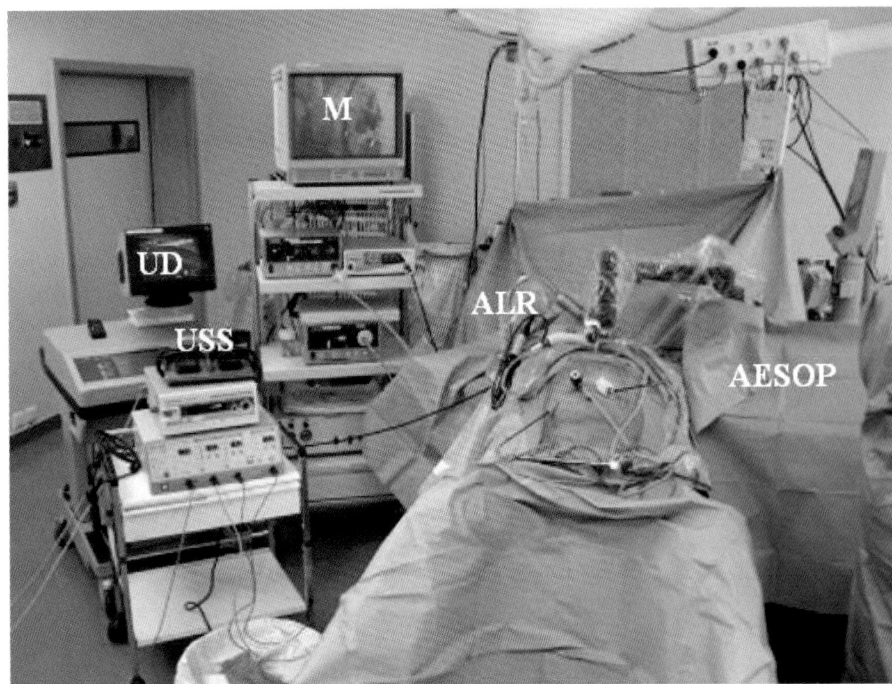

Fig. 36-2. Positioning of patient and operative equipment. AESOP, robotically controlled laparoscope holder placed on the left side of the patient; ALR, autostatic liver retractor, mounted to right side of operating table; M, high-definition monitor; UD, laparoscopic ultrasound device; USS, ultrasonic shear system.

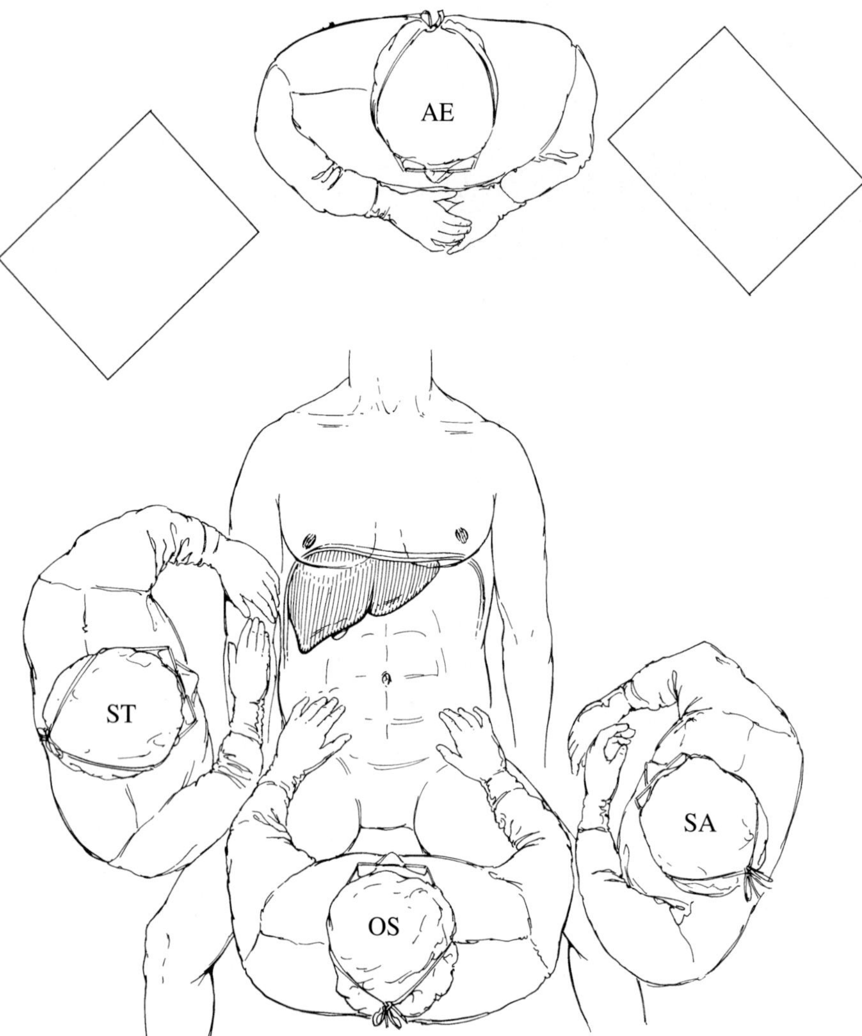

Fig. 36-3. Position of operating room personnel. The operating surgeon (OS) stands in between the patient's legs, the surgical assistant (SA) stands to the patient's left, and the surgical technician (ST) stands to the patient's right. The anesthetist (AE) is at the head of the table.

port is placed in the left upper quadrant along the subcostal line for use by the surgical assistant. If necessary, a final port can be placed along the right anterior axillary line below the costal margin specifically for liver retraction. When possible, subcostal incisions should be placed along a line so that they can be used to create a single subcostal incision should conversion to open surgery become necessary (Fig. 36-4).

Diagnostic Laparoscopy and Sonography

Once all ports are in place, a complete staging laparoscopy and ultrasonography are performed for all neoplasms. To do this all adhesions are lysed, and the peritoneal and hepatic surfaces are visually inspected with the laparoscope. The lesser sac is then entered by incising the gastrohepatic ligament. The portocaval and hepatic lymph nodes are visually inspected; any suspect nodes are removed and sent to pathology for intraoperative frozen section examination. A complete sonographic examination is then completed with a flexible tip laparoscopic ultrasound probe. Despite the flexible probe, it may be necessary to take down the falciform ligament to facilitate access to the dome and posterior segments of the liver. The attachment of the liver to the anterior abdominal wall via the round ligament, however, should be preserved to aid the suspension of the liver during the procedure. All known lesions are confirmed and their proximity to major vascular structures noted; any additional hepatic lesions are also sought.

MAJOR HEPATECTOMIES

Preparation of the Hepatic Pedicle

Once resectability is confirmed, the ligamentum teres (or round ligament) is retracted anteriorly by the surgical assistant to expose the porta hepatis. Using the round ligament as a handle, a suture can be passed with a suture passing device to retract the liver cephalad; otherwise the surgical assistant can provide retraction. This exposure can also be enhanced by retracting the liver cranially and laterally with the self-retaining liver retractor. If necessary the patient can also be placed in steeper reverse-Trendelenburg. The vascular pedicle is controlled by incising the pars lucida/flacida of the lesser omentum to fully expose the hepatoduodenal pedicle. An umbilical tape is then passed through the foramen of Winslow twice around the porta hepatis to permit rapid performance of the Pringle maneuver if needed. This is particularly useful if massive hemorrhage occurs during division of the hepatic parenchyma or the dissection of major hepatic and portal vein branches.

Technique of Parenchymal Division

For normal hepatic parenchyma, laparoscopic hepatotomy is performed with bipolar forceps until larger segmental vessels are encountered, in which case they are clipped or suture ligated. Ultrasonic shears are also useful for parenchymal division; however, they are less dependable for larger vessels. On the lowest setting and in the open position, the active blade of the ultrasonic shears works like the Cavitron ultrasonic dissector (CUSA; Radionics; Burlington, MA). In our hands the laparoscopic CUSA results in decreased visibility secondary to the irrigation fluid utilized and deflates pneumoperitoneum and is thus no longer used. For parenchymal division in cirrhotic patients, the LigaSure bipolar vessel sealing system (Valleylab; Boulder, CO) provides superior hemostasis.

Totally Laparoscopic Left Hepatectomy: Segments II to IV

Hilar Dissection and Control of Hepatic Inflow

The hepatoduodenal ligament is first incised and the portal triad dissected in a cranial fashion, starting from the confluence of the cystic and common hepatic duct. The common hepatic duct is followed until the confluence of the left and right hepatic ducts is found (Fig. 36-5). The entire

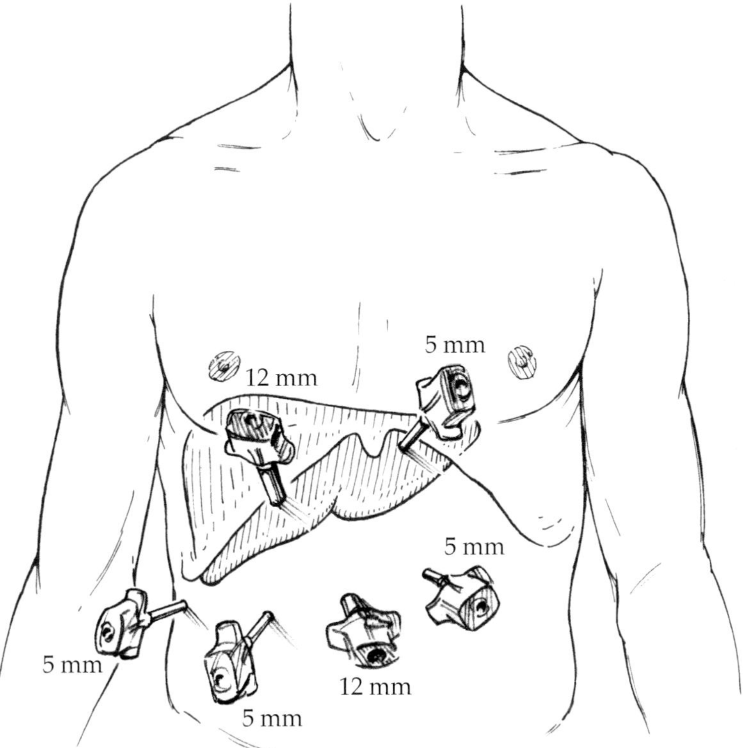

Fig. 36-4. Port placement. The 12-mm camera port is placed approximately 7 cm below the right costal margin along a line in between the midclavicular line and the midline. A second 12-mm port is placed just below the costal margin along the midaxillary line. Two 5-mm working ports are placed to the left and the right of the camera port. A fifth port (5-mm) is placed along the right anterior axillary line for liver retraction, and the final port (5-mm) is placed in the subxiphoid region.

biliary tree is retracted laterally and superiorly, exposing the left hepatic artery, which is skeletonized using bipolar cautery, clipped, and divided. Small vessels such as the cystic artery are simply cauterized with the bipolar forceps and divided (Fig. 36-6). The portal vein is then exposed and dissected cranially until it bifurcates into left and right branches. The left branch of the portal vein enters the umbilical fossa prior to entering into the left hepatic lobe and can be dissected for 1 to 2 cm to allow for transection with a laparoscopic vascular stapler or suture ligature. If some bleeding persists after application of the stapler device, the staple line can be reinforced with a running suture (Fig. 36-7). In some cirrhotic patients with portal hypertension and patients with large portal branches, two firings of the vascular stapler may be required. Lastly, the left bile duct is ligated with absorbable material and transected.

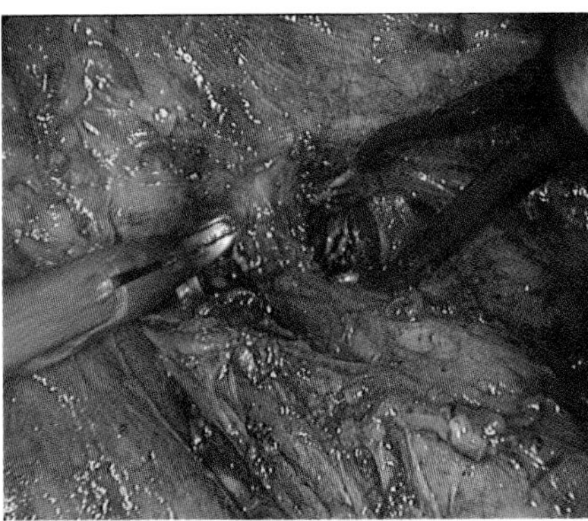

Fig. 36-5. Bifurcation of left hepatic artery. The left branch (supplying segments II and III) has been clipped and transected, and the paramedian branch (supplying segments IVa and IVb) is shown intact on the right.

Control of Hepatic Outflow and Mobilization of the Liver

To aid in visualization of the IVC and hepatic veins, the round, falciform, left triangular, and left upper aspects of the coronary and retrocaval ligaments above segment I are taken down sharply. The peritoneum above the ligamentum venosum is cut, enabling the left lobe of the liver to be retracted laterally. The IVC is then dissected in a cranial fashion until the diaphragm between the middle and left hepatic vein is visualized. If a segment IX is present, its connection with the caudate lobe may need to be transected to adequately visualize the IVC. Small perforating vessels can usually be controlled with the bipolar cautery; however, surgical clips may be necessary for larger vessels. After the left and middle hepatic veins are skeletonized, they are preserved until the liver parenchyma is completely divided. On occasion it is not possible to dissect out the hepatic veins from below the liver along the IVC, and they must be identified anteriorly after division of the hepatic parenchyma.

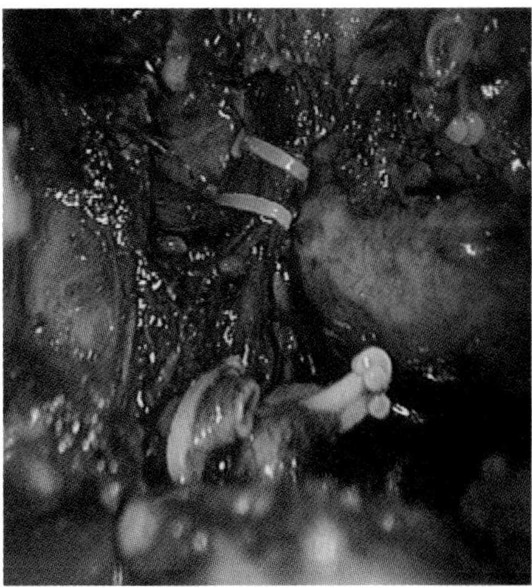

Fig. 36-6. The anterior and posterior pedicles of the right hepatic artery (highlighted in red) and of the right branch of the portal vein (highlighted in blue).

Parenchymal Division

Parenchymal division should be performed with as low a CVP as possible to allow for adequate visualization while minimizing hemorrhage from the divided liver parenchyma. Prior to parenchymal division, the intraabdominal pressure is decreased to 10 mmHg to decrease the risk of CO_2 gas embolism while at the same time maintaining adequate operating space and providing a counterpressure to minimize oozing. Once the arterial and portal blood flow to the left hepatic lobe have been transected, the retraction on the

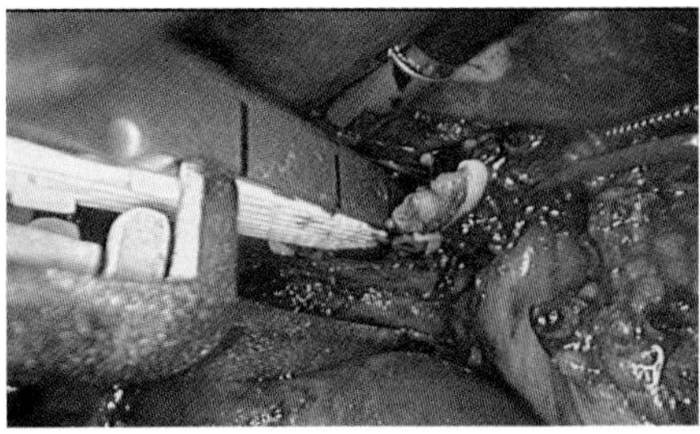

Fig. 36-7. Transection of the right branch of the portal vein with a laparoscopic vascular GIA stapler.

round ligament is released, exposing the anterior surface of the liver where a line of demarcation can be seen. For a totally laparoscopic left hepatectomy (TLLH), this line runs along the Cantlie line, which runs from the medial aspect of the gallbladder bed to the left side of the IVC. Along this line, the Glisson capsule can be incised with electrocautery or ultrasonic shears to divide the hepatic parenchyma. It is important to confirm adequate resection margins for lesions that are close to these lines of division with intraoperative ultrasound. Frequent use the ultrasound throughout the dissection to assess the plane of division, particularly with lesions close to the edge of resection, is helpful as it is difficult to maintain three-dimensional orientation with laparoscopy. A filter or smoke evacuation system will aid in improving visualization and speed of operation by reducing smoke in the abdomen.

The surgeon divides the parenchyma with the ultrasonic shears in the dominant hand and the bipolar forceps in the other one to provide retraction and simultaneously perform hemostasis of larger vessels. It is crucial to have meticulous hemostasis in laparoscopic hepatectomies in order to maintain visualization and to minimize operating room time. Constant suctioning of blood removes pneumoperitoneum and introduces cold air that can cause camera fogging, factors that can unnecessarily prolong surgery. It is important to completely dissect vascular and biliary structures to allow adequate ligation and transection. The Cantlie line dissection is continued to the medial aspect of the middle vein. Preoperative imaging and intraoperative ultrasound greatly assist in the identification of this structure.

Ligation of Hepatic Outflow

The left hepatic vein trunk is transected with a laparoscopic GIA vascular stapler proximal to its confluence with the middle vein (Fig. 36-8). Identification of the hepatic veins can be the most troublesome part of the procedure; if there is any uncertainty as to their identification, a small subcostal incision can be made and a hand port placed. This will allow for manual palpation of the fibrotic attachments to the hepatic veins and facilitate accurate application of the vascular staplers.

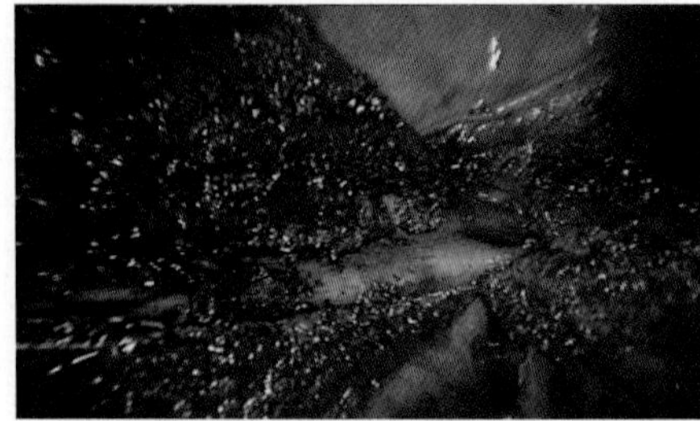

Fig. 36-8. Bifurcation of common bile duct into left and right hepatic ducts (highlighted in green).

Totally Laparoscopic Right Hepatectomy: Segments V to VIII

Mobilization of the Liver

Once resectability is confirmed, the falciform ligament may be left intact or taken down depending on how the liver hangs; it is usually beneficial to leave it intact. The ligamentum teres is retracted as mentioned above to expose the porta hepatis. As opposed to TLLH, in TLRH the liver is retracted cranially and medially with the self-retaining liver retractor after an umbilical tape is placed around the porta hepatis. The right lobe of the liver is mobilized by dividing the right aspect of the coronary ligament and the right triangular ligament.

Hilar Dissection and Control of Hepatic Inflow

As in a cholecystectomy, the cystic artery and duct are dissected and ligated, but the gallbladder is not initially dissected off of the liver bed, so that it can be used to retract the liver during the procedure. As for TLLH, the porta hepatis is dissected cranially starting from the origin of the cystic duct. The common hepatic duct is dissected until the convergence of the right and left hepatic ducts is found. Any arterial branches to the biliary tree are ligated and transected. The biliary tree is then retracted medially at the confluence of the right and left main hepatic ducts to expose the right hepatic artery, which often bifurcates early into anterior and posterior pedicles (Fig. 36-9). At this point the right hepatic artery and/or its branches are ligated and transected. The portal vein is then dissected until its bifurcation is found. The right portal vein is mobilized for several centimeters until a laparoscopic vascular stapler can be easily placed across it (Fig. 36-10). After the right trunk is transected, the portal vein is retracted medially and the right bile duct is identified above the confluence of the right and left main hepatic ducts. The right duct is then ligated and transected; care must be taken to identify its anterior and posterior branches if present.

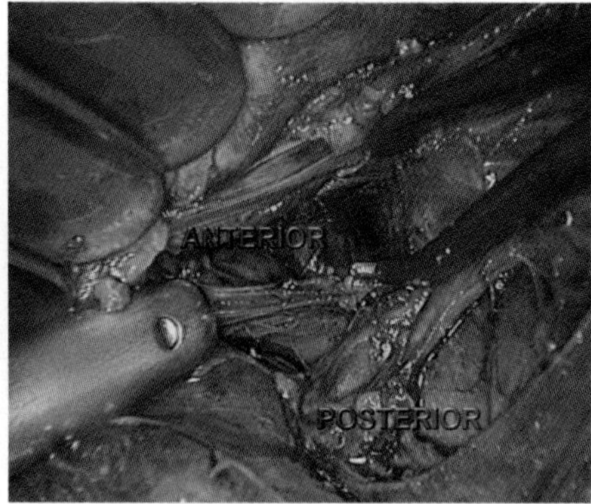

Fig. 36-9. The right aspect of right retrocaval ligament (highlighted in yellow). This structure needs to be transected in right and extended right hepatectomies. The inferior vena cava can be seen on the right of the image.

Control of Hepatic Outflow

The IVC is dissected in a cranial fashion towards the middle and right hepatic veins by retracting the liver medially if possible.

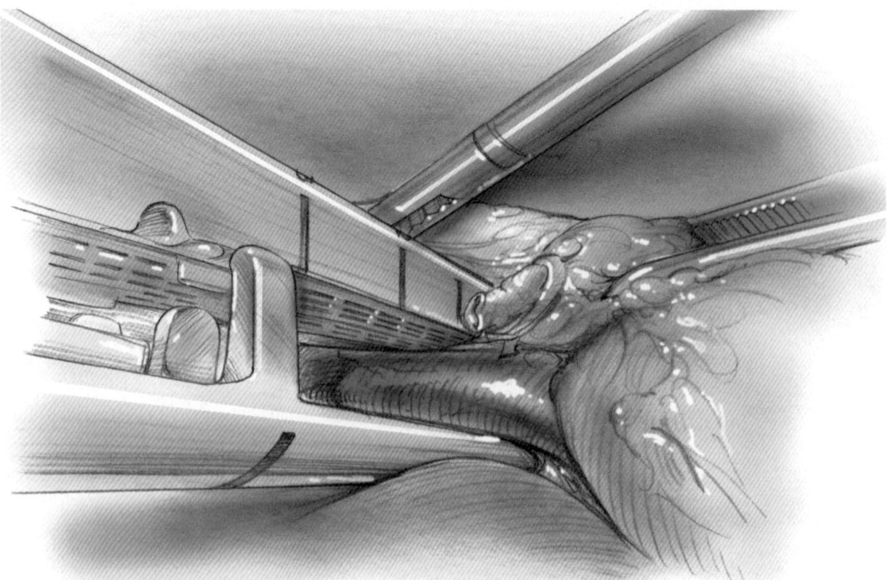

Fig. 36-10. Transection of the right branch of the portal vein.

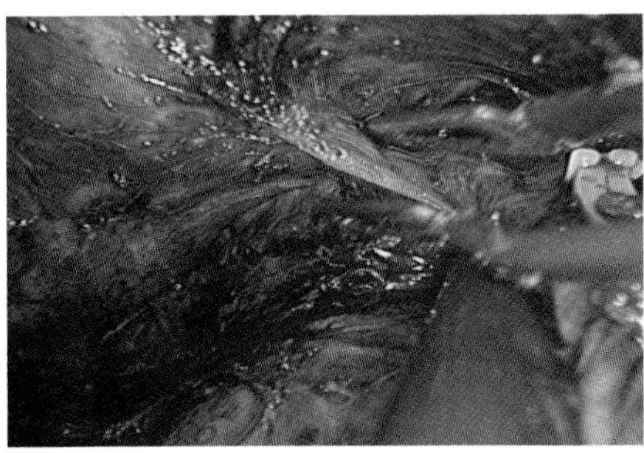

Fig. 36-11. Venous drainage of segment V, directly into the inferior vena cava. This structure has been clipped and can be seen on the left of the image, below the liver.

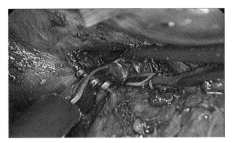

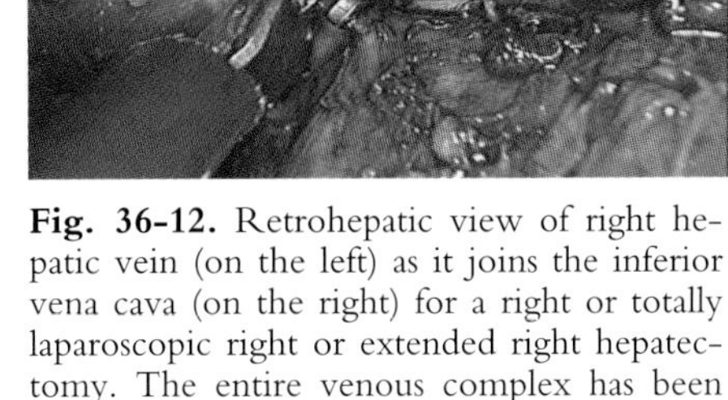

Fig. 36-12. Retrohepatic view of right hepatic vein (on the left) as it joins the inferior vena cava (on the right) for a right or totally laparoscopic right or extended right hepatectomy. The entire venous complex has been highlighted in purple.

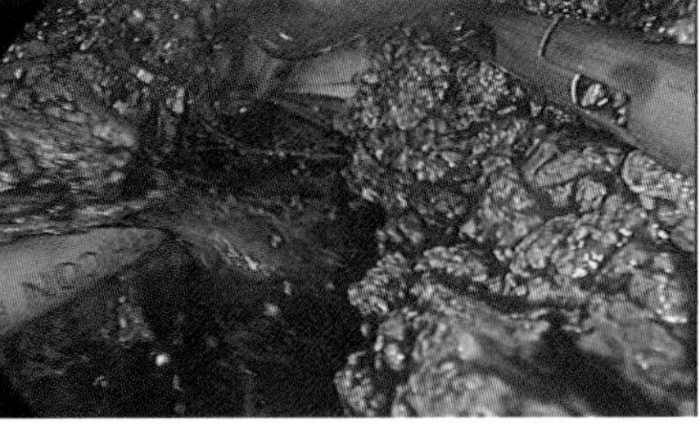

Fig. 36-14. Lateral transection line for a totally laparoscopic central hepatectomy (between the anterior and posterior segments of the right lobe of the liver). The line of demarcation can be seen superiorly.

All perforating vessels are controlled using bipolar cautery, LigaSure, clips, or ligation and then transected. Once the right hepatic vein is exposed posteriorly to the liver, the retrocaval ligament is incised to permit better access to the lateral aspect of the right hepatic vein (Fig. 36-11). First described by Gayet, the retrocaval ligament appears consistently in patients and attaches the posterior aspects of the liver to the tissues behind the IVC. Sometimes the ligament is replaced by vascular parenchyma, especially with hypertrophy of segment I, and transection of this structure can be extremely difficult. The dissection continues posterior to the liver to expose the medial side of the right hepatic vein. Ideally, the dissection is continued until the diaphragm can be seen between the right and middle hepatic veins.

Parenchymal Division

After division of the hepatic inflow, an area of ischemia is noted on the surface of the liver. Following the line of demarcation along the Cantlie line, the Glisson capsule is incised with the ultrasonic dissector. Again, the location of any lesions close to the line of transection is confirmed with the laparoscopic ultrasound, and the line of transection is adjusted accordingly. The hepatic parenchyma is transected down to the IVC. The segmental branches of segments V and VIII can be found within the parenchyma and are controlled with clips or monofilament non-absorbable suture ligation (Fig. 36-12). At the completion of the parenchymal division, the last remaining attachment is the right hepatic vein.

Sometimes a laparoscopic modification of the liver hanging maneuver as described by Belghiti et al. may be useful to enhance the visualization of the vascular structures and facilitate orientation for division of the parenchyma. This technique can be performed by passing an umbilical tape between the right and middle hepatic veins and between the posterior aspect of the liver and IVC and retracting laterally, thereby lifting the right hepatic lobe off of the patient's diaphragm. An advantage of performing this technique laparoscopically is that it can be performed under direct visualization, something that is not possible with an open procedure.

Ligation of Hepatic Outflow

As with TLLH, if the right hepatic vein cannot be adequately dissected via an extrahepatic approach posterior to the liver (Fig. 36-13), it can be approached intraparenchymally (Fig. 36-14, page 358). Either way, the right hepatic vein is transected after division of the portal structures to the right hepatic lobe.

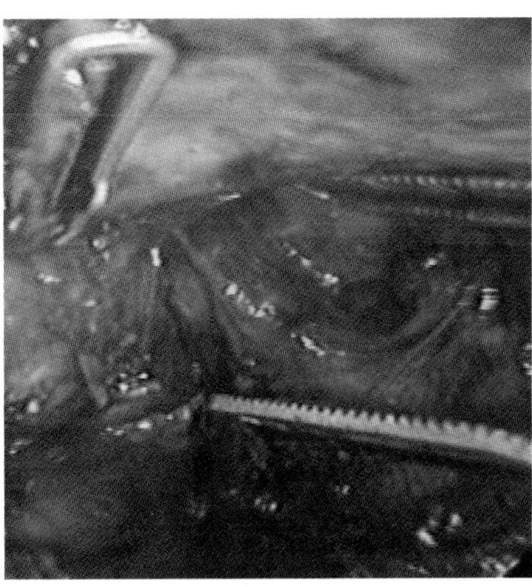

Fig. 36-13. Anterior identification of the right hepatic vein (RHV) after division of the hepatic parenchyma, in preparation for transection with a laparoscopic vascular stapler. The RHV has been highlighted in blue and the inferior vena cava in purple.

Totally Laparoscopic Extended Hepatectomies: Segments IV to VIII (Right) and Segments I to V and VIII (Left)

Totally laparoscopic extended right hepatectomy (TLERH) involves the additional en bloc resection of segments IVa and IVb. The porta hepatis is controlled as described above. The right hepatic artery and duct and right branch of the portal vein are also ligated and transected as described above. In addition, the right or paramedian branch of the left hepatic artery, which feeds segment IV, is ligated and transected (Fig. 36-6). This artery can also originate from the common hepatic artery, in which case it is known as the middle hepatic artery. The left branch of the portal vein is followed until the round ligament is reached, paying attention to staying on its upper side rather than its right side. During this dissection, the branches to segment IV, known as the paramedian branches of the pars umbilicus of the left portal vein, are found (Fig. 36-7). The pars umbilicus itself is a branch off of the pars transversus of the left portal vein. These vessels are either clipped or suture-ligated. A line of demarcation will be seen along the surface of the liver just lateral to the falciform ligament. The Glisson capsule is incised with the ultrasonic dissecting shears, and the division of the parenchyma is continued as described until the IVC is encountered. The dissection is then continued towards the IVC until the middle hepatic vein is reached. This in turn is skeletonized for 1 to 2 cm and divided with the vascular stapler. The rest of the technique is the same as that described for the poster-lateral TLRH.

For totally laparoscopic extended left hepatectomies (TLELH), the patients are placed supine on the operating table, but only five ports are necessary; the lateral liver retraction port is not necessary. The first steps are the same as those described for the TLLH. Then on the right, the anterolateral (V-VIII) and posterolateral (VI-VII) pedicles should be identified, so that the latter can be preserved (Fig. 36-6). The most difficult aspect of this dissection concerns the identification of the bile ducts; it is often safer to cut the anterior branches within the hepatic parenchyma using a vascular stapler after an en bloc dissection has been done. With this maneuver, the caudate lobe is often devascularized and has to be removed. In that case, the left aspect of the retrocaval ligament is incised, as is the coronary ligament. The caudate lobe is removed in this dissection because it receives its blood supply from the left portal vein.

The parenchymal division is started along the line dividing the anterolateral segments from the posterolateral segments of the right hepatic lobe. The sectoral branches from the right hepatic vein draining segments V and VIII must be taken down. The rest of the right hepatic vein will be followed until the IVC; it is imperative that its continuity be maintained. The right aspect of the coronary ligament is then incised from above the liver until the trunk of the hepatic vein is identified. At this point, the only attachment to the liver should be the left hepatic trunk, which is transected with a laparoscopic vascular stapler (Fig. 36-7).

Totally Laparoscopic Central Hepatectomy: Segments IV to V and VIII

Mobilization of the Liver

As opposed to other major resections, we do not mobilize the liver prior to beginning the dissection for totally laparoscopic central hepatectomy (TLCH). The suspensory action of the ligaments, particularly of the falciform, greatly aid in the laparoscopic performance of this procedure.

Hilar Dissection and Control of Hepatic Inflow

The hilar dissection is a combination of the TLERH on the left and the TLELH on the right.

Parenchymal Division

As in TLERH, the parenchyma just lateral to the falciform is scored with the ultrasonic shears, and the parenchyma is divided in a line down to the IVC. The parenchymal division is continued to the left aspect of the middle hepatic vein. The right lobe of the liver is then lifted superiorly to reveal the undersurface of the liver. A line of demarcation between segments V and VI and segments VII and VIII should be seen and scored (Fig. 36-15). This transection line is then completed with the ultrasonic shears. Again all large branches (VI and VII) are clipped or suture ligated as needed. The transection is continued laterally until the right hepatic vein is identified along its medial border and then preserved.

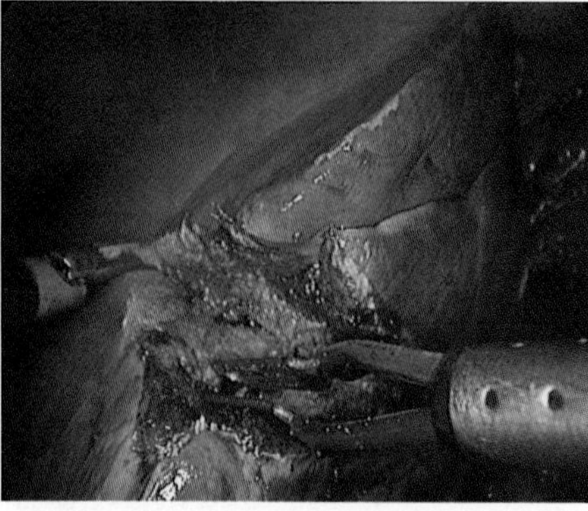

Fig. 36-15. Dissection of the middle hepatic vein in preparation for the completion of a totally laparoscopic central hepatectomy. The middle hepatic vein has been highlighted in purple, and the left hepatic vein and inferior vena cava have been highlighted in blue.

Control of Hepatic Outflow

Once the IVC is reached, the middle hepatic vein is skeletonized for 1 to 2 cm until a laparoscopic vascular GIA stapler can be placed around it (Fig. 36-8). Some variations are possible; most notably, a branch draining segment VIII may run directly into the IVC between the right and left vein and can be extremely dangerous if not recognized. This branch may require clipping or suture ligature prior to transection.

Totally Laparoscopic Trisegmentectomies

Resection of greater than three Couinaud segments is considered a major resection because of the potential postoperative derangements after these resections. Some of the totally laparoscopic trisegmentectomies (TLT) that we have performed include resections of segments IVb/V/VI, III/IV/V, and V/VI/VII. Using a combination of the above-mentioned techniques, along with some of the points noted below, allows virtually any combination of TLT to be performed. It is important to remember that patients need approximately 30% of functioning liver mass to live. Because of this, we consider cirrhotics and patients with liver failure who undergo totally laparoscopic bisegmentectomies (TLB) as major hepatectomies and discuss them as such. In this category we have performed TLBs for segments VI and VII.

SEGMENTECTOMIES AND BISEGMENTECTOMIES

To ensure adequate postoperative reserve in patients with normal liver function, the current limit to anatomical resections is approximately five segments. Below we discuss the technical issues involved in anatomical segmentectomies. Technical aspects of adjacent-segment bisegmentectomies and nonanatomic wedge resections are too numerous to discuss within the limits of this chapter; nonetheless, the principles described below will permit the performance of any combination of anatomic or nonanatomic minor hepatic resection.

Segment I

To approach the caudate lobe it is not necessary to isolate the portal triad with an umbilical tape. The caudate lobe is accessed through the pars lucida of the gastrohepatic ligament and isolated anteriorly with the ultrasonic shears. The hepatoduodenal ligament is dissected posteriorly to visualize the blood flow of the caudate lobe. The caudate lobe receives portal flow anteroinferiorly via left portal branches and drains into the IVC posteriorly via multiple Spigelian veins and usually a larger branch along its upper aspect. These vessels can either be ligated with the ultrasonic shears or suture-ligated, but we prefer to place clips prior to transection. Then you can very easily dissect between the IVC and the caudate lobe directly in front of you under the left lobe. Some authors consider any part of the caudate lobe that crosses the IVC laterally to be a segment IX. The principles of resection of this segment are the same for segment I, but a right portal branch is possible.

Segments II and III

For the left lateral segmentectomy, the falciform ligament can be preserved and the round ligament retracted superiorly and laterally. This retraction is enhanced by a self-retaining liver retractor. The inflow to the liver is isolated with an umbilical or umbilical tape again placed around the porta hepatis. Using the ultrasonic dissector and bipolar forceps the Glisson capsule medial to the falciform ligament is incised. The arterial and portal branches to the left lateral segment are identified on the left side of the round ligament in the umbilical fossa and clipped; the portal stumps are also oversewn. The division of the hepatic parenchyma is continued cranially and posteriorly towards the IVC, paying attention to the middle hepatic vein, which empties into the left hepatic vein. Once the left hepatic vein is identified before its confluence with the middle hepatic vein, it is skeletonized and transected with a laparoscopic vascular stapler. The specimen is then removed as described below. Though rarely necessary, solitary segmentectomies can also be performed by following the horizontal anatomic plane between these two segments. For resection of segment II, the ports can be placed in the left upper quadrant and the segment approached from the left; the portal pedicle is ligated intraparenchymally.

Segment IV

Segment IV or the quadrate lobe is bordered laterally by the Cantlie line and medially by the falciform ligament anteriorly and the umbilical fissure inferiorly. As with major hepatectomy, we isolate the portal triad prior to commencing resection. As with TLCH, the anterior aspect of the hepatoduodenal ligament is then dissected and the left paramedian branch of the left hepatic artery and the left paramedian branch of the portal vein identified and transected. The falciform ligament is preserved to suspend the liver, and the line of demarcation along the anterior aspect of the liver is scored laterally along the Cantlie line. The parenchymal division is started to the right of the falciform ligament within the umbilical fissure and is carried down to the IVC. The lateral division of the parenchyma is then undertaken along the previously scored line, remaining on the left side of the medial vein. For some posterior lesions it may be necessary to remove the middle vein.

Segment IV is divided into two sections: IVa and IVb. In cirrhotics and others with compromised liver function or multiple hepatic metastases to the extent that postoperative liver failure is a risk, it is advisable to resect only one of these sections when possible. For resection of IVb, the arterial branch from the right branch of the left hepatic artery can be found in the hilar plate. The portal blood supply to this section can be identified in the umbilical fissure and seen going directly into VIb. This vessel is a medioinferior branch of the paramedian branch of the pars umbilicus. In turn, section IVa receives its blood supply from the mediosuperior branch. Once the blood supply to IVb is ligated and transacted, the plane of transection is scored with an ultrasonic dissector along Cantlie line laterally and just lateral to the falciform ligament and umbilical fissure. Instead of continuing the transection superiorly, the junction between IVa and IVb is scored and the hepatic parenchyma dissection completed. A large branch of the middle vein will be encountered and should be clipped or oversewn. Using laparoscopic ultrasound can enhance the localization of this vessel.

For segment IVa, the arterial and portal blood supply cannot be ligated as easily as for section IVb. For this dissection, the portal triad is controlled. The round ligament is retracted on the left, and the superior half of the liver is transected from the anterior border. One has to stop far away from the pedicle of IVb. Laparoscopic ultrasound is absolutely necessary to find and mark the two pedicles. When the inflow is controlled, artery and veins, the demarcation is visible and the resection done in the direction of the middle vein. Again laparoscopic ultrasound is mandatory to find and avoid cutting the branch from IVb. At the end, we follow the middle hepatic vein on the right and the inferior vena cava posteriorly. The resection of IVa and IVb can usually be performed without having to transect the middle hepatic vein (Fig. 36-16). Wedge resections of the anterior segment of IVa close to the junction of the middle hepatic vein with the inferior vena cava are approached laterally, with control of the middle vein in case there is torrential hemorrhage.

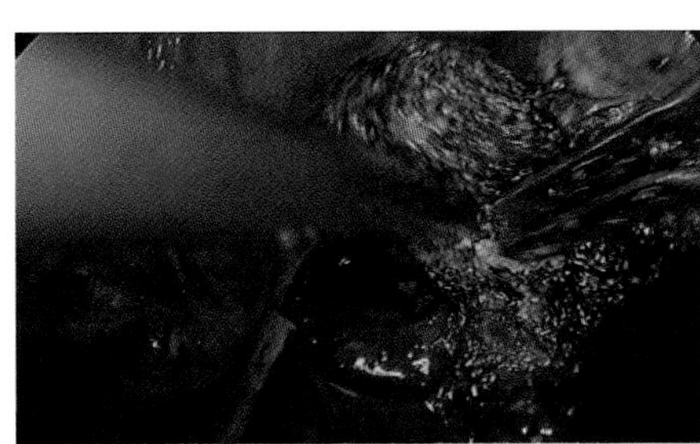

Fig. 36-16. Lateral view of the middle hepatic vein (MHV) as it drains into the inferior vena cava (IVC) for a lesion in segment IVa. The lateral approach has been used to approach this patient. The MHV has been highlighted in blue and the IVC in purple.

Segment V

The resection of segment V should begin by dissecting out the triangle of Calot and ligating the cystic duct and artery; the gallbladder can then be used as a retractor. The parenchymal dissection starts just medial to the gallbladder along the Cantlie line and continues inferiorly until the hepatic hilum is approached. During this dissection the pedicle to segment V will be encountered and is clipped and then transected with the ultrasonic shears or LigaSure device. The line dividing segments V and VI is then scored with the ultrasonic shears laterally until the border with segment VI is determined. In open surgery, this is often done by clamping the paramedian Glisson pedicles to see the line of demarcation between the lateral (VI and VII) and medial (V and VIII) segments of the right lobe. In laparoscopy, the lateral margin of segment V can be ascertained by intraoperative ultrasound and visual inspection. This lateral margin is divided with a combination of bipolar forceps and ultrasonic shears until segment V with and the gallbladder are completely resected from the remaining liver.

Segment VI

One should first control the porta hepatis with a vascular or umbilical tape prior to starting the parenchymal division. Segment VI is approached by mobilizing the right lobe of the liver (see TLRH). In addition, it is sometimes best to skeletonize the right hepatic vein prior to beginning the parenchymal dissection so that control of the right hepatic outflow can be easily obtained. Even with a Pringle maneuver, massive hemorrhage can obscure the retrohepatic space, making laparoscopic control of the hepatic outflow difficult and resulting in a conversion to open surgery.

The borders of resection are scored inferiorly and then anteriorly with ultrasonic shears, and the line connecting segment V and VI is divided as previously mentioned. Two lateral Glisson pedicles are often found feeding segment VI. Ultrasound is extremely useful in localizing the segmental branches and the efferent vein and verifying adequacy of resection margins.

Segments VII and VIII

Because of segment VII's lateral location just below the diaphragm, we approach this segment with the patient in the left

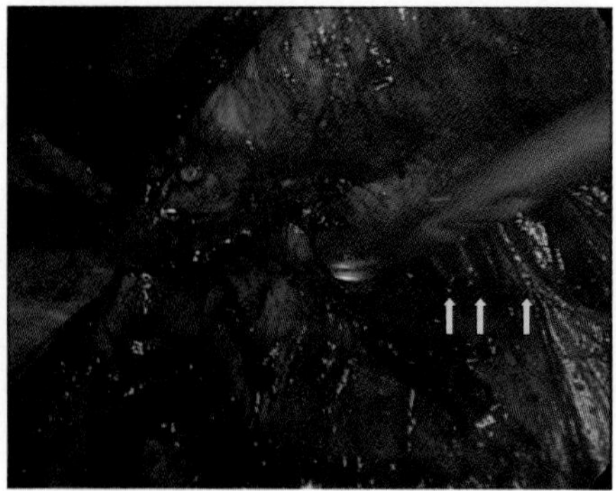

Fig. 36-17. Lateral view of the right hepatic vein (RHV) as it drains into the inferior vena cava (IVC) for a resection of segment VII. The lateral approach has been used to approach this patient. The RHV has been highlighted in blue and the IVC in purple; the arrows point to several small hepatic vessels draining directly into the IVC.

lateral decubitus position with the right arm suspended. Starting with three to four anterior ports, the entire right lobe is mobilized and the hepatic inflow to the liver controlled with an umbilical tape should a Pringle maneuver become necessary. The surgeon then places two more ports in the patient's flank in the same intercostal space as the more lateral one placed through the abdomen. A camera port is placed 5 cm more laterally than the abdominal one and one working 5-mm port is placed along the axillary line. This access enables the assistant standing between the patient's legs to retract the mobilized right liver medially, and the surgeon to dissect and visualize the suprahepatic IVC by cutting the remaining aspect of the right coronary ligament and to gain control of the right hepatic vein under direct vision (Fig. 36-17). An umbilical tape is placed around the right hepatic vein for control of the hepatic outflow, which, in addition to the hepatic inflow control offered by the Pringle maneuver, results in total vascular control.

The line dividing segment VII from VIII is then scored on the right side of the right hepatic vein and continued inferiorly until the efferent vein going to the right hepatic vein and the Glisson pedicle feeding segment VII are found with the help of IUS. These pedicles are controlled in the usual fashion, and the parenchymal dissection is continued laterally along the line dividing segments VI and VII. All large vessels and ducts are clipped or sutured closed. Because the trajectory of the two lateral working ports pass the pleural space, it is important to aspirate with the suction device upon removal of these ports. To date, none of our patients have been found to have a pneumothorax postoperatively.

The approach to segment VIII is the same as for segment VII. The intraoperative ultrasound (IUS) is indispensable in identifying the segmental branches draining segment VIII that run from the middle and right hepatic veins, comprising the lateral borders of the dissection. The inferior limit of the dissection is formed by the segmental branches to segment V; these veins need to be preserved to allow for the venous drainage of this more inferior segment.

REMOVAL OF SPECIMEN AND CLOSURE

When there are no adhesions from previous surgery or inflammatory process, the specimen is removed through a suprapubic incision. When dense adhesions are present in the pelvis, a subcostal incision is sometimes used as the extraction site. Prior to incising the extraction site, the pneumoperitoneum is released via the existing trocars. A retrieval bag is always used to reduce the risk of seeding at the extraction site.

After the specimen is removed, the wound is temporarily sealed and pneumoperitoneum re-established. The surface of the remaining liver is inspected, and vigorous hemostasis is obtained with bipolar electrocautery, surgical clips, or suture. All potential bile leaks are investigated with intraoperative cholangiography or with the transcystic tube air-tightness test. This latter test is performed by instilling air into the biliary tree via the cystic duct stump. The raw parenchymal surface is inspected for bubbles and the remaining main hepatic duct can be evaluated for air with laparoscopic ultrasound. We prefer this test to methylene blue because it can be performed multiple times. Any potential biliary fistulae are closed with absorbable suture. Additionally, fibrin glue or a carrier-bound fibrin sealant can be placed in an effort to reduce postoperative hemorrhage and bile leaks.

At the end of the procedure, the abdomen is irrigated with normal saline and aspirated. Drains are only used if there is a concern for postoperative bile leak or the adequacy of hemostasis. All ports are removed under direct vision, and the pneumoperitoneum is evacuated. The extraction site is irrigated and fascia closed, as are all port sites greater than 10 mm.

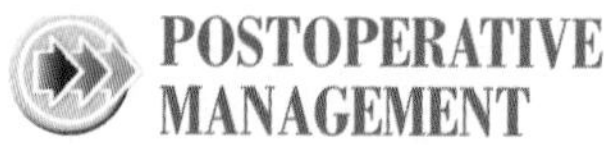

POSTOPERATIVE MANAGEMENT

Because of the need to maintain a low CVP during the division of the hepatic parenchyma, patients are given diuretics during the beginning of the procedure. As a result, it is important to rehydrate patients prior to the end of the procedure to prevent cardiovascular collapse when they are extubated. This rehydration may need to be continued in the postoperative period.

Postoperatively, patients who undergo regular laparoscopic hepatectomies are sent to the regular ward. Patients do not require as intensive monitoring after totally laparoscopic major hepatectomies as they do after open liver resections. They are only sent to the intensive care unit when they have preoperative comorbidities that require additional monitoring in the postoperative period. Furthermore, their length of hospital stay, analgesic requirements, and time to ambulation are significantly decreased. Patients are mobilized out of bed and encouraged to ambulate on postoperative day 1. Low molecular weight heparin is used for deep venous thrombosis prophylaxis until patients are ambulating without assistance. The urinary catheter is also removed unless concerns for fluid management exist; patients are started on a clear liquid diet, which is advanced as tolerated to a regular diet. Patients that undergo major hepatectomies are monitored for 24 hours in the intensive care unit. Complete blood counts and chemistries, including phosphorus levels, are checked daily. Liver function tests are followed, if they were elevated preoperatively, until they are normalized.

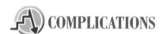

COMPLICATIONS

There has been no higher rate of ascites, bile leak, or postoperative hemorrhage in our series when compared to historical controls of open hepatic resection. In fact, we have noted decreased postoperative ascites. There have been no instances of port-site recurrences, and patient survival is similar in the treatment of liver primary and secondary tumors as compared to an open experience. Historically, the greatest impediment to the widespread adoption of laparoscopic techniques for hepatic resections has been the fear of CO_2 gas embolus. In the literature, mortality from this has only been documented in instances where the argon beam coagulator was in use; as a result, we do not use this device when performing a laparoscopic liver resection.

There has been a particularly low rate of pneumonia in patients treated laparoscopically; in fact, only 1 patient (<1%) developed a documented pulmonary effusion. Abscesses occur rarely (2%) and can usually be treated with antibiotics and percutaneous drainage. Postoperative ileus is also a rare occurrence (1%) that has always resolved with nonoperative management. We have had 2 mortalities (1%) in 206 patients due to postoperative hemorrhage on day number 8 and one patient who died of sepsis as a complication of a bile leak. These patients are also the only two who required reoperation (1%). In total 8 patients (4%) have required transfusions: 4 intraoperatively (2%) and 4 postoperatively (2%). We have diagnosed ascites in four patients (2%) after laparoscopic hepatectomy; all of these patients had a preoperative diagnosis of cirrhosis. When ascites presents, it has always been treated medically, but patients should remain in the hospital until it resolves.

CONCLUSIONS

Minimally invasive hepatectomy is particularly useful in cases of metastases, such as for colorectal cancer, because the laparoscopic approach results in fewer adhesions, and reoperation is much easier in these patients who may require it.

Minimally invasive techniques in hepatic resections are feasible, and high-volume centers that specialize in these techniques can have results similar to historical open series. Currently, only surgeons with advanced training in both laparoscopy and hepatobiliary surgery should attempt these complex procedures. Benefits to the patient include decreased hospital stay, analgesic requirements, and time to ambulation. For the surgeon, the advantages are superior visibility and the ability to visualize all aspects of the procedure. Disadvantages include a loss of palpation and the three-dimensional spatial localization of the tumors in relation to the hepatic structures. Relative contraindications include extrahepatic cholangiocarcinoma that will require extensive biliary reconstruction. Hand-port use may be of assistance when surgeons begin to use minimally invasive techniques for hepatic resections or as an aid in retraction or control of hemorrhage in difficult cases, although we prefer totally laparoscopic techniques. When difficulties arise intraoperatively, particularly in the case of a torrential hemorrhage, there should be no hesitation in converting to an open procedure.

The only absolute contraindications are surgeon ability and comfort level, rather than technical limitations of the laparoscopic approach. As experience grows, these procedures will certainly become more commonly performed.

SUGGESTED READING

Abdalla EK, Noun R, Belghiti J. Hepatic vascular occlusion: which technique? *Surg Clin North Am* 2004;84(2):563–585.

Barbare JC, Boige V, Boudjema K, et al. French guidelines for digestive cancers: hepatocellular carcinoma (primary cancer of the liver). *Gastroenterol Clin Biol* 2006;30:2S57–2S61.

Bouche O, Conroy T, Michel P, et al. French guidelines for digestive cancers: metastatic colorectal cancer. *Gastroenterol Clin Biol* 2006; 30:2S30–2S42.

Burpee SE, Kurian M, Murakame Y. The metabolic and immune response to laparoscopic versus open liver resection. *Surg Endosc* 2002; 16(6):899–904.

Cherqui D, Husson E, Hammoud R, et al. Laparoscopic liver resections: a feasibility study in 30 patients. *Ann Surg* 2000;232(6):753–762.

Cherqui D, Laurent A, Tayar C, et al. Laparoscopic liver resection for peripheral hepatocellular carcinoma in patients with chronic liver disease: midterm results and perspectives. *Ann Surg* 2006;243(4):499–506.

Descottes B, Glineur D, Lachachi F, et al. Laparoscopic liver resection of benign tumors. *Surg Endosc* 2003;17(1):23–30.

Dulucq JL, Wintringer P, Stabilini C, et al. Laparoscopic liver resections: a single center experience. *Surg Endosc* 2005;19(17):886–891.

Figueras J, Llado L, Ruiz D. Complete versus selective portal triad clamping for minor liver resections: a prospective randomized trial. *Ann Surg* 2006;243(1):137–138.

Fortner JG, Blumgart LH. A historic perspective of liver surgery for tumors at the end of the millennium. *J Am Coll Surg* 2001;193(2): 210–222.

Gagner M, Rogula T, Selzer D. Laparoscopic liver resection: benefits and controversies. *Surg Clin North Am* 2004;84(2):451–462.

Gigot JF, Glineur D, Santiago Azagra J, et al. Laparoscopic liver resection for malignant liver tumors: preliminary results of a multicenter European study. *Ann Surg* 2002; 236(1):90–97.

Lesurtel M, Cherqui D, Laurent A. Laparoscopic versus open left lateral hepatic lobectomy: a case-control study. *J Am Coll Surg* 2002;196(2):236–242.

Schmandra TC, Mierdl S, Hollander D, et al. Risk of gas embolism in hand-assisted versus total laparoscopic hepatic resection. *Surg Technol Int* 2004;12:137–143.

Vibert E, Perniceni T, Levard H, et al. Laparoscopic liver resection. *Br J Surg* 2006;93(1): 67–72.

COMMENTARY

At the dawn of laparoscopic general surgery in the late 1980s, the performance of major hepatectomies for cancer cure was simply inconceivable. The shear size of the organ, its vascularity, the invisibility of deep tumors, and the fear of CO_2 embolism seemed to exceed all parameters of laparoscopic abilities. Advances in technology, including improved instruments, novel energy and hemostasis devices, and retractors, etc., have not only enabled major organ resections like total colectomy, radical nephrectomy, and splenectomy, but have also made them commonplace. Major liver resection did require a few particular developments: the first of which was laparoscopic ultrasound. Few open surgeries rely on tactile input as much as major liver resections. Laparoscopic ultrasound has had to replace the hand of the surgeon in large part. For laparoscopic hepatectomy it is used throughout the procedure, from initial staging to checking for bile leaks at the end of the procedure. It is particularly key in the maintenance of margins during resection and for the localization of the major blood vessels. Expertise with the performance and interpretation of laparoscopic ultrasound is absolutely mandatory for those thinking of laparoscopic hepatectomy. Next, reassurance regarding the risk of CO_2 vascular embolism was needed before many surgeons felt comfortable performing liver resection in a positive pressure environment. Fortunately, as Drs. Gayet and Gumbs point out, both laboratory investigations and clinical outcomes from large series have shown that this is not a relevant concern, as long as the gas used is the well-tolerated CO_2. Alternative gases

(continued)

have no place in this surgery, and I would second the author's opinion that using the argon beam coagulator during laparoscopic liver surgery is not a good idea. Initially, the optimal technique and technology for parenchymal division was a mystery; open techniques like finger fracture or crush clamps were not feasible and devices like the CUSA were not useable in the laparoscopic milieu. Innovative new techniques such as the use of endoscopic linear cutters and use of energy sources like ultrasonic coagulation and saline coupled cautery have enabled the laparoscopic approach and are even beginning to influence how open resections are done. As mentioned by the authors, hand-assisted approaches can serve as a bridge technique for surgeons in their learning curve period. I would agree that it is unneeded after one is facile with the tools and techniques of the totally laparoscopic approach. A hand-assist device should always be available during these cases as it can be useful as an alternative to conversion to an open procedure if there are difficulties during the case.

Finally, it can't be stressed enough that the surgeon's skill level—with both advanced laparoscopic and liver surgery—is perhaps the most critical element for the safe and effective practice of minimally invasive liver surgery.

LLS

Diseases of the Pancreas and Spleen

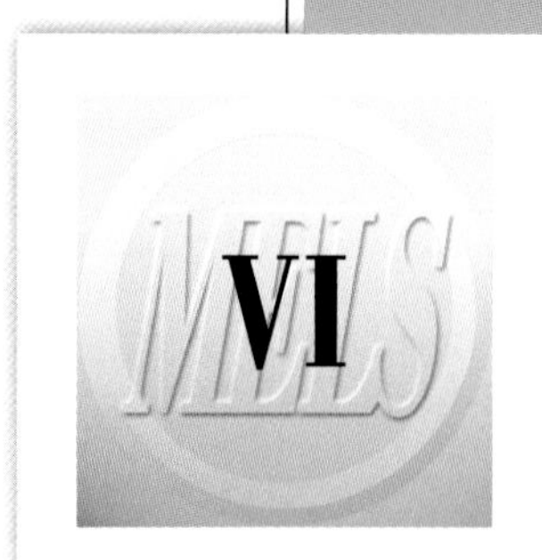

VI

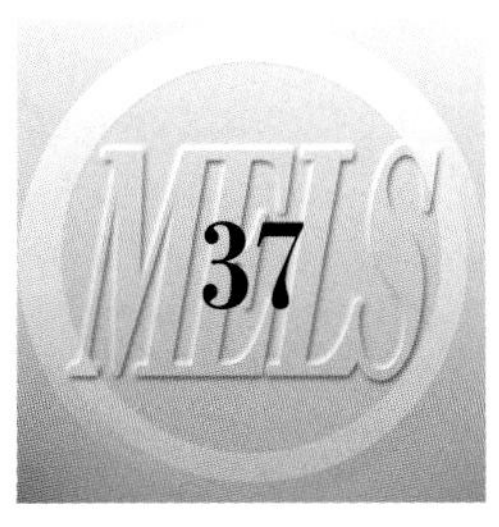

37

Endoscopic Techniques for Staging and Palliation of Pancreatic Masses

BORIS BRONFINE AND MAURICE ARREGUI

INTRODUCTION

A newfound mass in the pancreas is one of the typical pancreatic conditions referred for a surgical opinion. The discovery of such a lesion, often in the head of the pancreas, immediately raises the anxious concerns of a neoplasm, usually malignant. While, in fact, a variety of conditions may be responsible for this finding (Table 37-1, page 364), in a significant percentage of cases the suspicion will unfortunately be confirmed. Up to 70% of solid pancreatic masses are adenocarcinomas, and 30% are other pathology. The immediate questions expected to be answered by the surgeon are: (1) is this lesion likely a malignancy? (2) if yes, is it resectable? and (3) if this condition is symptomatic, is there any intervention that can alleviate the patient's symptoms? The simplification of the traditional approach to such a patient, in the absence of medical contraindication or an obvious, advanced unresectable disease, typically meant surgery as a first line of management. Surgical exploration would be expected to provide the diagnosis, staging, resection if the lesion was amenable to it, or palliation of the symptoms (if it wasn't). Nowadays, however, much of this process can be accomplished by minimally invasive modalities, without submitting patients to a major operation.

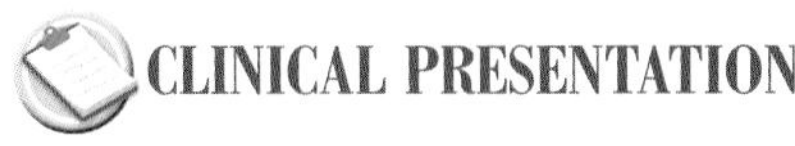

CLINICAL PRESENTATION

The most important factor determining the presentation of a pancreatic lesion, as well as the algorithm of its evaluation, is the location of the mass (Table 37-2, page 365). The classical presentation of a mass in the pancreatic head is painless obstructive jaundice, at the advanced stages complicated by pruritus. An enlarged, distended, and nontender palpable gallbladder (known as a Courvoisier gallbladder) sometimes is found on the physical examination; imaging studies confirm the dilatation of intrahepatic and extrahepatic bile ducts and indicate the level of obstruction at the level of the pancreatic head. Abdominal or back pain is a common symptom at presentation, correlating with a more advanced stage of the malignant disease. Duodenal obstruction is another well known manifestation of these tumors. Pancreatitis (often secondary to the duct obstruction) can occur. In contrast, the mass lesions located in the body or tail of the pancreas do not cause jaundice and can remain latent for a longer period of time, a well-known factor explaining their tendency to be more advanced and often unresectable at initial presentation. Weight loss, abdominal pain, nausea, vomiting, and changes in appetite can occur with tumors in any location. Ascitis, pancreatic insufficiency, and steatorrhea, unexplained thrombophlebitis, or sudden onset of diabetes can be found in some patients. In many cases, unfortunately, distant metastases are the first detected signs of a pancreatic neoplasm. With the increased use of modern medical imaging, more and more pancreatic lesions are found in the asymptomatic stage by an imaging study performed for an unrelated reason.

Once the mass is detected or suspected by clinical findings, a detailed imaging

TABLE 37-1. DIFFERENTIAL DIAGNOSIS OF THE PANCREATIC MASS

Neoplastic

Ductal adenocarcinoma of the pancreas
Ampullary adenocarcinoma
Osteoclast-like giant cell tumor
Acinar cell carcinoma
Cystic neoplasms of the pancreas:
- Serous cystadenoma and cystadenocarcinoma
- Mucinous cystadenoma and cystadenocarcinoma
- Intraductal papillary mucinous neoplasm (IPMN): benign or malignant
- Solid pseudopapillary cystic neoplasm: benign or malignant
- Cystic neuroendocrine neoplasms

Endocrine tumors of the pancreas
- Gastrinoma
- Insulinoma
- VIPoma
- Glucagonoma
- Somatostatinoma
- Carcinoid

Lymphoma
Anaplastic tumors
Adenosquamous carcinoma
Lipoma
Teratoma
Pancreatic sarcoma
Hamartoma
Gastrointestinal stromal tumor (GIST) neoplasms
Metastatic tumors of the pancreas (lung, colon, breast; melanoma; renal cell carcinoma)

Non-neoplastic

Simple cyst
Pancreatic pseudocyst
Chronic focal pancreatitis
Eosinophilic pancreatitis
Pancreatic abscess
Echinococcal cyst
Dermoid cyst
Pancreatic trauma
Intrapancreatic accessory spleen
Tuberculosis
Sarcoidosis
Vascular malformations

evaluation is necessary. Today, the first test of choice is a high-quality computed tomography scan. In our institution, "pancreatic protocol" CT includes helical thin-slice (2.5 mm) multi-detector high-speed three-phase (non-contrast, arterial, and venous phases) scan with sagittal and coronal reconstruction images. While the 16-slice CT scanners of the previous generation had the sensitivity of only up to 60% to 65%, current CT technology can detect a pancreatic mass (such as adenocarcinoma of the pancreas) with sensitivity up to 80% to 85%. This is due to the ability of the current 64-slice CT to obtain precise, thin (even 1-mm) cuts of the pancreas in the shortest time, to allow the exact imaging of arterial and venous phases, and to provide three-dimensional reconstruction images. The abdominal MRI usually doesn't add much to the information obtained by CT. On the other hand, magnetic resonance cholangiopancreatography (MRCP) can be very useful in delineating the relationship of the mass to the biliary and pancreatic ducts or other structures. The imaging may show a typical image of a mass in the pancreatic head associated with common bile duct (CBD) and/or pancreatic duct obstruction, or, quite often, an obstruction with no visible mass. Either way, an endoscopic intervention will be the next step for most of the patients. Currently, these interventions are based on two basic endoscopic approaches of imaging of the pancreas: radiographic visualization of the ducts via endoscopic retrograde cholangiopancreatography (ERCP) and endoscopic ultrasound imaging (EUS). Both these techniques have application for diagnosis and staging as well as for therapeutic interventions.

Endoscopic Techniques Available for the Diagnosis, Staging, and Preoperative Evaluation of Pancreatic Masses

ERCP

Endoscopic Retrograde Cholangiopancreatography (ERCP) has been widely used for the evaluation and treatment of pancreaticobiliary conditions since the 1980s. It's often the first test to be performed when a pancreatic lesion is suspected clinically but cannot be visualized radiologically or for the patient with obstructive jaundice requiring the relief of biliary obstruction. ERCP is useful to confirm the presence of a pancreatic mass, although it has a limited role in the staging of the mass and the assessment of its resectability. It can indirectly indicate the presence of the mass by demonstrating a bile duct or pancreatic duct stricture and its characteristics. It provides an excellent view of the duodenum and papilla and allows the biopsy of periampullary masses or the brush cytology of the biliary and pancreatic ducts. ERCP also has extensive applications in the management of CBD stones and biliary duct neoplasms, which are described in the other parts of this book.

Equipment and Technique

ERCP is typically performed on an outpatient basis with IV sedation using continuous monitoring of the patient's vital signs. General anesthesia may be used in the selective cases. The procedure should take place in a specially designated room with a fluoroscopy unit and mobile procedure table. The patient is placed in the prone position. ERCP is performed with a side-viewing endoscope (duodenoscope). That means that during the introduction of the scope into the esophagus, into the stomach, and then through the pylorus into the duodenal bulb, only a partial view of the lumen can be seen. This type of endoscope allows the perfect visualization of the papilla. Typically, it comes into the view at a 12 o'clock position. The pancreatic duct orifice is typically located at 9'oclock, and the common bile duct at the

TABLE 37-2. TYPICAL PRESENTATIONS OF A PANCREATIC MASS

Periampullary or ampullary mass	Obstructive jaundice GI bleeding and/or anemia Pancreatitis Duodenal obstruction Distant metastasis Incidental finding during GI endoscopy
Mass of the head of the pancreas	Obstructive jaundice Duodenal obstruction Weight loss Pancreatitis Distant metastasis Pain Pancreatic insufficiency Adult-onset insulin-dependent diabetes Endocrine manifestations (islet cell tumors) Incidental finding on imaging studies
Body and the tail of the pancreas	Pain Pancreatitis Weight loss Distant metastasis Pancreatic insufficiency Endocrine manifestations (islet cell tumors) Incidental finding on imaging studies

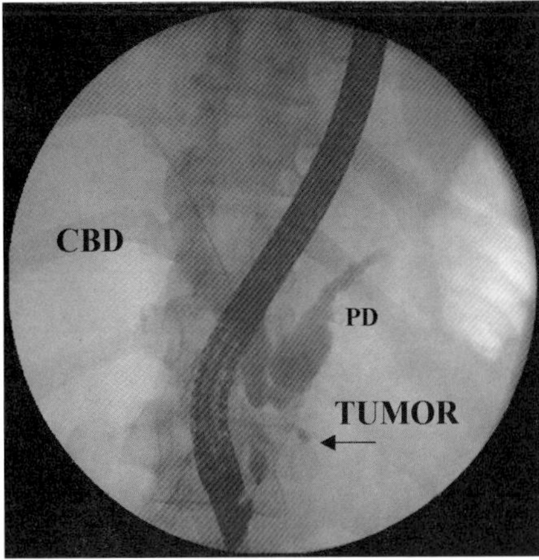

Fig. 37-1. Adenocarcinoma of the head of the pancreas. This ERCP displays a "double duct" sign, or dilated common bile duct (CBD) and pancreatic duct (PD).

11 o'clock position from the center of papilla. Selective cannulation of these ducts is performed. In addition to the usual steering controls, the duodenoscope has an elevator ever, allowing the adjusting of the angle of catheters or other accessories advanced through its instrument channel for precise selective cannulation. A variety of access catheters are used for cannulation, from a standard, slightly tapered catheter (usually the first choice), to smaller fine-tipped, tapered catheters, which can be easier to introduce in a stenotic opening but have a higher risk of creating a submucosal false track. A variety of guidewires, ranging from 0.018-inch to a standard 0.035-inch, are available to help in negotiating difficult strictures, including specialized guidewires, such as hydrophilic, angled or J-shaped, and steerable wires. If sphincterotomy is required, it can be performed by one of two techniques: traction-type sphincterotome or the needle-knife. Traction sphincterotomes such as the Apollo sphincterotome (CONMED; Utica, NY) are first advanced into the ampulla (if needed, over the wire), bent, and then withdrawn, allowing the monopolar current of the sphincterotome wire to divide the muscle of the sphincter of Oddi. If the cannulation is impossible because of the stenosis of the papilla, a small initial incision with the needle-knife may be required to facilitate the passage of papillotome (the so-called pre-cut procedure). The needle-knife sphincterotome is similar to a miniature monopolar cautery blader, which can be used to cut the papilla. It does not require introducing the catheter in the ampulla, but the cut is less precise and less controlled, potentially increasing the risk of complications. This technique is usually reserved for special circumstances: pre-cut of the stenotic papilla, incision over a stent, etc. Other appliances, such as retrieval baskets and balloon catheters, are also available for ERCP. Their appropriate use is described in other parts of this book.

A tissue diagnosis may be obtained during ERCP by the means of intraductal cytological brushing, but this method appears to be far less sensitive than EUS-guided biopsy (45% to 60% vs. about 90% sensitivity). The alternative is endoscopic intraductal biopsy, which when combined with intraductal ultrasound (see below) is reported to have higher sensitivity rates (up to 90%). The future use of DNA analysis assays to evaluate the specimens may increase the accuracy of the brush cytology.

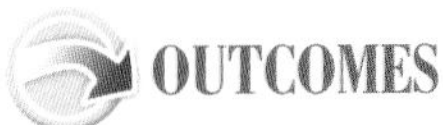

OUTCOMES

When used for the detection of pancreatic head masses, ERCP has a sensitivity and specificity of 90% to 95%. The typical ERCP findings suggesting the presence of a mass lesion in the pancreatic head are a "double duct" sign (strictures or obstruction of the pancreatic duct and distal common bile duct at the same level) or an abrupt cutoff of the duct (Fig. 37-1). Importantly, duct abnormalities with pancreatic tumors are focal and limited, as opposed to the more diffuse changes associated with benign chronic pancreatitis. However, the limitation of ERCP is its poor ability to detect mass lesions in the body, tail, and uncinate process of the pancreas, peripheral lesions located away from the pancreatic duct, and small lesions such as the majority of neuroendocrine tumors. ERCP also can not provide the information regarding the relation of the tumor to the vascular structures that is necessary to determine resectability.

ENDOSCOPIC ULTRASOUND

Endoscopic ultrasound (EUS) has been used for the evaluation of pancreatic masses since 1980s. In the 1990s this technique made a significant technical breakthrough with the development of linear array echoendoscopes, allowing guided biopsies or injections. Just like conventional transabdominal ultrasound, it uses the piezoelectric crystal (in this case, mounted on the tip of an endoscope), which generates high-frequency sound waves and detects their returning echoes to create an image of the biological tissues. The major advantage of the endoscopic ultrasonography, especially in regard to evaluating the pancreas, is that the ultrasound transducer is placed close to the examined organ. This eliminates the acoustic barrier effect of the abdominal wall and abdominal contents. The proximity also allows the use of higher frequencies of

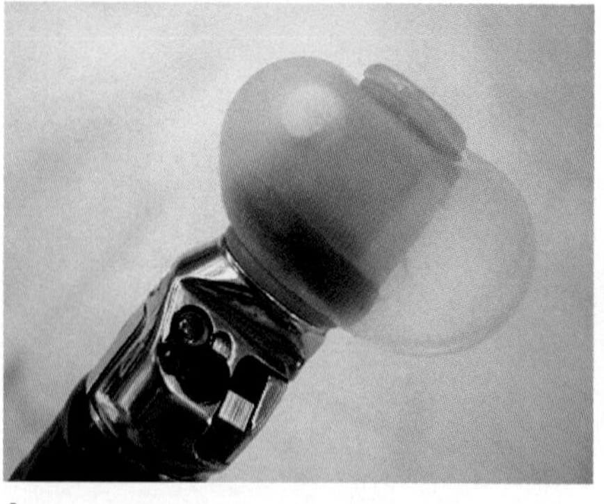

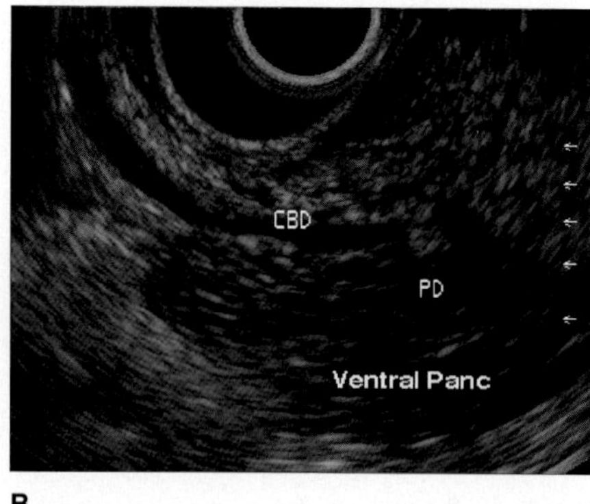

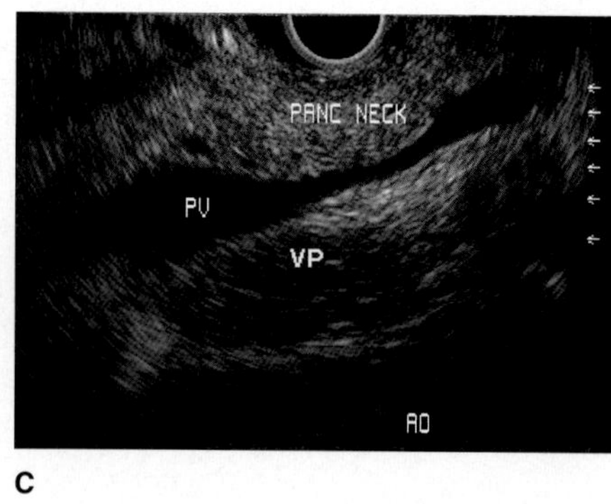

Fig. 37-2. Endoscopic ultrasound of a normal pancreas with radial array echoendoscope. **A.** Radial array echoendoscope. The acoustic balloon around the transducer is inflated with water. **B.** An EUS view of the head of the pancreas, with the scope positioned in duodenum. Note the hypoechogenic or "darker" appearance of the ventral pancreas. **C.** An EUS view of the pancreatic neck area. PD, pancreatic duct; CBD, common bile duct; PV, portal vein; VP, ventral part of the pancreas; AO, aorta.

ultrasound, which have limited depth of penetration but produce ultrasound images of better resolution and quality. EUS is nearly indispensable for diagnostic workup and staging of the pancreatic mass. It can detect small lesions unseen by CT, guide biopsy if needed, demonstrate a lesion's relationship to the duodenal wall, bile and pancreatic ducts, and vascular structures (for the planning of the resection), detect lymph node metastasis, and guide palliative procedures such as celiac ganglion block.

Equipment and Technique

The echoendoscope used to evaluate the pancreas is a fiber-optic endoscope similar to those used for gastroscopy. On its tip there is an ultrasound-emitting transducer connected to a unit similar to the one used in transabdominal ultrasound. Because of the position of the transducer at the tip of the scope, the optic is located slightly proximal to it and at an angle, somewhat in between the configuration of a standard gastroscope and a duodenoscope. The "picture in a picture" software technology allows the operator to see on the screen both the ultrasound image and the endoscopic view, facilitating the advancing and positioning of the scope.

Two main types of echoendoscopes exist today: radial and linear array endoscopes. The transducer of a radial echoendoscope is a piezoelectric crystal that revolves 360 degrees around the longitudinal axis of the endoscope's shaft, or a solid-state crystal producing a similar effect. It is surrounded by a water-filled inflatable balloon, which provides acoustic contact (Fig. 37-2A). The ultrasound frequency of the probe is 7.5 to 12 MHz. This scanhead gives a panoramic 360-degree view of the tissues surrounding it. The image is reconstructed by a processor and displayed as a two-dimensional view of the scanned tissue plane. Linear or curvilinear array echoendoscopes have the transducer oriented longitudinally along the axis of the endoscope. The transducer is immobile; its frequency may be from 5.0 to 12.5 MHz. The modern echoendoscope has a deflectable operating channel (2.0 to 3.8 mm depending on the model), with the angulation controlled by an elevating lever. This arrangement is designed for EUS-guided biopsy or injection, as the needle introduced through the operating channel of the scope can be guided to the target lesion (Fig. 37-3A). The latest models also have color Doppler capability (useful for identifying and avoiding vessels) and the capacity to vary the transducer frequency. The main disadvantage of linear array echoendoscopes is the limitation of the imaging field to 120 to 180 degress, as opposed to the 270- to 360-degree view of radial array endoscopes. Most of the currently available echoendoscopes are produced by Pentax-Hitachi Precision Instrument Corporation, (Orangeburg, NY) and Olympus Corporation (Center Valley, PA).

Recently, an ultrasound scanner capable of three-dimensional reconstruction images has been developed and suggested for the endoscopic use. This technology is based on the electronic tracking of the position of endoscope's tip (its advance and rotation) by a separate sensor system. These data are then integrated with the sonographic images to generate a 3-D picture on the screen.

The EUS evaluation of the pancreas with a radial scope starts with introducing the endoscope and locating the aorta at the level of the lower esophagus for future orientation. Upon advance of the scope in the stomach, the balloon is

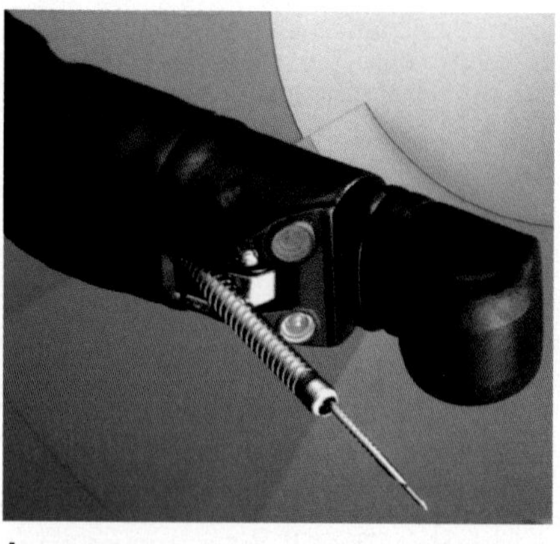

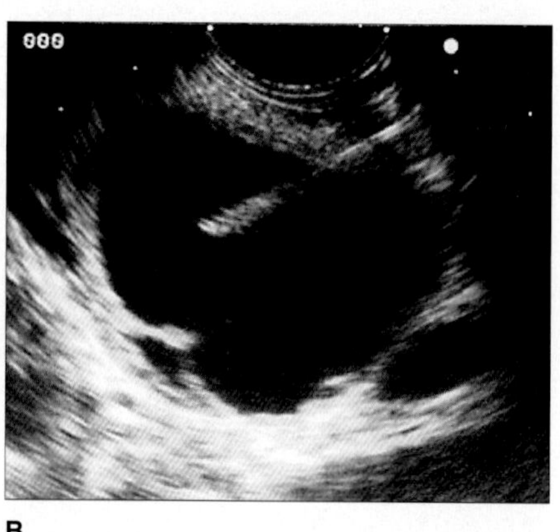

Fig. 37-3. Linear array EUS. **A.** Linear array echoendoscope with biopsy needle. Note the alignment of the needle axis in line with transducer and elevator mechanism of the instrument channel, allowing the adjustment of its angle. **B.** Fine needle aspiration of a cystic pancreatic mass under the linear array EUS guidance.

fully inflated and positioned against the posterior gastric wall. That allows the abdominal aorta, the celiac artery, and eventually the splenic vein and its entrance into the portal vein to be brought into view. The body of the pancreas is located between the splenic vein and the wall of the stomach. The pancreatic duct can be assessed in this position. By following the duct with the rotation of the endoscope, the body and tail of the pancreas can be visualized. By advancing the endoscope in the duodenum, the head of the pancreas and the ventral pancreas (uncinate process) can be seen (Fig. 37-2B to C). The ventral pancreas is often more hypoechoic ("darker") than the dorsal pancreas; this point should be kept in mind to avoid a false impression of pancreatic abnormality in this location. The distal CBD and the pancreatic duct can be seen in the head of the pancreas.

Although it is much more technically demanding for the operator, the diagnostic EUS is essentially not different from a usual upper endoscopy in terms of risks and contraindications. Typically, it is performed on the outpatient basis and under moderate IV sedation. The patients may resume immediately the usual diet, and are discharged home after the procedure.

EUS-Guided Biopsy

In the evaluation of a pancreatic mass, the major advantage of the EUS-guided biopsy, as opposed to a CT-guided percutaneous biopsy, for example, is that the former avoids the well reported complication of cancer seeding of the needle track. In the case of a potentially resectable malignancy, however, tumor seeding of the transduodenal biopsy track is not a concern, as this area will be resected.

EUS-guided fine needle biopsy is performed with a linear array echoendoscope. Usually, 22- or 25-gauge needle is used for the procedure (Fig. 37-3B). New commercially available needles have a Teflon-coated protective sheath to avoid damaging the endoscope channel and a safety mechanism to limit the distance of the advancement of the tip. The biopsy process starts by locating the lesion, evaluating its relation to the vascular structures, and positioning the tip of the endoscope to avoid their accidental puncture. The needle is then advanced under sonographic control into the tumor, with several back-and-forth movements. Aspiration with a 20-ml syringe is continuously maintained. At average, three to four passes of the needle are required to obtain adequate tissue for diagnosis.

Lesions located in the pancreatic body are often easier to sample than the ones in the head, and the lymph node adjacent to the tumor may be an easier target than the tumor itself (especially considering that three passes of the needle through a malignant lymph node are virtually always enough for diagnosis). A Tru-Cut needle biopsy device (Allegiance Healthcare Corporation; McGaw Park, IL) has become available in the last few years. Its theoretical advantage is the smaller number of passes needed to obtain the adequate sample. However, this needle is stiff and will not fire if the echoendoscope is angulated, which limits its use to more easily biopsied lesions accessible from the stomach. Preliminary data suggest that the fine needle aspiration (FNA) and Tru-Cut biopsy have similar sensitivity.

The obtained specimen should be expelled from the needle (for example, by using the stylet), fixed on the slide, and immediately passed to the pathologist. The presence of a cytotechnician in the endoscopy suite is strongly recommended. It allows the endoscopist to immediately know the diagnostic adequacy of the obtained sample. It addition to the cytological examination, immunochemistry and flow cytometry methods can be used; they are especially valuable in the diagnosis of lymphoma. Recently, the DNA analysis of pancreatic specimens started to gain popularity. This approach includes the microdissection of obtained cells with the extraction of DNA that is then amplified by polymerase chain reaction (PCR). Currently available comprehensive DNA testing assays, such as RedPath Integrated Pathology system (Pittsburgh; PA), include the quantitative analysis of mutant K-ras genes and identify the abnormal loci of allelic gains or losses. The preliminary data suggest that they may significantly improve the diagnostic accuracy of EUS samples, for example, in differentiating pancreatic cancer from focal chronic pancreatitis, and one type of cystic pancreatic neoplasms from another. The value of these new modalities is being evaluated, but they may prove highly beneficial for the subgroup of EUS-guided FNA or ERCP brush cytology samples that are deemed highly suspicious but not diagnostic of cancer.

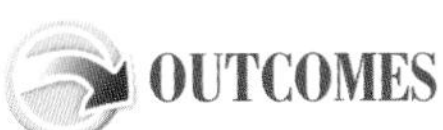

OUTCOMES

In general, EUS is more sensitive than CT, MRI, and ERCP in the detection of the pancreatic masses, especially small tumors less than 3 cm in size. It should be a next step if the CT and/or MRI fail to demonstrate a mass suspected by the clinical manifestations (such as obstructive jaundice without gallstones). In general, EUS should not compete with CT, MRI, or PET scan in the algorithm of evaluation of a pancreatic mass, as it has different capabilities and provides the surgeon with a different type of information. Moreover, the accuracy of EUS interpretation is improved if the endoscopist is familiar with the patient's previous imaging data, as studies of the interpretation of EUS tapes by experienced operators have demonstrated.

The main limitation of EUS in general is that this technique (as all ultrasound modalities) is very operator-dependent. Furthermore, EUS of the pancreas is technically one of the most complex areas of endoechosonography, requiring experience in both technical aspects of the procedure and interpreting of the findings. For example, normal differences in the sonographic appearance of the uncinate process and the dorsal pancreas may be falsely interpreted as the presence of a mass. In other cases, blood vessel involvement can be overestimated by the gastroenterologist without operative experience, a tumor can be declared unresectable based on its presumed invasion of the portal vein, and the patient not referred for surgical opinion.

Complications of EUS include bleeding, pancreatitis, perforation, and the infrequent complications related to sedation. The reported frequency of complications is 0.5% to 3% for EUS with biopsy, with most complications being minor and self-limited; it is even less for purely diagnostic procedures. Considering the value of the data obtained against the risks, the argument may be made that at least non-invasive EUS should be a routine part of the workup of any pancreatic mass considered for resection. It is also very helpful in the settings of an unresectable malignancy or symptomatic benign mass (see below).

EUS may have a role in the screening of high-risk individuals, such as patients with Peutz–Jeghers syndrome (up to 30% risk of pancreatic cancer) or those with a family history of the disease, which is found in up to 10% of pancreatic cancer patients. The best screening algorithm for this group is still unclear.

INTRADUCTAL ULTRASOUND

Intraductal ultrasound (IDUS) is more frequently applied to the evaluation of the biliary tree, but there is an evidence of its

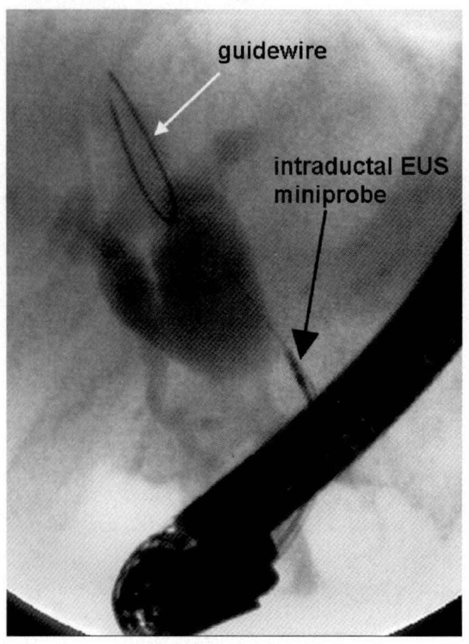

A

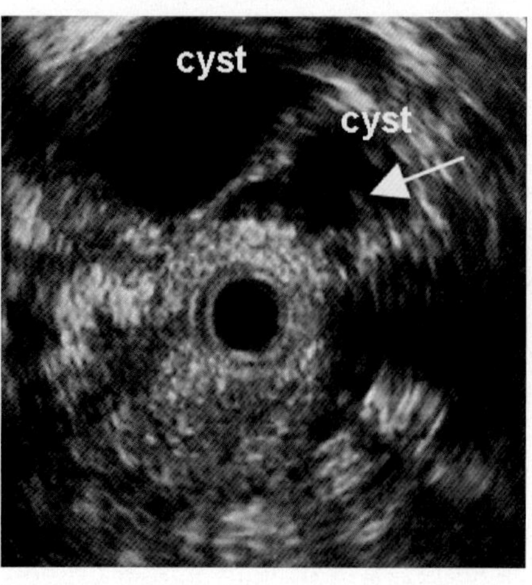

B

Fig. 37-4. Intraductal endoscopic ultrasound (IDUS). **A.** Fluoroscopic view of the mini-ultrasound probe inserted into the bile duct. **B.** Intraductal ultrasound with the probe in the proximal common bile duct. This view shows the area of the stricture caused by a malignant cystic tumor of the pancreas. Note the cysts with septations and irregular walls with projections. (From Machi J, Staren ED, eds., *Ultrasound for Surgeons*, 2nd ed., Philadelphia: Lippincott Williams & Wilkins, 2005.)

usefulness in evaluating pancreatic masses as well. This technique uses small-calibre (2.6 mm or less) ultrasound probes that can be passed through the operating channels of standard endoscopes into pancreatic or biliary ducts. The imaging produced by these probes is of a high quality, as the method takes advantage of excellent acoustic transmission through the fluid-filled ducts and the short distance between the probe and the examined anatomic structures. This allows the use of higher frequency probes (12 to 30 MHz), which produces images of better resolution. Radial, linear, and combined arrays have been developed, and single- or multiple-use designs are available. Some of the probes can be advanced over a wire, facilitating their placement into the duct. The advance of the probe in the distal pancreas may be difficult because of tortuosity of the pancreatic duct. The tail of the pancreas can be reached in only 35% to 55% of IDUS studies, which constitutes a certain limitation of this technique. Another limitation is the potential risk of pancreatitis, which, however, doesn't appear to be greatly increased in comparison to a standard ERCP. The technique appears particularly useful in differentiating pancreatic duct strictures (benign vs. malignant) and may be more sensitive and specific than EUS, CT, or ERCP. Another indication is the evaluation of cystic mucin-producing neoplasms of the pancreas (Fig. 37-4). Malignant tumors of this category and neoplasms with premalignant potential require surgical treatment, but the benign ones can generally be safely observed. The presence of mural nodules on an IDUS of the pancreatic ducts is highly indicative of malignancy; another important sign is the presence of papillary projections in the side branches of the duct. The detection rate for these findings is approaching 100%, according to the results of some studies. By some data, IDUS may be more sensitive than EUS in locating the small neuroendocrine tumors of the pancreas, especially the multifocal ones, such as in multiple endocrine neoplasia (MEN) syndrome.

Applications of Endoscopic Staging and Evaluation for Different Pancreatic Pathologies

DUCTAL ADENOCARCINOMA OF THE PANCREAS

Pancreatic adenocarcinoma is the fourth leading oncological cause of death in the U.S. and probably the most devastating of all gastrointestinal (GI) cancers. More than 30,000 new cases per year currently occur in the U.S., and almost all of these patients die of this disease. Most of these neoplasms present in the unresectable stage; even the 15% to 20% of the patients who have an apparently local and resectable tumor will develop recurrence, with an ultimate mortality in 85% to 90% of cases. The overall 5-year survival rate remains about 5%. The main issue in a case of suspected or proven pancreatic adenocarcinoma is differentiating between resectable and unresectable stages of the disease. It is critical to offer resection as the best chance to improve survival and quality of life to the appropriate patients in the first category and to avoid major and risky unnecessary surgery in patients in second group.

Endoscopic ultrasound plays an extremely useful role in this regard. The typical appearance of the pancreatic cancer on the EUS is a distinct hypoechoic ("dark") area (Fig. 37-5). The cancer can also appear as an irregular lesion with mixed hyper- and hypoechoic patterns. When the tumor is obstructing the pancreatic duct, the uninvolved pancreas may have a pattern of chronic pancreatitis (hypoechoic, with dilated distal pancreatic ducts). Overall, EUS is able to correctly determine the T-stage of cancer in 78% to 94% patients, and its accuracy is generally higher with the more advanced lesions (T3 and T4). Importantly, it is very helpful in determining the relation of the mass to the portal vein, splenic vein, hepatic artery, celiac trunk, and superior mesenteric vessels, as well as assessing their patency (Fig. 37-5C). This is of extreme importance if resection of the mass is considered. Direct invasion (as opposed to encasement) is suggested by loss of the normal border of the vessel. EUS is more accurate than CT, MRI, and probably arteriogram in detecting vascular invasion by the tumor, with the caveat that the portal and splenic vein are more easily seen by EUS than the superior mesenteric vessels, in which case the arteriogram performs better.

The adjacent lymph nodes can also be evaluated. Normal lymph nodes have an oval shape and a hyperechoic center or hilum with a thin hypoechoic rim, and are usually less than 1 cm in size. Abnormal lymph nodes (inflammatory or containing metastatic tumors) lose their hypoechoic center and often become round and enlarged. The status of peripancreatic lymph nodes, which are routinely included in a Whipple resection, is less important than the status of perihepatic, perigastric, celiac, or paraaortic nodes. If EUS-guided biopsy

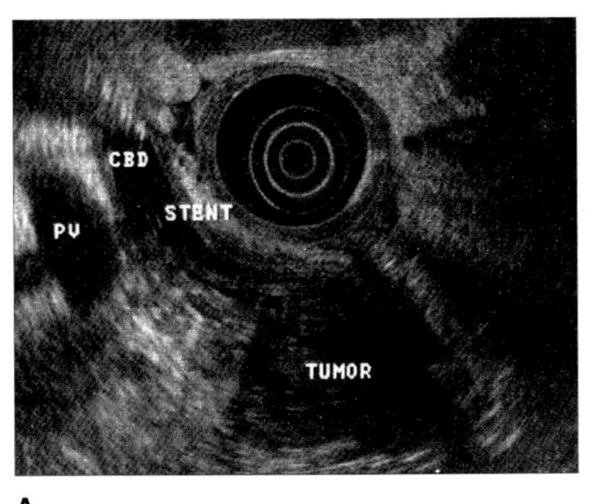

A

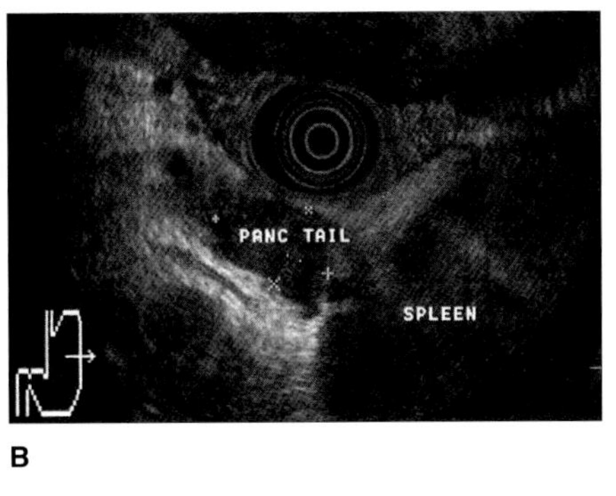

B

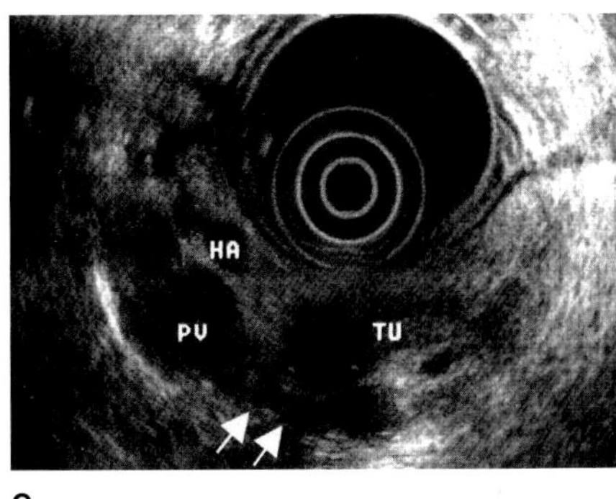

C

Fig. 37-5. An EUS evaluation of pancreatic cancer. **A.** Adenocarcinoma of the pancreatic head. View from the duodenal bulb. Note the previously placed stent in the common bile duct. **B.** Adenocarcinoma of the tail of the pancreas, near the spleen. View from the stomach. This lesion was not seen on CT scan. **C.** Adenocarcinoma of the neck of the pancreas (marked TU) with the impingement of the portal vein. This lesion is not invading the portal vein and is thus potentially resectable. PV, portal vein; CBD, common bile duct; HA, hepatic artery. (From Machi J, Staren ED, eds., *Ultrasound for Surgeons*, 2nd ed., Philadelphia: Lippincott Williams & Wilkins, 2005.)

of these groups of distant lymph nodes provides a positive diagnosis, it renders the cancer unresectable. The accuracy of EUS in determining the nodal (N) involvement is between 64% and 82%. Additionally, EUS partially visualizes the left lobe of the liver and can detect smaller metastatic liver lesions than the CT scan.

A separate area of controversy is the appropriate use of EUS-guided biopsy of the solid pancreatic mass itself. As described above, this procedure is technically feasible and reliable in experienced hands, with a sensitivity of 80% to 90% (and up to 96% to 99% in some series). That means, however, that even in the best hands the biopsy can miss up to 20% of pancreatic cancers. Therefore, the majority of experienced pancreatic surgeons believe that preoperative biopsy and tissue confirmation of the malignancy are not necessary if the mass otherwise appears resectable. The chance of a resected pancreatic lesion coming back as benign (5% to 10% of the specimens in several large studies from high-volume centers) is probably more acceptable than the risk of missing a resectable cancer because it didn't show on the biopsy. This is particularly true considering the improvement of mortality and morbidity of pancreatic resections in high-volume centers and the fact that many of these patients with benign disease will ultimately develop symptoms that require an intervention. Even the proponents of routine biopsy will concede that negative results should not be a contraindication to resection in cases of high clinical suspicion. This conclusion might change, of course, if the sensitivity of EUS-guided biopsy improves in the future to make the risk of missing a cancer acceptably low.

On the other hand, routine biopsy is clearly indicated in some settings, including:

1. Unresectable tumors, to prove the malignancy prior to nonsurgical treatment, such as chemoradiation therapy, especially for novel treatment protocols.
2. Suspicious or indeterminate lymph nodes outside of the field of resection, such as celiac, perigastric, paraaortic, or perihepatic lymph nodes. If these lymph nodes are positive, it makes the cancer unresectable for cure.
3. In appropriate clinical settings, to rule out a pathology that can be managed without surgical resection, such as pancreatic lymphoma, small

TABLE 37-3. STAGING OF DUCTAL ADENOCARCINOMA OF THE PANCREAS

TNM definition
Primary tumor (T)
Tis: Carcinoma in situ
T1 Tumor limited to the pancreas, 2 cm or less in greatest dimension
T2: Tumor limited to the pancreas, more than 2 cm in greatest dimension
T3: Tumor extends beyond the pancreas but without involvement of the celiac axis or the superior mesenteric artery
T4: Tumor involves the celiac axis or the superior mesenteric artery (unresectable primary tumor)
Regional lymph nodes (N)
NX: Regional lymph nodes cannot be assessed
N0: No regional lymph node metastasis
N1: Regional lymph node metastasis
Distant metastasis (M)
MX: Distant metastasis cannot be assessed
M0: No distant metastasis
M1: Distant metastasis
Stages
Stage 0: Tis, N0, M0
Stage IA: T1, N0, M0
Stage IB: T2, N0, M0
Stage IIA: T3, N0, M0
Stage IIB: Any T, N1, M0
Stage III: T4, any N, M0
Stage IV: Any T, any N, M1

American Joint Committee on Cancer, Chicago, Il. *AJCC Staging Manual*, 6th Edition (2002), published by Springer-Verlag, New York, NY.

cell carcinoma, tuberculosis, or an inflammatory mass.

4. In the situation where it might be preferable to accept a 10% to 15% risk of missing a malignancy rather than to proceed with major procedure without a confirmed cancer. The examples include a patient with significant comorbidities or when there is a high clinical suspicion that the lesion might be inflammatory and not malignant.

AMPULLARY NEOPLASMS

The endoscopy is very helpful in determining the diagnosis of an ampullary mass, its resectability, and the best approach to the resection (serial endoscopic excision vs. Whipple resection). ERCP is usually the best test to completely visualize and assess the lesion and to obtain a good biopsy sample. EUS, on the other hand, can reliably determine the T-stage of these neoplasms (with 80% accuracy) by detecting the invasion of separate layers of the duodenal wall. It is somewhat less precise in determining the N-stage of ampullary cancers (59% accuracy in assessing the nodal status).

Pancreatitis

Focal chronic pancreatitis and autoimmune pancreatitis are two benign entities that can most frequently mimic pancreatic cancer and should be considered in the differential diagnosis of a newly found pancreatic mass. They account for the majority of patients who are found to have a benign pathology after a radical pancreatoduodenectomy for presumed malignancy. In general, EUS findings suggesting pancreatitis are an irregular, inhomogeneous pattern with calcifications (seen as hyperechoic foci), diffuse and long duct strictures (as opposed to the focal ones), diffuse dilatation of the duct, and pancreatic duct stones. It is extremely difficult, if not impossible, however, to rule out cancer in these patients by endoscopic findings alone. A negative biopsy of the mass does not rule out malignancy with 100% certainty either.

CYSTIC NEOPLASMS OF THE PANCREAS

Cystic neoplasms of the pancreas represent a group of relatively uncommon lesions. Nevertheless, they cause significant diagnostic concerns, because the behavior and management of different tumors in this group is quite different. Some of them (e.g., serous cystadenoma) have a relatively benign natural history, while other ones, such as mucinous cystadenoma and intraductal papillary mucinous neoplasms (IPMN), have distinct premalignant potential and may contain cancer at the time of diagnosis. In total, about 1% of pancreatic malignancies originate from cystic neoplasms. Differential diagnosis between neoplastic cystic masses and non-neoplastic cystic masses (such as pseudocysts) and between different types of cystic neoplasms is not easy. It involves the both the assessment of CT and MRI and of ERCP, with pancreatography and sampling of the cyst's contents, and serological markers. EUS is an extremely useful modality in this setting, and different cystic neoplasms have some distinct EUS characteristics (Table 37-4). Serous cystadenomas are usually multilobulated multicystic masses with a honeycomb pattern. Mucinous cystadenomas are generally larger with fewer septations (Fig. 37-6A). In the case of IPMN, the EUS usually shows a diffusely dilated pancreatic duct with cystic dilatation of the side branches (Fig. 37-6B). EUS also allows the guided aspiration of a cystic mass with fluid analysis (amylase, CEA, mucin levels, and cytology). A high amylase level usually suggests benign cyst or pseudocyst. Serous cystadenoma fluid typically has a low viscosity and mucin level, low CEA and CA 19-9, and a positive periodic acid Schiff (PAS) stain for glycogen. The cyst-fluid CEA levels alone could yield a diagnostic accuracy of 75% to 90% using a level of CEA between 150 and 200 as a threshold, but at this point it is not possible to rely solely on this data to determine the benign or malignant character of a cystic mass. Newly available DNA analysis methods such as RedPath Integrated Pathology assay (RedPath Integrated Pathology, Inc.; Pittsburgh, PA) can detect key DNA abnormalities in aspirated samples; for example, microsatellite loss and k-ras point mutation. In the near future, such tests have a potential to become extremely valuable markers in distinguishing cystic neoplasms with the risk of malignancy from the benign ones.

TABLE 37-4. DIFFERENTIAL DIAGNOSIS OF PSEUDOCYSTS AND CYSTIC NEOPLASMS OF THE PANCREAS

Diagnosis	Risk of malignant transformation	Appearance on ERCP and EUS	Cyst fluid analysis	FNA Cytology
Pseudocyst	None	Single or multiple cysts, sometimes communicating with pancreatic duct; inflammatory changes in surrounding pancreas	• Low mucin content • High amylase • Low CEA levels	Inflammatory
Serous Cystadenoma	Only few cases reported	Multiple small (<2 cm) cystic areas in sponge-like pattern, sometimes with central scar or calcification	• Low mucin content • Variable amylase level • Low CEA	Variable
Mucinous Cystadenoma	Up to 45%	Large cystic lesions with intramural growth, without duct communication. No dilatation of the pancreatic duct	• Often high mucin content • Variable amylase level • High CEA	Positive in 50% (columnar epithelial cells)
Intraductal Papillary Mucinous Neoplasm (IPMN)	Up to 30%	Markedly dilated main and secondary pancreatic ducts, papillary and nodular projections	• High mucin content • Variable amylase level • High CEA	Usually positive

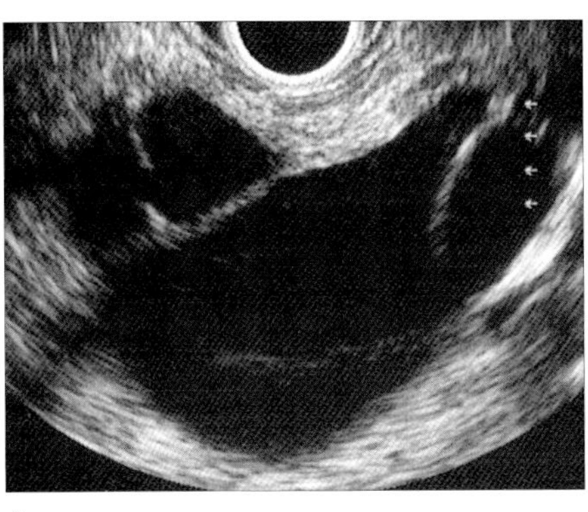

A

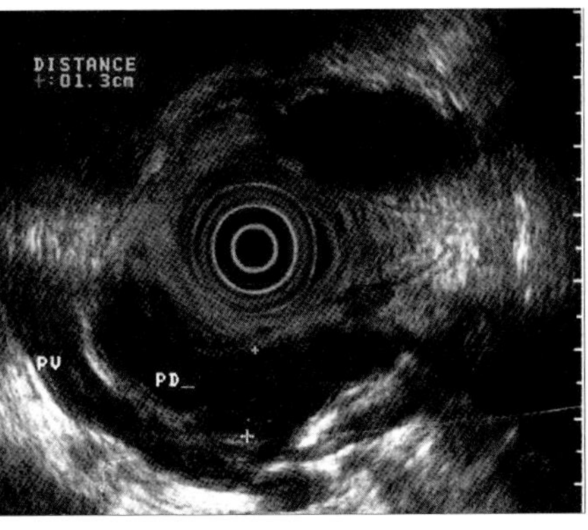

B

Fig. 37-6. Cystic neoplasms of the pancreas. **A.** The appearance of a mucinous cystadenoma of the pancreas on EUS. **B.** Intraductal papillary mucinous neoplasm of the pancreas. Note the dilated and irregular pancreatic duct. EUS, endoscopic ultrasound; PD, pancreatic duct; PV, portal vein. (From Machi J, Staren ED, eds., *Ultrasound for Surgeons*, 2nd ed., Philadelphia: Lippincott Williams & Wilkins, 2005.)

ISLET CELL TUMORS

The neuroendocrine tumors of the islet cells of the pancreas have two typical patterns of presentation. Functioning tumors usually manifest themselves by endocrine symptoms when the tumor is small and often undetectable by radiological studies. Nonfunctioning neoplasms present when the tumor is advanced enough to cause local symptoms (abdominal pain, biliary or duodenal obstruction, bleeding) or the symptoms of metastatic disease. Endoscopic modalities are often required to help locate the tumor in the first scenario. EUS is particularly useful, as it is the most sensitive preoperative method of locating small endocrine pancreatic neoplasms less than 2 cm in size, especially insulinomas. It can find neuroendocrine tumors as small as 3 mm in size and has an additional advantage of detecting tumors located within the duodenal wall or peripancreatic lymph nodes. Islet cell tumors usually present on EUS as small, smooth, discrete, homogeneous hypoechoic masses (Fig. 37-7). EUS can assess the proximity of the mass to the pancreatic duct or significant vessels and help in the planning of the surgical excision. Zimmer et al. found the overall sensitivity of EUS localization to be 93% for insulinomas and 79% for gastrinomas. In comparison, spiral CT has an overall sensitivity of only 17% for insulinomas (which are usually small). Generally, the recommendation is to proceed with EUS if the islet cell tumor can't be located by CT or MRI. In the case of gastrinomas, the alternative to EUS is somatostatin receptor scintigraphy (OctreoScan; Mallinckrodt Medical, Inc.; St. Louis, MO). ERCP and other endoscopic techniques have a limited role in the workup of islet cell tumors.

PANCREATIC METASTASES

Pancreatic metastases are typically large solitary masses, equally likely to be found in any part of the pancreas. Multifocal or diffuse involvement may also occur. The majority of these metastases are asymptomatic. The most common metastatic malignancy involving the pancreas is renal cell carcinoma, followed by lung, breast, and colon cancers, melanoma, and sarcomas. The endoscopic biopsy will establish the diagnosis.

PANCREATIC INCIDENTALOMA

A pancreatic mass incidentally found on the imaging study performed for unrelated reasons is an increasingly frequent scenario. The advent of a superior multi-slice CT technology since its coming to the market in the late 1990s has led to more CT studies being performed faster and with better resolution. Today, more than 50 million CT scans are performed in the U.S. every year. In addition to the CT, MRI, or ultrasound, pancreatic mass lesions are sometimes found during the workup of an asymptomatic elevation of serum pancreatic enzymes or incidentally during endoscopy. A recent study from Johns Hopkins Hospital reported that out of 1944 consecutive pancreatoduodenectomies performed in large U.S. centers over the last 8 years, 6% presented as an incidental finding. Of these incidentalomas, 31% were malignant, 47% had premalignant disease, and the remaining 22% were benign lesions with little or no risk of progression to malignancy (benign cystadenomas and inflammatory masses). The most common diagnosis was IPMN without malignant cancer (30%), followed by cystadenoma (17%), and pancreatic ductal adenocarcinoma (10%). Approximately 10% were neuroendocrine tumors of the pancreas. Predictably, incidentally found malignant tumors were discovered at an earlier stage than symptomatic ones (34.4% of stage I cancers vs. 10.4%) and these asymptomatic patients had a superior long-term survival after resection when compared to the patients who

A

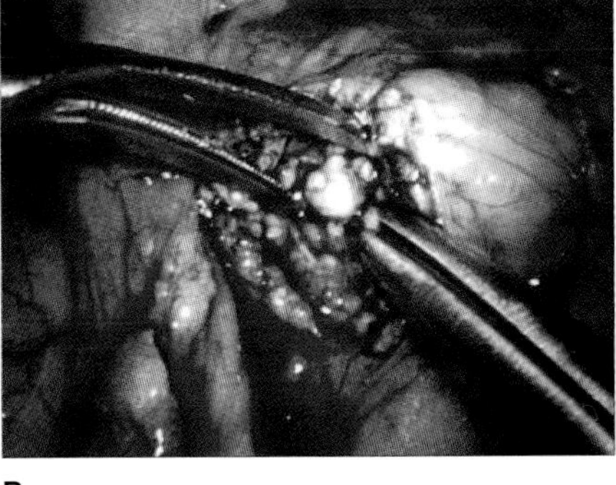

B

Fig. 37-7. Islet cell tumors. **A.** A 58-year-old nurse found to have hypoglycemia while at work. Workup was consistent with an insulinoma. EUS localized a small 3.6 × 2.8 mm insulinoma at the pancreatic neck adjacent to the pancreatic duct. **B.** The same patient while undergoing LUS-guided resection. Note the small insulinoma (small white arrow) held in the laparoscopic DeBakey clamp. EUS, endoscopic ultrasound; LUS, laparoscopic ultrasound; I, insulinoma; PD, pancreatic duct; PV, portal vein. (From Machi J, Staren ED, eds., *Ultrasound for Surgeons*, 2nd ed., Philadelphia: Lippincott Williams & Wilkins, 2005.)

presented with symptoms. It must be mentioned that the study only included lesions found in the area of the head of the pancreas and not ones that were managed conservatively, without operation. In general, there is insufficient data about the optimal management of this new, interesting problem. EUS evaluation should probably be recommended after imaging studies as the next step in the workup for unexplained, suspicious pancreatic incidentaloma. Solid lesions in the elderly patient should raise the concern of pancreatic adenocarcinoma and be addressed accordingly. Regarding asymptomatic cystic lesions, the trend is to observe them if they are less than 2 cm in size and without suspicious characteristics in a reliable patient without any risk factors. The analysis of such cysts demonstrates that only 3.5% harbor a malignancy, in contrast to 26% in larger asymptomatic lesions (the average rate was 17%). In addition, 40% contain premalignant epithelium. A recent study reported that approximately 78% of incidentally found cystic lesions were resected and 22% managed by observation.

Applications of Endoscopic Modalities for Palliation of Pancreatic Lesions

Most patients with malignant pancreatic conditions and many with benign ones will require a palliative intervention at some point. Historically this consisted of a surgical procedure: for example, hepaticojejunostomy or cholecystojejunostomy for biliary obstruction, gastrojejunostomy for duodenal obstruction, or celiac ganglion ablation for chronic pain. These procedures are still performed in patients found to be unresectable at the time of surgical exploration for pancreatic malignancy. Nevertheless, the majority of palliative interventions are nowadays performed endoscopically, percutaneously, or laparoscopically with excellent results.

PALLIATION OF BILIARY OBSTRUCTIONS

A malignant mass of the pancreatic head is the most common cause of malignant obstructive jaundice. This condition has the potential to be extremely disabling, as it is associated with severe pruritus, malabsorption, anorexia, and vitamin K deficiency. Therefore, relief of the biliary obstruction is an important palliative strategy. Biliary stents are a well established modality for palliation of obstructive jaundice, especially in patients with limited life expectancy. When compared with surgical bypass in several randomized studies, endoscopic stenting demonstrated similar long-term survival rates but shorter hospitalization, a lower rate of complications, and less procedure-related mortality. On the other hand, stented patients required more frequent readmissions for stent occlusion, stent migration, and cholangitis. Endoscopically placed biliary stents also appear to have a higher success rate (81% vs. 61%) and lower morbidity and mortality than the percutaneously placed ones, mostly by avoiding complications associated with liver puncture, such as bile leaks and bleeding.

There are two general types of biliary stents available for endoscopic placement: cheaper, simpler-to-place plastic stents and more expensive, expandable metal stents with a longer life. In general, plastic stents are more advantageous for patients with an expected survival of 6 months or less, and the metal expandable stents are for the patients expected to survive more than 6 months. The plastic stents selected for cases of malignant obstruction are usually 10 to 11.5F in size and should be 2 to 3 cm longer than the area of obstruction. The stents are placed over a guidewire positioned via ERCP. Correct positioning of the stent is verified by fluoroscopy and is usually confirmed by a free flow of bile after the stent is placed (Fig. 37-8). The average patency period of the standard large diameter plastic stent is 2 to 3 months. The usual explanation of a stent's malfunction is due to an obstruction formed from bacterial biofilm inside the stent with eventual occlusion of its lumen. In many cases, however, a stent with an obviously occluded lumen will not necessarily result in clinical biliary obstruction, so the exact mechanisms of the function—and malfunction—of the stent may be more complex. Attempts to prolong stent life by using larger stents, modifying the stent's design, and adding ursodeoxycholic acid or oral antibiotics so far have not been significantly successful. Unlike the primary jaundice caused by the pancreatic mass itself, jaundice associated with an occluded stent often leads to cholangitis because of the loss of the sphincter of Oddi's valve mechanism. Urgent ERCP with exchange of the stent is indicated in these patients.

Self-extendable metal stents (SEMS) are made of stainless steel, nitinol wire

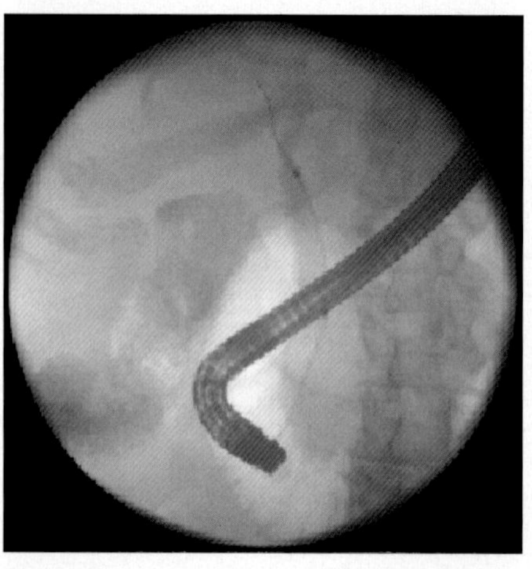
A

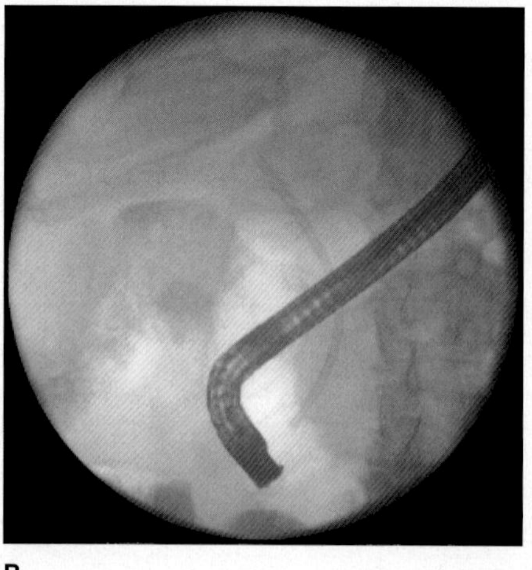
B

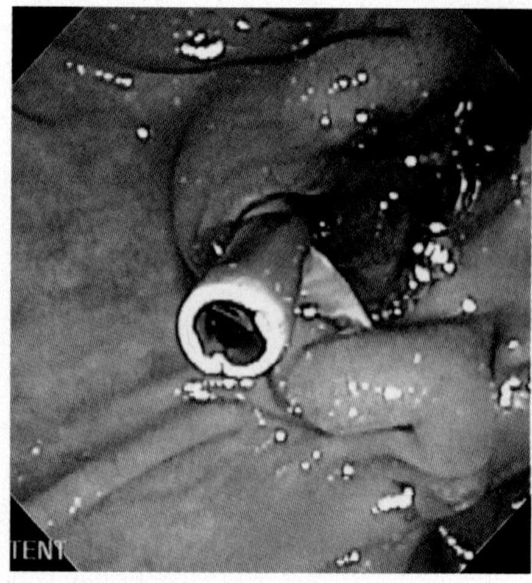
C

Fig. 37-8. Placement of a palliative plastic common bile duct stent. **A.** The endoscopic positioning of the stent delivery system in the common bile duct. **B.** Placement of the plastic stent. **C.** The placed stent as seen from the duodenum.

mesh, or spiral coil. They are mounted on a small-diameter delivery system that can be introduced through the operating channel of an ERCP scope and are deployed by withdrawing the protective sheath or releasing a trip wire. Various models of SEMS are available in 6- to 10-mm diameters and various lengths. The stents themselves are 20 to 30 times more expensive than their plastic counterparts, but their longer life is well documented. SEMS are not immune to obstruction, however, usually caused by the tumor ingrowth. The development of covered expandable metal stents has decreased the incidence of their obstruction. More recently, multiple-layer stents have been developed, such as the Double Layer stent (Olympus America Inc.; Center Valley, PA). It consists of a middle frame of stainless steel mesh covered with a water-repellent Teflon inner layer and an outer layer of polyamide elastomere. The hope is that these stents will have a patency rate comparable to extendable metal stents, while being much less costly.

As an alternative, the creation of choledochoduodenal anastomosis under EUS guidance has also been described in the literature. It consists of accessing the proximal CBD through the wall of the second part of duodenum with a needle, dilating the needle track over a guidewire, and placing a 10F plastic or a covered metallic expandable stent under ultrasound guidance. This method could become an alternative to surgery in the approximately 10% of patients in which an attempt of biliary stent placement by ERCP is unsuccessful for a variety of reasons.

THE PALLIATION OF A DUODENAL OBSTRUCTION

A pyloric or duodenal obstruction caused by pancreatic masses is often underdiagnosed and not recognized until an advanced stage of malnutrition has been reached, with a near-complete cessation of oral intake. By the data of classic studies, up to 15% to 20% of patients with malignant pancreatic masses will develop duodenal obstruction at some point. Based on that, a prophylactic duodenal bypass was recommended by many surgeons for patients with unresectable pancreatic cancer initially presenting without this condition (as is usually the case). This recommendation, however, was questioned as some series showed that the need for this intervention may indeed be much smaller, and that the benefits did not justify routine prophylactic laparotomy. The development of extendable duodenal stents offered a third option. The data showed that the stents were able to effectively relieve obstruction 80% to 90% of the time and were associated with shorter hospitalization, lower costs, and a lower rate of complications than surgical gastrojejunostomy.

A preoperative assessment with contrast GI studies is often very helpful in preparing for the procedure, although it is not an absolute requirement. The procedure is typically performed under conscious sedation in the endoscopy suite equipped with fluoroscopy. Usually the patients can be discharged the same day without need for hospitalization. In the case of existing or expected biliary obstruction, the expandable biliary stent should be placed before the duodenal stent, as the latter procedure interferes with future ERCP access to the papilla. Currently, the enteral WALLSTENT (Boston Scientific; Natick, MA) is the only stent approved by the Food and Drug Administration (FDA) for the treatment of duodenal obstruction. It exists in 18- to 22-mm diameters, with lengths of either 6 cm or 9 cm, and may be either mounted on a separate delivery system (160 to 255 cm long) or adapted to placement through the therapeutic channel of the endoscope. The first technique requires placement over a previously placed guidewire. The wire can sometimes be placed across the area of obstruction under direct visual control, if the endoscope can be passed beyond the area of stenosis. Otherwise, a stiff guidewire is passed through the stricture under fluoroscopic control. The position is then confirmed by injecting Gastrograffin through a catheter advanced over the wire to document the patency of the lumen. The scope is then removed, leaving the guidewire in place. The stent is advanced over the wire, positioned, and deployed under fluoroscopic guidance. If the stent is adequate in length and position, the stricture produces a "waist" in the contour of the stent, which flares at its ends. An additional second overlapping stent may be placed beyond the first one if the length was too short to cross the whole stricture. The newer stent delivery systems can be placed through the instrument channel of the endoscope, eliminating the need to exchange the scope over the wire and allowing better visual control of the stent's deployment (Fig. 37-9, page 374).

Technically successful placement of stents has been achieved up to 97% of the time. The successful placement of the stent produces at least partial relief of duodenal obstruction in 90% of patients or more. Complications may include stent obstruction by ingrowing tumor (17% of patients), perforation (1%), or distal migration (5%). Re-intervention after the stent is initially placed usually consists of the placement of an additional stent if the obstruction progresses and procedures to relieve biliary obstruction, which can develop as much as 44% of the time; a percutaneous transhepatic approach is the procedure of choice in this circumstance.

THE PALLIATION OF A PANCREATIC DUCT OBSTRUCTION

There is growing evidence that malignant pancreatic duct obstruction is a contributing factor in steatorrhea and pain (especially postprandial pain) in cancer patients. Traditionally, these symptoms were treated by analgesics and enzyme supplementation. Pancreatic duct stenting improves symptoms in certain patients with pancreatic malignancy. However, the associated risks of pancreatitis and stent obstruction limit the use of interventional modalities in managing this condition.

PALLIATION OF PAIN

EUS-guided celiac plexus neurolysis is widely used for the palliation of abdominal and back pain related to the pancreatic pathology. The rationale behind this procedure is the disruption of the afferent splanchnic nerves passing through the celiac plexus. This method has been used to treat pain from chronic pancreatitis and pancreatic malignancies. Celiac plexus neurolysis can be performed surgically (at the time of laparotomy or laparoscopy) or percutaneously, via CT or fluoroscopic guidance. The latter method is the most widely used, with several variations of technique. Success rates of up to 70% to 90% at 3 months have been described.

Unlike percutaneous techniques, the EUS-guided bloc offers the most direct access to the celiac plexus as well as the best way to visualize and avoid the celiac artery and its branches during injection. It also allows one to avoid puncturing the diaphragm and pleura and its potential risks. The unusual major neurological complications of the percutaneous technique, such as paraplegia, have not been reported with the EUS-guided method. In addition, a simultaneous biopsy of the tumor can be obtained if it is needed for palliative chemoradiation treatment. EUS-guided celiac ablation is performed using linear

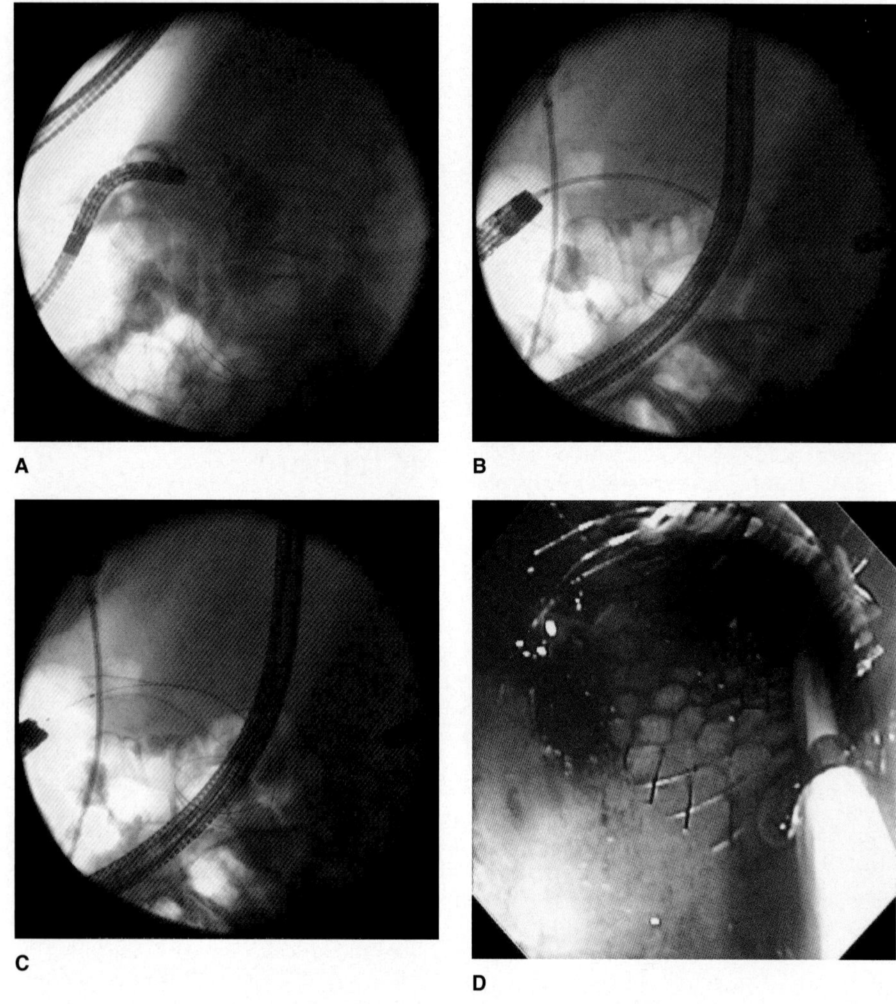

Fig. 37-9. Placement of palliative extendable Wallstent for duodenal obstruction. **A.** Endoscopic placement of the guidewire across the stricture. **B.** The stent delivery system is positioned. **C.** Deployment of the stent. **D.** Deployed duodenal Wallstent in position.

array echoendoscopes. As the endoscope is inserted in the esophagus, the aorta is identified and followed distally. The crus of the diaphragm is seen, and the celiac trunk can be identified using this landmark as the first major branch off the aorta. The celiac ganglions are located on both sides of the trunk, several millimeters below its origin (Fig. 37-10). The injection is performed via the posterior gastric wall with a 22-gauge needle. Aspiration is necessary prior to injection to avoid intravascular puncture. If no blood is aspirated, 10 ml of 98% ethanol is introduced on both sides of the celiac axis. There is evidence that this technique is more effective than a single injection. An injection of 0.25% bupivacaine solution prior to ethanol has been advocated by some authors to minimize the discomfort of alcohol injection. Usually it is possible to observe the formation of a "cloud" around the celiac axis as the solution infiltrates the tissues. In the case of benign pancreatic disease, the injection of a total 30 ml 0.25% or 0.5% bupivacaine with or without the addition of 40 mg methylprednisolone is commonly used instead of ethanol.

The reported success rate of EUS-guided neurolysis varies, with up to 88% reported in some series. However, the pain is usually not completely eliminated by the neurolysis, and the effects—even when successful—are temporary. Almost all patients will continue opioid use, albeit sometimes at a decreased dose. This circumstance should be discussed with the patient as the realistic goals of the procedure are determined. The most common complications include transient hypotension (thought to be due to sympathetic blockade), diarrhea (usually subsiding in 24 to 48 hours), a temporary increase of the pain, and hematomas. Infectious complications are uncommon, probably because of the bactericidal action of ethanol. If bupivacaine is used, an accidental intravascular injection may lead to a devastating complication such as ventricular fibrillation or other arrhythmias extremely resistant to resuscitation attempts. Meticulous precautions must be used, such as careful sonographic confirmation of the needle's position and careful aspiration prior to injection.

NEW, EXPERIMENTAL, AND PROSPECTIVE DEVELOPMENTS IN ENDOSCOPY FOR PANCREATIC DISEASES

One recently developed ERCP-based technique is the use of miniature fiberoptic probes, which can be advanced into ducts like a tiny choledochoscope. The SpyGlass Direct Visualization System, developed by Boston Scientific (Natick, MA), utilizes a miniature 6000-pixel fiber-optic probe inserted via a single-use access and delivery catheter that has steering capability in four directions. The

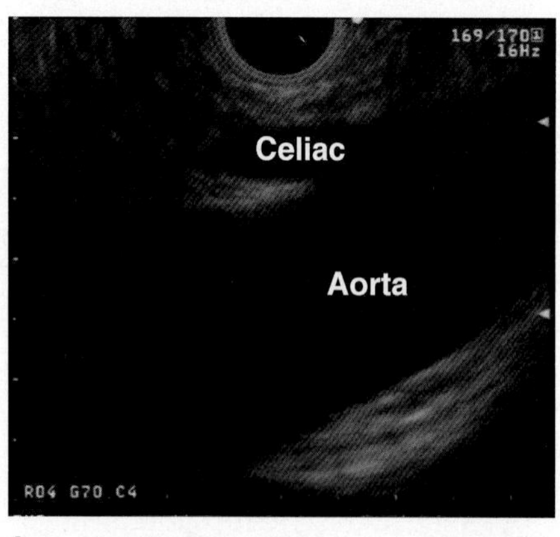

A

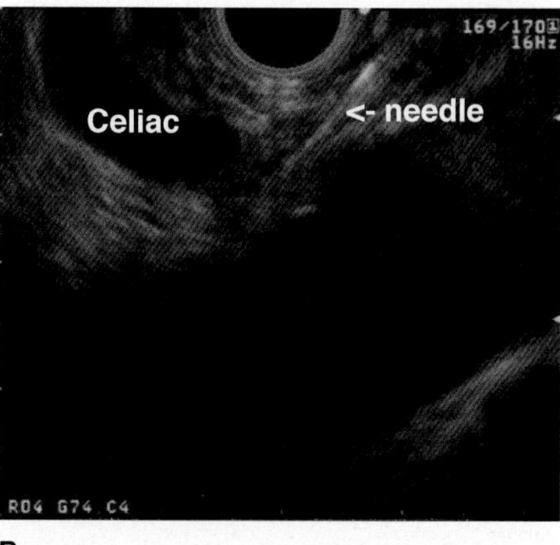

B

Fig. 37-10. EUS-guided celiac plexus neurolysis. **A.** EUS view of the abdominal aorta and celiac artery with linear array echoendoscope. EUS, endoscopic ultrasound.

system attaches directly to a standard duodenoscope and passes through its instrument channel. It allows the direct visualization of the ductal lumen and precise biopsy under vision. In the future, this technology will likely also be used for therapeutic interventions such as stone retrieval, electrohydraulic lithotripsy, or the treatment of strictures.

Ultrasound contrast agents such as SonoVue (Bracco Diagnostics, Inc.; Princeton, NJ) may become valuable for the endoscopic ultrasound. They are designed to help visualize vascular structures. The agent is a preparation of microscopic bubbles of sulfur hexafluoride gas in phospholipidic shells. This preparation is injected intravenously, and its presence in the bloodstream enhances the Doppler signal, improving the imaging of the blood vessels and therefore the delineation of the vascular characteristics of a lesion. SonoVue is rapidly (within minutes) excreted via the pulmonary route. Its value and safety in transabdominal ultrasound (such as cardiac, cerebrovascular, and hepatic imaging) is being evaluated. If confirmed, it could potentially help EUS to detect hypovascular pancreatic cancers or hypervascular neuroendocrine tumors and to distinguish between chronic pancreatitis and pancreatic cancer and between cystic pancreatic neoplasms and benign cysts on the basis of their different vascular patterns.

The EUS-directed injection of chemotherapy agents or allergenic lymphocyte culture ("cytoimplant") has been used as an experimental modality to control locally advanced unresectable carcinomas of the pancreas. Another novel type of therapy is gene therapy, using adenoviruses as vectors in genetic transfer. Preliminary studies using EUS for successful intratumor delivery of such vectors have been reported. The endoscopic placement of radioactive seeds (Iridium-192) has also been attempted for the palliation of the malignant biliary strictures in hope of controlling local tumor growth; the results of this method are being studied.

EUS-guided radiofrequency ablation (RFA) of pancreatic lesions has been successfully performed in animal models. There are also reports of ablating the pancreatic metastases of renal cell carcinoma. In the future, this modality could be of potential use in cases of unresectable pancreatic malignancy or for the ablation of small neuroendocrine tumors of the pancreas. The EUS-guided ethanol lavage of cystic lesions of the pancreas has also been described.

SUGGESTED READING

Baron TH, Dunn GP, eds. Palliative gastroenterology. *Gastroenterol Clin North Am* 2006;35.

Domingues-Munos EJ, ed. *Clinical pancreatology for practicing gastroenterologists and surgeons*, Malden, MA: Blackwell Publishing, 2005.

Ingram M, Arregui M. *Endoscopic ultrasonograph* in "An update in surgeon-performed ultrasound," *Surg Clin North Am* 2004;84: 1035–1060.

Jacobson IM, ed. *ERCP and its applications*, Philadelphia, PA: Lippincott Williams & Wilkins, 1998.

Machi J, Staren ED, eds. *Ultrasound for surgeons*, 2nd ed., Philadelphia, PA: Lippincott Williams & Wilkins, 2005.

Vilmann P, Saftoiu A. Endoscopic ultrasound-guided fine needle aspiration biopsy: equipment and technique. *J Gastroenterol Hepatol* 2006;21(11):1646–1655.

Wolfson D, Barkin J, Chari S, et al. Management of pancreatic masses (Controversies in clinical pancreatology. *Pancreas* 2005;31(3): 203–217.

COMMENTARY

Drs. Bronfine and Arregui have written a new chapter for this textbook covering the endoscopic techniques that can be used to stage and palliate pancreatic masses. Evaluation of the pancreatic mass has evolved over the last decade. Refinements in CT, MRI, and PET scanning have all led to a more accurate diagnosis of pancreatic masses. Unfortunately, most cases of pancreatic malignancy are not resectable for cure and may require only palliative therapy. Furthermore, not an insignificant number of cases remain a diagnostic dilemma after even the most modern diagnostic imaging modalities are performed. It is in these situations that flexible endoscopy with endoscopic ultrasound, biopsies, or the deployment of palliative devices play such a critical role.

ERCP remains a mainstay for the diagnosis and palliation of pancreatic masses. ERCP can provide an accurate roadmap of the biliary and pancreatic ducts, demonstrate the position of obstructing lesions, allow for brushings and other means of obtaining histologic diagnoses, and enable the deployment of stents for those with high-grade obstruction. More recently, endoscopic ultrasound (EUS) has been used for the diagnosis and biopsy of pancreatic masses. EUS is far more sensitive for demonstrating small pancreatic masses than are traditional imaging modalities. As with ultrasound performed for other applications, however, the interpretation of EUS images is very operator-dependent and requires significant expertise. The "new kid on the block" is the use of very small diameter ultrasound probes that can be inserted into the ducts themselves for high-resolution imaging.

Many patients initially present for the evaluation of pancreatic masses that are then deemed unresectable by imaging tests. These pancreatic masses may cause obstruction of the duodenum, bile duct, or pancreatic duct or lead to severe, unrelenting pain. Endoscopic techniques may be used to place stents in the pancreatic or bile ducts or even in the duodenum to improve the quality of life in these patients, whose expected survival is measured in months. The use of the echoendoscope to perform neurolysis of the celiac plexus is very helpful in providing short-term relief of incapacitating pain.

Other newer technologies will further expand the armamentarium of the flexible endoscopist, who should be poised to play a role in the development of these new technologies to allow comprehensive treatment of patient with pancreatic masses.

NJS

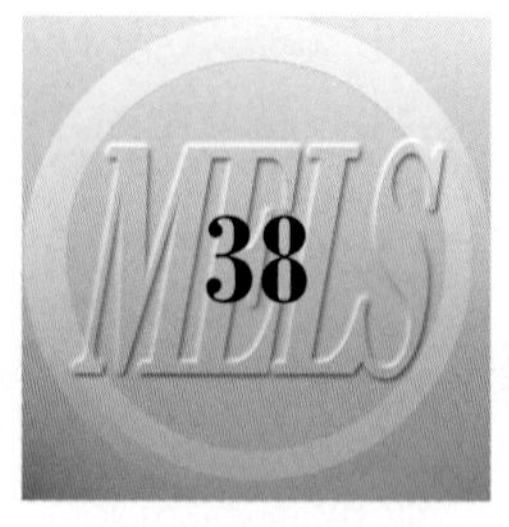

Endoscopic and Laparoscopic Management of Pseudocysts and Pancreatitis

KHASHAYAR VAZIRI AND FRED BRODY

INTRODUCTION

Currently, endoscopic and laparoscopic techniques are used to treat a variety of pancreatic pathology including pseudocysts, abscesses, and neoplasms. Some of these operations mirror their open counterparts, while others incorporate novel laparoscopic and flexible endoscopic techniques. All of these techniques require careful preoperative consideration, advanced endoscopic skills, two-handed laparoscopic dissection, advanced suturing skills, and a systematic stepwise approach.

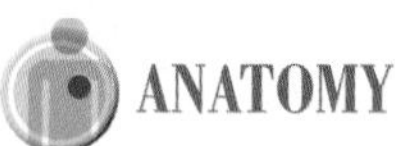

ANATOMY

The pancreas lies in the retroperitoneum, posterior to the stomach and lesser omentum. The organ has four portions: the head is nuzzled in the C-loop of the duodenum while the neck, body, and tail extend obliquely to the splenic hilum. The uncinate process is an inferior extension of the head that passes posterior to the superior mesenteric vessels. The neck of the pancreas lies directly anterior to the superior mesenteric vessels. The body and tail lie to the left of the superior mesenteric vessels and extend into the splenic hilum. The splenic artery courses along the cephalad border of the pancreas, while the splenic vein is adherent to its posterior surface. The arterial supply of the pancreas originates from multiple sources. The superior and inferior pancreaticoduodenal vessels comprise the two major arterial arcades that supply the head, neck, and uncinate process. These vessels arise from the celiac and superior mesenteric arteries respectively. Branches of the splenic and left gastroepiploic arteries feed the body and tail of the pancreas (Fig. 38-1).

PANCREATITIS

Acute pancreatitis is defined as an acute inflammatory process of the pancreas that may involve surrounding organs and tissues. In severe forms, pancreatitis can lead to multisystem organ failure and death. Although there are many etiologies of pancreatitis, alcohol abuse and gallstones account for over 80% of cases in the western hemisphere. Many theories of alcohol-induced pancreatitis exist, but the exact mechanism remains unknown. Gallstones, in turn, theoretically migrate and cause transient obstruction of an anatomical common channel that is shared by the distal common bile and pancreatic duct near the ampulla of Vater.

The clinical presentation of acute pancreatitis can identify its underlying etiology. The majority of patients present with abdominal pain, nausea, vomiting, fever, tachycardia, and distention. The onset of epigastric pain 12 to 48 hours after an episode of binge drinking usually implicates alcohol-induced pancreatic injury. Conversely, epigastric pain in the setting of recurrent right upper quadrant pain and cholelithiasis suggests gallstone-associated pancreatitis. The diagnosis of pancreatitis is confirmed by laboratory and radiographic tests. These tests may include a serum amylase, lipase, and liver function tests along with a right upper quadrant ultrasound and/or a computed tomography (CT) scan of the abdomen with intravenous contrast (Fig. 38-2). These tests, along with the clinical presentation, help determine the severity of the disease. The majority of patients with acute pancreatitis have a mild, self-limited clinical course. Approximately 10% to 15% of patients, however, develop complications of pancreatitis, including pseudocysts, abscesses, and necrosis.

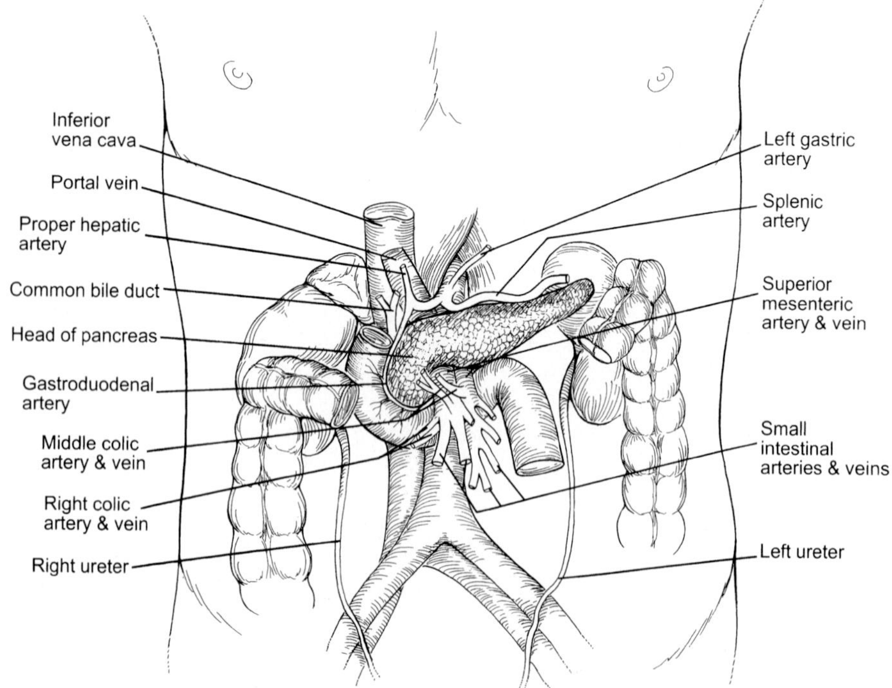

Fig. 38-1. The anatomy of the pancreas and its relationship to adjacent structures.

PANCREATIC PSEUDOCYSTS

Pancreatic pseudocysts are fluid collections of pancreatic secretions surrounded by visceral structures and fibrous tissue that define a cyst wall. By definition, the cyst wall lacks true epithelial cells. Fluid collections with pancreatic enzymes occur in approximately 50% of patients with acute pancreatitis. Those collections that persist beyond 4 weeks are no longer referred to as acute fluid collections and are considered pseudocysts. A pseudocyst occurs from pancreatic duct disruption with leakage of

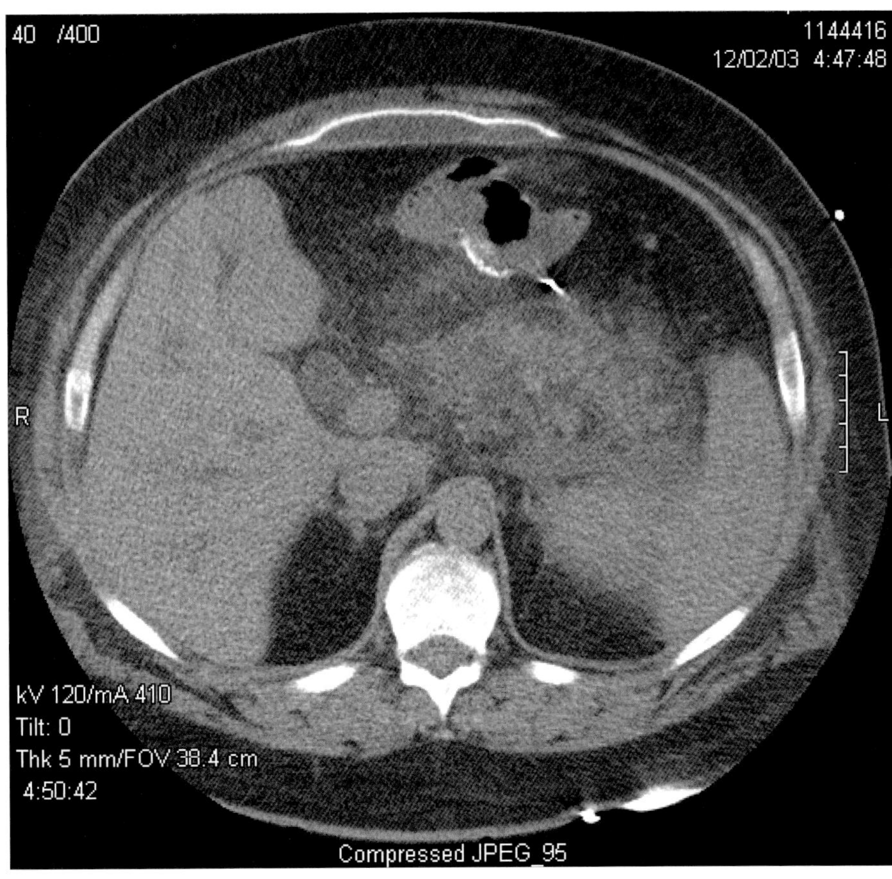

Fig. 38-2. A computed tomography (CT) scan showing an edematous pancreas consistent with acute pancreatitis.

pancreatic enzymes into the surrounding tissue. Subsequently, the enzymes cause a localized inflammatory and fibrous reaction that result in an encapsulated collection of pancreatic fluid.

The most common clinical presentation of a pancreatic pseudocyst is epigastric pain and a sensation of "fullness." This may be accompanied by nonspecific symptoms including nausea, vomiting, and weight loss. Radiographic confirmation of the pseudocyst is accomplished with ultrasound or a CT scan, the latter is preferred as it delineates the relationship between the cyst and surrounding viscera (Fig. 38-3). Ultrasound evaluation is particularly helpful for serial examination to follow patients with known pseudocysts for interval changes in size and possible resolution.

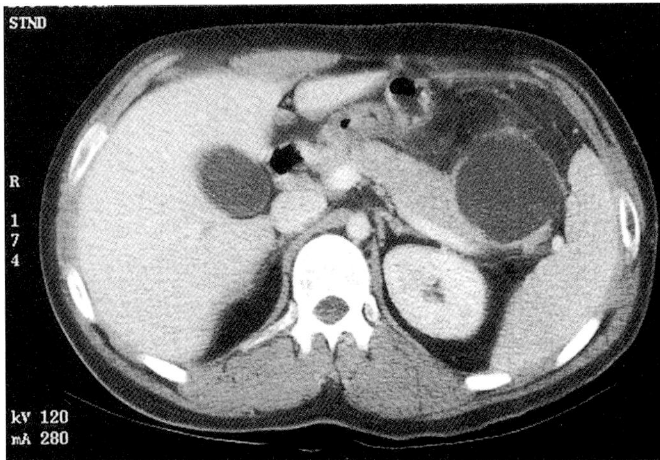

Fig. 38-3. Computed tomography (CT) scans are highly accurate at delineating pancreatic pseudocysts and detecting findings suspicious for malignancy.

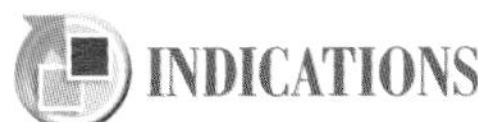

INDICATIONS

Over 90% of pseudocysts resolve spontaneously. Expectant management can be achieved safely as long as the patient remains asymptomatic. Close clinical follow-up of even large cysts is associated with exceedingly low morbidity. Operative intervention is necessary for symptomatic cysts or complications of pseudocyst formation including infection, bleeding, rupture, and obstruction. The major goal in the management of pancreatic pseudocysts is symptomatic relief with definitive drainage of the fluid collection.

PREOPERATIVE PLANNING

Prior to treating a pancreatic pseudocyst, two key characteristics must be established. First, the anatomical location and relationship to other abdominal viscera must be accomplished radiologically, usually with a CT scan. Findings on the CT define the maturity of the cyst, thickness of the cyst wall, heterogeneity of cystic contents, presence of septae, and location of the cyst. These factors influence the appropriate technique for a cystenteric anastomosis. Secondly, the pancreatic ductal anatomy and its relationship to the pseudocyst must be identified. Recent studies show that pancreatic duct anatomy dictates the appropriate drainage modality in order to successfully treat pancreatic pseudocysts. Pancreatic ductal anatomy is evaluated using endoscopic retrograde cholangiopancreatography (ERCP) or magnetic resonance cholangiopancreatography (MRCP). Although MRCP is less invasive and does not confer the risks of endoscopy (pancreatitis and possible infection), it may lack the clarity of ERCP. Regardless of technique, either test should identify the duct–cyst communication and associated ductal abnormalities. In order to prevent unnecessary complications, delineation of ductal anatomy with an ERCP should be performed prior to any type of operative intervention if MRCP is not available or inadequate. Unless the patient is symptomatic or manifests signs and symptoms of infection, recent studies propose that patients with normal ducts with or without duct–cyst communication can be managed without any intervention. Overall, patients with pseudocysts in the setting of chronic pancreatitis and abnormal ductal anatomy should be drained surgically or endoscopically. In the absence of chronic pancreatitis, there is considerable debate as to the management of the remaining group of patients with abnormal ductal anatomy with or without duct–cyst communication. This debate is beyond the scope of this chapter. Operative management of pseudocysts includes percutaneous drainage, endoscopic drainage, internal surgical drainage, and pancreatic resection.

SURGICAL TECHNIQUE

Percutaneous Drainage

Percutaneous drainage (PD) is appropriate in two specific patient populations. The first group consists of patients with normal ductal anatomy with or without duct–cyst communication in the absence of chronic pancreatitis. These patients are treated successfully without prolonged drainage times, hospital stay, and pancreaticoenteric fistulae. The second group consists of morbid patients that cannot tolerate other invasive procedures associated with deep intravenous sedation or general anesthesia. Patients who are not amenable to operative drainage due to systemic effects of pseudocyst infection or malnutrition can be treated with PD as a bridge to formal operative drainage. Overall, PD has a success rate of 60% to 90%, with a complication rate of less than 10%. The primary complication is the creation of a pancreatic fistula that may be hard to control.

Endoscopic Drainage

Using transpapillary or transmural techniques, endoscopic drainage (ED) is successful in the majority of selected patients. The transpapillary approach is technically demanding but can be successful in patients with duct–cyst communication. This approach drains the pseudocyst via a transpapillary stent placed in the pancreatic duct. This allows free drainage of the cyst across the papilla and into the duodenum (Fig. 38-4). Essentially, the stent provides the path of least resistance to engender duct–cyst closure. Transampullary ED shows comparable results to operative drainage in selected patients. Vitale et al. demonstrated a success rate of 83% for transampullary ED of pancreatic pseudocysts.

Anatomical considerations for endoscopic transmural cystogastrostomy and cystoduodenostomy are similar to open operative drainage. The position of the pseudocyst and thickness of the pseudocyst wall are important considerations for ED. Patients with cysts adherent to the posterior wall of the stomach or the duodenum and with relatively thin cyst walls (<1 cm) are best suited for ED. Endoscopic ultrasound (EUS) and CT scan can easily identify this subset of patients. Once the cyst position is confirmed with EUS, a needle-knife cautery is used to puncture the cyst and a sphincterotome used to enlarge the cystogastrostomy (Fig. 38-5). A 7F to 10F stent is placed to bridge the cystogastrostomy. Optimally, multiple stents are left in a "pack of cigarettes" configuration to ensure patency of the cyst–enteric communication. Endoscopic cystduodenostomy is performed in a similar fashion. A drawback to the ED technique is that it is difficult to adequately evaluate the cyst wall. Although brushings can be obtained, a large biopsy of the cyst wall to adequately rule out malignancy is difficult to achieve. Patients with CT findings that may point to malignancy (septations, inhomogeneous cyst contents, or atypical presentations) are best suited for surgical drainage. Cysts with thick debris and septae may also not be adequately drained with an ED procedure. Finally, patients with varices and associated coagulopathies may not be ideal candidates for ED.

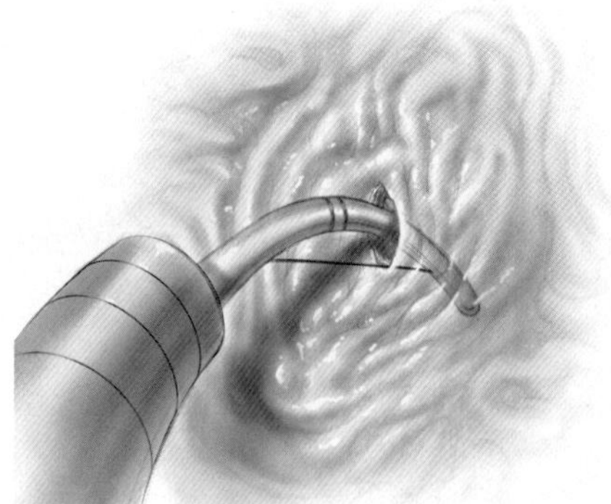

Fig. 38-5. Endoscopic cyst gastrotomy is performed by identifying the best drainage area by endoscopic ultrasound (EUS) and marking the spot, using a needle-knife cautery to penetrate the cyst and enlarging the defect with a pull sphincterotome.

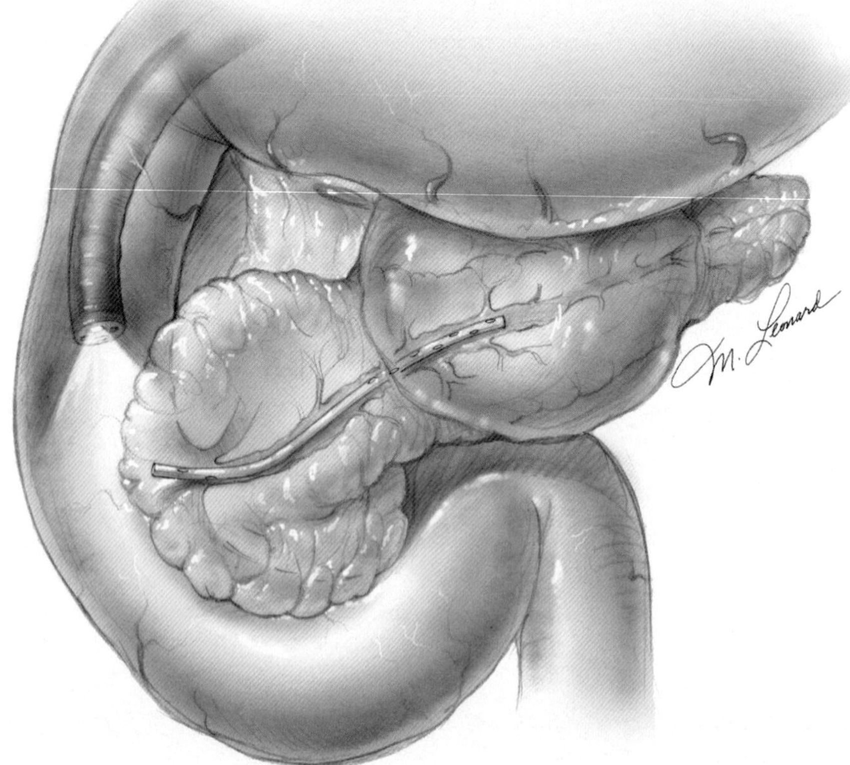

Fig. 38-4. The endoscopic placement of a pancreatic duct stent can occasionally help resolve pseudocysts with a ductal connection.

Operative Drainage

The pseudocyst location, its the relationship to surrounding viscera, and the possibility of malignancy dictate operative drainage (OD). These cases are ideally approached laparoscopically. Cystogastrostomy or cystoduodenostomy are preferred in patients with pseudocysts that bulge into the posterior wall of the stomach or duodenum, respectively. Cytogastrostomy is performed using either an intragastric or transgastric technique. The intragastric technique avoids a large anterior gastrotomy and is best for patients with alcohol-induced pancreatitis, as a concomitant laparoscopic cholecystectomy is not warranted. A Roux-en-Y cystojejunostomy is useful in patients with pseudocysts located at the base of the mesocolon or tail of the pancreas. Although more versatile than cystogastrostomy, it is technically more demanding to perform laparoscopically. Pancreatic resections are reserved for patients with multiple pseudocysts or pseudocysts confined to the pancreatic tail. Due to the advances in ED, OD is performed rarely today. Usually, OD is reserved for patients that have failed ED or performed at institutions that lack endoscopic expertise.

Laparoscopic Transgastric Drainage

Transgastric laparoscopic drainage of a pancreatic pseudocyst is accomplished by modifying the four-port technique for a laparoscopic cholecystectomy. A Hasson trocar is placed through the umbilicus and a 10-mm epigastric port is placed to the right of the falciform ligament. Two 5-mm ports are positioned at the midclavicular and anterior axillary lines, approximately 6 cm below the right costal margin. This configuration facilitates removal of the gallbladder for patients with gallstone pancreatitis while permitting drainage of the pseudocyst (Fig. 38-6).

After successful removal of the gallbladder, the 10-mm epigastric port is retracted and repositioned to the left of the falciform ligament. A 30- or 45-degree, 5-mm laparoscope is inserted through the anterior axillary port and the laparoscopic ultrasound probe is used to identify the pseudocyst. After localization, the ultrasound probe is removed and a 6-cm anterior gastrotomy is performed using a 5-mm ultrasonic dissector. Ultrasound localization of the pseudocyst is performed directly against the posterior gastric wall. The splenic artery and vein can be intimately associated with the pancreatic pseudocysts. These structures are identified easily using simultaneous color duplex scanning. The site of cyst decompression is marked with the electrocautery.

Retracting the anterior gastrotomy with two Keith needles optimizes operative exposure. Each needle is introduced through the anterior abdominal wall and placed full thickness through each side of the gastrotomy. The needle traverses the abdominal wall again and is removed. The two ends are tightened gently and secured with a hemostat at the skin level (Fig. 38-7). The medial stay suture also retracts the lateral segment of the liver. Alternatively, another 5-mm port can be placed along the left flank for retraction.

At the previously marked location, the hook cautery is inserted through the posterior gastric wall and into the adjacent cyst cavity. The cystic contents are evacuated with suction. Two instruments are placed side-by-side through the tiny posterior gastrotomy and the opening is enlarged bluntly to approximately 1 cm to accommodate an endovascular stapler. The stapler is fired and hemostasis is verified (Fig. 38-8, page 380). Cautery, clips, or suture ligatures are used to control any bleeding from the staple line. A biopsy of the cyst wall is obtained at the apex of the staple line. A second stapler is fired, incorporating the previous biopsy site to control any oozing. Utilizing the reticulating staplers, a wedged or diamond-shaped cystogastrostomy is formed to ensure patency. This wedge suffices for an adequate biopsy. A blunt grasper and suction catheter are introduced through the cystogastrostomy and any debris is irrigated copiously and removed. After verifying hemostasis, the anterior gastrotomy is reapproximated using sutures or endoscopic staplers (Fig. 38-9, page 380). Additional ports are introduced based on patient anatomy, intraoperative complications, and overall laparoscopic experience.

Laparoscopic Intragastric Drainage

An intraluminal cystogastrostomy is accomplished using a combined endoscopic and laparoscopic transgastric approach. A flexible gastroscope is introduced and the

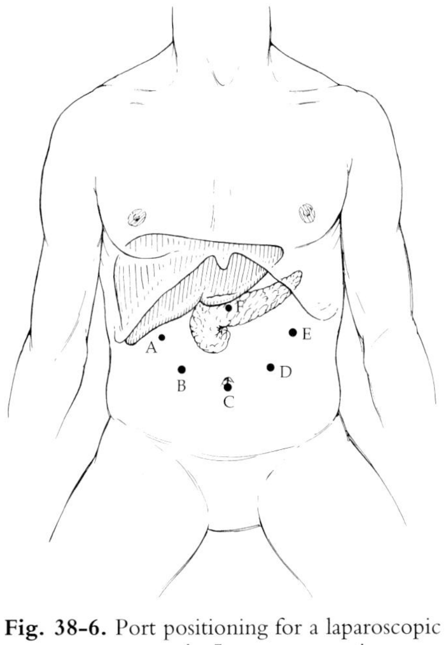

Fig. 38-6. Port positioning for a laparoscopic cystogastrostomy: A, 5-mm pancreatic resection; B, 10-mm exploration and resection; C, camera port; D, 12-mm exploration and resection; E, 10-mm exploration and resection; F, 5-mm resection.

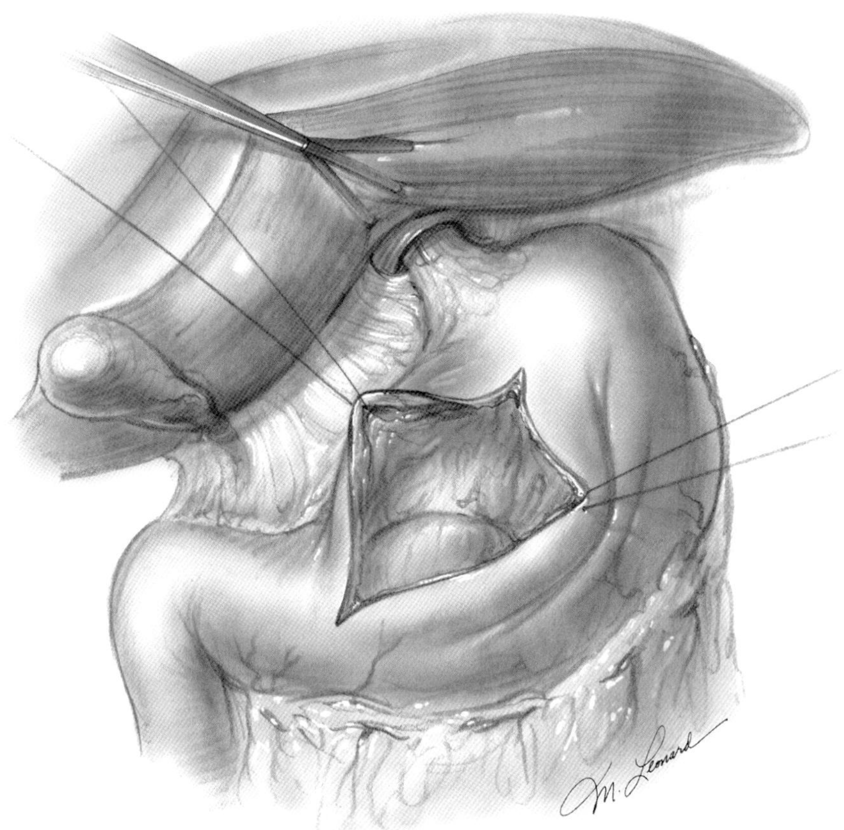

Fig. 38-7. Percutaneous stay sutures expose the posterior gastric wall.

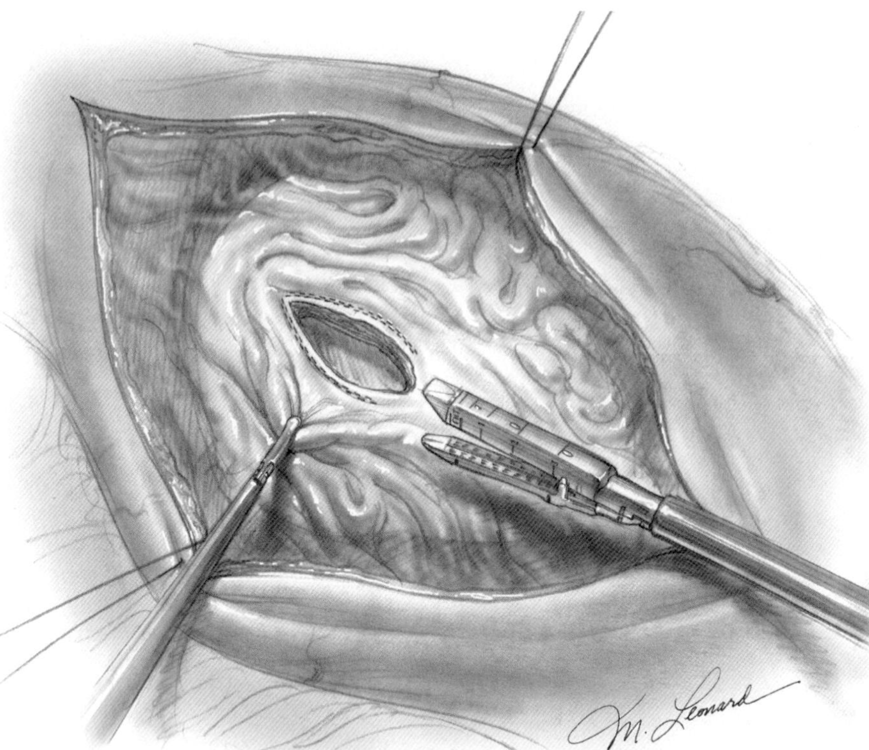

Fig. 38-8. An endoscopic linear stapler is inserted and fired to create the cystogastrostomy.

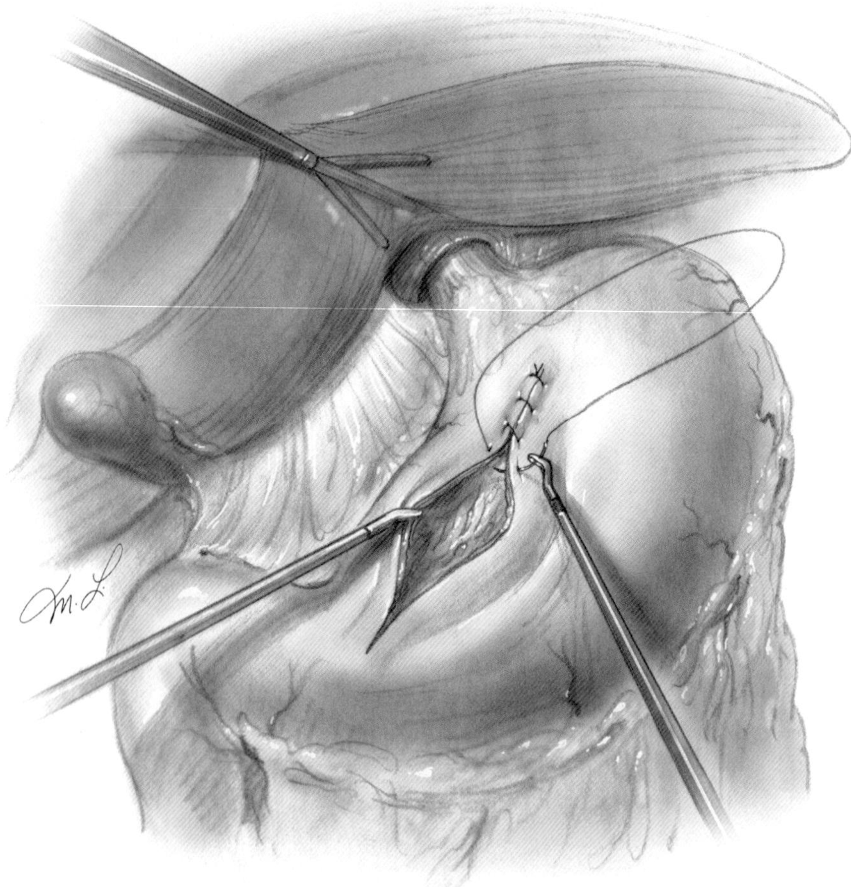

Fig. 38-9. The anterior gastrotomy is closed with a running suture or linear stapler.

stomach is insufflated. Under endoscopic visualization, a 5- to 12-mm balloon-tipped trocar is placed into the stomach using a direct puncture technique similar to a percutaneous endoscopic gastrotomy. The balloon is inflated and snugged against the abdominal wall. The laparoscopic ultrasound is inserted and localizes the pseudocyst through the posterior wall of the stomach. Two additional 5-mm balloon-tipped trocars are similarly introduced under direct endoscopic vision. A 5-mm laparoscope is inserted and the laparoscopic ultrasound reverifies cyst location. Using the ultrasonic dissector or electrocautery, a small posterior gastrotomy is performed overlying the pseudocyst (Fig. 38-10). The endoscopic stapler with a vascular load is placed through this small gastrotomy and fired, creating the cystogastrostomy. The cyst contents are removed with the suction-irrigator. A small sample of the pseudocyst wall is removed as described previously to rule out malignant disease. A series of reticulating staplers is fired, extending and widening the cystogastrostomy as noted above. After verifying hemostasis, the balloon trocars are removed from the stomach. However, the deflated trocars remain in the peritoneal cavity and the anterior gastric wall port sites are closed with interrupted silk sutures (Fig. 38-11).

Laparoscopic Cystojejunostomy

A laparoscopic cystojejunostomy is performed for pseudocysts located at the base of the transverse mesocolon. Room setup and port placements are similar to that for a gastrectomy (Fig. 38-12, page 382). The patient is placed in slight reverse-Trendelenburg and the omentum is retracted up to the right upper quadrant. After the pseudocyst is located, the small bowel is divided 40 cm distal to the Treitz ligament. A Roux limb measuring at least 45 cm is made and a jejunojejunostomy is formed using staplers or sutures. These anastomotic techniques are prevalent today with the explosion of bariatric surgery and are reviewed in other chapters. Finally, the Roux limb is secured to the base of the mesocolon with two or three tacking sutures. A side-to-side anastomosis is formed by placing an enterotomy in the small bowel followed by an enterotomy through the mesocolon and into the pseudocyst. The enterotomy should be located at the inferior border of the pseudocyst to promote dependent drainage. A stapler is used to approximate the anastomosis by delicately placing one leg of the stapler through each of the enterotomies (Fig. 38-13, page 383). The

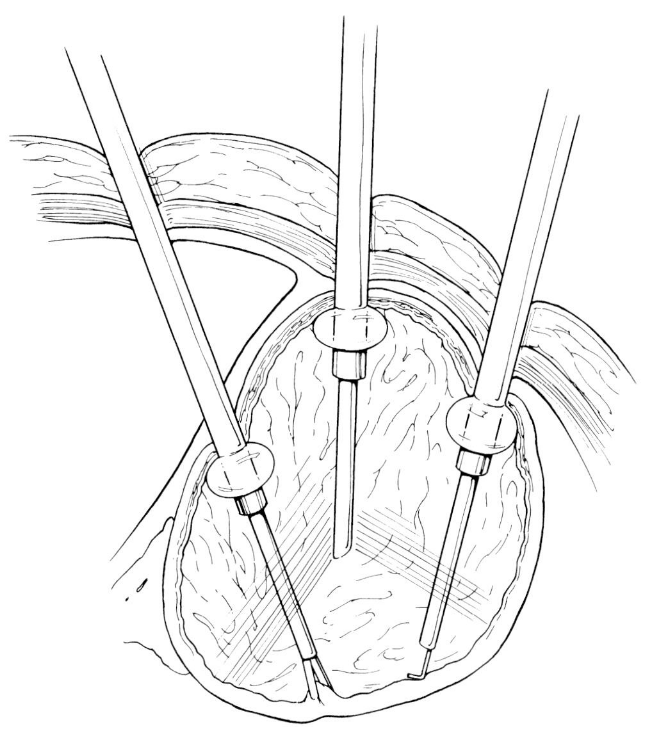

Fig. 38-10. Endoluminal trocars provide excellent exposure to create the cystogastrostomy.

stapler is fired once or twice depending on the size of the pseudocyst. Hemostasis is verified and the pseudocyst contents are suctioned and debrided. Finally, the enterostomy is closed with a running suture. One or two layers are appropriate, depending on surgical technique (Fig. 38-14, page 384).

Laparoscopic Pancreatic Resection

In some clinical scenarios, internal pseudocyst drainage is not possible due to the pseudocyst characteristics or pancreatic duct anatomy. The pseudocyst wall may be too thick to accommodate internal or external drainage or the pseudocyst may be associated with a gross infection or necrosis. In other scenarios, the main pancreatic duct may be completely divided and the pseudocyst nestled distally along the pancreatic tail adjacent to the splenic hilum. This scenario is not amenable to endoscopic drainage. Although a long Roux limb may be an option, pseudocyst resection may be an easier option without the concurrent morbidity associated with two anastomoses. Laparoscopic pancreatic resections are reviewed in Chapter 39.

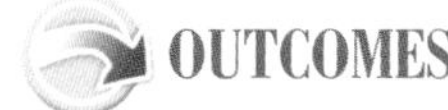

OUTCOMES

The authors have experience with 13 patients utilizing all of the various techniques. One patient was converted to an open procedure due to the lack of laparoscopic ultrasound early in the series. A recurrent pseudocyst developed in one patient secondary to a proximal duct stricture. This only reiterates the importance of examining the ductal anatomy prior to intervening with any modality. Postoperative bleeding developed in one patient on postoperative day three and required an open exploration with oversewing of an anastomotic bleeding vessel at the cystgastrostomy site. Three patients underwent resections as opposed to drainage procedures due to ductal anatomy and distal pseudocysts. These patients showed a cutoff sign of their main pancreatic ducts coupled with distal pseudocyst location. There were no leaks or mortalities.

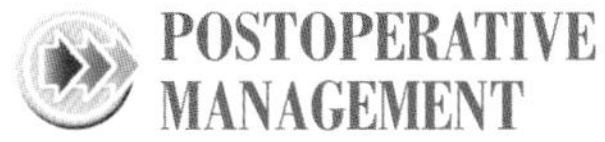

POSTOPERATIVE MANAGEMENT

In most cases, a clear liquid diet may be started on postoperative day one following endoscopic pseudocyst surgery. The diet is advanced to a regular diet as tolerated. Postoperative antibiotics are not given routinely with the exception of infected pseudocysts. Percutaneous drains remain until postoperative radiographic imaging (CT or ultrasound) demonstrates cyst resolution. Furthermore, drains are not removed until output is approximately 30 to 50 cc per day, amylase levels are less than three times serum levels, and the patient is tolerating a solid diet.

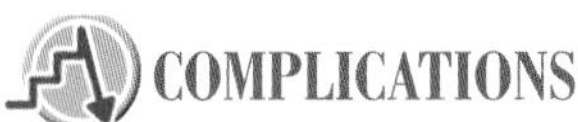

COMPLICATIONS

Complications of PD include inadvertent visceral injuries, bleeding, infection, pseudocyst recurrence, prolonged drainage,

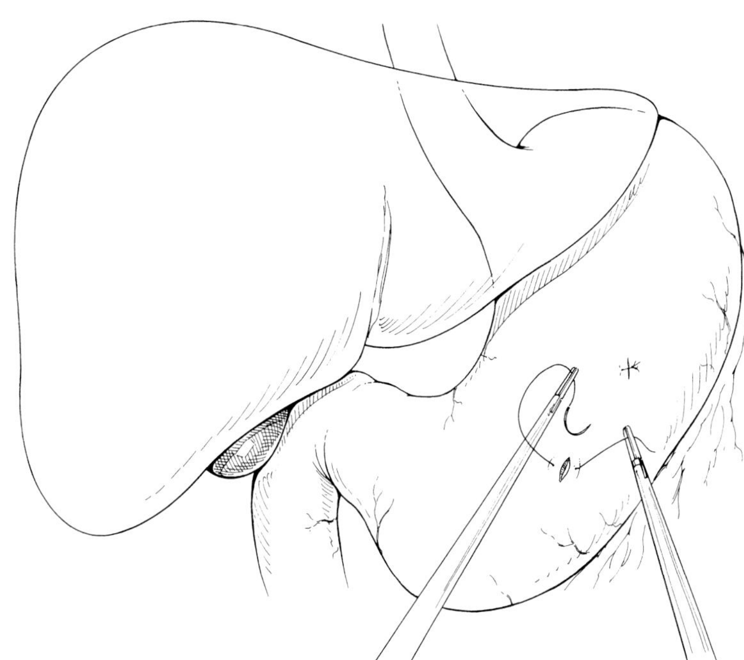

Fig. 38-11. The same ports are used to close the gastric perforations with sutures.

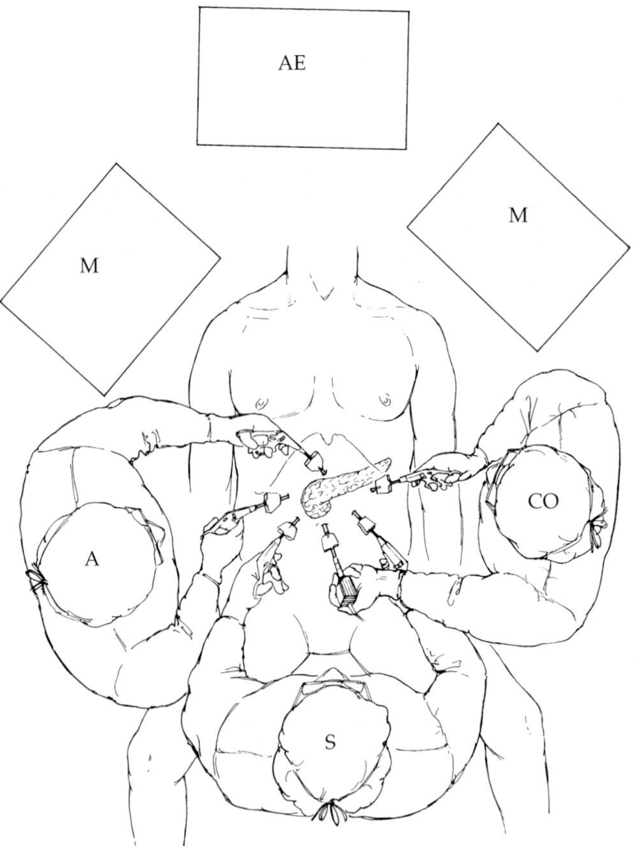

Fig. 38-12. The room setup and port placement for laparoscopic cystojejunostomy. S, surgeon; A, assistant; M, monitor; AE, anesthesia; CO, camera operator.

and pancreatic-cutaneous fistulae. Persistent drainage, failure of cyst resolution, and pseudocyst recurrence warrant re-evaluation of ductal anatomy, cyst communication, and parenchymal status. Major complications of ED include visceral perforation, stent blockage, stent migration, bleeding, and recurrence. Complications encountered in laparoscopic pancreatic surgery mirror those of the analogous open procedure. Postoperative bleeding can occur hours to days after pseudocyst decompression. These patients are resuscitated and coagulation factors assessed. Persistent bleeding is managed initially with esophagogastroduodenoscopy (EGD) to evaluate for anastomotic bleeding. Endoscopic control of bleeding can be attempted initially but occasionally may require angiography and embolization. Operative re-exploration is reserved for refractory cases.

Pancreatic fistulae occur in approximately 10% to 15% of cases after pancreatic resection. Persistent drainage is best managed, traditionally, by decreasing pancreatic stimulation with cessation of oral intake and initiation of parenteral or jejunal nutrition. However, many fistulae close even with oral intake. Somatostatin is not given routinely, but can be used in the setting of persistent drainage.

NECROTIZING PANCREATITIS

Severe acute pancreatitis can affect multiple organ systems and can be complicated by infection, necrosis, and abscess formation. The pathophysiology of pancreatic necrosis mirrors diffuse acute pancreatitis but results in selected regions of apoptosis with subsequent tissue death. This leads to sterile fluid collections, nonviable tissue, and a pancreatic phlegmon. Contrast-enhanced CT scan remains the gold standard for pancreatic necrosis (Fig. 38-15, page 384). Its sensitivity is high, approaching 90% when approximately one-third of the pancreas is necrotic. The preferred treatment of sterile pancreatic necrosis and associated fluid collections is nonoperative supportive care with acceptable mortality rates of 5% to 10%. Secondary pancreatic infections develop from sterile necrosis and carry a considerable increase in mortality of close to 100% without appropriate debridement and drainage. Pancreatic abscesses, infected pancreatic pseudocysts, and infected pancreatic necrosis usually require operative intervention. A definitive diagnosis is based on clinical manifestations and aided by radiographic diagnostic procedures. Clinical manifestations of secondary pancreatic infections include deterioration of clinical status, fever, tachycardia, and bacteremia. Contrast-enhanced CT scans will show the presence of necrotic pancreatic tissue identified by the absence of uniform uptake of intravenous contrast throughout the parenchyma. Furthermore, the presence of air bubbles and abscesses are diagnostic of pancreatic infections. Differentiation of sterile necrosis and infected necrosis is accomplished by percutaneous guided-needle aspiration. Infected pancreatic necrosis shows overt organisms on gram stain or bacterial growth on culture medium. However, none of these tests is 100% sensitive and in all cases sound clinical judgment prevails. The fundamental treatment of infected pancreatic necrosis includes broad-spectrum antibiotics, wide debridement, and drainage.

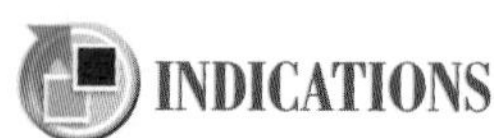

INDICATIONS

Operative intervention in acute pancreatitis is indicated for secondary pancreatic infections, recurrent biliary tract disease, and clinical deterioration despite supportive care. Cholecystectomy with intraoperative cholangiogram or ERCP may be performed in patients with gallstone-associated pancreatitis in order to relieve biliary and pancreatic duct obstruction. The presence or absence of associated cholangitis may dictate the need for either of these procedures. However, infected pancreatic necrosis with peripancreatic and pancreatic abscesses should be treated promptly with drainage and debridement.

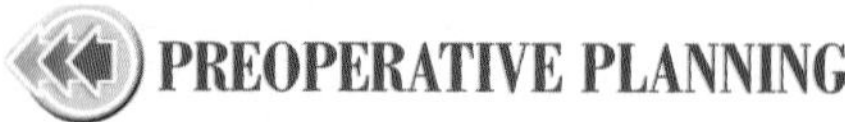

PREOPERATIVE PLANNING

The treatment of biliary disease depends upon the acuity and severity of the pancreatitis. The majority of patients with acute pancreatitis have a mild and self-limited disease course. At this time, most surgeons perform a laparoscopic cholecystectomy and intraoperative cholangiogram during the same hospital admission as the acute episode of pancreatitis resolves. Deferring the definitive operation to a second hospital admission with an 8-week interval time period often results in recurrent pancreatitis, a longer length of stay, and a second hospital admission. A minority of

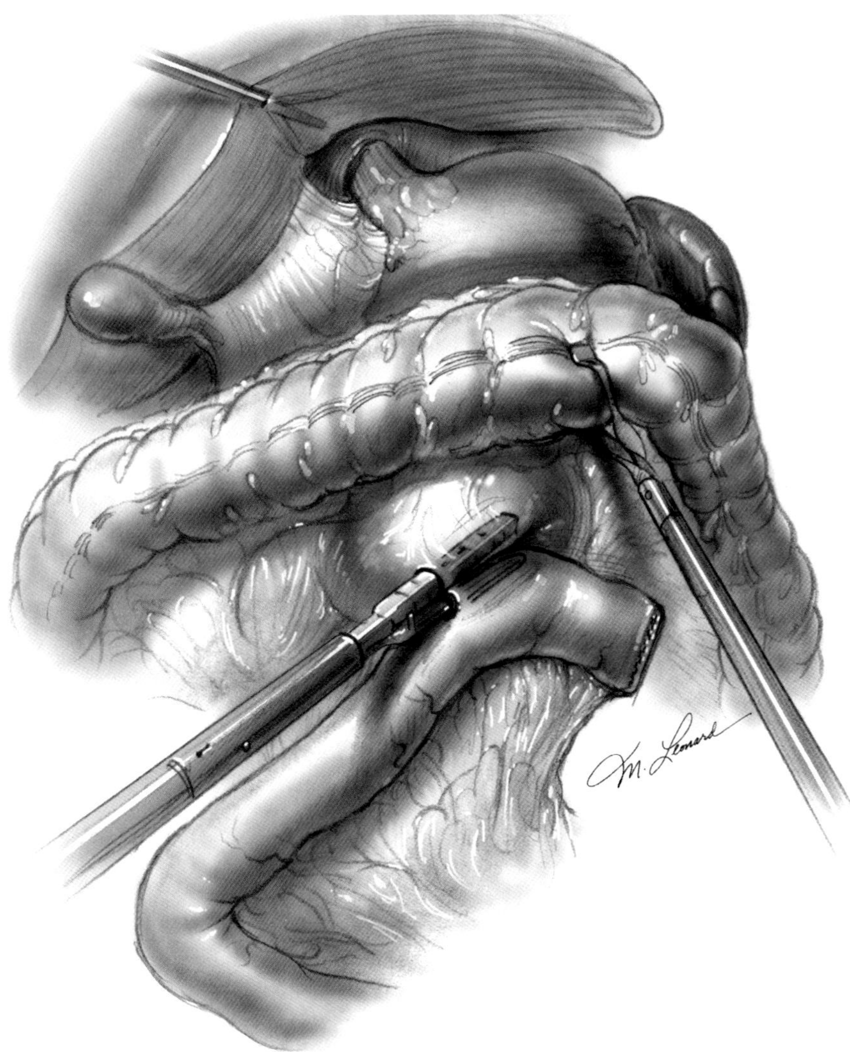

Fig. 38-13. The Roux limb is fastened to the transverse mesocolon overlying the cyst, the enterotomy and cystotomy made, and a linear stapler used to create the anastamosis.

patients with severe acute pancreatitis and associated complications including fluid collections, necrosis, and phlegmon may benefit from delayed treatment of their biliary disease. The timing of surgical intervention to treat the biliary disease associated with pancreatitis requires an analysis of each patient and his or her respective disease severity.

The operative indications and timing are debatable for infected pancreatic necrosis. Some studies demonstrate that patients operated after 4 weeks from the onset of pancreatitis have a decreased mortality compared to those patients operated within 3 weeks from the date of onset. Other studies advocate early operative intervention. Optimal timing of surgical intervention remains controversial; sound bedside clinical judgment should prevail.

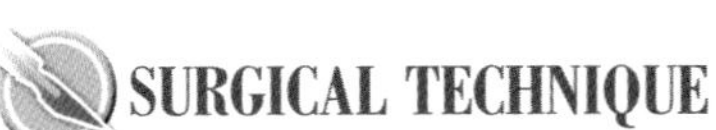

SURGICAL TECHNIQUE

Pancreatic abscesses and peripancreatic abscesses can sometimes be managed successfully with PD. Successful treatment depends on a paucity of particulate debris from the abscess cavity and aggressive catheter management. Usually, these patients have frequent radiologic evaluations and multiple drains are placed. The drains are monitored closely and upsized to allow adequate drainage of large particulate debris. However, patients with extensive necrosis and large particulate debris usually fail PD. Conventional therapy for infected pancreatic necrosis entails open necrosectomy with wide drainage. Laparoscopic approaches have been described with some success. Transabdominal laparoscopic necrosectomy and drainage have been performed successfully, but have been criticized for seeding the peritoneal cavity. Other techniques such as retroperitoneal laparoscopy and laparoscopic-assisted PD are described as well. These techniques involve laparoscopic access to the retroperitoneum and the use of percutaneous drains to guide other ports. Currently, Horvath et al. utilize a technique called videoscopic-assisted retroperitoneal debridement (VARD). Briefly, this method uses two flank incisions for access to the retroperitoneum. A laparoscope is inserted in one incision while the other is used for debridement, hydrodissection, irrigation, and drainage (Fig. 38-16, page 385). The VARD technique is feasible and somewhat successful in a small series of patients, but the safety and efficacy have not been definitively documented. Currently, this technique is undergoing further study. While laparoscopic techniques continue to improve, they remain novel and difficult for inexperienced surgeons. If patient safety is jeopardized, conversion to open laparotomy should be performed for infected pancreatic necrosis.

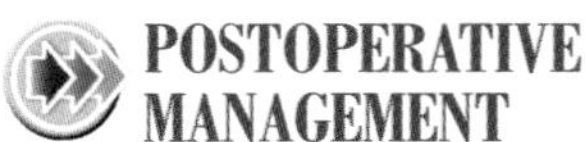

POSTOPERATIVE MANAGEMENT

Postoperative management of secondary pancreatic infections involves supportive care, antibiotics, and patent drainage. Computed tomography scans are used in conjunction with the patient's clinical status to evaluate any new collections and adequate debridement of necrotic tissue. The management of these patients is complex and may require multiple trips to the operating room for subsequent debridement. Despite aggressive resuscitation and repeated operative debridement, mortality is approximately 30%.

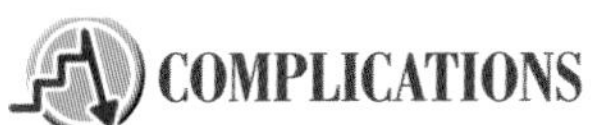

COMPLICATIONS

The main intraoperative complication of necrosectomy is bleeding. Conversion to an open procedure should be performed promptly with uncontrolled bleeding, as these patients have little physiologic reserve. Other complications of laparoscopic necrosectomy include colonic and pancreatic fistulae, splenic injury, pancreatic insufficiency, pseudoaneurysms, and enterotomies.

CONCLUSION

The armamentarium of the pancreatic surgeon should include minimally invasive techniques. Currently, laparoscopic

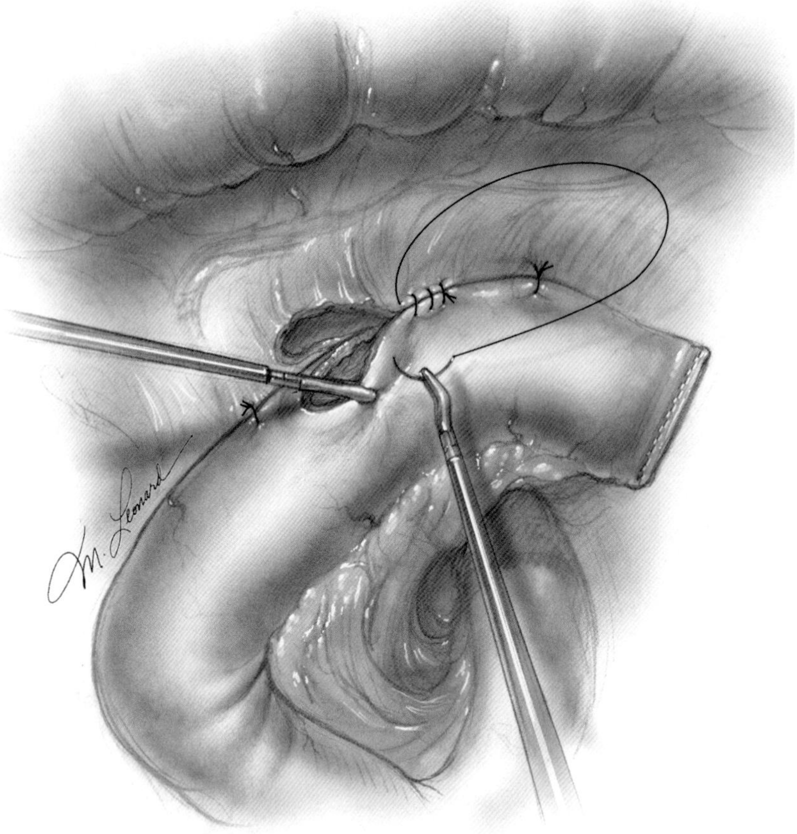

Fig. 38-14. After debriding the interior of the cyst under laparoscopic vision, the enterostomy is sutured closed.

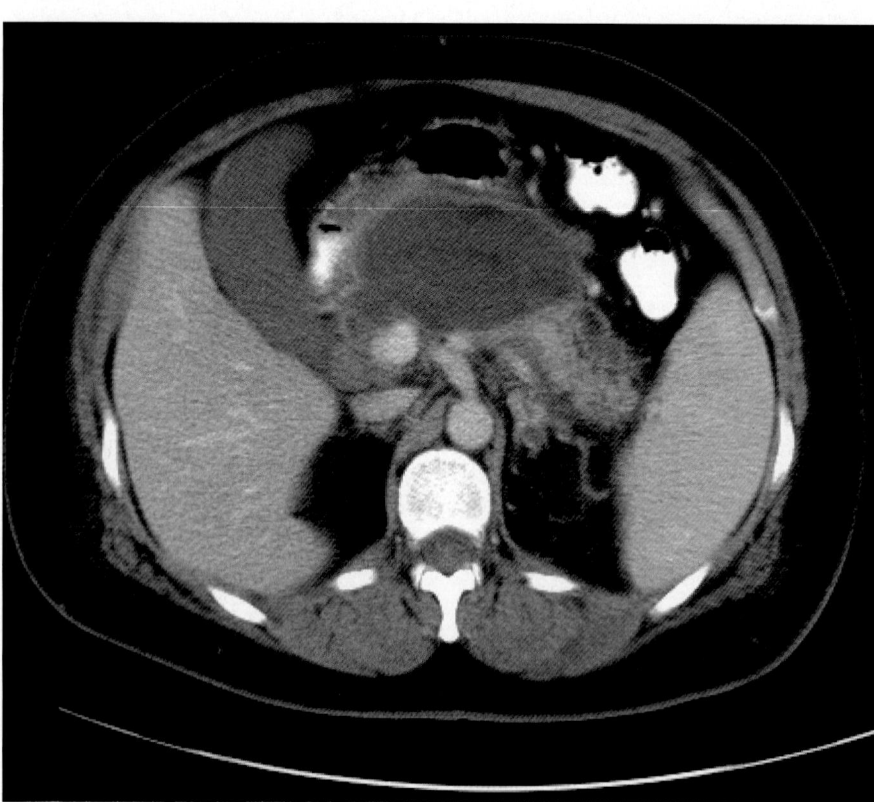

Fig. 38-15. A computed tomography (CT) scan showing pancreatic necrosis.

and endoscopic approaches are used for pancreatic pathology ranging from pseudocysts to necrosis. Although these modalities are technically demanding, careful preoperative consideration and appropriate patient selection produces successful results. These minimally invasive techniques follow the same principles and steps of their open counterparts. Regardless of technique, long-term follow-up of these patients will be necessary to justify the use and effectiveness of minimally invasive methods.

SUGGESTED READING

Bhattacharya D, Ammori BJ. Minimally invasive approaches to the management of pancreatic pseudocysts. *Surg Laparosc Endosc Percutan Tech* 2003;13(3):141–148.

Horvath KD, Kao LS, Ali A, et al. Laparoscopic-assisted percutaneous drainage of infected pancreatic necrosis. *Surg Endosc* 2001;15:677–682.

Horvath KD, Kao LS, Wherry KL, et al. A technique for laparoscopic-assisted percutaneous drainage of infected pancreatic necrosis and pancreatic abscess. *Surg Endosc* 2001;15:1221–1225.

Kellogg TA, Horvath KD. Minimal-access approaches to complications of acute pancreatitis and benign neoplasms of the pancreas. *Surg Endosc* 2003;17:1692–1704.

Nealon WH, Walser E. Main pancreatic ductal anatomy can direct choice of modality for treating pancreatic pseudocysts (surgery versus percutaneous drainage). *Ann Surg* 2002;235(6):751–758.

Nealon WH, Walser E. Surgical management of complications associated with percutaneous and/or endoscopic management of pseudocyst of the pancreas. *Ann Surg* 2005;241(6):948–960.

Vitale GC, Davis BR, Tran TC. The advancing art of endoscopy. *Am J Surg* 2005;190:228–233.

Vitale GC, Lawhon JC, Larson GM, et al. Endoscopic drainage of the pancreatic pseudocyst. *Surgery* 1999;126(4):616–623.

Zong-Guang Z, Yang-Chun Z, Ye S, et al. Laparoscopic management of severe acute pancreatitis. *Pancreas* 2003;27(3):e46–e50.

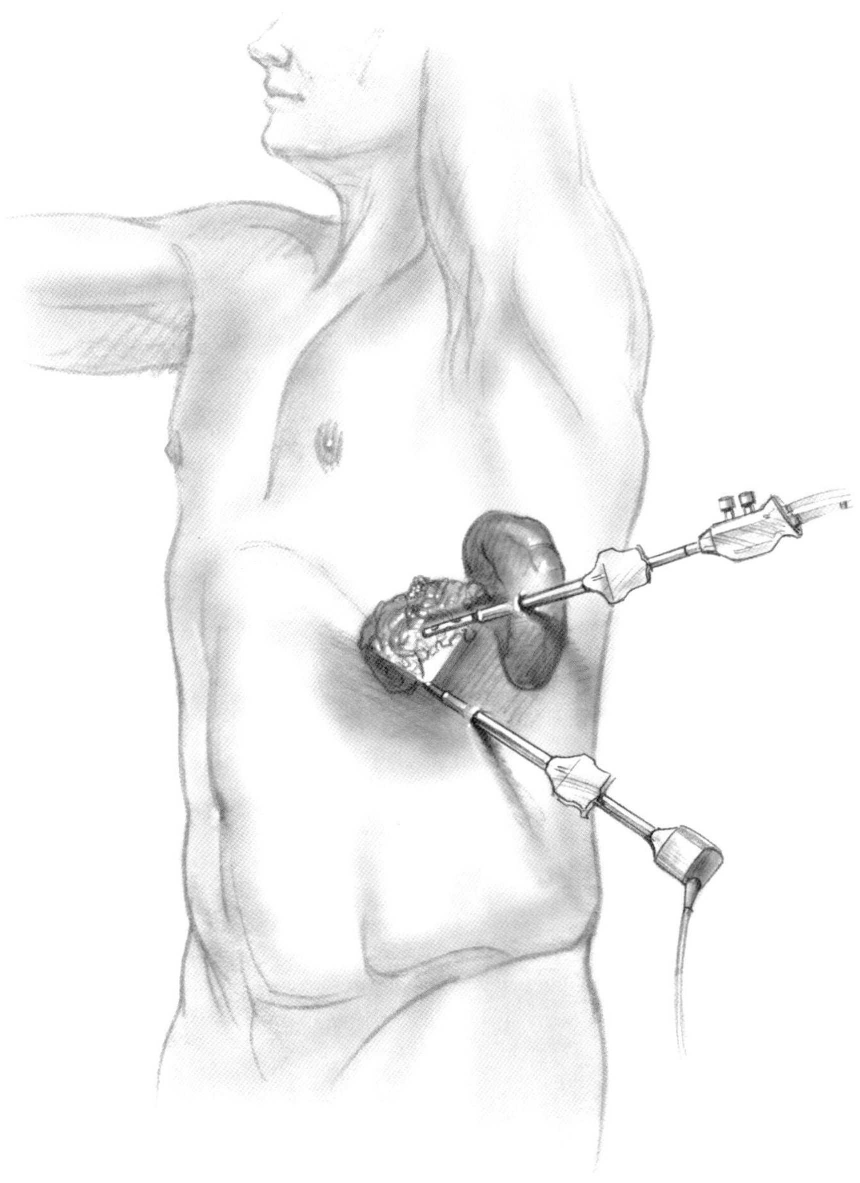

Fig. 38-16. Videoscopic-assisted retroperitoneal debridement (VARD) is a new, less-invasive way to perform pancreatic necrosectomy.

COMMENTARY

Today's surgeon has many treatment modalities available for dealing with the sequelae of pancreatitis: improved supportive care, easy availability of accurate imaging modalities, image-guided percutaneous drainage techniques, endoscopic ultrasound, pancreatic stenting, endoscopic ultrasound, and, should all this fail to solve the problem, the full panoply of endoscopic and laparoscopic surgical procedures. Decision-making becomes complex and it is not surprising that treatment of these patients has developed into a multidisciplinary team effort. The pancreatic surgeon should take an active role in decision-making; I would argue that he or she should be the one to perform the more aggressive interventions, whether endoscopic or laparoscopic. Certainly, except in the direst circumstances of vascular collapse or pancreatic hemorrhagic shock, the treatment of choice should be endoscopic or laparoscopic. These patients are at high risk of complications from open surgery: wound infection, inability to close the fascia and subsequent ventral hernias, dehiscence, and adhesion caused by small bowel obstructions are all more common in these malnourished, sick,

(continued)

and immunocompromised patients. Anything that *can be* done to minimize access trauma should obviously *be* done.

Pseudocyst drainage, whether laparoscopic or endoscopic, is an enjoyable and satisfying procedure—when it goes right. On rare occasions bad things happen and the surgeon must be prepared to rapidly intervene in the case of the cyst wall separating from the stomach wall or massive bleeding. This can occur with laparoscopic cyst enterostomies but can also happen during endoscopic drainage. We certainly know that when it comes to endoscopic drainage, the more aggressive the approach (with regards to a large cyst enterostomy and thorough debridement of cyst contents), the better the success rate. Obviously a more aggressive approach translates into a higher potential for the aforementioned complications. This is why I feel that the surgeon should be the one to do any endoscopic drainage, so that the procedure is not compromised by fear of complication and any severe complications can be immediately and definitively dealt with. This of course implies that the surgeon is a skilled endoscopist, flexible and laparoscopic, which is, unfortunately, somewhat rare now but perhaps will be less so with the new interest in natural orifice transluminal endoscopic surgery (NOTES) and surgical endoscopy in general.

Laparoscopic pancreatic necrosectomy is a new development but it certainly deserves attention. Intuitively it sounds impossible but several centers have now reported amazing results with retroperitoneoscopy and debridement. The benefits of CO_2 insufflation to define tissue planes and precise dissection seem to translate into better outcomes and certainly fewer wound care issues. This may become the future treatment of choice.

LLS

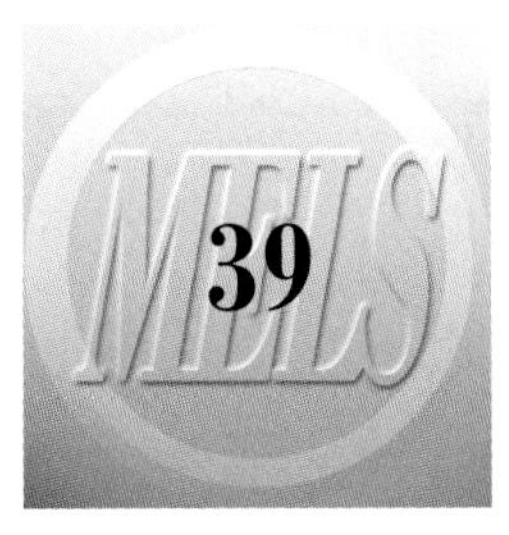

Laparoscopic Resection of the Pancreas

W. STEVEN EUBANKS

INTRODUCTION

Laparoscopic pancreatic resections comprise a small percentage of all laparoscopic procedures performed. The topic remains important, however, due to the importance of the pancreas and the potential for devastating complications. The techniques described are intended as a guide and not a dogmatic step-by-step instruction to approach these operations.

Debate currently exists regarding the appropriateness of performing pancreatic resections in hospitals with a low volume of experience. Adding laparoscopy as a factor into the best treatment of curable surgical diseases of the pancreas serves to heighten the tension surrounding the debate. Opponents of the use of laparoscopy for resections of the pancreas cite higher fistula rates, the inadequacy of some operations, and longer operative times for laparoscopic techniques. Proponents of laparoscopic pancreatic surgery report equivalent results from an oncologic and disease-control perspective.

Proponents of laparoscopic pancreatic resections also claim shorter hospital stays, fewer wound complications, and the avoidance of unnecessary laparotomy in the patient thought to have resectable disease but is found to have previously undetected metastatic disease.

PANCREATIC NEUROENDOCRINE TUMORS

A variety of types of neuroendocrine cells is dispersed throughout the parenchyma of the pancreas. These cells produce hormones; tumors that form from these cells can produce excess hormones that escape or override normal feedback mechanisms. Both the classic syndromes and the excess hormones produced are used to categorize these functional tumors.

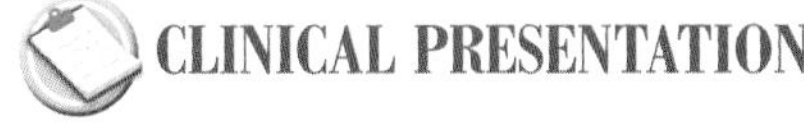

CLINICAL PRESENTATION

The patient who presents with symptoms that lead the physician to evaluate for a functional neuroendocrine tumor of the pancreas should be approached with a logical, stepwise algorithm for assessment and management. The initial step in evaluation of the patient is to establish the diagnosis biochemically. Proven biochemical excess without other causes leads to an evaluation for familial syndromes. Functional neuroendocrine tumors of the pancreas can be a component of a Multiple Endocrine Neoplasia (MEN) syndrome.

The next step in the management of this patient population involves medical management and, occasionally, dietary control of the excess hormones.

Tumor localization with computed tomography (CT) scans, magnetic resonance imaging (MRI), angiography, or endoscopic ultrasound (EUS) is next in the ideal situation. Due to liberal and widespread current use of imaging technologies in the United States, many tumors are identified incidentally and are localized prior to testing for biochemical excess. Preoperative localization allows the patient to become prepared for pancreatic resection or enucleation of the tumor. Preparation of the surgical team is likewise of importance so that the appropriate skill sets and technology (e.g., laparoscopic ultrasound) are available at the time of the procedure.

The major types of neuroendocrine tumors of the pancreas include: insulinoma, gastrinoma, glucagonoma, somatostatinoma, and VIPoma. This chapter will focus only on the management of insulinoma among the neuroendocrine tumors.

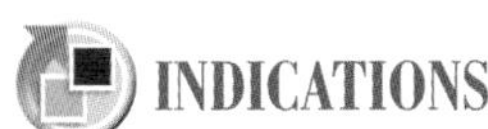

INDICATIONS

Insulinomas are usually diagnosed while small (<1.5 cm) and not metastatic. They usually present with neuroglycopenic symptoms and are usually benign, solitary, and located within the pancreatic parenchyma at the time of diagnosis. Fifty to 70% of insulinomas are found in the body and tail of the pancreas.

A multicenter study from France published by Ayav et al. reported the results of 36 patients who underwent laparoscopic pancreatic surgery for insulinoma. Nineteen of the 39 were managed with laparoscopic enucleation of the insulinoma while 12 patients underwent distal pancreatectomy. Three of the 36 patients required splenopancreatectomy. The remaining two patients were treated with one duodenopancreatectomy and one central pancreatectomy. This study demonstrated the feasibility of using a laparoscopic approach for insulinomas. The 30% reported complication rate is high but comparable to reported complication rates from open series.

Preoperative localization is advised prior to planning a laparoscopic resection. With or without preoperative localization, intraoperative ultrasonography is strongly recommended and in some cases essential for intraoperative confirmation of the location of the tumor. Additionally, intraoperative laparoscopic ultrasonography can demonstrate the relation of the mass to the pancreatic duct(s).

Patients presenting with neuroglycopenic symptoms can suffer permanent central nervous system (CNS) injury if subject to prolonged hypoglycemia. Many insulinoma patients carry a psychiatric or neurologic diagnosis (e.g., anxiety or seizure disorders) related to behaviors exhibited during hypoglycemic events. Whipple triad is a classic presenting symptom complex consisting of hypoglycemia, neuroglycopenia, and symptom relief with the administration of glucose. Fasting hypoglycemia is the classic finding for a diagnosis of insulinoma but the findings of the Whipple triad are required for a diagnosis. It is necessary to measure C-peptide and proinsulin levels to eliminate the diagnosis of exogenously administered insulin. Urine testing can eliminate the possibility of administered sulfonylureas, which can cross-react, as a cause of symptoms.

Only 5% to 10% of insulinomas are large, malignant, or metastatic. In fact, insulinomas are the least likely to be malignant of the neuroendocrine tumors mentioned in this chapter.

Surgical removal of insulinomas can be performed by enucleation or distal pancreatic resection. Tumor location, proximity to the pancreatic duct, and proximity to the large vessels is determined using laparoscopic ultrasound. Pre- and intraoperative imaging aids the surgeon in determining whether resection or enucleation is optimal.

ADENOCARCINOMA OF THE PANCREAS

There were approximately 37,000 new cases of pancreatic cancer diagnosed and 33,000 deaths attributed to pancreatic cancer in the U.S. in 2007. Ductal adenocarcinomas constitute more than 90% of diagnosed cases of pancreatic cancer. Approximately 10% of patients will survive 1 year or longer after being diagnosed with pancreatic cancer.

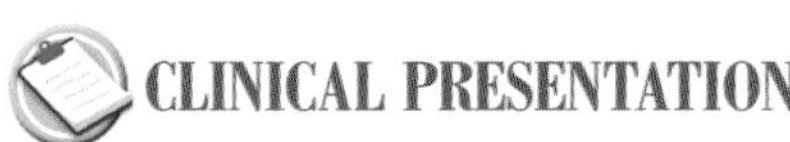

CLINICAL PRESENTATION

Patients may present with a nonspecific clinical picture. Many patients complain of abdominal pain, weight loss, and jaundice. Seventy-five percent of patients with pancreatic cancer complain of both abdominal pain and weight loss. Eighty percent of patients are jaundiced at the time of diagnosis of pancreatic cancer. Other presenting findings can include pruritis, enlargement of the liver and gallbladder, and changes in bowel habits. Pancreatic adenocarcinoma is found most commonly in the head of the pancreas. Those patients who have cancer in the body or tail of the pancreas may present with splenomegaly or thrombophlebitis.

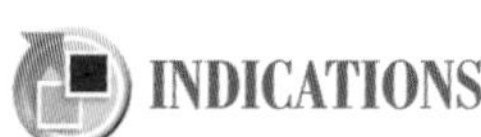

INDICATIONS

Laparoscopic pancreaticoduodenectomy has not reached widespread acceptance in the surgical community. There is a small number of centers around the world where minimally invasive techniques are offered routinely for the resection of cancer located in the head of the pancreas. The feasibility of the laparoscopic techniques for pancreaticoduodenectomy has been clearly established. Unfortunately, several authors have reported excessive morbidity and unacceptable length of operation with laparoscopic pancreaticoduodenectomy. Other reports document the safety of the procedure, but with a small number of patients. The initial report of a laparoscopic pancreaticoduodenectomy was in 1994 by Gagner and Pomp. Much discussion followed this report (including comments by those same authors) regarding the appropriateness of routinely performing pancreaticoduodenectomy via laparoscopic techniques. Variations on the total laparoscopic approach have been reported, including a hand-assisted laparoscopic (HAL) technique and a laparoscopic resection combined with a minilaparotomy for reconstruction.

TABLE 39-1. COMPLICATIONS OF LAPAROSCOPIC PANCREATIC SURGERY

- Bleeding
- Pancreatic leak or fistula
- Anastomotic leak or stricture
- Small bowel obstruction
- Delayed gastric emptying
- Wound complication
- Urinary tract infection
- Deep venous thrombosis
- Pulmonary embolus

Authors experienced with laparoscopic pancreaticoduodenectomy emphasize the necessity for the surgeon to possess exceptional laparoscopic skills. The operating room team must also be well prepared and have available several types of instrumentation and technology that usually include: laparoscopic clips, energy sources (ultrasonic dissection equipment and/or electrocautery), and angled laparoscopes.

Complications of laparoscopic pancreaticoduodenectomy can be significant and occur frequently (Table 39-1). Bleeding is the most frequently reported complication of laparoscopic pancreatic resection, and it can occur from multiple sources, including the anastomosis, the pancreatic parenchyma, vessels supplying the pancreas, adjacent organs, and other sites. Other reported complications include: small bowel obstruction, delayed gastric emptying, pancreatic leak, fistulae, anastamotic stricture or leak, and wound complications. Major complications that occur with laparoscopic pancreatic resection are the same experienced with open procedures.

SURGICAL TECHNIQUE

Access and Exposure

Laparoscopic pancreatic resection is usually performed with the patient in the supine position. While many experienced surgeons prefer to stand between the patient's legs for this and other upper abdominal procedures, a supine approach without the use of stirrups provides the surgeon with comparable access, less frustration during setup locating and placing secure stirrups, less concern regarding intraoperative injury to the patient's legs or hips, and greater physical comfort for the surgeon (Fig. 39-1).

Four or five ports are routinely used (Fig. 39-2, page 390), and access is obtained via an open or Hasson approach. Carbon dioxide pneumoperitoneum is maintained at 12 to 15 mmHg. An angled (30-degree) laparoscope is inserted, and a careful 360-degree survey of the peritoneal cavity is undertaken with initial close attention to the surfaces of the liver, diaphragm, peritoneum, and visible surfaces of the omentum and other organs.

Three ports are placed in addition to the Hasson port, and a suture through the upper abdominal wall is used to elevate the stomach (Fig. 39-3, page 390). An additional port can be placed in the subxiphoid region or lateral subcostal area for a retractor in lieu of the epigastric suture.

Pancreaticoduodenectomy

A window is created through the gastrocolic ligament using harmonic dissection and locking clips in attempt to eliminate bleeding or oozing that could later compromise optimal visualization. Other forms of energy, scissors and titanium clips, or linear cutting staplers can also be used in dividing the gastrocolic ligament. The right colon is then fully mobilized and a Kocher maneuver performed to fully mobilize the duodenum and head of the pancreas. The pancreas is then evaluated visually and with laparoscopic ultrasound to confirm resectability (Fig. 39-4, page 391). The laparoscopic ultrasound probe can be placed behind the uncinate process for an excellent view of the head of the pancreas and the pathologic lesion. It also allows the surgeon to once again confirm resectability by ruling out vascular invasion. The anterior surface of the head of the pancreas can also be well seen by dividing the gastrohepatic ligament. The superior surface of the pancreas is dissected and the right gastric and gastroduodenal arteries are divided between locking clips. The distal stomach is dissected with division of the vessels along the lesser curvature. The distal third of the stomach is divided using the linear cutting stapler (Fig. 39-5, page 391). Two or more firings of the stapling device are usually needed for complete transection. The staple line should be examined for hemostasis, and any bleeding found should be controlled prior to proceeding. The proximal jejunum is isolated and then transected with a linear cutting stapler. Dissection of the jejunal mesentery is taken cephalad to the level

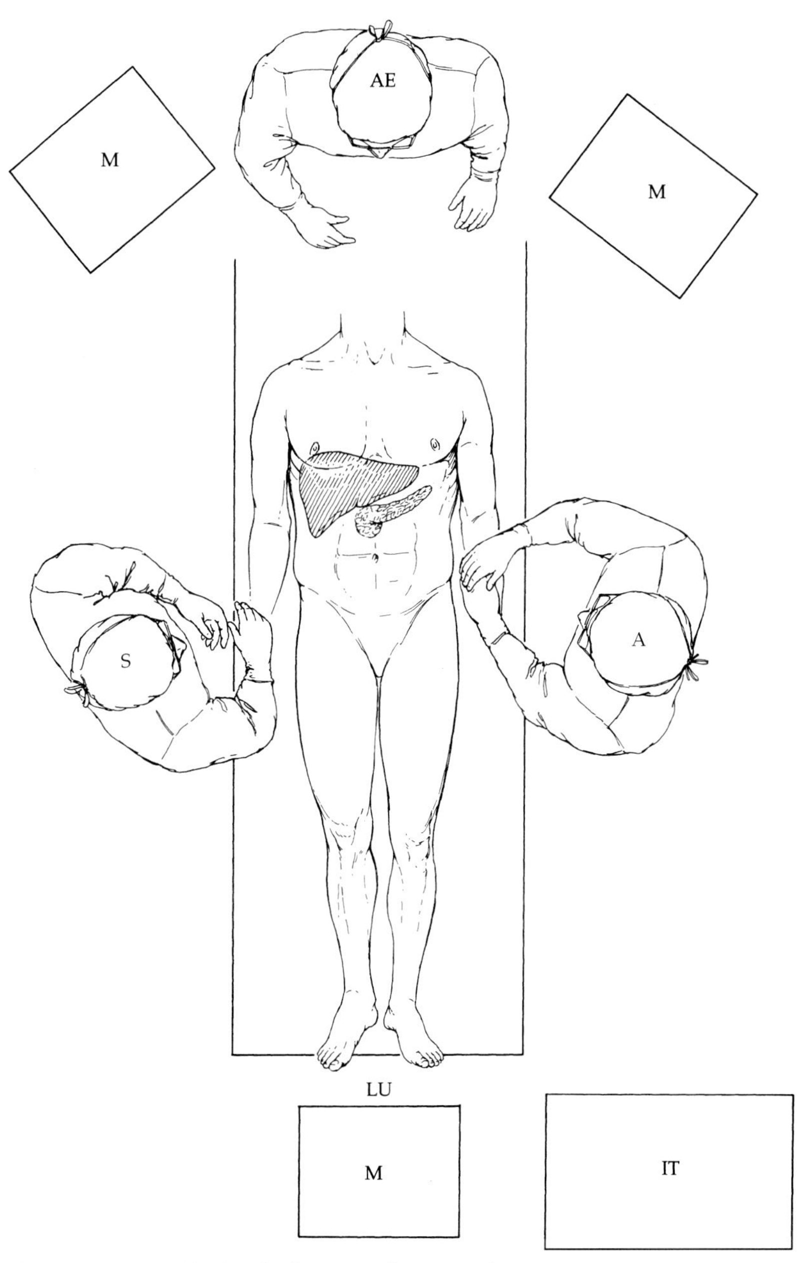

Fig. 39-1. Patient positioning for laparoscopic pancreatic surgery.

of the previous duodenal mobilization. Attention is then turned to dissection of the inferior edge of the pancreas, leading to posterior dissection. Gentle elevation and precise division of the multiple small posterior pancreatic branches is best performed with the ultrasonic coagulation shears. Dissection of the pancreas from the portal vein must be executed with skill and caution. The pancreas is transected from caudad to cephalad at the selected location as mapped out with laparoscopic ultrasound. Transection of pancreatic parenchyma is now accomplished with an ultrasonic coagulating shears (Fig. 39-6, page 392). A linear cutting stapler was used in the past, but problems with the mismatch between the thickness of the pancreatic parenchyma and the gap between the closed jaws of the stapler caused a crushed line of tissue adjacent to the staple line on the pancreatic remnant that lead to necrosis and pancreatic fistula in an unacceptably high number of cases.

The remaining mesenteric branches to the uncinate process are divided to completely mobilize the specimen. Finally, the bile duct is transected approximately three centimeters away from the head of the pancreas. The transected jejunum is passed through a window in the transverse mesocolon to allow the specimen to be placed in a specimen bag for removal.

Reconstruction occurs through a small abdominal incision in the upper midline, where specimen extraction can also occur. Approximately 50% of reported laparoscopic pancreaticoduodenectomy operations include reconstruction via a minilaparotomy. Reconstruction includes a pancreaticoduodenectomy, hepaticojejunostomy, and gastrojejunostomy. The totally laparoscopic reconstruction is performed in the same sequence and manner as the open reconstruction but usually requires significantly more time (Fig. 39-7, page 392). The end-to-end pancreaticoduodenectomy is performed initially. An end-to-side hepaticojejunostomy is sutured ten to 15 cm away from the initial anastomosis. A stapled side-to-side gastrojejunostomy is performed using jejunum 40 to 50 cm distal to the hepaticojejunostomy. One or two closed suction drains are placed near, but not touching, the pancreatic and biliary anastamoses. The drain(s) exit the abdomen at the 5-mm port site(s).

Distal Pancreatectomy

Resection of the distal pancreas by laparoscopy is performed far more frequently than laparoscopic pancreaticoduodenectomy. The resection of the distal pancreas is usually much easier technically than resection of the head of the pancreas. Furthermore, anastomoses and reconstruction are not usually required.

Indications for distal pancreatectomy are numerous and include pancreatic adenocarcinoma, neuroendocrine tumors, chronic pancreatitis, cystadenoma, cystodenocarcinoma, cysts, and pseudocysts.

Access to the peritoneal cavity is gained, pneumoperitoneum is established, ports are placed, and an initial survey is executed as previously described in this chapter.

The gastrocolic ligament is divided using ultrasonic dissection and clips are applied to larger vessels. The lesser sac is opened, the stomach is elevated with sutures or a retractor, and the pancreas is examined. Laparoscopic ultrasound can be very helpful in identifying the pancreatic duct, vessels, tumors, and desired lines of parenchymal dissection (see Figs. 39-3 and 39-4).

The decision to perform the procedure in a spleen-sparing fashion is based

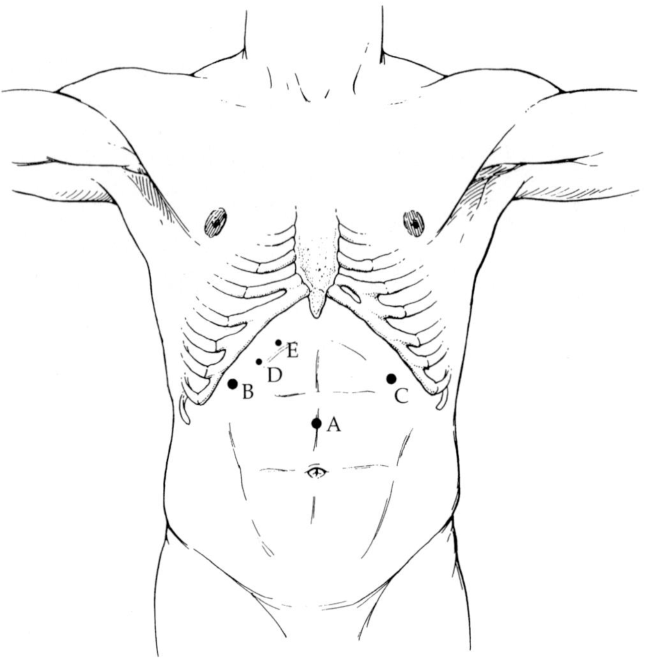

Fig. 39-2. Port placement for laparoscopic pancreatic resections.

upon the surgeon's judgment, the size and location of the mass, and splenic viability after completion of dissection. The inferior border of the pancreas to the left of the mesenteric vessels is mobilized using the ultrasonic dissector (Fig. 39-8, page 393). If the spleen will be sacrificed, it can be mobilized initially. Inferior mobilization of the pancreatic border allows posterior dissection. Attention is turned to the cephalad border where the splenic artery is isolated. Individual branches of the splenic artery feeding the pancreas are divided with the ultrasonic dissector or clips and scissors when the splenic artery is spared (Fig. 39-9, page 393). When dividing the splenic artery, the artery and splenic vein are usually divided individually with the linear cutting stapler using a vascular cartridge. Once again, the pancreatic parenchyma is divided with the ultrasonic dissector (see Fig. 39-6). One should attempt to identify the major pancreatic duct and ligate it near the transaction point at the cut surface with a single figure-eight suture. The specimen is placed in a bag for removal through the enlarged Hasson trocar site. A soft closed-suction drain is routinely placed in a dependent position near the cut surface of the pancreas. Fibrin glue or other tissue sealant products are not routinely used.

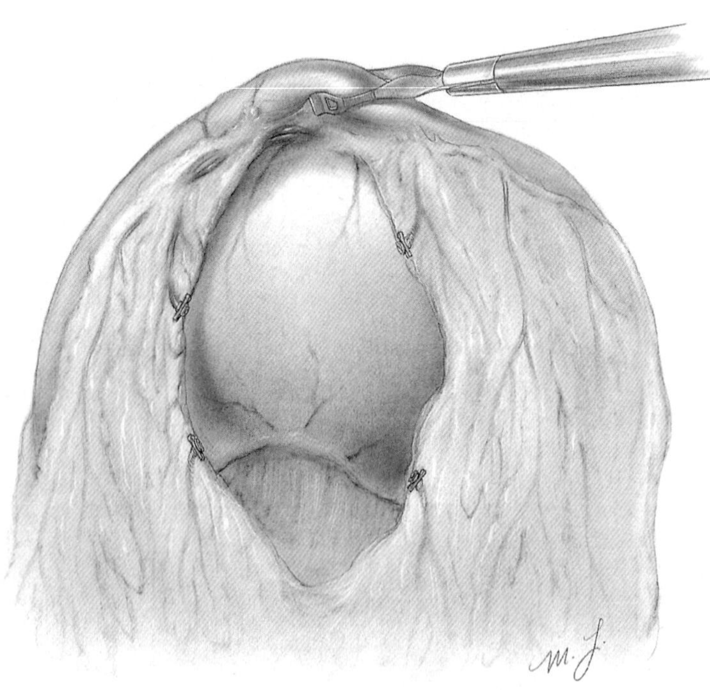

Fig. 39-3. The stomach is suspended with a percutaneous transfixion stitch.

Enucleation

Access and exposure of the pancreas are obtained as previously described within this chapter. The pancreas is evaluated visually and with the laparoscopic ultrasound. The mass is identified and its relation to the major pancreatic duct and vessels determined. Enucleation is usually performed using an ultrasonic dissection or hook cautery (Fig. 39-10, page 394). Hemostasis is carefully maintained and injury to the pancreatic duct is avoided. Caution is exercised in avoiding entering the mass during mobilization. The mass is removed from the pancreas, placed in a bag, and removed through the Hasson port site.

SUMMARY

The feasibility and safety of laparoscopic pancreatic resections have been reported in several small case series. Pancreaticoduodenectomy is not performed currently in the vast majority of hospitals as it requires excellent laparoscopic skills and a thorough understanding of pancreatic surgery in order to obtain good results on a routine basis. On the other hand, tumor enucleation and distal pancreatectomy are feasible with a combination of high-volume laparoscopic and pancreatic surgical experience.

SUGGESTED READING

Ayav A, Bresler L, Brunand L, et al. Laparoscopic approach for solitary insulinoma: a multicentre study. *Langenbecks Arch Surg* 2005;390: 134–140.

Corcione F, Marzano E, Cuccurullo D, et al. Distal pancreas surgery: outcome for 19 cases managed with a laparoscopic approach. *Surg Endosc* 2006;20:1729–1732.

Cuesta MA, Meijer S, Borgstein PJ, et al. Laparoscopic ultrasonography for hepatobiliary

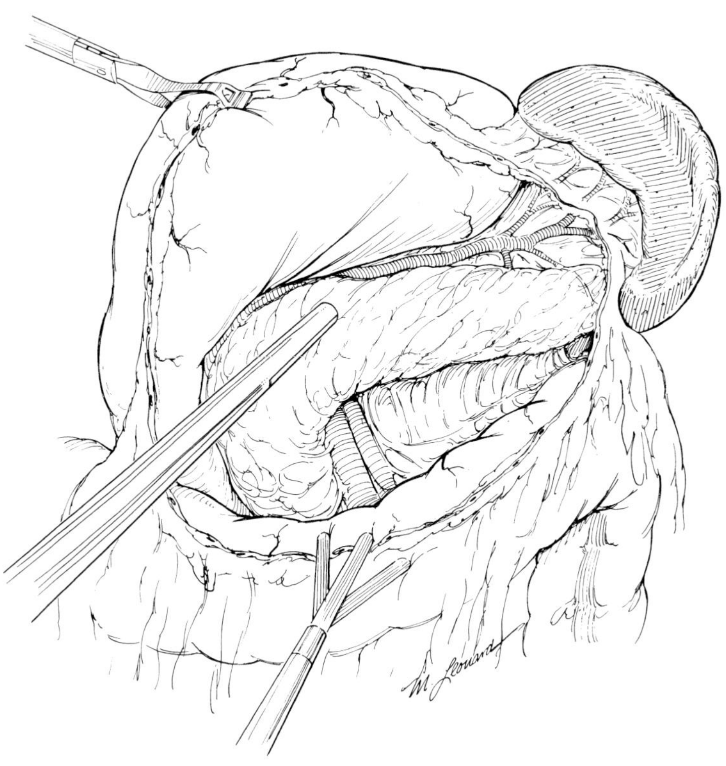

Fig. 39-4. A Kocher maneuver allows the head of the pancreas to be elevated.

and pancreatic malignancy. *Br J Surg* 1993;80:1571–1574.

Dulucq JL, Wintringer P, Mahajna A. Laparoscopic pancreaticoduodenectomy for benign and malignant diseases. *Surg Endosc* 2006;20: 1045–1050.

Dulucq JL, Wintringer P, Stabilini C, et al. Are major laparoscopic pancreatic resections worthwhile? *Surg Endosc* 2005;19: 1028–1034.

Gagner M, Inabnet WB, Biertho L, et al. Laparoscopic pancreatectomy: a series of 22 patients. *Ann Chir* 2004;129:2–7.

Gagner M, Pomp A, Herrera MF. Early experience with laparoscopic resection of islet cell tumors. *Surgery* 1996;120:1051–1054.

Iihara M, Kanbe M, Okamoto T, et al. Laparoscopic ultrasonography for resection of insulinomas. *Surgery* 2001;6:1086–1092.

Lillemoe KD, Kaushal S, Cameron JL, et al. Distal pancreatectomy: indications and outcomes in 235 patients. *Ann Surg* 1999;5:693–700.

Mabrut JY, Boulez J, Peix JL, et al. Laparoscopic pancreatic resection. *Ann Chir* 2003;128: 425–432.

Mabrut JY, Fernandez-Cruz L, Azagra JS, et al. *Surgery* 2005;6:597–605.

Underwood RA, Soper NJ. Current status of laparoscopic surgery of the pancreas. *J Hepatobiliary Pancreat Surg* 1999;6:154–164.

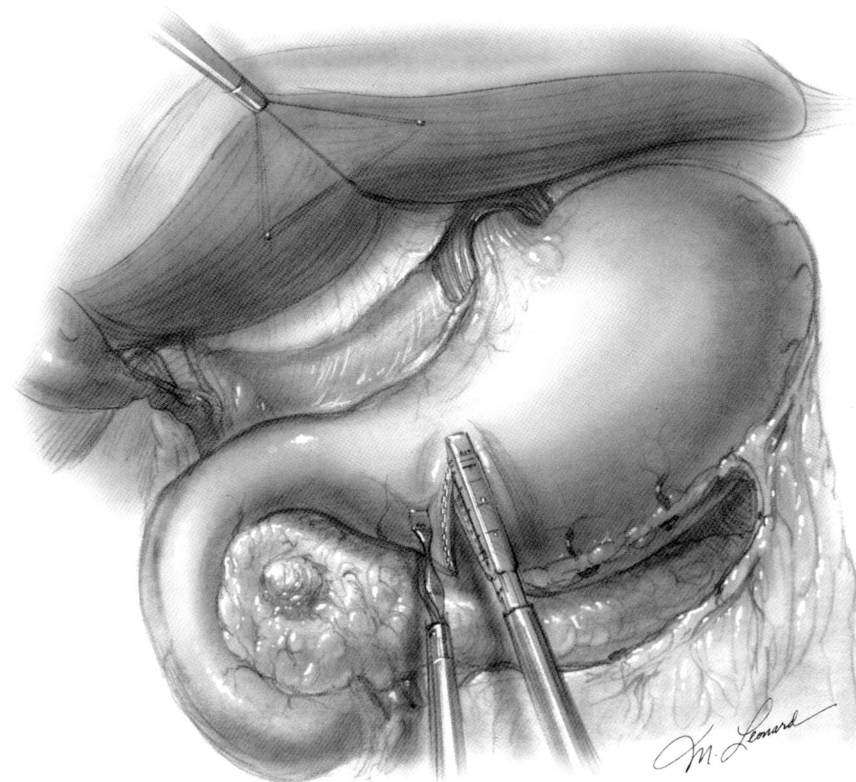

Fig. 39-5. The distal stomach is divided with multiple firings of the endoscopic stapler.

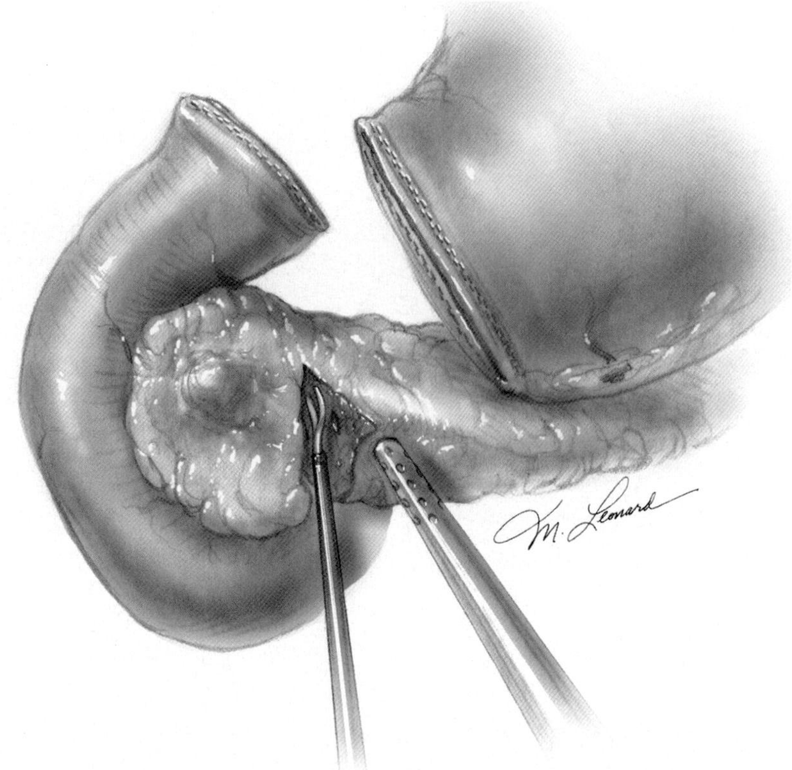

Fig. 39-6. The ultrasonic coagulating shears are used to divide the body of the pancreas.

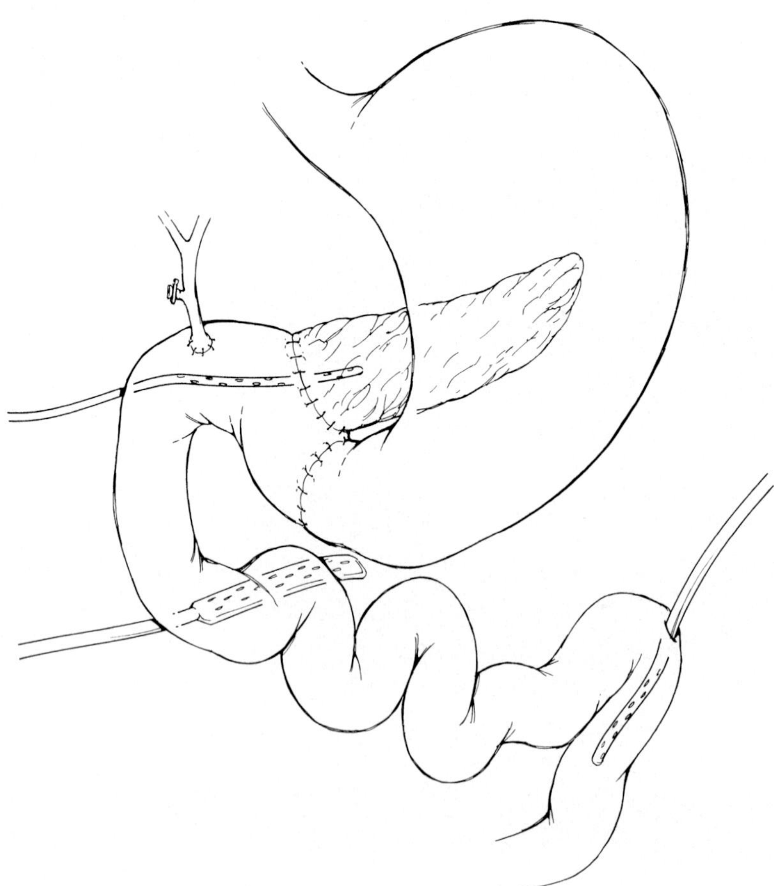

Fig. 39-7. A classic Whipple reconstruction is performed through a mini-laparotomy.

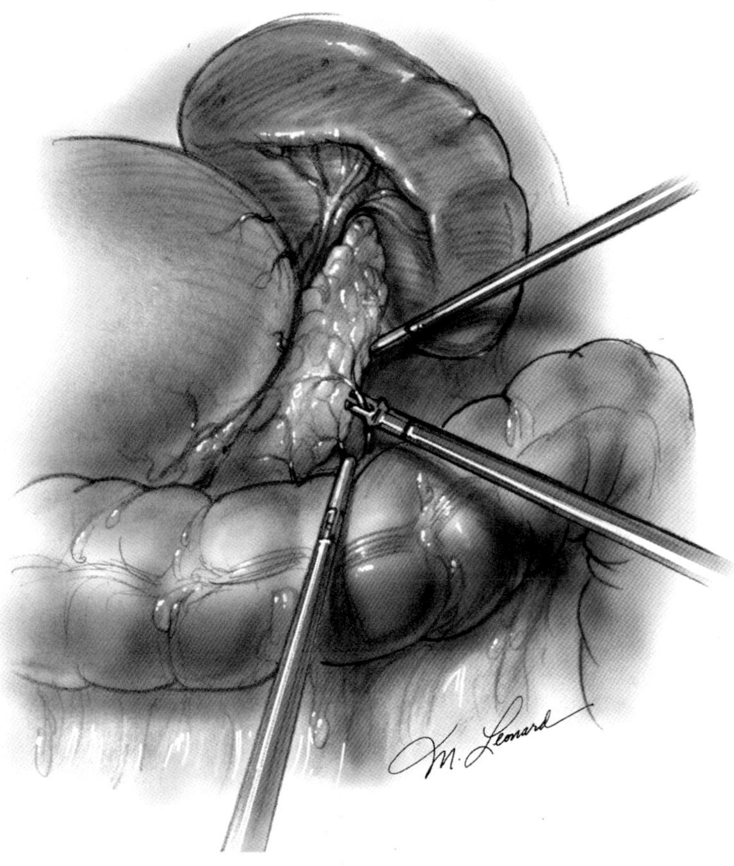

Fig. 39-8. The inferior margin of the pancreas is mobilized using the ultrasonic coagulating shears.

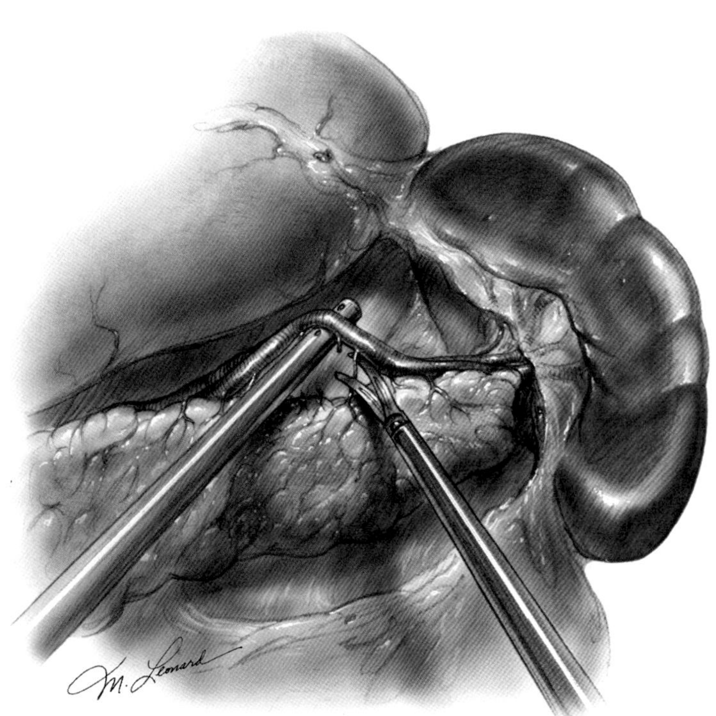

Fig. 39-9. Separating the splenic artery from the dorsal pancreas is tedious.

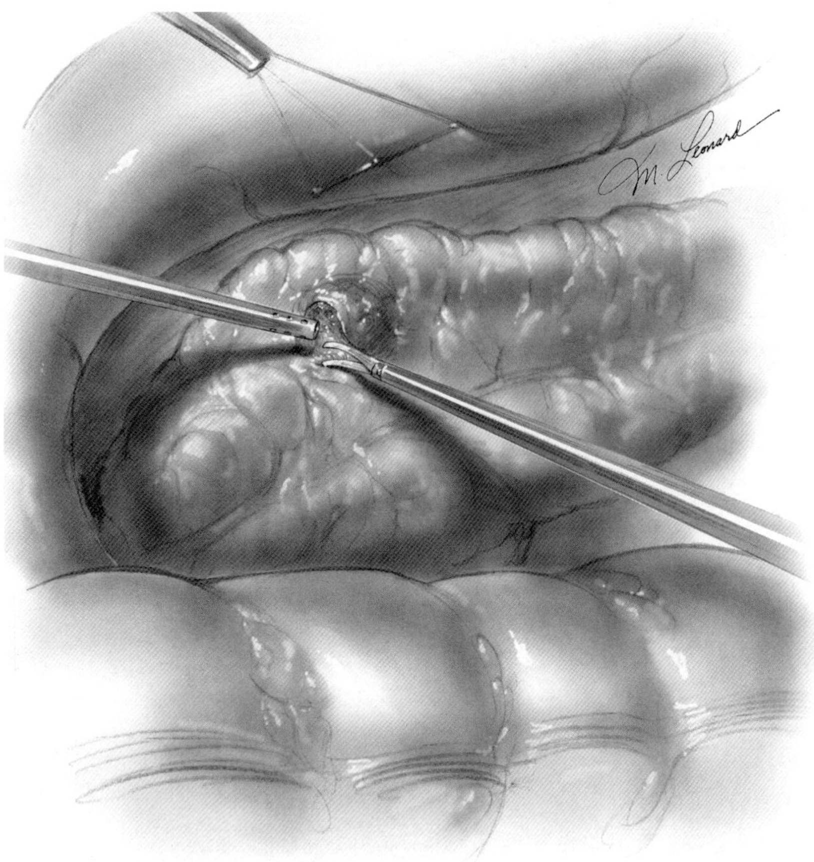

Fig. 39-10. Enucleating a pancreatic neuroendocrine tumor.

COMMENTARY

A truism of surgery has been that one should not lightly "mess with the pancreas." Dr. Eubanks nicely outlines the current status of laparoscopic pancreatic resections, which basically includes every surgery done open. Emphasis is placed on the fact that caution must be used, and it comes across clearly that laparoscopic resections are no place for the inexperienced; either in pancreatic surgery or advanced laparoscopy. That being said, this does represent one of the final frontiers of laparoscopic surgery and is therefore worthy of scrutiny.

While enucleation of neuroendocrine tumors has been shown to be safe and feasible and not a technically complex procedure, it does require an extensive and knowledgeable preoperative workup and evaluation. It also requires a facility with laparoscopic ultrasound, which is not a common skill. For that reason, the somewhat more complex distal pancreatectomy is the closest to achieving universal adoption. Technological tools such as ultrasonic dissectors or bipolar cautery devices have really enabled a laparoscopic approach even to the difficult splenic preserving pancreatectomy. This is true even to the point of surgeons using the laparoscopic tools for open pancreas resection! While early series had a disappointing incidence of pancreatic fistula, most pancreatic surgeons have stopped using the endoscopic stapler alone and supplement it either with sutures or biologic glue, with corresponding improvements in the leak rate. With care even difficult cases like chronic pancreatitis can be approached laparoscopically.

The laparoscopic Whipple procedure remains problematic and little performed. This is due to the multiple steps involved, which, though they are not individually difficult to do laparoscopically, have to be done sequentially and therefore take a lot of time and energy. Recent descriptions of using a mini-laparotomy after the resection to perform the multiple anastomoses have led to a mini-renaissance in laparoscopic Whipple procedures. It will, however, take a significant evolution in technology, perhaps some sort of single-shot anastomotic device, to make laparoscopic pancreatoduodenectomy an everyday occurrence.

LLS

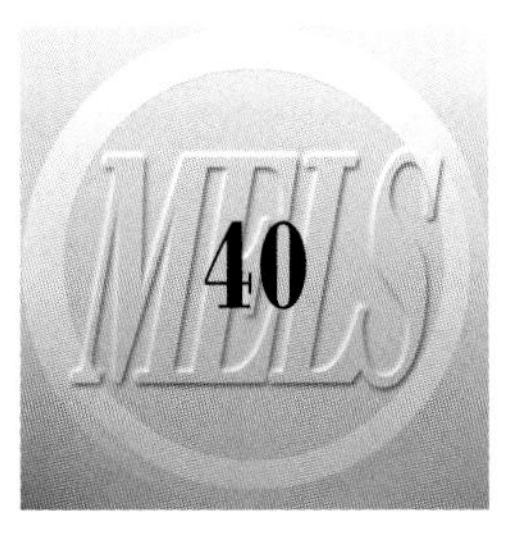

Laparoscopic Surgery of the Spleen

ERIC C. POULIN

INTRODUCTION

Laparoscopic surgery of the spleen presents the special challenge of removing a fragile and richly vascularized organ situated close to the stomach, colon, pancreas, and kidney as well as having to plan an extraction strategy that ensures proper histologic confirmation of the pathology while maintaining the objectives of minimal access surgery. This is made even more complicated when a large spleen or a partial splenectomy is involved.

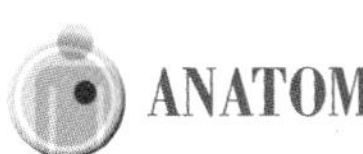

ANATOMY

A thorough appreciation of splenic anatomy is essential to the smooth performance of laparoscopic splenic surgery, with particular focus on optimal hemostatic control and preservation of the integrity of the spleen and pancreas during the procedure (Table 40-1). Whereas most anatomy texts imply that the splenic artery is constant in its course and branches, the classic essay by Michels demonstrates the fact that each spleen has its own peculiar pattern of terminal artery branches. Michels divides splenic artery topography into two types: *distributed* and *bundled* (magistral). He reports that the distributed type is found in 70% of dissections. By definition, the splenic trunk is short, and many long branches (6 to 12) enter over three-fourths (75%) of the medial surface of the spleen. The branches originate between 3 and 13 cm from the hilum (Fig. 40-1, page 396). The bundled type, present in the remaining 30% of specimens, is characterized by the presence of a long main splenic artery that divides into short terminal branches near the hilum. In this type, the splenic branches enter over only one-fourth to one-third (25% to 33%) of the medial surface of the spleen. These branches are large and few (3 to 4), originate 3.5 cm on average from the spleen, and reach the center of the organ as a compact bundle (Fig. 40-2, page 396).

The splenic branches exhibit so many variations in number, length, size, and origin that no two spleens have the same anatomy. Outside the spleen, the arteries also present frequent transverse anastomoses with each other, which, according to Testut, arise at a 90-degree angle between the involved arteries, as with most collaterals (Fig. 40-1). This means that the application of hemostatic clips or the embolization of coils occluding a branch of the splenic artery before such an anastomosis may fail to devascularize the corresponding splenic segment. Before it divides, the splenic trunk usually gives off a few slender branches to the tail of the pancreas. The most important, called the pancreatica magna, is familiar to vascular radiologists. It is an important landmark in selective angiography of the splenic artery. Severe pancreatitis has been reported following its occlusion during embolization procedures or while attempting to ligate the splenic artery in the lesser sac. The number of arteries entering the spleen is not determined by the organ's size, but rather by the presence of notches and tubercles, which usually correlates well with a greater number of entering arteries.

The splenic artery in the hilum can include up to seven branches at various division levels and in various anatomic arrangements: the superior terminal artery, the inferior terminal artery, the medial terminal artery, the superior polar artery, the inferior polar artery, the left gastroepiploic artery, and the short gastric arteries (Fig. 40-3, page 397). Veins are usually behind arteries except at the ultimate division level, where they may be anterior or posterior. According to Lipshutz, 72% of spleens have three terminal branches (superior polar, superior, and inferior terminal), and 28% have two, the other remaining branches being collaterals. When the superior terminal is excessively large, the inferior terminal is rudimentary, and more blood supply often comes from the left gastroepiploic and polar vessels. Up to six short gastric arteries may arise from the fundus of the stomach, but usually only those opening into the superior polar artery of the spleen (generally one to three) need to be ligated during laparoscopic splenectomy (Figs. 40-1 and 40-2). Despite the fact that no two spleens have the same anatomy, most specimens have two or three terminal branches entering the hilum (superior polar, superior, and inferior terminal). Two-colored corrosion casting and anatomic dissection have defined splenic lobes and segments that correspond to the entering terminal arteries, confirming the terminal nature of splenic blood supply. Relative avascular planes are identified between lobes and segments. When one considers the superior pole, fed by the short gastric vessels, and the inferior pole, fed by the gastroepiploic branches, there can be anywhere from three to five splenic lobes for most patients. The simple fact is that the

TABLE 40-1. SURGICAL FEATURES OF SPLENIC ANATOMY

No two spleens have the same anatomy.
Two types of splenic blood supply exist: the bundled (magistral) and the distributed types.
Transverse anastomoses exists between the splenic artery branches outside the hilum.
The gastrosplenic ligament contains short gastric and gastroepiploic vessels.
The lienorenal ligament contains the hilar vessels and the tail of the pancreas.
Other suspensory ligaments are avascular except in portal hypertension and myeloid metaplasia.
The tail of the pancreas lies within 1 cm of the inner surface of the spleen in 73% of cases.
The tail of the pancreas is in direct contact with the spleen in 30% of cases.
The size of the spleen does not determine the number of entering arteries.
The presence of notches and tubercles correlates with a greater number of entering arteries.
If splenic artery embolization is used, it should be done distal to the pancreatica magna artery.

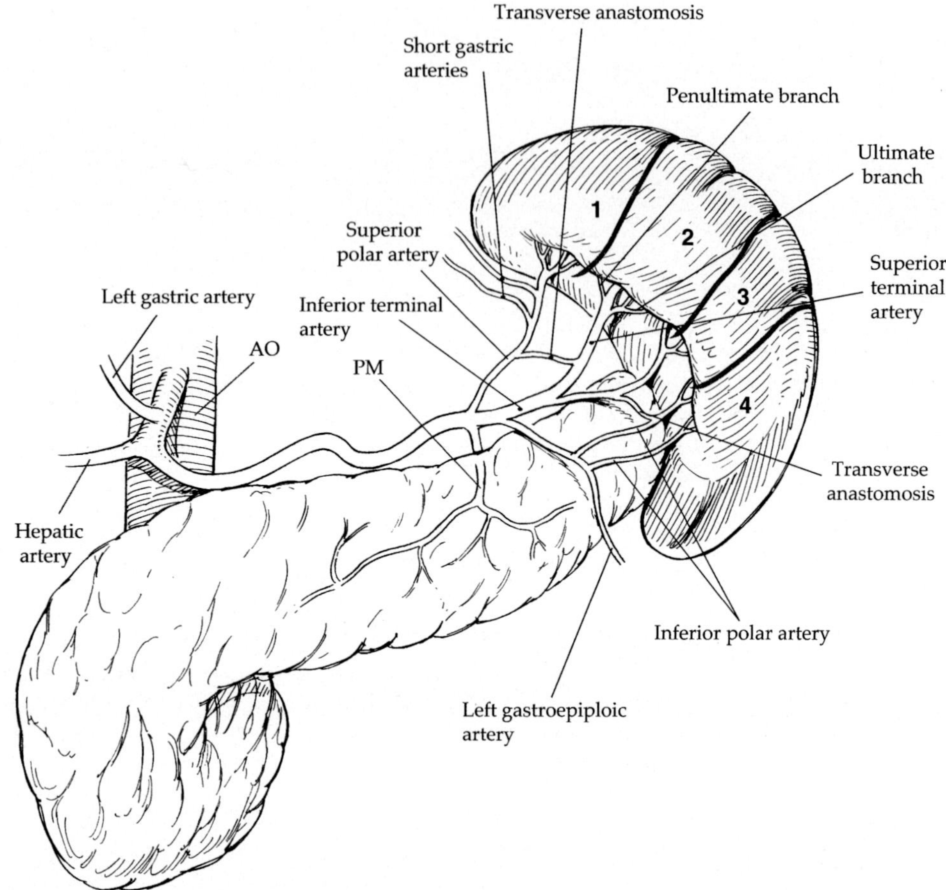

Fig. 40-1. Distributed type of vascularization. PM, pancreatica magna. (Reproduced with permission from Poulin EC, Thibault C. The anatomical basis for laparoscopic splenectomy. *Can J Surg* 1993;36:484–488.)

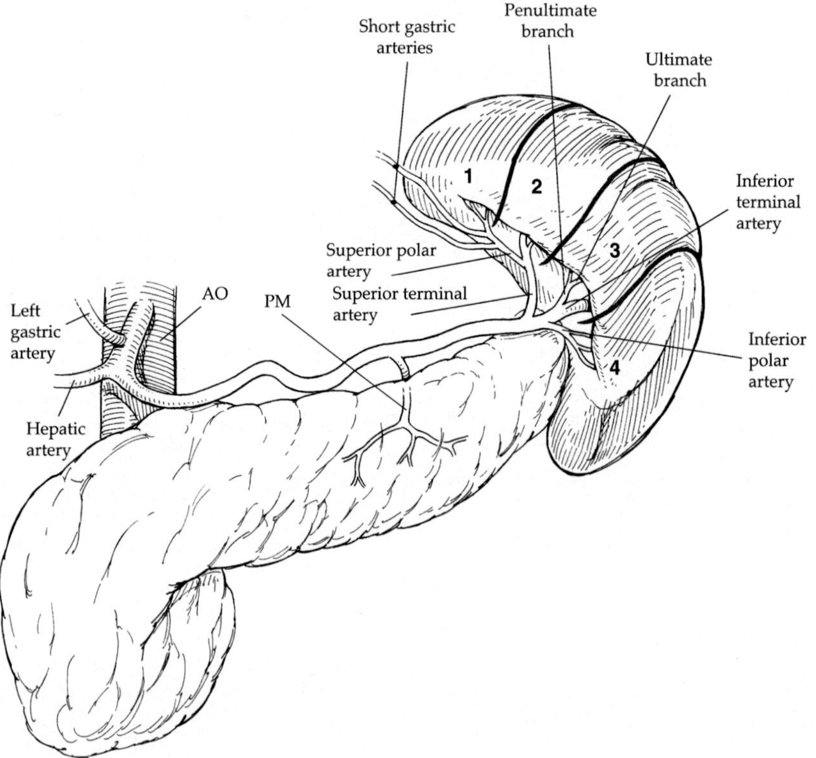

Fig. 40-2. Bundled (magistral) type of vascularization. PM, pancreatica magna. (Reproduced with permission from Poulin EC, Thibault C. The anatomical basis for laparoscopic splenectomy. *Can J Surg* 1993;36:484–488.)

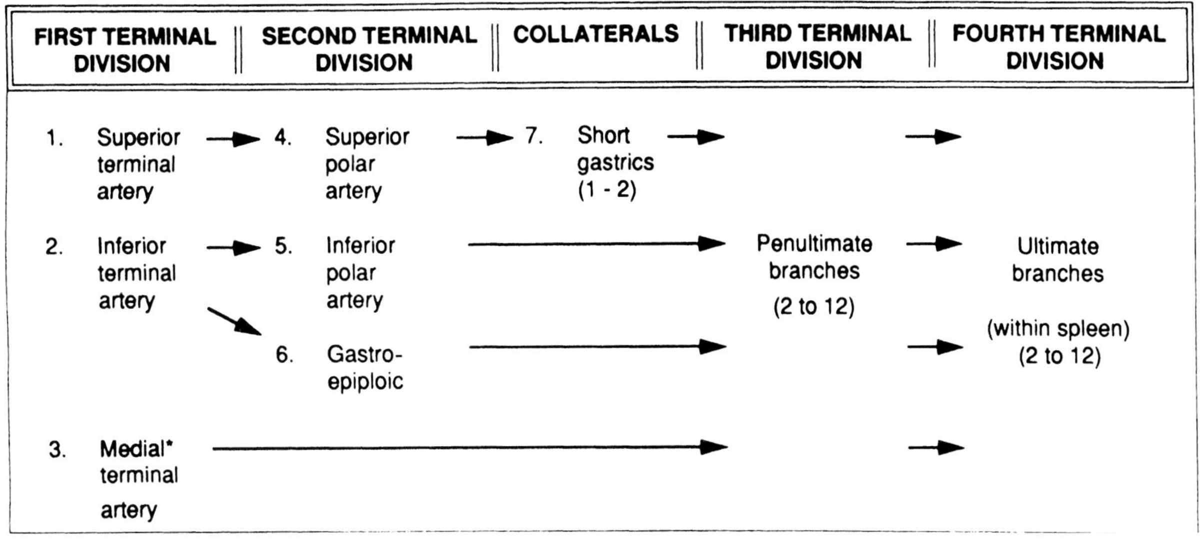

Fig. 40-3. General scheme of splenic artery branches. *present in only 20% of cases (Reproduced with permission from Poulin EC, Thibault C. The anatomical basis for laparoscopic splenectomy. *Can J Surg* 1993;36:484–488.)

surgical unit of the spleen is based on the surgically accessible vessels at the hilum (Figs. 40-1 and 40-2).

Duplications of the peritoneum form the many suspensory ligaments of the spleen. On the medial side, posteriorly, the lienorenal ligament contains the tail of the pancreas and the splenic vessels. Anteriorly, the gastrosplenic ligament contains the short gastric and the gastroepiploic arteries. The remaining ligaments are usually avascular except in patients with portal hypertension or myeloid metaplasia. The longest is the phrenicocolic ligament, which courses laterally from the diaphragm to the splenic flexure of the colon; its top end is called the phrenosplenic ligament. The attachment of the lower pole on the internal side is called the splenocolic ligament. Between the phrenicocolic and the splenocolic ligaments, a horizontal shelf of areolar tissue is formed on which rests the inferior pole of the spleen. It is often molded into a sac that opens craniad called the sustentaculum lienis, which acts as a brassiere to the lower pole of the spleen (Fig. 40-4).

Scoson-Javoschewitsch found the tail of the pancreas to be in direct contact with the spleen in 30% of cadavers. Baronofsky confirmed this finding and added that the distance was less than 1 cm in 73% of these patients.

PREOPERATIVE PLANNING

Before undergoing laparoscopic splenectomy, patients undergo the same hematologic preparation as for open surgery; that is, steroids, gamma globulins, fresh frozen plasma, cryoprecipitate, or platelets when required by the patients' hematologic disorder. Polyvalent pneumococcal vaccine is administered 2 weeks before surgery with boosters every 5 to 10 years as dictated by the levels of antibody titers. There should also be immunization for *Haemophilus influenzae* type B and meningococcal serogroup C. An annual influenza vaccination should also be offered. An ultrasound examination or computed tomography

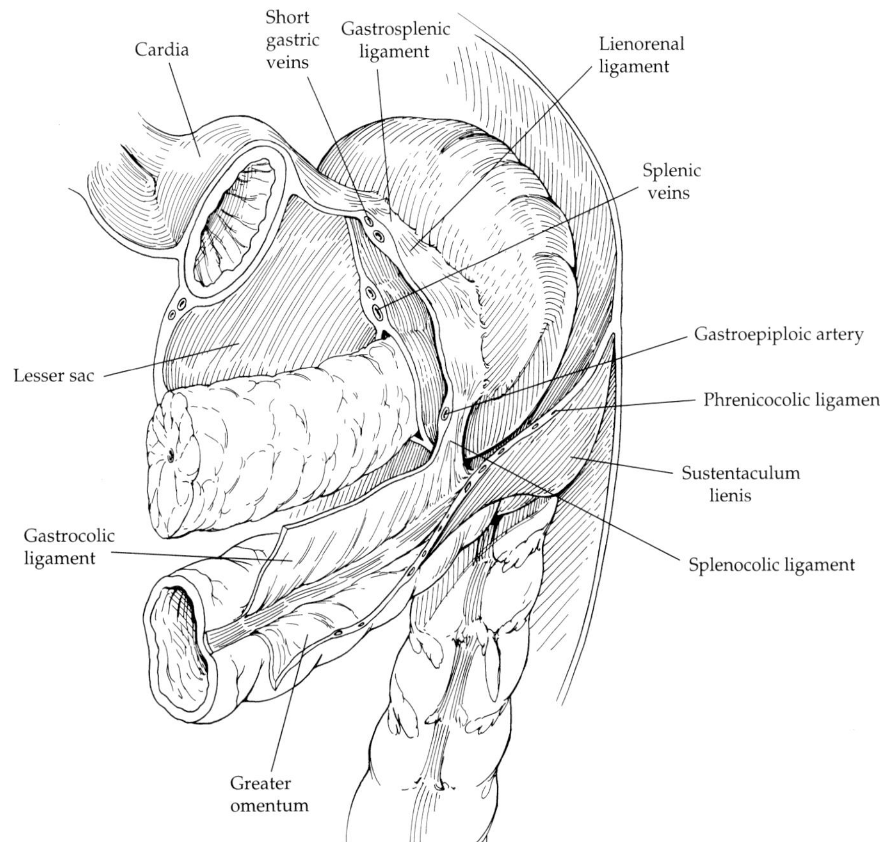

Fig. 40-4. Suspensory ligaments of the spleen. (Reproduced with permission from Poulin EC, Thibault C. The anatomical basis for laparoscopic splenectomy. *Can J Surg* 1993;36:484–488.)

(CT) scan is obtained to assess spleen size (maximum pole length), measured as the joining line between the two organ poles and divided into four categories: normal spleen (less than 11 cm long), moderate splenomegaly (11 to 20 cm), severe splenomegaly (21 to 30 cm); and megaspleens (exceeding 30 cm). More recently multi-detector row spiral computed tomography (CT) has been shown to accurately determine spleen volume, splenic vascular anatomy, presence and size of accessory spleens, and parenchymal lesions in patients who were undergoing laparoscopic splenectomy. The radiologist is also asked to try to identify accessory spleens. The choice between the anterior or lateral surgical approach is often decided from the preoperative determination of spleen size.

Preoperative splenic artery embolization is now very rarely used as an adjuvant procedure to help reduce blood loss and makes laparoscopic splenectomy easier to perform. Although it was useful to reduce the conversion rate when laparoscopic splenectomy was first attempted, its role is now confined to a few cases of laparoscopic splenectomy for very large spleens or for some cases of laparoscopic partial splenectomy. Some see an increasing role for embolization in selected cases of splenic trauma with or without total or partial laparoscopic splenectomy. However, it is worthwhile to describe this technique, which should be part of the skill set of any center with an interest in splenic surgery. It involves launching 3- to 5-mm microcoils or absorbable gelatin sponge fragments in each hilar branch of the splenic artery through a 3F or 5F Cobra catheter (Anthron; Toray Medical Co. Ltd; Tokyo, Japan) and a coil plunger. The catheter is then pulled back 2 to 4 cm, and one or two 5- to 8-mm microcoils are launched in the main trunk of the splenic artery distal to the pancreatica magna artery (known as the double embolization technique) to avoid pancreatitis or pancreatic necrosis (Fig. 40-5). The surgical plane of dissection is therefore situated between the proximal and distal embolization sites. The procedure is ended when it is estimated radiologically that 80% or more of the splenic tissue or the area containing the lesion to be removed has been successfully embolized.

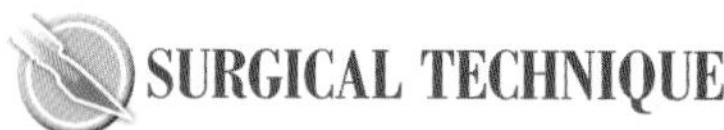

SURGICAL TECHNIQUE

There are two major surgical approaches to laparoscopic splenectomy: lateral and anterior.

Lateral

This approach was first described for laparoscopic adrenalectomy and has become the approach of choice for most cases of laparoscopic splenectomy. The patient is put on a beanbag mattress in right lateral decubitus, a position similar to that used for left-side posterolateral thoracotomy. The operating table is flexed, and the bolster is raised to increase the distance between the lower rib and the iliac crest. Usually four 12-mm trocars are used around the costal margin to allow maximum flexibility for the interchange of camera, clip applier, linear stapler, and other instruments. Three trocars are located anteriorly along the rib margin, and one is located in the left flank. Enough distance between trocars is required to preserve good working angles and easy triangulation. Some advantage exists in slightly tilting the patient backward, because doing so allows more freedom to move the instruments placed along the left costal margin, especially for lifting movements, when the instrument handles can come too close to the operating table. For the same reason, it is advantageous to place the anterior or abdominal side of the patient closer to the edge of the operating table. Using some reverse-Trendelenburg positioning also allows the spleen to move away from the diaphragm (Fig. 40-6).

An open approach is now favored for direct first trocar entry and creation of a symmetric 15-mmHg pneumoperitoneum. The camera is inserted, and a thorough search is made for accessory spleens, which should be removed when they are found, if possible. Placement of the remaining trocars is determined by patient configuration in relation to the size of the spleen to be excised. Usually the fourth posterior trocar cannot be inserted until the splenic flexure of the colon or sometimes the left kidney is mobilized. Therefore, the procedure is started with three trocars. The splenic flexure is partially mobilized by incising the splenocolic ligament, the lower part of the phrenicocolic, and the sustentaculum lienis to allow access to the gastrosplenic ligament, which can be readily separated from the lienorenal ligament in this position. Incising the splenocolic ligament and the sustentaculum lienis is the most productive move of this approach. Gentle upward retraction of the lower pole of the spleen then creates a tent-like structure with the gastrosplenic ligament making up the left panel and the lienorenal ligament the right panel of the tent. The stomach makes up the floor of the tent. All the pertinent splenic anatomy is then readily seen in one exposure. Surgeons performing laparoscopic splenectomy through the lateral approach should always try to reproduce this maneuver to separate the gastrosplenic from the lienorenal ligament and clearly

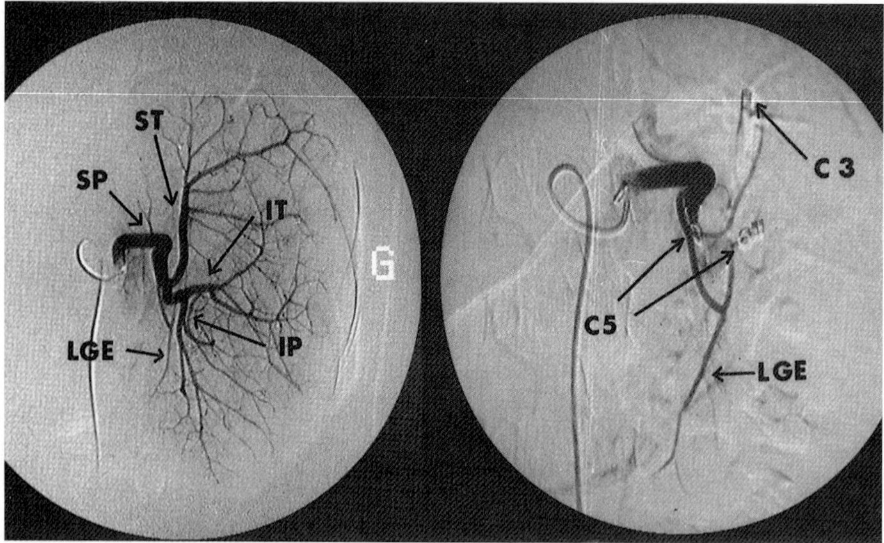

Fig. 40-5. Left: An 18-cm spleen, enlarged due to spherocytosis, with a distributed type of blood supply. Spherocytosis. SP, superior polar artery; ST, superior terminal artery; IT, inferior terminal artery; IP, inferior polar artery LGE, left gastroepiploic artery. **Right:** After embolization with microspheres (not visible). The 3-mm (C3) and 5-mm coils (C5) and the left gastroepiploic artery (LGE) are now clearly visible. (Reproduced with permission from Poulin EC, Thibault C, Mamazza J, et al. Laparoscopic splenectomy: clinical experience and the role of preoperative splenic artery embolization. *Surg Laparosc Endosc* 1993;3:445–450.)

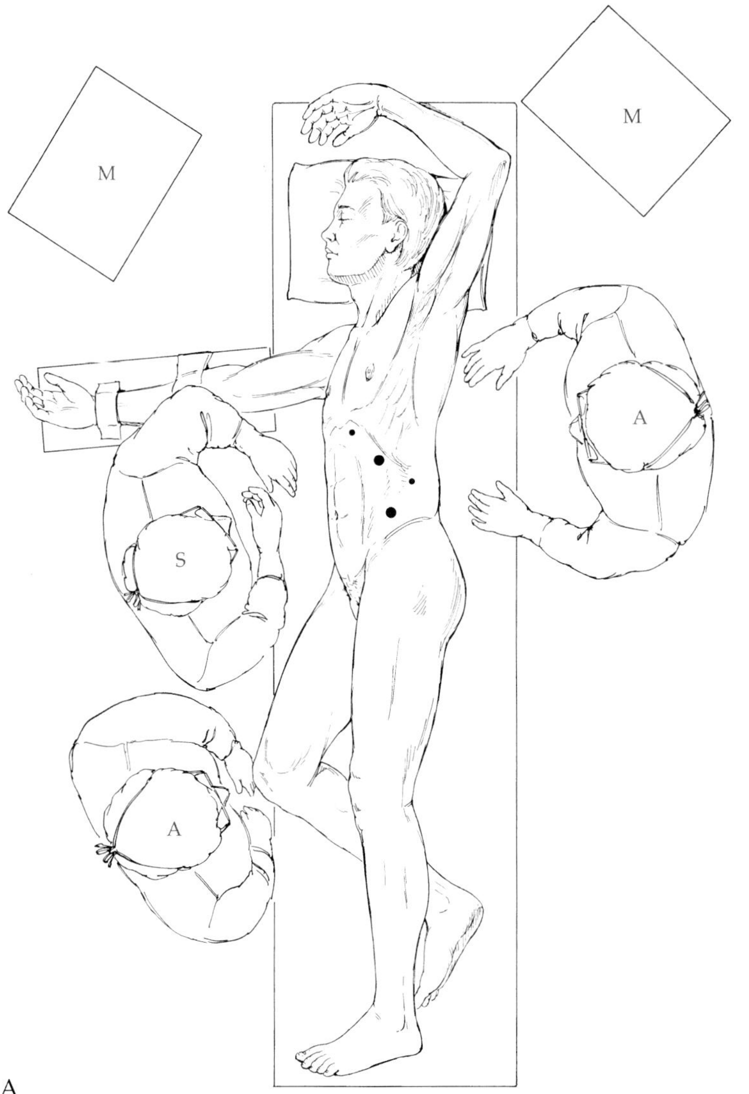

Fig. 40-6. The lateral approach. Patient positioning and operating room setup. Three 12-mm trocars are used anteriorly along the left costal margin. A fourth (5-mm or 12-mm) trocar is placed posterior to the iliac crest.

demonstrate all the noteworthy anatomic structures. Both the vessels contained in each ligament and the tail of the pancreas are easily identified and dissected (Fig. 40-7, page 400). The branches of the left gastroepiploic artery are taken with the cautery or clips, depending on the size of such branches. The avascular portion of the gastrosplenic ligament is then incised sufficiently to allow exposure of the hilar structures in the lienorenal ligament; this is done with gentle elevation of the lower pole. With the patient in the lateral position, the spleen almost retracts itself as it naturally falls toward the left lobe of the liver. The role of the assistant in retracting the spleen is therefore much less critical in this approach. At this point, the surgeon can usually assess the geography of the hilum and have an idea of the degree of difficulty of the operation. Then, the fourth trocar is placed posteriorly under direct vision, taking care to avoid the left kidney. In easier cases, one or two 5-mm trocars can be substituted for the usual 12-mm trocars. Care must also be taken in the choice of placement for the trocars situated immediately anterior and posterior to the iliac crest. The iliac crest can impede movements to mobilize structures upward if the trocars are placed over it rather than in front and behind it (Fig. 40-6).

The incision of the phrenicocolic ligament is then carried toward the diaphragm. A 2-cm-wide portion of the ligament is left attached to the spleen, making a long structure from which the spleen can be manipulated with graspers. With the camera in the lower or posterior trocar site, the tail of the pancreas is then dissected from the structures of the hilum in the areolar avascular tissue of the retroperitoneum. It is important to locate the tail of the pancreas and dissect it away from its position close to the splenic hilum to avoid injury during control of the vessels. If a *distributed type* of anatomy is present with its wide hilum, the splenic branches will usually be dissected and clipped. The *bundled type* lends itself more to a single use of the linear stapler as long as the tail of the pancreas is identified and dissected away when required. When possible, a window is created above the hilar pedicle in the lienorenal ligament so that all structures can be included within the markings of the linear stapler under direct vision (Figs. 40-7 and 40-8, pages 400 and 401). The viewing angles provided by moving the camera into the various trocars make this maneuver much easier in the lateral position than in the anterior approach (Fig. 40-9, page 402). The dissection is continued with individual dissection and clipping of the short gastric vessels. Occasionally these vessels can also be taken en masse with the linear stapler. Sutures are rarely necessary during laparoscopic splenectomy and have been used only occasionally to control a short gastric vessel too short to be clipped safely. This portion of the operation is performed while the spleen hangs by the upper portion of the phrenicocolic ligament. The experienced surgeon also learns to move the spleen back and forth so that it can be observed from both the anterior and posterior perspectives. The surgeon will then decide whether vessels are more easily approached from the back or the front for dissection and ligation. At this point in the operation, the spleen is inserted in a plastic bag; this is often simplified by preserving the upper portion of the phrenicocolic ligament during its initial dissection. After final section of the phrenicocolic ligament and of diaphragmatic adhesions when they are present, extraction is performed through one of the anterior ports. Extraction through the posterior port is made more difficult by the thickness of the muscle mass at this level and will usually require opening the incision and fulgurating more muscle than is necessary.

For specimen bagging purposes, a medium or large heavy-duty plastic home freezer bag that has been sterilized is folded and introduced into the abdominal cavity through one of the 12-mm trocars. The bag is unfolded and the spleen slipped inside to avoid splenosis from the

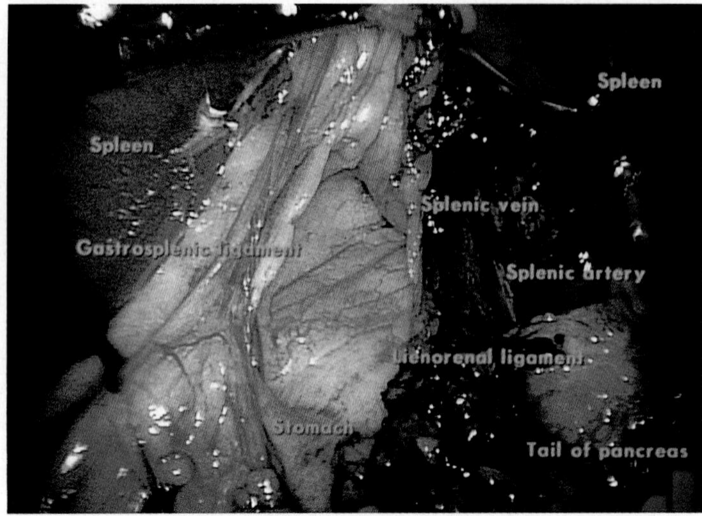

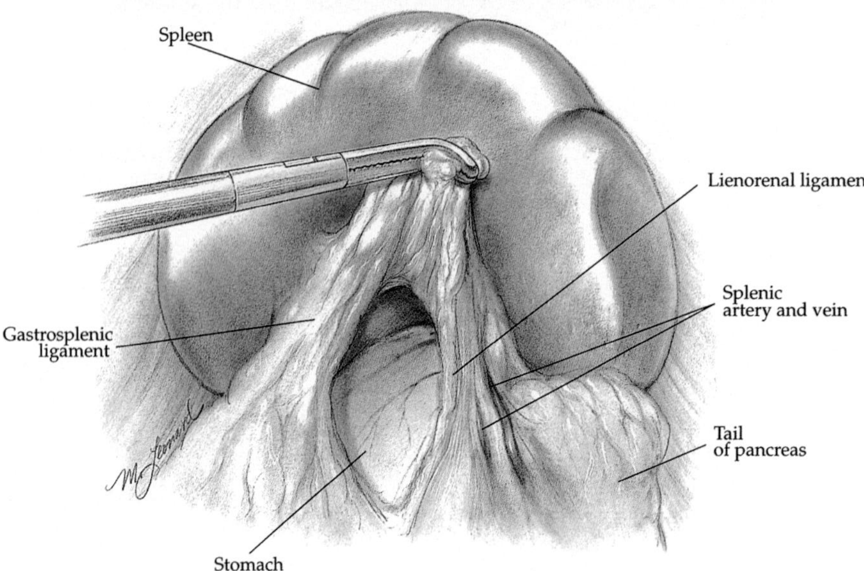

Fig. 40-7. Top: Color plate. **Bottom:** The "splenic tent," with separation of the gastrosplenic and lienorenal ligaments, demonstrating all anatomic elements as seen in the lateral approach after section of the ligaments attached to the lower pole of the spleen.

manipulations necessary for extraction (Fig. 40-10A, page 403). Grasping forceps are used to hold the two rigid edges of the bag and effect partial closure (Fig. 40-10B). It is difficult to insert the spleen into the plastic bag before unfolding and opening the bag completely. Bagging the resected spleen requires patience and imagination and at first can be frustrating. The 10-mm jaw forceps holding the edges at the lower end of the bag inside the abdomen is pushed through one of the mid anterior trocar sites, and the tip of the bag is grasped and brought out of the wound. Gentle traction on the bag from the outside brings the spleen close to the peritoneal surface of the umbilical incision. It is important during this maneuver to pull out only the ridged edges of the plastic bag while keeping a finger inside. Otherwise it is easy for the spleen to flip out of the bag, and the maneuver has to be repeated. The use of sterilized home freezer bags is the most cost-effective means of bagging and extracting the spleen. The thick freezer bags should not be confused with other plastic bags that are thinner and too prone to tearing during fragmentation and other manipulations, making them improper for extraction purposes.

A biopsy of a size suitable for pathologic identification is obtained by incising the splenic tip. Subsequently, the spleen is fragmented with finger fracture and the resulting blood is suctioned. The remaining stromal tissue of the spleen is then extracted through the small incision, hemostasis again verified, and all trocars removed (Figure 40-10C and D, page 403). Trocar sites are closed with resorbable sutures and paper strips. No drains are used.

Anterior

The anterior approach was the first procedure described for laparoscopic splenectomy. Nowadays, it is only used in special circumstances, mainly for very large spleens with the hand-assist technique or when other procedures need to be performed concomitantly, especially in pediatric patients. In this approach, the patient is under general anesthesia and placed in a modified lithotomy position to allow the surgeon to operate between the patient's legs and for the assistants to be positioned on each side of the patient. Surgery is performed through five trocars in the upper abdomen in a steep Fowler position with left-sided elevation. A 12-mm trocar is introduced through an umbilical incision using an open approach under direct vision, and a 10-mm laparoscope (0-degree or 30-degree) is connected to a video system. Two 12-mm trocars are placed in each upper quadrant, and two 5-mm trocars are inserted close to the rib margin on the left and right sides of the abdomen. Careful selection of all trocar sites is made to optimize working angles. As needed, the 12-mm ports are used to introduce clip appliers, staplers, or a laparoscope from a variety of angles. Trocars can also be placed in a half-circle facing the left upper quadrant (Fig. 40-11, page 405). The left hepatic lobe is retracted with a palpator or retractor through the right lateral 5-mm trocar site. While retracting the liver, the tip of the instrument should lie against the diaphragm to avoid lacerations and nuisance bleeding. A toothed grasping forceps placed on the diaphragm at the apex of the crura can also be used for this purpose. The stomach is retracted medially through the left 5-mm trocar to expose the spleen after the omentum has been displaced inferiorly. Then a fairly standard sequence is followed. First, a search is made for accessory spleens. When found, they are removed immediately, for they can be much harder to locate after the spleen has been removed. Then the phrenicocolic, the splenocolic, and the sustentaculum lienis are incised near the lower pole using electrocautery and hook probe or scissors through the left 12-mm port. Some vascular adhesions, which are frequently found on the medial side of the spleen, are

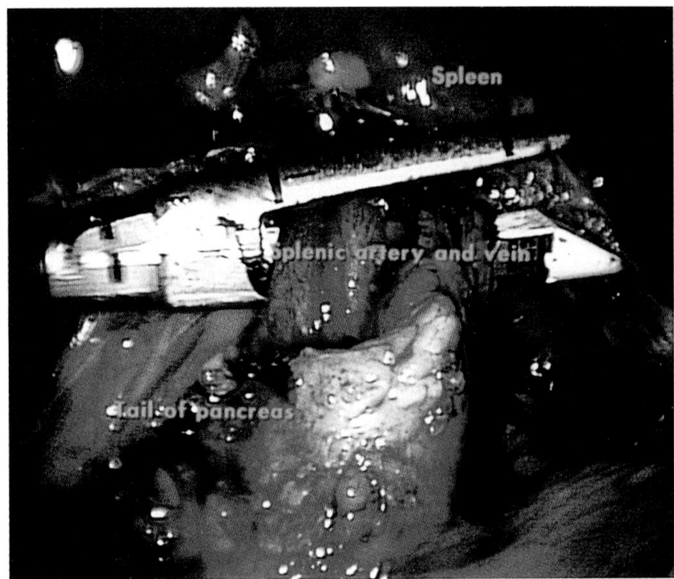

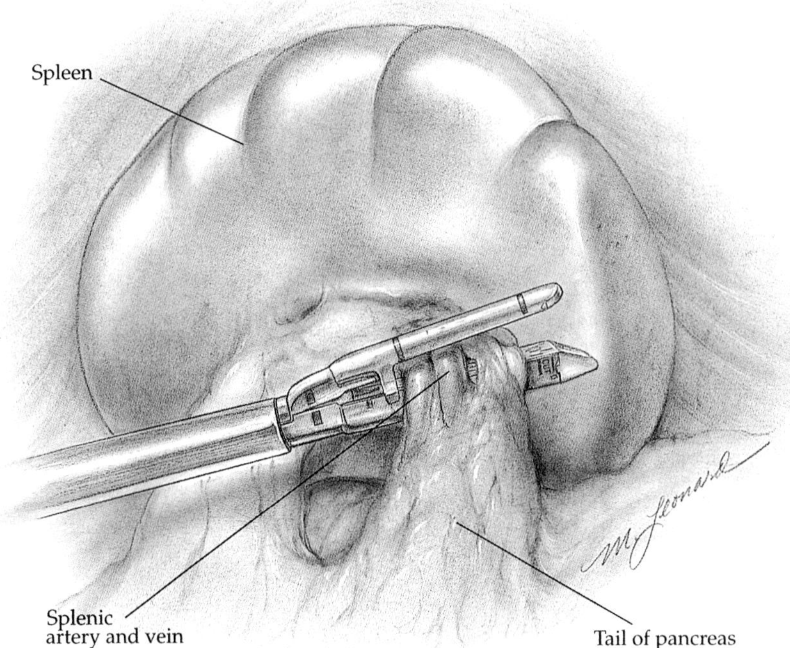

Fig. 40-8. Top: Color plate. **Bottom:** The lateral approach. En bloc stapling of hilar structures after creation of a window above the tail of the pancreas.

cauterized. These have also been called *criminal folds* for their tendency to be pulled off the spleen during dissection and cause nuisance bleeding from capsular injury. The gastrocolic ligament is carefully dissected close to the spleen, and the left gastroepiploic vessels are ligated one by one with metallic clips or simply cauterized if they are small. The lower pole of the spleen is gently lifted with one palpator through a 5-mm port to expose the splenic hilum and the tail of the pancreas within the lienorenal ligament. This maneuver must be done with great care; it requires constant concentration by the assistants to avoid lacerations of the spleen and troublesome bleeding. The tip of the instrument used for lifting the lower pole should therefore rest against the left lateral abdominal wall. Lifting the lower pole facilitates the individual dissection and clipping of all branches of the splenic artery and vein as close as possible to the spleen. Staying close to the spleen decreases the likelihood of causing trauma to the tail of the pancreas. In the anterior approach, the gastrosplenic and the lienorenal ligament and the vessels they contain lie on top one another. Their separation is not always easily performed and requires experience with the anatomy. The operation can also differ depending on the type of vascular anatomy. Surgery on a spleen with a distributed type of blood supply will usually mean dissection of more blood vessels that are, however, spread over a wider area of the splenic hilum, making individual dissection of the vessels easier. Operation on a spleen with a bundled-type blood supply will usually mean fewer vessels. The hilum is more compact and narrower, and the dissection of each vessel is thereby more troublesome. Using the anterior approach, it is difficult to create safely a window above the tail of the pancreas to permit the application of a stapling device and to control all hilar vessels, a maneuver more easily performed using the lateral approach. It is dangerous to apply a stapling device across the hilum in the anterior approach without ascertaining that the tip is free of tissue or making sure that the tail of the pancreas has been identified and dissected away; it can lead to serious hemorrhage or pancreatic trauma. After control of the hilar vessels, the short gastric vessels are then identified and ligated with clips or occasionally with a stapler. No sutures are used.

When preoperative splenic artery embolization is used, the dissection plane is situated between the sites of distal embolization of splenic artery branches and the site of proximal embolization of the splenic artery itself. Because of the segmental and terminal distribution of splenic arteries, it is easy to determine the devascularized portions of the spleen by a characteristic grayish color; vascularized segments retain a pinkish hue. When the organ is completely isolated, it is left in its natural cavity and hemostasis is verified.

The umbilical trocar is then removed and the umbilical incision extended to 2 cm for specimen extraction. The extraction technique is similar to the one used in the lateral approach. No drains are used unless damage to the tail of the pancreas has occurred. If so, a closed suction drain is left in place.

Hand-Assisted Laparoscopic Splenectomy

Hand-assisted laparoscopic surgery (HALS) refers to laparoscopic procedures performed with the aid of a plastic device inserted in a 7.5- to 10-cm wound. Although several variations exist, the hand port

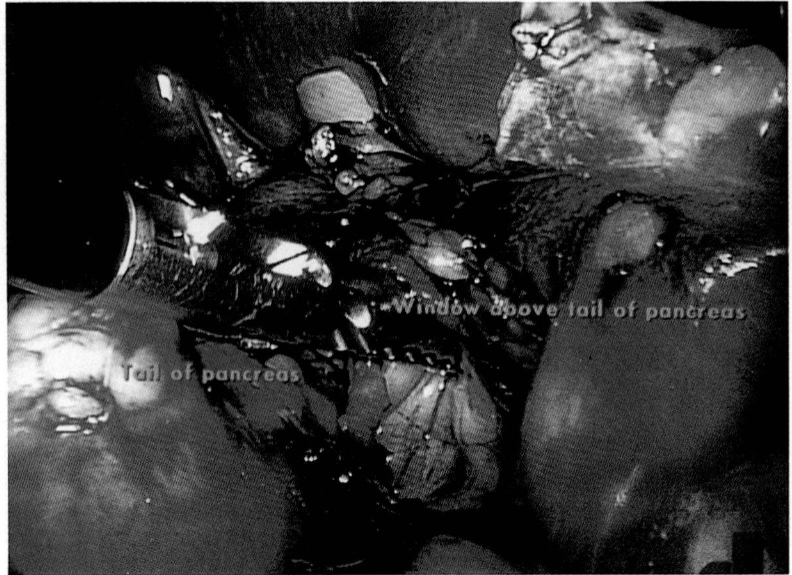

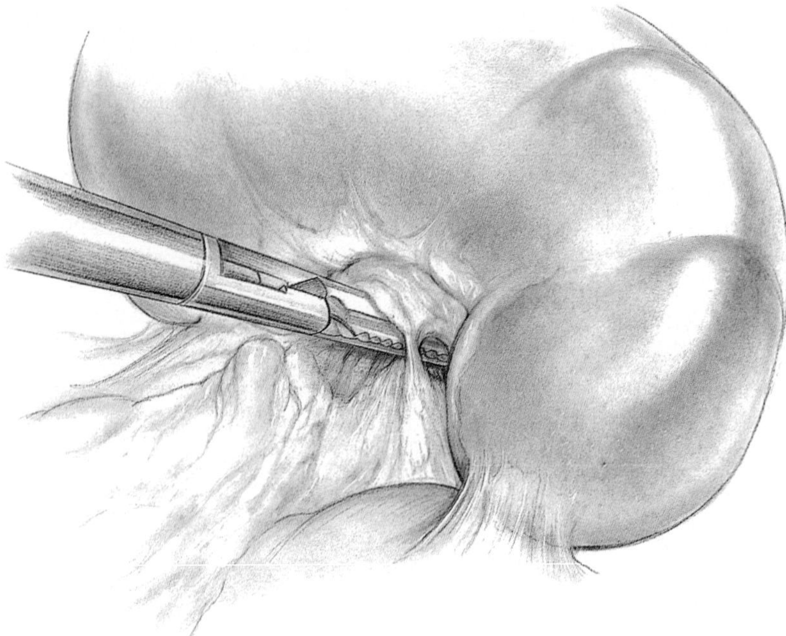

Fig. 40-9. Top: Color plate. **Bottom:** The lateral approach. The tail of pancreas as seen from the lateral approach in the areolar tissue of the retroperitoneum. Note the window created above the hilar vessels, making en bloc stapling easy.

consists of a sealed cuff that enables insertion and withdrawal of the operative hand within the abdomen without loss of pneumoperitoneum during the operation, thus recovering the haptic sensation lost in conventional laparoscopic surgery. A few different models exist and use either an inflatable sleeve clipped to an O-ring, a spiral inflatable valve, or a flap valve to maintain pneumoperitoneum (Fig. 40-12, page 406).

In the case of laparoscopic splenectomy, debate persists where the incision is best placed, depending on whether the surgeon is left- or right-handed. It has been described in the upper midline, the right upper quadrant, the left iliac fossa, and, for very large spleens, in a Pfannenstiel position. Most surgeons agree that the nondominant hand should be used in the device. There are obvious advantages and drawbacks to this technique. The most apparent disadvantage is the cosmetic cost of a longer abdominal incision, except in the Pfannenstiel position. Moreover, this technique would seem to defeat the goal of developing surgical techniques that further decrease surgical trauma. However, comparative studies of laparoscopic splenectomy for large spleens (those exceeding 700 g) seem to indicate outcomes similar to conventional laparoscopic techniques.

Although the final role of HALS splenectomy is still being defined, it will probably find a place in laparoscopic splenectomy for large spleens, with the threshold yet to be determined. It will also probably be helpful to surgeons performing laparoscopic splenectomy during the early part of their learning curves. It has also curtailed the role of preoperative splenic embolization for most very large spleens.

Needlescopic Splenectomy

The term needlescopic surgery is a loosely defined one that serves to describe a laparoscopic procedure performed with as many small (<3 mm) trocars and instruments as possible. The obvious limiting factors in end-organ excisional surgery are that the smallest available clip applier is 5 mm in diameter and that the linear stapler is a 12-mm instrument. Currently available formats include a 5-mm multifire disposable metallic clip applier and a reusable 5-mm locking plastic clip applier. The standard reusable clip appliers are usually 10 and 12 mm in diameter for medium-large and large clips. Hence, this surgery is only possible when using one or more "escape hatches" that would preserve the desired outcomes of needlescopic surgery and allow the use of clip appliers or linear staplers to control the blood supply. In needlescopic splenectomy, the umbilicus is therefore used for placement of a 12-mm or 5-mm trocar so that clips or stapler cartridges can be fired from the umbilical incision, whereas a 3-mm laparoscope is used to illuminate the operative field. Therefore, performance of this surgery requires the use of 3- and 10-mm laparoscopes sequentially with the obvious attendant sacrifice in vision with the small diameter laparoscope, another limiting factor. In needlescopic splenectomy, the plastic specimen bag needs to be introduced into the umbilical trocar site and extracted from the *same* site. All this increases the level of difficulty of laparoscopic splenectomy.

Numerous technical variations on this theme are in current use. Needlescopic splenectomy can be performed with one 12-mm trocar in the umbilicus and two subcostal 3-mm trocars (Fig. 40-13, page 406). Alternatively, an additional 3-mm trocar can

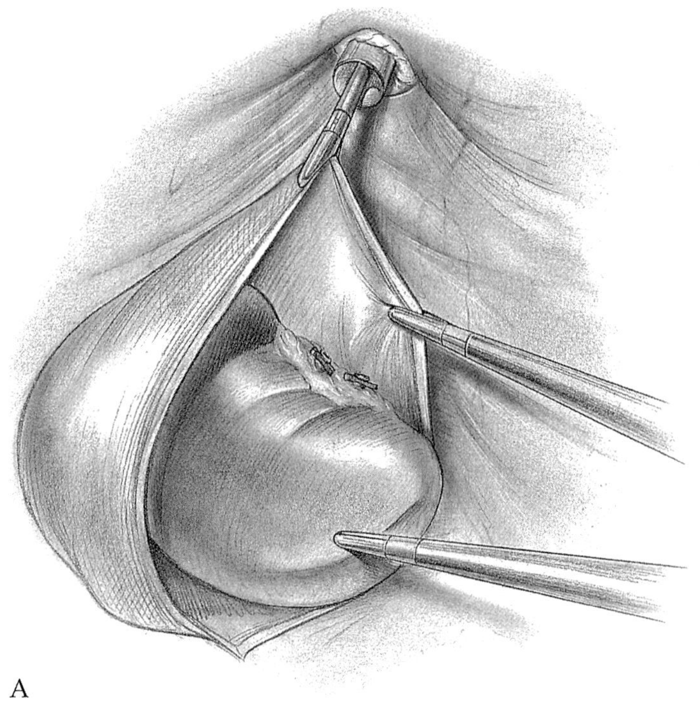

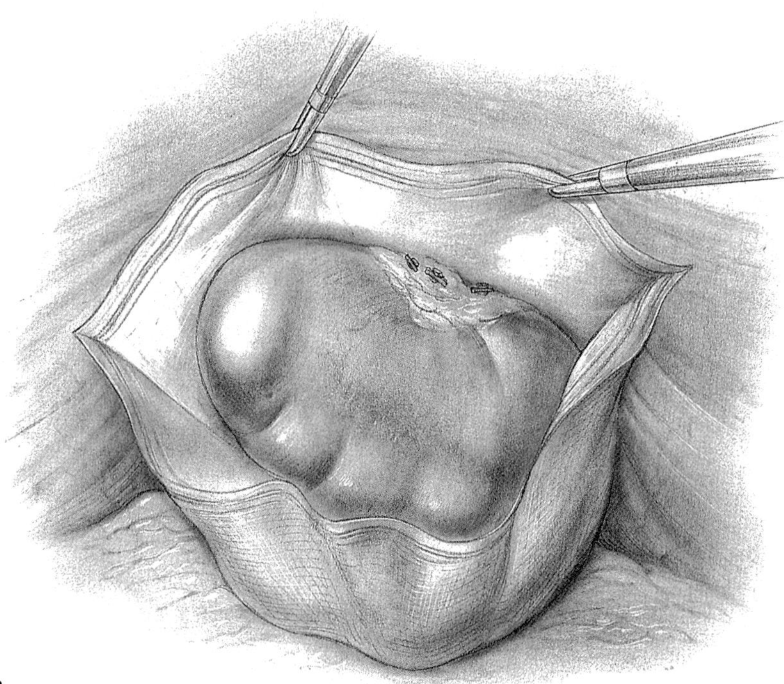

Fig. 40-10. A. Placing the resected spleen in a sterile plastic freezer bag. **B.** The spleen in the bag before extraction.

be added in the left flank. A 5-mm trocar can be substituted for the 3-mm flank trocar because this scar is less obvious than an abdominal scar. The addition of a 5-mm trocar also gives an extra site through which a slightly larger 5-mm laparoscope and a 5-mm clip applier can be used.

Case selection and surgeon experience for needlescopic splenectomy are obviously important. The ideal patient is thin, has a small spleen, suffers from immune thrombocytopenic purpura, and has a preoperative platelet count above 50,000. Whereas no randomized trial has yet confirmed better outcomes with needlescopic splenectomy with regard to the usual outcomes of morbidity, pain, and length of hospital stay, there are some obvious advantages. Cosmesis is definitely improved with the 12-mm vertical incision hidden in the depth of the umbilicus and the 3-mm sites becoming almost invisible over time. Furthermore there are, as yet, no reports of incisional hernias or infections in 3-mm wounds. Whether it is justifiable to pursue pushing the limits of minimally invasive surgery to this level for mainly cosmetic reasons remains debatable.

Partial Laparoscopic Splenectomy

Arguable elective indications for partial splenectomy include rare selected isolated trauma in a stable patient, resection of nonparasitic cysts, hamartomas, inflammatory pseudotumor of the spleen, some splenic hydatid cysts, other benign splenic tumors, type I Gaucher disease, cholesteryl ester storage disease, chronic myelogenous leukemia, single metastasis, thalassemia major, spherocytosis, and staging of Hodgkin disease in children. It has also been suggested for some cystic fibrosis patients with hypersplenism.

For partial laparoscopic splenectomy, the standard set-up for the lateral position is used and trocar placement is the same. Several types of 5-mm and 12-mm trocars can be adapted to the individual case. Initially, splenocolic and phrenicocolic ligaments are partially incised with monopolar cautery to expose the lower pole. Then the phrenicocolic ligament is incised to the diaphragm to allow full mobilization of the spleen as required by the spleen segment to be resected. Care must be taken to leave a 2-cm portion of the phrenicocolic ligament on the spleen side to allow for easier spleen mobilization. Attention is then given to the gastrosplenic ligament anteriorly. It contains the short gastric arteries to the superior pole and the branches of the gastroepiploic artery (up to five branches) to the lower pole. A relatively avascular space exists between the vessels to both poles. Opening this space allows definition of the type of splenic blood supply and the number of splenic branches entering the medial aspect of the hilum, thus helping determine the number of splenic lobes.

After the surgeon has determined which lobe(s) needs resection, tedious dissection of the involved splenic branch or branches is undertaken and the involved artery or arteries clipped. This dissection can also be performed from the front or the back of the spleen, because the spleen can be mobilized fairly easily. In the lateral decubitus position, gravity does most of the work. The spleen is allowed to demarcate in the chosen region. After the devascularized area has been determined

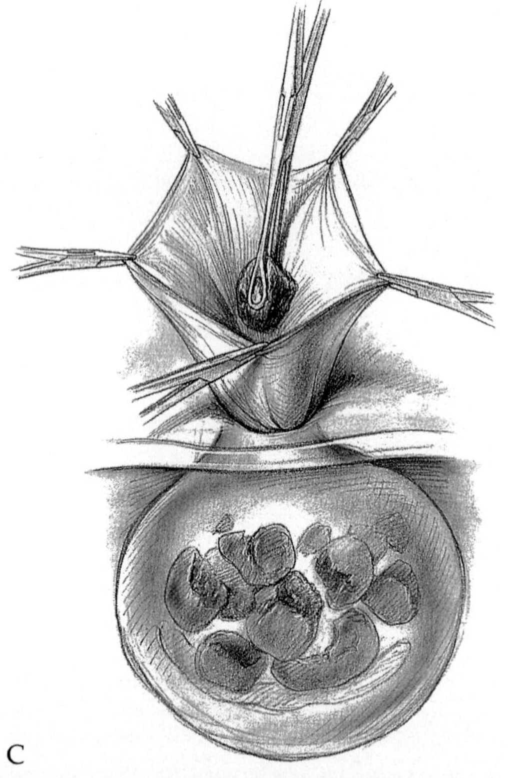

C

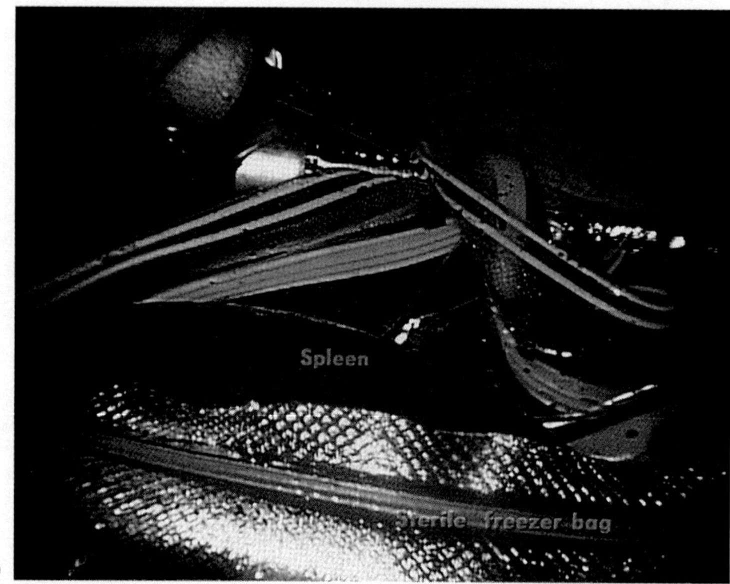

D

Fig. 40-10. (Continued). **C.** Mannal morcellation of spleen within the entrapment sac. **D.** Appearance of spleen within the entrapment sac.

to contain the lesion that needs resection, attention is turned to the corresponding venous drainage, using a similar technique. In splenic anatomy, veins are situated closely behind arteries, except at the level of penultimate and ultimate branches (usually within the spleen itself), where they can be either anterior or posterior.

The capsule of the spleen is then scored with monopolar cautery on coagulating current circumferentially, ensuring that a 5-mm rim of devascularized splenic tissue remains in situ (Fig. 40-14, page 406). After the splenic pulp has been penetrated, noncrushing intestinal graspers are used to fracture the splenic pulp. A laparoscopic hook and scissors can also be used. If a 5-mm rim of devitalized spleen is intentionally left, this procedure remains noticeably bloodless (Fig. 40-15, page 407). Spot coagulation with monopolar cautery on coagulation or spray current can be used for the remaining hemostasis. No drains are used.

The specimen is then placed in a sterile commercially available freezer bag for removal. One of the anterior 12-mm ports is enlarged to 2 cm and used as an extraction incision. The handling of the specimen in the plastic bag is determined by the underlying pathology and prior agreement with the pathologist. It will be based on the need to have tissue showing the pathologic structure preserved for diagnosis. Alternatively the specimen can be morcellated by the clinician's fingers, cut into intact pieces with scissors within the bag, or retrieved in its entirety.

The keys to success with partial laparoscopic splenectomy are experience with advanced laparoscopy, case selection, ability to dissect branches of the splenic artery close to the hilum, and foremost the realization that leaving a 5-mm margin of devitalized spleen in situ greatly simplifies hemostasis. We have not had to use argon beam coagulators or other hemostatic technology because ultrasonic shears, bipolar tissue welding instruments such as LigaSure (Valleylab; Boulder, CO), or radio frequency ablation probes can be useful in more difficult cases.

The most frequent intraoperative complication requiring immediate conversion to open surgery and possibly jeopardizing the completion of a partial splenectomy is hemorrhage. For this reason, all efforts should be directed at the prevention of intraoperative mishaps during the laparoscopic approach as in all advanced laparoscopic procedures.

Extraction of Specimen

Spleens removed through the anterior or lateral approach are extracted after finger fragmentation in a plastic bag from the umbilical or subcostal trocar site. It is rarely necessary to enlarge this incision to more than 2 or 3 cm. A small subcostal incision has been used as the extraction site during laparoscopic splenectomy through the anterior approach to better deal with diaphragmatic adhesions. When the lateral approach is used, extraction is more easily performed through an anterior port. This extraction site also requires little or no enlargement. On occasion, such as for a spleen longer than 20 cm, a 7.5- to 10-cm Pfannenstiel incision is used, and the forearm is introduced in the abdomen to deliver the spleen in the pelvis for extraction in large fragments under direct vision (Fig. 40-12A). The surgeon can also use this incision to inspect

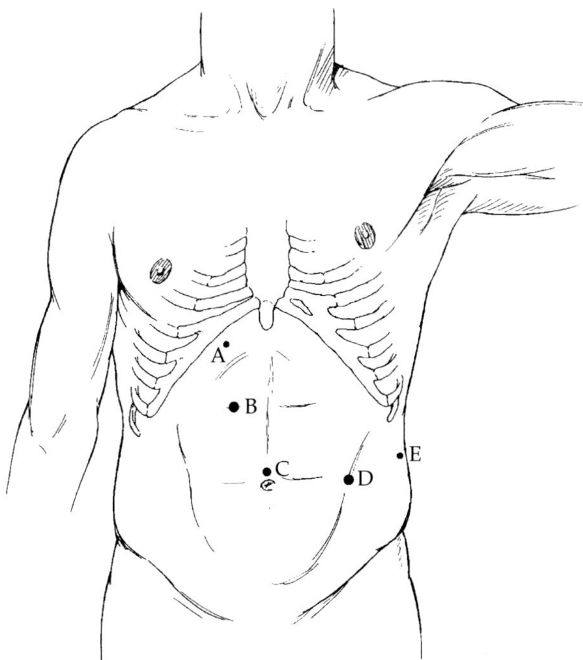

Fig. 40-11. The anterior approach. Positioning of the trocars A and E: 5-mm trocars; B: 10- or 12-mm trocar; C: camera; D: 10- or 12-mm trocar). (Modified from Thibault C, Mamazza J, Poulin EC, et al. Laparoscopic splenectomy: operative technique and preliminary report. *Surg Laparosc Endosc* 1992;2:248–253.)

the hilum manually using the view afforded by the videoscope to ensure that all vascular structures have been properly identified and controlled. The abdomen is copiously irrigated before closure. At this point, the largest spleen we have been able to bag was 24 cm long, and the largest spleen removed laparoscopically was 32 cm long.

Special notice should be given of laparoscopic splenectomy's role in malignant disease. In cases where lymphoma or Hodgkin disease is suspected, preoperative splenic artery embolization or finger fragmentation in a plastic bag is not used out of concern about making the histologic diagnosis more difficult. Extraction of intact spleens through a small left subcostal or median incision has also been described when it is required to preserve tissue architecture. The various techniques of fragmentation and extraction of splenic tissue during laparoscopic splenectomy should be discussed and agreed on with the pathologists to ensure that proper pathologic diagnoses are not missed by necrotic tissue in the case of preoperative splenic artery embolization or altered tissue architecture through finger fragmentation, especially if the diagnosis of malignancy is suspected but not proved. The choice of the appropriate extraction technique therefore largely depends on the type of splenic pathology or the size of the spleen.

Choice of Surgical Approach

The description by Gagner et al. of the lateral approach to laparoscopic splenectomy has been a useful addition to the set of techniques necessary to undertake successfully laparoscopic splenectomy for various hematologic conditions and for differently sized spleens. This approach is especially useful for excision of normal or moderately enlarged spleens safely without earlier splenic artery embolization. There are many reasons for this. First, it allows dissection of the splenic vessels in the relatively avascular areolar tissue of the retroperitoneum, which provides easier access than the anterior approach. Second, it almost eliminates inadvertent trauma from instruments usually held by assistants to lift the lower pole of the spleen as done in the anterior approach. In the lateral approach, little force is necessary to retract the spleen. Gravity is almost all that is required, because the spleen naturally will fall toward the left lobe of the liver and out of the way to permit identification of the vessels and the tail of the pancreas after the lower portion of the phrenicocolic ligament is sectioned. Because the phrenicocolic ligament is so accessible in this approach, it can be dissected early, leaving a generous portion on the splenic side that can be grasped easily to manipulate the spleen. Third, with this approach, it is much easier to distinguish and separate the gastrosplenic and lienorenal ligaments to identify the anatomic structures they contain. It is also easy to safely create windows through the ligaments to place clips or staples, especially above the tail of the pancreas (Figs. 40-7 and 40-8). Fourth, the tail of the pancreas is more accessible to dissection, especially in its superior and posterior aspects, than in the anterior approach (Fig. 40-9). Fifth, when one refrains from cutting the last portion of the phrenicocolic ligament at the end of the procedure, there is more room in this position to insert the spleen in a plastic bag before extraction. Finally, one major advantage of the lateral approach is that if blood loss occurs, it will tend to flow away from the hilum and not obscure dissection. (In the anterior approach, blood will pool in the hilum, decreasing illumination and impairing safe dissection.) All these advantages translate into a procedure that can take 30 to 60 minutes less to perform.

There are some disadvantages, however. First, the anterior approach is probably better suited to a situation in which concomitant surgery is intended, such as cholecystectomy. Second, dealing with a very large spleen is probably safer using the anterior approach and possible prior splenic artery embolization. Third, performing a complete exploration for accessory spleens is possibly more difficult by the lateral approach. The splenic hilum, gastrocolic ligament, tail of the pancreas, descending colon, and its mesentery are readily visualized, but structures within the pelvis, the right side of the colon, the small bowel, and its mesentery are more difficult to evaluate. This may be more theoretical than real, because the literature states that more than 80% of accessory spleens are located in areas accessible to the lateral approach (Fig. 40-16, page 407). Moreover, in our experience so far, accessory spleens were as readily found regardless of surgical approach. For example, they are found 30% of the time in cases of immune thrombocytopenic purpura. This compares most favorably with the 15% to 30% rate cited in the literature on open splenectomy. A report of eight cases of recurrent hematologic disease after splenectomy, all successfully treated by removal of accessory spleens, serves as a reminder that searching for and excising accessory spleens is an essential step in this procedure, whether the site access is conventional or laparoscopic.

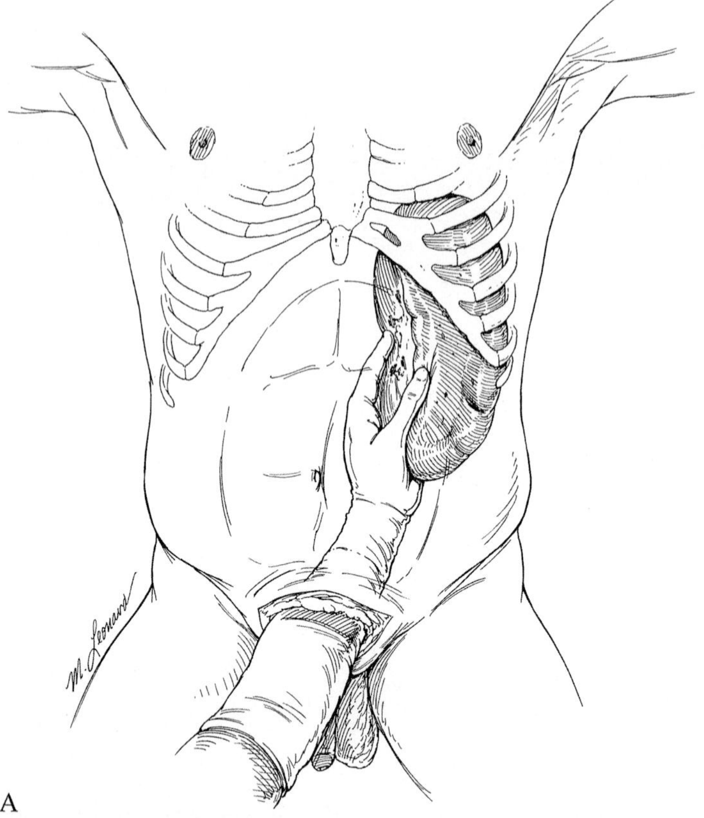

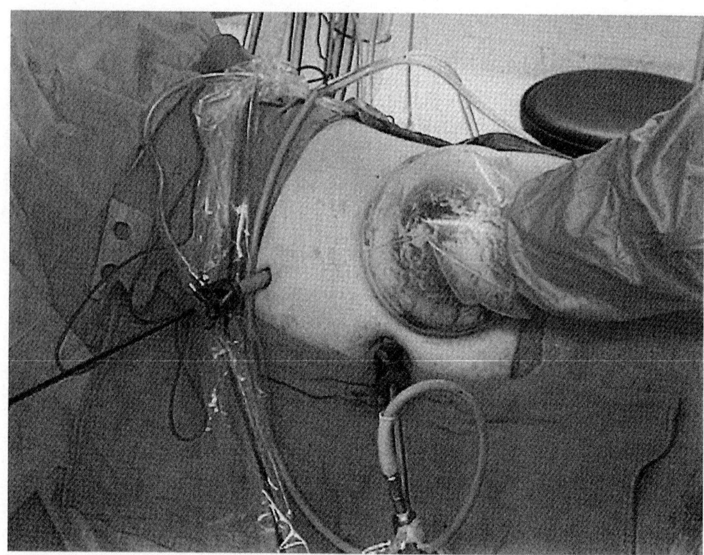

Fig. 40-12. A. Extraction method for laparoscopic splenectomy in massive splenomegaly. Diagram demonstrating final examination of operating field under laparoscopic control after division of ligaments and vessels. (From Poulin EC, Thibault C. *Can J Surg* 1995;38:69–72.) **B.** Use of a hand port in the left lower quadrant to assist in splenectomy for a large spleen.

Most patients treated by splenectomy suffer from immune idiopathic purpura, and most have a normal-sized spleen; therefore, the lateral approach without prior embolization currently remains the technique of choice for these patients.

Alternate Strategies and Tools

There is an emerging literature concerning many technological advances and operative strategies that may find a place in laparoscopic surgery of the spleen. First,

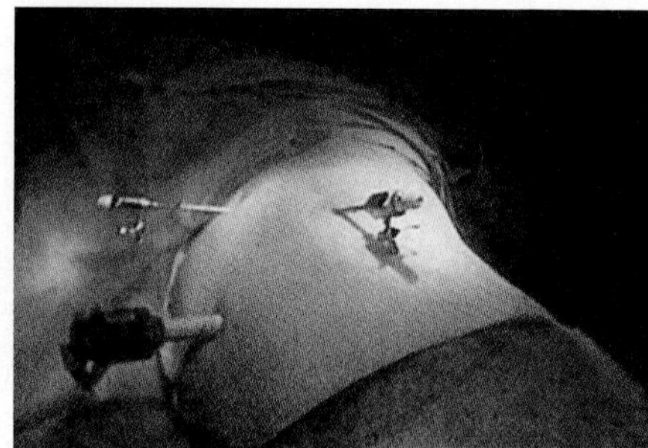

Fig. 40-13. Needlescopic splenectomy performed with a 12-mm trocar in the umbilicus and two subcostal 3-mm trocars.

the strategy of in situ splenectomy, where all vessels are identified and controlled prior to incision of the supporting ligaments, can be a useful adjunct in dealing laparoscopically with very large spleens, partial splenectomy, or selected trauma. Second, while robotic splenectomy undoubtedly increases the elegance of laparoscopic splenectomy, its high cost, different room set-up, and similar clinical outcomes have limited its adoption so far. Third, some authors have started using handheld gamma probes in an attempt to locate accessory spleens at the primary or revision surgery mainly in operations for immune purpura. Fourth, the use of an energy-based device (LigaSure; Valleylab: Boulder, CO), which works by applying a precise amount of bipolar energy and pressure to the tissue and achieving a permanent seal of vessels up to 7 mm, is frequently reported. Laparoscopic splenectomy can then be achieved with few or no application of clips or linear staplers. Finally, the use of radiofrequency needles has been suggested as an adjunct in some cases of blunt trauma of the spleen.

It is too early to tell to what degree these adjuncts will find a niche in laparoscopic surgery of the spleen, but they all have one goal in common: the simplification of a delicate laparoscopic procedure.

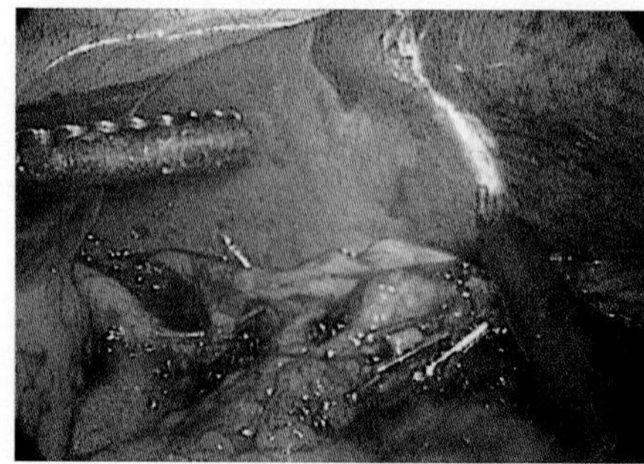

Fig. 40-14. Scoring of the splenic capsule and leaving behind a 5-mm strip of devitalized tissue.

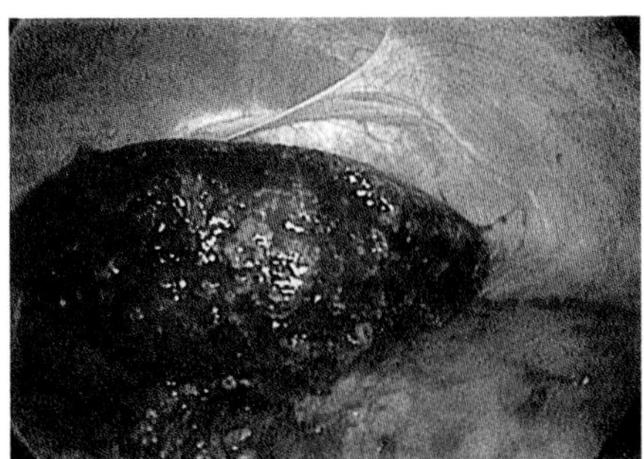

Fig. 40-15. Raw surface of remaining spleen after laparoscopic partial splenectomy.

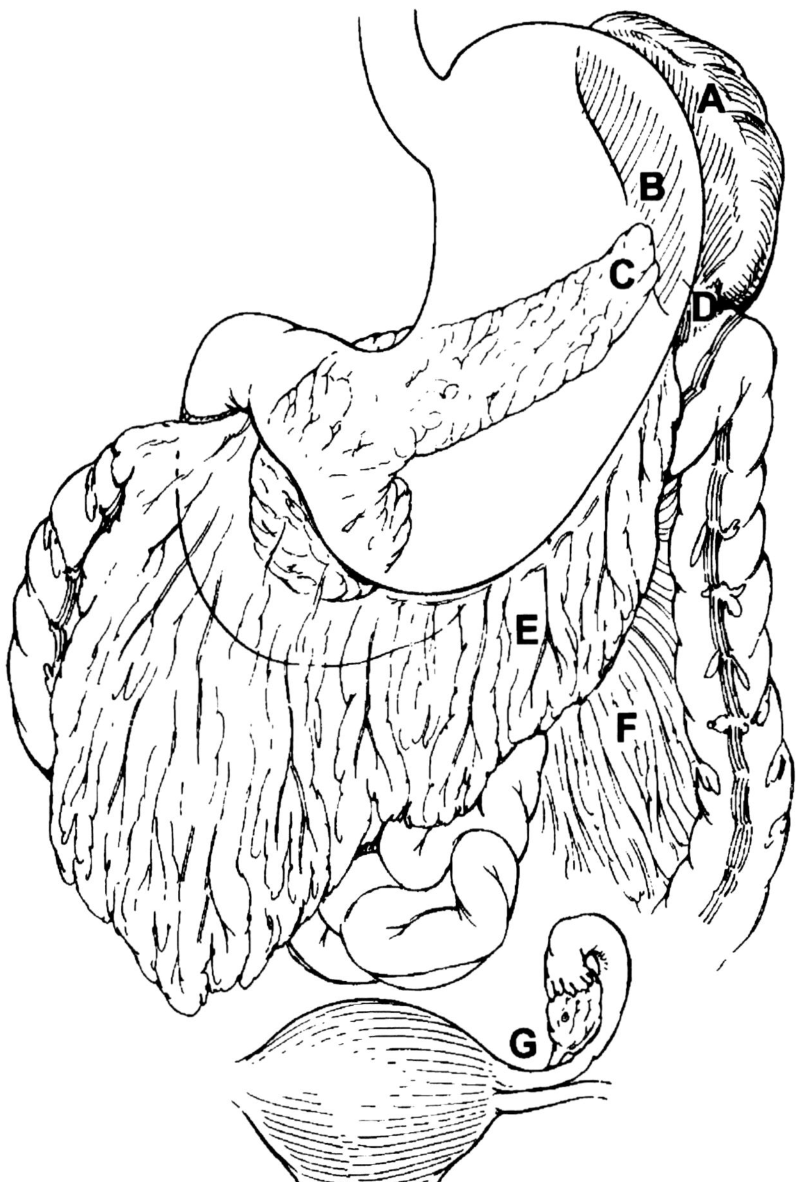

Fig. 40-16. Sites where accessory spleens are found in order of importance. (From Curtis GM, Movitz D. The surgical significance of the accessory spleen. *Ann Surg* 1946;123:276–298.)

POSTOPERATIVE MANAGEMENT

Postoperative care of a laparoscopic splenectomy patient is usually straightforward. The nasogastric tube is either removed in the recovery room after making sure that the stomach has been emptied or the next morning, depending on the duration and the difficulty of the procedure. The urinary catheter is usually removed before the patient is discharged from the recovery room. The patient is permitted clear fluids the next day and, when this is well tolerated, allowed to move to a preferred diet.

Postoperative pain medication is individualized with a view of ensuring complete patient comfort. This can start with Celecoxib, a Cox-2 non-steroidal anti-inflammation drug preoperatively, as there is no effect on platelet function. Alternatively 50 mg of ketorolac, an NSAID drug, can be administered 30 minutes before the end of the case. All trocar sites are infiltrated with local anesthetic at the start of the procedure. This is done to prevent the establishment of peripheral and central sensitization ("wind-up"), conditions that lead to an augmented response to pain stimuli.

Ketorolac or its equivalent is administered regularly in the postoperative period following the "first in, last out" principle of NSAID administration for pain control. NSAIDs have been shown to have a 30% to 50% opioid-sparing effect. Morphine-based patient controlled analgesia (PCA) is used the first night after surgery. The following morning, acetaminophen and NSAIDs generally suffice. 2 to 4 mg of oral hydromorphone hydrochloride is reserved for breakthrough pain. The patient is discharged with prescriptions for these three oral drugs. Meperidine injections can be used during the first night, followed by an oral acetaminophencodeine preparation or acetaminophen alone. Alternatively, provided there is no history of ulcer or dyspepsia, the patient is administered naproxen 500 mg by mouth on the morning of surgery and every 12 hours for a total of three to five doses or rofecoxib 50 mg by mouth once daily starting on the day prior to surgery. Then, depending on the intensity of postoperative pain, several meperidine injections are used for the first 12 to 24 hours, followed by oral acetaminophen. This combination has produced the best results. Because of its adverse effects of nausea, vomiting, abdominal fullness, and constipation, codeine therapy should be avoided if possible. Furthermore, increased awareness of codeine intoxication associated with ultrarapid CYP2D6 metabolism makes it a poor choice.

When indomethacin is used, prophylactic doses of subcutaneous heparin should not be used, especially when the platelet count is low or a platelet function abnormality is present. Oral steroids are started on the first postoperative day after an overlap intravenous injection if steroid coverage is required. Thereafter, steroid dosage is gradually decreased. Patients are allowed to shower on the first day following surgery as long as they dry the paper strips covering the trocar sites. They are advised to keep the paper strips covering trocar incisions in place for 8 to 10 days. No drains have been required by patients in this series, with the possible exception of injury to the tail of the pancreas. No limitation of physical activity is imposed, and the patient is allowed to tailor his or her activities to the degree of asthenia or discomfort, except for cases of laparoscopic partial splenectomy where, as a general rule, patients are asked to refrain from strenuous activity for a month.

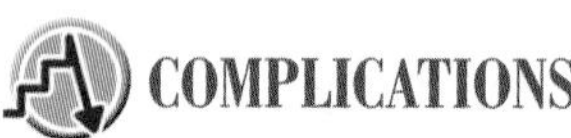

COMPLICATIONS

Laparoscopic Splenectomy

The complications of splenectomy include intraoperative and postoperative hemorrhage; left lower lobe atelectasis and pneumonia; left pleural effusion; subphrenic collection; iatrogenic pancreatic, gastric, and colonic injury; and venous thrombosis.

Success with laparoscopic splenectomy depends largely on proper preparation and avoiding complications and technical misadventures. Recognition of anatomic elements and their arrangement is paramount. Vascular structures should be cleanly isolated and dissected from surrounding fat. Most can then be controlled safely and cheaply using two clips placed proximally and distally. Staplers should be used with care and should not be applied without visual input. The stapler tip should be verified to be free of tissue by the clinician's visual inspection before it is closed. Otherwise, significant hemorrhage from a partial section of a major splenic branch might occur after release of the instrument. Blind application of the stapler may also damage the tail of the pancreas, often lying close to the inner surface of the spleen, especially in the anterior approach.

Improper use of the cautery can cause iatrogenic injury to the stomach, colon, and pancreas. Structures close to the lower pole in the gastrocolic ligament can be approached aggressively with the cautery, but blind fulguration of fat in the hilum can result in serious bleeding. The instrument should be activated only in proximity to the target organ to avoid arcing and spot necrosis, which may result in delayed perforation and sepsis.

The role of the assistants is also important in the prevention of complications. All instruments, including those handled by assistants, should be moved only under direct vision. Retraction of the liver and stomach and elevation of the spleen require constant concentration to avoid lacerations with subsequent hemorrhage or perforation, especially when using the anterior approach. There should be no iatrogenic trauma to the spleen during the surgery to eliminate the possibility of subsequent splenosis. For the same reason, if splenic trauma occurs intraoperatively or intraabdominal fragmentation is required for extraction of a large spleen, copious irrigation should be used before closure.

Portal Vein Thrombosis

Because of its potential lethality and increased reports in the literature, a special mention of portal vein thrombosis (PVT) needs to be made. Although the true incidence of PVT is unknown, it has been reported to occur in anywhere from 1% to 10% of the cases after splenectomy. Presenting symptoms include anorexia, abdominal pain, ileus, low-grade fever, and elevated leukocyte and platelet counts. Diagnosis is usually made by contrast-enhanced computed tomography (CT) scan, and anticoagulation is the treatment. The complication can occur months after splenectomy. It is more often reported in patients with splenomegaly, myeloproliferative disorders, or hemolysis, in which case the incidence of PVT increases to 25% to 75%. It has also been seen in patients on prophylactic subcutaneous heparin injections.

A recent report in which patients were routinely scanned after splenectomy raises more questions than it answers. When actively looked for, a PVT incidence of close to 20% was found. In 9% of cases, PVT was asymptomatic. In some cases the thrombosis involved the main portal system venous effluents, in others only secondary branches. One study even suggests a higher incidence of PVT in laparoscopic splenectomy. Further studies are needed to define the appropriate duration of heparin prophylaxis in patients undergoing splenectomy and the best recommendation for postoperative follow-up with CT scans for early diagnosis. Guidance is also needed for asymptomatic patients and cases involving only secondary branches of the portal system.

Preoperative Splenic Artery Embolization

Selective embolization of splenic artery branches demands appropriate equipment and expertise from the radiologist because many variations in arterial splenic blood supply complicate the technique. Moreover, the only acceptable embolic material should be gelatin sponge fragments and 3- to 8-mm coils, because serious complications can occur when microspheres or gelatin powder are used. Selective embolization should also be performed distal to the pancreatica magna artery to avoid causing pancreatitis. Preoperative splenic artery embolization can be performed with little morbidity and is a useful adjunct for some cases of laparoscopic splenectomy.

SUGGESTED READING

Fujitani RM, Johs SM, Cobb SR, et al. Preoperative splenic artery occlusion as an adjunct for high-risk splenectomy. *Am Surg* 1991;54:602–608.

Gagner M, Lacroix A, Bolte E, et al. Laparoscopic adrenalectomy. The importance of a flank approach in the lateral decubitus position. *Surg Endosc* 1994;8:135–138.

Hiatt JR, Gomes AS, Machleder HI. Massive splenomegaly. Superior results with a combined endovascular and operative approach. *Arch Surg* 1990;125:1363–1367.

Ikeda M, Sekimoto M, Takiguchi S, et al. High incidence of thrombosis of the portal venous system after laparoscopic splenectomy: a prospective study with contrast-enhanced CT scan. *Ann Surg* 2005;241(2):208–216.

Michels NA. The variational anatomy of the spleen and splenic artery. *Am J Anat* 1942;70: 21–72.

Poulin EC, Mamazza J, Schlachta CM. Splenic artery embolization before laparoscopic splenectomy. An update. *Surg Endosc* 1998;12: 870–875.

Poulin EC, Thibault C. Laparoscopic splenectomy for massive splenomegaly: operative technique and case report. *Can J Surg* 1995; 38:69–72.

Poulin EC, Thibault C. The anatomical basis for laparoscopic splenectomy. *Can J Surg* 1993; 36:485–488.

Seshadri PA, Poulin EC, Mamazza J, et al. Technique for laparoscopic partial splenectomy. *Surg Laparosc Endosc* 2000;10:106–109.

Targarona EM, Balague C, Cerdan G, et al. Hand-assisted laparoscopic splenectomy (HALS) in cases of splenomegaly: a comparison analysis with conventional laparoscopic splenectomy. *Surg Endosc* 2002;16:426–430.

Winslow ER, Brunt LM, Drebin JA, et al. Portal vein thrombosis after splenectomy. *Am J Surg* 2002;184(6):631–635.

COMMENTARY

Dr. Poulin has described the basic technique of laparoscopic splenectomy along with a number of variations on the theme. Several of his points bear amplification. In regard to patient positioning, we have generally employed a 45-degree right lateral decubitus position using a beanbag mattress and appropriate placement of tape across the hips and shoulders. After the body is padded and stabilized, it is possible to not only tilt the patient into a full right lateral decubitus position, but also to then bring the patient back to a supine position for portions of the operation that are more appropriately performed supine, such as during the initial abdominal entry and exploration. The search for accessory spleens must be performed as the first part of the operation. Waiting until the end of the case is risky because, if there has been a problem intraoperatively, there may be an urgency to complete the procedure. Alternatively, if the case has gone well, the operating team may be "flush with victory" and may inadvertently forget this necessary step.

Dr. Poulin has pointed out an inexpensive alternative to the usual off-the-shelf entrapment sacks. If one of the thinner commercially available bags is used, great care must be taken to prevent rupture with spillage of splenic tissue. The author also discusses some of the technical tips for performing splenectomy in the presence of marked splenomegaly. I would caution surgeons to stick to removing normal or near-normal sized spleens early in their experience until comfortable with the basic technique.

The author mentions the use of splenic artery embolization in several areas of the narrative. Over the last few years preoperative embolization has virtually disappeared completely from our clinical practice. This procedure can lead to significant patient discomfort and potential complications. For the current edition, the author has added a section on the potential for postoperative development of portal vein thrombosis. This is an increasingly recognized complication and must be considered as a possibility in patients with untoward symptoms developing in the postoperative interval. I would also add one final note regarding the use of postoperative drains. Although it is generally accepted that a left upper quadrant drain is not required after an uncomplicated laparoscopic or open splenectomy, I will place a closed suction drain in patients in whom I suspect trauma to the tail of the pancreas. As Dr. Poulin notes, the tail of the pancreas lies within one centimeter of the spleen in the vast majority of patients and may be at risk. I would rather deal with a well-drained pancreatic fistula than a postoperative peripancreatic abscess.

NJS

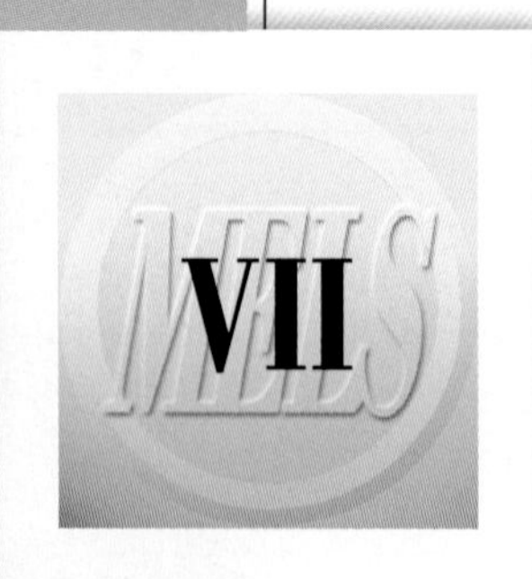

VII Endocrine Disorders

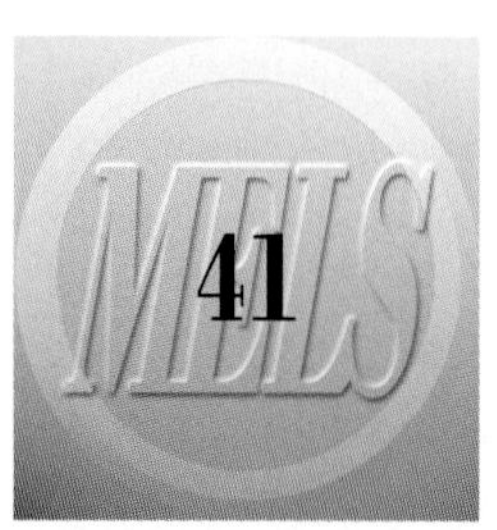

41 Laparoscopic Adrenalectomy

DERON J. TESSIER AND L. MICHAEL BRUNT

INTRODUCTION

Since the first laparoscopic adrenalectomy was reported in 1992, the safety and efficacy of this approach has been demonstrated by several groups. Laparoscopic adrenalectomy has also been shown to have several advantages over open adrenalectomy, including decreased pain, a shorter duration of postoperative ileus, earlier hospital discharge, fewer complications, and a more rapid recovery. Most adrenal gland tumors should be amenable to laparoscopic excision because most adrenal neoplasms are small and pathologically benign. This chapter reviews the basic principles of laparoscopic adrenal surgery including anatomy, diagnostic considerations, indications for operation, and the technical aspects of the procedure. Partial adrenalectomy and the controversial issues of large and malignant tumors will also be addressed.

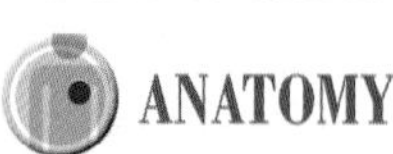

ANATOMY

The adrenal glands are retroperitoneal organs located along the superomedial aspect of each kidney. The normal adrenal gland in adults weighs 4 to 6 g, measures 3 to 5 cm in length, and is 4 to 6 mm thick. The adrenal glands are composed of a cortex and a medulla, each of which has distinct endocrine functions and separate embryologic origins. The adrenal cortex is derived from the coelomic mesoderm and is the site of the synthesis and secretion of steroid hormones: cortisol, the adrenal androgens, and aldosterone. Cortisol secretion is regulated through a classic negative-feedback pathway involving the hypothalamic-pituitary-adrenal axis and adrenocorticotropic hormone (ACTH). The major physiologic regulator of aldosterone secretion is the renin-angiotensin-aldosterone system. The adrenal medulla is derived from cells of the neural crest and synthesizes the catecholamines: norepinephrine and epinephrine. Catecholamines may also be synthesized in extraadrenal chromaffin tissue, most commonly in the paraaortic and paravertebral regions and in the organ of Zuckerkandl.

Precise knowledge of the normal adrenal anatomy and the relationship of the adrenals to surrounding structures is essential for successful adrenalectomy, regardless of whether a laparoscopic or open technique is used. Each adrenal gland is embedded in Gerota's fascia and is surrounded by retroperitoneal fat. The adrenal gland has a fibrous capsule and is colored golden yellow due to the high lipid content of the adrenal cortex. The right adrenal gland is somewhat pyramidal and lies superior to the right kidney, whereas the left adrenal is more flattened and is in intimate contact with the medial aspect of the superior pole of the left kidney. On the right side, the adrenal gland is bordered medially by the inferior vena cava, and often a portion of the anteromedial border of the gland actually lies beneath the vena cava. The right triangular ligament of the liver crosses the anterior surface of the adrenal gland superiorly, which means that the upper portion of the gland has no peritoneum covering its surface. The lower portion of the right adrenal may be overlapped or partially covered by the duodenum. Posteriorly, the right adrenal rests on the diaphragm superiorly and on the anteromedial aspect of the upper portion of the right kidney inferiorly. The left adrenal gland is bounded superiorly by the peritoneum of the posterior omental bursa, the stomach, and the superior pole of the spleen. Inferiorly, the left adrenal is covered by the pancreas and splenic vein and is closely related to the renal hilar vessels. Posteriorly, the left adrenal rests on the left crus of the diaphragm medially and the medial aspect of the left kidney laterally.

The adrenal glands are highly vascularized and derive their blood supply from numerous branches of the inferior phrenic, aortic, and renal arteries (Fig. 41-1). Each adrenal gland has a single central vein, which is one of the keys to adrenalectomy. The right adrenal vein is short (0.5 to 1 cm in length) and drains from the medial aspect of the gland directly into the posterolateral aspect of the inferior vena cava. A second right adrenal vein that enters either the vena cava or right hepatic vein is occasionally encountered. The left adrenal vein is usually 2 to 3 cm in length and exits the anteromedial aspect of the gland, where it runs obliquely to empty into the left renal vein. The inferior phrenic vein frequently joins the left adrenal vein proximal to its entry into the renal vein.

TABLE 41-1. INDICATIONS AND CONTRAINDICATIONS FOR LAPAROSCOPIC ADRENALECTOMY

Indications	Contraindications
Aldosteronoma	Any locally invasive adrenal tumor
Cushing syndrome	Large benign adrenal mass (>10–12 cm)*
Cortisol-secreting adrenal adenoma	Large adrenocortical cancer
Adrenal hyperplasia after failed treatment of pituitary Cushing syndrome	Existing contraindication to laparoscopic surgery
Primary adrenal hyperplasia	Prior nephrectomy, splenectomy, liver resection on affected side*
Nonfunctioning cortical adenoma (>4–5 cm or suspicious radiographic appearance)	
Pheochromocytoma (sporadic or familial)	
Adrenal metastases	

*Relative contraindications that depend on surgeon experience and patient selection

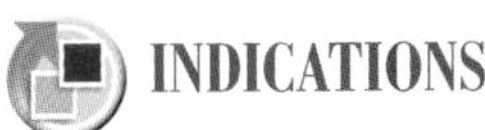

INDICATIONS

Adrenalectomy is indicated for any biochemically functional adrenal tumor and for all suspected primary adrenal malignancies. Most adrenal tumors are benign and may be considered for laparoscopic excision (Table 41-1).

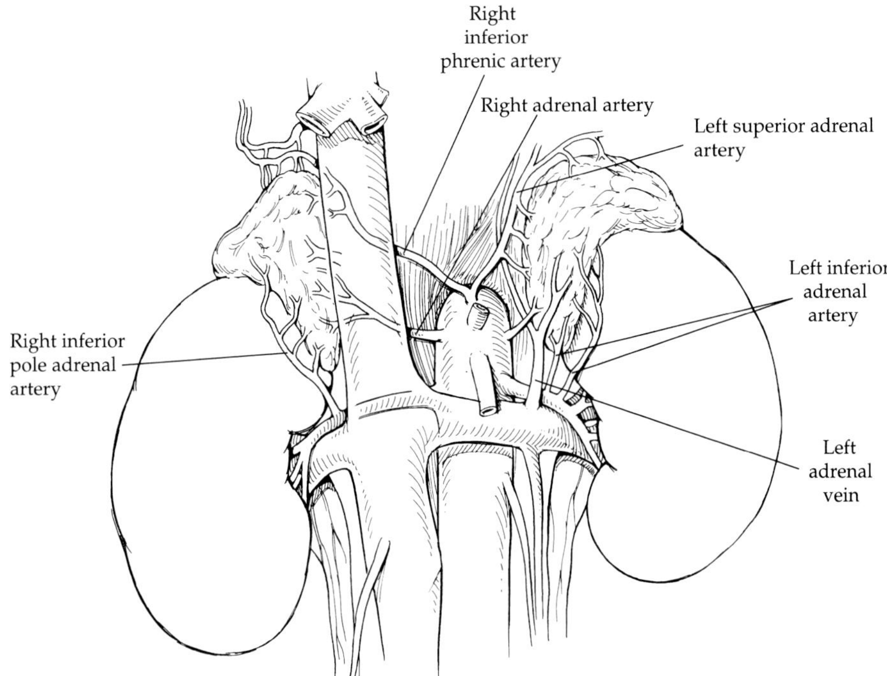

Fig. 41-1. Adrenal anatomy and blood supply.

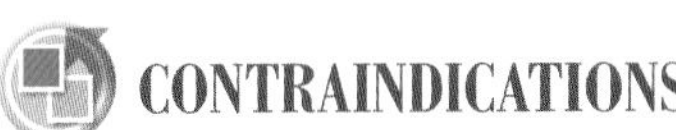

CONTRAINDICATIONS

The only absolute contraindication to laparoscopic adrenalectomy is the presence of a locally invasive tumor, because of the need to resect contiguous structures. Large primary adrenocortical tumors (larger than 6 cm) should also be considered for an open approach because of the likelihood that such lesions are malignant. Small, isolated adrenal metastases may be appropriate for laparoscopic surgical resection in carefully selected patients, provided the tumor is well circumscribed. No clear-cut size limitation has yet been identified for considering laparoscopic adrenalectomy; however, caution should be exercised on attempting a laparoscopic approach for adrenal masses larger than 10 to 12 cm because of the difficulty in manipulating such masses with current laparoscopic instrumentation and the possibility of spillage of a potentially malignant tumor. Prior nephrectomy, splenectomy, or liver resection on the affected side of the adrenal lesion may also contraindicate a laparoscopic approach.

CUSHING SYNDROME

Cortisol-producing adrenal neoplasms account for 15% to 20% of all cases of Cushing syndrome. ACTH-secreting pituitary tumors comprise 60% to 70% of cases, and ectopic ACTH-secreting tumors account for about 15%. Rarely, the source of Cushing syndrome is primary adrenal hyperplasia (pigmented micronodular adrenal hyperplasia or macronodular adrenal hyperplasia). The diagnosis of Cushing syndrome is confirmed by demonstration of elevated 24-hour urine-free cortisol levels or by failure to suppress plasma cortisol levels to lower than 3 to 5 μg per dl after administration of 1 mg of dexamethasone. After a diagnosis of Cushing syndrome is established biochemically, further diagnostic tests (e.g., plasma ACTH and diagnostic imaging) may be used to determine the cause. Patients with primary adrenal tumors usually have elevated cortisol levels, low plasma ACTH levels, and radiographic evidence of an adrenal mass on computed tomography (CT) or magnetic resonance imaging (MRI). Unilateral adrenalectomy is the treatment of choice for patients with a cortisol-producing adenoma. Bilateral adrenalectomy is indicated for patients with persistent Cushing syndrome due to either failed treatment of pituitary tumors or primary adrenal hyperplasia.

Subclinical Cushing syndrome is an increasingly recognized entity in patients with adrenal incidentaloma in which there is absence of normal suppressibility of glucocorticoid function. These patients fail to suppress cortisol secretion with dexamethasone and may also exhibit loss of diurnal variation of cortisol levels and low plasma ACTH. However, classic Cushing features are typically lacking, although they may have associated obesity, osteoporosis, hypertension, or diabetes. Patients with subclinical Cushing may benefit from adrenalectomy, although most patients do not appear to progress to overt Cushing syndrome.

ALDOSTERONOMA

Primary hyperaldosteronism is the most common cause of secondary hypertension and has been reported in 8% to 12% of the hypertensive population. The classic presentation is one of hypertension and hypokalemia; however, the serum potassium is normal in many individuals. The initial biochemical screening for primary hyperaldosteronism should consist of measurement of plasma aldosterone concentration (PAC) and plasma renin activity (PRA). A plasma aldosterone level greater than 15 ng/dl and suppressed plasma renin activity (aldosterone-to-renin ratio exceeding 20 to 30) is highly suggestive of the diagnosis and should be confirmed by placing the patient on a high-sodium diet and demonstrating a urine aldosterone level greater than 12 μg/dL.

The next step in the evaluation is to determine the subtype of primary hyperaldosteronism. The most common cause is an aldosterone-producing adenoma (65% to 70% of cases). Bilateral idiopathic adrenal hyperplasia accounts for about 20% to 30% of cases and is treated medically rather than by adrenalectomy. The initial differentiation of these two disorders is made radiographically with a thin (3-mm) section abdominal CT. If the patient is young (under age 40), and CT shows a unilateral macroadenoma (adrenal adenoma greater than 1 cm and a normal contralateral gland), then an aldosteronoma is highly likely, and one can proceed with adrenalectomy. In all other patients (microadenoma <1 cm; bilateral nodules; bilateral normal glands; age >40 to 50 years), adrenal vein sampling should be used to determine if there is a lateralizing source for increased aldosterone production. Adrenal vein sampling consists of the measurement of aldosterone and cortisol from both adrenal veins and the inferior vena cava. A gradient in the aldosterone-to-cortisol ratio of 4.0 or greater between sides indicates a lateralizing source and is appropriate for adrenalectomy. Adrenal vein sampling is a technically demanding procedure and should be performed by interventional radiologists who are skilled with this technique.

Preoperatively, hypokalemia should be corrected, and the patient's blood pressure should be adequately controlled, which may be facilitated by administration of the aldosterone antagonist spironolactone (Aldactone). Spironolactone should not be given to patients until biochemical testing has been completed, because it will interfere with interpretation of test results.

ADRENAL CORTICAL CARCINOMA

Adrenal cortical carcinomas are rare tumors with an incidence of approximately 1 per 1.7 million. This malignancy should be suspected in any patient with a large adrenal mass (>6 cm) or who presents with virilizing features. Approximately 60% of patients with adrenal cortical carcinomas have virilizing features due to an overproduction of cortisol. En bloc resection of all gross tumors with negative surgical margins at the initial operation offers the best potential for cure. Computed tomography or MRI is helpful in distinguishing benign from malignant lesions. Imaging characteristics that are worrisome for malignancy include local invasiveness, tumor necrosis, heterogeneity of the mass, and regional lymphadenopathy. On CT, adenomas typically have low attenuation values (<10 HU) while carcinomas are higher in attenuation. On MRI, adenomas have a lipid-rich composition compared to nonadenomatous lesions and show a loss of signal with chemical shift sequences due to their high lipid content. Further discussion of the role of laparoscopy for malignant lesions will be discussed at the end of the chapter.

ADRENAL INCIDENTALOMA

Incidentally discovered adrenal masses are detected in approximally 0.6% to 4% of abdominal CT scans. Most are small, nonfunctioning cortical adenomas that do not require adrenalectomy. Patients with functional or potentially malignant lesions should undergo surgical resection. The evaluation of the patient with an incidentally discovered adrenal mass begins with a complete history and physical examination. Biochemical screening should be carried out, which should include measurement of plasma fractionated metanephrines to screen for pheochromocytoma and an overnight dexamethasone test to screen for hypercortisolism. Patients with hypertension and/or hypokalemia should also be evaluated for primary hyperaldosteronism with measurement of plasma aldosterone concentration and plasma renin activity. Large, solid masses larger than 4 to 5 cm in size should probably be removed regardless of functional status because of their malignant potential; exceptions to this indication would be asymptomatic adrenal cysts and adrenal myelolipomas. For nonfunctioning adrenal masses, MRI may provide additional discrimination between benign and malignant lesions. Benign adrenal adenomas have greater lipid content than malignant lesions and show a loss of signal intensity on MRI opposed-phase gradient-echo images compared to in-phase images. In contrast, malignant lesions do not have high lipid content and maintain similar signal intensities on both imaging sequences. Fine-needle aspiration (FNA) is not useful in distinguishing benign from malignant primary adrenal tumors and is rarely indicated. FNA should never be performed unless a pheochromocytoma has first been excluded biochemically because of the risk of precipitating a hypertensive crisis. Patients with benign, nonfunctional tumors smaller than 4 to 5 cm should be reevaluated in 4 and 12 months, at which point adrenalectomy should be performed if there is any growth in the mass or evidence of biochemical function.

PHEOCHROMOCYTOMA

Pheochromocytoma should be suspected in any patient with hypertension and an adrenal mass. The initial evaluation of a patient with suspected pheochromocytoma should consist of measurement of plasma fractionated metanephrines. Alternatively, the clinician may measure 24-hour urinary catecholamine and metanephrine levels. Radiographically, pheochromocytomas can be demonstrated by CT or MRI, but MRI is more specific for this tumor because T2-weighted images typically show tumor enhancement relative to the liver. Pheochromocytomas may be removed laparoscopically, provided that they are confined to the adrenal gland and the patient has been adequately prepared pharmacologically for surgery. Pheochromocytomas develop in extraadrenal sites in 10% to 15% of cases; although laparoscopic removal of extraadrenal pheochromocytomas has been described, this approach should probably be reserved for carefully selected cases. Preoperatively, an alpha (α-adrenergic receptor blockade with phenoxybenzamine hydrochloride (Dibenzyline) should be implemented with the goal of controlling hypertension and other symptoms. Failure to prepare patients adequately pharmacologically may result in a severe hypertensive crisis and even sudden death intraoperatively. Beta (β-blockade is reserved for patients with tachyarrhythmias or predominantly epinephrine-secreting tumors.

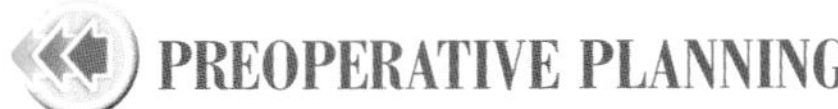

PREOPERATIVE PLANNING

Patients with a functional adrenal mass and hypertension should have preoperative control of their blood pressure and correction of any electrolyte abnormalities. Patients with a pheochromocytoma should undergo α-adrenergic receptor blockade 7 to 10 days prior to surgery. The goal of the pharmacologic blockade should be to control hypertension and to achieve mild orthostasis. If tachycardia persists after α blockade, or if the patient has a tumor that is largely epinephrine secreting, then β-adrenergic blockade should be instituted as well. However, β blockade should never be implemented without first achieving α blockade because of the potential for unopposed α stimulation, leading to marked hypertension. All patients with hypercortisolism should receive stress doses of corticosteroids intravenously before and after surgery. A urinary catheter is placed intraoperatively in all patients, and an arterial line should be inserted in hypertensive patients with pheochromocytomas. A central venous catheter is rarely necessary. A type and screen of the patient's blood should be done routinely, but crossmatching of blood is usually reserved for patients with large, vascular tumors.

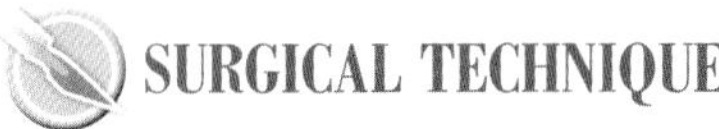

SURGICAL TECHNIQUE

The retroperitoneal location of the adrenal glands makes them surgically accessible with a variety of operative approaches: through the abdomen, flank, or retroperitoneum. As a result, laparoscopic approaches to adrenalectomy have been designed to mimic their open counterparts. The most widely used approach to laparoscopic adrenalectomy is a transabdominal lateral flank approach that provides excellent exposure in the retroperitoneum by allowing gravity retraction of adjacent organs. This technique also permits examination of other intraabdominal organs, although it does not allow access to the contralateral adrenal gland. The adrenal gland may also be removed laparoscopically using an anterior transabdominal approach with the patient supine or slightly rotated. This approach provides a conventional view of abdominal anatomy and may allow access to both adrenal glands. However, operative exposure is more difficult because additional effort must be expended to maintain exposure and retraction of overlying organs, including the spleen, pancreas, stomach, liver, and colon. Operative times have generally been longer with this approach than with other techniques. Finally, a retroperitoneal endoscopic approach to adrenalectomy has been successfully used in some centers. This approach uses a totally extraperitoneal technique and may be especially useful in patients who have had previous abdominal surgery or who require bilateral adrenalectomy. Disadvantages of the retroperitoneal endoscopic approach include a smaller working space that may complicate the removal of larger tumors, difficulties with dissecting the retroperitoneal fat, and less familiar anatomic relationships that make it more difficult to learn. The transabdominal lateral flank approach is the most commonly used technique and is described in detail later in this chapter.

General Principles of Dissection

Laparoscopic adrenalectomy should follow the general principles of open adrenalectomy regardless of the approach employed. Dissection should remain extracapsular to the gland both to avoid injury to and bleeding from the friable adrenal parenchyma and to prevent fracture and spillage of tumor cells. Grasping the adrenal gland or tumor with the laparoscopic instruments should be avoided. Exposure is obtained by pushing or elevating the gland with a blunt instrument or by gently grasping periadrenal fat. Meticulous hemostasis is essential to maintain a clear field of view and to avoid damaging adjacent structures. Isolation of the adrenal vein should be attempted early in the dissection in cases of pheochromocytoma in order to reduce the release of catecholamines into the systemic circulation. Small arterial branches can be secured with an ultrasonic coagulator, electrocautery, or endoscopic clips. Vascular branches may retract into the retroperitoneal fat if inadequately controlled and thereby cause troublesome or delayed hemorrhage. Finally, the gland should be removed using an impermeable entrapment sac.

Patient Positioning and Operating Room Setup

The first key to success in this operation is proper patient positioning. Before general anesthesia is induced, a well-padded beanbag mattress is placed beneath the patient. General anesthesia is induced with the patient supine. An orogastric tube and urinary catheter are inserted. An arterial line is placed in the patient with a vasoactive pheochromocytoma, as indicated clinically. The patient is then rolled into a lateral decubitus position, with the side that contains the adrenal tumor facing up, and then secured with a combination of the beanbag mattress, safety straps, and tape. A roll is placed under the chest wall to protect the axilla, and all other pressure points (including the hips) must be padded to prevent nerve compression injuries. The operating table is flexed at the patient's waist area to increase flank exposure (Fig. 41-2, page 414). Placement of the table in a reverse Trendelenburg position also facilitates endoscopic exposure and allows fluid and blood to drain away from the operative field.

Video monitors are positioned on each side at the head of the operating table. For both right and left adrenalectomy, the surgeon usually stands to the patient's right, and the assistant should be on the opposite side. The camera operator is usually stationed on the same side as the surgeon for left adrenalectomy and opposite the surgeon for right adrenalectomy. However, these positions may be interchangeable, if necessary, according to the exposure required in any individual patient and whether the surgeon is right- or left-hand dominant.

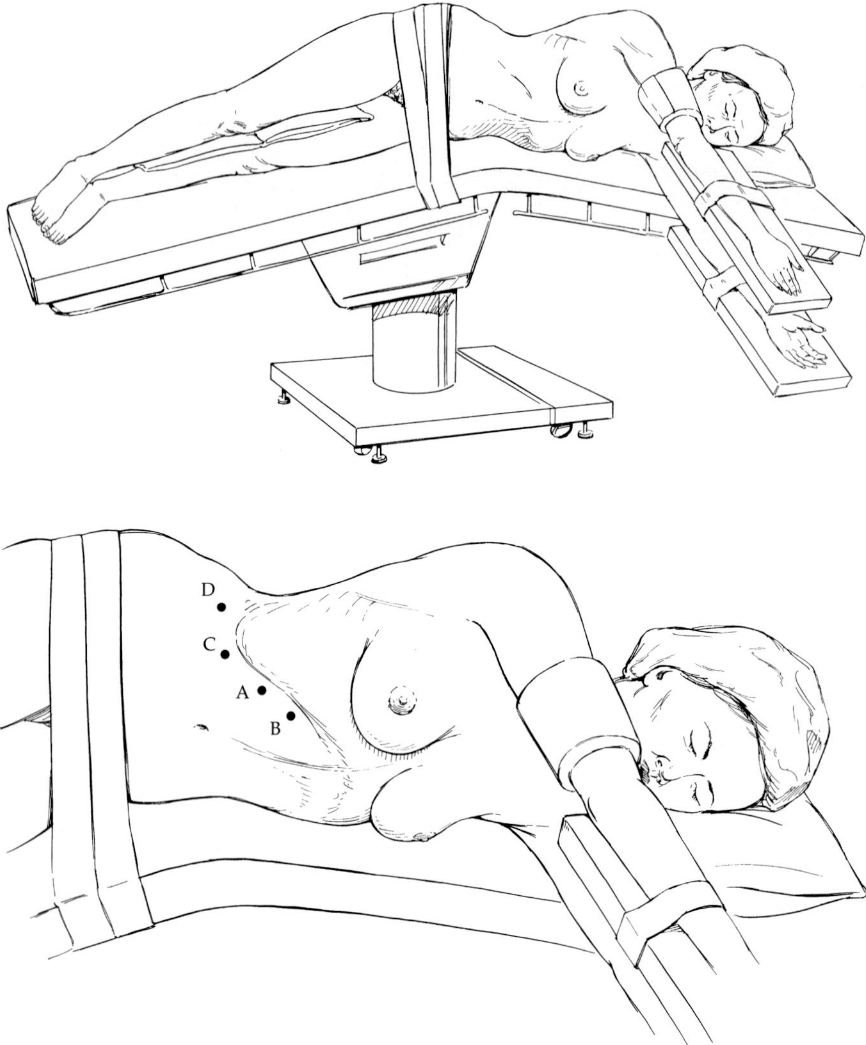

Fig. 41-2. Patient positioning (above) and port-site placement (below) for laparoscopic right adrenalectomy using the lateral flank approach. The letters adjacent to the sites marked in the lower figure reflect the sequence in which the ports are generally inserted (**A:** 5 mm; **B:** 5 mm; **C:** 11 mm; **D:** 5 mm). Further details regarding positioning and port placement are given in the text.

Initial Access and Port Placement

With the patient in the lateral decubitus position, initial access to the peritoneal cavity is most easily accomplished using a closed technique with a Veress needle. Alternatively, open insertion of a blunt-tipped cannula may be used, but this technique is somewhat more difficult because of the thickness of the lateral abdominal wall musculature. The first port should be inserted along the anterior axillary line two finger-breadths below the costal margin. Subsequent ports are then placed as shown in Figure 41-2 from the subcostal region to a point near the posterior axillary line. All ports can be 5 mm in size (if a 5-mm laparoscope is used), except for one 11-mm working port for placement of the endoscopic clip applier. An angled 30- or 45-degree laparoscope is used to provide improved viewing angles. The ports are spaced at least 5 to 7 cm apart to avoid clashing of the instruments and the ports both externally and within the abdomen. Some retroperitoneal dissection is usually necessary before the most dorsal fourth port can be inserted on the left side. A two-handed dissection technique is mandatory for this operation, and the surgeon must be comfortably situated relative to the ports because of the time required to complete the procedure. After the first three ports have been inserted, the next step is to expose the retroperitoneum and adrenal gland, as described subsequently for right and left adrenalectomy.

Right Adrenalectomy

Removal of the right adrenal gland is somewhat easier than the left because of the shape and location of the gland. Right adrenalectomy is potentially more hazardous, however, due to the anatomy of the adrenal vein and its drainage into the inferior vena cava. Indeed, proper dissection of the right adrenal gland involves dissection of the lateral border of the vena cava, which it abuts. Adequate exposure and meticulous dissection and hemostasis are, therefore, critical to a successful procedure. After access to the peritoneal cavity has been accomplished, a 5-mm flexible retractor is inserted through the subcostal port and is used to elevate the right lobe of the liver. The right triangular ligament is then incised from the inferior border of the liver superiorly to the diaphragm (Fig. 41-3). This maneuver allows medial rotation of the right hepatic lobe and exposes the adrenal gland and inferior vena cava. It is not necessary to mobilize or retract the hepatic flexure of the colon or duodenum.

After division of the right triangular ligament and elevation of the right hemiliver, the adrenal gland and tumor should be visible in the retroperitoneum superior to the kidney (Fig. 41-4). Extracapsular dissection is usually begun adjacent to the medial border of the adrenal gland. Using a combination of blunt dissection and L-hook electrocautery, the medial border of the gland and the lateral border of the inferior vena cava are further delineated by dividing connective tissue fibers and small vessels in this area. The surgeon should be aware of the location of the vena cava at all times during the dissection. The adrenal vein is usually visible at this stage in the dissection and is isolated by blunt dissection posterior to it and then by using a right angle dissector to encircle the vein (Fig. 41-5, page 416, and see Fig. 41-4). The vein is ligated with two endoscopic clips placed proximally on the inferior vena cava side and one or two clips distally depending on the length of the adrenal vein. Minimal traction should be placed on the vein during dissection and clipping because of the risk of tearing the adrenal vein—vena cava junction.

After the adrenal vein has been ligated, the adrenal attachments, including arterial branches to the adrenal inferiorly, medially (crossing behind the vena cava), and superiorly, are divided. A combination of techniques is used for this portion of the dissection, including blunt dissection, electrocautery, and ligation of vessels with endoscopic clips. Alternatively,

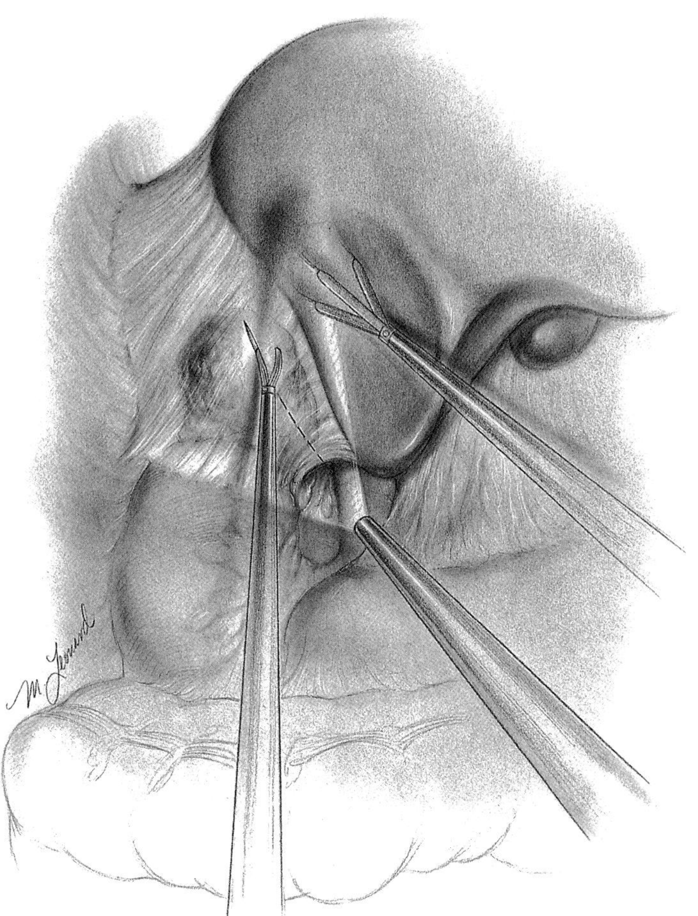

Fig. 41-3. Anatomic relationships as viewed during laparoscopic right adrenalectomy with the transabdominal lateral flank approach. The first phase in the operation entails retraction of the liver medially and division of the right triangular ligament.

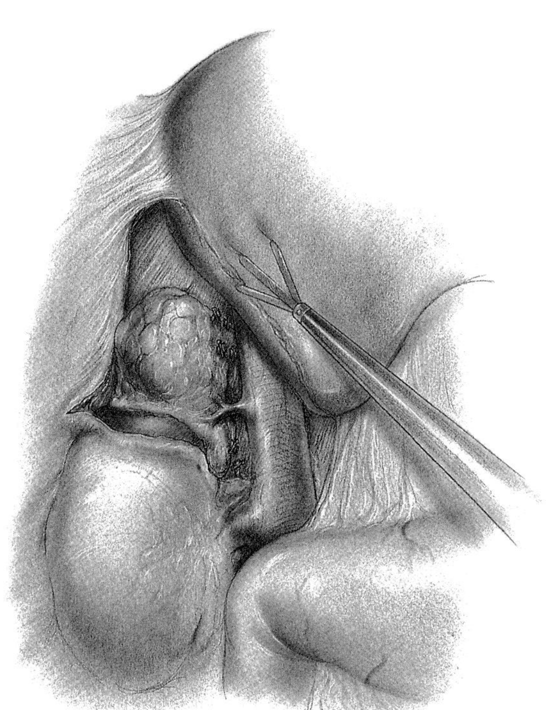

Fig. 41-4. A schematic view of the right adrenal gland as exposed laparoscopically. The triangular ligament has been divided, and the medial border of the adrenal gland has been partially dissected free, exposing the adrenal vein and inferior vena cava.

an ultrasonic dissector may be used for coagulation of the periadrenal vessels. Retraction on the gland is accomplished by gently pushing or elevating the tumor with a blunt instrument. One may also retract the gland by grasping the periadrenal fat but should avoid grasping the adrenal gland or tumor itself because the gland is friable and will bleed, or tumor itself may be spilled into the retroperitoneum. Finally, the lateral border of the adrenal gland is mobilized from the surrounding retroperitoneal fat. The surgeon should remain close to the adrenal gland throughout the dissection to avoid injury to the inferior vena cava medially, diaphragm and hepatic veins superiorly, and kidney and renal vein inferiorly. After the specimen has been freed through dissection, it is placed in an impermeable entrapment bag inserted through the 11-mm port site. It is usually necessary to enlarge the incision somewhat to remove the specimen. Large pheochromocytomas, in which the pathologic evaluation is less important, may be morcellated before removal to avoid extending the incision much.

After the specimen has been removed, the abdomen is reinflated with CO_2 and the retroperitoneum irrigated and inspected for hemostasis. The clips on the adrenal vein should also be examined. Each 10-mm or larger port site is closed with a fascial suture, and the skin is closed with absorbable subcuticular suture. 5-mm ports may be closed with steri-strips or a tissue glue. A closed suction drain may be inserted into the retroperitoneum through one of the ports, if deemed necessary, but this is not often indicated.

Left Adrenalectomy

Mobilization of the splenic flexure of the colon is the first step in left adrenalectomy. Following this maneuver, a more dorsally located fourth port can be inserted if necessary. Dissection lateral to the kidney should be avoided, because this will result in medial rotation of the kidney and a compromised exposure of the adrenal gland. The next step in the operation—and the key to laparoscopic left adrenalectomy—is complete division of the splenorenal ligament superiorly to the diaphragm and medial rotation of the spleen (Fig. 41-6, page 416). This maneuver allows access to the superior retroperitoneum and minimizes the need to retract the spleen. The next step is to develop the plane between the kidney and the tail of

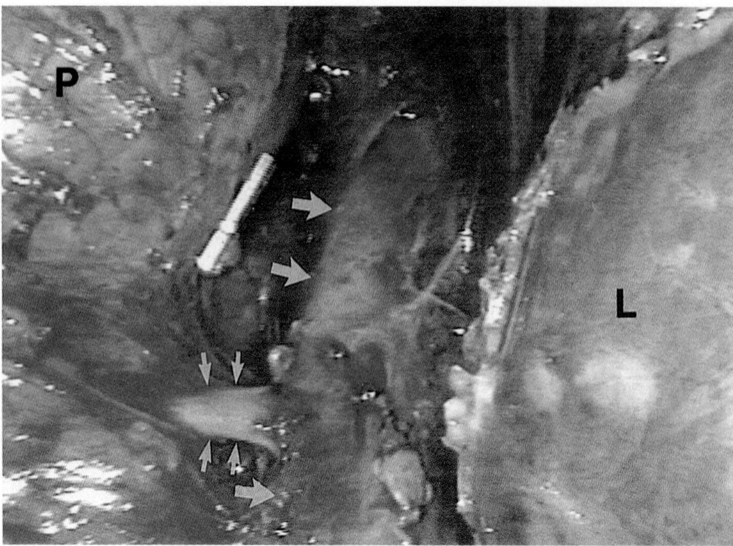

Fig. 41-5. Endoscopic view of the right adrenal vein (small arrows) and inferior vena cava (large arrows). A 4-cm pheochromocytoma (P) is seen to the left, and the liver (L) is on the right.

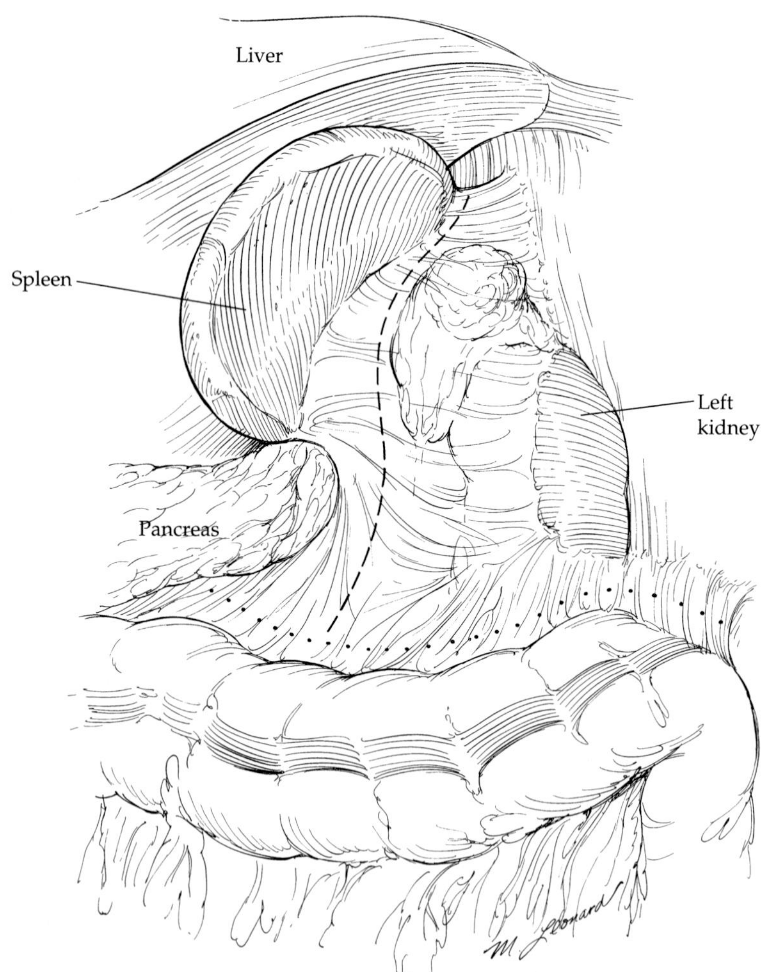

Fig. 41-6. Sequential steps in laparoscopic exposure of the left adrenal gland (lateral flank approach). The splenic flexure of the colon is mobilized first (dotted line), followed by complete division of the splenorenal ligament (dashed line).

the pancreas and to rotate the pancreas medially to expose the inferior portion of the adrenal gland and the left adrenal vein. Minimal retraction is usually needed if the spleen and pancreas have been adequately mobilized. As the dissection continues within the retroperitoneal fat, the adrenal gland should be found closely applied to the superomedial aspect of the kidney.

Locating the left adrenal gland may be difficult at first, especially in a patient with extensive retroperitoneal fat or with either a small tumor or adrenal hyperplasia. Laparoscopic ultrasonography can facilitate localization of the adrenal gland and tumor and help define the relationship of the gland to adjacent vascular structures in difficult cases. Laparoscopic ultrasound (LUS) is most useful in obese patients during left adrenalectomy because of the difficulty in localizing the gland in the retroperitoneal fat. It may also be used to define the limits of the adrenal gland and its relationship to surrounding structures in such patients, and it can also be useful in patients with large or potentially malignant adrenal lesions to confirm that there is no extracapsular extension of the tumor.

After the adrenal gland has been located, its borders should be clearly defined. In most patients, it is possible to approach the inferomedial border of the gland directly early in the operation and expose the adrenal vein (Fig. 41-7). In our experience it is easiest to first define the medial and lateral borders of the gland and then follow these caudally to the inferior margin of the adrenal where the adrenal vein lies. One must be aware of the inferior phrenic vein medially, which frequently joins the adrenal vein prior to the latter's entry into the renal vein. The left renal vein should be visible at this point; the adrenal is gently elevated off this vessel, using a hook cautery or ultrasonic coagulator.

The dissection methods for isolation and division of the blood supply to the left adrenal gland are identical to those for the right side. The relationships of the relevant structures and the position of the laparoscopic instruments during ligation of the left adrenal vein are illustrated schematically in Figure 41-8. After the adrenal vein has been ligated and the inferior and medial borders of the gland have been cleared, the dissection continues laterally and posteriorly, and superiorly. Arterial branches from the renal artery are frequently encountered along the medial and lateral borders of the left adrenal gland. The left adrenal is usually closely applied to the superior pole of the kidney

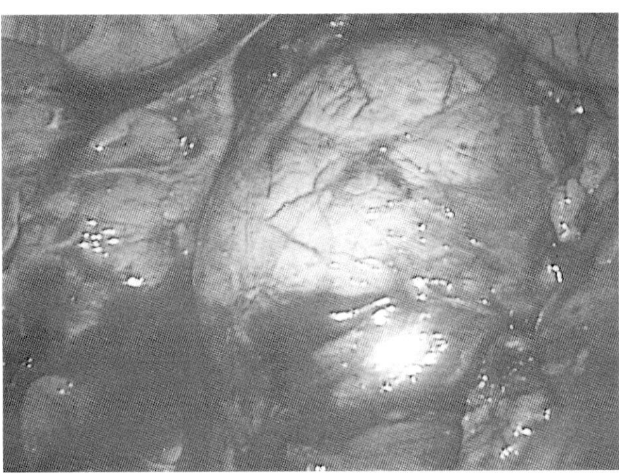

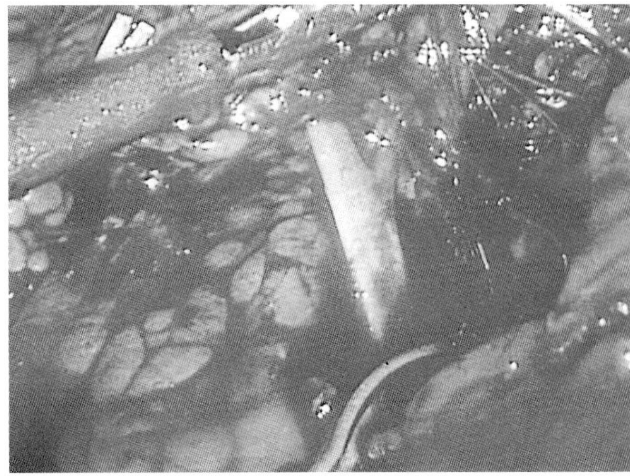

Fig. 41-7. Laparoscopic views. **A.** A 3.5-cm cortical adenoma of the left adrenal gland. **B.** The left adrenal vein. The vein is usually 2- to 3-cm long and runs obliquely from the inferomedial aspect of the adrenal to its junction with the left renal vein.

with left adrenalectomy, so that one must be careful not to damage the renal capsule and incur bleeding. Other structures that may be injured include the renal vessels, the tail of the pancreas, the diaphragm, and the spleen. Once the specimen is free, the concluding steps are the same as for right adrenalectomy. If any concern exists that the pancreatic parenchyma has been injured, a closed suction drain should be placed.

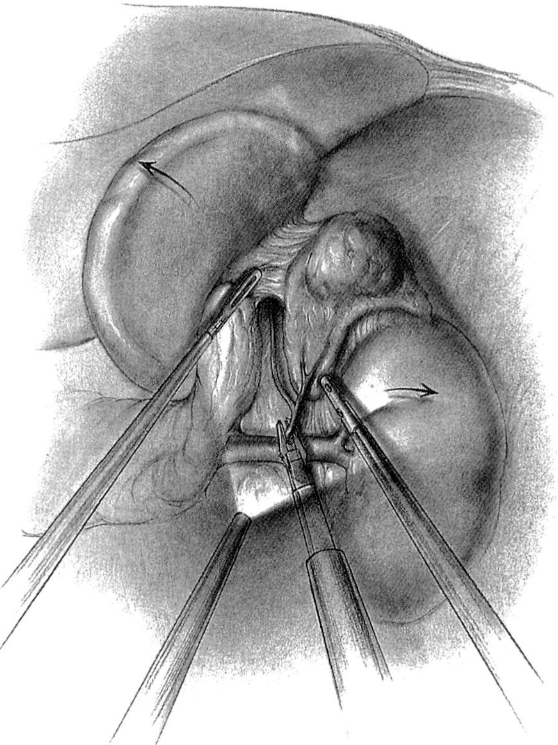

Fig. 41-8. Exposure and ligation of the left adrenal vein. The spleen has been rotated medially and the kidney retracted laterally. The vein is ligated at the anteromedial border of the adrenal gland with endoscopic clips. Note the inferior phrenic vein entering the left adrenal vein proximal to the latter's entry into the renal vein.

Bilateral Adrenalectomy

The most common indication for bilateral adrenalectomy is adrenal hyperplasia due to failed treatment of pituitary Cushing disease. Other indications in patients with Cushing syndrome include ectopic ACTH production refractory to medical treatment, primary pigmented micronodular hyperplasia, and macronodular adrenal hyperplasia. Bilateral pheochromocytomas may also be an indication for laparoscopic bilateral adrenalectomy.

With the lateral flank approach, bilateral adrenalectomy is carried out as two separate procedures with repositioning of the patient between sides. The technical aspects to the operation are identical to those described for right and left adrenalectomy. Alternatively, a retroperitoneal endoscopic approach can be used, which may eliminate the need to reposition the patient.

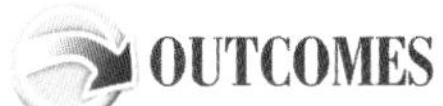

OUTCOMES

Several centers have reported results of large series of patients treated by laparoscopic adrenalectomy. The results from these various centers show conversion rates to open adrenalectomy of about 3.5%. Operative times typically average between 1.5 to 2 hours for uncomplicated cases. Laparoscopic adrenalectomy has been compared with open adrenalectomy in numerous retrospective studies. Although operative times have generally been longer for the laparoscopic approach, laparoscopic adrenalectomy has been consistently shown to require less pain medication and to result in less pain, shorter postoperative hospitalization, and a faster return to full activity compared with open anterior or posterior adrenalectomy. Another important advantage of laparoscopic adrenalectomy is a reduction in the complication rate. In one meta-analysis of complications reported by Brunt derived from laparoscopic and open adrenalectomy series published from 1980 through 2000, a significant reduction in the complication rate was seen with the laparoscopic approach. In this analysis, the complication rate in 50 studies of laparoscopic adrenalectomy performed in 1522 patients was 10.9% compared with a complication rate of 25.2% in 48 reports involving 2273 patients undergoing open adrenalectomy. This benefit was principally due to a reduction in the incidence of wound, pulmonary, and infectious complications. Laparoscopic adrenalectomy was also associated with a lower incidence of associated organ injury, primarily due to a reduction in the incidence of incidental splenectomy. As a result, laparoscopic adrenalectomy should now be considered the standard procedure for removal of benign adrenal lesions smaller than 6 cm.

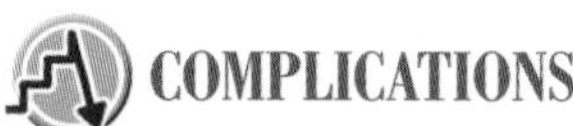

COMPLICATIONS

Patients who undergo laparoscopic adrenalectomy are subject to the same potential risks as with open adrenalectomy. Bleeding is the most likely complication and has been the most common cause for conversion to open adrenalectomy. The conversion rate to open adrenalectomy in over 176 consecutive laparoscopic adrenalectomies carried out at the Washington University Medical Center was 2.3%, with an additional three cases converted to a hand-assist approach. The best approach is a preventive one with a careful, meticulous dissection technique. Intraoperative hemorrhage can usually be managed laparoscopically if it comes from small retroperitoneal vessels, such as the adrenal arteries or the adrenal gland. Bleeding from the adrenal veins is potentially more serious, because this may also involve the inferior vena cava on the right or the renal vein on the left. The surgeon must clearly visualize these structures before attempting to dissect around them and must be prepared to convert rapidly to an open operation in the event of major uncontrolled hemorrhage. In our experience, there have been no instances of uncontrolled bleeding from the adrenal veins or vena cava. Another potential site of hemorrhage is the right lobe of the liver, which may be lacerated by the retractor during right adrenalectomy. Bleeding from this area is usually self-limited and does not require any specific treatment. The operative field, however, must be kept clear of blood to visualize the dissection adequately laparoscopically. Injuries to the liver, kidney, or bowel may also occur with insertion of the Veress needle and initial trocars into the abdomen. These risks are inherent in any laparoscopic surgical procedure, and a closed insertion technique should be avoided in any patient with extensive previous abdominal surgery or abdominal distention. Fracturing the tumor and spillage of tumor cells should be preventable events during laparoscopic adrenalectomy if one adheres to the precautions described above.

Hypertensive exacerbations may occur during laparoscopic removal of pheochromocytomas. These episodes are best controlled by adequate preoperative α-adrenergic receptor blockade, by intravenous administration of labetalol or esmolol (or alternatively sodium nitroprusside) intraoperatively, and by early ligation of the adrenal vein.

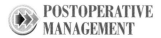

POSTOPERATIVE MANAGEMENT

After laparoscopic adrenalectomy, most patients can be cared for in a regular nursing unit. The intensive care unit is reserved for patients at higher risk because of unstable hemodynamics or advanced cardiopulmonary disease. Patients are started on oral liquids once they are fully awake, and the diet is advanced as tolerated. A parenteral narcotic may be required in some patients during the first 24 hours postoperatively, but most patients are taking oral analgesics exclusively by the first postoperative day. A complete blood count is obtained the morning after surgery, and electrolytes are monitored as clinically indicated. Most patients can be discharged from the hospital within 24 to 48 hours of the operation. Patients are discharged home without restrictions in physical activity and should be able to return to work within 7 to 14 days of surgery. A follow-up examination should be performed in the office 2 to 3 weeks after discharge. Wound healing problems are rarely seen postoperatively, even in patients with Cushing syndrome.

Stress doses of a steroid should be administered intravenously in the perioperative period to patients with Cushing syndrome or subclinical Cushing and to all patients who undergo bilateral adrenalectomy. Once the patient resumes oral food intake, oral corticosteroid replacement therapy should be instituted at a dose of 5 to 15 mg per day of prednisone in divided doses. Patients with Cushing syndrome due to an adrenocortical adenoma may require replacement therapy up to 6 to 12 months or longer to allow the contralateral adrenal gland to completely recover. In most cases, corticosteroid replacement is tapered gradually according to patient tolerance. Symptoms of headache, nausea, and fatigue may indicate inadequate replacement and require adjustments in dosaging. Evaluation of the hypothalamic-pituitary-adrenal axis with an ACTH-stimulation test may be useful in patients who are difficult or slow to wean.

Patients who have undergone bilateral adrenalectomy also require lifelong mineralocorticoid replacement with fludrocortisone acetate (Florinef Acetate) in a dose of 0.1 mg per day. Acute adrenal insufficiency may develop postoperatively in any patient with hypercortisolism or following bilateral adrenalectomy. Acute adrenal insufficiency often presents as cardiovascular collapse with hypotension and shock; if not recognized and treated promptly, it may be fatal. Patients may also experience abdominal pain, weakness, fever, nausea, and vomiting; leukocytosis may also develop. One must have a high index of suspicion for this diagnosis and institute prompt therapy by administration of intravenous hydrocortisone.

Patients with a pheochromocytoma may develop hypotension and require large amounts of intravenous fluids postoperatively due to intravascular volume expansion from loss of α-adrenergic receptor–mediated sympathetic tone. Rebound hyperinsulinemia and hypoglycemia may also develop in these patients, from the loss of inhibition of insulin secretion by circulating catecholamines. Following resection of a pheochromocytoma, all patients should have plasma fractionated metanephrines measured postoperatively and then on an annual basis.

CONTROVERSIES IN LAPAROSCOPIC ADRENAL SURGERY

Primary and Metastatic Adrenal Malignancies

The ability to remove the adrenal gland laparoscopically for benign disease with minimal morbidity and mortality has led some surgeons to liberalize their indications for laparoscopic adrenalectomy to include malignancies, both primary and metastatic. Initial recommendations were that laparoscopy should only be used for tumors that were less than 6 cm and not suspected of malignancy. As experience has grown, however, these two absolute contraindications have become more relative contraindications. Several groups have reported removal of tumors over 6 cm and up to 15 cm with good results. The conversion rate appears to be higher with these patients (5% to 14%), however. As mentioned previously, in considering laparoscopic adrenalectomy for potential malignancy, the preoperative evaluation is of paramount importance to minimize the potential for a suboptimal cancer operation.

Primary adrenal malignancies may be either adrenal cortical carcinomas or malignant pheochromocytoma. Both of these tumors are rare, and large single-institution experiences with laparoscopic excision are lacking. Two important risk factors for primary adrenal malignancy include older patient age and virilizing tumors. Additionally, tumors larger than 6 cm have an increased potential for malignancy for adrenal cortical carcinoma but not necessarily for pheochromocytoma. The diagnosis of malignant pheochromocytoma can only be made by the findings of local invasion or nodal metastases, and up to 26% can be malignant. Approximately 50% of adrenal cortical carcinomas are functioning tumors. Functioning adrenal cortical carcinomas may secrete excess cortisol (30%), androgens (20%), estrogens (10%), aldosterone (1% to 2%), or a combination thereof (35%).

Several studies have now been published of laparoscopic adrenalectomy for large and primary adrenal malignancies. Short-term follow-up (9 to 39 months) would suggest that the recurrence rate ranges from 0% to 50%. In one study, in three out of six patients clinically unsuspected adrenocortical carcinomas removed laparoscopically subsequently recurred. In another report at the MD Anderson Cancer Center (University of Texas) of 170 patients with adrenocortical carcinoma, six patients underwent laparoscopic resection and all had recurrences, with 83% having peritoneal carcinomatosis. This is in sharp contrast to 153 patients who underwent open anterior adrenalectomy, with a 35% local recurrence rate and an 8% carcinomatosis rate. Other isolated reports of recurrences after laparoscopic adrenalectomy for both benign and malignant lesions have appeared in the literature. In most cases, these recurrences were due more likely due to the biology of the primary tumor rather than surgical technique. Indeed, open adrenalectomy for malignancy has been shown to have a recurrence rate up to 70% in some series.

Tumors that commonly metastasize to the adrenal gland include melanoma, lung, breast, colon, and renal cell cancers. Lymphoma can also involve the adrenal gland. The majority of these metastases do not occur in isolation, and therefore it is a rare patient for whom adrenalectomy is indicated. In reported series, an adrenal incidentaloma in the setting of a patient with a history of malignancy represents metastatic disease in up to 32% to 73% of cases. As a result, metastasis should be considered for any adrenal lesion that is larger than 2 cm in a patient with a history of cancer. The workup for these patients is similar to that for an adrenal incidentaloma, with the addition of PET imaging to evaluate for extraadrenal disease. In the setting of an isolated metastasis, biopsy should be avoided as this may potentially result in seeding of tumor cells.

It would appear from reported series that metastatic disease is more amenable to laparoscopic removal due to the smaller size of metastases. Such patients should have well circumscribed lesions, and the surgeon should be highly experienced in laparoscopic adrenalectomy. While isolated metastases are usually confined to the capsule, the adjoining fatty tissue should be removed along with the gland to minimize the risk of a positive margin. As with laparoscopic resection for large primary tumors, the conversion rate for metastatic disease is higher than for benign disease. In one study from the Memorial Sloan-Kettering Cancer Center comparing open to laparoscopic adrenalectomy for metastatic disease, there were no differences in the incidence of positive margins or survival; however, laparoscopic adrenalectomy conferred a shorter hospital stay. Survival after resection of isolated metastases has ranged from 20 to 30 months.

Laparoscopic adrenalectomy for primary malignant disease should be undertaken with great caution until more definitive long-term results become available. If a laparoscopic approach for a suspected malignancy is being considered, a few points should be emphasized. The lesion should be well circumscribed on preoperative imaging, and these features should be confirmed intraoperatively with laparoscopic ultrasound. The surgeon performing the operation should be highly experienced with laparoscopic adrenalectomy and have a low threshold to convert to an open operation if the dissection becomes difficult. Finally, because tumors greater than 6 cm in size may be difficult to manipulate laparoscopically, a hand-assist approach may be useful in selected cases. Regardless of the approach, minimal tumor manipulation should be the goal to minimize the risk of tumor recurrence.

Partial Adrenalectomy

Open partial adrenalectomy had been performed by a number of groups as a cortical sparing procedure for bilateral disease in the setting of bilateral pheochromocytoma in order to avoid the lifelong consequences of adrenal insufficiency and steroid replacement. Indeed, patients who have undergone bilateral adrenalectomy have a 25% to 33% lifetime risk of an Addisonian crisis. The first laparoscopic adrenal sparing procedure was described in 1997, and since that time several groups have advocated its use for partial resection of adrenal tumors. Laparoscopic partial adrenalectomy has been described for bilateral aldosterone producing adenomas, bilateral Cushing syndrome, and bilateral pheochromocytomas in MEN 2A and von Hippel-Lindau syndrome. In series comparing open to laparoscopic bilateral partial adrenalectomy, the mean blood loss and length of postoperative stay were less with laparoscopy while the operative time was longer. The rate of recurrent pheochromocytoma after laparoscopic bilateral partial adrenalectomy has ranged from 7% to 23% in larger series.

Some groups have recently extended the indications for partial adrenalectomy to include unilateral disease. In the largest series reported by Walz et al. in 2004, 96 patients underwent laparoscopic unilateral partial adrenalectomy for pheochromocytoma, aldosteronomas, Cushing adenoma, and nonfunctioning tumors. There were no differences in tumor size, operating time, and blood loss for patients undergoing partial compared to complete adrenalectomy. All patients undergoing partial adrenalectomy had resolution of biochemical disease and no recurrence at 51 months follow-up. Sasagawa et al. demonstrated comparable results in 47 patients with unilateral solitary adenomas (13 aldosteronomas, 10 Cushing, 3 pheochromocytomas, 2 myelolipomas, 1 ganglioneuroma, and 18 nonfunctioning tumors). The operating time dropped significantly from the first 20 cases (270 minutes) to the last 27 cases (198 minutes). Increasing experience did not result in a decreased blood loss, however. No patients needed steroid supplementation. In some smaller reported series, the recurrence rates for laparoscopic partial adrenalectomy ranged from 0% to 25%. Despite these reports, the use of laparoscopic partial adrenalectomy for patients without an inherited predisposition to adrenal neoplasia represents a departure from the well-established principles of adrenal surgery. The advantages to partial adrenalectomy in these patients should be minimal because there is very low risk of developing contralateral disease. Furthermore, this technique should never be used for unilateral primary malignancy or metastatic disease because of the potential for tumor seeding. In addition, its use for aldosteronoma is also highly questionable because of the potential for a nodule other than the dominant-sized nodule to be the primary source of increased aldosterone production.

Several technical aspects of partial adrenalectomy must be considered. While the patient preparation, positioning, and trocar placement are the same as with total adrenalectomy, the need for hemostasis, accurate tumor localization with intraoperative ultrasound, and precise surgical technique is paramount. Ultrasonic coagulating shears, metal clips, fibrin glue, bipolar coagulation, and argon beam coagulation have all been used to maintain hemostasis along the divided adrenal parenchyma. If partial resection is contemplated, the dissection should attempt to preserve the adrenal vein and limit dissection of normal adrenal tissue to preserve the arterial supply. A rim of normal tissue should be left on the specimen to allow adequate margins for pathologic evaluation. In no case should resection of the primary lesion be compromised by efforts to perform a partial resection. To preserve adrenal function, 15% to 30% of normal cortex must be left in situ if the central adrenal vein is taken.

CONCLUSION

In summary, laparoscopic adrenalectomy is the preferred method for removing the vast majority of adrenal tumors. With growing experience the indications for adrenalectomy are being broadened to those with large tumors and metastatic disease. Caution should be used when addressing potentially large primary adrenal malignancies, as the risk of tumor recurrence may be substantially increased. In experienced hands, laparoscopic adrenalectomy can confer improved patient outcomes compared to open adrenalectomy.

SUGGESTED READING

Bonjer HJ, Berends FJ, Kazemier G, et al. Endoscopic retroperitoneal adrenalectomy: lessons learned from 111 consecutive cases. *Ann Surg* 2000;232:796–803.

Brunt LM, Moley JF. Adrenal incidentaloma. *World J Surg* 2001;25:905–913.

Brunt LM. Minimal access adrenal surgery. *Surg Endosc* 2006;20:351–361.

Brunt LM. The positive impact of laparoscopic adrenalectomy on complications of adrenal surgery. *Surg Endosc* 2001;16:252–257.

Cobb WS, Kercher KW, Sing RF. Laparoscopic adrenalectomy for malignancy. *Am J Surg* 2005;189:405–411.

Gagner M, Lacroix A, Bolte E, et al. Laparoscopic adrenalectomy: the importance of a flank approach in the lateral decubitus position. *Surg Endosc* 1994;8:135–138.

Gagner M, Pomp A, Heniford BT, et al. Laparoscopic adrenalectomy: lessons learned from 100 consecutive cases. *Ann Surg* 1997;226: 238–247.

Henry J-F, Defechereux T, Raffaelli M, et al. Complications of laparoscopic adrenalectomy: results of 169 consecutive cases. *World J Surg* 2000;24:1342–1346.

Kebebew E, Siperstein AE, Clark OH, et al. Results of laparoscopic adrenalectomy for suspected and unsuspected malignant adrenal neoplasms. *Arch Surg* 2002;137:948–953.

Li ML, Fitzgerald PA, Price DC, et al. Iatrogenic pheochromocytomatosis: a previously unreported result of laparoscopic adrenalectomy. *Surgery* 2001;130:1072–1077.

MacGillivray DC, Whalen GF, Malchoff CD, et al. Laparoscopic resection of large adrenal tumors. *Ann Surg Oncol* 2002;9:480–485.

Sarela AI, Murphy I, Coit DG, et al. Metastasis to the adrenal gland: The emerging role of laparoscopic surgery. *Ann Surg Oncol* 2003; 10:1191–1196.

Sturgeon C, Kebebew E. Laparoscopic adrenalectomy for malignancy. *Surg Clin N Am* 2004; 84:755–774.

Thompson GB, Grant CS, van Heerden JA, et al. Laparoscopic versus open posterior adrenalectomy: a case-control study. *Surgery* 1997;122: 1132–1136.

Walz MK, Peitgen K, Diesing D, et al. Partial versus total adrenalectomy by the posterior retroperitoneoscopic approach: Early and long-term results of 325 consecutive procedures in primary adrenal neoplasia. *World J Surg* 2004;28:1323–1329.

COMMENTARY

Drs. Tessier and Brunt have provided an update on the technique and results of laparoscopic adrenalectomy. They discuss the anatomy, physiology, and evaluation of the patient with an adrenal mass. It must be emphasized that surgeons performing adrenal surgery be well versed in the physiology of the pituitary adrenal cortical axis. The appropriate perioperative preparation of the patient for surgery is also of key importance, particularly in the presence of a pheochromocytoma. At present, the use of laparoscopic techniques to perform adrenalectomy in the presence of known malignancy remains controversial. One of the most critical factors in performing laparoscopic adrenalectomy, whether for benign or malignant disease, is to maintain an extracapsular dissection of the adrenal gland. There have been several reports of recurrence of adrenal tumors following laparoscopic removal, presumably due to an inadvertent disruption of the capsule with seeding of adrenal tissue.

The authors have carefully outlined the laparoscopic approach to the left and right adrenal glands using the transabdominal technique with the patient in the lateral decubitus position. This is the primary approach used by most surgeons today. Others have reported laparoscopic adrenalectomy using a posterior retroperitoneal approach, which may have value in patients with bilateral tumors. However, the anatomy is much more difficult to ascertain using this approach, which should only be used by those with extensive experience in adrenal surgery and retroperitoneal access.

Of the many operations performed laparoscopically, adrenalectomy is one of the ideal procedures to be performed minimally invasively, because the adrenal gland and its tumor are usually small and located in an area that is difficult to access. Laparoscopic adrenalectomy has rapidly become the standard of care for most patients with adrenal masses. Using the information contained in this excellent chapter should facilitate the safe performance of laparoscopic adrenalectomy in the clinical setting.

NJS

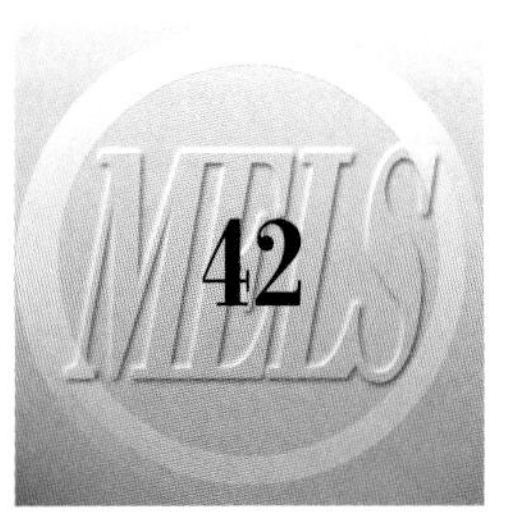

Endoscopic Approaches to the Thyroid and Parathyroid Glands

LEAQUE AHMED AND WILLIAM B. INABNET

INTRODUCTION

Traditional thyroid and parathyroid surgery is performed through a 4- to 6-cm transverse cervical incision, necessitating the creation of myocutaneous flaps to gain access to the thyroid compartment. This approach to thyroid and parathyroid surgery will leave a scar on the anterior surface of the neck in a cosmetically unfavorable location.

The description of endoscopic parathyroidectomy in 1996 led to the development of several innovative approaches to the thyroid and parathyroid glands. With improvement in endoscopic instrumentation and increased understanding of endoscopic cervical anatomy and physiology of carbon dioxide insufflation of the neck, several new minimally invasive techniques for performing thyroid and parathyroid operations have been developed. The minimally invasive endoscopic procedure offers better magnification of anatomy, improves illumination of the operative field, leads to quicker recovery, is less painful, and has better cosmetic results. This chapter details the vast array of approaches that are available to the endocrine surgeon, including the development of totally endoscopic and video-assisted techniques. Endocrine surgeons today should be facile in each of the minimally invasive techniques so that the operative approach can be individualized on the basis of any given patient's situation.

Endoscopic Parathyroidectomy

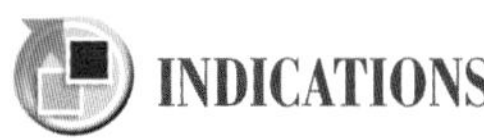

INDICATIONS

Bilateral neck exploration with the identification of all four parathyroid glands and the removal of enlarged parathyroid glands has been considered the gold standard surgical approach for the treatment of primary hyperparathyroidism. With this approach, the decision to excise a parathyroid gland is based on gland appearance, color, shape, and size without any knowledge of the gland's metabolic activity. For most large adenomas, this approach is straightforward; when parathyroid glands are only slightly enlarged or multiple abnormal glands are encountered, however, functional information is invaluable when making intraoperative decisions. Because 80% to 90% of patients with primary hyperparathyroidism have a solitary parathyroid adenoma, resection of one gland leads to cure in most cases. The development of high-resolution ultrasonography and sestamibi scintigraphy has greatly improved the accuracy of preoperative localization of diseased parathyroid glands and has laid the foundation for minimally invasive, or focused, parathyroidectomy. A unilateral approach for solitary parathyroid adenomas was first reported by Tiblin et al., who concluded "unilateral parathyroidectomy . . . is advocated in hyperparathyroidism due to single adenoma because it offers . . . reduced operation time, decreased risk for complication, reduced early hypocalcemia and a more favourable technical conditions for re-operation." The development and availability of intraoperative parathyroid hormone (IOPTH) monitoring has allowed for narrowing unilateral neck exploration to a focused approach for parathyroid adenoma. Because parathyroid hormone (PTH) has a half-life of 3.5 minutes, the surgical team can confirm during surgery that the patient will be eucalcemic after surgery by demonstrating an appropriate reduction in intraoperative PTH levels after excision of all hypersecreting parathyroid tissue (an IOPTH drop of 50% or more from the highest of either preoperative baseline or preexcision level at 10 minutes after gland excision).

The diagnosis of primary hyperparathyroidism is established by demonstrating hypercalcemia in the setting of an elevated intact PTH level. Familial hypocalciuric hypercalcemia and vitamin D deficiency must be ruled out by measuring the 24-hour urine calcium and serum vitamin D levels as surgery will not be needed in these patients. Parathyroidectomy rather than surveillance is currently recommended for most patients with primary hyperparathyroidism for several reasons: a better appreciation of overt symptoms such as fatigue and depression, an earlier diagnosis of parathyroid-induced osteopenia/osteoporosis because of a more frequent use of bone densitometry, and an increased risk of premature cardiovascular death. Parathyroidectomy will lead to reversal of bone loss in patients with low bone mass and it will also correct the metabolic abnormalities associated with hyperparathyroidism.

Patients with sporadic primary hyperparathyroidism with an adenoma localized by preoperative imaging studies are candidates for endoscopic parathyroidectomy. In some patients the endoscopic approach is not indicated. Absolute contraindications for endoscopic parathyroidectomy are the presence of parathyroid carcinoma and/or a voluminous goiter. Relative contraindications for endoscopic parathyroidectomy are evidence of multigland disease, the presence of large goiter, previous neck surgery or irradiation of the neck, equivocal preoperative localization studies, and large (>3 cm) parathyroid adenomas.

PREOPERATIVE PLANNING

Primary hyperparathyroidism is caused by a solitary adenoma in 80% to 90% of cases, and preoperative imaging studies will localize the adenoma in many patients. Sestamibi scan and cervical ultrasound are the usual initial imaging studies performed on patients with hyperparathyroidism. Technetium-99m-sestamibi, which is retained by mitochondria of enlarged parathyroid glands, accurately predicts the correct quadrant of the neck in more than 90% of patients, thereby permitting a targeted approach (Fig. 42-1, page 422). The addition of single-photon emission computed tomography reconstruction can provide important information on the location of parathyroid adenomas, particularly in the

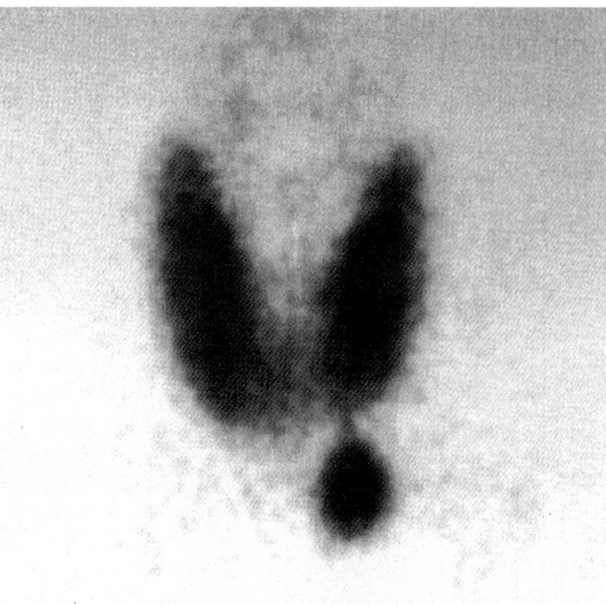

Fig. 42-1. A sestamibi scan showing a left inferior parathyroid adenoma.

anterior/posterior axis of the neck. Cervical ultrasonography is another useful test that allows not only assessment of the size and location of enlarged parathyroid glands but also of the relationship to surrounding structures. The thyroid gland is also easily evaluated by ultrasonography, which can help diagnose thyroid nodular disease or thyroiditis, conditions that may alter surgical recommendations. As preoperative localization plays an important role in patient selection, other imaging studies such as CT scan, MRI, or selective venous sampling could be performed to properly localize the disease process when sestamibi scan and ultrasound do not provide adequate information.

Endoscopic Thyroidectomy

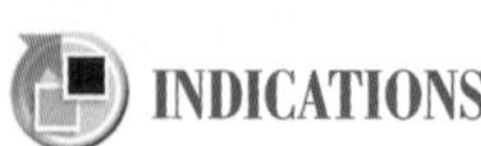

INDICATIONS

Endoscopic neck surgery involves creating and maintaining a working space in the subplatysmal tissue plane. A thyroid nodule less than 3 cm will not obliterate the working space, and so patients with small thyroid nodules are considered candidates for the endoscopic approach. Relative contraindications for an endoscopic approach include thyroid nodules greater than 3 cm, large goiters, and morbid obesity. Severe Graves' disease is also a relative contraindication, in that the thyroid gland is often markedly enlarged and may be more likely to bleed during thyroidectomy. Previous neck surgery and radiation are also contraindications for the endoscopic approach. Small well-differentiated thyroid cancers are amenable to an endoscopic approach as long as there is no clinical or radiographic evidence of gross invasion. As assessment and excision of involved lymph nodes is important in the treatment of thyroid cancer, all patients with large well-differentiated cancer or medullary thyroid cancer should undergo an open, conventional thyroidectomy with appropriate lymph node dissection. Recently however some authors have reported the feasibility of performing both central neck and lateral neck dissection with the minimally invasive approach.

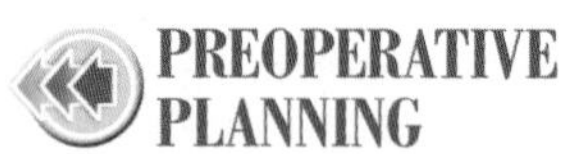

PREOPERATIVE PLANNING

Preoperative planning will include a complete history and physical exam, laboratory tests, imaging studies, and fine needle aspiration of suspected thyroid nodules. Small, solitary thyroid nodules are most amenable to an endoscopic approach. Thus the physical examination should help characterize the size, location, and texture of the thyroid nodule as well as the presence or absence of cervical adenopathy. Previous neck radiation and surgery are contraindications for endoscopic approach and so this history should be obtained from the patient. Indirect laryngoscopy should be performed on all patients undergoing thyroid surgery to assess vocal cord function given the fact that ipsilateral vocal cord paresis can be asymptomatic and indicative of a malignant process. Thyroid-stimulating hormone levels are measured to determine whether thyroid nodules are functioning or nonfunctioning. Fine needle aspiration also plays an important role in the preoperative evaluation. The widespread use of fine needle aspiration has decreased the number of unnecessary thyroid operations while dramatically increasing the percentage of patients with thyroid cancer undergoing thyroid surgery. The procedure is safe, cost-effective, and accurate, with a positive predictive value approaching 95%.

Ultrasonography is useful in the evaluation of patients with thyroid nodules and should be considered an extension of the physical examination. A complete neck survey, which can be performed in 10 minutes, includes an evaluation of the thyroid gland and lymph node basins in the central and lateral compartments of the neck. Ultrasound provides useful information on the size, shape, and location of thyroid nodules and can be used to monitor the precise dimensions of a nodule during suppressive therapy. In addition, ultrasound can detect nonpalpable nodules, especially because up to 50% of the population may have nonpalpable thyroid nodules. Fine needle aspiration of these nonpalpable thyroid lesions has increased the number of small nodules that require surgery. Such patients will be excellent candidates for endoscopic thyroidectomy.

Endoscopic Neck Surgery

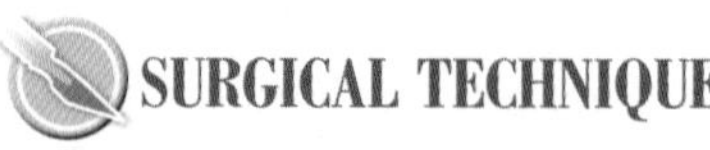

SURGICAL TECHNIQUE

The minimal access approaches to the thyroid compartment can be broadly classified into three groups:

1. The open approach through a small incision placed either centrally or laterally.
2. A totally endoscopic approach through a cervical, axillary, or chest wall incision.
3. A video-assisted approach through a central or lateral incision.

Here we will discuss the latter two techniques.

TOTALLY ENDOSCOPIC CERVICAL APPROACH

After the induction of general endotracheal anesthesia, the neck is extended slightly but much less so than with conventional thyroidectomy. The initial incision is made along the anterior border of the sternocleidomastoid (SCM) muscle in a superior location. Sharp dissection is used to identify the carotid artery. The space medial to the carotid artery but lateral to the strap muscles is developed with blunt dissection either by using a blunt instrument or by inserting a sponge to dissect the perithyroid tissue plane. During endoscopic thyroidectomy, the superior pole vessels are identified, isolated, and divided using ultrasonic energy by working directly through the small incision. A purse-string suture is inserted in the subcutaneous tissue, and a 10-mm trocar is inserted. Carbon dioxide (CO_2) insufflation is initiated to a pressure of 10 mmHg, and initially a 5-mm 0-degree endoscope is used to better develop the working space. Once an adequate working space has been developed, a 5-mm 30-degree endoscope is used for the remainder of the procedure. Under direct vision, two 3-mm trocars and one 5-mm trocar are inserted to allow retraction of the thyroid gland, and a two-handed technique is used to dissect the pertinent cervical anatomy (Fig. 42-2). The inferior thyroid artery and recurrent laryngeal nerve are immediately identified and dissected (Fig. 42-3).

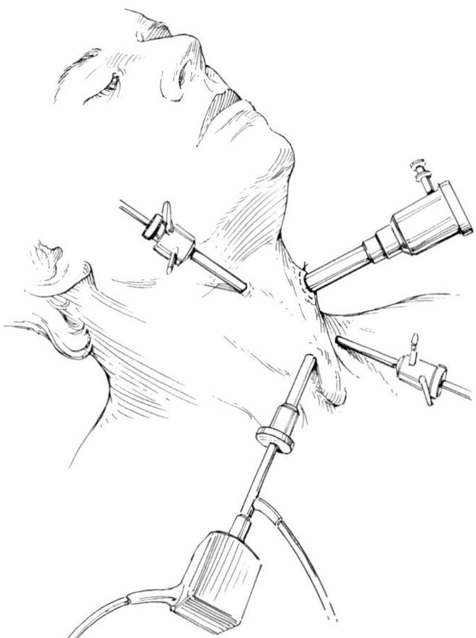

Fig. 42-2. Trocar placement for endoscopic thyroidectomy. (Reprinted with permission from Elsevier Science.)

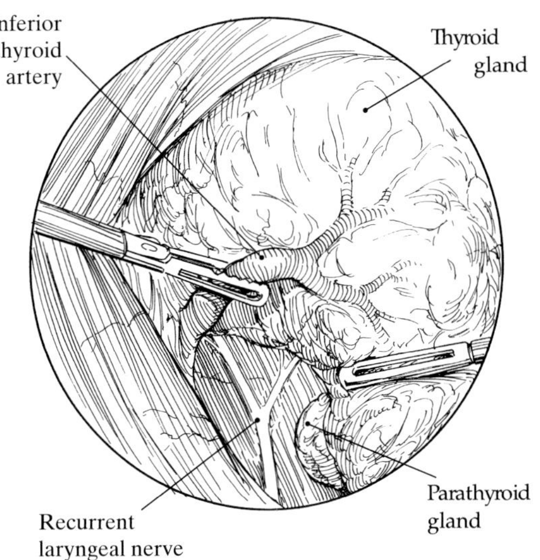

Fig. 42-3. An endoscopic view of the recurrent laryngeal nerve and inferior thyroid artery. (Reprinted with permission from Elsevier Science.)

During endoscopic parathyroidectomy, a focused neck exploration is performed on the basis of the preoperative imaging. For example, if the preoperative imaging has identified a left inferior parathyroid adenoma, the left lower quadrant of the neck is explored. Once the adenoma is visualized, the vascular pedicle is isolated and divided (Fig. 42-4). This can be accomplished with a 5-mm clip applier, endoloops, or ultrasonic coagulating forceps. The adenoma can be removed directly through the 10-mm trocar or by placing it in a small retrieval bag. No attempt is made to identify the ipsilateral parathyroid gland unless there is an inappropriate reduction in intraoperative PTH levels, although this maneuver can be easily accomplished if desired.

When surgeons perform endoscopic thyroidectomy, the inferior thyroid artery is divided with ultrasonic energy, taking great care to carefully preserve the recurrent laryngeal nerve. The inferior and superior parathyroid glands are easily identified and dissected off of the capsule of the thyroid gland. The inferior pole vessels are divided with ultrasonic energy, as is the isthmus of the thyroid gland (Fig. 42-5, page 424). Finally, the ligament of Berry is divided and the specimen is placed in a small bag, which can be made from the thumb of a surgical glove with the suturing of a nylon purse-string

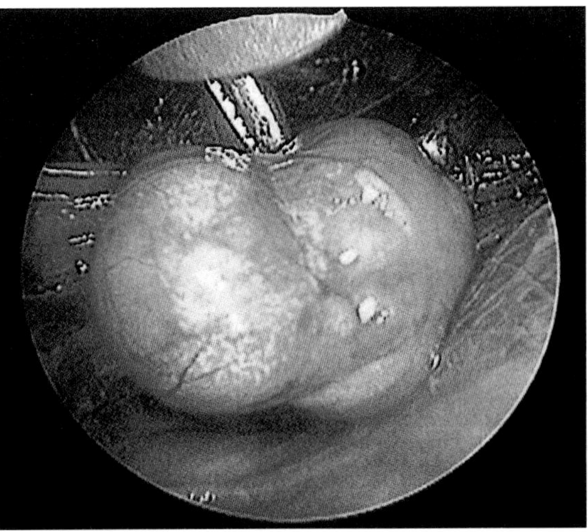

Fig. 42-4. An endoscopic view of a parathyroid adenoma.

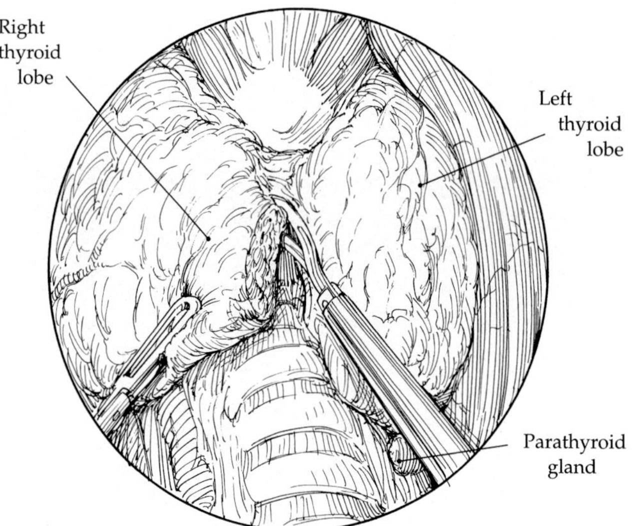

Fig. 42-5. The isthmus of the thyroid can be easily divided with a 5-mm ultrasonic scissor.

VIDEO-ASSISTED CENTRAL APPROACH

Both the thyroid and parathyroid glands are easily approached with this technique. A small 1- to 2-cm incision is made immediately superior to the sternal notch, and the strap muscles are identified and separated at the midline. Small narrow retractors are inserted directly into the incision, allowing retraction of the strap muscles and the carotid sheath laterally and the thyroid gland medially (Fig. 42-7). A 5-mm angled endoscope is inserted directly into the incision. Special spatulated instruments are used to bluntly dissect the pertinent cervical anatomy under video-assisted control. During video-assisted thyroidectomy, the superior pole vessels are ligated with ultrasonic energy, as is the inferior thyroid artery. The thyroid lobe

around the opening. This allows easy retrieval through the initial incision, although often it must be slightly enlarged.

The totally endoscopic cervical approach is the most difficult to master but has the best cosmetic results.

TOTALLY ENDOSCOPIC AXILLARY OR ANTERIOR CHEST WALL APPROACH

The axillary and anterior chest wall endoscopic approaches, which were developed and popularized in Asia, are similar to the cervical approach except that the neck is approached from a remote location (Figs. 42-6A and B). The ipsilateral arm is placed in an abducted position above the head with the elbow flexed. The first incision is placed either in the axilla or on the anterior chest wall. The initial dissection is performed by using blunt dissection with either a blunt instrument or an endoscopic vein dissector. Low-pressure CO_2 insufflation is initiated to a pressure of 4 mmHg through a 10-mm trocar, and additional trocars are inserted. One key difference from the cervical approach is that the axillary or anterior chest wall approach requires the use of a flexible endoscope to allow maximal maneuverability over the clavicle. Moreover, the strap muscles are divided to improve exposure of the thyroid basin, which increases the risk of postoperative bleeding. The remainder of the procedure is identical to that described for the cervical approach.

The axillary or anterior chest wall approach is not widely practiced in the western world.

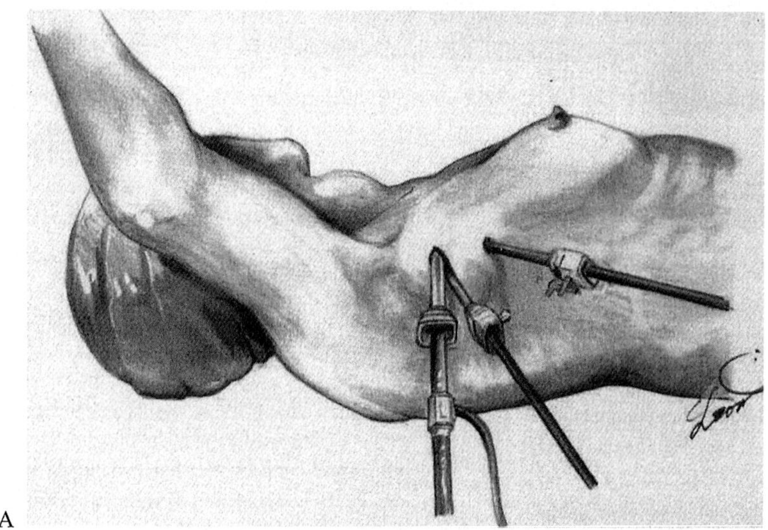
A

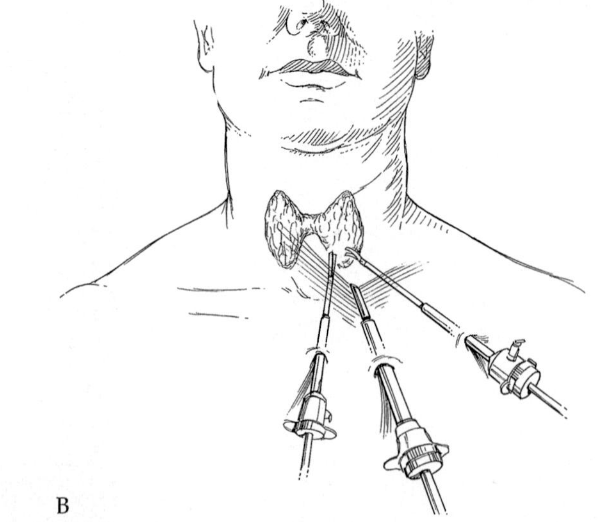
B

Fig. 42-6. A. Axillary approach. **B.** Anterior chest wall approach. (Reprinted with permission from Inabnet WB. Radioguided parathyroidectomy. In: Gagner M, Inabnet WB, eds. *Minimally Invasive Endocrine Surgery*. Philadelphia: Lippincott Williams & Wilkins, 2002:103–110.)

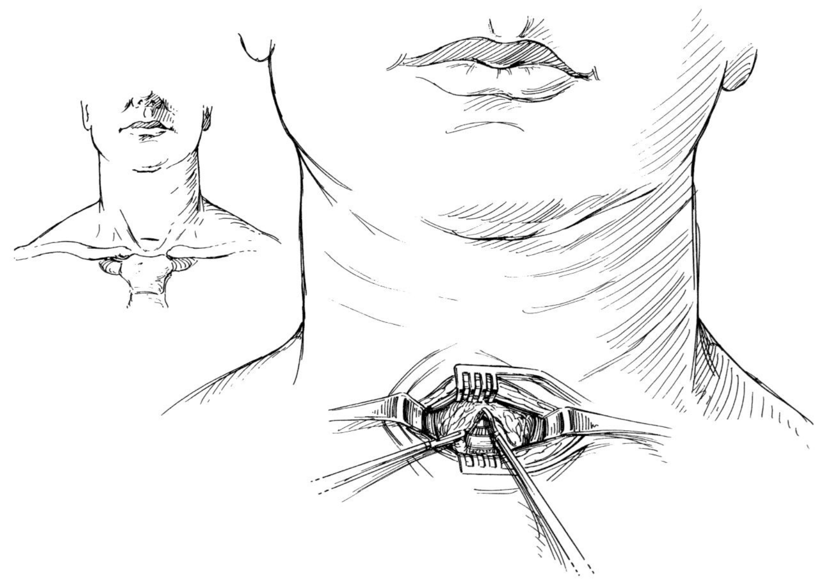

Fig. 42-7. Anterior or "suprasternal" approach using a combination of special retractors and laparoscopic instruments.

is then extracted through the small incision permitting division of the isthmus and ligament of Berry directly through the small incision in a conventional manner.

During video-assisted parathyroidectomy the diseased gland is located and dissected without disrupting the capsule using spatulas. The pedicle of the gland, which is well visualized under optical magnification, is then clipped. The adenoma is then retrieved through the skin incision. All four quadrants of the neck can be explored using this approach.

This approach is the most versatile because the sides of the neck can be explored, total thyroidectomy can be performed, and the procedure can be converted to a conventional operation by extending the incision.

VIDEO-ASSISTED LATERAL APPROACH

The video-assisted lateral approach is a modification of the standard endoscopic approach that has been described for parathyroidectomy and recently for thyroidectomy. The initial incision, which is approximately 1 to 1.5 cm in length, is made at the midportion of the ipsilateral SCM, and the parathyroid basin is entered laterally to the strap muscles by using sharp and blunt dissection. A 10-mm trocar is inserted and secured with a purse-string suture in the subcutaneous tissue. CO_2 is insufflated to a pressure of 10 mmHg and a 10-mm 0-degree scope is used to visualize the operative field. Two 3-mm trocars are inserted along the anterior border of the SCM, one being placed superiorly and the other inferiorly. This approach best allows a unilateral neck exploration to be performed under endoscopic control. The parathyroid adenoma is located and mobilized until the vascular pedicle is isolated. The 10-mm port is then removed, and the vascular pedicle is clipped directly through the small incision, thereby permitting removal of the enlarged gland through the small incision. While waiting for the post-excision PTH levels to be determined, the surgeon can easily identify the remaining ipsilateral gland to rule out the presence of hyperplasia.

During endoscopic thyroidectomy using the lateral approach, the posterior surface of the thyroid gland is completely mobilized and the superior and inferior thyroid vessels are skeletenized but not divided. The recurrent laryngeal nerve is identified and traced along its entire length. The superior and inferior parathyroid glands are identified and preserved. The trocars are removed, the gland is exteriorized, and the superior vascular pedicle is divided with harmonic scalpel followed by the division of the isthmus. The inferior thyroid vessels are divided, and finally the ligament of Berry is divided, and the specimen is removed.

The lateral approach is most suited for posteriorly placed parathyroid adenomas, particularly when the recurrent laryngeal nerve has to be visualized.

VIDEO-ENDOSCOPIC APPROACHES TO ECTOPIC, MEDIASTINAL PARATHYROID GLANDS

Ectopic parathyroid adenomas are estimated to occur in 4% to 20% of patients with primary hyperparathyroidism. Possible sites of ectopic parathyroid location include the parapharyngeal space at the level of the mandible, intrathyroidal, the carotid sheath and the mediastinum. Ectopic inferior parathyroid glands are commonly found in the anterior mediastinum in an intrathymic location, but they can rarely be extrathymic. Mediastinal parathyroid adenomas can also occur rarely in the middle mediastinum in the aortopulmonary window or in the precarinal location. Posterior mediastinal parathyroid adenomas are essentially superior parathyroid adenomas that have descended into the posterior mediastinum, always posterior to the recurrent nerve.

Mediastinal parathyroid adenomas must be well localized prior to surgery in order to determine the best operative approach. Ideally, the lesion should be visualized and/or located on two different tests, which most commonly include sestamibi scanning, CT scanning with 2.5-mm cuts, MRI, and/or selective venous sampling (SVS) for PTH. If the parathyroid adenoma is not visualized on CT or MRI, SVS is an excellent confirmatory localizing study. Most patients who undergo mediastinal exploration for parathyroid adenoma do so after failed neck exploration. However, due to the increasingly frequent use of sestamibi scanning in patients with primary hyperparathyroidism, patients who are found to have a mediastinal parathyroid adenoma are now undergoing direct mediastinal exploration without neck exploration.

Videoendoscopic exploration of the mediastinum is most commonly performed via thoracoscopy, but video-assisted cervical approaches have been described for lesions located in the anterior mediastinum. Flexible laryngoscopy is performed to rule out vocal cord injury in patients with prior neck exploration. The thoracoscopic approach is performed under general anesthesia using a double-lumen endotracheal tube to ventilate the opposite lung. The patient is placed in a full lateral position (Fig. 42-8, page 426). Three trocars are utilized: a 10-mm trocar placed in the third interspace in the midaxillary line for the camera and two 5-mm trocars in the fifth or sixth interspace. A fourth 5-mm trocar may be utilized for lung retraction. The

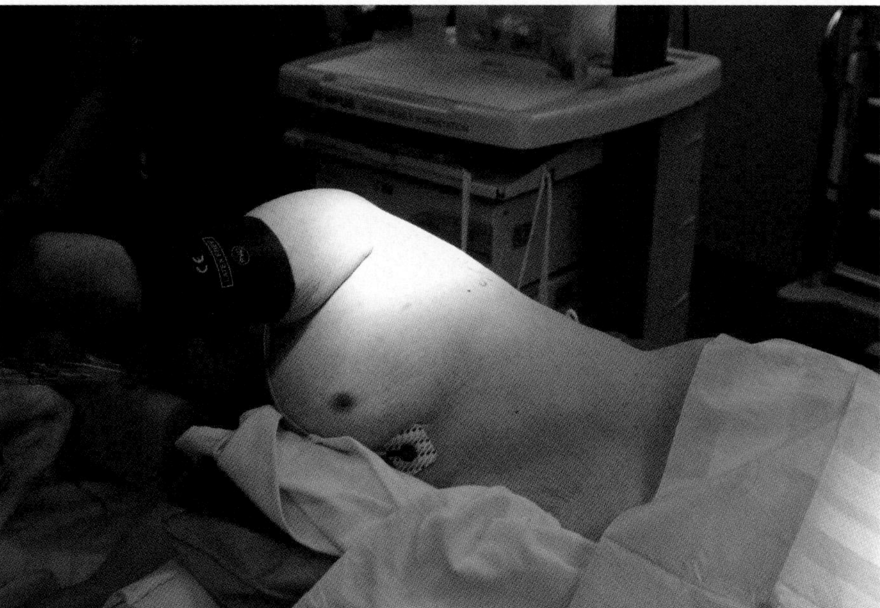

Fig. 42-8. Patient positioning for left thoracoscopic parathyroidectomy.

procedure is begun by identifying the vagus and phrenic nerves, both of which are preserved. The pleura is incised anterior to the phrenic nerve to permit exposure of the thymus. Dissection is performed with the harmonic scalpel, LigaSure Vessel Healing System (Valleylab; Boulder, CO), or hook cautery. For intrathymic lesions, the thymus is excised en bloc, but for lesions in the aortopulmonary window the adenoma is excised after incising the overlying pleura (Fig. 42-9). In either case, the specimen is first placed in a retrieval sac and then extracted through the 10-mm trocar site to prevent accidental spillage of parathyroid tissue. Intraoperative PTH levels are monitored to confirm excision of all hyperfunctioning parathyroid tissue. A small chest tube is left in place and removed after one day. Patients are usually discharged on postoperative day 1.

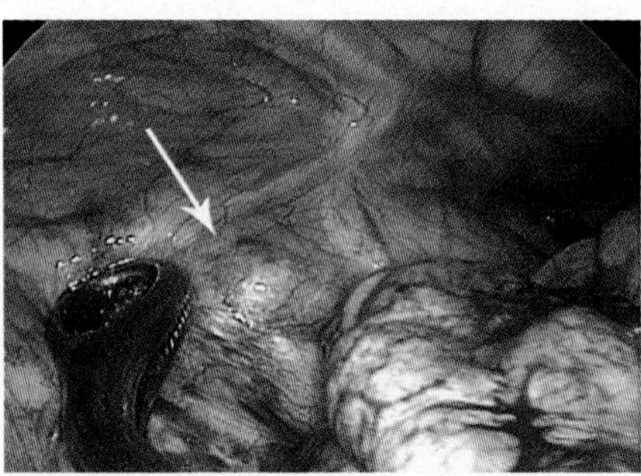

Fig. 42-9. A thoracoscopic view of the parathyroid adenoma overlying the aortic arch.

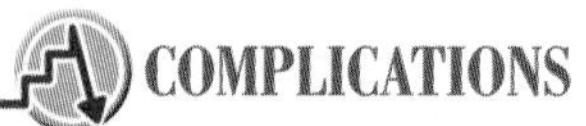

COMPLICATIONS

All of the endoscopic approaches to the thyroid and parathyroid glands have been shown to be safe, feasible, and efficacious. The incidence of recurrent laryngeal nerve injury ranges from 1% to 2%. Great care must be taken to avoid applying ultrasonic energy too close to the recurrent laryngeal nerve; one case of a permanent palsy has been reported from collateral energy transmission. With the cervical endoscopic approach, subcutaneous emphysema is common in the postoperative period; however, this always resolved within 8 to 12 hours and is of no clinical significance. Hypercarbia has been reported, but this complication is rare if the insufflating pressures are maintained less than 12 mmHg and the duration of surgery is shortened. Only minor complications have been reported after thoracoscopic excision of mediastinal adenomas.

CONCLUSION

There is a definite role for endoscopic techniques in thyroid and parathyroid surgery. The main advantages of endoscopic approaches when compared to the conventional approach are better cosmetic results, superior magnification and illumination of the operative field, and less postoperative pain. The major disadvantages are a need for specialized equipment (more expense) and the need for general anesthesia. Endocrine surgeons should be facile in each technique so that the operative approach can be individualized. Surgeons who perform endoscopic neck surgery should begin with parathyroidectomy before attempting endoscopic thyroidectomy.

SUGGESTED READING

Gagner M. Endoscopic subtotal parathyroidectomy in patients with primary hyperparathyroidism. *Br J Surg* 1996;83:875.

Gagner M, Inabnet WB. Endoscopic thyroidectomy for solitary thyroid nodules. *Thyroid* 2001;11:161–163.

Haber RS. Ultrasound-guided fine-needle aspiration of thyroid nodules. *Endocr Pract* 2002; 8:5–9.

Inabnet WB, Gagner M. How I do it: endoscopic thyroidectomy. *J Otolaryng* 2001; 30:1–2.

Inabnet WB, Rogula T, Gagner M. The safety and efficacy of alternative energy sources in endoscopic thyroidectomy. *Surg Endosc* 2003; 17:S304.

Kido T, Hazama K, Inoue Y, et al. Resection of anterior mediastinal masses through an infrasternal approach: *Ann Thorac Surg* 1999; 67:263–265.

Lombardi CP, Raffaelli M, Princi P, et al. Minimally invasive video-assisted functional lateral neck dissection for metastatic papillary thyroid carcinoma. *Am J Surg* 2007 Jan;193(1): 114–118.

Lombardi CP, Raffaelli M, Princi P, et al. Video-assisted thyroidectomy: report on the experience of a single center in more than four hundred cases. *World J Surg* 2006 May;30(5): 794–800.

Medrano C, Hazelrigg SR, Landreneau RJ, et al. Thoracoscopic resection of ectopic parathyroid glands. *Ann Thorac Surg* 2000;69:221–223.

Miccoli P, Bellantone R, Mourad M, et al. Minimally invasive video-assisted thyroidectomy: multiinstitutional experience. *World J Surg* 2002;26:972–975.

Miccoli P, Elisei R, Donatini G, et al. Video-assisted central compartment lymphadenectomy in a patient with a positive RET oncogene: initial experience. *Surg Endosc* 2007 Jan; 21(1):120–123.

Pasieka JL, Parsons LL, Demeure MJ, et al. Patient-based surgical outcome tool demonstrating alleviation of symptoms following parathyroidectomy in patients with primary hyperparathyroidism. *World J Surg* 2002;26: 942–949.

Sebag F, Palazzo FF, Harding J, et al. Endoscopic lateral approach thyroid lobectomy: safe evolution from endoscopic parathyroidectomy. *World J Surg* 2006 May;30(5):802–805.

Tibblin S, Bondeson AG, Ljungberg O. Unilateral parathyroidectomy in hyperparathyroidism due to a single adenoma. *Ann Surg* 1982;195:245–252.

Vestergaard P, Mollerup CL, Frokjaer VG, et al. Cardiovascular events before and after surgery for primary hyperparathyroidism. *World J Surg* 2003;27:216–222.

COMMENTARY

Endoscopic thyroid and parathyroid surgery are currently performed by relatively few laparoscopic surgeons. However, many endocrine surgeons who have not mastered these techniques have seen a decrease in their volume of patients. Not every patient with thyroid disease or parathyroid surgical conditions will be an optimal candidate for endoscopic surgery. Many patients, however, seek out surgeons who can and will offer the least invasive option when appropriate.

The authors provide the reader with multiple approaches and an overview of patient preparation for endoscopic thyroid and parathyroid surgery. This chapter is presented in a manner that will also be extremely helpful to the surgical trainee who has limited or no experience in these techniques.

The advances in patient care from a minimally invasive approach are rarely as dramatic as was witnessed with the introduction of laparoscopic cholecystectomy. Many could view endoscopic surgery in the neck as an approach that provides minimal advances or advantages over an open approach. There is validity to such an argument, but not without reasonable counter arguments. Advances that provide enhanced visualization, better light in the surgical field, enhanced differentiation of structures in close proximity, and improved cosmesis should be given careful consideration before being dismissed. The group of surgeons now emerging from training have been immersed in minimally invasive techniques and are well prepared to adapt to these types of procedures and are likely to improve upon these early advances.

WSE

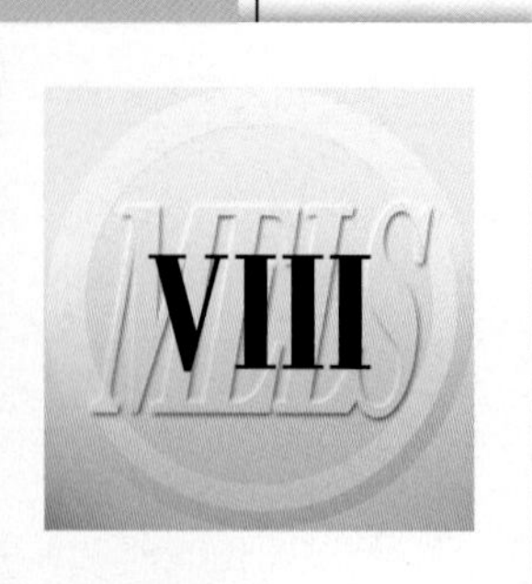

Diseases of the Small and Large Bowel

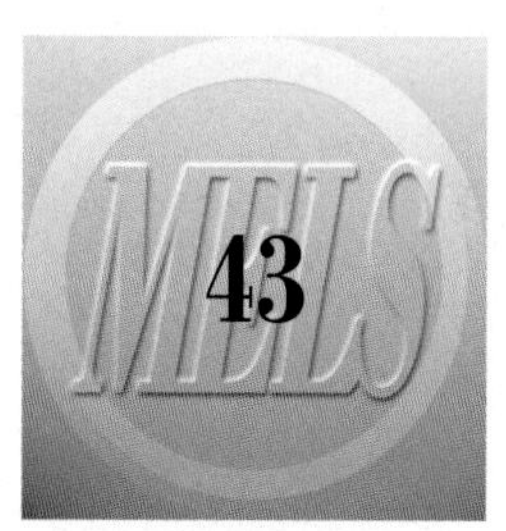

The Endoscopic Diagnosis of Small Intestinal Diseases

AMR M. EL SHERIF AND CHARLES J. FILIPI

INTRODUCTION

For many decades, there has been a need to study the small intestine for a variety of diseases. The small bowel has been, however, the most difficult portion of the gastrointestinal tract to evaluate due to its length, location, redundancy, and complexity of loops. With advances in technology, different modalities have become available for the diagnosis of small intestine pathologies. The barium small bowel follow-through (SBFT), enteroclysis studies, and computed tomography (CT) scanning with contrast are most commonly used. These techniques involve infusion of contrast medium into the small bowel and static intermittent radiological imaging. Precise radiological documentation and careful interpretation are essential steps in obtaining a reliable examination.

Unfortunately, no gold standard technique for the diagnosis of small intestinal disease has been established. An ideal test would require no more than moderate sedation, allow proper visualization of the entire small intestine, and make it possible to obtain biopsies and to perform therapeutic interventions.

Endoscopy has played an important role in the diagnosis and treatment of many alimentary tract diseases. New endoscopic techniques, endoscopes, wireless capsule cameras, and better quality video processors have improved direct visualization and biopsy capability as they have led to more aggressive therapeutic procedures. In this review we describe new endoscopic modalities that more effectively achieve the diagnostic accuracy and interventional capabilities required.

Techniques of Endoscopy

VIDEO CAPSULE ENDOSCOPY

The first commercially available video capsule endoscope was developed by Dr. Paul Swain in collaboration with Given Imaging, Ltd (Yoqneam, Israel). It was introduced in Europe in 2001 and subsequently approved for use in the U.S. by the Food and Drug Administration in 2002. To date, this technology has been used in more than 50,000 patients. Several studies comparing the diagnostic yield of video capsule endoscopy (VCE) to the other traditional methods of small bowel investigation showed that VCE had a diagnostic yield of 83% vs. 41% for small bowel series and 85% vs. 53% for push enteroscopy.

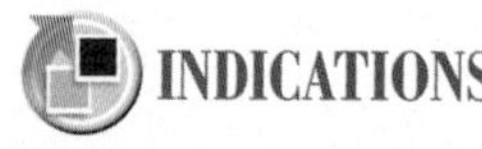

INDICATIONS

Gastrointestinal Bleeding

The primary indication for VCE is obscure gastrointestinal bleeding (OGIB) after a negative upper and lower endoscopy. Obscure gastrointestinal bleeding usually is the result of arteriovenous malformation, angiodysplasia, telangiectasia, or ulcerations. The diagnostic yield for this condition with VCE is 55% to 70%; if applied to those who have active bleeding, it may be as high as 92%. Sachdev et al. demonstrated in a recent study that VCE can be effectively used to investigate nonhematemesis acute gastrointestinal bleeding in the emergency room setting. They found that VCE halved the time needed to establish a diagnosis and that its diagnostic yield was higher (54%) as compared to esophagogastroduodenoscopy (11%).

Crohn Disease

Video capsule endoscopy is helpful in the diagnosis of suspected Crohn disease, especially in patients who present with atypical symptoms and nonspecific findings on conventional imaging. Video capsule endoscopy has the ability to visualize aphthoid ulcers and other superficial ulcers up to only 0.1 cm in diameter. The International Conference for Capsule Endoscopy (ICCE) held in 2005 approved the use of VCE for Crohn disease.

Indeterminate Colitis

Video capsule endoscopy can also be used for indeterminate colitis (colitis in which the distinction between ulcerative colitis and Crohn disease is difficult both pathologically and clinically), as effective management is dependent on an accurate diagnosis. Lo et al. and Mow et al. have demonstrated in two separate studies utilizing VCE that 33% to 49% of patients with indeterminate colitis have small bowel ulcerations, indicating they have Crohn disease.

Small Intestinal Neoplasms

Video capsule endoscopy is superior to other methods in assessing tumors such as carcinoids or gastrointestinal stromal tumors. Video capsule endoscopy is able to detect these lesions earlier, thus making it possible to cure such lesions by early removal. However, VCE has a limited capacity to detect the size of large tumors because they may be only partially visualized. It can also be difficult to assess submucosal tumors that have an intact mucosal covering.

Celiac Disease

This disorder is the result of a hypersensitivity reaction to gluten in genetically susceptible patients. The prevalence of celiac disease among the general population of North America and Western Europe ranges between 0.5% and 1.26%. Preliminary studies have shown that VCE can replace conventional upper endoscopy in patients with serologically positive disease. Confirmation of villous atrophy is the hallmark of this condition, although indeterminate cases still require biopsy to make the diagnosis.

Abdominal Pain

The use of VCE in acute abdominal pain is controversial. In a recent study Carey et al. showed that when VCE was used as a diagnostic tool, only one case was proven to have pain due to an organic cause. Barden et al. demonstrated no significant abnormalities when VCE was used in 20 patients with chronic abdominal pain.

Inherited Polyposis Syndrome

Video capsule endoscopy can be used as a surveillance tool for small bowel polyps in patients with the inherited familial polyposis syndrome. The procedure has a diagnostic yield of 90% and is able to detect various size polyps. This allows early management and possibly a better patient outcome.

Additional Indications

Video capsule endoscopy has been described for surveillance in patients with small bowel transplantation to detect graft rejection, for gastrointestinal disorders due to graft versus host reaction in bone marrow transplant patients, for the diagnosis of radiation enteritis, for the detection of small intestinal hypertensive enteropathy, for small intestine varices in portal hypertensive patients, and for the surveillance of drug-induced injury. For instance, Graham et al. demonstrated that nonsteroidal anti-inflammatory drugs (NSAIDs) are associated with small bowel lesions as evidenced by erythema, erosions, ulcerations, and stricture formation in 71% of long-term users.

CONTRAINDICATIONS

Patients with implanted cardiac pacemakers and defibrillators are often excluded. The initial concern was that signals produced by the VCE might alter heart device functionality. However, subsequent studies have shown that VCE can be used safely in cardiac patients dependent on cardiac electrical aide devices. In patients with swallowing problems, particularly those with obstructing esophageal pathology, the capsule can still sometimes be introduced into the duodenum using a special delivery device. Video capsule endoscopy avoidance during pregnancy has no supportive literature but remains a relative contraindication. See Table 43-1 for other contraindications.

TABLE 43-1. EXCLUSION CRITERIA FOR SMALL BOWEL CAPSULE ENDOSCOPY

- Demented patients
- Patients with known small bowel obstruction or strictures
- Pregnant women
- Children under 10 years of age
- Patients with cardiac defibrillators and pacemakers
- Patients with esophageal strictures, diverticula, motility disorders
- Patients who have undergone gastric bypass surgery
- Patients who would be scheduled for magnetic resonance imaging before the excretion of the capsule

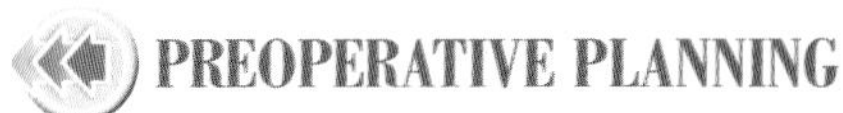

PREOPERATIVE PLANNING

Preparation

The need for small bowel preparation before VCE is controversial. The International Conference on Capsule Endoscopy 2005 consensus panel could not recommend a particular bowel preparation. The simplest approach is for the patient to fast for 12 hours before the procedure. Some investigators have suggested the use of laxatives, purgatives, prokinetics, and even simethicone to remove air bubbles, based on studies that support their use. The patient is allowed to drink clear liquids 2 hours after swallowing the VCE capsule and can have a light meal after another 2 hours.

Equipment

The VCE system has four main components: the capsule, eight sensors similar to electrocardiographic leads pasted to the patient's abdomen, a data recorder worn on the patient's belt, and a computer workstation (Fig. 43-1, page 430). The PillCam SB video capsule endoscope (Given Imaging, Ltd.; Yoqneam, Israel) is a wireless capsule measuring 11 mm by 27 mm (Fig. 43-2, page 430) composed of a light source (six illuminating light-emitting diodes), a lens, a complementary metal oxide

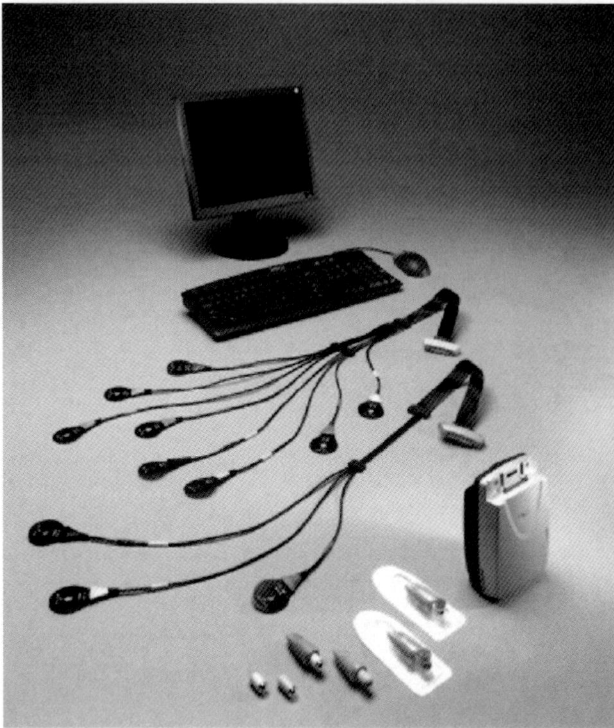

Fig. 43-1. The paraphernalia necessary for video capsule endoscopy.

semiconductor imager, two batteries, a wireless transmitter, and an antenna. The capsule has a lubricious coating that allows easy ingestion and grants steady flow by propulsive peristalsis of the gastrointestinal tract. The batteries provide 8 hours of working time, during which the capsule photographs two images per second (a total of 50,000 to 60,000 images) in a 140-degree field of view with a magnification power of 8:1. This generates approximately 600 Mb of data, which is transmitted through eight sensors to the recording system fixed at the side of the patient (Fig. 43-3). The data is then downloaded on a computer work station for interpretation by special software that can display the images as a video film. The downloading of data initially took 3 hours but now has been reduced to 30 minutes. The video film can be viewed in a variety of ways, ranging from display of single and sequential images to showing several images simultaneously. Relevant images can be selected, including key landmarks such as the first image of the duodenum and the cecum (Fig. 43-4, page 432). Additional complementary software includes localization capability (which has proved to be somewhat disappointing) and a "suspected blood indicator," which marks appropriate images for interrogation by automatically detecting areas of red color and has been helpful with a sensitivity of 37% and 81% and a positive predictive value of 50% and 81% for active bleeding.

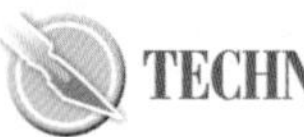

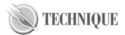

TECHNIQUE

After fasting for 12 hours, the patient has the eight sensors attached to the abdomen with the data recorder attached to the patient's belt. The capsule is ingested with water, after which it starts transmission of images to the recorder through the sensor array. There is some evidence that placing the patient in the right lateral decubitus position for 1 hour after ingestion will decrease the gastric transit time. During the remainder of the procedure the patient is free to carry out normal daily activities. Eight hours later the sensors and the recorder are removed from the patient, and the data is downloaded to a computer workstation. The disposable capsule eventually passes per rectum and is not recovered.

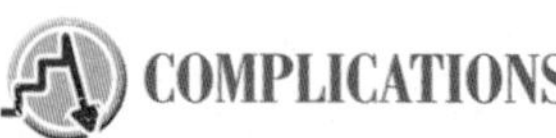

COMPLICATIONS

Video capsule endoscopy is a safe technique, with over 200,000 capsules used worldwide. There have been no reported deaths. Abnormal capsule retention, defined as prolonged presence of the capsule in the small bowel, has a reported rate of up to 0.75% in over 10,000 endoscopic procedures. Retention can sometimes lead to symptomatic obstruction. The incidence of retention depends on the indication. Patients with OGIB have a retention incidence of 5%, while in those with suspected Crohn disease the incidence is 1.4%. The incidence of retention in patients with confirmed Crohn disease may reach up to 8%. Once retention is confirmed, intervention should be performed using either open surgery or small intestine endoscopy.

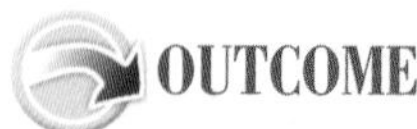

OUTCOMES

Video capsule endoscopy has proven to be an effective, noninvasive diagnostic tool for investigation of the small intestine. Pennazio et al. reported to have used VCE to examine the entire length of the small bowel in 79% of patients. The diagnostic yield of VCE is high and has been shown to be superior to both enteroclysis and standard push endoscopy. Data from several preliminary studies suggest that VCE has a 25% to 87% impact in clinical decision making. The major disadvantage of the procedure is the inability to obtain histopathology and to perform therapeutic maneuvers. Video capsule endoscopy is in its infancy: new indications, new devices, and new interpretation software are anticipated in the coming years.

ENTEROSCOPY

Endoscopy plays an essential role in the diagnosis and management of diseases of the esophagus, stomach, duodenum, and large intestine. However, the satisfactory diagnosis and treatment of small intestinal disease has been suboptimal as a result of difficulty introducing the endoscope completely, from the mouth to the cecum. Enteroscopy that refers to evaluation of the distal duodenum, the jejunum, and ileum was initially a concept without adequate technology. With the development of video processing technology and magnification, a better image quality of the small intestine became available. Enteroscopy has the advantage of directability and of allowing biopsies and therapeutic interventions.

Push Enteroscopy

Push enteroscopy (PE) is the most commonly used method of examination of the proximal small intestine. This

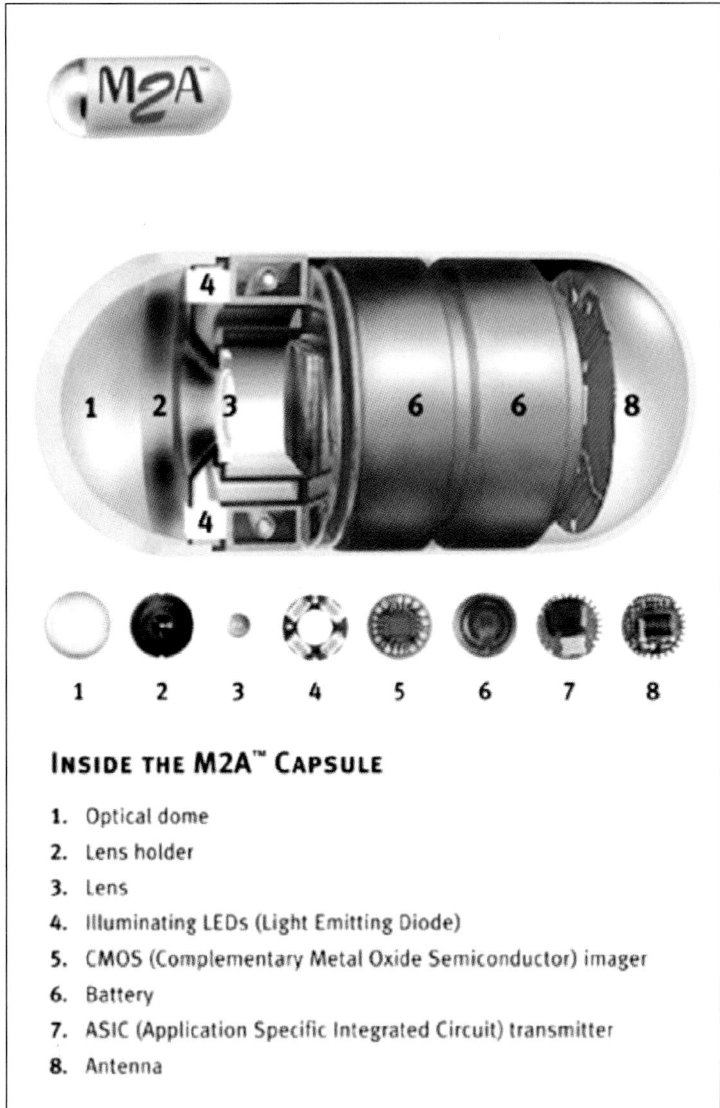

Fig. 43-2. The video capsule endoscope is an intricate device with many components, as shown.

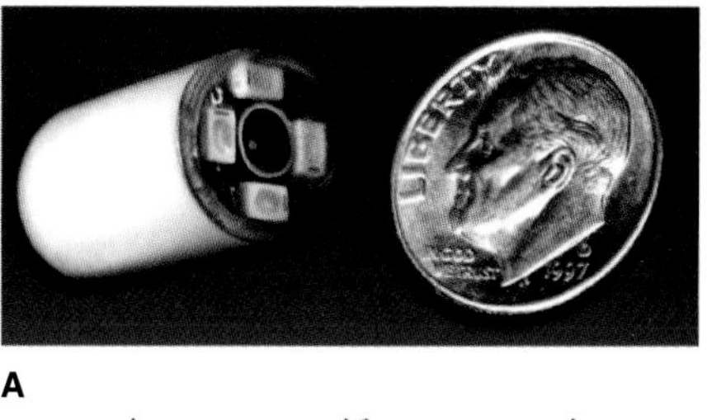

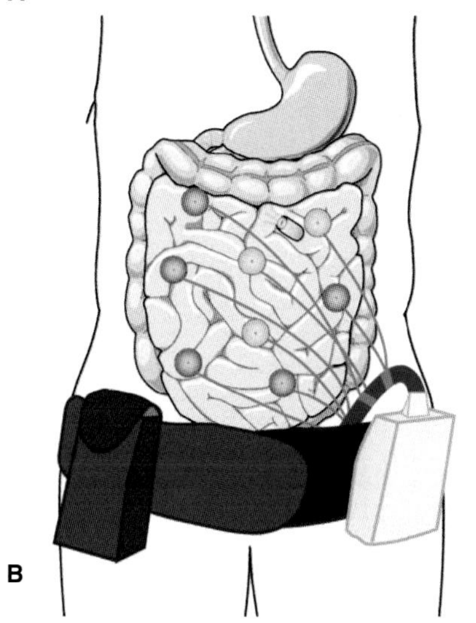

Fig. 43-3. A. The size of the endoscopy capsule relative to a dime. **B.** The diagram shows the sensors attached to the abdomen and the recorder and battery attached to a belt.

procedure represents an extension of esophagogastroduodenoscopy in which the endoscope is pushed beyond the ligament of Treitz. Push enteroscopy can be performed in ambulatory patients but is best done using CO_2 as the insufflation gas.

INDICATIONS

Common Indications

The most common indication for PE is OGIB. Push enteroscopy has a diagnostic yield that ranges from 38% to 75% (Table 43-2, page 432). Push enteroscopy allows therapeutic intervention in the form of polypectomy for familial polyposis and biopsies for chronic diarrhea and malabsorption.

Other Indications

Pennazio et al. reported the use of PE in 72 patients. Of these patients, 12 had intestinal neoplasms and two were studied as a follow-up to lymphoma chemotherapy. Davies et al. reported the use of PE for the diagnosis of iron deficiency anemia in seven patients on NSAIDs. They also reported therapeutic percutaneous endoscopic jejunostomy in 15 patients, polypectomy in patients with Peutz-Jeghers syndrome, placement of nasojejunal feeding tubes, dilation of strictures, and cautery for angiodysplasias. Foutch et al. were able to control bleeding in eight of eleven patients who underwent fulguration of angiodysplasias. Gowen used a pediatric colonoscope placed transorally for the insertion of a specialized long (9-ft) tube into the jejunum for decompression in 23 small bowel obstruction patients. The procedure achieved rapid resolution of intestinal obstruction in 90% of the cases.

Equipment

The Olympus SIF-B fiber-optic push endoscope was first used by Ogoshi et al. in 1973. The instrument was 162 cm in length and had a 1-cm outer diameter. With fluoroscopy, the instrument had an estimated introduction length of 30 cm beyond the ligament of Treitz. Further development of the PE lead to longer enteroscopes, ranging from 200 to 300 cm in working length. Although deep intubation can be achieved by this instrument, some investigators use it with an overtube (also known as stiffening tube) first described by Shimizu et al. in 1987. The course of PE changed in 1983 when Parker and Agayoff reported the use of a colonoscope for enteroscopy. Like PE, colonoscopes provide four-way directional tip deflection (up to 160 to 180 degrees in one direction), which makes

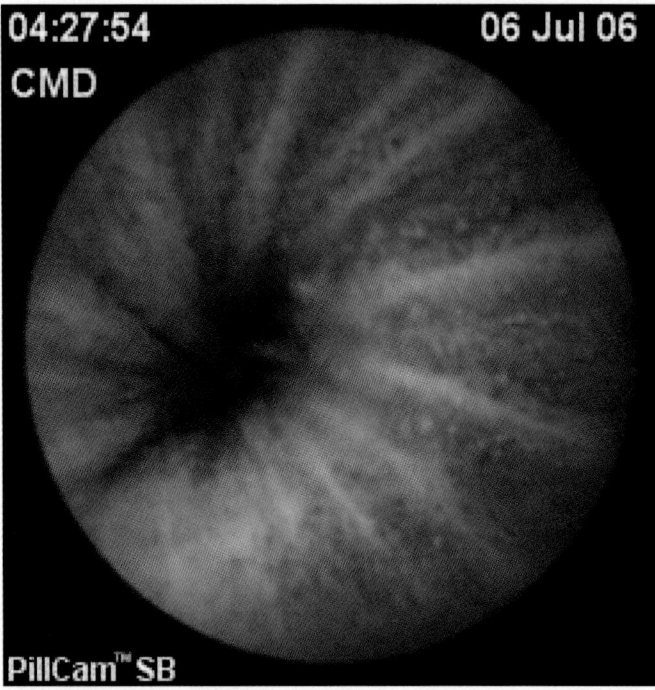

Fig. 43-4. A. The endoscopic capsule camera allows a well-illuminated view of the small bowel. **B.** The capsule has sufficient resolution to document fine detail of the mucosa.

them ideal for enteroscopy. Pediatric colonoscopes are now routinely used for PE. Cleaning was initially an issue, as it was believed that a colonoscope should not be passed per os (by the mouth) despite routine cleaning.

Overtubes are semiflexible tubes that assist in insertion, by limiting intragastric and intraduodenal looping, thus facilitating deeper jejunal intubation (up to 120 cm beyond the ligament of Treitz). Overtubes may have metal bands at intervals to assist in fluoroscopic localization. Overtubes range from 11 to 15 mm in diameter and they are 60 to 100 cm in length. Some overtubes have a Goretex 10-cm tip, which is soft and pliable and decreases the chance of mucosal injury while the overtube is being advanced over the enteroscope. More recently, overtubes called ShapeLock (USGI Medical; San Clemente, CA) have been developed that are flexible during insertion but can be "rigidized" once past the ligament of Treitz (Fig. 43-5).

New Pentax enteroscopes (Pentax Optical Co.; Tokyo, Japan) are available for use without an overtube, thus preventing overtube complications. Instead, these enteroscopes feature a polyurethrane coating, which has been applied homogeneously on the surface of the working shaft. Concomitantly, there is a continuous change in the components of the endoscope shaft such that there is a gradual increase in distal-to-proximal stiffness.

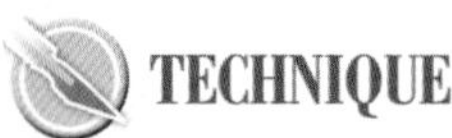

TECHNIQUE

With the patient under conscious sedation and lying in the left lateral decubitus position or a semiprone position, the enteroscope is passed transorally in a similar fashion to standard esophagogastroduodenoscopy. A complete examination of the esophagus and stomach is completed before the enteroscope is introduced into the duodenum. The patient may feel discomfort during advancement of the instrument as it distends the greater curvature of the stomach. Paradoxical or arrested tip motion can be noted if the instrument loops within the fundus. The ligament of Treitz is usually encountered 80 to 100 cm from the incisors and always requires extreme deflection of the tip to localize the lumen. Then the enteroscope is actively advanced into the small intestine with alternating push-pull movements and the hooking of the enteroscope on the bowel with withdrawal to pleat the small intestine. The enteroscope's recurrent tendency is to coil into concentric loops, the mesenteric attachments of the intestine representing fixed points around which the enteroscope coils. The large gastric reservoir represents another contributing factor to coil formation as the enteroscope naturally loops against the greater curvature. Changing patient positioning and palpating the abdomen are maneuvers that can be used to facilitate deeper intubation. In conjunction, or for known distal disease, a colonoscope can be introduced transanally until it reaches the cecum and then advanced across the ileocecal valve to examine the ileum (a retrograde examination). A full bowel preparation is required for this.

An overtube is commonly used to minimize intragastric loop formation. The well-lubricated overtube is backloaded over the working shaft of the enteroscope prior to intubation. When the enteroscope is within the jejunum, the overtube is advanced until the distal tip rests within the second portion of the duodenum (for the 60-cm overtube) or at or beyond the ligament of Treitz (for the 100-cm overtube). Fluoroscopy can be used during the procedure to localize the position of the overtube, to detect the best location for abdominal pressure to minimize looping, and to determine the depth of intubation on reaching the point of maximal insertion (Fig. 43-6). Whether the overtube is used or not, the wall of the small bowel is examined first upon intubation and later upon withdrawal of the enteroscope. Biopsies and other therapeutic intervention can be achieved using a variety of devices such as snares, laser probes, and bipolar forceps. Glucagon may be used to decrease peristaltic movements. Patients typically tolerate the procedure well and can be discharged on the same day.

TABLE 43-2. DIAGNOSTIC YIELD OF PUSH ENTEROSCOPY FOR OGIB

Author	Number of patients	Diagnostic yield
Rossini 1996	61	25/61 (41%)
Schmit 1996	83	49/83 (59%)
Barkin 1992	28	21/28 (75%)
Fouch 1990	39	15/39 (38%)

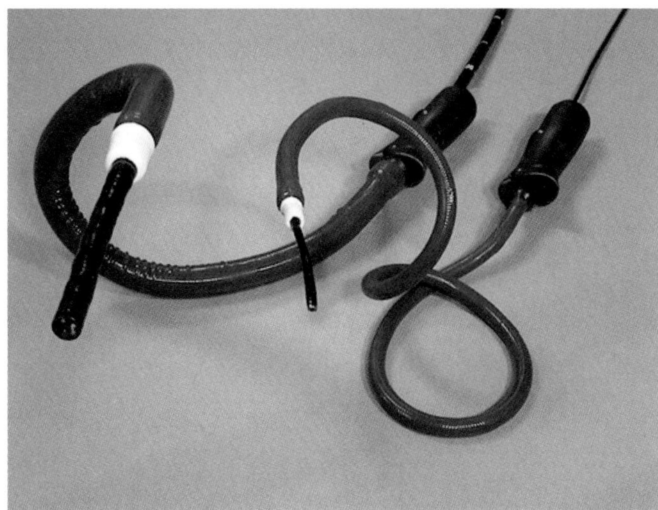

Fig. 43-5. The ShapeLock device is a stiffening overtube designed to enable transcolonic or transgastric enteroscopy.

Several methods of enteroscopy that involve patients swallowing their own GI peristalsis to propel the scope into the distal small bowel, such as the ropeway enteroscopy described by Classen et al. in 1972 and the Sonde enteroscopy described by Tada et al, have been largely abandoned due to the complexity of the technique, patient discomfort, and the long time needed to complete a procedure.

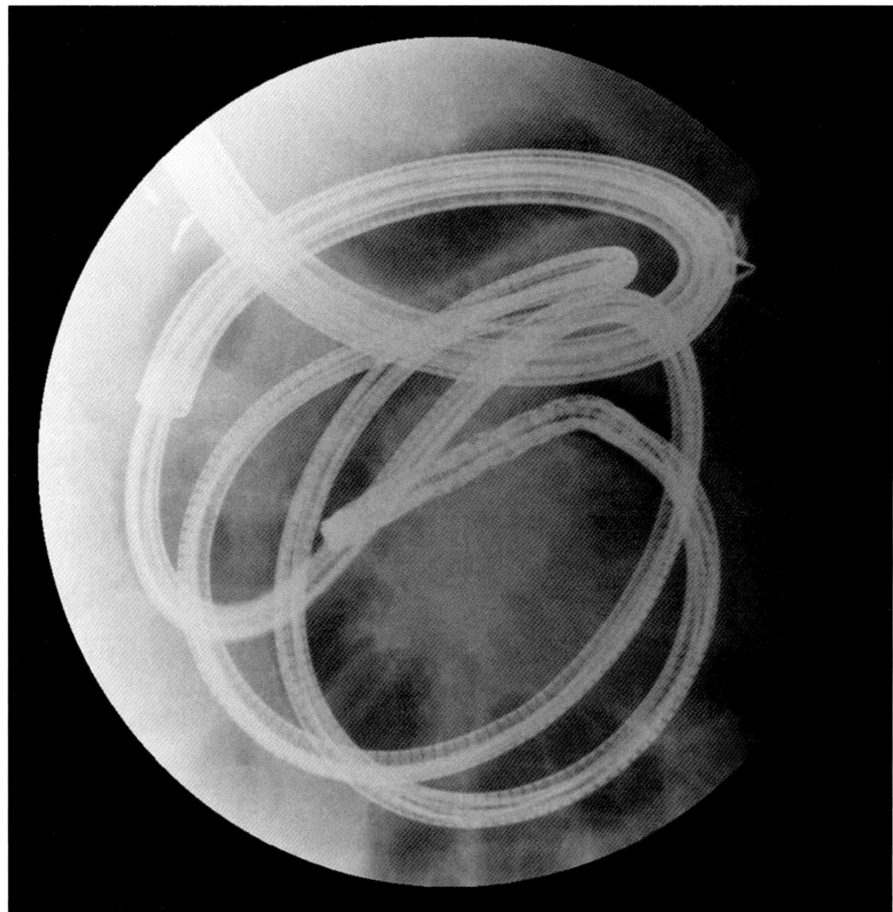

Fig. 43-6. Fluoroscopy is useful when performing push enteroscopy in order to observe the formation and elimination of loops.

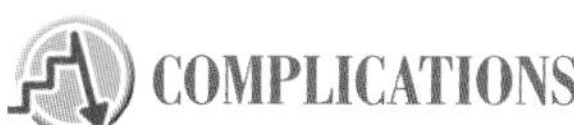

COMPLICATIONS

Complications are uncommon with enteroscopy. Extreme patient discomfort was reported by Barkin et al. in 34% of patients who were examined using an overtube. Patients do need to be heavily sedated, and propofol is a good adjunct to enteroscopy. Mallory-Weiss tears and pancreatitis, have been reported, most probably due to papillary trauma. Overtubes have also been associated with complications, including pharyngeal tears, duodenal perforation, cases of gastric mucosal stripping during advancement of the overtube, due to entrapment of the tissue between the overtube orifice and the enteroscope, and rare cases of small bowel perforation

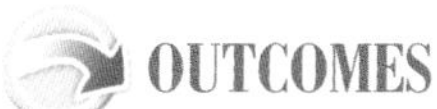

OUTCOMES

The technical success of PE is determined by the depth of intubation beyond the ligament of Treitz. Most studies confirm that PE facilitates the examination of 40 to 150 cm of the small intestine. Push enteroscopy rarely allows an entire small bowel examination; however, the diagnostic yield of PE ranges between 47% and 72% for all the conditions in which for is used. In OGIB patients, PE has a diagnostic yield of 17% to 89%.

DOUBLE-BALLOON ENDOSCOPY

In 2001, Yamamoto et al. developed an endoscopic diagnostic technique with higher insertability and maneuverability, a double-balloon method that was capable of observing the entire length of the small bowel. A dedicated double-balloon endoscopy system became available commercially in November of 2003.

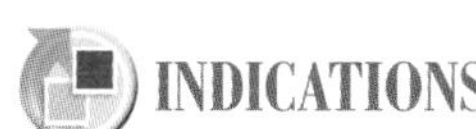

INDICATIONS

Diagnosis

In Yamamoto's study of 178 cases, sources of bleeding for OGIB were identified in 76% of patients. This diagnostic yield is comparable to that of VCE, which ranges from 30% to 80%. In the same study, small intestinal tumors were detected in 17 patients. Sun et al. studied the diagnostic yield and therapeutic impact of double-balloon endoscopy in a large cohort of patients (n = 152) with OGIB and were able to identify the source of bleeding in 75.7% of cases. They also reported the use of double-balloon endoscopy in suspected cases of Crohn and celiac disease. Nishimura et al. reported the use of double-balloon endoscopy for the diagnosis of gastrointestinal stromal tumors, while Yoshida et al. were able to diagnose ileal mucosal ulcers secondary to lymphoma. Miyata et al. used double-balloon endoscopy to perform selective-contrast enhanced X-ray examinations of the intestine by occluding the lumen of the intestine proximal to the lesion to prevent reflux of contrast medium.

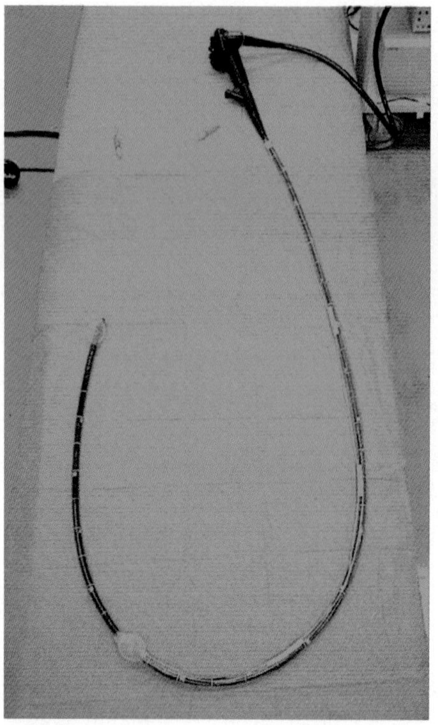

A

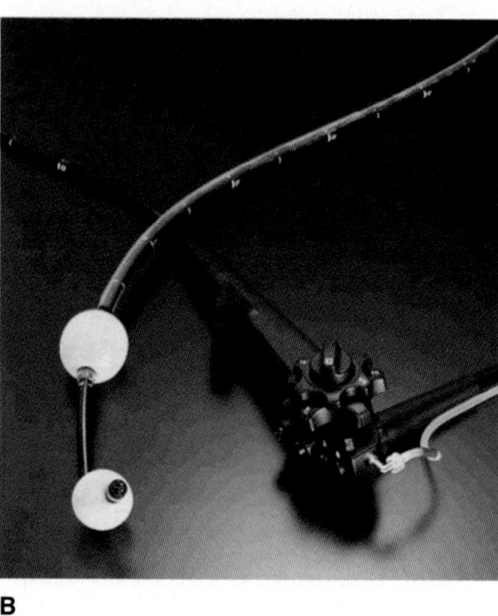

B

Fig. 43-7. A double-balloon Fujinon endoscope: A soft latex balloon is attached at the tip of the endoscope, and a soft overtube with a distal balloon is loaded onto the endoscope.

Therapeutic Intervention

Double-balloon endoscopy can also be used for endoscopic treatment of the small intestine. Yamamoto et al. were able to successfully perform therapeutic interventions, including hemostasis (n = 12), polypectomy (n = 1), endoscopic mucosal resection (n = 1), balloon dilation (n = 6), and stent placement (n = 2). Ohmiya et al. used a double-balloon endoscopic technique to perform polypectomy along the entire length of the small intestine in patients with Peutz-Jeghers syndrome without bleeding or perforation, while Perez et al. performed argon plasma coagulative ablation for angiodysplasias of the small bowel (n = 19).

Equipment

The double-balloon endoscope is available only from Fujinon (Saitama, Japan). It consists of an endoscope with a balloon at the tip of the intubation shaft, an overtube with a balloon at its distal end (Figs. 43-7 and 43-8), and an air pump controller to inflate or deflate the balloons (Fig. 43-9). Two types of endoscopes are available: the EN-450P5 endoscope, which is for general use and the EN-450T5, which is used for treatment. The EN-450P5 has an outer diameter (OD) of 8.5 mm and a forceps channel diameter of 2.2 mm; it is used with an overtube that has an OD of 12.2 mm and an inner diameter (ID) of 10 mm. The EN-450T5 has an OD of 9.4 mm and a forceps channel diameter of 2.8 mm; the overtube has an OD of 13.2 mm and an ID of 11 mm. The length of the intubation shaft of both endoscopes is 200 cm, while that of the overtubes is 145 cm. The inner and outer surfaces of the overtube are hydrophile-coated. The balloons are synthesized from latex (0.1-mm thickness) and monitored for air pressure. The lowest pressure needed to hold the intestine for insertion is 45 mmHg. This pressure does not seem to create patient discomfort.

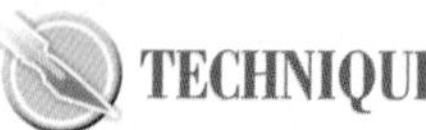

TECHNIQUE

The main impediment for small intestine enteroscopic introduction and advancement is the stretching of the intestine and

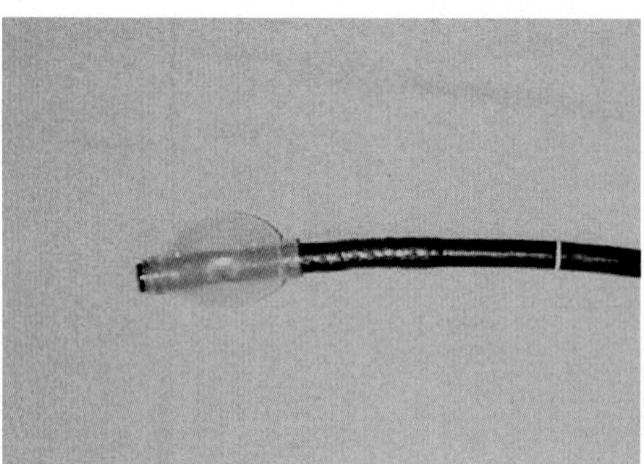

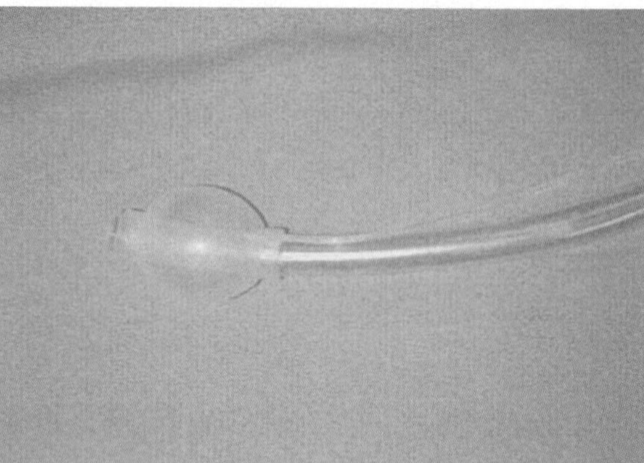

Fig. 43-8. Balloons attached to the tip of the endoscope (left) and distal end of the overtube (right).

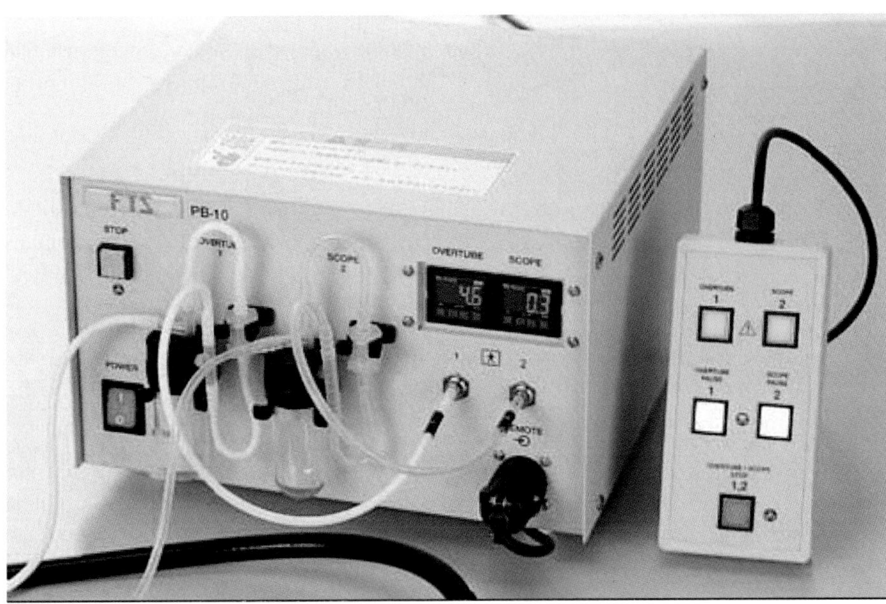

Fig. 43-9. A specially designed Fujinon air pump controller for inflation of the balloons.

its mesenteric attachment when a push force is applied. This leads to the bending of the enteroscope and to non-transmission of the pushing force. The overtube, with the balloon inflated at its distal end, holds the intestine from within and prevents stretching, thus allowing the transfer of force to the distal end of the enteroscope, resulting in distal advancement (Fig. 43-10). The overtube is back-loaded onto the endoscope before patient intubation and after adequate lubrication of its inner surface.

During the insertion process, the wall of the intestine is held alternatively by the endoscope balloon and the overtube balloon. With the wall of the intestine held by the inflated enteroscope balloon, the overtube is advanced. Then, with the two balloons inflated and holding the wall of the intestine, the overtube and the enteroscope are pulled back slowly to pleat the intestine onto the overtube and to straighten the more distal intestine. This is followed by deflation of the enteroscope balloon and deeper insertion of the enteroscope, after which the enteroscope balloon is re-inflated. The overtube balloon is deflated again and the overtube is advanced over the enteroscope (Fig. 43-11, page 436). As shown in the figure, double-balloon endoscopy can be performed either per os or via the anal approach. Each technique reaches an average of one-half to two-thirds of the small intestine length; it is possible to examine the entire small intestine by combining both routes.

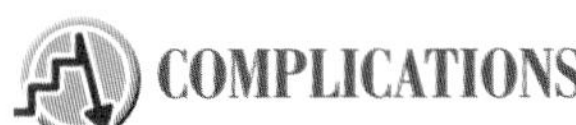

COMPLICATIONS

Few complications have been reported with double-balloon endoscopy. Yamamoto et al. reported two problems in 178 patients. One patient with Crohn disease developed a fever and abdominal pain requiring fasting and antibiotic administration. The other patient sustained a perforation after endoscopy for post-chemotherapeutic evaluation of a malignant lymphoma. Laparotomy revealed multiple perforations in the region of the lymphoma and perforations distal to the reach of the endoscope, suggesting that chemotherapy was the offending agent. Sun et al. reported mild self-limited mucosal bleeding from the push-pull action of the overtube. Perez et al. reported one case of colonic perforation, which required surgical intervention, during transanal double-balloon endoscopy.

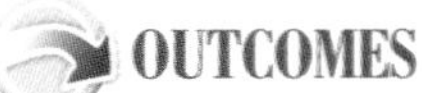

OUTCOMES

In 178 patients, Yamamoto et al. succeeded in observing the entire length of the intestine in 86% of the cases in which total enteroscopy was attempted. Their results for OGIB were comparable to the 79% success rate of VCE. Sun et al. reported that double balloon endoscopy altered therapeutic management in 83.5% of their patients.

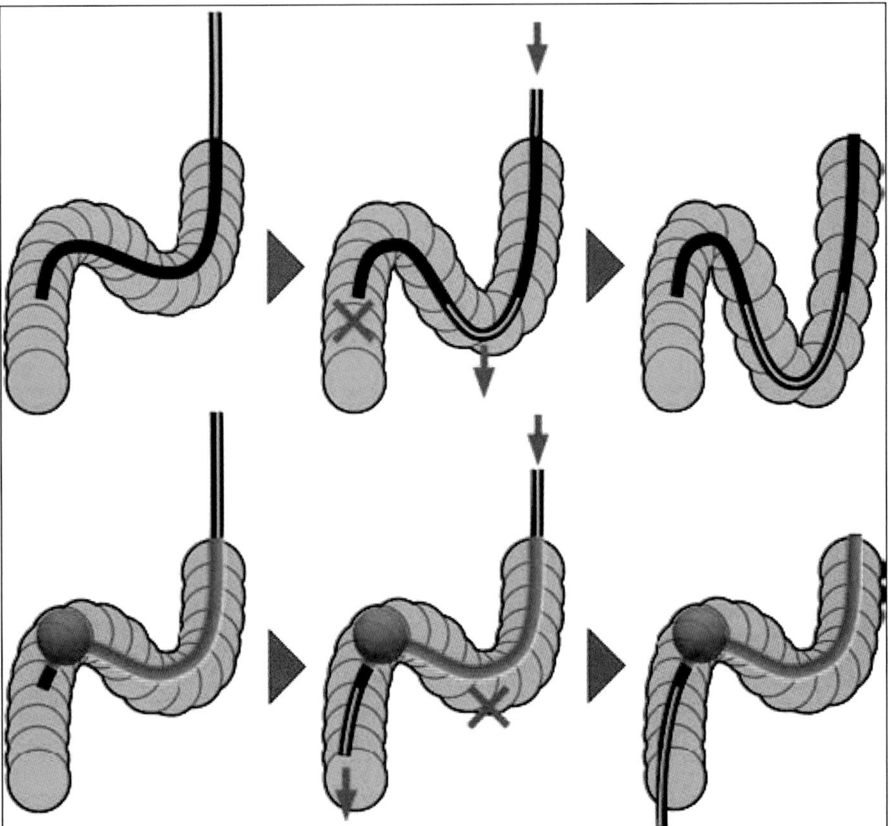

Fig. 43-10. The overtube prevents stretching of the intestine when a push force is applied, thus allowing advancement of the endoscope.

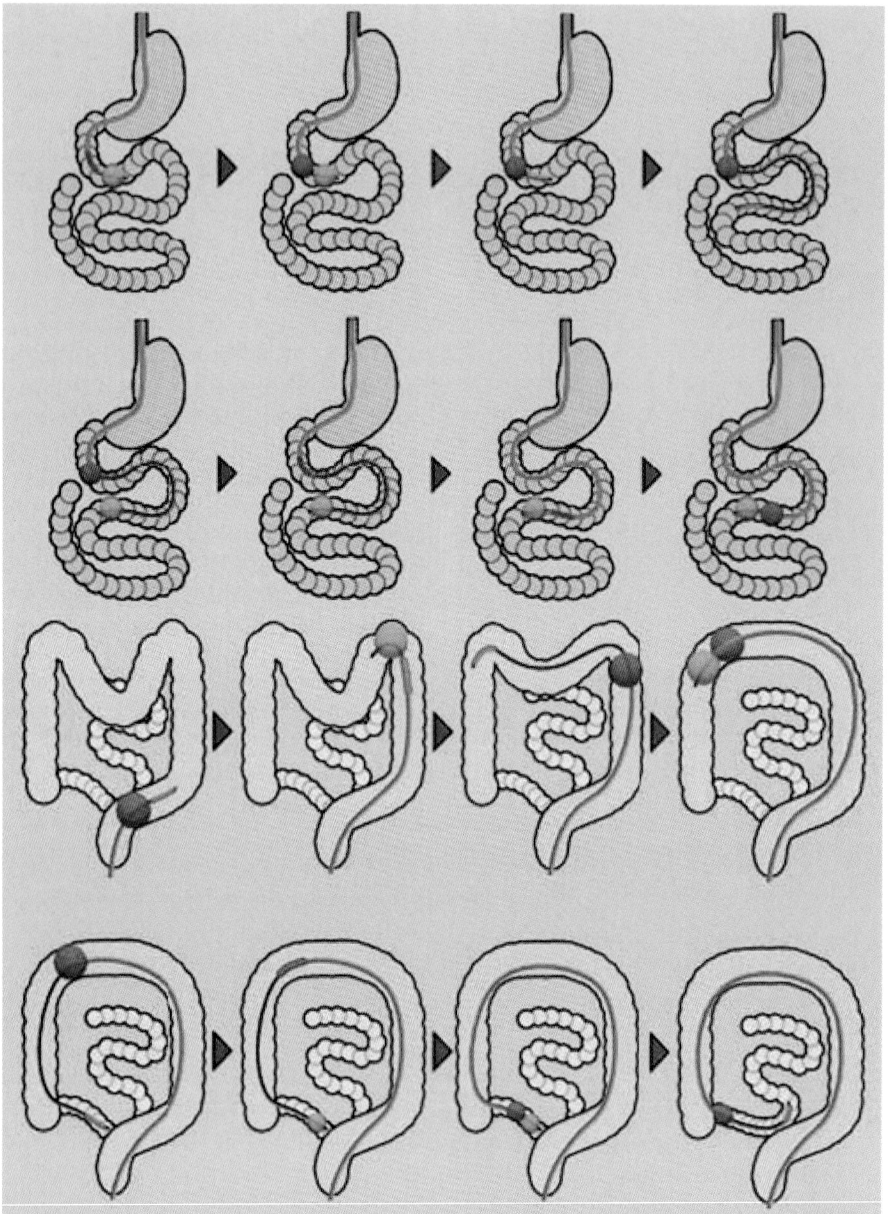

Fig. 43-11. The diagram shows the technique of double-balloon endoscopy. The alternating inflation-deflation of both balloons at the tip of the endoscope and the overtube allows transoral (above) or transanal (below) advancement of the endoscope.

Double-balloon endoscopy is a safe technique that has the potential to become the standard of care for diagnostic and therapeutic endoscopy of the small bowel. In addition to its high diagnostic yield, it provides real-time imaging, multiple biopsy capability, and the opportunity for therapeutic maneuvers. Moreover, double-balloon endoscopy can be performed in the presence of intestinal stenosis, as shown by Sunada et al. in 17 patients. All the procedures were performed safely, including balloon dilations in four cases.

INTRAOPERATIVE ENTEROSCOPY

The small intestine is the source of OGIB in up to 5% of patients. Most of these patients will have undergone an extensive diagnostic evaluation. Intraoperative enteroscopy (IE) is a consistent method for localizing and treating small bowel lesions that are neither palpable nor visible at laparotomy. Intraoperative enteroscopy allows the evaluation of the entire small bowel in the majority of patients. Because of its invasive nature, the decision to perform IE requires careful evaluation of risks and benefits as compared to the other available modalities.

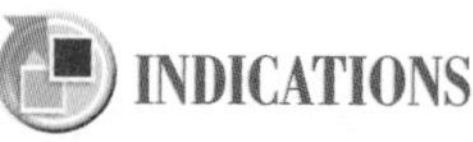

INDICATIONS

Intraoperative enteroscopy is mainly indicated in patients with OGIB for whom the other enteroscopic evaluations and radiological imaging techniques were unable to establish a definitive diagnosis. Intraoperative enteroscopy is used also for the evaluation of patients with Crohn disease, small intestinal tumors, ulcers, Meckel diverticulum, and familial polyposis. It can be used for therapeutic interventions such as endoscopic ablation of angiodysplasias, snare polypectomy, and surgical resection of small intestinal tumors and large diverticula.

Patient Selection and Preparation

Open intraoperative enteroscopy is performed in the operative room under general anesthesia; thus the selected patients should be physically suitable for surgical intervention. Patients usually do not require colon preparation unless concomitant colonoscopy is planned.

Equipment

There is no dedicated enteroscope needed for IE. A push enteroscope, a Sonde enteroscope, or an adult or pediatric colonoscope can be used. The enteroscope does not need to be sterile.

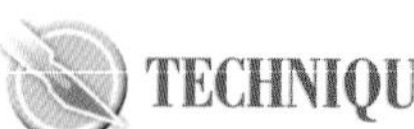

TECHNIQUE

Intraoperative enteroscopy is not a difficult procedure but it requires the collaboration of the surgeon and the endoscopists. The enteroscope is introduced transorally until it reaches beyond the ligament of Treitz. This is done prior to laparotomy as it may be difficult to advance the instrument beyond the ligament of Treitz due to the extra non-opposed bowing of the endoscope against the greater curvature of the stomach. After the endoscope is in the proximal jejunum, the abdomen is accessed, and the ileocecal valve is occluded with a non-crushing clamp to prevent distention of the colon during air insufflation. Exploration of the small intestine by both direct vision and palpation should be accomplished before the endoscope is advanced. Enteroscopic examination is then conducted by the surgeon grasping the endoscopic tip and straightening a segment of the intestine to allow luminal inspection. Dimming of the overhead lights provides the best view as the surgeon can examine the intestine through the transilluminated bowel wall. Once examined internally and externally, the loop is pleated onto the shaft of the endoscope and the next section of bowel is examined. Generally, the examination is performed during intubation as mucosal trauma usually occurs with pleating, causing an artifact that may be mistaken for an angiodysplasia. In this situation, a *reverse transillumination technique* can be used to recognize the feeding vessels and to distinguish trauma from angiodysplasias. Identified lesions are marked with a serosal suture. At the end of examination the endoscope may be used to perform argon plasma coagulation or a polypectomy. Alternatively the enteroscope is withdrawn and a resection of the intestine is performed at the sites marked by sutures.

Other techniques of IE have been described. Some authors introduce the enteroscope via the transanal approach, then across the ileocecal valve. Others perform an enterotomy in the middle third of the small bowel, through which a sterile endoscope or a clean one covered by a sterile plastic sheath is introduced. This is followed by proximal and distal intestinal intubation and inspection.

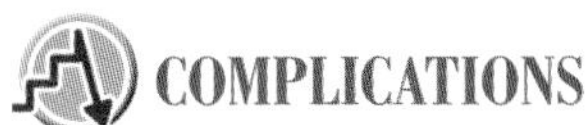

COMPLICATIONS

Intraoperative enteroscopy is associated with anesthesia-related complications, postoperative complications including a paralytic ilues, mucosal trauma associated with pleating of the small bowel loops onto the endoscope, perforation, and avulsion of mesenteric vessels. The enterotomy entrance site is subject to considerable trauma, spillage of intestinal fluid, and contamination of the peritoneal cavity. Postoperative deaths have been reported. Desa et al. reported two deaths in 12 patients who had IE for OGIB. One patient died intraoperatively, while the other died in the late postoperative period. Lewis et al. had four postoperative deaths in 53 patients who underwent IE for OGIB.

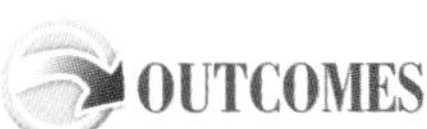

OUTCOMES

Intraoperative enteroscopy is the most effective procedure for examination of the entire length of the small bowel in patients requiring blood transfusions and in whom the other methods of enteroscopy and radiological imaging were unrewarding. The diagnostic yield of IE in patients with OGIB ranges between 50% and 100%, as reported by several authors. In spite of its high diagnostic yield and its superiority to other enteroscopic approaches, IE should be cautiously utilized as it is invasive and associated with a higher rate of mortality.

LAPAROSCOPICALLY ASSISTED PANENTEROSCOPY

The first laparoscopically assisted panenteroscopy (LAPE) in humans was reported by Reddy et al. in 1996. They used LAPE for the diagnosis and endoscopic excision of a jejunal lipoma. This was followed shortly by other published cases.

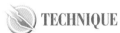

TECHNIQUE

Laparoscopically assisted panenteroscopy is also performed under general anesthesia. After a pneumoperitoneum is established, three ports are inserted in the upper abdomen: one port for the laparoscope and two for atraumatic bowel forceps. A PE or a colonoscope can be used. Laparoscopic exploration of the abdomen and the intestine is followed by introduction of the enteroscope. Several techniques have been described. Reddy et al. introduced the endoscope through a 12-mm port and into an enterotomy performed in a jejunal loop. The 12-mm port was then negotiated into the jejunal loop. Examination was completed by advancing the endoscope through the intestine while telescoping the bowel loops over the endoscope using atraumatic bowel graspers. Matsushita et al. performed a 5-cm incision in the lower abdominal wall (after initial laparoscopic observation) through which a loop of the ileum was exteriorized. A 1-cm enterotomy was performed in the ileal loop, and the endoscope was introduced for examination. Ingrosso et al. used a "double-way" technique of combined transoral and transrectal retrograde enteroscopy. They performed peroral PE followed by transrectal pancolonoscopy with retrograde ileoscopy assisted by laparoscopy. Lesions detected during enteroscopy were marked by surgical clips or sutures. This was followed by surgical or endoscopic therapeutic intervention.

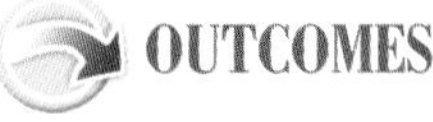

OUTCOMES

Laparoscopic assisted panenteroscopy was associated with a 100% success rate in all of 31 patients reported on by Reddy et al. They were able to complete the examination of the entire small intestine and established a diagnosis in all patients, with or without therapeutic intervention. Endoscopic electrocautery for arteriovenous malformation (n = 14), endoscopic snare polypectomy (n = 6), resection of a lipoma (n = 4), and resection of a leiomyoma (n = 2) were performed. The study concluded that LAPE is safer and less invasive than IE and not as associated with complications.

Several questions are still under investigation for LAPE: what is the best endoscope and what is the best approach (peroral, transanal, or enterotomy)? In addition, the instruments currently used for manipulation of the intestine and pleating are suboptimal.

CONCLUSION

Significant advances in the examination of the small intestine have recently occurred. Nevertheless further advances in capsule endoscopy to allow insufflation, independent movement, and biopsy capability are necessary. In addition, a different or refined mechanism of per oral enteroscope introduction is still needed for 100% intubation.

SUGGESTED READING

Cave DR. Technology insight: current status of video capsule endoscopy. *Nature Clinical Practice Gastroenterology and Hepatology* 2006; 3(3):158–164.

Iddan G, Meron G, Glukhovsky A, et al. Wireless capsule endoscopy. *Nature* 2000; 405–417.

Keizman D, Brill S, Umansky M, et al. Diagnostic yield of routine push enteroscopy with a graded-stiffness enteroscope without overtube. *Gastrointest Endosc* 2003;57(7): 877–881.

Lewis BS. Enteroscopy. *Gastrointest Endosc Clin N Am* 2000;10(1):101–116.

Lewis MP, Khoo DE, Spencer J. Value of laparotomy in the diagnosis of obscure gastrointestinal haemorrhage. *Gut* 1995; 37(2): 18–90.

Matsushita M, Hajiro K, Takakuwa H, et al. Laparoscopically assisted panenteroscopy for small bowel diseases: transenterotomy versus peroral approach. *Gastrointest Endosc* 2000; 51(6):771–772.

Ohmiya N, Taguchi A, Shirai K, et al. Endoscopic resection of Peutz-Jeghers polyps throughout the small intestine at double-balloon enteroscopy without laparotomy. *Gastrointest Endosc* 2005;61: 140–147.

Pennazio M, Santucci R, Rondonotti E, et al. Outcome of patients with obscure gastrointestinal bleeding after capsule endoscopy: report of 100 consecutive cases. *Gastroenterol* 2004;126(3):643–653.

Sriram PV, Rao GV, Reddy DN. Laparoscopically assisted panenteroscopy. *Gastrointest Endosc* 2001;54(6):805–806.

Sunada K, Yamamoto H, Kita H, et al. Clinical outcomes of enteroscopy using the double balloon method for strictures of the small intestine. *World J Gastroenterol* 2005;11(7):1087–1089.

Sun B, Rajan E, Cheng S, et al. Diagnostic yield and therapeutic impact of double-balloon enteroscopy in a large cohort of patients with obscure gastrointestinal bleeding. *Am J Gastroenterol* 2006;101(9):2011–2015.

Swain P, Fritscher-Ravens A. Role of video endoscopy in managing small bowel disease. *Gut* 2004;53:1866–1875.

Yamamoto H, Kita H. Enteroscopy. *Am J Gastroenterol* 2005;40:555–562.

COMMENTARY

The small bowel remains the final frontier of GI endoscopy, but, as this chapter details, that barrier is rapidly falling as well. Capsule endoscopy (CE) has now become a routine diagnostic aid in many types of GI pathology. While it hasn't totally supplanted small bowel X-rays, it certainly has advantages over radiologic exams—especially for obscure bleeding. CE is, however, still in the infancy of its technologic development and has several drawbacks of yet: It is contraindicated for obstructive disease, though some have advocated that it could be used to lodge an obstruction in to facilitate subsequent surgical exploration and treatment. It is currently a non-directable modality, which means that it is impossible to slow down in areas where there is greater interest or the initial findings are obscure, or even to "back up" and take another look at something. This will eventually change, as there are currently prototypes of CE that are self-propelled or externally steerable using radio control or magnets. Finally, there is, to date, no capability to perform biopsies or therapeutics such as injection or cautery. This too will undoubtedly change; when it does this important diagnostic tool will essentially become the endoscope of the future.

Because of the lack of therapeutic ability with CE and of the increased diagnosis of small bowel pathology with it, enteroscopy is currently undergoing somewhat of a renaissance. Newer devices and aids have dramatically increased the capability of small bowel endoscopy, which is now becoming almost routine at some endoscopy centers. Improvements in overtube technology have allowed the use of standard pediatric colonoscopes and extended the range and usability of push enteroscopes. An example of this is the ShapeLock technology (USGI Medical, San Clemente, CA), which is a flexible overtube that can be placed and then "locked" or stiffened to straighten loops or to give stability for insertion. This has proven especially useful to facilitate ERCP in patients who are postoperative from a gastrectomy or, as is increasingly common, following a gastric bypass.

Perhaps an even more important development is the design of single- and double-balloon enteroscopes which, as described in this chapter, almost seem to propel the scope forward. When lesions are seen with the enteroscope, it is important to mark the lesion with an India ink tattoo as subsequently finding it again, either endoscopically or surgically, can be very difficult. Intraoperative enteroscopy is occasionally indicated and can be either open or laparoscopically assisted, but is not an easy procedure due to the complex logistics of scoping during surgery.

LLS

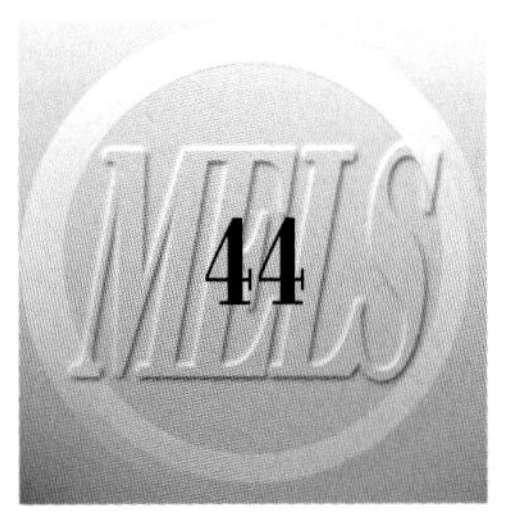

Laparoscopic Treatment of Diseases of the Small Bowel

TRACEY D. ARNELL AND DENNIS L. FOWLER

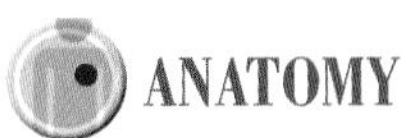

ANATOMY

The anatomy of the small bowel is quite suitable for the laparoscopic approach. It is approximately 700 cm in length, is very mobile, and can be examined in its entirety without mobilization in most cases. It begins at the Treitz ligament under the middle of the transverse mesocolon and terminates in the right lower quadrant at the ileocecal valve. The terminal ileum is easily recognized as it is the only portion of the small intestine with antimesenteric fat. The root of the mesentery is approximately 15 cm long and is attached to the retroperitoneum from the origin of the superior mesenteric artery to the terminal ileum.

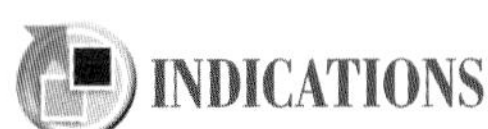

INDICATIONS

In general, the indications for laparoscopic surgery of the small bowel are the same as for open. Small intestinal diseases (other than adhesive disease) requiring operative intervention are relatively rare but quite varied and include Crohn disease, neoplasms, traumatic injury, and ischemia. Table 44-1 lists indications for which the laparoscopic approach may be employed. The ability to diagnose small intestinal disorders preoperatively has improved with new technologies as described in Chapter 43, including capsule endoscopy and small intestinal endoscopy. Despite this, because there can be difficulty in evaluating the small intestine adequately preoperatively, the indication for surgery may be based upon the clinical presentation such as obstruction or occult bleeding without a known preoperative diagnosis.

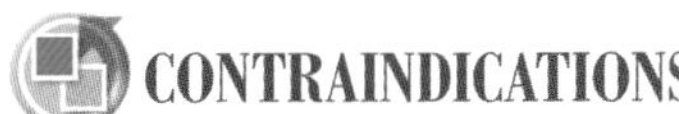

CONTRAINDICATIONS

As experience has grown with the use of laparoscopic techniques in complex cases, the contraindications have decreased. They include inability to undergo insufflation either because of bowel distention and loss of domain or patient comorbidities such as severe pulmonary or cardiac disease. In the hemodynamically unstable patient, laparoscopy may be too time-consuming and the physiologic effects may be deleterious, in which case open surgery should be given strong consideration.

Previous abdominal surgery is not a contraindication to laparoscopy, but individual patient and surgeon factors should be considered. Regarding surgeon factors, the most important is experience. Reoperative surgery is more challenging and associated with an increased risk of complications and should be undertaken with caution. With respect to the individual patient, the type and number of previous surgeries, any history of prior adhesive small bowel obstructions, and, when available, a review of operative reports can be helpful in deciding if the laparoscopic approach is appropriate.

Presently, the role of laparoscopic surgery for adenocarcinoma of the small bowel is unclear. The completion of the Nelson et al. Clinical Outcomes of Surgical Therapy (COST) trial evaluating laparoscopy in colon cancer did not demonstrate an increased risk of cancer recurrence or wound implantation. The recommendations for laparoscopy in colon cancer may be extrapolated to small bowel adenocarcinoma and include avoidance of direct manipulation of the tumor, avoidance of venting gas through the trocar sites, and use of this approach by experienced surgeons only.

TABLE 44-1. INDICATIONS FOR LAPAROSCOPY IN SMALL INTESTINAL DISEASE

Inflammatory
Crohn disease
Neoplasm
Benign
Adenoma
Lipoma
Gastrointestinal stromal tumor (GIST)
Hamartoma
Hemangioma
Fibroma
Mesenteric cyst
Malignant
Adenocarcinoma
Carcinoid
Malignant GIST
Lymphoma
Congenital
Meckel diverticulum
Malrotation
Duplication
Vascular
Ischemia
Angiodysplasia
Other
Radiation stricture
Trauma
Foreign body (e.g., gallstone, toothpick)
Endometriosis

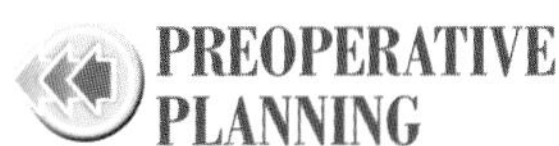

PREOPERATIVE PLANNING

Most patients with small bowel disorders requiring an operation present with symptoms; the cause is then found during the evaluation of these symptoms. Occasionally, as use of the computed tomography (CT) scan has expanded, incidental findings may lead to laparoscopy. Intestinal obstruction, abdominal pain, and occult gastrointestinal (GI) bleeding are the most common symptoms associated with small intestinal pathology. Beyond review of any previous operative reports, preoperative preparation and evaluation is problem-based.

In the case of occult GI bleeding, if upper and lower endoscopy is unrevealing, small bowel evaluation should be carried out with capsule endoscopy, bleeding scan, small bowel follow-through (SBFT), or balloon endoscopy. If bleeding is ongoing and remains unlocalized, operative exploration may be required. In this case, plans for intraoperative push endoscopy can be made. In the case of massive bleeding, if a small intestinal source is not identified, the colon is the most likely location and the patient should be prepared for a possible total abdominal colectomy.

Small bowel obstruction is most commonly related to adhesive disease and prior surgery. In a patient without prior surgery or a hernia with a documented small bowel obstruction, suspicion for a small bowel lesion must be high. Occasionally, intraabdominal tumors with known patterns of peritoneal spread and non-GI cancers such as melanoma and small-cell lung cancer may lead to small bowel obstruction. In those not requiring immediate surgical intervention, evaluation by CT, SBFT, or capsule endoscopy may be carried out. If these do not reveal the source of obstruction, operative exploration is likely required. Assessment of the degree of distention and the feasibility of laparoscopy in terms of obtaining domain with insufflation should be made.

Crohn disease deserves special mention as the preoperative preparation is extremely important. Findings at the time of exploration may be difficult to interpret unless the extent of disease is known. Preoperative "staging" includes colonoscopy and SBFT to document location of disease. In this way, if an enteric fistula is found at surgery, only the diseased bowel is resected and not bowel that is secondarily involved with extrinsic inflammation. Review of previous operative reports in cases of small intestinal disease to assess length of resected intestine may help guide the decision of resection versus bowel conservation when possible.

The use of bowel preparation as a means of preventing infectious complications is being questioned based on several large reviews of prospective trials in elective colon resections and should be decided on an individual basis. When used in cases of partial obstruction, some authors advocate small-volume preparations to prevent retention in the proximal small bowel. It is critical to know that the use of Phosphosoda preparations can lead to elevated phosphate and potassium levels and, rarely, renal failure and/or cardiac arrest; their use is thus contraindicated in cases of known obstruction. If push endoscopy is planned, bowel preparation is necessary for visualization of the small-bowel mucosa.

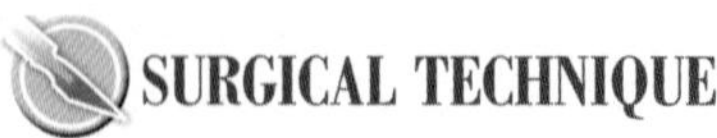

SURGICAL TECHNIQUE

Patient Positioning

Unless there is suspicion that access to the perineum may be required, the supine position with both arms tucked to the side is the preferred position. It is important to pad the bony prominences of the elbow to prevent injury to the ulnar nerve. Both arms are tucked, as mobility to all quadrants of the abdomen may be necessary. Monitors should be placed on both sides of the patient.

Instrumentation

It is extremely helpful to have the ability to manipulate the table to various side-down and Trendelenburg positions. If an automatic table is available it should be used after it is verified to be functioning properly. A 5-mm camera can be moved between ports and should be used if available. Most commonly, a 30-degree angled scope is used, although a 0-degree scope is adequate. During manipulation of the bowel, direct grasping of the intestine is avoided unless necessary, especially in cases of cancer. Although any grasper can be made traumatic, there are several that are considered atraumatic and these should be used. A source of energy is chosen based on surgeon experience and preference but may be bipolar, monopolar, or ultrasonic shears. For the anastomosis either staplers or sutures are chosen. If push endoscopy is to be performed, a standard colonoscope (for length) or an enteroscope is used. It is now possible to use carbon dioxide insufflation, which prevents ongoing bowel distention as it is absorbed and may facilitate intraoperative endoscopy.

The specific details of the surgical procedure will vary based on the findings, but can generally be divided into several phases. These are access, exploration, mobilization and mesenteric division, and anastomosis or ostomy.

Access

Access is dependent on surgeon preference and previous surgery. Both the Hasson cutdown and inserting a Veress needle at either umbilical or alternative sites such as the left upper quadrant may be employed. There has been no definitive study demonstrating superiority of one approach over the other for reducing insertion injuries. Whichever technique is selected, the avoidance of access attempts through previous scars, willingness and ability to change the type of access if initial attempts fail, and close inspection of the area once pneumoperitoneum is established are basic tenants. Ultrasound may aid in finding areas free of adhesions by identifying a "visceral slide" of bowel loops during respiration or a "peritoneal reflection band sign," which relies on the presence of tethering bands to the abdominal wall. These are obviously specialized techniques that are very operator-dependent and not used in most institutions. Once access and pneumoperitoneum are obtained, additional trocars are placed. Trocar positions vary widely but they are generally placed laterally to prevent them from being on top of the working area. If the intracorporeal use of staplers is planned, a 12-mm trocar must be placed.

Exploration

Throughout the procedure the surgeon must be cognizant of the injuries that can occur to the small bowel either by grasping and tearing or by the inappropriate use of diathermy. When possible, grasping the mesentery instead of the bowel or using the graspers as a blunt retractor is advised. Diathermy instruments should be checked for intact insulation and proper functioning.

In cases of suspected cancer, the peritoneal surfaces, the liver, and, in women, the adnexa should be visualized. Suspicious nodules should be biopsied and any ascites should be aspirated and sent for cytology. Frozen section does not usually impact the operative procedure as most patients are undergoing an operation because of symptoms. The small intestine should be examined in its entirety. It may be helpful to place the patient in slight reverse-Trendelenburg. If this is too steep, the transverse colon may obscure the small bowel. The Treitz ligament is identified by elevating the mesentery of the transverse colon and looking at the base of the transverse mesocolon in the midabdomen. The bowel is evaluated in a hand-over-hand manner. As the small intestine is visualized from section to section, repositioning of the table can be used to allow the small bowel to fall away and improve exposure. Once the terminal ileum is reached, generally the patient is in mild Trendelenburg, left side-down.

If the pathology has not been localized, especially in cases of occult GI bleeding, push endoscopy is used. Most reports describe creating a mini laparotomy to allow guidance of the scope when necessary. An alternative to a mini laparotomy is provided by telescoping the bowel over the scope intracorporeally. This approach is technically challenging and the minimal benefits of avoiding a small incision may not be warranted.

Mobilization and Mesenteric Division

Once the pathology has been identified, operative treatment may then be carried out. Some surgeons choose to make a mini laparotomy and exteriorize the diseased small intestine at this time. Other surgeons complete the mesenteric division intracorporeally, but enlarge the incision for specimen extraction only after the resection and anastomosis have been completed laparoscopically. The technique of mesenteric division and anastomosis are the same as for an open procedure when performed extracorporeally.

As in open surgery, consideration of the friability of the bowel and mesentery must be considered. This is especially true in conditions requiring emergency surgery such as bowel obstruction and ischemia or chronic inflammatory conditions such as Crohn's disease. The bowel and mesentery can be injured intracorporeally with manipulation or when being exteriorized. If the extraction site is quite small, significant tension and force may be necessary to remove the intestine. This can result in injury to the mesentery or perforation of the intestine with contamination.

Overall nutritional status of the patient and the use of immunosuppressants such as steroids and transplant medications have implications in terms of healing of anastomoses and abdominal incisions. This is not unique to laparoscopic surgery and must be accounted for in the operative technique.

For intracorporeal mesenteric division, the surgeon should use a familiar energy source. In many patients, the vascular arcade can be visualized by elevating the bowel to be resected and fanning out the mesentery (Fig. 44-1). Locations of the proximal and distal lines of resection of the bowel are chosen and the mesentery divided between the two. The amount of mesenteric resection depends on the surgical indication. For example, in cases of malignant disease, a broader mesenteric resection may be required.

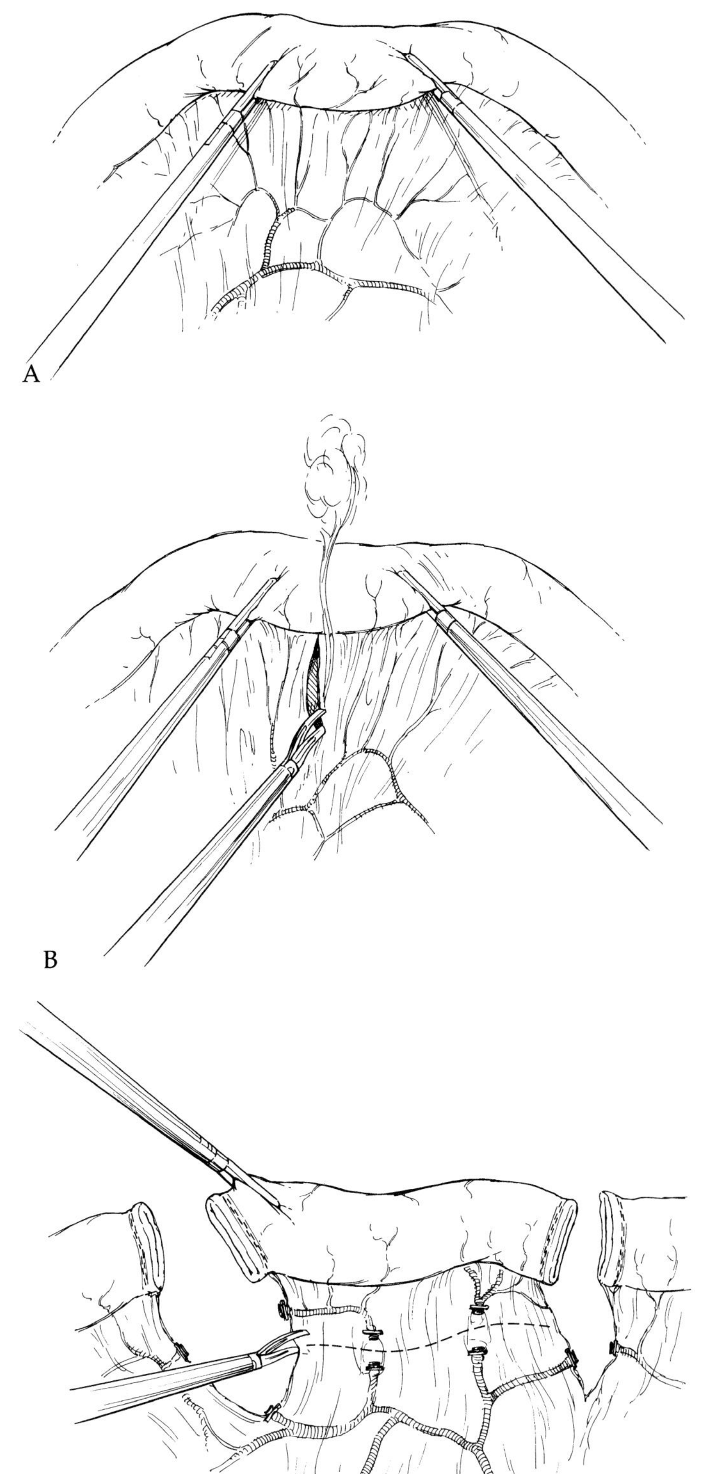

Fig. 44-1. For small-bowel resection, the area of interest is displayed, the overlying peritoneum opened, and the vascular arcades divided.

Anastomosis or Ostomy

A stapled or sutured intracorporeal anastomosis can be performed, and there are variations for both methods. We describe the most common here. For either technique, the small bowel is divided proximally and distally with a laparoscopic stapling device. The specimen may be placed in a bag or left in the abdomen (usually above the liver or in the pelvis). The proximal and distal ends are approximated in a side-to-side manner and held in place with stay sutures (Fig. 44-2, page 442). For the stapled anastomosis, enterotomies are created in the ends of both staple lines. The stapler is passed through both enterotomies and fired while elevating the proximal and distal stay sutures. The enterotomy is then closed with an additional firing of the stapler. For the sutured anastomosis, after placing the bowel side to side, enterotomies are created in the antimesenteric side of the small bowel and a sutured anastomosis performed.

CROHN DISEASE

The most common indications for surgery in isolated, non-ileocolonic small bowel Crohn disease are fistula and stricture. The treatment of Crohn disease with small intestinal fistula is very challenging as the

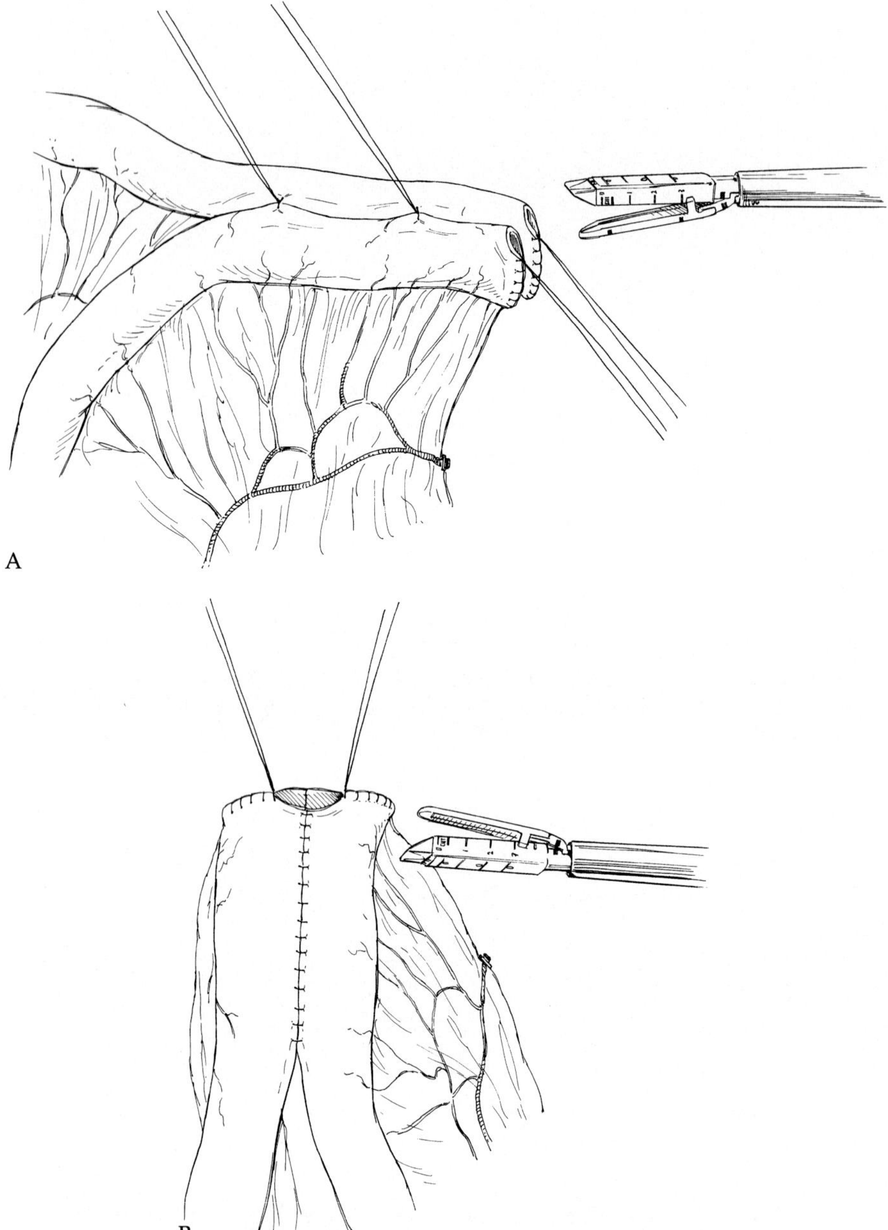

Fig. 44-2. In creating a stapled side-to-side anastomosis, the bowel is aligned along the antimesenteric border. A stay stitch helps to maintain alignment and can provide countertraction as the two blades of the linear stapler are introduced into the adjacent lumina. The resultant confluent enterotomy is closed with a second firing or with sutures.

areas of disease are often fibrotic and/or inflamed. Blunt dissection can be helpful to separate loops of bowel. Careful inspection of these adjacent loops must be performed to assess for injury. Regarding the mesenteric division, the mesentery may be very foreshortened and thickened. Careful, slow division of the mesentery in these cases is critical. Also, staying near the bowel edge will prevent retraction of a vessel in the inflamed mesentery towards the root of the mesentery, where it may be difficult to control.

In cases of stricture, either from Crohn disease or radiation, it is important to recognize that strictures may be present beyond the proximal one. The simplest way to evaluate this is to place a catheter with a balloon inflated through an enterotomy. This is done just past the proximal stricture and the catheter is then passed distally. If resistance is encountered, these areas should be addressed as well. In Crohn disease, stricturoplasty may be performed. In radiation enteritis, resection is recommended because radiated bowel heals poorly. The technique is the same for laparoscopic and open procedures and is done as a Heineke-Mikulicz closure. Long strictures may be stapled with a linear stapler. This can be very difficult in the presence of inflamed bowel and may be most expeditiously performed extracorporeally.

Malignancy

For primary neoplasms, except for lymphoma, a broad mesenteric resection is necessary for oncologic treatment. Additionally, as stated previously, it is important to be aware of the risk of tumor aerosolization and implantation when performing laparoscopy in patients with cancer, especially adenocarcinoma. During exteriorization of the specimen in malignant disease, the gas should be suctioned from the peritoneal cavity prior to enlarging the abdominal incision. This prevents "venting" of the carbon dioxide and potential aerosolization of tumor cells through the wound.

A wound protector should be placed prior to decrease the risk of tumor cell shedding and potential implantation in the wound during removal of the specimen. After handling of the specimen, gloves are changed.

Carcinoid may be a challenge because of its multicentric nature in the small intestine, and the possibility of a severe desmoplastic reaction in the mesentery. Complete exploration and careful division of the mesentery as described for Crohn disease is important.

Meckel Diverticulum

A Meckel diverticulum that does not require a small bowel resection because of inflammation is easily removed intracorporeally with an endoscopic stapler. The diverticulum is elevated, its vascular supply divided with an energy source or a clip, and a linear endoscopic stapler used for transection (Fig. 44-3).

Ischemic Enteritis

If the diagnosis of arterial mesenteric occlusion has been made prior to surgical exploration and revascularization was not performed by endovascular techniques, laparotomy will be required for establishing arterial flow. If flow has been reestablished, or if the diagnosis of ischemic

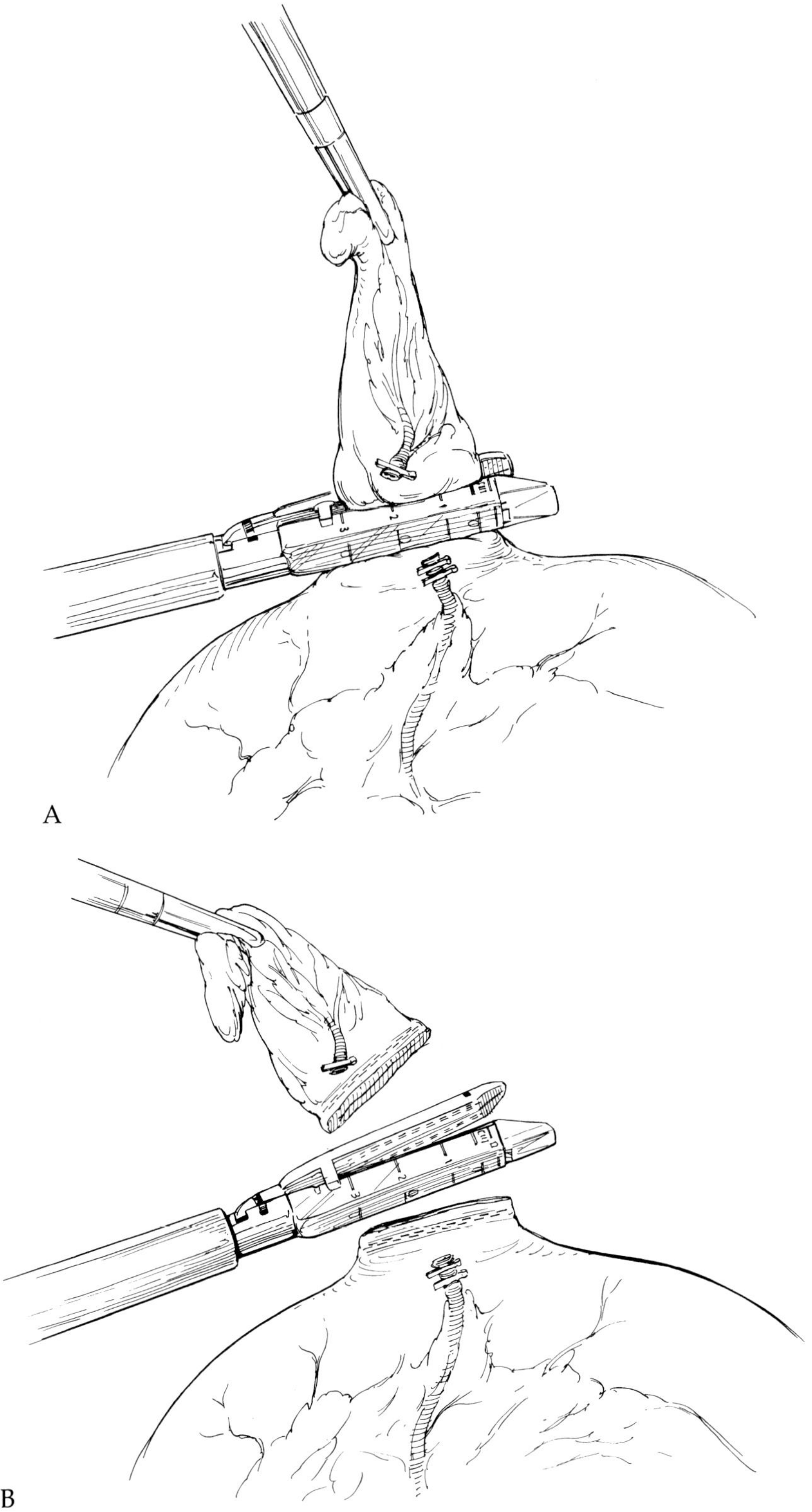

Fig. 44-3. A Meckel diverticulectomy with close apposition of the gastrointestinal anastomosis endoscopic cutting stapler to the intestinal lumen.

enteritis has not been established, diagnostic laparoscopy is useful. This can be performed in some institutions at the bedside in the intensive care unit. If ischemia is found, patients are most often too ill to undergo laparoscopic resection and a laparotomy is done. Laparoscopy can be performed for the second look, even when a laparotomy was the prior operation. It has been described leaving the trocars in place at the conclusion of the first operation. At the subsequent "second look", these trocars may be used avoiding the need for obtaining access.

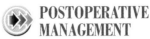

POSTOPERATIVE MANAGEMENT

Postoperative management is as typical for gastrointestinal surgery. Deep vein thrombosis prophylaxis continues throughout the hospitalization. Diet advancement is based on the clinical parameters of subjective complaints (e.g., nausea, belching) and objective findings (e.g., distention). Nasogastric tubes are used only when they were placed preoperatively for obstruction or in patients who develop significant vomiting or distention after surgery. Discharge occurs when the patient requires no intravenous fluids or pain medications, is tolerating a diet, and has no evidence of ongoing infection.

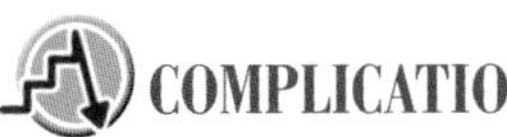

COMPLICATIONS

Unique complications to laparoscopic small bowel surgery are unrecognized intestinal injury as a result of obtaining access, use of the energy source, or mechanical injury from bowel manipulation. Otherwise, the most common surgical complications include incisional infection, anastomotic leak, fistula, recurrence of the disease, and hernia. By adhering to accepted indications for surgery and using judgment regarding the appropriateness of conversion, complications may be minimized.

SUGGESTED READING

Casillas S, Delaney C. Laparoscopic surgery for inflammatory bowel disease. *Dig Surg* 2005; 22:135–142.

Craigie RJ, Forrest N, Nanthakumaran S, et al. Case report: Laparoscopy in diagnosis and management of Meckel's diverticulum. *J Laparoendosc Adv Surg Tech* 2006;16:70–73.

Kim J, Kim YS, Hoon JC, et al. Laparoscopy-assisted exploration of obscure gastrointestinal bleeding after capsule endoscopy: The Korean experience. *J Laparoendosc Adv Surg Tech* 2005; 15:365–373.

Nguyen SQ, Divino CM, Wang JL, et al. Laparoscopic management of gastrointestinal stromal tumors. *Surg Endosc* 2006;20:713–716.

Pei K, Zemon H, Venbrux, et al. Case report: Laparoendoscopic techniques for occult gastrointestinal bleeding. *J Laparoendosc Adv Surg Tech* 2005;15:615–619.

COMMENTARY

The use of laparoscopy for the treatment of diseases of the small bowel covers the full spectrum of technical difficulty of an operation. A straightforward Meckel diverticulectomy can be one of the simplest of laparoscopic procedures and lysis of adhesions for small bowel obstruction might require a single snip of the scissors to divide an offending band. At the other end of the spectrum one might encounter a complex fistula in a Crohn disease patient who has chronically used steroids and has terrible tissue quality. Furthermore, a difficult adhesiolysis can challenge even experienced and gifted surgeons.

Many laparoscopic operations lend themselves to an approach that limits the number and size of the tumors. A single large site might be needed for extraction of a specimen, but usually up to three additional sites, which can be small in size, will be necessary. No consensus exists regarding the use of energy for the lysis of adhesions. Some surgeons hold the position that the use of energy sources for adhesiolysis increases the risk of immediate or delayed bowel injury and that dissection must be accomplished with sharp or blunt dissection. Those surgeons who favor the judicious use of energy sources for adhesiolysis hold the position that the hemostasis maintained by using energy sources offers excellent visualization and thereby reduces the risk of bowel injury and results in less blood loss.

Most laparoscopic surgeons will agree that the majority of small bowel diseases can be treated effectively with minimally invasive surgical techniques. The patient undergoing laparoscopic small bowel surgery can expect equivalent or better rates of surgical complications to an open procedure. When the procedure is accomplished without complication the laparoscopic patient usually enjoys a faster return to normal activities, less pain, shorter hospital stay, and decreased need for narcotics compared to one who undergoes the same procedure via an open technique.

WSE

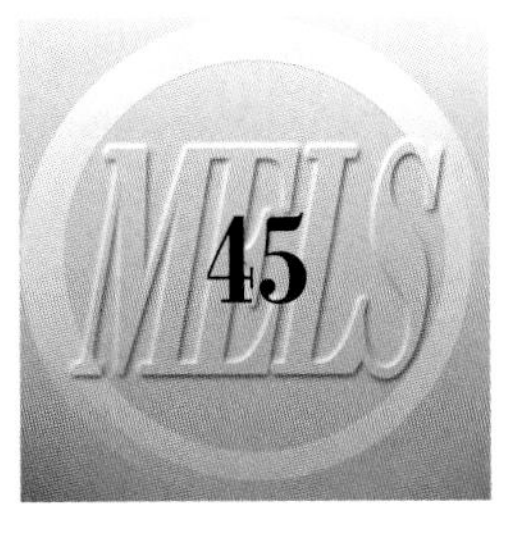

Flexible Endoscopy of the Lower Gastrointestinal Tract

CHRISTOPHER J. BRUCE AND JOHN A. COLLER

INTRODUCTION

Flexible endoscopy of the lower gastrointestinal (GI) tract, which includes flexible sigmoidoscopy and colonoscopy, is an essential tool for surgeons for the diagnosis and management of disorders of the colon and rectum. Although colonoscopy may seem to be simply an extension of flexible sigmoidoscopy, it is in fact a considerably more complex procedure. Flexible sigmoidoscopy is performed in the office setting without the need for sedation or a complete bowel preparation. In contrast, colonoscopy is technically more demanding, is associated with increased risks, and requires supervised training and certification for competence. However, the techniques of intubation of the rectum and sigmoid are similar for both procedures, and experience in one complements the other. Whether the flexible sigmoidoscope or colonoscope is used, redundancy and acute angulations of the colon can pose problems requiring skills in scope manipulation that often frustrate even the most resourceful endoscopist. A thorough knowledge of the anatomy of the colon and an understanding of the mechanics of the flexible endoscope and its interaction with the bowel are necessary for the performance of a safe and expeditious examination.

INSTRUMENTATION

Flexible endoscopes are available from a wide variety of vendors. Most of these instruments use similar optical devices and differ mainly in length, diameter, and maneuverability. Diameters vary from 10 to 15 mm, while flexible sigmoidoscopes range from 60 to 71 cm in length and colonoscopes from 115 to 180 cm. Pediatric colonoscopes (10 mm) can prove invaluable when a tight stricture prevents access with a standard instrument, but their inferior maneuverability and greater flexibility limit their routine use. Maneuverability has improved greatly from the prototype instruments developed in the 1960s that provided only two-way tip deflection, compared to modern-day devices that allow a full 360-degree articulation. Variable stiffness colonoscopes allow the endoscopist to change the flexibility of the shaft, which can be useful to control loop formation and lessen patient discomfort, especially in patients with a redundant colon or those who have adhesions from previous surgery. All endoscopes have buttons for air insufflation and aspiration, as well as a water jet directed at the distal lens to clean away debris and mucus. Various devices such as biopsy forceps, diathermy snares for polypectomy, baskets for the removal of foreign bodies, grasping forceps, laser fibers, needle injectors, and balloon dilators may be inserted through the suction/accessory channel of the scope. Colonoscopes designed with two instrument channels are available for specialized procedures such as a difficult polypectomy or acute bleeding, but these are somewhat stiffer than the standard, smaller-diameter, single-channel scopes and have a greater potential to cause patient discomfort.

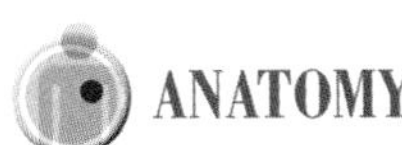

ANATOMY

Each segment of bowel has its own distinct endoscopic characteristics. The anal canal and distal rectum may be evaluated with a retroflexion maneuver of the flexible instrument; however, the role of anoscopy and rigid proctosigmoidoscopy should not be overlooked. The rectum is recognized by its ample lumen and prominent semicircular valves. The rectosigmoid junction is approximately 15 to 20 cm from the anal verge, and this is the first major angulation that is encountered (Fig. 45-1, page 446). The sigmoid colon turns toward the left and follows the convexity of the sacrum. Effectively negotiating the sigmoid colon is key to a successful colonoscopy. Different processes may limit the mobility of the sigmoid, namely scarring from previous surgery, pelvic sepsis, or irradiation. The descending colon–sigmoid junction is commonly an acute angle, but once past this obstacle, intubating the descending colon is usually not difficult. The typical muscular rings help in negotiating the lumen as it runs a relatively straight course before turning medially and anteriorly at the splenic flexure. Not infrequently, a bluish discoloration may be seen here as the spleen is viewed through the relatively thin colonic wall. A distinctive gate-like fold is commonly seen just below the splenic flexure. Once around the splenic flexure, the characteristic triangular folds of the transverse colon are seen (Fig. 45-2, page 446). Advancing the scope through the transverse colon is usually uneventful unless a deep pelvic bend or gamma loop is present. The hepatic flexure is identified by a widening of the lumen and the presence of prominent arcuate folds that do not fully encircle the lumen. The blue color of the liver can be seen through the colonic wall where the right lobe of the liver causes a flattened impression on the superior aspect of the flexure. The ascending colon is usually short and dilated with prominent arcuate folds that do not fully encircle the lumen. The ileocecal valve is pointed toward the base of the cecum, and its orifice is usually not identifiable during colonoscopy. The location of the ileocecal valve can usually be seen as an indentation of a colonic valve approximately 4 to 6 cm above the appendiceal orifice or the blind end of the cecum. The appendiceal orifice and the ileocecal valve are the most reliable landmarks for confirming the position of the tip of the scope in the cecum (Fig. 45-3, page 447).

Fluoroscopy during colonoscopy is an invaluable tool in the training of young endoscopists to gain an appreciation of both normal colonic anatomy and its variations. The colon is usually fixed at the rectum, descending colon, and ascending colon, allowing the sigmoid and transverse colon to move freely on their mesenteries. The amount of movement depends on the length of colon and the elasticity of the mesenteries. The sigmoid colon may take the shape of the Greek letter α, while a redundant transverse colon occasionally conforms to a γ configuration. Both the splenic and hepatic flexures may have a reversed configuration; these are important to recognize because a straightening maneuver to convert them to a normal orientation is often required. The mobility of the cecum is variable and depends on the extent of its posterior attachments. During

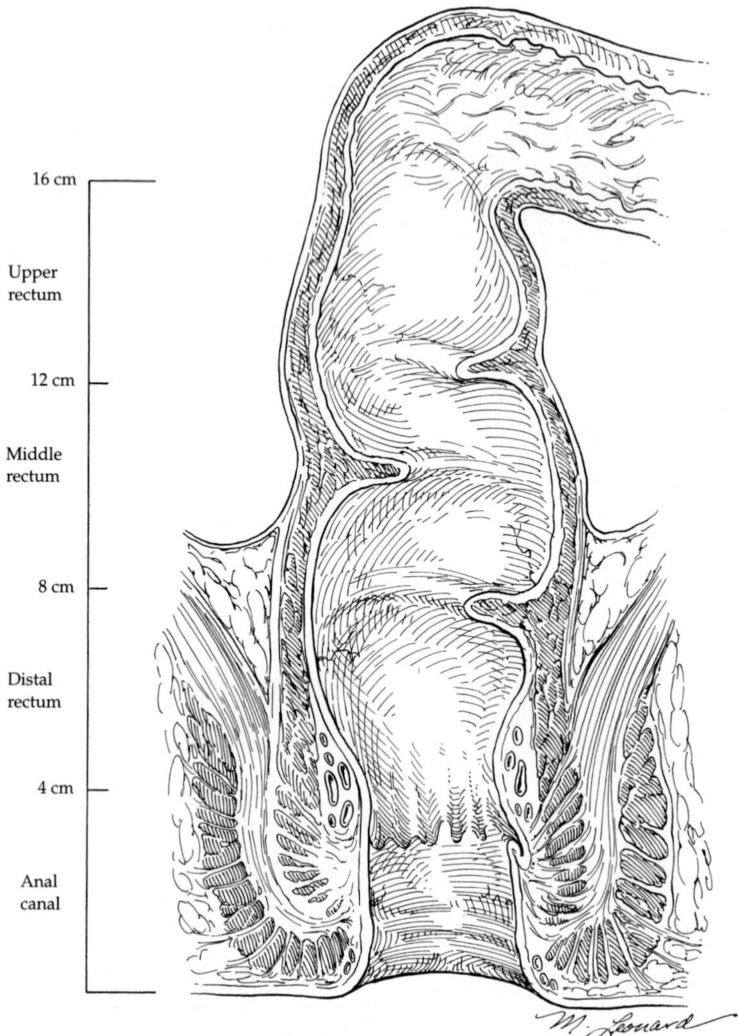

Fig. 45-1. The complex anatomy of the rectum and sigmoid colon can make endoscopy difficult.

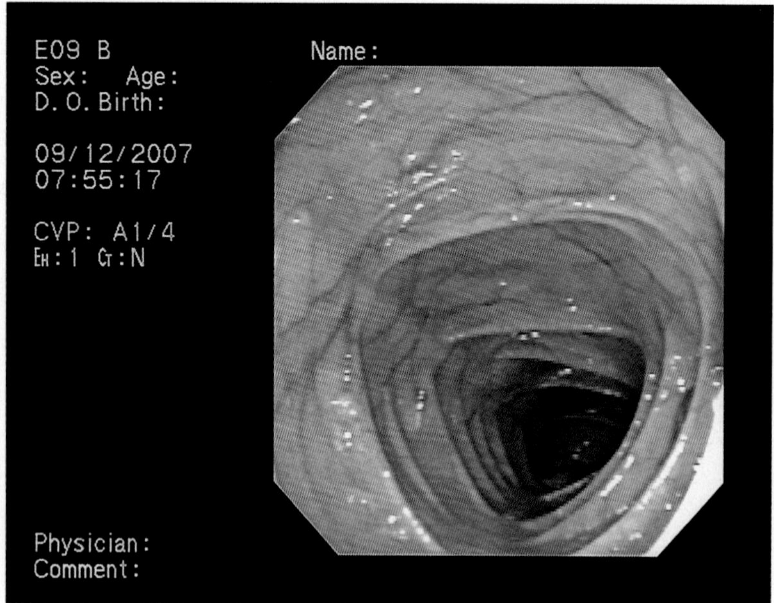

Fig. 45-2. The transverse colon is easily identified due to its triangular configuration.

negotiation of these difficult formations, it is often prudent to take advantage of this mobility, rather than trying to counter it.

Only by understanding the anatomy of the colon and its variations will one appreciate the complexity of the scope–colon interaction. The ease with which intubation of the colon can be accomplished depends on the smooth integration of several independent control mechanisms. In this chapter, each of the various maneuvers—tip deflection, shaft torquing, advancement/withdrawal (dithering), and insufflation/aspiration of gas—are discussed separately and then collectively applied to intubation techniques.

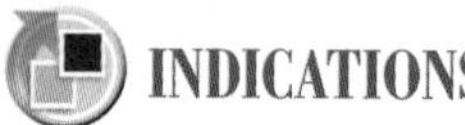

INDICATIONS

Flexible Sigmoidoscopy

The indications for flexible sigmoidoscopy are similar to those for rigid proctosigmoidoscopic examination, but the flexible scope has been shown to be superior in terms of the length of colon examined, diagnostic yield, and patient compliance. In contrast, examination with the rigid scope is associated with fewer complications, is less time-consuming, requires less training to perform, and is more accurate in assessing the distance of a rectal lesion from the anal verge. Furthermore, flexible instruments are more expensive and require greater maintenance. Flexible sigmoidoscopy has been found to yield pathology three times more often than rigid sigmoidoscopy. However, the length of bowel that can be examined with the flexible endoscope is often overestimated. By placing a clip marking the point at which 60 cm of the flexible sigmoidoscope was inserted and then confirming its position with a barium enema examination, Lehman and colleagues found that in only 81% of patients was the entire sigmoid colon visualized. This study emphasizes the importance of utilizing various straightening maneuvers when negotiating the sigmoid colon.

Flexible sigmoidoscopy is not a substitute for colonoscopy or radiologic evaluation of the colon when a complete assessment of the entire colonic mucosa is indicated, such as when occult blood is present or when polyps have been documented. Flexible sigmoidoscopy indications can be divided into two main groups: diagnostic and therapeutic.

Diagnostic

- Polyp or cancer screening
- Evaluation of GI complaints when colonoscopy is not indicated

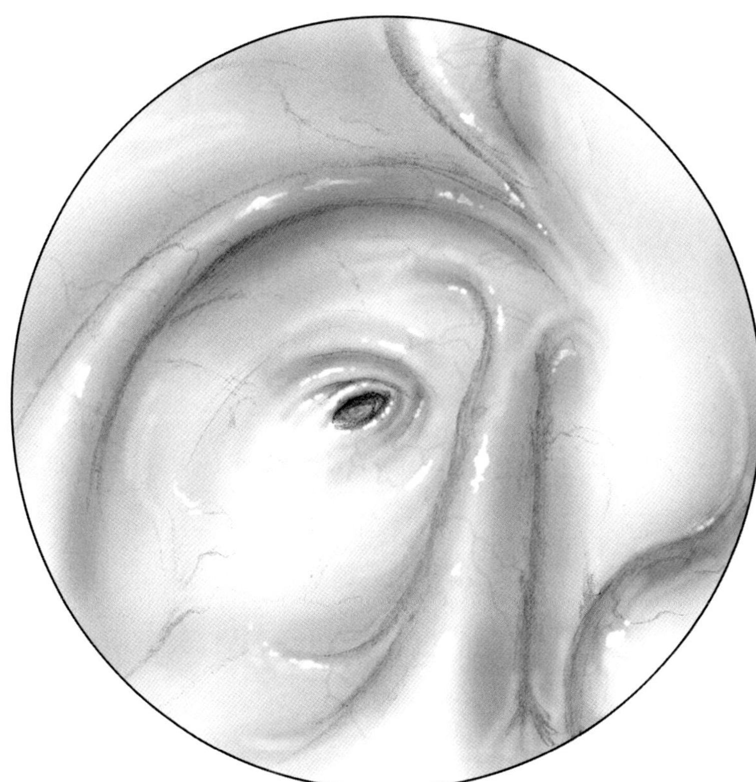

Fig. 45-3. The characteristic endoscopic landmarks that identify the cecum.

- Interim polyp and cancer surveillance between colonoscopic examinations
- Evaluation of questionable radiographic findings within the range of the instrument
- Confirmation of radiographic findings within the range of the instrument
- Follow-up examination in patients with inflammatory bowel disease
- Diagnosis of colonic ischemia
- Differential diagnosis of diverticular disease and malignancy
- Inspection of colonic anastomoses within the range of the instrument

Therapeutic

- Detorsion of a sigmoid volvulus
- Decompression of a over-distended bowel
- Removal of a foreign body within the range of the instrument
- Dilation of a stricture within the range of the instrument

It should be specifically noted that electrocautery should not be used during flexible sigmoidoscopy unless the patient has undergone a complete purgative preparation as used for colonoscopy. Explosive mixtures of methane and hydrogen may be present if the colon has not been adequately cleansed.

Colonoscopy

There is a long-standing debate about the relative merits of contrast radiography versus colonoscopy; each examination has its benefits and limitations. The advantages of double-contrast barium enema (DCBE) include its general availability, quick completion, lower cost, and low morbidity. In diverticular disease, a DCBE is actually superior at defining the number and anatomic distribution of the diverticula. For neoplastic disease, however, one study by Saito et al. showed that DCBE alone missed almost 50% of the lesions in the rectosigmoid region that were detected by endoscopy. In addition, DCBE inevitably results in considerably more radiation exposure, requires a cooperative patient, and is not without potential complications such as perforation, bleeding, or barium peritonitis. Virtual colonoscopy, or computerized tomography (CT) colonography, is a relatively new method of imaging the colon in which thin-section helical CT is used to generate high-resolution, two-dimensional axial images of the colon following a standard bowel preparation. Air or carbon dioxide is insufflated per rectum without sedation, and three-dimensional images of the colon are reconstructed offline (Fig. 45-4). Although comparative studies between virtual and conventional colonoscopy are still being conducted, a meta-analysis of data from 16 studies showed that virtual colonoscopy misses 18% of lesions greater than 1 cm. Advocates of virtual colonoscopy proclaim lower complication rates, less patient

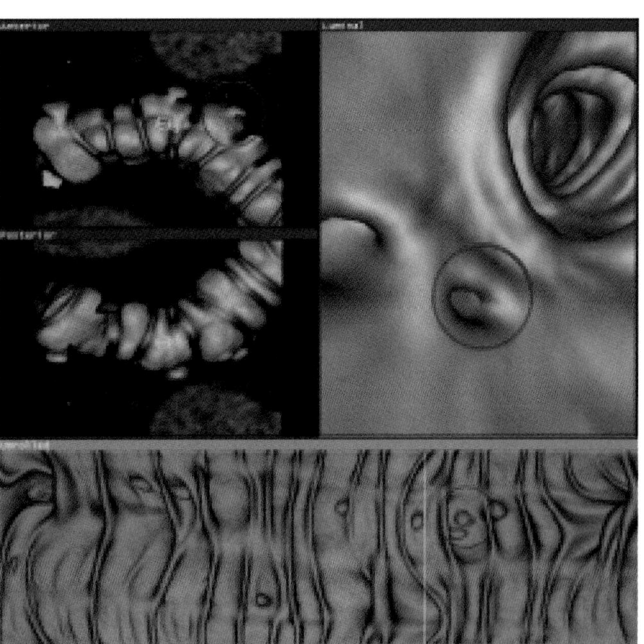

Fig. 45-4. A three-dimensional reconstruction of an abdominal computed tomography colonography (virtual colonoscopy).

discomfort, and concomitant evaluation for metastatic disease. However, colonoscopy demonstrates greater surface detail for determining mucosal vascular patterns in inflammatory conditions or the presence of arteriovenous malformations. Moreover, colonoscopy permits the performance of other diagnostic and therapeutic maneuvers, such as the biopsy of abnormal mucosa and removal of polyps and foreign bodies. The role of virtual colonoscopy as an effective screening tool for colorectal neoplasia is still under investigation. Primary colonoscopy without a preceding DCBE is indicated in specific clinical situations, such as when a patient has lower GI bleeding or when an index adenoma is discovered on rigid or flexible proctosigmoidoscopy. Primary colonoscopy is also indicated for patients at high risk for the development of colon and rectal neoplasia. This group includes patients with a strong family history of colon cancer and those with longstanding inflammatory bowel disease. It is generally agreed that colonoscopy supplements but does not replace DCBE in the evaluation of most colonic disorders. Indications for colonoscopy are outlined below.

Diagnostic

- Evaluation of suspected (or equivocal) abnormalities on DCBE
- Presence of a polyp on sigmoidoscopy or DCBE
- Unexplained GI bleeding, either overt or occult
- Unexplained iron deficiency or anemia
- Colorectal cancer screening (age greater than 50, family history of colorectal cancer)
- Surveillance of colonic neoplasia
- Follow-up evaluation after prior colorectal surgery
- Evaluation and follow-up of inflammatory bowel disease
- Clinically significant diarrhea of unexplained origin
- Intraoperative colonoscopy for localization of a lesion (e.g., polyp, bleeding source)

Therapeutic

- Treatment of a bleeding lesion
- Excision of colonic polyps
- Reduction of a sigmoid volvulus
- Foreign body removal
- Decompression of a dilated colon
- Balloon dilation of a stenotic lesion (e.g., anastomotic stricture)
- Palliative treatment of a stenosing or bleeding neoplasm

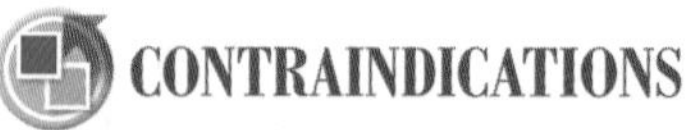

CONTRAINDICATIONS

There are relatively few absolute contraindications to endoscopic examination of the lower GI tract. Both flexible sigmoidoscopy and colonoscopy should not be performed in patients suspected of having a perforated viscus, severe acute diverticulitis, or fulminant colitis. Relative contraindications to performing these procedures include patients who are uncooperative, have a poor or inadequate bowel preparation, or have a poor general medical condition, such as a recent myocardial infarction or pulmonary embolism. Caution should be exercised in the presence of coexisting abdominal pathology, such as hypersplenism or aortic aneurysm.

PREOPERATIVE PLANNING

The success of an endoscopic procedure is not entirely dependent on the technical skills of the endoscopist. In addition to an adequate bowel preparation, the patient's understanding of the procedure is very important. Experience has shown that well-informed patients who fully comprehend the implications, circumstances, and potential risks and benefits of the endoscopy show less apprehension and less anxiety during the actual procedure.

Conscious sedation is generally not required for flexible sigmoidoscopy but may be advantageous for certain patients, including children, extremely anxious patients, or those with painful perianal disease. Although recent studies question the need for the routine use of conscious sedation for colonoscopy, most endoscopy centers still use a combination of an opiate analgesic plus a benzodiazepine administered intravenously for this procedure. There has been a trend toward having anesthesiologists or nurse anesthetists administer sedation with agents such as propofol or fentanyl. In some states, registered nurses under strict protocol have been administering propofol or fentanyl in order to reduce costs. More recently, patient-controlled sedation, where patients administer their own medication, has been touted as being safe and effective and with potentially less risk of overdosing. The American Society for Gastrointestinal Endoscopy (ASGE) has developed guidelines for the use of monitoring devices during conscious sedation, but mechanical monitoring techniques such as pulse oximetry and continuous electrocardiography are not a substitute for an alert and competent endoscopy assistant. It is also imperative that the endoscopist have thorough knowledge of the pharmacology, indications and contraindications, recommended dosages, duration of action, side effects, and methods of reversal for each of the drugs used.

For flexible sigmoidoscopy, one or two saline or phosphate enemas are usually satisfactory for adequate visualization. Colonoscopy, on the other hand, requires a more complete bowel-cleansing program including dietary restriction and purgation. Because colonoscopy is usually performed as an outpatient procedure in a hospital, clinic, or office setting, most patients undergo bowel preparation at home. However, frail, elderly, and mentally disabled patients may require hospitalization for supervised bowel preparation. The extent of preparation required depends on the clinical indication; for example, a patient who has profuse diarrhea or has undergone a subtotal colonic resection will require much less preparation than an elderly patient with chronic constipation. According to ASGE guidelines, patients with active colitis and diarrhea should not receive enemas or lavage.

Diagnostic accuracy and therapeutic safety of colonoscopy depends on the quality of the colonic preparation. The most widely used bowel preparation for colonoscopy utilizes an electrolyte solution containing with polyethylene glycol (PEG) as an additional osmotic agent; examples are Colyte (Schwarz Pharma; Milwaukee, WI), GoLYTELY, and, NuLYTELY (both Braintree Laboratories Inc; Braintree, MA). Due to problems with patient compliance, other, more palatable preparations have been sought. Low-volume PEG preparations such as HalfLytely or MiraLAX (both Braintree Laboratories Inc) contain two liters of PEG compared to the standard four liters, and patients are instructed to use stimulant tablets prior to ingesting the PEG solution. Aqueous sodium phosphate in the form of Fleet Phosphosoda ACCU-PREP (Fleet Pharmaceuticals; Lynchburg, VA) is a low-volume hyperosmotic solution that has been shown to be safe, effective, less expensive, and better tolerated than the standard PEG preparations. Alternatively, sodium phosphate monobasic/dibasic is available in the tablet form Visicol (InKine Pharmaceutical Co., Inc.; Blue Bell, PA). Because of the osmotic mechanism of action of these two preparations, significant fluid and electrolyte shifts can occur and caution is advised in pediatric and elderly patients, patients with congestive heart failure, or those with renal or liver disease. Acute phosphate nephropathy, a form of acute renal failure, has been reported. Individuals at risk for acute phosphate nephropathy include elderly patients, those with underlying kidney disease or decreased intravascular volume, and those using medications that affect renal perfusion or function. All bowel preparations require a no-residue or low-residue diet 24 to 48 hours prior to colonoscopy.

Practice parameters have been published by the American Society of Colon and Rectal Surgeons regarding the use of prophylactic antibiotics. In general, a prophylactic antibiotic is not routinely indicated because lower GI endoscopy carries a low risk of significant bacteremia. However, in certain high-risk individuals, such as those with a prior history of infective endocarditis or with a prosthetic heart valve, surgically created systemic pulmonary shunt, or recent (within 1 year) insertion of a prosthetic vascular graft, broad-spectrum prophylaxis is recommended. Medications such as aspirin, nonsteroidal anti-inflammatory agents, anticoagulants, and iron-containing compounds should ideally be discontinued at least 1 week prior to colonoscopy.

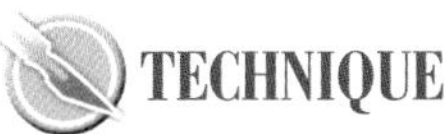

TECHNIQUE

Colonoscopic intubation is a marvelous example of the interaction between human and machine. Most examinations are rather straightforward, while a good many require at least some manipulations of note and a sufficient number of procedures challenge the examiner to draw from his or her bag of tricks. It is vital that the endoscopist have a thorough understanding of the relationship between the relatively unforgiving scope and the variably compliant colon. If the colon were an absolutely fixed structure, a totally different instrument would have been constructed to afford optimal intubation. There would be no manipulation of the organ itself; the instrument would simply be advanced and would follow the contour of the organ. But the colon is not rigid and it is not fixed in position. Although there are areas of the colon that are relatively fixed, the wall of the colon at these points is usually still quite compliant. Consequently, unlike intubation of other structures such as the esophagus, the ureter, and the aorta, successful colon intubation depends in great part on appropriate manipulation of the compliant structure.

Successful intubation makes use of a number of individual maneuvers. These include tip deflection, shaft torquing, and shaft dithering. Combinations of these maneuvers are used, along with gas insufflation and deflation, patient positioning, and abdominal pressure.

Tip Deflection

Clearly it is not difficult to see how the articulating deflection tip is the essential element of the colonoscope, the one that makes retrograde examination of the colon possible. Deflection permits the endoscopist to look around a bend or fold to see in the direction he or she needs to go. Folds can be pressed against the wall so that small lesions that might otherwise stay hidden are exposed. This articulation is essential during therapeutic maneuvers to aim a snare or biopsy forceps in the proper direction.

This very characteristic, the articulating tip, becomes what is probably the single biggest impediment to intubation. For the novice endoscopist, it is also the most likely source of injury. This occurs because a gentle curve forms along the distal 10 to 12 cm of the scope as the tip is deflected from a straight position,. As deflection increases to beyond the 90-degree level, the radius of this curve becomes shorter, and the distribution of forces against the colon wall changes abruptly. The application of extreme deflection to both dial controls does not have the effect that one would predict. This can be observed with any scope before the procedure is started. Maximum application of the up/down dial will give a 180-degree deflection in the up direction (Fig. 45-5). Similarly, maximum application of the left/right dial will give 180 degrees to the right. One would think that maximum application of both dials would give 180-degree deflection halfway between up and right. Instead, there is only a little movement of the tip between the two quadrants, but there is a much more dramatic overtightening of the deflection bend to well beyond 180 degrees. Longitudinal advancement of the scope no longer follows the tip of the scope but is instead distributed along the side of the deflection bend against the bowel wall. At a deflection of 180 degrees, which can usually be achieved with extreme application of a single deflection dial, the force to the bowel wall is distributed over a relatively small surface area (Fig. 45-6, page 450). This can easily lead to serosal injury or frank perforation of the bowel. The fact that the bowel under view seems to be getting farther away rather than closer as the scope is advanced should alert the operator that he or she is using extreme deflection. It is impossible for the scope to advance along the axis of the colon with this configuration. On occasion, extreme deflection must be used to find the lumen; once it is found, the deflection should be eased, preferably to less than 90 degrees, before attempting further advancement of the scope.

The following generalizations relative to deflection control can be made:

- Use the least amount of tip deflection possible.
- Use the up/down dial alone for most deflection needs and resist applying both controls.
- Release deflection when the lumen is found.

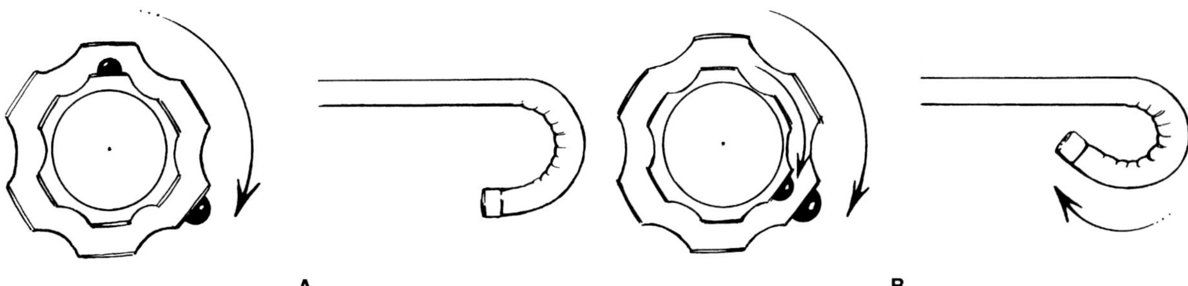

Fig. 45-5. Dual coaxial control knobs determine the degree of tip deflection. **A.** Full deflection of the up/down or left/right controls results in approximately 180 degrees of deflection. **B.** Full deflection of both controls results in overdeflection.

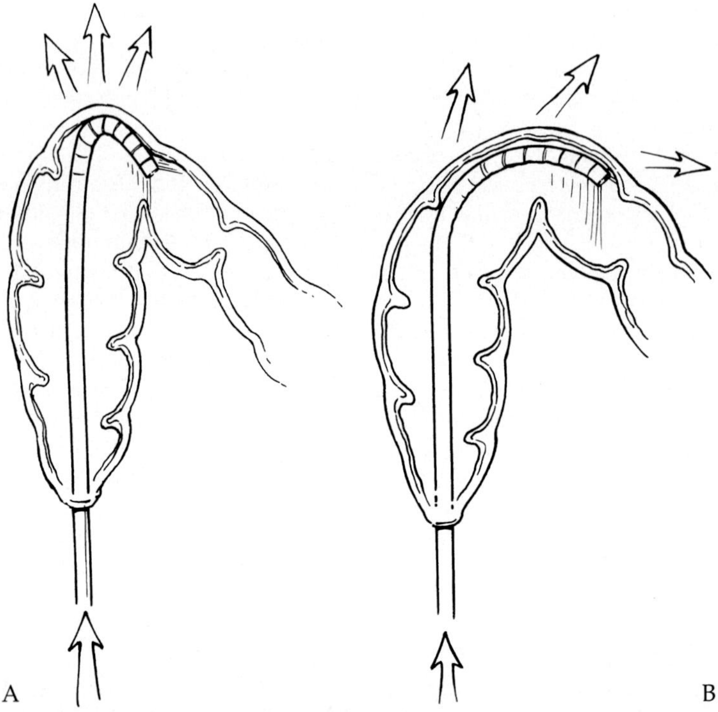

Fig. 45-6. Tip deflection. **A.** If severe tip deflection is applied around a flexure, the bend in the deflection tip becomes the leading edge of the scope pushing against the bowel wall. **B.** Once the lumen is visualized, the deflection tip should be flattened to transmit advancement force in a forward direction.

Shaft Torquing

Torquing the colonoscope shaft is an essential maneuver for effective intubation and good surface visualization during extubation. If the shaft is straight and there is a modest deflection to the scope's tip, the lumen can most easily be located by twisting or torquing against the inside surface of the bend in the colon. This torquing into the lumen is often more effective than searching for the lumen with the deflection tip.

As more scope is introduced, the response to torquing becomes more complex. If there is a simple alpha loop in the sigmoid, the effect of clockwise torquing, especially when combined with withdrawal, is to reduce the loop and to accordion the sigmoid onto the scope without loss of intubation distance. Once reduced, this sigmoid loop will usually have a tendency to reform, particularly if counterclockwise torque is applied during scope advancement. Therefore, if a reduced, redundant sigmoid loop tends to reform, it is best to advance the scope while maintaining clockwise torque. One can readily sense this tendency to reform the loop in the following way: Apply clockwise torque and the scope will appear to advance; apply counterclockwise torque and the scope will tend to lose ground.

On occasion, the sigmoid will have two major complete loops that are created during intubation. Both of these loops are almost always reducible. However, in this situation, the first loop is removed by counterclockwise rotation and the second by clockwise rotation. Removing both loops is usually essential before intubation proximal to the descending colon can be accomplished. Once both loops are removed, the sigmoid is once again most likely to stay straightened by maintaining clockwise torque. This is not always compatible with the task to be accomplished at the distal end of the scope.

Torque also becomes very important in manipulations around the hepatic flexure. If the transverse colon is able to be held in the upper abdominal cavity (e.g., the scope takes a straight line to the hepatic flexure), clockwise torque is usually beneficial as the gently deflected tip is directed down the ascending colon. If the transverse colon is redundant, stretching down toward the pelvis, the hepatic flexure is then approached from below. By the time the ascending colon is viewed, there is a rather sharp deflection of the tip. Once again, gentle scope withdrawal combined with clockwise torquing and intermittent desufflation work together to broaden the hepatic flexure and drop the scope down into the ascending colon and cecum.

During extubation, torquing is an extremely important manipulation for efficient examination of the colon surface. As the scope is withdrawn, the right hand should remain on the shaft while the left hand supports the scope head, with the thumb free to move the up/down control to make small deflections. Torquing while the scope is withdrawn and readvanced 10 to 20 cm at a time affords a thorough view of the entire colon surface. This permits the colon that has been accordioned onto the scope to be dropped off a bit at a time. If the scope is simply withdrawn while both hands of the dial controls are used and no torquing is applied, the view behind prominent folds is likely to be insufficient. In addition, if the colon is quite redundant, it will likely fly off the scope at an uncontrollable rate.

The following generalizations relative to shaft torquing can be made:

- Clockwise torque straightens the sigmoid; counterclockwise torque promotes loop formation.
- Torquing is more effective than tip deflection for negotiating bends and for surface examination.

Scope Advancement/Withdrawal (Dithering)

If the colon were a simple noncompliant tube without redundancy or irregularity, colonoscopic intubation would be a rather simple endeavor of advancing the scope while following the tip. Occasionally, especially if there has been a prior sigmoid resection, colonoscopy may demand no more than simple scope advancement. However, straight advancement in an intact colon usually promotes the development of loops, stretching the colon. When progression of the scope is not impeded by severe tip deflection, the colon can be encouraged to accordion along the length of the scope. This is most likely to occur if the scope is repeatedly advanced and withdrawn. In some areas, particularly distally, this is most effective if it is performed with short, rapid strokes, referred to as "dithering" the scope. Elsewhere, such as in the transverse colon, this maneuver is often performed with long, gentle strokes of 30 to 50 cm.

Gas Insufflation

Insufflation of gas is essential to the effective visualization and safe performance of a colonoscopy. However, insufflation should be used sparingly. Excess gas, especially filtered room air, can cause distention that results in extreme discomfort and vasovagal reaction. If the examination is taken into the distal ileum, even a very short period of insufflation may result in a great deal of small-bowel gas accumulation. For this reason, it is becoming more common to use CO_2 as the insufflating gas as it is quickly desorbed from the intestinal lumen. Excessive intraluminal gas often works against intubation progress, particularly at a flexure or during negotiation of a loop. The distention effectively pushes the more proximal side of the loop or flexure away. The corner to be negotiated becomes more acute and consequently harder to negotiate. This is most apparent at the hepatic flexure, where the deflection tip is sharply angulated into the distal ascending colon. As air is introduced, the ileocecal valve in the distance is seen to move farther away. Consequently, the endoscopist should take advantage of this while removing air during clockwise torque. The ascending colon will collapse back onto the scope, bringing the cecum into closer proximity to the end of the scope.

Patient Positioning

Although no single patient position is distinctly preferable to others, the construction of most endoscopes and the right-handedness of most physicians favor a left lateral position. Colostomy and ileostomy patients may be examined in the lateral or supine position. In patients with poor or absent abdominal wall muscle tone, such as patients with paraplegia or prior dehiscence, examination in the prone position may overcome this disadvantage. An elastic abdominal binder can also provide artificial abdominal wall resistance.

Changing the position of the patient during the examination when forward advancement of the scope becomes difficult is often very helpful. After all, rotating the patient 90 degrees to the left is similar to torquing the scope 90 degrees to the right. After an excessively redundant sigmoid loop has been reduced, broad pressure from just right of the umbilicus and directed toward the left iliac fossa will discourage its reformation. Likewise, in the case of a redundant transverse colon dipping deeply into the pelvis, abdominal pressure from just below the umbilicus and directed cephalad will assist entry into the ascending colon.

Abdominal Pressure

An alternative is to apply a more generalized abdominal pressure by rolling the patient into the prone position once the sigmoid has been negotiated and is felt to be reduced. This rotation is not performed unless intubation progress is hung up. Most frequently, this position change is made at the hepatic flexure. If there is no need to change patient position, the entire examination is performed in the left lateral decubitus position. If there is difficulty with entry into the ascending colon in the prone position, the patient is rotated into the right lateral decubitus position. This is frequently the last additional maneuver that one has to perform in the case of a recalcitrant hepatic flexure. It is presumed that in this position, pressure from the liver may encourage the flexure to be flattened just enough to allow the scope to slip down to the ascending colon.

Many endoscopists prefer to perform much of the examination with the patient in the supine position. We find that this position is somewhat difficult for the endoscopist. If the scope is brought out between the legs, there is minimal working room between the anus and the bed for shaft manipulation. If the scope is brought out beneath the raised right leg, one continually has to reposition the leg, unless there is an assistant to attend to this.

General Approach to the Examination

Before the start of the procedure, it is important to check that the scope is working properly, that the suction line is attached and switched on, and that air insufflation and water for lens washing are adequate. During the procedure, the expert colonoscopist is able to perform an expedient and thorough examination by avoiding the formation of bowel loops that interfere with intubation while utilizing loops that facilitate intubation. The experienced colonoscopist detects that a loop is starting to form from subtle cues: the loss of one-to-one correspondence of instrument insertion and image movement, a gradual increase in resistance to forward motion, and signs of patient discomfort. Withdrawing the scope and losing ground to gain more proximal intubation on subsequent attempts is almost always a prudent initial maneuver.

Advancement of the scope should nearly always be under direct or nearly direct vision. The "slide-by" technique, whereby the tip of the scope is burrowed into the colon wall, should be avoided. Although it is often necessary to have less than a totally clear view of the lumen, insertion for any distance when the endoscopist is blind to lumen orientation is strongly discouraged. One may be treading on dangerous ground if the colon surface blanches or the patient experiences pain.

There is a strong desire to not lose ground. During a difficult colonoscopy, one may have spent some time getting to an area that seems to have no outlet. Because of an abrupt bend, the next segment eludes identification. The endoscopist may persist in vain, searching for a way out and not wanting to give up what has already been accomplished. Instead, it is more likely that the difficulty is being accentuated by failure to ease the scope. One should never be reluctant to withdraw shaft length when progress is arrested. Often, withdrawal is the very maneuver that is needed to advance. This point cannot be overemphasized. Examination of the mucosa for abnormalities and therapeutic interventions for polyps, tumors, etc. should usually be performed when the scope is slowly withdrawn after maximum intubation.

Although not required for most examinations, fluoroscopy is invaluable in the training of new colonoscopists and often helpful during difficult cases. Although flexible sigmoidoscopy and colonoscopy will usually be performed in the outpatient setting, it is worthwhile observing a few examinations under fluoroscopic control to appreciate the various configurations assumed by the sigmoidoscope.

Sedation

Without sedation, colonoscopic manipulation of the entire colon is often uncomfortable and sometimes frankly painful. Although it has clearly been shown that a modest proportion of patients can undergo colonoscopy without sedation, many endoscopists prefer to initiate the examination after administration of a minimal intravenous dose of a short-acting narcotic and a benzodiazepine such as midazolam hydrochloride (Versed). Supplementation of this base dose, if required, is determined by the patient's sensory and physiologic reactions. The primary objective is not to avoid medication but rather to provide a safe and comfortable examination. All hospitals and outpatient endoscopy suites should have rules and procedures for conscious sedation that usually include CPR training of the staff, a monitoring person to record vital signs during the procedure, and monitoring equipment to record blood pressure an oxygen saturation. If necessary, naloxone hydrochloride (Narcan) can be used after the procedure to expedite recovery.

EXAMINATION PERFORMANCE

Rectal Examination

A digital rectal examination is an essential starting point in every patient. To begin with, it is not unusual to find significant local pathology, such as large hemorrhoids, anal fissures, or prostatic nodules or masses. In addition, digital rectal examination allows one to gauge anal sphincter tone; poor tone will make it difficult to retain insufflated air. A tight or strictured anus may require some gentle dilation to accommodate the scope. Third, the examination mentally prepares the patient to have the instrument inserted and provides lubrication for tube insertion.

Anorectal Intubation

After lubricating the instrument tip but not the lens, the scope is inserted with lateral (not end-on) pressure. Insertion requires two hands: one to separate the buttocks and the other to hold the tip of the scope. It is helpful to have an assistant hold the control section or place it over the endoscopist's right shoulder. Due to anatomic and technical factors, it is often difficult to initially visualize the rectal ampulla. The anal canal is oriented in the direction of the umbilicus for a short distance, at which point it joins the rectal ampulla, whose axis is abruptly posteriorly oriented toward the sacrum. However, the tip deflection mechanism may respond poorly at this level, because the greater portion of the deflecting system is still outside the anorectum and has nothing to work against. It is not until the bulk of the deflecting section has traversed the sphincter mechanism that the examiner starts to have control of tip deflection. Once the scope is inserted approximately 10 cm above the anal verge, tip deflection responds properly, and the middle and upper rectum can be clearly visualized. An understanding of the limitations of tip deflection when restricted by the sphincter mechanism can avoid this initial problem. Proximal intubation for the next few centimeters into the rectosigmoid and distal sigmoid colon does not generally represent a problem even to the most inexperienced, but once the rectosigmoid is reached (15 to 20 cm), the stage is set for the technique of sigmoid intubation.

With the instrument tip seated in the rectosigmoid, one takes the control section with the left hand while the right hand is positioned on the scope shaft. Throughout the rest of the examination, this hand placement will be the basic posture used.

Sigmoid-Descending Colon Intubation

Properly negotiating the sigmoid colon is often challenging and sets the stage for the remainder of the examination. Avoidance of bowel-loop formation not only is more comfortable for the patient but also allows a more expeditious examination of a greater length of colon with less length of scope. The three methods of intubating the sigmoid colon are elongation, looping (alpha maneuver), and accordioning (dithering/torquing). Although these are distinctly different techniques, they are not mutually exclusive solutions to the same problem. In recognizing these basic differences in technique, the operator can more deliberately and effectively control the process of intubation.

Intubation by Elongation

Intubation by elongation merely means that the scope is inserted until either the scope no longer advances or no more endoscope is available. One relies on the deflection tip to lead the way as long as the lumen is in view. This is the simplest and most perfunctory approach: no fancy maneuvers, just doing what appears obvious. Indeed, this is probably the most common approach undertaken with flexible fiberoptic sigmoidoscopy. Most often, this technique merely stretches a redundant sigmoid until the first major angulation is encountered. If there is only a single sigmoid loop and the sigmoid-descending junction is reached, further intubation may be accomplished with clockwise torquing, shaft withdrawal, and flattening of the deflection tip (Fig. 45-7).

Intubation by Looping (Alpha Maneuver)

The relative mobility of the sigmoid colon, which is fixed proximally and distally, is best appreciated under fluoroscopy, where a loop resembling the Greek letter α is intentionally created to permit passage of the tip of the scope into the distal descending colon, followed by reduction of this loop for further advancement. The alpha loop is promoted by counterclockwise rotation of the scope while it is advanced through the sigmoid until the tip is securely within the descending colon. By encouraging the mid to proximal sigmoid, through counterclockwise torque, to occupy the right lower quadrant, the sigmoid-descending junction is flattened, providing a less acute angle to negotiate. Next, the loop is reduced by withdrawing the scope while maintaining clockwise rotation on the shaft (Fig. 45-8, page 454). One can assume that this reduction is working when the image advances despite considerable scope withdrawal. Once derotation has been accomplished, the scope can be advanced toward the splenic flexure by maintaining clockwise torque during advancement of the shaft. This technique is an expeditious way to negotiate the entire sigmoid colon when only a moderate degree of redundancy is present and multiple, tightly adherent loops are absent. If several adherent loops are present, this technique is technically impossible and only serves to increase the level of discomfort for the patient. If the loop cannot be reduced on entry into the descending colon, then one should maintain the loop, traverse the splenic flexure, and attempt derotation after the scope is well into the transverse colon. No effort should be made to derotate with the deflection tip hooked around the splenic flexure.

Intubation by Accordioning the Bowel (Dithering/Torquing)

This approach most consistently enables the examination of the greatest length of colon with the least amount of scope. In contrast to the first two techniques, in which the scope is advanced up into the colon, the accordionization method should be viewed as bringing the colon down onto the scope.

This technique employs simultaneous application of both dithering and torquing. While the shaft is being advanced approximately 6 to 10 cm, a small amount of counterclockwise torque of about 45 to 60 degrees is applied. The process is reversed by applying clockwise torque and simultaneous withdrawal of the scope for the same length. This cycle is repeated in a rhythmic manner at a rate of about one cycle per second, but without net advancement of the shaft. It is useful to hold the shaft of the scope close to the anus to avoid overadvancing. Although the first few dithering/torquing cycles may appear to accomplish little, by rhythmically continuing this motion the cumulative effect is to pleat a short segment of sigmoid colon

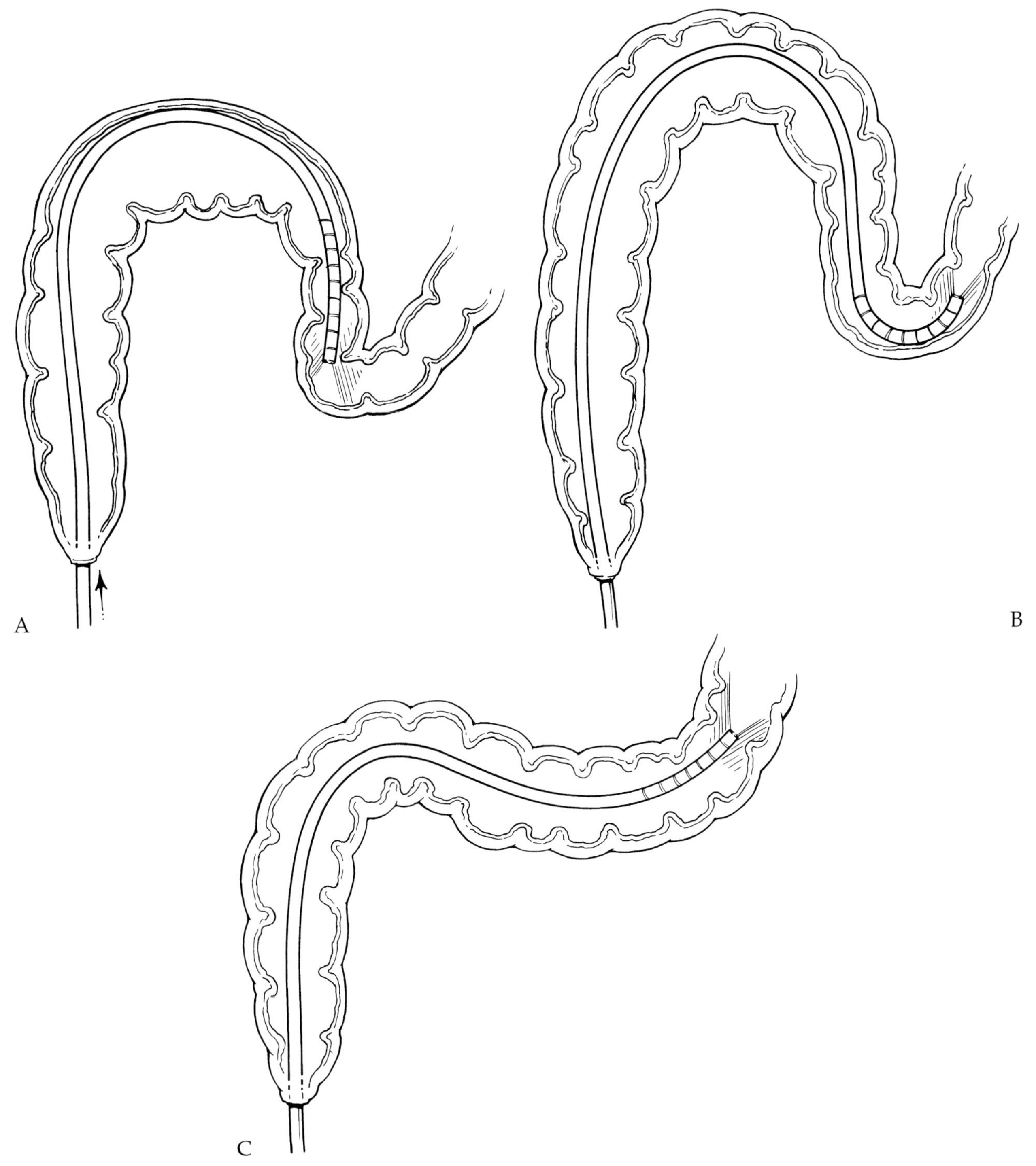

Fig. 45-7. Intubation by elongation. **A.** The scope is advanced into the proximal sigmoid. **B.** The deflection tip is turned into the distal descending colon. **C.** The sigmoid is accordioned onto the scope by simultaneous clockwise torquing, shaft withdrawal, and flattening of the deflection tip.

onto the scope. As one acquires experience with this technique, it soon becomes apparent that the cyclic rhythm, amount of torque, degree of tip deflection, and shaft advancement distance are all variables that can by altered to achieve maximum effect. If this technique is successful, the descending colon can be readily intubated as far as the splenic flexure by applying clockwise torque during shaft advancement with minimal deflection of the tip. With this approach, the endoscopist is attempting to straighten the colon as he or she progresses, rather than intentionally creating a loop that has to be removed later. Several principles should be kept in mind when this technique is performed:

- This method should be started early in the process of intubation in the rectosigmoid to minimize the deflection angle.

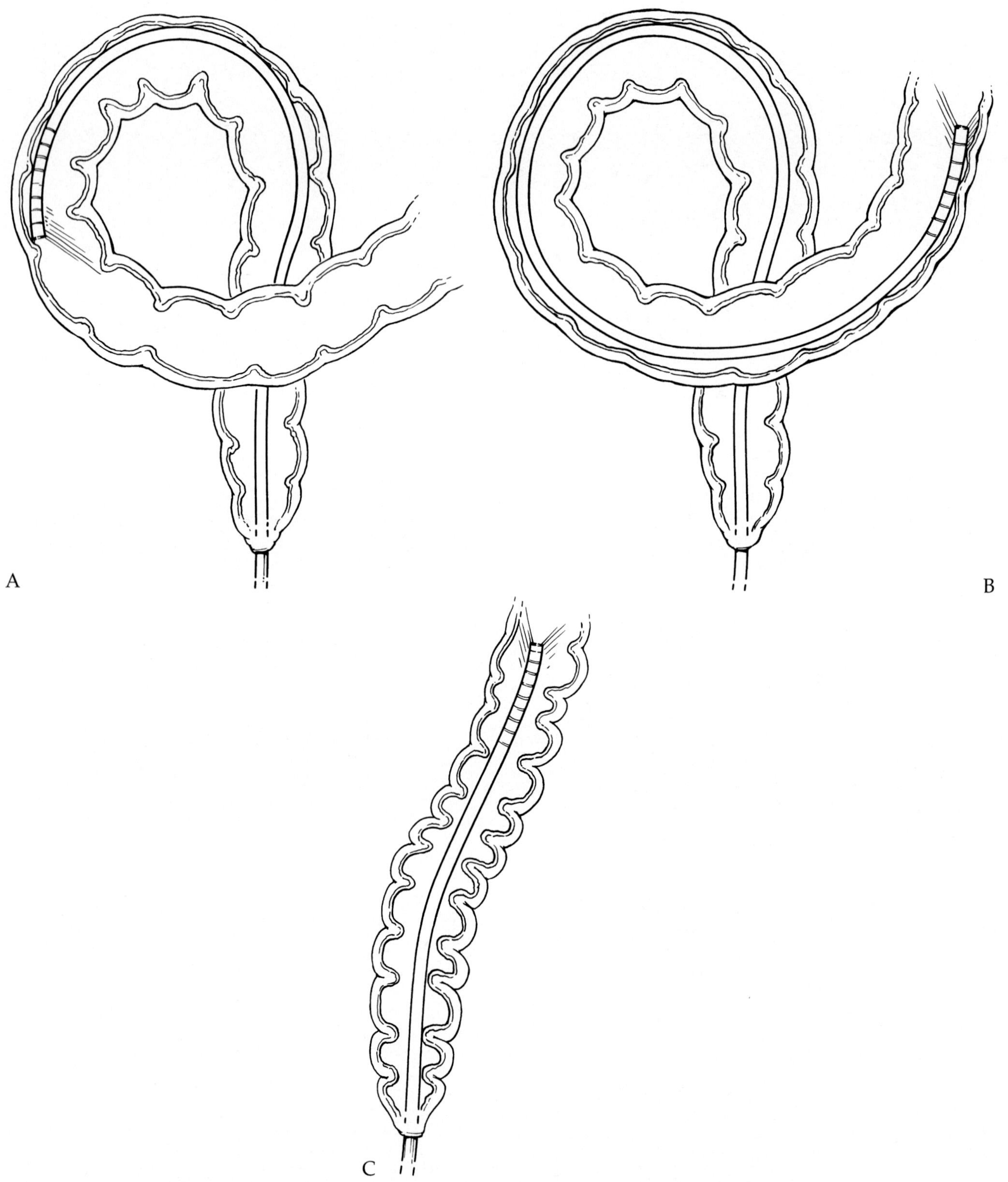

Fig. 45-8. Intubation by looping. **A.** The scope is inserted into the sigmoid with counterclockwise torquing during shaft advancement. **B.** The broad loop in the sigmoid flattens the sigmoid–descending colon junction. **C.** Clockwise rotation of the scope with shaft withdrawal accordions the sigmoid onto the scope.

- It is not always necessary to see the entire lumen, but the endoscopist should avoid pushing directly into the colonic wall.
- The endoscopist should resist the temptation to advance the scope as soon as the lumen is seen and instead continue with this process to maximize the accordioning of the entire sigmoid colon.
- Excessive gas insufflation is a deterrent to accordioning.

- If this technique is not successful, the endoscopist can then proceed with intentional looping.

Splenic Flexure and Transverse Colon Intubation

If the sigmoid colon has been accordioned onto the scope and is straightened into a gentle smooth curve, negotiating the splenic flexure is usually not difficult. Even if the flexure is quite high, the deflection can be rotated into the distal transverse colon without much difficulty. It is at this point that the hazard of excess deflection bend should be remembered. As soon as there is visual acquisition of the transverse colon, the degree of deflection must be eased to provide a gentle bend of less than 90 degrees. The lumen may be somewhat obscured by the outside wall, but it need not be entirely lost from view. However, in approximately 5% of individuals, there is reversal of the splenic flexure, which turns to the patient's left due to medial migration of the flexure on a false mesentery. This anomaly can cause difficulty in intubating the transverse colon and hepatic flexure. A straightening maneuver is required that involves counterclockwise rotation of the instrument shaft to convert the splenic flexure to a normal orientation. Entry into the transverse colon typically reveals a well defined triangular lumen.

Advancing the colonoscope through the transverse colon is usually uneventful. Difficulty may arise, however, if the transverse colon is redundant and assumes the configuration of the Greek letter γ. Changing the patient's position, using external pressure above the umbilicus, and/or dithering/torquing are useful techniques when progress is impeded. In the transverse colon, dithering/torquing is often best performed with long, 30- to 50-cm strokes rather than the short strokes used in the sigmoid.

Hepatic Flexure and Ascending Colon Intubation

The hepatic flexure is recognized by a widening of the lumen and a bluish discoloration of the wall superiorly, where the liver is in close proximity. The lumen to the ascending colon may be readily apparent or sharp angulation may lead one to believe that the cecum has been reached. Inability to proceed without also identifying specific cecal landmarks is nearly always evidence of incomplete intubation.

If the transverse colon can be negotiated straight across or straight down from a high splenic flexure, then intubation into the ascending colon can usually be accomplished by clockwise torquing, flattening of the deflection tip, and simultaneous gas aspiration (Fig. 45-9, page 456). These three mechanisms combine to drop the scope directly into the cecum. If the transverse colon is excessively redundant, it may not be possible to maintain it in the upper abdomen, even with abdominal pressure. In such cases, the midtransverse colon will have to be intentionally moved toward the pelvis, and the scope will approach the hepatic flexure from below rather than from across. Effectively, the deflection will have a 180-degree bend to negotiate. Once again, clockwise torquing, flattening deflection, and gas aspiration now combined with shaft withdrawal will be required for entry into the ascending colon. Negotiation of redundant proximal bowel is facilitated by the removal of sigmoid colon loops. If the hepatic flexure is not readily passed, then the patient should be positioned onto the abdomen. For hepatic flexures that continue to defy intubation, it is most helpful to place the patient in the right lateral decubitus position.

Cecal and Distal Ileum Intubation

The most reliable landmarks for visual confirmation of reaching the cecum are the appendiceal orifice, the tenia confluence, and the ileocecal valve (see Fig. 45-3). Palpation of the right lower quadrant with concomitant movement of the colon endoscopically and transillumination of the abdominal wall in the right iliac fossa are less dependable signs. Fluoroscopy is quite helpful but it must be kept in mind that the cecum is not always in the right iliac fossa.

On occasion, it is important to intubate the distal ileum, especially in the evaluation of inflammatory bowel disease. The success rate for this maneuver increases with experience. The tip of the colonoscope should be partially deflected toward the ileocecal valve, which lies 5 to 7 cm proximal to the base of the cecum. By slow withdrawal of the colonoscope, the tip of the scope is pressed against the valve orifice, prying on the upper lip of the valve. With gentle air insufflation, a view of the distal ileum is apparent by the ground-glass appearance of the mucosa. Insufflation should be kept to a minimum, as small-bowel gas rapidly extends proximally and is difficult to remove, leading to considerable postprocedure discomfort. Once again, using CO_2 as the insufflating gas for colonoscopy helps eliminate this problem.

Withdrawing the Scope

Inspection of the mucosa for abnormalities is usually best performed on withdrawal of the scope. Residual debris will have been removed from the colon, and the endoscopist will already have obtained an overview of the work that has to be performed. A systematic survey of the entire colonic mucosa is mandatory, and this is more easily and completely performed on withdrawal than on insertion. Reinspection of areas behind haustra and around flexures may be required. The instrument may have to be advanced and withdrawn intermittently over varying distances to ensure that abnormalities have not been overlooked. This is best performed by keeping the right hand on the scope shaft and torquing a slightly bent deflection tip first against one fold and then the next. If a considerable length of colon has been accordioned onto the scope, it will have to be removed a small amount at a time. Steady withdrawal will result in the colon flying off the scope without adequate evaluation.

Retroflexion of the Endoscope

Retroflexion of the endoscope within the rectum has been shown to increase the diagnostic yield of polyps by 1% to 2% without imposing much risk of perforation. However, retroflexion can lead to significant patient discomfort, especially as the maneuver is generally performed at the end of the procedure when sedation is wearing off. With the tip of the endoscope in the mid to proximal rectum (10 to 15 cm), both the up/down and right/left dials are maximally turned while torquing the shaft 45 to 90 degrees to visualize the most distal rectum. Here the scope can be seen emanating from the anal canal while the scope "looks back at itself." With gentle torquing of the scope, the entire distal rectum can be visualized, including the internal hemorrhoids and dentate line. Therapeutic maneuvers such as polypectomy can be difficult due to the acute angulation of the scope. Prior to removal, the scope should be straightened and as much insufflated air as possible should be removed with the suction.

Biopsy

Biopsy of a polyp or mass may be performed with (hot) or without (cold) the use of electrocautery. Electrocautery should only be used in patients who have undergone a complete bowel preparation to

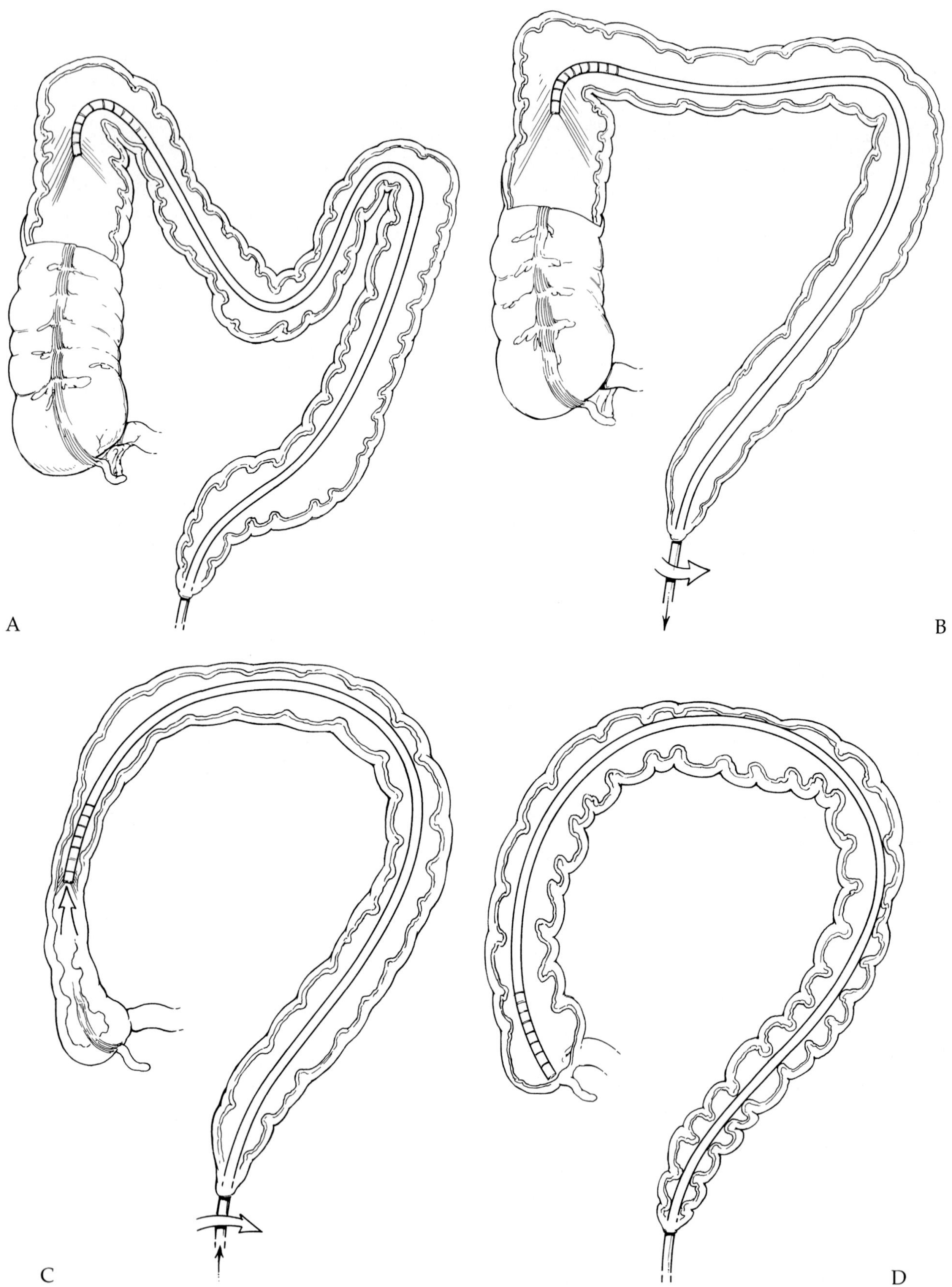

Fig. 45-9. Intubation of the ascending colon. **A.** The ascending colon is in view with sharp angulation at the hepatic flexure. **B.** The transverse colon is elevated into the upper abdomen during clockwise torquing and shaft withdrawal. **C.** Shaft advancement is accompanied by clockwise torquing, flattening of the deflection tip, and evacuation of air from the distended colon. **D.** Complete intubation to the cecum.

avoid the potential for explosion. All colonic biopsy tools should be inserted under direct vision, with the tip of the scope centered within the lumen at all times to reduce the risk of perforation. Keeping the scope as straight as possible with minimal tip deflection will allow easier passage of the catheter.

Hot biopsy is a useful technique that destroys small polyps by coagulating the base of the lesion to provide hemostasis while preserving the tissue inside the forceps for pathologic evaluation. The tip of the polyp is grasped by the forceps and pulled into the lumen, with care taken to avoid injury to the surrounding bowel. This process is facilitated by placement of the lesion in the 5 o'clock position prior to its being grasped. Only a brief application of coagulating current is necessary to cause blanching at the base of the polyp, and with gentle traction the lesion is removed.

Snare Polypectomy

One of the most significant advances in colon surgery during the past few decades has been the development of endoscopic polypectomy. The contrast between an 8-day hospitalization for an open or laparoscopic colotomy/polypectomy and a colonoscopy polypectomy performed in less than 1 hour is dramatic.

Several disposable snares are available for polyp excision. A hexagonal snare is preferred for most polyps. This configuration is most likely to hold its shape during difficult positioning or multiple excisions. For small lesions too large for hot biopsy management, a minisnare is convenient.

Prior to snare application, it is best to rotate the scope so that the polyp base is located at about 5 o'clock in the field of view. This will ensure that the polyp stays in view while the snare loop is positioned over it. In the case of a pedunculated polyp, the snare loop can be snugly tightened on the stalk under direct view. For a sessile polyp that has to be removed in a piecemeal fashion, each lobule excised can be clearly visualized.

Several techniques may be used for removing larger sessile lesions. A two-channel scope permits the endoscopist to combine both a snare and a grasper to manipulate the polyp. The snare is passed through one channel. A grasper or large biopsy forceps is placed in the second channel and passed out through the open loop of the snare. In this fashion, the recalcitrant polyp can be encouraged into the snare. On occasion, when removing a sessile polyp it is helpful to elevate it above the plane of the colon wall by injecting saline into the submucosa. This provides a greater margin between the muscularis propria and the polyp base. In addition, the greater tissue hydration makes for more efficient electrocoagulation.

Proper application of electrocautery is essential for a effective and safe polypectomy. There is no single combination of cutting and coagulation current or wattage that has to be used. A colonoscopist gradually develops confidence in his or her own electrosurgery method; it is surprising how varied these techniques may be. A generally effective approach involves using short bursts of monopolar blended cutting current while squeezing on the snare. By the use of intermittent bursts, deep tissue cooling is permitted, minimizing the likelihood of a full-thickness burn. Average-size polyps are suspended within the lumen to avoid collateral injury. If the polyp is too large to avoid wall contact, then surface contact should intentionally be maximized to avoid pinpoint areas of high current density (Fig. 45-10, page 458). At no time should electrosurgery be undertaken in the absence of a thorough colon preparation.

Removal of small tissue segments with the hot biopsy forceps requires a somewhat different technique. The hot biopsy forceps presents a very small surface area and consequently results in high current density with rapid, deep injury. Consequently, the grasped tissue should be well tented into the lumen. Two or three short bursts of current are usually sufficient to provide homeostasis and tissue destruction at the base. This can be seen as the development of pallor for a couple of millimeters around the jaws. At that point, the tissue specimen is abruptly drawn back into the scope channel. If one waits for the forceps to cut through on its own, an excess amount of wall damage will result.

Blood vessel lesions, such as vascular ectasia, are best treated with a bipolar electrode. Complete destruction can be accomplished with minimal risk of full-thickness wall injury.

Malignant polyps, even if technically removable at colonoscopy, may require subsequent resection. Such lesions are unlikely to be palpable at the time of operation. Accurate localization is important, particularly if intraluminal landmarks are absent and fluoroscopic control is unavailable. An injection of sterile particulate India ink can be applied submucosally with a sclerotherapy needle. This marker will persist indefinitely.

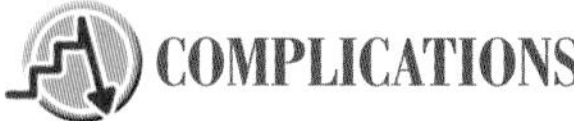

COMPLICATIONS

Complications following flexible sigmoidoscopy from eight collected series of more than 29,000 examinations between 1979 and 1988 reported no deaths, three perforations, and ten patients with rectal bleeding. The most common problems following flexible sigmoidoscopy were syncope and persistent abdominal pain. Following colonoscopy, the reported overall complication rate is higher when therapeutic maneuvers are employed, but the mortality remains low (0% to 0.02%) in large series. The most common complications after diagnostic colonoscopy are perforation (0.16%) followed by bleeding (0.03%), while bleeding is more common (0.66%) than perforation (0.33%) following polypectomy.

Hemorrhage is usually from a biopsy site but may also occur from a laceration to the mucosa by the endoscope or, less commonly, from tearing of the mesentery or splenic capsule. It is usually more common after resection of a large polyp or from inadequate coagulation of the stalk. Management depends on the timing and severity of the bleeding. Bleeding evident at the time of colonoscopy can usually be controlled by reapplication of the snare to the pedicle, if present, with electrocautery or by strangulation of the bleeding point for 5 to 10 minutes if additional electrocautery is deemed unsafe. Delayed hemorrhage typically occurs 10 to 14 days later due to sloughing of the coagulum, but most of these bleeds are self-limited and respond to conservative management. The incidence of delayed hemorrhage is increased in patients who have a coagulopathy or take anticoagulant or antiplatelet therapy. Repeat endoscopy with sclerotherapy or epinephrine injection, electrocautery, bipolar cautery, or heater-probe application may be necessary to control delayed hemorrhage. Rarely, angiographic techniques and/or operative intervention may be the only solution.

Perforation may be the result of excessive mechanical force or pneumatic pressure. Most perforations are located in the sigmoid colon and occur in patients with preexisting colonic disease. Perforation is diagnosed during the endoscopic procedure

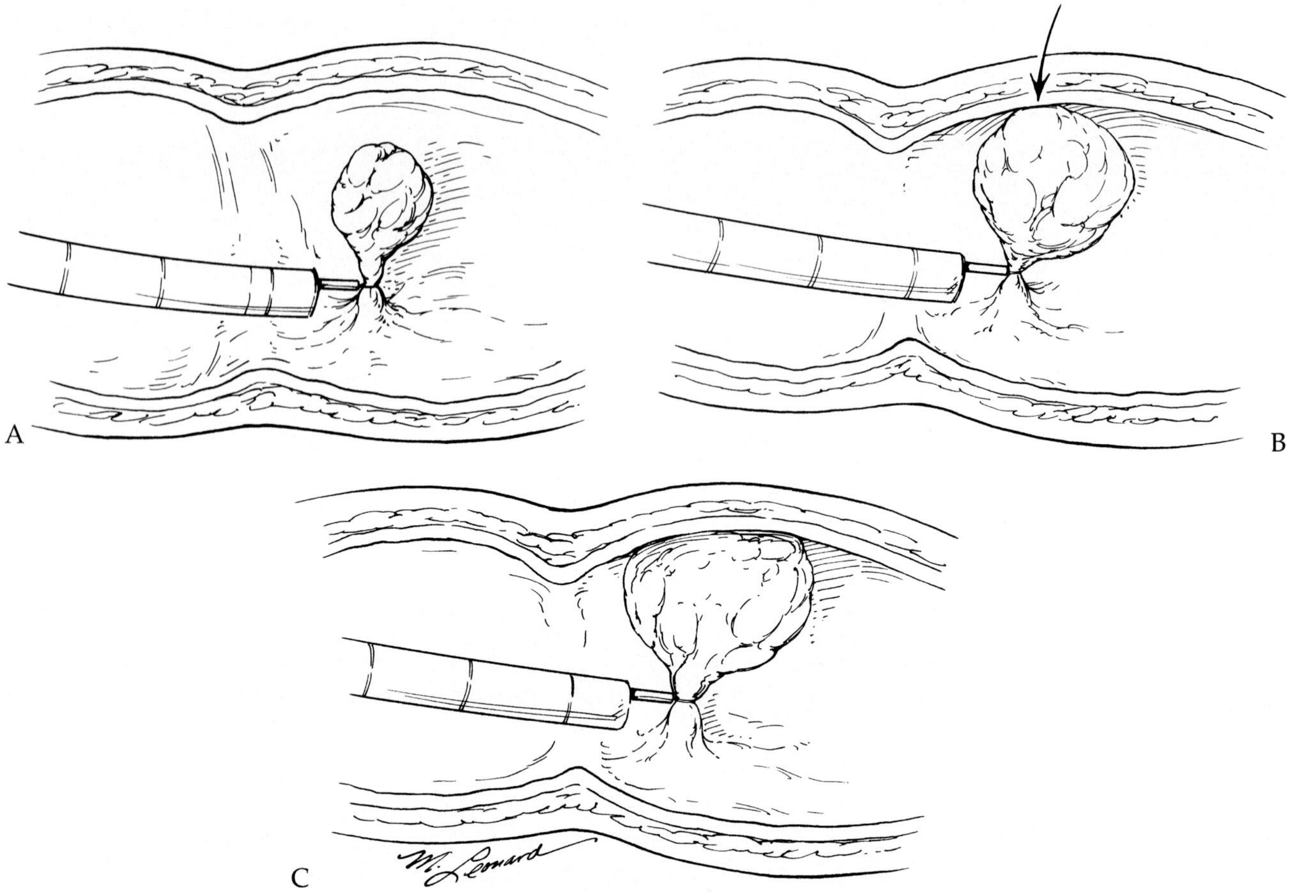

Fig. 45-10. Polypectomy. **A.** A pedunculated polyp is freely suspended in lumen, resulting in a safe excision. **B.** A polyp with a small contact area to the bowel wall (arrow) will result in high current density, leading to an unsafe excision. **C.** A polyp with a large contact area means a safe excision.

if intraperitoneal structures are visualized or should be suspected if the inability to maintain insufflation is encountered. Following endoscopy, perforation is suspected on the basis of symptoms and physical findings and confirmed by the presence of free intraperitoneal air on abdominal radiographs. The management of patients with perforation depends on the timing of presentation and the clinical status of the individual. If perforation is recognized immediately, surgical intervention is warranted and usually consists of primary repair. The approach to symptomatic patients with pneumoperitoneum should also be operative, especially when it is associated with underlying colonic disease. Controversy exists in the management of asymptomatic or minimally symptomatic patients with delayed presentation and pneumoperitoneum. There are reports of successful nonoperative therapy in selected stable patients with a well-prepared bowel and without peritonitis or obstruction. Management in these individuals consists of bowel rest and the administration of broad-spectrum antibiotics with careful observation for deterioration in clinical status.

Postpolypectomy coagulation syndrome or transmural burn syndrome occurs from a full-thickness thermal injury to the colon that is sealed by adjacent organs or omentum. Patients usually present with abdominal pain, fever, and leukocytosis without pneumoperitoneum 6 to 24 hours later. Care should be taken during polypectomy to avoid damaging the colonic wall opposite the lesion by minimizing contact time with the wall during application of the diathermy current. Bowel rest and broad-spectrum antibiotics with careful clinical follow-up are usually sufficient treatment for these patients.

Less frequently reported complications following colonoscopy with or without polypectomy are listed in Table 45-1. Despite these potential problems, flexible endoscopy of the lower GI tract can be undertaken with a very low morbidity. Awareness of these morbidities serves as a reminder to all endoscopists, particularly those in the learning phase, to maintain a high level of suspicion in all cases because many of these complications occur in seemingly innocuous procedures.

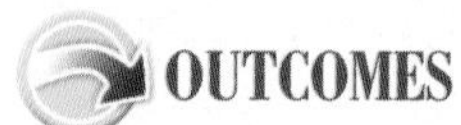

OUTCOMES

In an effort to determine the safety and efficacy of colonoscopy as performed by surgeons, the Society of American Gastrointestinal Endoscopic Surgeons (SAGES) Colonoscopy Outcomes Study Group orchestrated a prospective outcomes

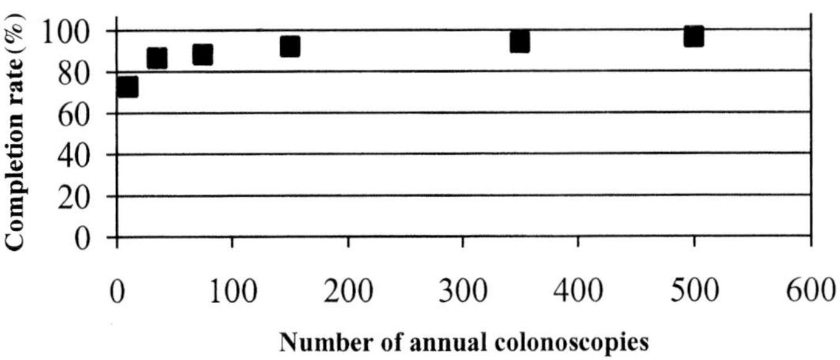

Fig. 45-11. Colonoscopy completion rate as a function of the number of colonoscopies performed per year.

study. Between April 1998 and September 1999, 13,580 colonoscopies performed by surgeons were prospectively entered into a database. For the 207 participating surgeons, consecutive case entry was required. Surgical residents contributed 1368 cases, fellows in specialty training contributed 879 cases, and staff with a median of slightly more than 20 years in practice performed 11,333 cases. Targeted end points included frequency of exam completion, duration of examination, and complications versus experience as measured in terms of prior or annual colonoscopy experience.

The likelihood of exam completion increased in proportion to the number of annual colonoscopies performed by the surgeon. Although there was rapid improvement up to the less than 50 exams/year level, there continued to be a steady improvement up through the greater than 500 exams/year level (Fig. 45-11).

In a similar fashion, the time required to perform the colonoscopy was inversely proportional to the number of annual colonoscopies performed by the surgeon. The mean completion time was nearly 30 minutes for surgeons who do fewer than 10 examinations per year. The time is cut by nearly one-half (16.3 ± 9.8 minutes) for those who perform more than 500 annual colonoscopies (Fig. 45-12).

Of considerable interest is the finding that the complication rate did not correlate with prior colonoscopy experience (ranging from <10 to >1000), annual colonoscopy experience (ranging from <10/year to >500/year), or level of training (resident, fellow, or staff). Bleeding and perforation complications each occurred at a 0.07% rate, which is very respectable when compared to other studies.

Based upon the findings from this large prospective study, in a surgical setting, efficiency and effectiveness improve with experience and performance volume. However, adverse encounters leading to significant complications are not experience dependent. Consequently, for surgeons, there does not appear to be a specific number of cases that should be mandated before credentialing is permitted. This speaks strongly against the requirement for "numbers" in the surgical setting.

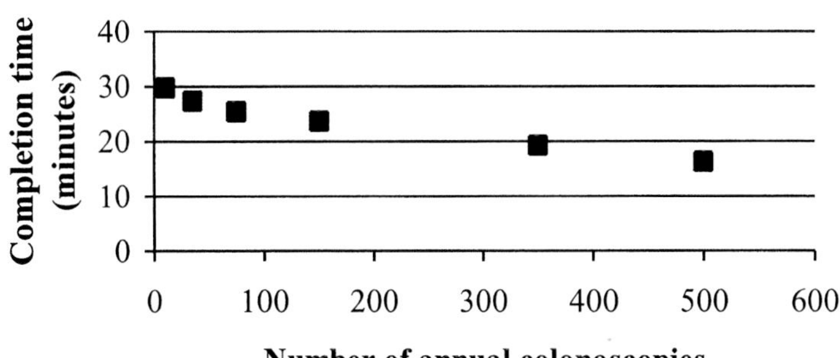

Fig. 45-12. Examination completion time as a function of the number of colonoscopies performed per year.

SUGGESTED READING

American College of Gastroenterology 68th Annual Scientific Meeting: Abstract 701.

A consensus document on bowel preparation prior to colonoscopy: Prepared by a task force from the ASCRS, ASGE, and SAGES. *Gastrointestinal Endoscopy* Volume 63, Nov. 7, 2006.

Baillie J. *Gastrointestinal endoscopy: basic principles and practice.* Oxford: Butterworth-Heinemann, Ltd, 1992.

Berk JE, ed. *Bockus gastroenterology,* 4th ed. Philadelphia: W.B. Saunders, 1985.

Coller JA. Technique of flexible fiberoptic sigmoidoscopy. *Surg Clin North Am* 1980;60: 465–479.

Corman ML. *Colon and rectal surgery.* 5th ed. Philadelphia: J.B. Lippincott Co, 2004.

Hunt RH, Waye JD, eds. *Colonoscopy: techniques, clinical practice and color atlas.* Cambridge: Chapman and Hall, Ltd., 1981.

Lehman GA, Buchner DM, Lappas JC. Anatomical extent of fiberoptic sigmoidoscopy. *Gastroenterology* 1983;84:803–808.

Mazier WP, Levien DH, Luchtefeld MA, eds. *Surgery of the colon, rectum, and anus.* Philadelphia: W.B. Saunders, 1995.

Saito Y, Slezak P, Rubio C. The diagnostic value of combining flexible sigmoidoscopy and double-contrast barium enema as a one-stage procedure. *Gastrointest Radiol* 1989;14: 357–359.

Silvis SE, ed. *Therapeutic gastrointestinal endoscopy,* 2nd ed. New York: Igaku-Shoin, 1990.

The Standards Task Force. American Society of Colon and Rectal Surgeons. Practice parameters for antibiotic prophylaxis—supporting documentation. *Dis Colon Rectum* 1992;35: 278–285.

Wexner SD, Garbus JE, Singh JJ. The SAGES Colonoscopy Outcomes Study Group. A prospective analysis of 13,580 colonoscopies, reevaluation of credentialing guidelines. *Surg Endosc* 2001;15:251–261.

Yamada T, ed. *Textbook of gastroenterology,* 2nd ed. Philadelphia: J.B. Lippincott Co, 1995.

COMMENTARY

Colonoscopy is by far the most common endoscopic procedure done today. Numbers of colonoscopies have dramatically increased due to a concerted effort by regulatory agencies and physicians (using popular media and media stars) to educate the public on the value of screening for colon cancer. This public campaign appears to be succeeding, as there has been a dramatic decrease in the number of deaths from colorectal cancer in the last 10 years. The popularity of colonoscopy however, has placed a strain on the medical system to provide adequate numbers of well-trained endoscopists to perform all of these studies. The advent of waiting lists for screening colonoscopy has given rise to several unexpected phenomena: The rise of high-volume outpatient endoscopy units, a push to have non-GI (surgeon or gastroenterologist) practitioners perform colonoscopy, and the development of rival technologies including virtual (CT scan) colonoscopy, capsule endoscopy, and fecal marker testing. The future of screening colonoscopy may therefore be limited if a more cost-effective alternative becomes apparent. Therapeutic colonoscopy on the other hand, which is practiced by both surgeons and gastroenterologists, seems to be safe from obsolescence and in fact is evolving into an increasingly surgical tool. Stenting of malignancies, piecemeal polypectomy, ultrasound staging of lesions and even closure of perforations are routinely practiced and are certainly an important adjunct to colorectal surgery. With the advent of natural orifice surgery on the horizon, surgeons have been mandated to bolster their endoscopy numbers during training; this is mainly accomplished through experience with screening colonoscopy. The question arises, then, of how sufficient expertise for these advanced procedures will be obtained by physicians if screening colonoscopy goes away. Obviously only time will tell.

Drs. Bruce and Coller give excellent tips on performing expeditious and high quality colonoscopy—borne from their vast experience as endoscopists. It is a fortunate surgeon who has the opportunity to work with master endoscopists to learn all the myriad small tricks that make colonoscopy safe, easy on the patient, and fun for the endoscopists. While there are virtual-reality simulators that can help learners gain some degree of expertise, there is still no substitute for direct observation and the instruction of an endoscopic mentor. Likewise, there are no established metrics that determine when someone learning colonoscopy is truly competent to actually perform it. The Society of American Gastrointestinal and Endoscopic Surgeons (SAGES) is working to create such a tool, which would provide cognitive knowledge, training in a simple trainer for manual skills, and a certifying exam.

LSS

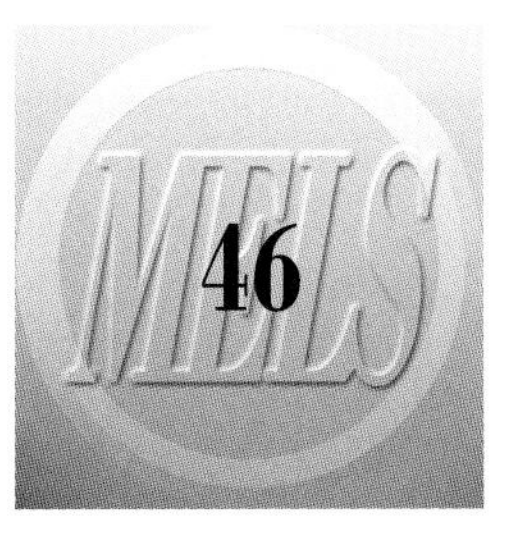

Laparoscopic Surgery of the Appendix

NAMIR KATKHOUDA

INTRODUCTION

In 1982, almost exactly 300 years after the first description of appendicitis by Heister (1683), Semm performed the first laparoscopic incidental appendectomy by transecting the appendix between two endoloops. Laparoscopic surgery has subsequently evolved and firmly established itself in the surgical practice and routine. While there is still ongoing debate about what the best indications for and technical aspects of the procedure are, there has been ample documentation in the literature that laparoscopic appendectomy for acute appendicitis is at least equally safe as conventional open appendectomy (see Table 46-1). Despite the initial lack of a clear-cut statistical advantage of the laparoscopic approach as compared to the open appendectomy, there is growing evidence that the laparoscopic approach provides a faster recovery, fewer complications, and improved cosmesis compared to open appendectomy. This benefit is seen for all age groups, but elder patients in particular seem to benefit from the minimally invasive approach.

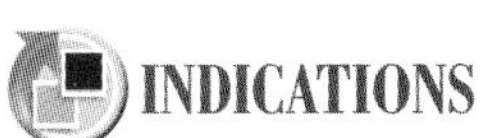

INDICATIONS

The laparoscopic approach should not result in a change of the indications for appendectomy. Any patient who, based on the overall assessment, requires and qualifies for a surgical exploration for suspected acute appendicitis is a likely candidate for the laparoscopic procedure. In addition, there are a number of patients in whom a diagnostic uncertainty persists despite multiple tests; in these patients, a diagnostic laparoscopy with a *possible* appendectomy may be indicated to clarify and treat the causative pathology. A final group of patients are those whose initial acute episode was treated nonoperatively, such as the percutaneous drainage of an appendiceal abscess combined with antibiotics, and who now need an interval appendectomy.

Absolute contraindications are few and mainly are related to the physiologic condition of the patient and the potential effects of the pneumoperitoneum (for example, a severe CO_2-retaining pulmonary cripple). The most common reason for not performing an indicated "lap appy" is lack of institutional preparedness for emergency laparoscopies. The increasing popularity of dedicated minimally invasive surgical suites makes this "late night" resistance less common.

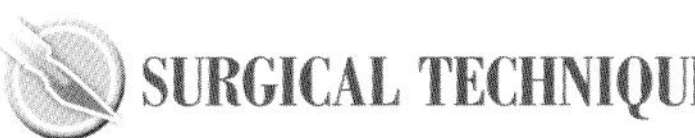

SURGICAL TECHNIQUE

Operating Room Setup and Port Placement

After induction of general anesthesia, the patient is placed in supine position with both arms, or at least the left arm, tucked alongside the body to give both the surgeon and the assistant comfortable space. A Foley catheter and lower-extremity sequential pneumatic compression devices are placed routinely. Insertion of an oral-gastric tube for decompression depends on the patient's presentation and degree of abdominal distension. The abdomen is prepared and draped in sterile fashion exposing the entire abdomen from the epigastrium to the pubic bone and both groins. Standard laparoscopic equipment is usually sufficient, as long as it includes some atraumatic graspers, Babcock clamps, scissors, suction/irrigation, and a specimen retrieval bag.

While the surgeon's assistant initially stands on the opposite side until the ports have been inserted and the pneumoperitoneum established, eventually both the surgeon and the assistant will be on the left side of the patient facing the monitor placed on the right side (Fig. 46-1, page 462).

A pneumoperitoneum is created in standard fashion, using either the Veress needle technique, the open Hasson technique, or by insertion of a nontraumatic bladeless OptiView port (Ethicon Endo-surgery, Inc; Cincinnati, OH).

"Port planning" refers to the steps and considerations taken before inserting the actual ports in order to optimize the usability of the placed ports, to maximize safety, and to minimize patient morbidity and negative aesthetic impact. Considerations include the patient's habitus (such as obesity) and anatomic landmarks (such as epigastric vessels), the presence and location of scars from previous abdominal operations, and potential aesthetic expectations. As a result of this planning, the surgeon should have a clear concept about each port's location, size, and intended use. For example, the insertion of a stapling device or specimen retrieval will typically require a larger port than the insertion of grasping instruments or endoloops alone. The laparoscope is typically inserted at the umbilicus, although the position can be altered according to the patient's anatomy. Preferably, insertion of the other two ports should be in a symmetric triangulated pattern that will avoid a "knitting needle" effect between the working instruments and the laparoscope. In effect, all ports should be placed in such a way that they have free movement and do not interfere with each other. Options

TABLE 46-1. RESULTS OF A RANDOMIZED PROSPECTIVE STUDY COMPARING LAPAROSCOPIC AND OPEN APPENDECTOMY

	Patient numbers	Operative time P = .001	Complications NS (%)	LOS NS	Pain scores NS
Open appendectomy	123	60 minutes	18.5	=	=
Laparoscopic appendectomy	124	80 minutes	17	=	=

LOS, length of stay; NS, nonsignificant.

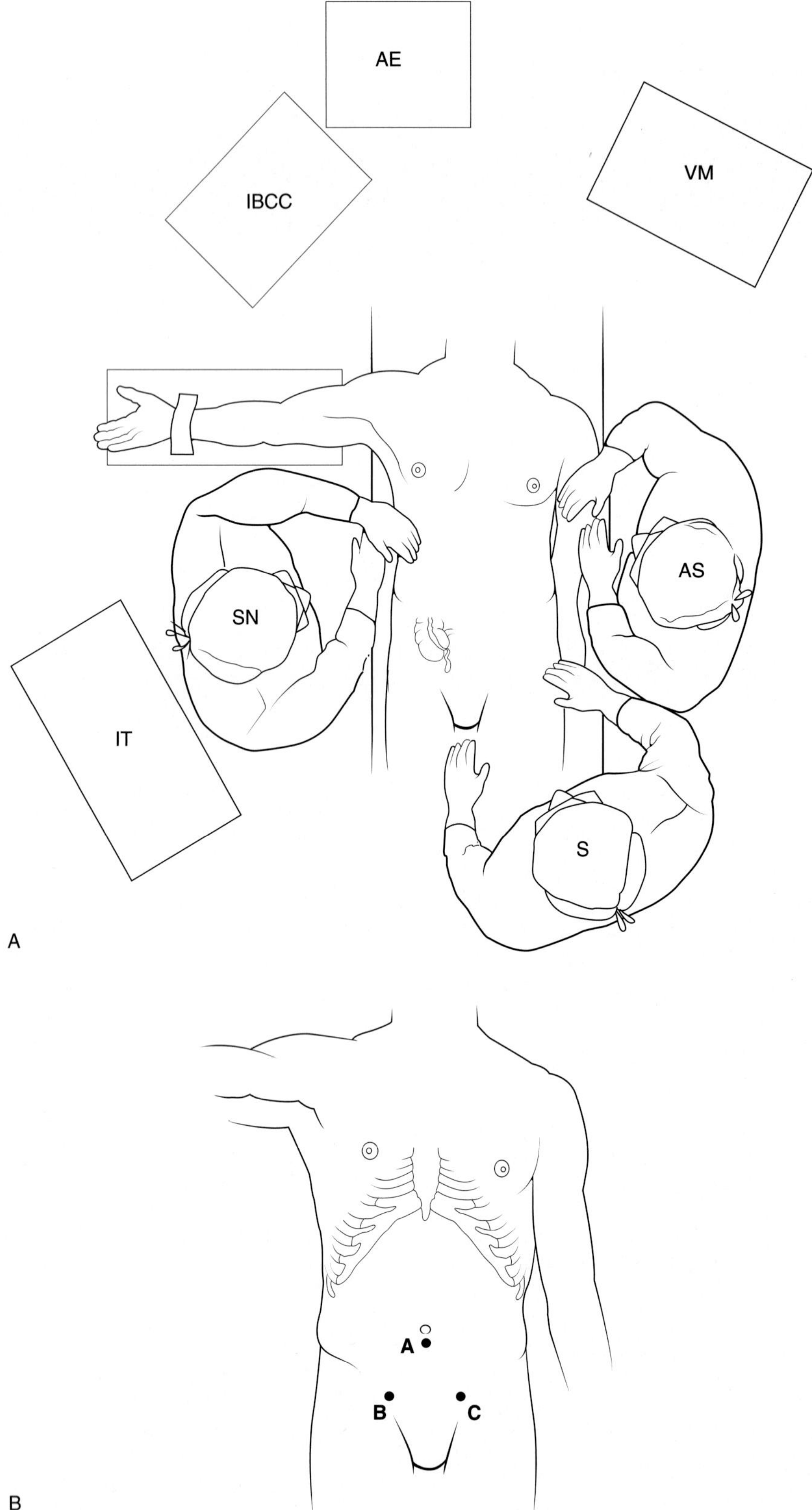

Fig. 46-1. A. Patient positioning and trocar placement for a laparoscopic appendectomy, showing the surgeon (S), assisting surgeon (AS), surgical nurse (SN), instrument table (IT), endoscopic instrument control console (EICC), anesthesia (AE), and video monitor (VM). **B.** Trocar positioning: A is a 12-mm trocar and B and C are 5-mm trocars.

for placement include placing the working ports at the McBurney point and at the corresponding point on the left side (Fig. 46-2A). For cosmetic reasons the port positions can be moved down towards the pubic hair line (Fig. 46-2B). Other settings (e.g., left lower quadrant plus suprapubic midline port or a port right under the right costal margin) are possible if indicated by previous incisions but may have functional disadvantages or be less cosmetically appropriate.

Exposure of the Appendix

After insertion of the ports, a quick diagnostic laparoscopy is performed in order to confirm the diagnosis and assess other pathologies, such as diverticulitis, inguinal hernias, liver or gallbladder disease, and carcinomatosis. The surgeon's assistant and camera holder then moves to the patient's left side, cephalad to the surgeon. The patient is brought into Trendelenburg position with the right side elevated in order to facilitate the exposure of the right lower quadrant.

The surgeon's left hand operates a Babcock grasper to retract the cecum and subsequently expose the appendix (if the appendix is in its usual paracecal position). Particularly if the appendix is significantly inflamed and friable, it is advisable not to grasp the appendix itself but rather to place the Babcock around it or at the level of the mesoappendix (Fig. 46-3, page 464). Occasionally, an endoloop can be placed around the appendix and mesoappendix in order to create a handle to hold a particularly inflamed appendix. Cautery scissors can be used to incise the retroperitoneal attachments of the cecum to allow it to be pulled anteriorly, which will optimize access to the appendix and its mesentery. The surgeon's right hand operates a dissecting instrument or cautery scissors, which are used to create a window in the mesoappendix at the base of the appendix. If the appendix is retrocecal and not clearly identifiable, additional dissection of the cecum needs to be performed to allow it to be retracted medially (Fig. 46-4, page 464).

Transection Techniques

Once the appendix has been completely mobilized, it is amputated at the base. While in general there is no need for inversion of the appendiceal stump, it is of crucial importance to divide it in healthy

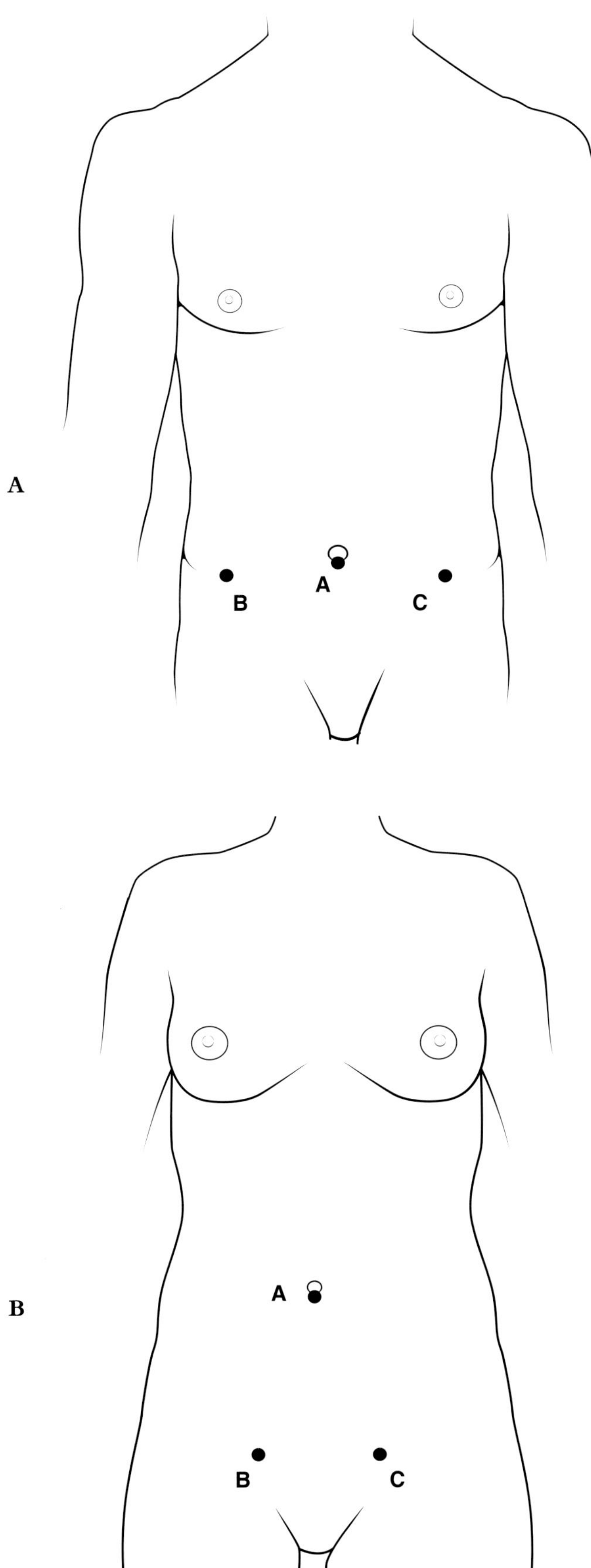

Fig. 46-2. Trocar placement. **A.** Male patient. **B.** Female patient.

appearing tissue, if necessary even across the cecum, to avoid a breakdown of the ligation or stapler line.

Either suture ligation or staplers can be used to divide the appendix and the mesoappendix. Suture ligation, either with free ties or pre-tied endoloops, is inexpensive and only requires a 5-mm port, but it demands more skill and may initially take more time. The stapling technique requires less skill and is initially time-saving, but it is more expensive and requires a 12-mm port.

Endoloop Technique

In this technique, the mesoappendix is first divided by means of cautery and the appendix is subsequently divided between two endoloops. The appendix should be clearly visible from tip to base. Special bipolar cautery forceps can be used to cauterize and "crush" the mesoappendix. Alternately ultrasonic coagulating shears can be used, although it is an additional expense. Care has to be taken not to touch and burn adjacent loops of bowels with cautery devices. Portions of the mesoappendix are cauterized and subsequently cut with the scissors until the base of the appendix is identified and completely freed. Two endoloops or free ties are inserted and tied at the base, leaving sufficient space to transect the appendix. Transection should be done sharply without cautery to prevent late stump necrosis at the ligated base. After transection, the appendiceal stump mucosa can be carefully cauterized (Fig. 46-5, page 464).

Stapling Technique

In this technique, a 30-mm vascular (white load) endoscopic stapler is used to divide the mesoappendix, and a 30-mm blue load is then used to divide the appendix as close as possible to the cecum leaving only a very short stump. A window is bluntly created in the avascular plane between the base of the appendix and the appendiceal artery. The first stapler with its appropriate cartridge (white for vasculature and blue for the appendix) is inserted and fired (Fig. 46-6, page 465), followed by a second stapler for completion of the transection (Fig. 46-7, page 465). Care should be taken to avoid creating a "junkyard" by releasing unused staples into the surgical field. Therefore, the staplers should be opened very carefully after firing, just enough to release the tissue, but then immediately be closed again before dropping the unused staples.

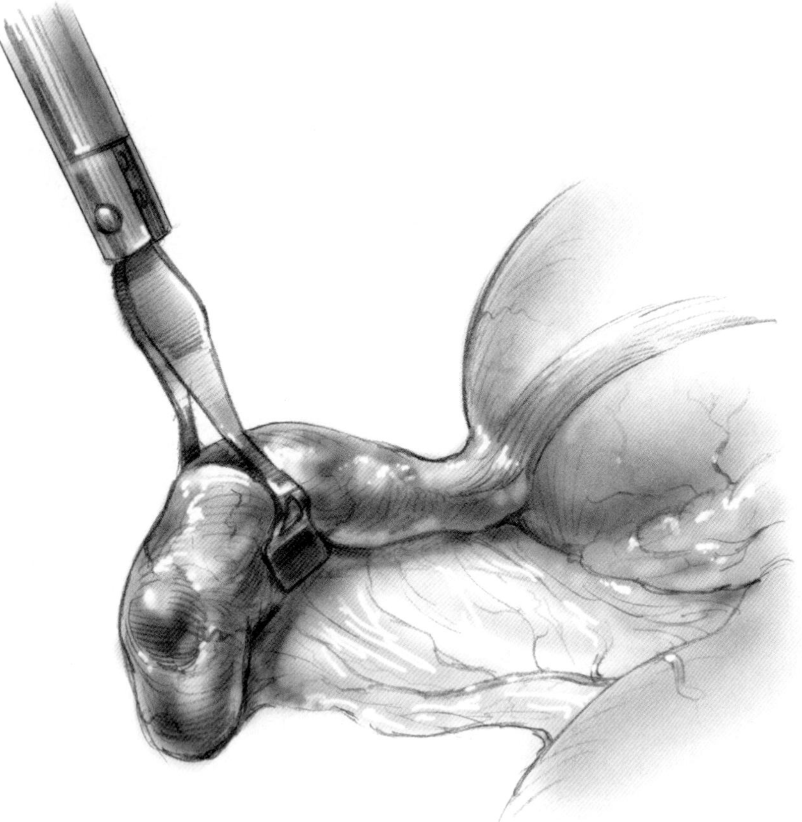

Fig. 46-3. Exposure of the appendix and creation of a window in the mesoappendix.

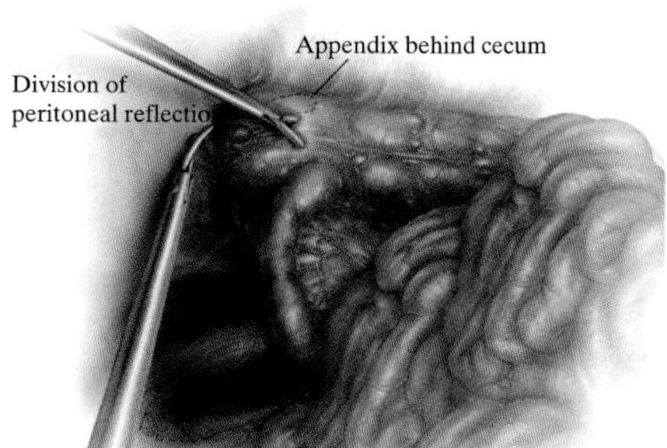

Fig. 46-4. Mobilization of the cecum for retrocecal location of the appendix.

aspirated and irrigated out by retracting the sigmoid colon and exposing the Douglas pouch.

In the majority of cases, a drain is not necessary. However, if residual contaminated fluid is to be left in the peritoneal cavity, a mature abscess was drained, or if the appendiceal/cecal stump is of suboptimal quality, placement of a small closed-suction drain may be prudent. It should be brought in through a separate 4- to 5-mm incision in the right lower quadrant, not through one of the trocar sites, and laid along the cecum into the pelvis in order to drain those dependent areas. The drain can be removed after a

Specimen Retrieval

As care is needed to avoid contamination of the abdomen and port site wounds, the appendix is placed in an impermeable retrieval bag before it is removed from the abdomen. Alternatively, if the appendix is not too large, it can be pulled into one of the larger ports and withdrawn with the whole port. Rupture of the retrieval bag within the abdominal wall because of an inadequate fascial gap should be avoided under any circumstances. If delivery of the endobag is difficult, it is advisable to widen the fascial incision.

Irrigation and Drainage

The purpose of irrigation is to remove all debris, purulent fluid collections, and blood from the surgical area. In early phlegmonous appendicitis without any pus, there is no advantage of irrigation and, in fact, there may be a risk of spreading contaminated fluid throughout the abdomen. Otherwise, with the appendix removed, a thorough lavage of the area is performed. In particular the pelvis has to be well exposed and any residual contaminated fluid should be

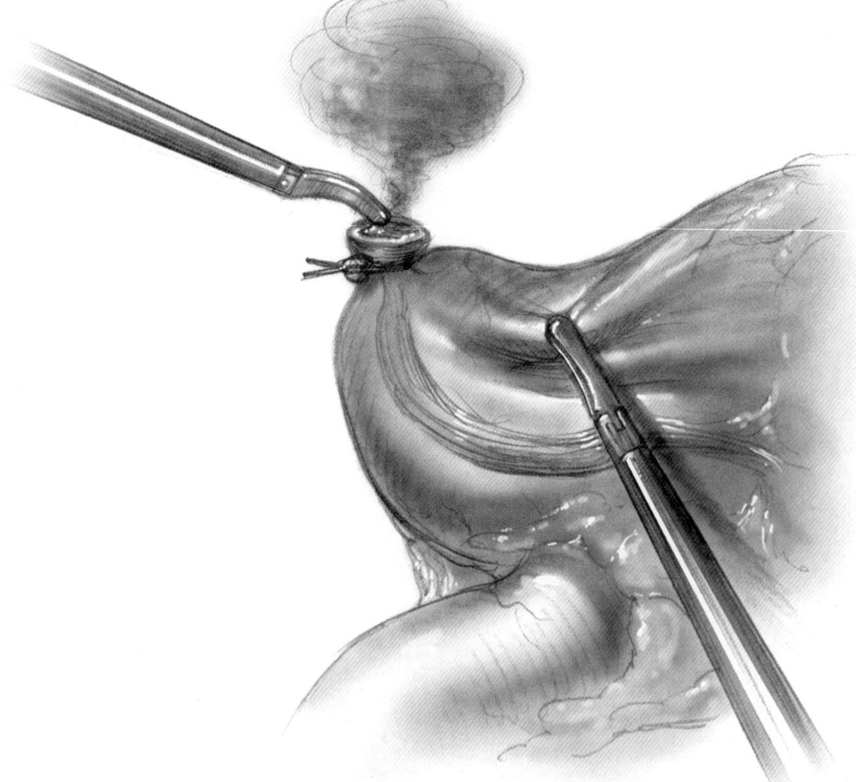

Fig. 46-5. Endoloop technique: the transection of the appendix between two loops.

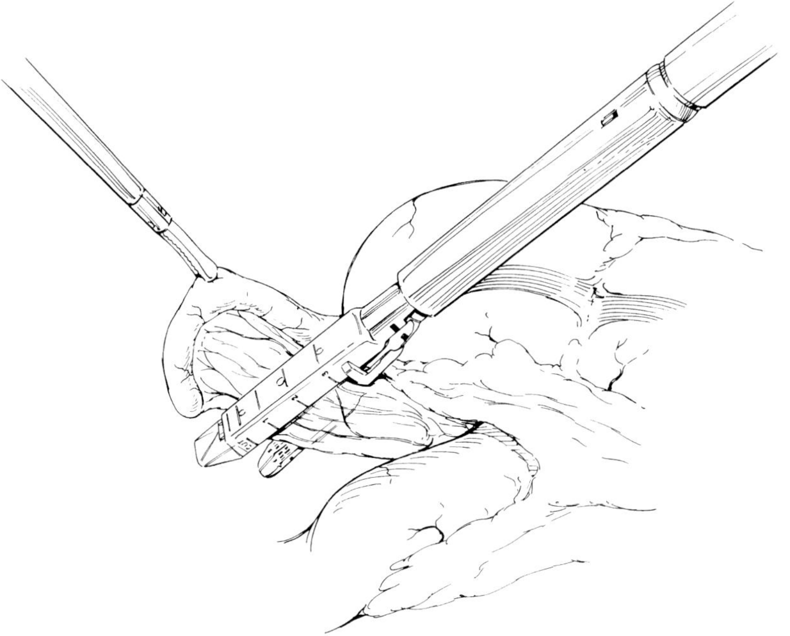

Fig. 46-6. Stapler technique: the transection of the mesoappendix.

few days, once the quality of the fluid is serosanguinous.

Technical Variations

Retrograde Appendectomy

When the tip of the appendix is not clearly visible, a retrograde appendectomy can be performed (Fig. 46-8, page 466). The visible base of the appendix is transected after the creation of an appropriate window, followed by the transection of the mesoappendix, and finally the whole appendix is progressively dissected from the base to the tip. This is done as in open surgery and does not require specific skills.

Difficult Appendicitis

When the surgeon encounters a gangrenous or perforated appendicitis or a large appendiceal phlegmon, it can initially be difficult to recognize the appendix. In these circumstances it may be necessary to completely mobilize the cecum. This mobilization should be as conservative as possible to avoid opening and contaminating retroperitoneal cellular spaces. The cecum can then be flipped over and the appendix visualized. If this is still not possible, a "fingeroscopy" or conversion to an open procedure have to be considered. The former technique involves removal of the port from the right lower quadrant and insertion of the index finger in order to restore tactile sensation. A blunt, atraumatic mobilization is performed, similar to the open procedure but under laparoscopic guidance. This speeds up the procedure and should be considered in situations where conversion seems inevitable. "Fingeroscopy" can only be performed if the right lower quadrant incision is close enough to the surgical area (see the section on port placement). If the base of the appendix is necrotic, it may be necessary to staple across a portion of the cecum to achieve viable tissues (Fig. 46-9, page 466).

If satisfactory progress can't be made, conversion to an open operation may be required. The projection of the cecum is marked on the abdominal wall using transillumination of the laparoscope, and an incision is made appropriate for the operation to be carried out.

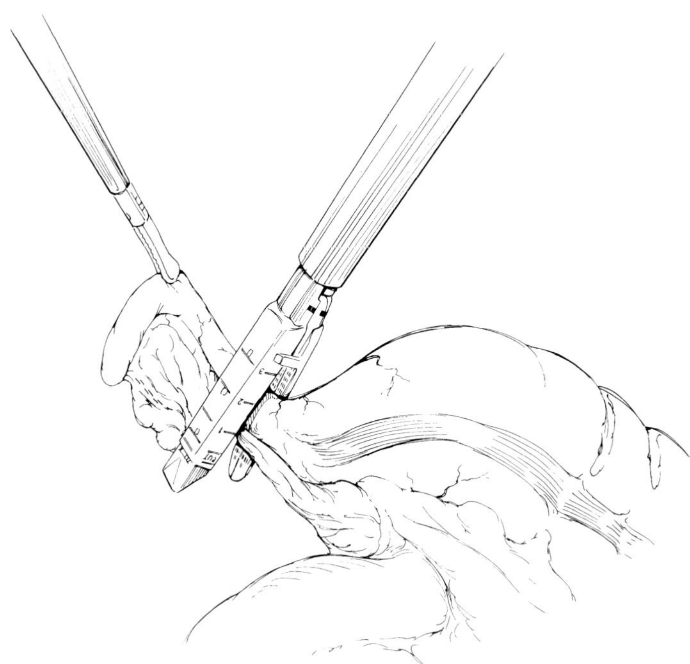

Fig. 46-7. Stapler technique: the transection of the appendix.

Laparoscopically Assisted Appendectomy

In some cases, especially in children where the appendix is extremely long and the working space small, the "assisted" technique is an easy way of performing an appendectomy. The mesoappendix is first controlled by means of bipolar electrocautery. The right lower quadrant port is then removed with the appendix inside. The whole appendix is exteriorized and ligated outside the abdomen before the cecum is pushed back inside the abdomen.

SPECIAL PROBLEMS

Diagnostic Uncertainty and Normal Appendix

Encountering a normal appendix occurs either in patients in whom preoperative studies and assessment were inconclusive or proved to be falsely positive. A careful assessment has to be performed of the whole peritoneal cavity, including running the small bowel. If a different intraabdominal pathology is found, that disease process should be appropriately treated and the ap-

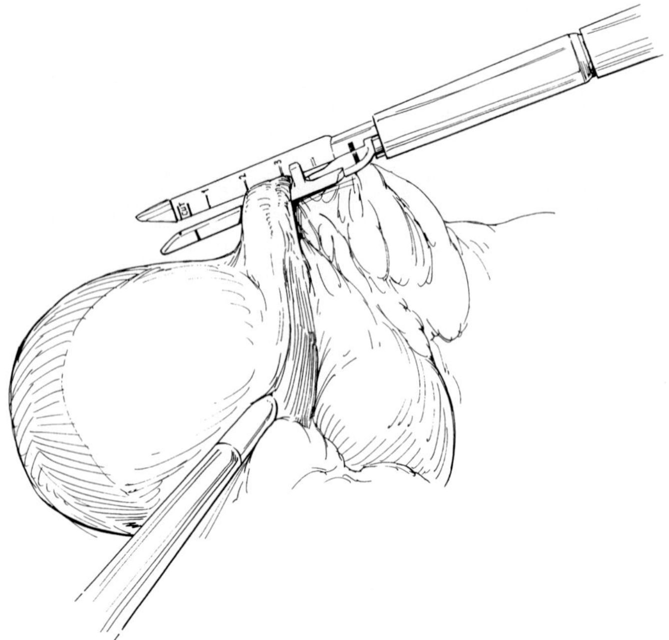

Fig. 46-8. Retrograde dissection with transection of the appendix base, followed by its mobilization towards the tip.

pendix left in place. If no other pathology is found, we recommend removing the appendix and having it assessed by the pathologist.

Pregnancy

Acute appendicitis with any type of appendectomy carries a risk for the pregnant patient and for her unborn fetus. While pregnancy in and of itself is not necessarily a contraindication for the laparoscopic approach, the following requirements have to be respected: the surgeon must be an experienced laparoscopist, the operation should under no circumstances be prolonged, and the trocars should always be placed in an open access technique. Consultation by the obstetric department is advisable and fetal monitoring may be prudent as well.

Control of Intraoperative Bleeding

While bleeding complications are relatively rare, they most commonly arise from the appendiceal artery. Bleeding related to the trocar placement (e.g., epigastric or iliac vessels) should be avoided by careful and visually controlled insertion of the ports. If appendiceal bleeding occurs, a prompt and controlled reaction to localize the bleeder and stop it is required. A suction in one hand and a fine dissector in the other should be used to expose the bleeder and grasp the vessel. Diffuse and uncontrolled cautery to arrest bleeding should be avoided. Adding an additional port may be needed to provide retraction. It may be helpful to insert a 2 by 2-cm radiopaque-labeled gauze to temporarily compress the area. Once the vessel is grasped, a clip or figure of eight stitch may be placed. If the bleeding cannot be stopped in a timely fashion, the procedure should be converted to an open operation.

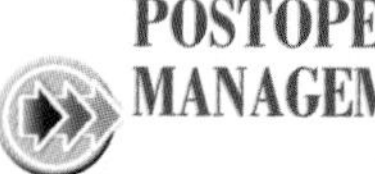

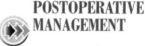

POSTOPERATIVE MANAGEMENT

The post-surgical management depends on the intraoperative findings as well as the patient's symptoms. The duration of antibiotics, in contrast, is determined by the extent of the inflammation and the presence of perforation, rather than by the surgical approach. Early ambulation and resumption of an oral diet are encouraged; the latter should be advanced as tolerated. Patients who have undergone non-perforated laparoscopic appendectomies can often go home the following day.

SUGGESTED READING

de Perrot M, Jenny A, Morales M, et al. Laparoscopic appendectomy during pregnancy. *Surg Lap Endosc Perc Techn* 2000;10: 368–371.

Guller U, Hervey S, Purves H, et al. Laparoscopic versus open appendectomy: outcomes comparison based on a large administrative database. *Ann Surg* 2004;239: 43–52.

Guller U, Jain N, Peterson ED, et al. Laparoscopic appendectomy in the elderly. *Surgery* 2004;135:479–488.

Kaiser AM, Corman ML. History of laparoscopy. *Surg Oncol Clin N Am* 2001;10: 483–492.

Katkhouda N, Mason RJ, Mavor E, et al. Laparoscopic finger-assisted technique (fingeroscopy) for treatment of complicated appendicitis. *J Am Coll Surg* 1999;189: 131–133.

McKinlay R, Mastrangelo MJ, Jr. Current status of laparoscopic appendectomy. *Curr Surg* 2003;60:506–512.

Semm K. Endoscopic appendectomy. *Endoscopy* 1983;15:59–64.

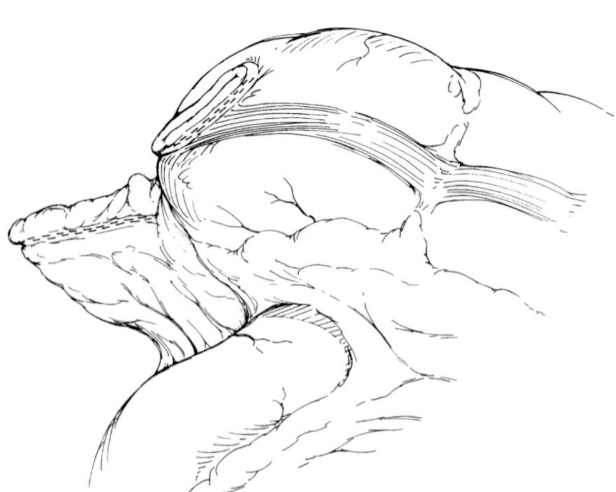

Fig. 46-9. If the appendiceal base is necrotic, a stapler should be used to transect a portion of the cecum in order to achieve viable tissues.

COMMENTARY

Dr. Katkhouda presents a very thorough review of the technique of laparoscopic appendectomy. Appendectomy is usually considered to be the "most minor" of the intraabdominal surgeries and as such it frequently is relegated to the surgical intern, with little attention paid to the finer technical points of the procedure. Yet, in severe cases, it can represent a major challenge to even experienced laparoscopists. Certainly, mastery of this commonly presenting disease is a great stepping stone to laparoscopic colectomy and the handling of intraabdominal complications such as perforated peptic ulcer disease, iatrogenic or inflammatory perforations of the colon, or postoperative anastomotic complications. As mentioned, the endoscopic stapler makes the procedure relatively quick and easy, but I always encourage surgeons, both trainees and those introducing more advanced laparoscopic techniques into their repertory, to use ligation as it provides a frequent opportunity to use endoloops or intracorporeal tying. The other issue for surgeons to consider is the cost of using devices such as staplers or ultrasonic coagulating shears.

It is estimated that around 27% of appendectomies in the United States are currently done with the laparoscope, an appreciable number but still no where near the ubiquity of cholecystectomy. Why is that? One hears arguments that it makes "no clinical difference" or that "it takes too long" but in fact, for the most part, it comes down to an infrastructure issue more than anything else. Hospitals without dedicated minimally invasive operating rooms or a specially trained core nursing group find these emergency cases stressful and inconvenient. After opening MIS suites in each of our hospitals, we have seen the incidence of laparoscopic appendectomy go from 18% to 88%. It has, in fact, become the default approach; if an open appendectomy is desired, one must expressly ask for it when calling down to schedule. This is a good thing for patients: while studies show length of stay and degree of pain are about the same as with the open technique, most studies don't assess the benefits of a rapid return to normal activity, the absence of wound complications, or the potential reduction in the long-term risk of adhesive bowel obstructions. Cosmetic concerns can also not be ignored; there is no doubt that patients prefer the scars left from laparoscopy over that of a classic incision.

LLS

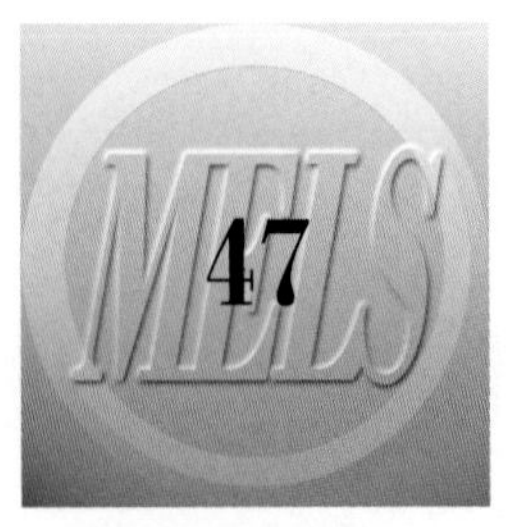

Laparoscopic Surgery for Benign Diseases of the Colon

KARIN HARDIMAN AND MARK WHITEFORD

INTRODUCTION

Much attention has been directed at the role of the laparoscopic colectomy for cancer treatment, particularly regarding the patterns of recurrence and long-term survival. Laparoscopic surgery for benign disease, however, has its own challenges. It covers a broader spectrum of disease processes including diverticulitis, inflammatory bowel disease, colonic inertia, volvulus, ischemic colitis, infectious colitis, and lower gastrointestinal hemorrhage. Inflammatory processes such as peritonitis, abscess, phlegmon, and fistula, as well as the scar tissue that these processes induce, can significantly alter the normal anatomy by obliterating tissue planes, which in turn can make mobilization more difficult and increase the risk of injury to adjacent organs or structures during surgery. The extent and complexity of resection can also vary from segmental colectomy focused on one to two quadrants of the abdomen to restorative proctocolectomy, which requires operating in all four quadrants as well as the pelvis. Proper patient selection and an advanced laparoscopic skill set acquired over time will enable a surgeon to tackle these challenges and become facile with these complex procedures. Many studies have found that laparoscopic management of benign diseases of the colon is safe, with similar or better outcomes when compared to open surgery. This chapter will review indications and technical perspectives for the laparoscopic management of benign diseases of the colon.

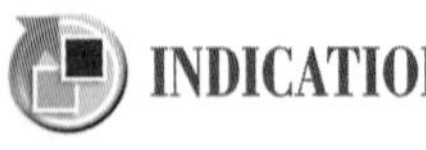

INDICATIONS

Diverticulitis, a micro- or macroperforation of a colonic pseudodiverticulum, is one of the most common indications for laparoscopic colectomy. Surgery is indicated for cases of diverticulitis complicated by an abscess, fistula, stenosis, or diffuse peritonitis or cases that fail to respond to bowel rest and antibiotics. Every effort should be made to convert an urgent situation into an elective one. Most abscesses can be drained with image-guided or laparoscopic techniques. Definitive one-stage surgery can then be postponed 6 or more weeks to allow for resolution of the inflammatory process and optimization of patient nutrition and comorbidities.

Traditionally, elective surgery has also been recommended following resolution of two or more episodes of uncomplicated diverticulitis. Several recent studies are revisiting this recommendation. It appears that the natural history of uncomplicated diverticulitis may be more indolent than previously reported, with recommendations trending toward conservatism. Postponing surgery until after four or more attacks may be less morbid and more cost-effective than operating sooner. This issue is in evolution and the answer is yet to be determined.

Mucosal ulcerative colitis and Crohn colitis are chronic inflammatory diseases of the colon and rectum. Goals of medical therapy include induction of remission, maintenance of remission, enhancement of quality of life, and minimizing complications of the disease itself and the therapy directed at the disease. Indications for surgery include symptoms refractory to medical management, intolerance of medical management, perforation, bleeding, or neoplastic transformation. A thorough gastrointestinal evaluation is necessary to differentiate between these two forms of inflammatory bowel disease, as restorative proctocolectomy is generally contraindicated in patients with Crohn disease.

Restorative proctocolectomy is the surgical procedure of choice for ulcerative colitis and familial adenomatous polyposis. It achieves the goals of removing the diseased organ and preserving transanal defecation. This operation is most commonly performed in two stages, beginning with total proctocolectomy with ileal pouch anal anastomosis and protecting loop ileostomy, with subsequent ileostomy reversal once the pouch has healed. Patients requiring surgery in the setting of fulminate ulcerative colitis, toxic megacolon, malnutrition, or high-dose immunosuppression may be best served by total abdominal colectomy with an end ileostomy, with postponement of restorative procedures until health and nutrition returns. Patients with Crohn colitis and a small proportion of patients with ulcerative colitis will choose a one-stage total proctocolectomy with permanent ileostomy.

While constipation is a common condition in North America, it is rarely a surgical condition. Patients with severe constipation should undergo a thorough gastroenterological evaluation to exclude other medically or surgically correctable causes. The extent of this workup is significant and is beyond the scope of this chapter. Colonic inertia, also known as slow transit constipation, should be confirmed objectively with a colonic transit time test such as a Sitzmarks test (KONSYL PHARMACEUTICALS, INC.; Easton, MD). Obstructed defecation syndrome should also be excluded by history, physical examination, and video defecography. Once confirmed, the surgical treatment of choice for colonic inertia is a total abdominal colectomy with ileorectal anastomosis or ileostomy.

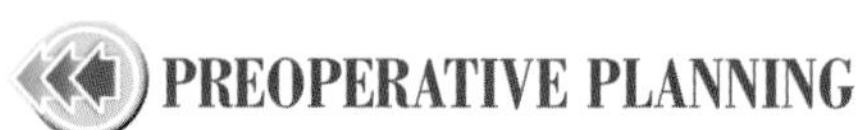

PREOPERATIVE PLANNING

In addition to standard history, physical, and continence evaluations, a patient's suitability for laparoscopic colectomy is determined by a combination of patient factors and the surgeon's experience. Challenging patient factors include pulmonary or cardiac conditions that limit his or her ability to tolerate pneumoperitoneum, morbid obesity (BMI >30 to 35), prior abdominal surgery or radiation, inflammatory process, abscess, or fistulizing disease. Surgeon factors include the laparoscopic skill set and experience in the laparoscopic management of challenging conditions such as extensive adhesions, fistulizing disease, inflammatory conditions, transverse colon and flexure mobilizations, and nerve-sparing pelvic dissection. Conversion rates are always higher under these circumstances and should be discussed with the patient during the informed consent process. Conversions are best performed for proactive reasons such as extensive adhesions, unclear anatomy, and failure to progress rather than for reactive reasons such as hemorrhage, inadvertent enterotomy, or transected ureter. A patient is better served by a well performed open operation than a poorly performed laparoscopic operation.

Preoperative consultation with a wound ostomy continence (enterostomal therapy) nurse should be obtained for patients who may require a temporary or permanent ostomy. Patients will receive valuable teaching, counseling, and siting advice that will continue in the postoperative setting.

Mandatory bowel preparation prior to elective colorectal surgery has recently been called into question. Several randomized prospective trials show no benefit of cathartic antegrade bowel lavage over administration of broad spectrum intravenous preoperative antibiotics alone with regard to wound infection and anastomotic leak rates. Of note, these studies did include a preoperative rectal enema for patients requiring a colorectal anastomosis. For technical reasons, there are some situations in which full bowel preparation would be preferred, such as the need for intraoperative colonoscopic localization or when the added weight of the unprepped colon may overwhelm the delicate laparoscopic instrumentation.

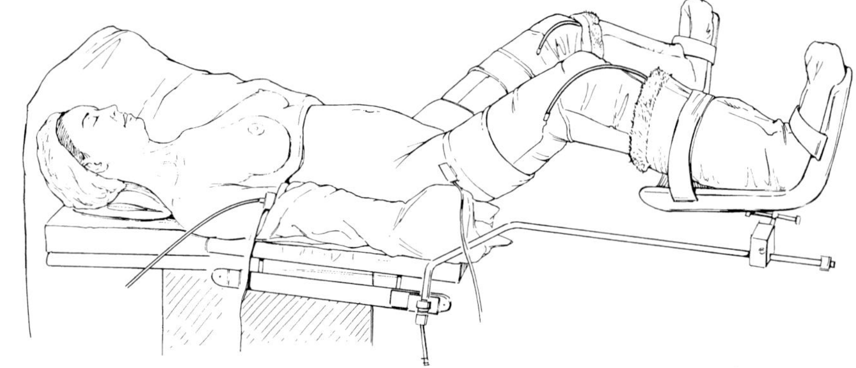

Fig. 47-1. Patient positioning for a standard laparoscopic approach.

SURGICAL TECHNIQUE

Initially, the majority of minimally invasive surgeons performed laparoscopic-assisted colectomy in the same fashion as the conventional open technique, by starting at the lateral peritoneal reflection (the white line of Toldt) and then progressing medially to mobilize the colon off of the retroperitoneum. An alternate method of colon mobilization, the medial-to-lateral approach, has gained considerable favor, becoming a preferred approach for many surgeons who perform laparoscopic colorectal surgery. The benefits of this approach include (1) early identification and avoidance of retroperitoneal structures (ureter, gonadal vessels, and duodenum), (2) simplified dissection along the avascular embryonic fusion plane between the colonic mesentery and the retroperitoneum, (3) early identification and control of the vascular pedicle or pedicles, and (4) important countertraction and minimal manipulation of the colon, by leaving division of the lateral peritoneal attachments until the end of the case. This approach is particularly beneficial when operating for diverticulitis, a condition in which the inflammatory and technically demanding portion of the procedure occurs during the lateral portion of the dissection. The medial approach, which begins in an uninflamed field, tends to be easier to dissect.

In order to displace the small bowel and provide adequate visualization, laparoscopic colorectal surgery requires extremes of operating table tilt and positioning. The patient is secured to the operating room table with straps, tapes, beanbags, or similar devices and placed in a low lithotomy position with arms carefully padded and tucked at the sides to prevent pressure points and positioning injuries, which may occur during these several-hour operations (Fig. 47-1). Preoperative deep venous thrombosis and antibiotic prophylaxis

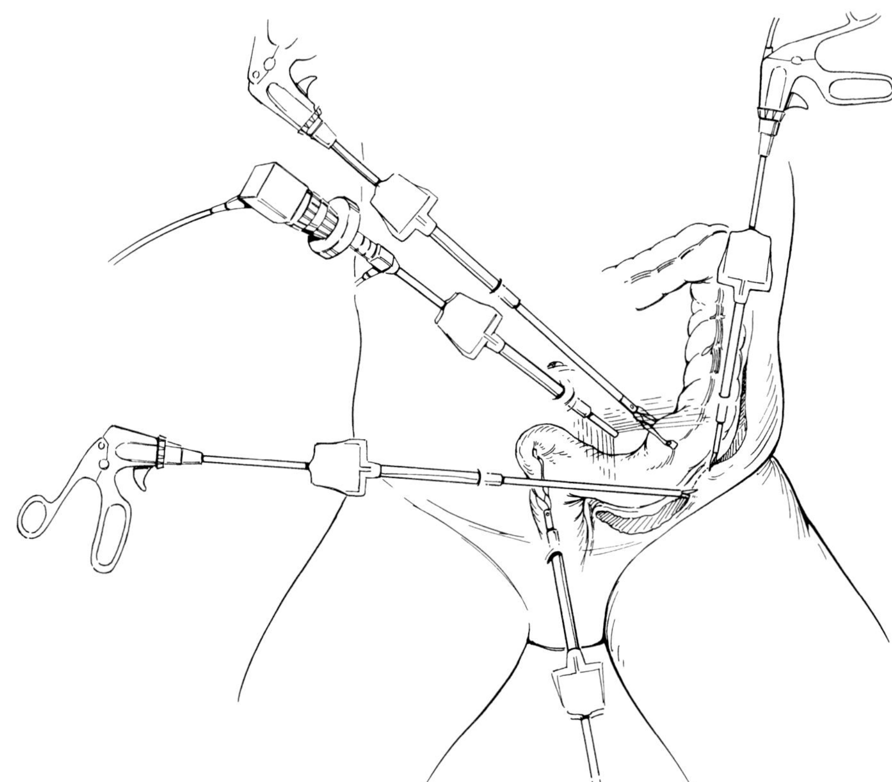

Fig. 47-2. Setup for dissection of the sigmoid colon. The surgeon stands on the patient's right side, and the assistant stands on the patient's left side.

should be confirmed. Urinary and orogastric catheters and rectal irrigation are utilized per surgeon preference. Standard laparoscopic instruments, including Hunter or Glassman graspers, Maryland dissector, 5-mm vessel sealing devices, suction irrigator, and a 30-degree laparoscope are utilized. The 12-mm working ports are necessary to accommodate the endoscopic GIA staplers or larger-diameter vessel-sealing devices. Normothermia should be maintained perioperatively through the use of warming blankets and warmed insufflation gas.

Port placement, specimen extraction sites, and the use of hand-assist devices for laparoscopic surgery are at the discretion of the surgeon. They may vary based on the section(s) of the bowel to be resected, whether the dissection is medial or lateral, the size of the patient, preexisting incisions, and planned ostomy sites. For left-sided and total colectomy operations we start out with a 12-mm supraumbilical Hasson cannulation for the camera port and 5-mm working ports in the right lower quadrant, the right mid-abdomen, and the left midclavicular line at the level of the umbilicus (Fig. 47-2, page 469). Early on in a surgeon's experience, the hand-assist and specimen extraction sites should be a lower midline incision, as this can easily be extended for open surgery. As a surgeon's experience increases and conversion rates plateau, a Pfannenstiel or left lower quadrant muscle-splitting transverse incision is preferred. For right-sided operations, the same camera port is used along with 5-mm working ports in the left lower quadrant and left mid-abdomen. An optional port in the right iliac fossa or left upper quadrant may facilitate lateral or hepatic flexure mobilization (Fig. 47-3). The specimen is extracted through an upper midline or alternatively a right lower quadrant muscle-splitting incision.

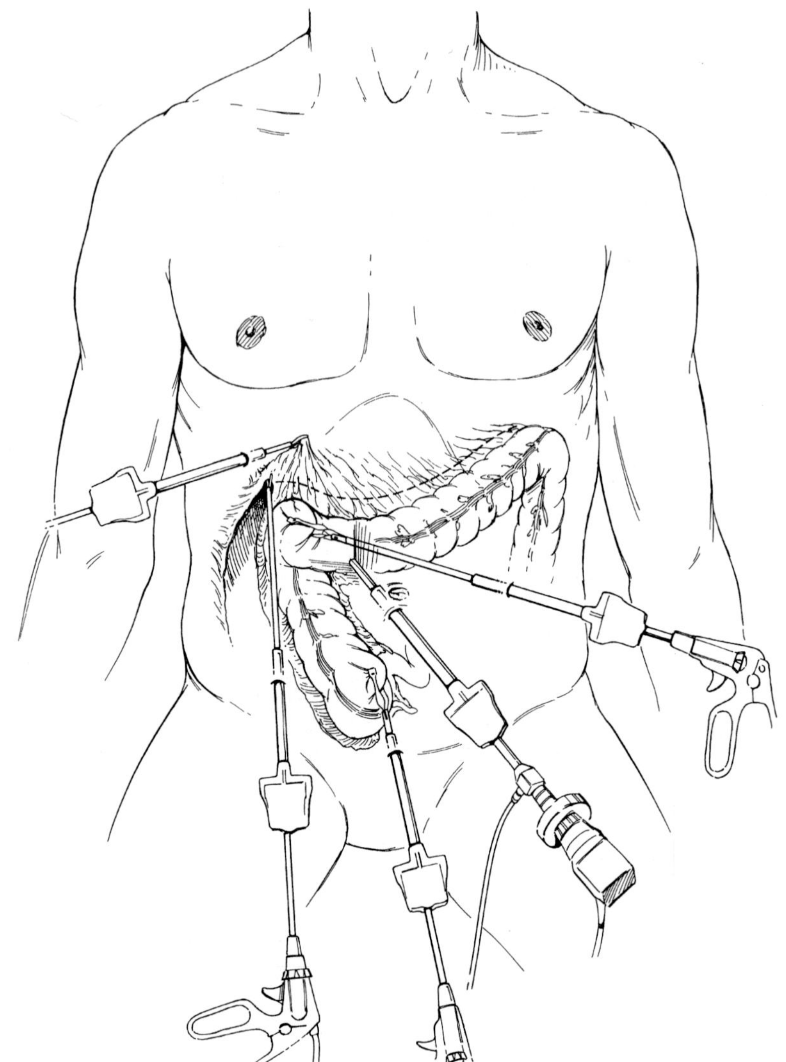

Fig. 47-3. Setup for dissection of the hepatic flexure and transverse colon. The surgeon stands on the patient's left side, and the assistant stands between the patient's legs.

SEGMENTAL COLECTOMY

Right Hemicolectomy: Medial-to-Lateral Approach

Table 47-1 presents the steps for a medial-to-lateral right hemicolectomy. Following port placement, laparoscopic exploration, and any necessary adhesiolysis, the patient is tilted into steep Trendelenburg and left-side down position. This allows gravity to displace the small bowel away from the surgical field. All remaining small bowel should be swept up out of the pelvis. Gentle inferolateral traction is applied to the ileocolic vascular pedicle where it enters the mesenteric border of the ascending colon (1 to 2 inches cephalad/distal to the ileocecal valve). The embryonic retroperitoneal fusion plane between the colonic mesentery and the Gerota fascia is entered through the mesenteric window between the ileocolic vessels and the ileal branches of the superior mesenteric artery (SMA). The peritoneum at the base of this window is scored parallel to the ileocolic vessels, and the avascular plane behind them is entered by using two blunt instruments. Care is taken to identify the duodenum near the base of the mesentery and the marginal artery within

TABLE 47-1. STEPS FOR MEDIAL-TO-LATERAL RIGHT HEMICOLECTOMY

1. Exploration
2. Establishment of the retroperitoneal plane from a medial approach
3. Identification and division of the ileocolic vascular pedicle
4. Mobilization of the colonic mesentery off of the Gerota fascia and duodenum
5. Mobilization of the terminal ileum mesentery and cecum off of the retroperitoneum
6. Division of the white line of Toldt, mobilization of the hepatic flexure
7. Specimen exteriorization, resection, and anastomosis

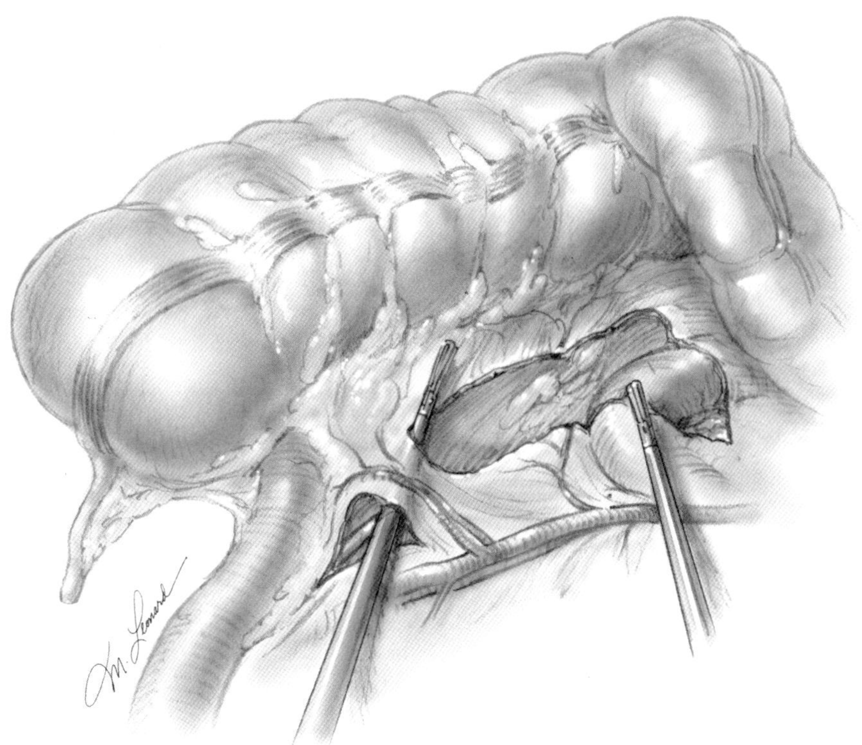

Fig. 47-4. A window is created on either side of the ileocolic vascular pedicle, and blunt dissection used to mobilize the right colonic mesentery of the retroperitoneum. The duodenum and ureter remain posterior.

the mesentery adjacent to the ileocecal junction.

The proper retroperitoneal dissection plane appears laparoscopically as a blue or purple areolar interface. One or two blunt instruments are used to tent up the ileocolic vessels while a third instrument sweeps down the retroperitoneum and duodenum (Fig. 47-4). Once the third portion of the duodenum has been swept down, a mesenteric window of peritoneum between the ileocolic and the right colic vessels is identified and bluntly opened. The ileocolic vessels, now isolated, are divided with a vessel-sealing device or an endoscopic GIA stapler (Fig. 47-5). The dissection continues in the retroperitoneal plane out to the abdominal sidewall, up under the liver, and then turns the corner up and over the second portion of the duodenum and into the lesser sac.

At this point in the operation, a high vascular ligation has been performed, the duodenum has been dissected free, and the ureter has been left undisturbed in its native retroperitoneal location. Attention is then directed to the cecum and terminal ileum. They are elevated cephalad to expose and then release the medial and lateral retroperitoneal attachments of the terminal ileal mesentery then up the white line of Toldt (see Fig. 47-3). To facilitate the hepatic flexure mobilization, the patient may be repositioned in a reverse-Trendelenburg position. The lesser sac is then entered by detaching the omentum off of the mid transverse colon and mesocolon. This plane of dissection is then continued in a retrograde fashion up and around the hepatic flexure to complete the right colon mobilization (Fig. 47-6). The right branch of the middle colic artery can be identified and divided intracorporeally or extracorporeally.

An upper midline or periumbilical extraction incision is preferred. This site allows access to the mesenteric root and can be used in a hybrid fashion to complete the hepatic flexure, transverse colon mobilization, or anastomosis. A wound protector is placed and the terminal ileum and right colon are delivered and inspected. The resection and anastomosis is completed extracorporeally using traditional techniques (Fig. 47-7, page 472). The specimen should be opened on the back table to confirm the presence of the intended pathology. The anastomosed bowel is returned to the abdomen and the incisions closed.

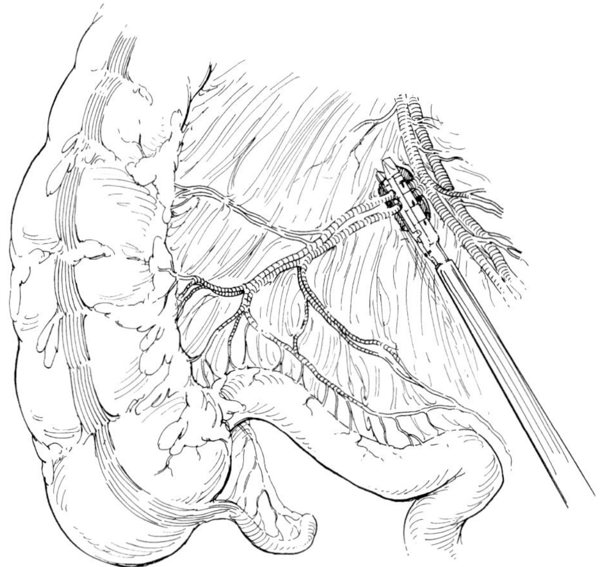

Fig. 47-5. Division of the ileocolic artery and vein. To avoid injuring the superior mesenteric vessels, the ileocolic vascular pedicle should be traced distally to the cecum.

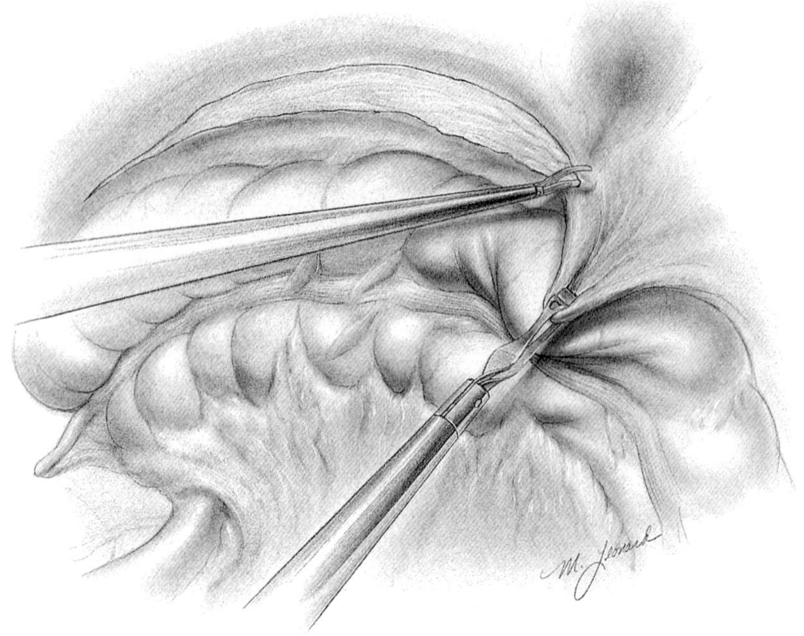

Fig. 47-6. Mobilization of the right colon is begun by incising the peritoneum lateral to the cecum.

TABLE 47-2. STEPS FOR MEDIAL-TO-LATERAL LEFT HEMICOLECTOMY

1. Exploration
2. Establishment of the plane between the superior hemorrhoidal artery and the sacral promontory
3. Identification and preservation of the hypogastric nerves, left ureter, and gonadal vessels
4. Identification and ligation of the inferior mesenteric artery and vein
5. Retroperitoneal mobilization of the left colon mesentery behind the splenic flexure
6. Division of the colonic attachments laterally, around the splenic flexure, and the omentum
7. Division of the mesorectum and rectum
8. Specimen exteriorization, resection, and colorectal anastomosis

Left Hemicolectomy: Medial-to-Lateral Approach

Table 47-2 lists the steps to a medial-to-lateral left hemicolectomy. Following port placement, laparoscopic exploration, and any necessary adhesiolysis, the patient is

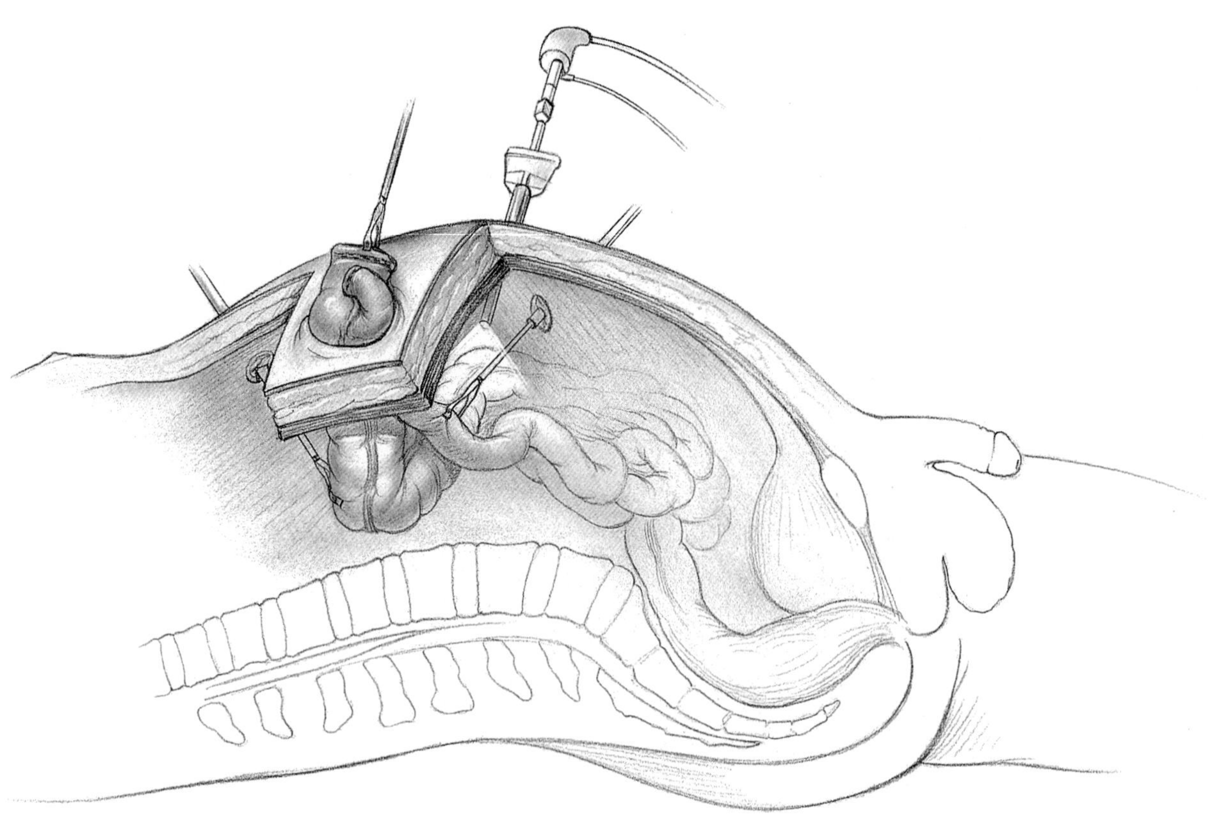

Fig. 47-7. Side-to-side anastomosis at the skin level.

tilted into steep Trendelenburg and right-side down position. The base of the medial sigmoid mesentery over the sacral promontory is exposed by sweeping the small bowel out of the pelvis and off to the right and then placing the sigmoid mesocolon on tension by retracting it anterolaterally to the left. The root of the sigmoid mesentery is scored parallel to and just posterior to the superior hemorrhoidal artery as it courses over the sacral promontory. This plane is gently dissected using a blunt spreading technique in an anterior-to-posterior direction to establish the avascular retroperitoneal plane and preserve the hypogastric nerves (Fig. 47-8). Generally two blunt instruments are used to suspend the mesentery and a third instrument (in the surgeon's dominant hand) pushes the areolar tissue down. If dissection is initiated too high in the mesentery (close to the bowel), the sigmoidal vessels will be encountered as they course in an anterioposterior direction off of the superior hemorrhoidal artery. The proper dissection plane should be reestablished further posterior. Once established, the purplish areolar plane between the sigmoid colon mesentery and the retroperitoneal structures are swept down, creating a "cave." The left ureter can be identified coursing over the left iliac vessels. Dissection is continued out to the lateral abdominal sidewall.

With the plane established, ureter identified, and dissection complete out to the white line of Toldt, the next step is to continue the plane cranially and medially to identify the inferior mesenteric artery (IMA). The inferior mesenteric vein (IMV) runs anterior and parallel to the aorta, cephalad to the IMA; an avascular window exists between the two. This window is entered to allow complete access to and isolation of the root of the IMA, which can then be divided with a vessel-sealing device or an endoscopic GIA stapler (Fig. 47-9). The IMV is then dissected free and divided in a similar fashion. The remainder of the retroperitoneal plane can now be visualized and dissected up behind the splenic flexure to the tail of the pancreas.

The sigmoid colon is then retracted medially and the white line of Toldt divided using cautery or ultrasonic shears starting at the sigmoid colon and progressing proximally (Fig. 47-10, page 474). Splenic flexure mobilization can be facilitated by repositioning the patient in reverse-Trendelenburg. The plane of dissection is established between the omentum and the colonic

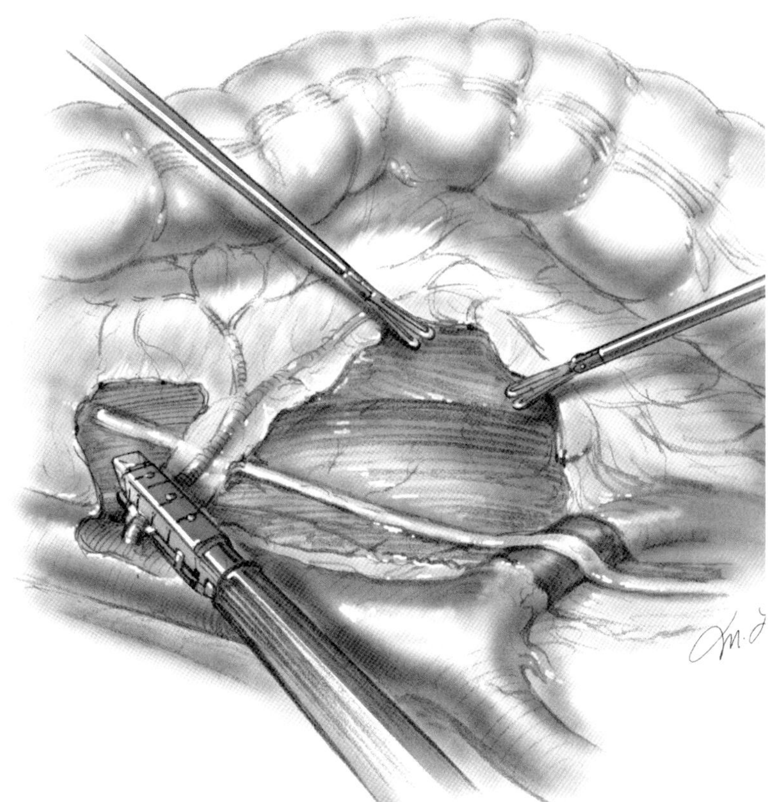

Fig. 47-8. The inferior mesenteric artery is isolated using the endoscopic shears prior to transection with the vascular stapler.

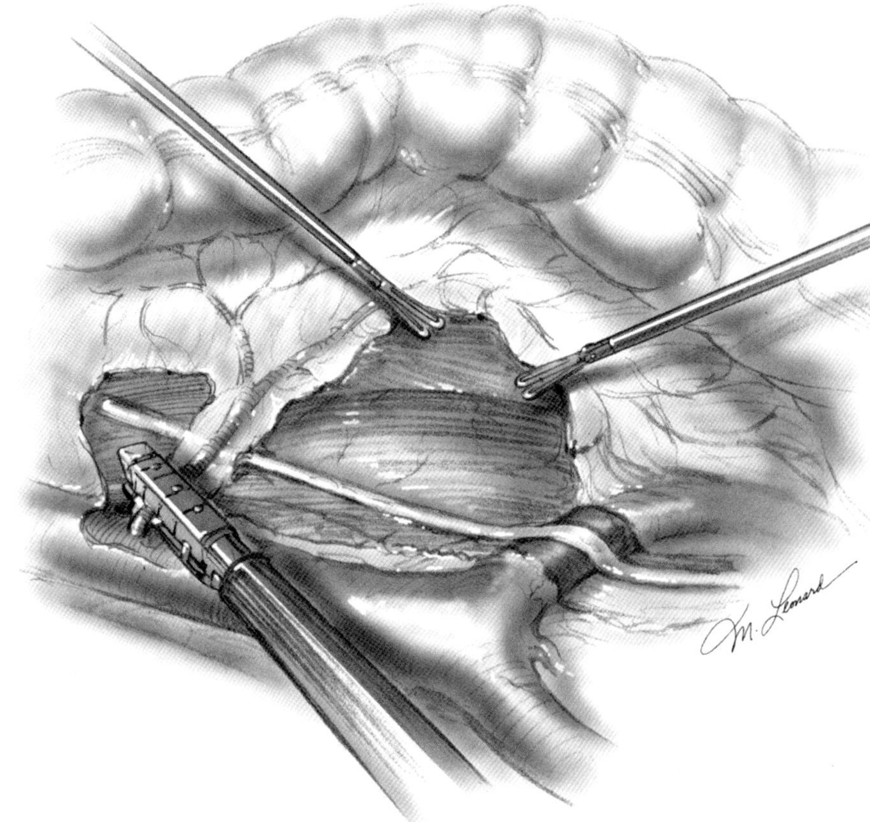

Fig. 47-9. High ligation of the inferior mesenteric artery is performed after mobilizing the left colon off the retroperitoneum.

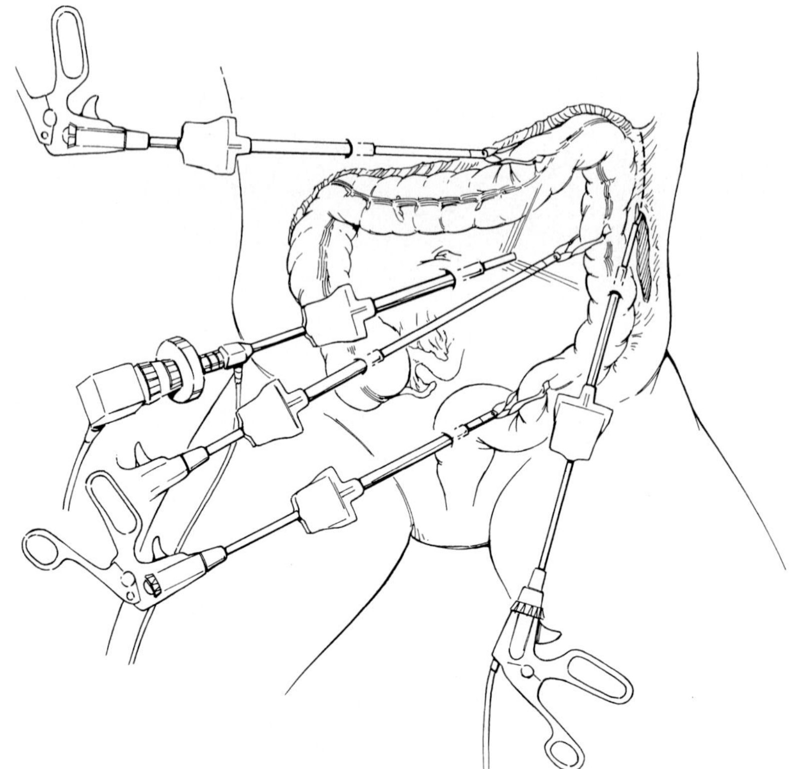

Fig. 47-10. Setup for dissection of the splenic flexure and descending colon. The surgeon stands between the patient's legs, and the assistant stands on the patient's left side.

Total Abdominal Colectomy with Ileoproctostomy

The steps to performing a medial-to-lateral total abdominal colectomy are listed in Table 47-3, page 476. Port placement and initial steps of a total abdominal colectomy are similar as for a left hemicolectomy. Following medial-to-lateral dissection and intracorporeal mesenteric ligation of the left colon, the splenic flexure mobilization continues as far proximally as possible into the lesser sac and towards the hepatic flexure. The mesentery of the transverse colon should be freed from its superior attachments to the spleen, omentum, and stomach. The middle colic vessels are then isolated and divided intracorporeally. The now-freed left colon should be transposed and placed anterior to the small bowel. This will facilitate extraction later during the operation.

The patient is then tilted in steep Trendelenburg with the left side down. Right colon mobilization and mesenteric division is then completed as described above. The patient is then tilted back to

wall and continues proximally into the lesser sac up to the level of the mid-transverse colon (Fig. 47-11). This should provide adequate length of colon to reach the pelvis for an anastomosis.

The patient is repositioned back into steep Trendelenburg. Distal dissection is continued down to the rectum along the previously established planes (Fig. 47-12). Once the distal margin of resection is chosen, the mesorectum is divided using either a vessel-sealing device or endoscopic GIA stapler (Fig. 47-13). The rectum can then be divided with one or more applications of an articulating endoscopic GIA stapler (Fig. 47-14, page 476).

The colon is now delivered through a 6- to 8-cm extraction site in the lower abdomen. The specimen is resected proximally, an end-to-end anastomosis (EEA) anvil is secured, and the bowel returned to the abdomen. A transanal EEA is monitored directly through the extraction site or alternatively the extraction site closed, pneumoperitoneum reestablished, and the anastomosis performed through laparoscopic techniques (Fig. 47-15, page 476).

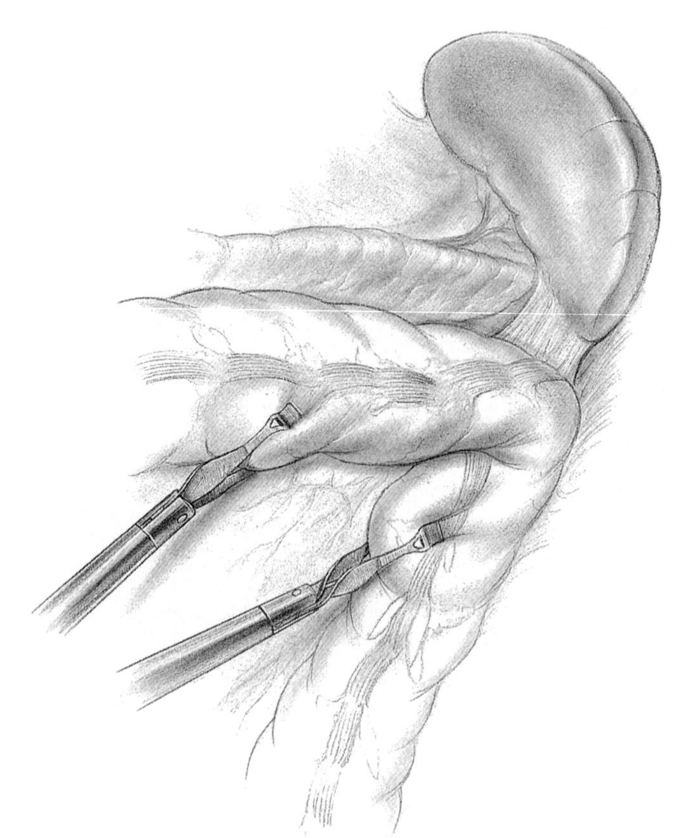

Fig. 47-11. The splenic flexure is dissected with the patient in the right-side down Trendelenburg position. The mobilized omentum is draped over the stomach, out of the surgical field, and the colon is retracted downward.

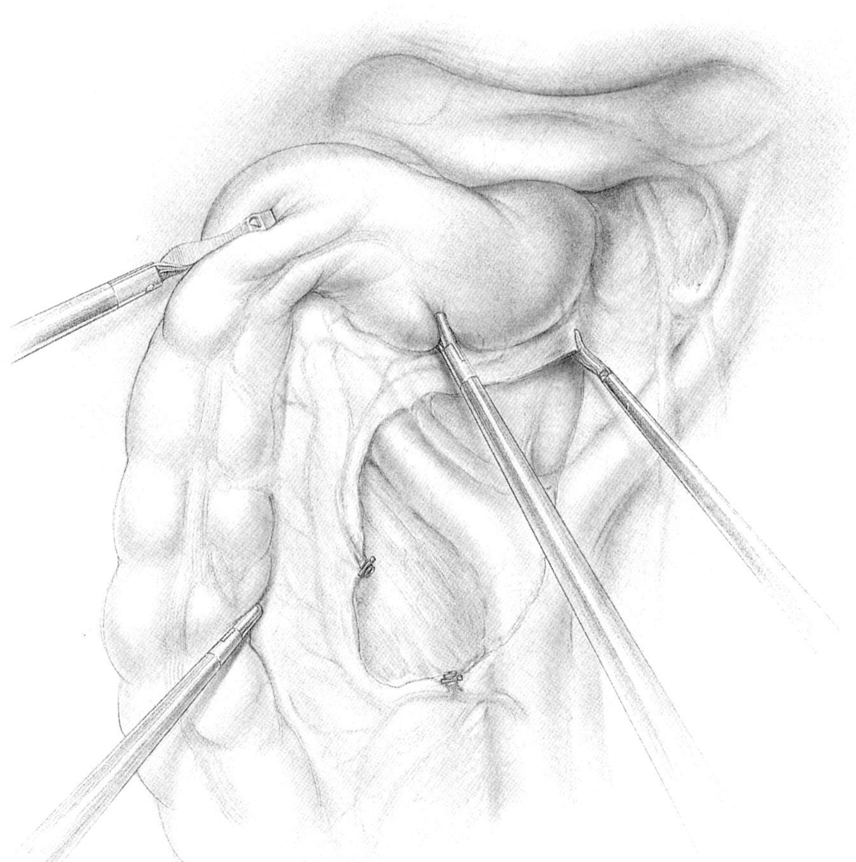

Fig. 47-12. The rectum is dissected from the sacral promontory to the levator ani muscles in the avascular retrorectal plane.

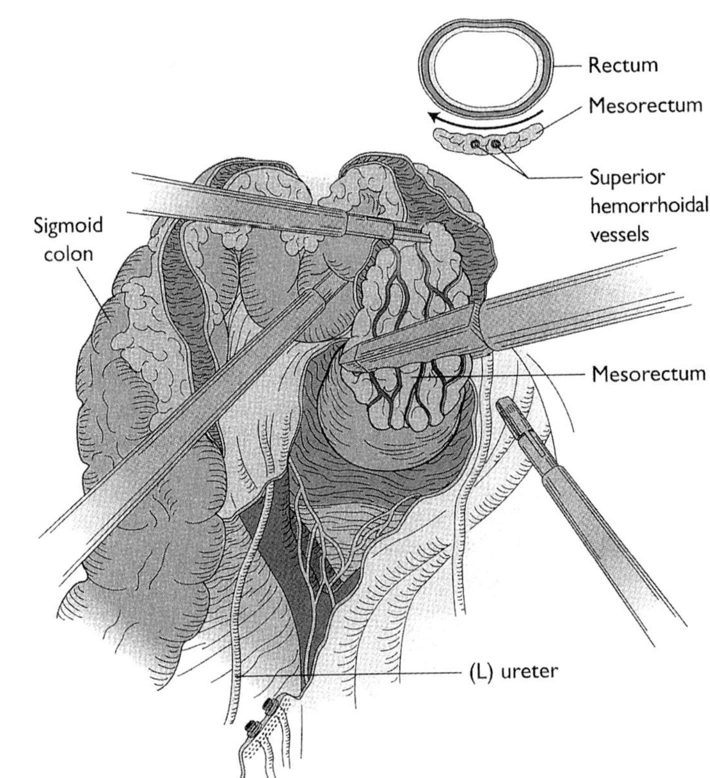

Fig. 47-13. Mobilization of the rectum.

the right. The upper rectum is identified and an appropriate transaction point identified. The bowel is transected with an endoscopic GIA stapler and the mesorectum transected with a vessel-sealing device. Alternatively, these transaction steps may be performed via a Pfannenstiel extraction site.

The colon is then exteriorized, with care taken not to twist the ileal mesentery. The ileocolic junction is divided along with its mesentery. An EEA anvil is secured in the ileal lumen and then returned to the abdomen. Anastomosis is created via the extraction site or following reestablishment of pneumoperitoneum.

Restorative Proctocolectomy

The steps to a medial-to-lateral restorative proctocolectomy are shown in Table 47-4, page 476. The surgical treatment of choice in most cases of ulcerative colitis and familial adenomatous polyposis is a restorative proctocolectomy (total proctocolectomy with ileal pouch–anal anastomosis). This is considered one of the most challenging laparoscopic colorectal procedures because it requires release of the omentum, mobilization and resection of the entire colon and rectum, creation of an ileal reservoir to be anastomosed to the anal canal, and, in most cases, creation of a loop ileostomy. While most surgeons perform a double-stapled ileoanal anastomosis, the patient should be positioned low enough on the table for available access to the perineum in the event that a hand-sewn ileoanal anastomosis is necessary.

Following the steps to mobilize the abdominal colon as listed previously, the small bowel mesentery is freed off of the retroperitoneum, up and over the duodenum to the inferior edge of the pancreas. Attention is then directed towards the pelvis for the rectal dissection. Because laparoscopic pelvic dissection is challenging and has several inherent dangers such as nerve injury, proctotomy, and hemorrhage, many surgeons perform a "hybrid" operation, completing the pelvic portion of the operation with open instruments through the 6- to 10-cm extraction site. With accumulated experience and a coordinated operating room team, straight laparoscopic dissection of the rectum may be safely and effectively performed.

Location of hypogastric nerves and ureters should be confirmed as the pelvis is entered. The dissection should progress in the embryonic fusion plane along the

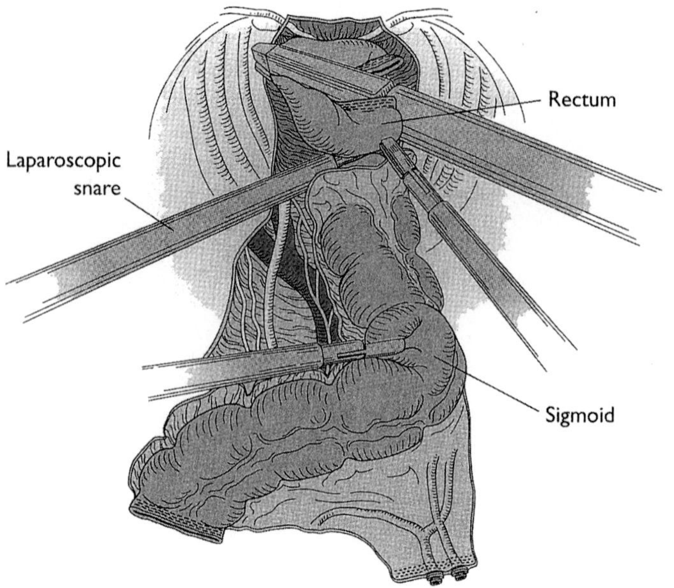

Fig. 47-14. Division of the rectum.

TABLE 47-3. STEPS FOR A MEDIAL-TO-LATERAL TOTAL ABDOMINAL COLECTOMY

1. Exploration
2. Medial-to-lateral left colon mobilization and mesenteric ligation
3. Splenic flexure mobilization
4. Transverse colon mobilization and mesenteric ligation
5. Right colon mobilization and mesenteric ligation
6. Specimen extraction, resection, and ileorectal anastomosis

fascia propria of the mesorectum. This plane is most easily identified posteriorly, then laterally, and finally anteriorly. This pattern is repeated as deeper and deeper dissection is obtained. An experienced first assistant is critical to maintain adequate traction and countertraction. The dissection and division of the lateral stalks can be performed with cautery or a vessel-sealing device. We prefer a hook cautery as this allows for an additional degree of countertraction to facilitate dissection. Care is taken throughout the dissection to avoid autonomic nerves, the pelvic sidewall, seminal vesicles, the prostate, or the vagina. Dissection must continue down into the upper anal canal. This should be confirmed by digital rectal examination.

Laparoscopic division of the distal rectum is challenging because it is difficult to manipulate current stapling devices into the deep pelvis. Two options are available: first, an endoscopic GIA stapler may be placed via a right lower quadrant or suprapubic port and then maneuvered onto the low rectum under laparoscopic guidance. Second, operating via a Pfannenstiel or lower midline extraction site, a rectal division can be performed using the traditional open TA 45 (United States Surgical; Norwalk, CT) or Contour Curved Cutter (Ethicon Endo-Surgery, Inc.; Cincinnati, OH) staplers.

The specimen is then exteriorized via the extraction site. In very thin patients,

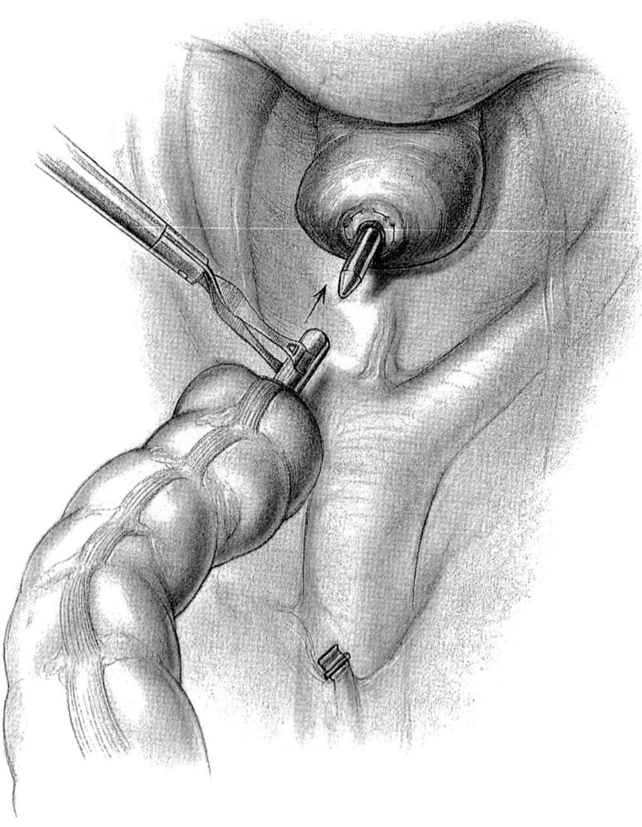

Fig. 47-15. Anastomosis of the colon and rectum with a double-stapling technique.

TABLE 47-4. STEPS FOR A MEDIAL-TO-LATERAL RESTORATIVE PROCTOCOLECTOMY

1. Exploration
2. Total abdominal colectomy
3. Complete mobilization of small bowel mesentery off of the retroperitoneum
4. Proctectomy down to the pelvic floor and anus
5. Specimen extraction, resection, creation of ileal J-pouch, anastomosis
6. Loop ileostomy

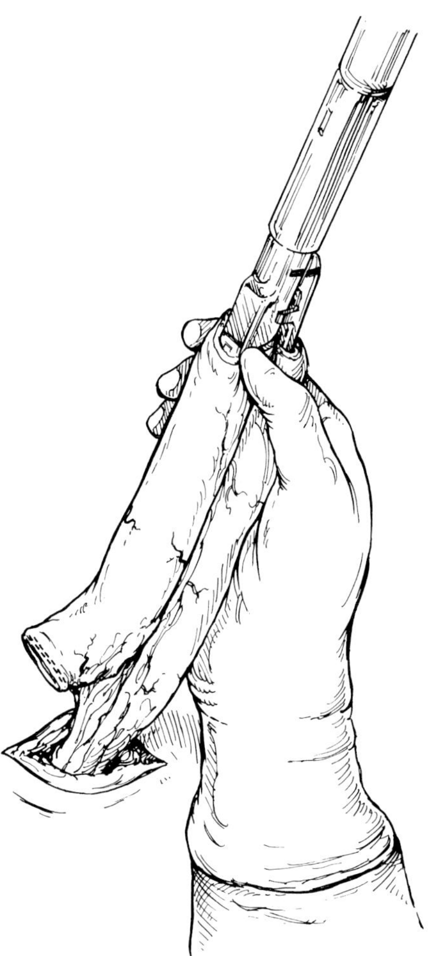

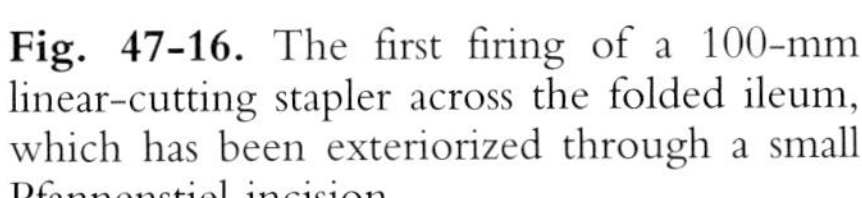

Fig. 47-16. The first firing of a 100-mm linear-cutting stapler across the folded ileum, which has been exteriorized through a small Pfannenstiel incision.

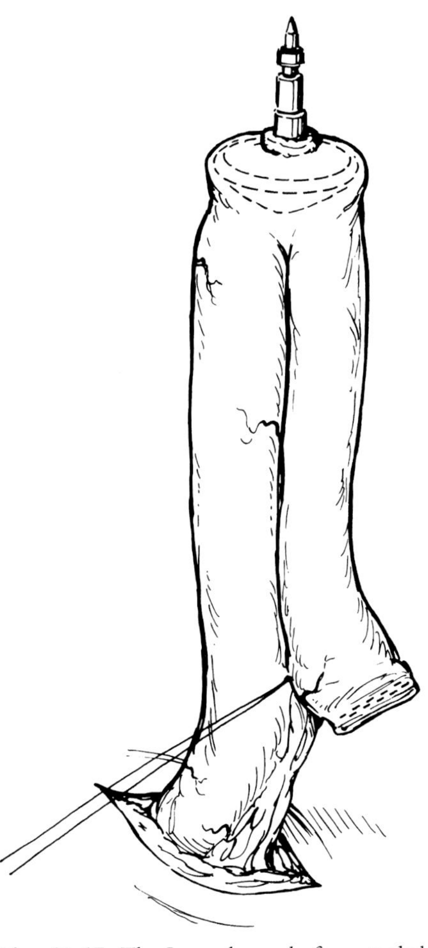

Fig. 47-17. The J-pouch, ready for a stapled anastomosis.

the ileostomy site may be sufficient for extraction. The small bowel is inspected to exclude Crohn disease. The ileocolic junction is divided with a GIA stapler. The specimen is handed off the table and then opened to inspect the mucosa for disease pattern and signs of neoplasia.

The most dependent portion of the terminal ileum is chosen to create a 15- to 20-cm J-pouch, which will reach 1 to 2 cm below the pubic symphysis. Mesenteric lengthening maneuvers such as peritoneal scoring or the division of vascular arcades may be necessary. A 2-cm enterotomy is created in the apex of the pouch, through which the GIA stapler is placed to create the pouch (Fig. 47-16). Multiple firings of the GIA stapler will be necessary to obtain the desired length. A purse-string suture is then placed around the enterotomy site to secure an EEA stapler anvil in the apex of the pouch (Fig. 47-17). The pouch is returned to the abdomen for double-staple EEA anastomosis creation using either laparoscopic or hybrid techniques. The anastomosis and pouch are assessed using rigid proctoscopy with an air-leak test. A loop ileostomy is fashioned via a rectus-splitting abdominal wall fenestration at the previously chosen site on the right abdomen. Care is taken to avoid creating undue tension on the J-pouch during ileostomy creation. Incisions are then closed and the ileostomy is matured.

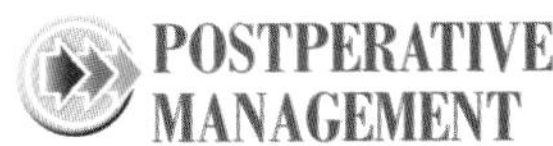

POSTPERATIVE MANAGEMENT

Early postoperative mobilization and feeding are encouraged. Orogastric tubes are removed in the operating room and patients are allowed to have clear liquid diet once fully awake. Patients are offered a soft diet once they are tolerating clear liquids and showing no signs of abdominal distention. Analgesia is provided with intravenous ketorolac and opioid patient-controlled analgesia, transitioning to oral analgesia once the patient is tolerating a soft diet. Urinary catheters are removed postoperative day 1 for colectomy patients and postoperative day 3 for patients with rectal dissections. Ambulation is encouraged on the first postoperative day. Physical therapists are utilized liberally for elderly, obese, and frail patients. Patients are discharged when they are able to provide adequate self-care and are tolerating soft diet and oral analgesics.

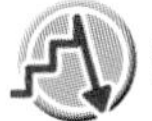

COMPLICATIONS

Complications are best avoided through careful planning and safe surgical technique. They still occur, however, even in the most skilled and experienced hands. Fortunately, most complications in colorectal surgery are not life-threatening. For example, the mortality from a colectomy is reported to be less than or equal to 1%. The exact frequency and severity of complications are difficult to determine due to heterogeneous definitions, patient populations, procedures, comorbidities, and intensity of follow-up. Some perspective on the incidence of complications can be gleaned from four recent randomized controlled trials comparing laparoscopic to open colon resections for cancer (Table 47-5, page 478).

CONCLUSION

Laparoscopic approaches and benign colorectal diseases are a perfect marriage; matching nonlethal conditions with minimal invasion and trauma. It must be remembered, however, that the spectrum of disease is very broad for the benign diagnoses and, therefore, the degree of surgical difficulty can vary widely. The practitioner should therefore be a skilled laparoscopist and a knowledgeable colon surgeon and well acquainted with a full repertory of approaches and techniques as a "one-approach-fits-all" philosophy will only lead to trouble.

TABLE 47-5. COMPLICATION RATES FOLLOWING LAPAROSCOPIC AND OPEN COLON RESECTIONS

	Trials			
Complications	**Barcelona trial (%)**	**COST trial (%)**	**CLASICC trial (%)**	**COLOR trial (%)**
Wound infection	11.9	2.5	8.7	3.3
Persistent ileus	5.5	2.8	NA	NA
Evisceration	0.9	NA	NA	0.8
Bleeding	0.5	1.2	4.8	1.9
Anastomotic leak	0.9	NA	6.0	2.3
Pneumonia	0	NA	6.5	1.9
UTI	0.5	1.2	NA	2.3
ARF	1.4	NA	NA	NA
DVT	NA	NA	1.0	NA
Cardiac	NA	2.6	NA	1.2

UTI, urinary tract infection; ARF, acute renal failure; DVT, deep venous thrombosis; NA, no answer.

SUGGESTED READING

Clinical outcomes of surgical therapy study group. A comparison of laparoscopically assisted and open colectomy for colon cancer. *N Engl J Med* 2004;350:2050–2059.

Guillou PJ, Quirke P, Thorpe H, et al. Short-term endpoints of conventional versus laparoscopic-assisted surgery in patients with colorectal cancer (MRC CLASICC trial): multicentre, randomised controlled trial. *Lancet* 2005;365:1718–1726.

Hassan I, Pemberton JH, Young-Fadok TM, et al. Ileorectal anastomosis for slow transit constipation: long-term functional and quality of life results. *J Gastrointest Surg* 2006;10:1330–1336.

Lacy AM, Garcia-Valdecasas JC, Delgado S, et al. Laparoscopy-assisted colectomy versus open colectomy for treatment of non-metastatic colon cancer: a randomised trial. *Lancet* 2002;359:2224–2229.

Larson DW, Dozois EJ, Piotrowicz K, et al. Laparoscopic-assisted vs. open ileal pouch-anal anastomosis: functional outcome in a case-matched series. *Dis Colon Rectum* 2005;48:1845–1850.

Senagore AJ. Laparoscopic sigmoid colectomy for diverticular disease. *Surg Clin North Am* 2005;85:19–24.

Senagore AJ, Duepree HJ, Delaney CP, et al. Results of a standardized technique and postoperative care plan for laparoscopic sigmoid colectomy: a 30-month experience. *Dis Colon Rectum* 2003;46:503–509.

Young-Fadok TM, Nelson H. Laparoscopic right colectomy: five-step procedure. *Dis Colon Rectum* 2000;43:267–271.

COMMENTARY

Drs. Whiteford and Hardiman present a comprehensive review of the reasons for and minimally invasive techniques of laparoscopy for benign colorectal pathologies. This may seem like rather "low-hanging fruit" to the casual reader, who may be focused on the more common and controversial laparoscopic colectomy for colon cancer, but it is critical to the adoption of laparoscopic colorectal surgery. Benign indications are the ideal way for the surgeon new to laparoscopic colectomy to develop the technical skills needed to safely perform oncologic resections. For the most part, a minimally invasive approach is also more appreciated by patients with benign disease, as cancer patients are generally more concerned with survival and less with cosmetics and length of recovery. This is certainly not to say that these are *easier* cases. Benign indications present the full spectrum of difficulty to the laparoscopic approach: from very easy localized segmental resections for a polyp, to complex dissections of obscured anatomy as seen with chronic inflammatory conditions, and finally to extensive anatomical resections as for a total proctocolectomy. Obviously the novice laparoscopic surgeon should carefully triage early cases according to their difficulty.

The authors are strong advocates of the "medial-to-lateral" approach, which represents somewhat of a paradigm shift in the laparoscopic world. Maintaining the lateral attachments as long as possible provides an automatic retraction of the colon and facilitates the mesenteric dissection. This technique has dramatically decreased the operative times for the procedures and has proven an excellent approach for cancer resections as well. It does require some time and experience on the part of a surgeon however; laboratory practice with cadaver models and/or the presence of a knowledgeable proctor are invaluable aids in mastering this approach. As spelled out in this chapter, there is little need for hand-assisted approaches unless one is in the early learning curve with advanced laparoscopic dissection or as an intermediate alternative to conversion to open surgery when difficult situations are encountered.

While laparoscopic colectomy for benign disease may not represent the easiest spectrum of cases to deal with, the ability to offer patients a less-invasive surgery remains a true benefit to these patients. A rapid return to normal activity and dramatically decreased wound complications are the primary benefits; once past their learning curve surgeons find that these cases are often an elegant and more enjoyable alternative to open colon resection.

LLS

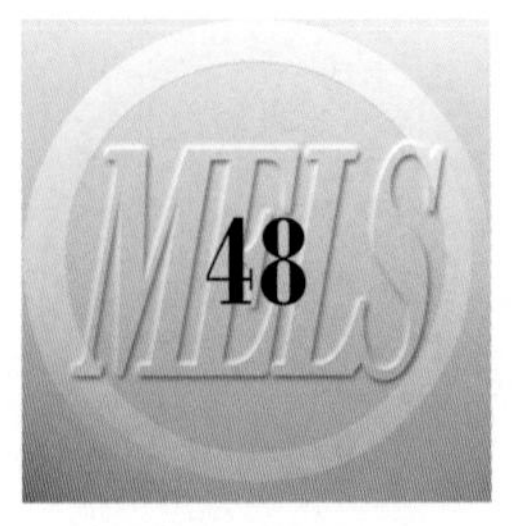

Laparoscopic Resection for Carcinoma of the Colon

DANIEL A. LAWES AND TONIA M. YOUNG-FADOK

INTRODUCTION

Laparoscopic procedures have been performed for colonic malignancy since 1991. Initial enthusiasm for the procedure was tempered by doubts about its safety. Reports of metastatic disease in the port sites and questions regarding the adequacy of the oncologic resection lead to several large randomized controlled trials to evaluate the merits of laparoscopic versus open colectomy for cancer. The majority of these trials included only right- and left-sided lesions, excluding malignancies of the transverse colon and rectum, and many of the procedures were undertaken by surgeons, who were considered adequately trained at the time, but would now be considered to have limited laparoscopic experience. This relative lack of initial training is highlighted by the reduction in the conversion rate seen in most trials as time progressed. It became clear that with the use of appropriate oncologic techniques, port site metastases were extremely uncommon, with an incidence of less than 1%, similar to that of wound recurrence in open colectomy. Oncologic results appear to be similar to those obtained for open surgery, with no differences detected in the resection margins and numbers of lymph nodes harvested. Although only limited long-term data are available, meta-analysis of the existing studies does not demonstrate any significant difference in cancer-related mortality or recurrence rates between open and laparoscopic groups. Complication rates for common complications such as wound infection and ileus are also similar for both groups, albeit with conversion rates in the randomized trials of up to 29% in the laparoscopic groups. The benefits of laparoscopic surgery are seen in reduced blood loss, reduced post operative pain and decreased use of analgesia, faster return of bowel function, faster return to independent activity, and reduced hospital inpatient stay (by an average of between 0.5 to 2.7 days). These advantages are offset by an increased operative time (142 to189 minutes for laparoscopic vs. 95 to 144 minutes for open) and although the cost of the procedure may be greater than traditional surgery, this is offset by a reduction in length of hospital stay.

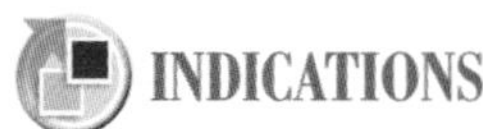

INDICATIONS

A resection of the colon that conforms to oncologic principles is indicated by several clinical scenarios. The most obvious is the diagnosis of colon cancer, but the same principles apply to resection for a polyp not amenable to colonoscopic removal. Such polyps often cannot be removed because of their size and extent; these characteristics are associated with an increased risk of malignant degeneration, thus mandating an oncologic resection. Similar principles may also apply in the event of syndromes such as hereditary nonpolyposis colorectal cancer (HNPCC) and familial adenomatous polyposis (FAP), if there is any concern that there may be an associated malignancy. Patients with ulcerative colitis with high- or low-grade dysplasia should also be approached with an appropriate oncologic resection, as a malignancy may already be present.

An oncologic resection requires adherence to certain surgical principles. There should be adequate proximal and distal margins. The vascular pedicle(s) should be divided at the base. These two factors then ensure an appropriate lymphadenectomy. If the tumor is adherent to an adjacent organ, an en bloc resection is required to minimize the risk of recurrence.

The indications for performing a laparoscopic colon resection for cancer are similar to those of an open resection. Obesity and the presence of previous surgical incisions increase the risk of conversion to an open operation, but are not contraindications to attempting laparoscopic resection. An initial diagnostic laparoscopy should be performed to assess the feasibility of a laparoscopic approach in cases where there is doubt, with a plan for early conversion to an open procedure should adhesions prove too dense to divide safely or the patient's intraabdominal adipose tissue renders exposure difficult.

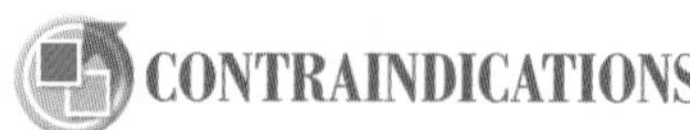

CONTRAINDICATIONS

The main relative contraindications to laparoscopic colonic resection include intestinal obstruction, bulky tumors, cancer invasive into adjacent organs, and pregnancy. In the case of uncompensated intestinal obstruction, the small intestine and/or colon are distended, reducing the ability to obtain an adequate pneumoperitoneum and sufficient intraabdominal space in which to operate. In addition the intestine is often very edematous and friable and may tear or perforate when manipulated with laparoscopic instruments. Large masses of 8 cm or more tend to be difficult to manipulate safely and often obscure the correct tissue planes; furthermore the incisions required to remove the specimen are equivalent to those required for a conventional laparotomy, thus reducing the benefits of a laparoscopic resection. Cancers that invade adjacent organs or the abdominal wall may not be resectable laparoscopically; unless the surgeon has the necessary skills to perform an en bloc resection laparoscopically, the tumor should be removed by a planned laparotomy. In addition laparoscopic resection should not be attempted in the rare case of a pregnant patient requiring colonic resection for a colonic neoplasm, particularly in the first and third trimesters, because of concerns regarding fetal injury and inability to achieve adequate working space respectively. The procedure may be technically feasible in the second trimester but there is no supporting data regarding the safety of laparoscopy for colon cancer during pregnancy.

The experience of the surgeon is highly important in determining if a laparoscopic resection should be undertaken. For that reason, more straightforward cases should be attempted early in a surgeon's learning curve so that experience is gained. Similarly, a potentially curative resection should not be performed by an inexperienced laparoscopic surgeon due to risks such as inadequacy of oncologic resection and perforation of the tumor. The joint position statement from the American Society of Colon and Rectal Surgeons (ASCRS) and the Society of American Gastrointestinal and Endoscopic Surgeons (SAGES) states that data from clinical trials supports a minimum experience of 20 laparoscopic colorectal resections with anastomosis should be obtained for benign disease or in those with metastatic cancer before curative resection is undertaken.

PREOPERATIVE PLANNING

Preoperative evaluation remains essentially the same as for the open procedure. Patients should undergo standard history, physical examination, and laboratory tests, including blood typing and screening, with further evaluation guided by these findings as appropriate. The local extent of the tumor can be assessed by CT scan of the abdomen and pelvis, especially in the case of bulky tumors, to ensure that there is no invasion into the abdominal wall, retroperitoneum, or other organs that would require en bloc resection to remove.

If the tumor is resectable laparoscopically, care should be taken to ensure that it is adequately localized. This is particularly important in the case of small cancers or polyps, which are often not apparent from the serosal surface of the colon. As localization by colonoscopy is often inaccurate and tactile sensation is not available to the laparoscopic surgeon, there is a risk of removing the wrong section of colon. To minimize this risk, there are several options available to localize the tumor either pre- or intraoperatively. Our preference is for Indian ink tattooing at the site of the lesion during the endoscopy; we encourage our gastroenterological colleagues to tattoo any lesion identified that they believe may require surgical intervention and certainly all polyps greater than 1 cm in diameter. Submucosal injection of dye should be performed at the distal border of the lesion to ensure that division of the bowel beyond this point will not include diseased tissue and in at least three places around the circumference of the colon, to ensure that even if one of the tattoos is obscured by either the mesocolon or retroperitoneum and thus invisible to the surgeon, the position of the remaining tattoos remains visible. Tattoos reliably last up to 3 months in the colon and frequently longer. If the tumor has not been marked during colonoscopy, CT colonography or contrast enema can accurately depict the site of the lesion. CT colonography is thus useful both for localization of the lesion and also for staging the tumor.

In our experience, the above measures have been sufficient to avoid problems with intraoperative localization. If, however, preoperative localization has been inadequate and the lesion is not identifiable at the time of surgery, two options are available. A hand port can be introduced, allowing palpation of the colon, but this may not be 100% sensitive; small lesions can still be missed as they may not be distinguishable from pericolonic fat. Another option is intraoperative colonoscopy. To minimize intestinal insufflation an atraumatic grasper should be placed across the terminal ileum prior to insertion of the scope. On localization of the lesion the intestinal wall should be marked with a laparoscopically applied suture and as much gas as possible removed from the colon prior to removal of the colonoscope. The problem of colonic distension is avoided if carbon dioxide is available for colonoscopic insufflation, as the gas is rapidly absorbed.

SURGICAL TECHNIQUE

We employ a standardized, reproducible approach for patient positioning and port placement for all laparoscopic colorectal procedures.

Patient Positioning in the Operating Suite

The patient lies on the operating table on foam "egg-crate" padding that is secured to the table, as this prevents the patient from slipping during steep position changes. It is essential that the operating table can be moved easily into extremes of Trendelenburg, reverse Trendelenburg, and right and left inclines, because this facilitates access to different areas of the abdomen by using gravity to move the small intestine away from the operative field. Right colectomy is performed with the patient supine on the operating table (Fig. 48-1); all other colonic procedures are performed in modified synchronous position with the legs in stirrups (Fig. 48-2, page 482). The patient's distal sacrum is positioned at the end of the table in order to gain access for stapled colorectal anastomosis or intraoperative colonoscopy, should they be necessary. Knee- or thigh-length pneumatic compression devices are applied to the legs, which are placed in padded Lloyd-Davies stirrups and secured with padded foot straps. It is important to position the patient's thighs parallel to

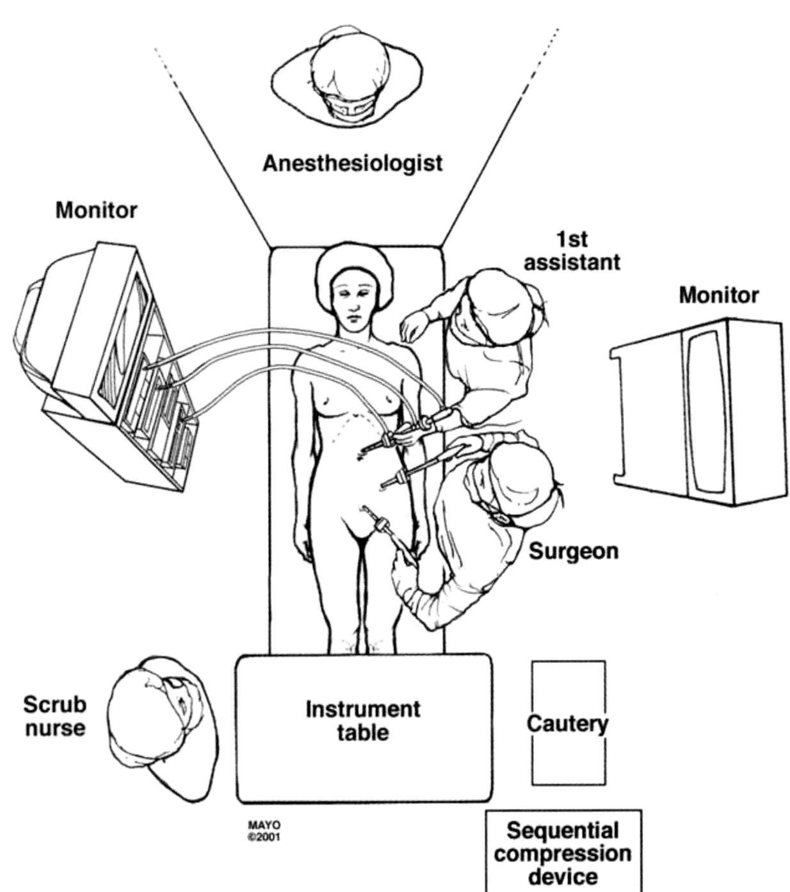

Fig. 48-1. Positioning of patient, staff, and OR equipment for right colectomy.

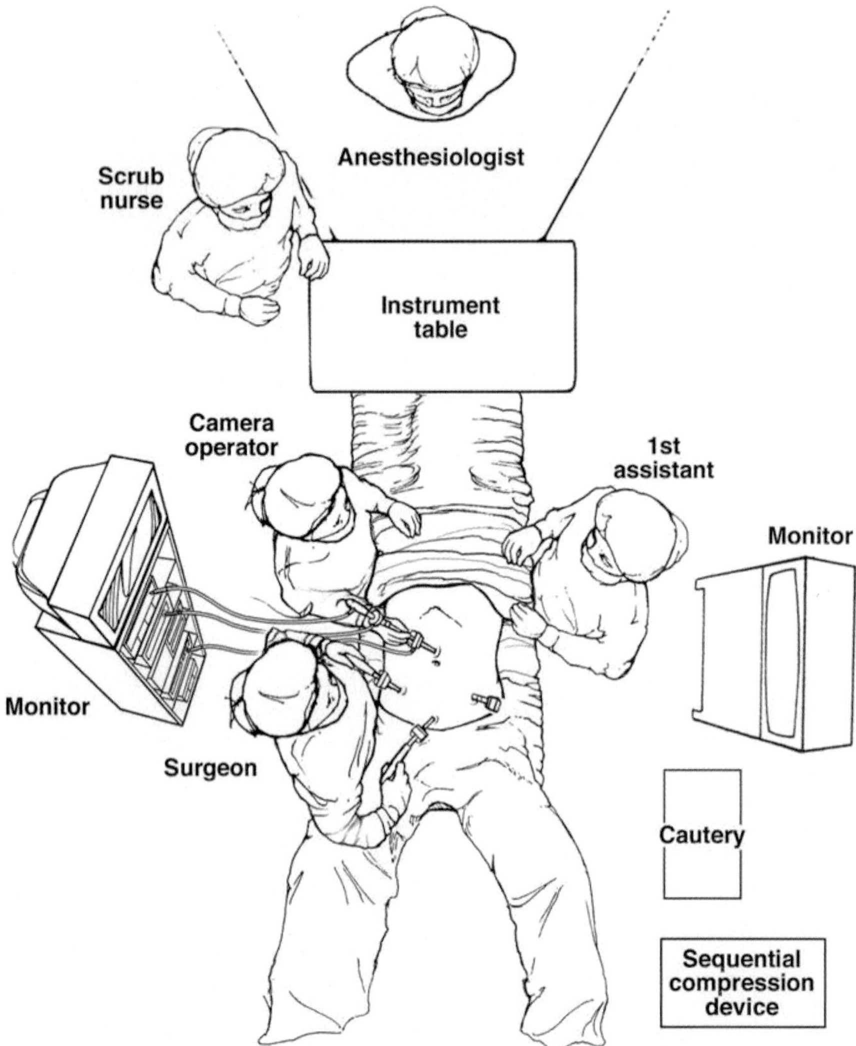

Fig. 48-2. Positioning of patient, staff, and OR equipment for left colectomy.

the abdomen to prevent interference with the movements of instruments deployed in the lower abdominal ports. The patient's hands are protected with further foam padding, and the arms secured alongside the patient with sheets that are wrapped around the arms and folded beneath the torso. Additional "egg-crate" padding is laid on the patient's chest and secured with a chest strap to further reduce the risk that the patient will slip during position changes.

The patient is catheterized, and the skin is prepared and draped in a standard manner with sterile leggings and adhesive drapes to expose the abdomen. Prior to insertion of the trocars the laparoscopic equipment is placed and checked. The laparoscopic "stack," containing the light source, camera, and insufflator, are positioned on whichever side allows for least interference of the cords with the progression of the case. A 30-degree, 10-mm laparoscope is used throughout the procedure. Two video screens are utilized, positioned on either side of the patient to allow the surgeon, assistant, and scrub nurse adequate visualization. It is important that the screens can be moved during the procedure to facilitate operating in different areas of the abdominal cavity and to ensure all members of the operative team have a good view of the procedure. Other instruments that we routinely use are two 5-mm Babcock graspers, laparoscopic scissors with a finger-operated cautery button attached to the scissors, a power source that allows division of vessels up to 7 mm in diameter, a selection of laparoscopic staplers including articulated staplers with 30- and 45-mm cartridges and staple heights appropriate for bowel and vessels, suction irrigation, and a smoke evacuator.

Positioning and Placement of Trocars

For almost all colonic procedures the ports are placed in a standard diamond configuration. The first port inserted is a supraumbilical 12-mm blunt port. The trocar is inserted by a cut-down method and secured to the fascia with two sutures. This acts as the camera port throughout the procedure, and is the site subsequently extended periumbilically and used for specimen extraction. A periumbilical extraction site facilitates delivering the transverse colon compared to a Pfannenstiel incision. Following insufflation to a pressure of 13 mmHg, the camera is introduced and the abdominal cavity inspected. Subsequent ports are then inserted under direct vision. For the majority of colonic resections a 5-mm port is inserted in the left lower quadrant, lateral to the rectus sheath, a second 5-mm port is placed in the suprapubic region, and a 12-mm port is inserted in the right lower quadrant also lateral to the rectus sheath. This port is used for deployment of the stapler for the inferior mesenteric vessels and intracorporeal division of the upper rectum. During dissection, a 5-mm reducer is used in conjunction with this port. The only alteration in this configuration would be for a right hemicolectomy, in which case the right lower quadrant port is 5 mm. Division of the ileocolic vessels is usually performed with an energy source, but if the vessels are calcified or particularly large a 5-mm camera is placed via the left lower quadrant port with the stapler placed via the supraumbilical port to allow division of the ileocolic vessels by means of a stapler. We utilize this standard diamond-shaped position of the trocars for all laparoscopic colorectal operations and find that it allows good access to the entire abdominal cavity. On occasion, in a particularly difficult case, an additional 5-mm port is introduced, its position being dictated by the specific requirements of the case.

LEFT HEMICOLECTOMY/ SIGMOID COLECTOMY

This procedure can be divided into five distinct steps: (1) mobilization of the sigmoid and descending colon, (2) mobilization of the splenic flexure, (3) division of the inferior mesenteric vessels, (4) division of the colon, and (5) exteriorization of the specimen, resection, and anastomosis.

Mobilization of the Sigmoid and Descending Colon

The patient is positioned in a steep Trendelenburg with the left side elevated. The surgeon and assistant stand on the

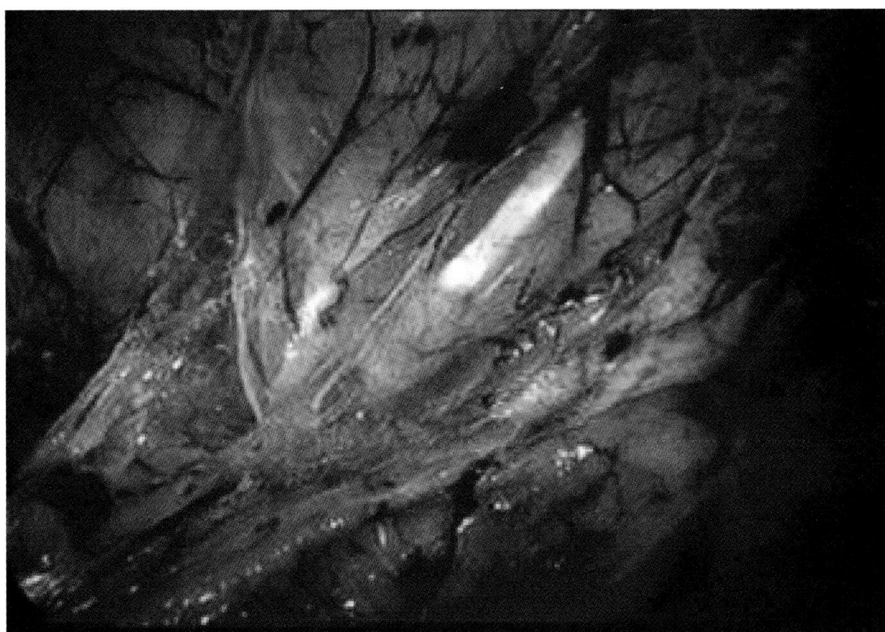

Fig. 48-3. As the sigmoid is mobilized medially, the left ureter, gonadal vessels, and psoas tendon are exposed and identified.

right side of the patient facing the left so that hands, instruments, operative site, and video screen are aligned. The surgeon holds a grasper in the left hand through the right lower quadrant port and cautery scissors in the right hand via the suprapubic port. The first maneuver is to ensure that the small bowel is swept out of the pelvis towards the patient's right upper quadrant and that any adhesions tethering the intestine are divided. It is usually unnecessary to grasp the bowel as the steep positioning of the operating table allows gravity to move the bowel and maintain its position. The sigmoid colon is identified and retracted medially to expose the peritoneal reflection, or white line of Toldt. The peritoneum immediately medial to this line is incised. It is important to identify the left ureter, which is usually visible once the sigmoid mobilization has commenced, running medial to the gonadal vessels and over the left iliac vessels (Fig. 48-3). Remaining in the correct plane involves dissection of the colon off the retroperitoneum, leaving the white line *with the patient*. We prefer the use of cautery for mobilization of the colon as it mirrors the use of cautery in open cases, it is faster, and ensures that the correct bloodless dissection plane is maintained. Dissection is continued cephalad between the sigmoid mesocolon and retroperitoneum. Medial traction is maintained on the colon allowing the correct plane to be opened with a combination of gentle blunt dissection and cautery. Dissection continues towards the splenic flexure along the peritoneal reflection, and again traction is important to allow the correct plane to be identified (Fig. 48-4). This may be facilitated by the assistant, who can use a grasper via the right lower quadrant port whilst the surgeon uses the cautery scissors through the left lower quadrant port and a grasper through the suprapubic port. By carefully delineating the plane one avoids dissecting in a plane lateral to the true peritoneal reflection, which runs the risk of mobilization of the kidney or pancreas.

Mobilization of the Splenic Flexure

When the descending colon has been mobilized to the level of the spleen, attention is turned to mobilizing the greater omentum from the colon. This can be achieved in one of two ways: mobilizing the omentum off the distal transverse colon thus leaving the omentum behind, or entering the lesser sac and dividing the splenocolic attachments and thus taking the omentum with the splenic flexure. The patient is repositioned in reverse Trendelenburg, still with the left side of the operating table planed upwards. The surgeon moves to stand between the patient's legs to facilitate splenic flexure mobilization. The assistant uses a grasper via the right lower quadrant port in order to elevate the omentum cephalad so that it exposes the transverse colon. The surgeon retracts the transverse colon downwards, and the peritoneum joining the colon and omentum is divided to gain entry into the lesser sac (Fig. 48-5, page 484). Dissection continues along the superior border of the colon until the spleen is reached and the distal transverse colon is free from omentum. In patients who are obese it may be difficult to enter this plane, in which case the lesser sac may be entered by dividing the omentum, leaving it attached to the

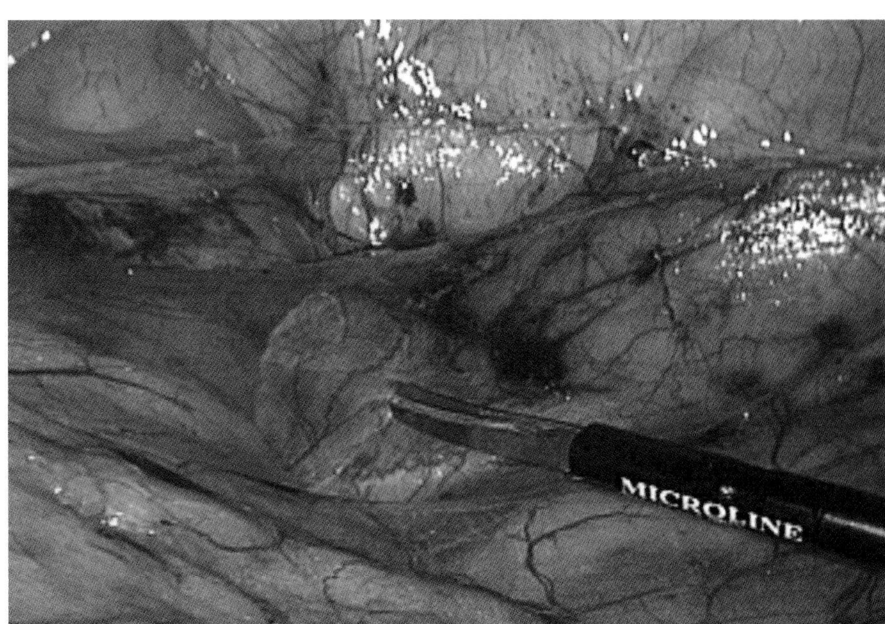

Fig. 48-4. Mobilization of the descending colon. In the Trendelenburg position, with the left side tilted up, the left lateral peritoneal reflection is clearly seen as the descending colon is mobilized medially.

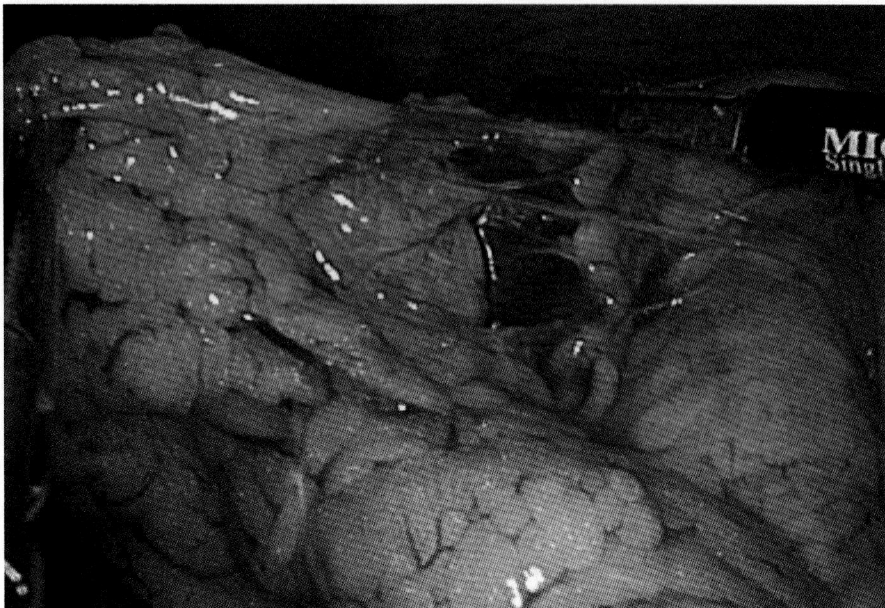

Fig. 48-5. The splenic flexure is mobilized by exposing the peritoneal attachment between the undersurface of the omentum and the distal transverse colon.

colon. Again with the assistant providing traction on the omentum pulling it inferiorly, the area between the stomach and colon to the left of the midline can be safely divided until the lesser sac is entered. Dissection proceeds towards the spleen with the assistant grasping the superior cut edge of the omentum whilst the surgeon provides countertraction on the inferior edge using a grasper in the right hand placed through the left lower quadrant port, as the power source is used in the surgeon's left hand via the suprapubic port. Once the omentum has been divided, the splenic flexure is retracted inferiorly and any further retroperitoneal attachments divided. Mobilization is considered to be satisfactory when the splenic flexure can be easily pulled below the level of the umbilicus. Care taken achieving adequate mobilization at this time will ensure that exteriorization of the colon will be achieved smoothly. Even if subsequent dissection in the pelvis is not possible (e.g., for a bulky tumor) and conversion is required, the remainder of the procedure can often be completed via a Pfannenstiel incision instead of requiring a midline incision, as the splenic flexure has already been fully mobilized.

Division of the Inferior Mesenteric Vessels

In order to isolate and divide the inferior mesenteric artery, the operating table is returned to steep Trendelenburg, with the left side still inclined up. The assistant stands on the right side and, using a grasper via the right lower quadrant port, retracts the left side of the rectosigmoid mesentery medially to expose the left pelvic brim and left pararectal tissues. The surgeon, on the left side, uses a grasper in the left hand via the suprapubic port and scissors in the right hand via the left lower quadrant port. The incision along the left lateral peritoneal fold at the pelvic brim is now extended over the pelvic brim and along the right pararectal tissues. This allows entry into the presacral space, which is developed medially and distally as far as necessary, to the anticipated distal margin of transection. Dissection of the presacral space is facilitated by the assistant placing the grasper behind the mesorectum where the presacral space has been entered and elevating the tissues anteriorly.

The operating table is then placed with slight right side inclination upwards. The rectosigmoid mesentery is again elevated and the right pararectal peritoneum is scored. The correct line of dissection is often indicated by air in the presacral space from the previous left-sided dissection. Once the peritoneum is scored, the presacral space is entered and developed to the chosen distal resection margin. The dissection in the presacral space is continued cephalad until the undersurface of the inferior mesenteric artery (IMA) is reached. The peritoneal window superior to the IMA is opened and in this manner the base of the vascular pedicle is isolated. The vessel can now be divided; our choice is for a linear stapler with vascular cartridge in heavier patients, and energy sealing device (which can close vessels up to 7 mm) in patients with normal body mass index. We do not routinely divide the inferior mesenteric vein when performing left or sigmoid colectomy, unless potential tension on the anastomosis requires it, which is less likely than with rectal resection.

Division of the Colon

With the assistant on the left elevating and exposing the right side of the rectosigmoid, the surgeon stands on the right. At the chosen distal resection margin, usually at the rectosigmoid for a sigmoid cancer, the mesorectum/sigmoid mesentery is divided with the energy device, until the posterior wall of the rectosigmoid is reached. The rectosigmoid can then be divided with a linear stapler deployed via the 12-mm right lower quadrant port. By elevating the cut edge of the rectosigmoid, the sigmoid mesentery is exposed. Starting at the already opened peritoneal window superior to the IMA, the sigmoid mesentery is divided close to the retroperitoneum, moving proximally until the chosen level of the proximal resection margin is reached. At this point, the specimen is ready for exteriorization.

Exteriorization of the Specimen, Resection, and Anastomosis

For sigmoid colectomy our preferred anastomotic method is a stapled end-to-end colorectal anastomosis. Prior to extending the supraumbilical cutdown incision to 3 to 5 cm, a grasper is placed on the divided end of the colon to facilitate delivery of the specimen. The fascia is opened, a wound protector is introduced (we use a sterilized plastic bag with the bottom edge cut off), and the divided end of the rectosigmoid colon is passed up to the incision. A proximal resection margin in the descending colon is chosen, and the small amount of remaining mesentery is divided and ligated. After dividing the descending colon, a purse-string suture of 2/0 polypropylene is used to secure the cut distal end around the anvil of a circular stapling device. The bowel is returned to the abdominal cavity, the wound closed with the blunt port between interrupted fascial sutures, and a pneumoperitoneum reestablished. The stapler is advanced to the top of the rectum, the spike brought out adjacent to the staple line, and the anvil docked onto the handle taking care to ensure the bowel is not twisted, by checking the cut edge of the mesentery. On closure of the stapler, the surgeon again checks that nothing has been caught in the staple line before the gun is fired. All ports are removed under direct vision and the 12-mm port site is closed prior to release of the pneumoperitoneum.

If the tumor is situated in the descending colon, the distal resection margin will be more proximal and can often be exteriorized, which facilitates a hand-sewn rather than a stapled anastomosis. Following mobilization and vessel and mesenteric division, the colon containing the tumor can be exteriorized, the mesentery and colon divided at an appropriate place, and intestinal continuity is re-established using a hand sewn end-to-end anastomosis in the traditional fashion.

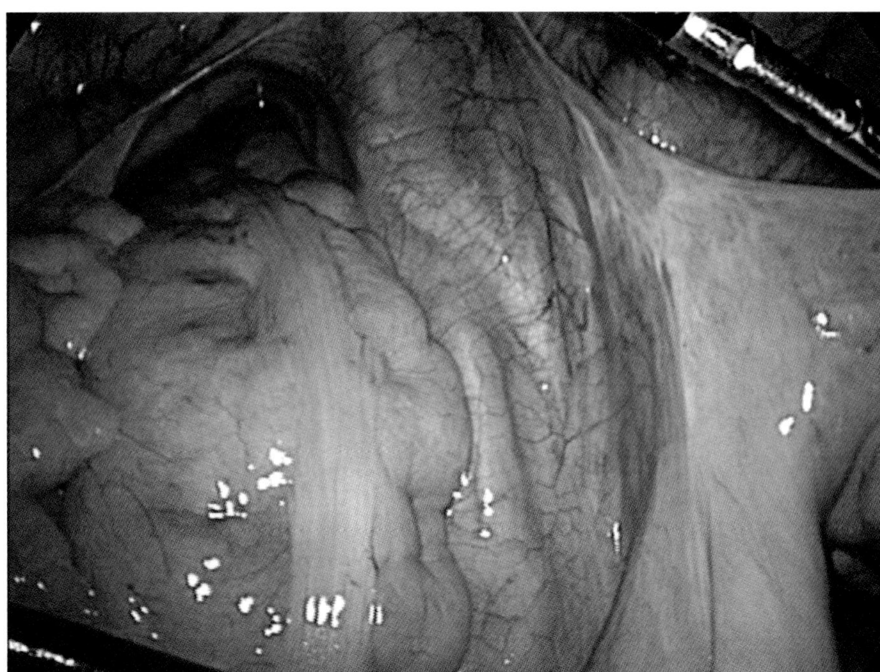

Fig. 48-6. Mobilization of the cecum. In the Trendelenburg position, with the right side tilted up, the peritoneum around the base of the cecum and terminal ileal mesentery is scored to enter the retroperitoneal plane.

RIGHT HEMICOLECTOMY

This procedure can be divided into four distinct steps: (1) mobilization of the cecum and ascending colon, (2) mobilization of the hepatic flexure, (3) division of the ileocolic pedicle and mesentery, and (4) exteriorization of the specimen, resection, and anastomosis. A diamond-shaped configuration of ports is again used, with a cut-down for a 12-mm supraumbilical blunt port and three 5-mm ports in the right and left lower quadrants and the suprapubic midline.

Mobilization of the Cecum and Ascending Colon

The patient is placed in steep Trendelenburg with the right side elevated. After port placement, both surgeon and assistant stand on the left side of the patient. The grasper is in the surgeon's right hand via the left lower quadrant (LLQ) port and cautery scissors in the left hand via the suprapubic port, preventing crossing of the instruments. The small intestine is swept out of the pelvis towards the left upper quadrant. The peritoneum inferior to the junction of the cecum and terminal ileum is grasped and lifted anteriorly and cephalad (that is, towards 2 or 3 o'clock on the screen). This exposes the "valley," that runs roughly parallel to the iliac artery, where the mesentery of the colon meets the retroperitoneum (Fig. 48-6). In a patient with normal body mass index, the right ureter can be seen though the peritoneum, but in a heavier patient, it must be identified after opening the peritoneum. The peritoneum is scored along this valley, allowing gas to enter the tissues and helping to identify a layer of filmy connective tissue and delineate the correct bloodless plane. By maintaining traction on the cecum the peritoneum is divided and this plane is developed medially and superiorly. Once the cecum and terminal ileum are mobilized, the right lateral peritoneal reflection alongside the ascending colon is divided and the colon mobilized medially. It is important to recognize that the plane of dissection turns medially and obliquely between the posterior aspect of the ascending colon mesentery and the retroperitoneum. The "white line" at the junction of these two planes should be visualized and dissection continued just medial to this layer. This prevents the surgeon straying laterally and avoids inadvertent mobilization of the right kidney. As dissection continues medially, care must be taken to identify and protect the duodenum. Adequate mobilization of the cecum and ascending colon has been achieved when the duodenum, inferior vena cava, and right ureter are all exposed and protected and the lateral peritoneal fold has been divided up to the hepatic flexure.

Mobilization of the Hepatic Flexure

The patient is moved to reverse Trendelenburg position, still with the right side of the table elevated. The surgeon switches the instruments so that the cautery scissors are in the surgeon's right hand via the LLQ port and the grasper is in the left hand through the suprapubic port. The small intestine is swept down towards the patient's pelvis and away from the operative field. To divide the omentum either cautery or other energy device may be employed, depending on surgeon preference and habitus of the patient. The hepatocolic attachments are grasped between the colon and the liver and the correct plane is sought by elevating the tissues and looking for an area where the tissues can be seen to slide over the retroperitoneum (Fig. 48-7, page 486). The hepatocolic attachments are divided, and this plane is developed laterally until it meets with the dissection already performed inferiorly and laterally. Again, the duodenum should be exposed and protected. At this point, the entire right colon can be pulled across to the left side of the abdominal cavity, ensuring that full mobilization has been performed to the midline. Any remaining attachments to the retroperitoneum or duodenum are cleared at this time. Mobilization of the hepatic flexure is considered adequate when it can reach below the level of the umbilicus. Time spent ensuring complete mobilization facilitates exteriorization of the colon later.

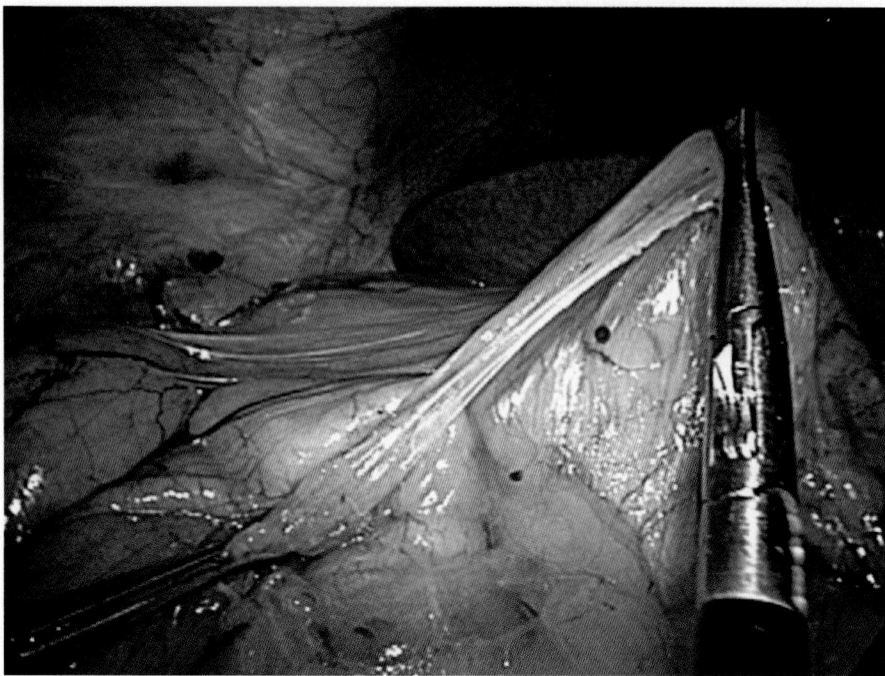

Fig. 48-7. Mobilization of the hepatic flexure. In reverse Trendelenburg, with the right side up, the plane is found between the gastrocolic ligament and the retroperitoneum.

Division of the Ileocolic Pedicle and Mesentery

The colon is placed back in its normal anatomical position. The patient is positioned in slight Trendelenburg again with the right side elevated. The surgeon uses the grasper in the left hand via the suprapubic port and the energy source in the right hand via the LLQ port. The small intestine is swept towards the patient's left upper quadrant. Via the RLQ port, the assistant grasps the mesentery adjacent to the ileocolic junction and elevates it towards the anterior abdominal wall, creating a bowstring effect on the ileocolic vessels (Fig. 48-8). The surgeon then opens the mesenteric windows caudad and cephalad to the base of the ileocolic pedicle. The vessels are isolated and divided with the energy source (Fig. 48-9). If the pedicle is bulky secondary to obesity or the vessels are calcified, the 10-mm camera in the 12-mm supraumbilical port is switched to a 5-mm camera via the LLQ port, a vascular stapler is introduced via the 12-mm port, and the vessels divided. Division of the colonic mesentery is continued cephalad up to the duodenum.

Exteriorization of the Specimen, Resection, and Anastomosis

When the colon has been adequately mobilized, the cecum is grasped, the pneumoperitoneum is evacuated through the ports, and the periumbilical incision opened to 3 to 5 cm. With wound protection in place, the bowel is exteriorized from the distal ileum to the mid-transverse colon (Fig. 48-10). The remaining mesentery is divided and ligated extracorporeally and the bowel divided, followed by a side-to-side stapled anastomosis (our preference). As the anastomotic configuration lies over the mesenteric defect, no attempt is made to close the mesentery, and the bowel is returned to the abdominal cavity. The abdominal cavity is irrigated; if the irrigant is clear the ports are visualized via the periumbilical incision and the sites checked for hemostasis as they are removed. If the irrigant is blood-tinged, the periumbilical incision is closed, the pneumoperitoneum re-established, the abdomen inspected for bleeding, and ports are removed under direct vision.

TRANSVERSE COLECTOMY

True transverse colectomy is rarely required. Mobilization of the transverse colon, however, is a component of more extensive procedures such as total colectomy and proctocolectomy. In a patient with normal body mass index, it is frequently sufficient to mobilize right and left colon as described, and fully mobilize both flexures to the point that they may be drawn to reach a point below the umbilicus. This facilitates exteriorization of the entire colon, including the transverse colon. As the periumbilical incision overlies the base of the middle colic pedicle, the pedicle can readily be divided at the base via this incision in a normal weight patient. This approach is the

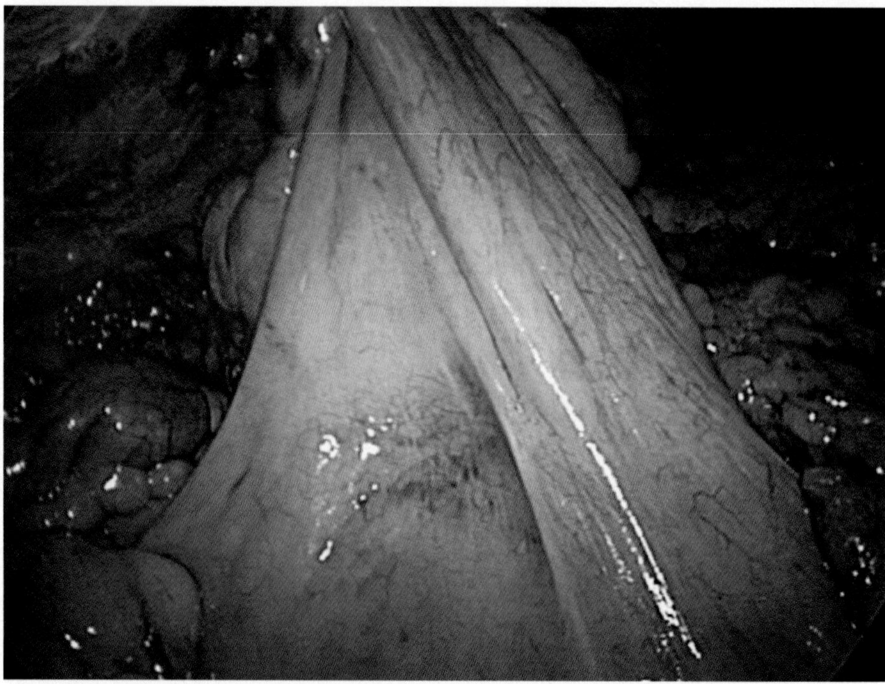

Fig. 48-8. The ileocolic pedicle is placed under tension, creating a bowstring effect on the vessels and allowing the mesenteric windows caudad and cephalad to the base of the pedicle to be identified.

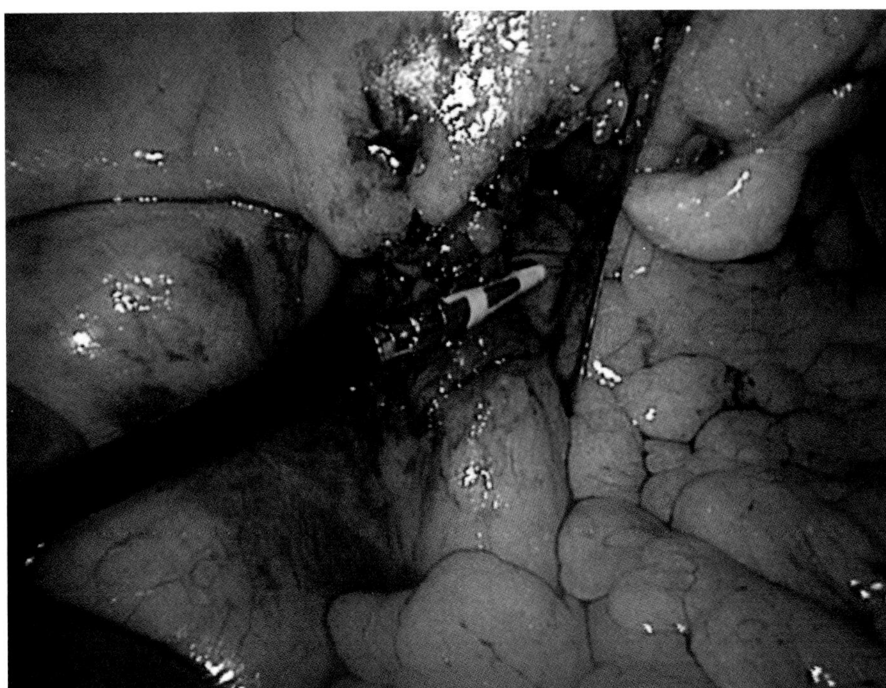

Fig. 48-9. The vessels are isolated at the base of the ileocolic pedicle and individually divided.

simplest technique for the transverse colon and middle colic vessels. In order to facilitate exteriorization of the transverse colon, it is helpful to approach the omentum in similar fashion at both flexures, either leaving the omentum behind at both sites or taking it with the colon at both flexures.

In the obese patient, it may not be possible to reach the base of the middle colic pedicle via the periumbilical incision. Then the most direct approach is to mobilize the right colon and hepatic flexure as described and divide the ileocolic and (if present) the right colic vessels. The omentum is placed in the upper abdomen, exposing the transverse colon, which is elevated, placing the middle colic pedicle under tension. This allows continuation of the division of the right colon and hepatic flexure mesentery distally, until the middle colic pedicle is reached, isolated, and divided.

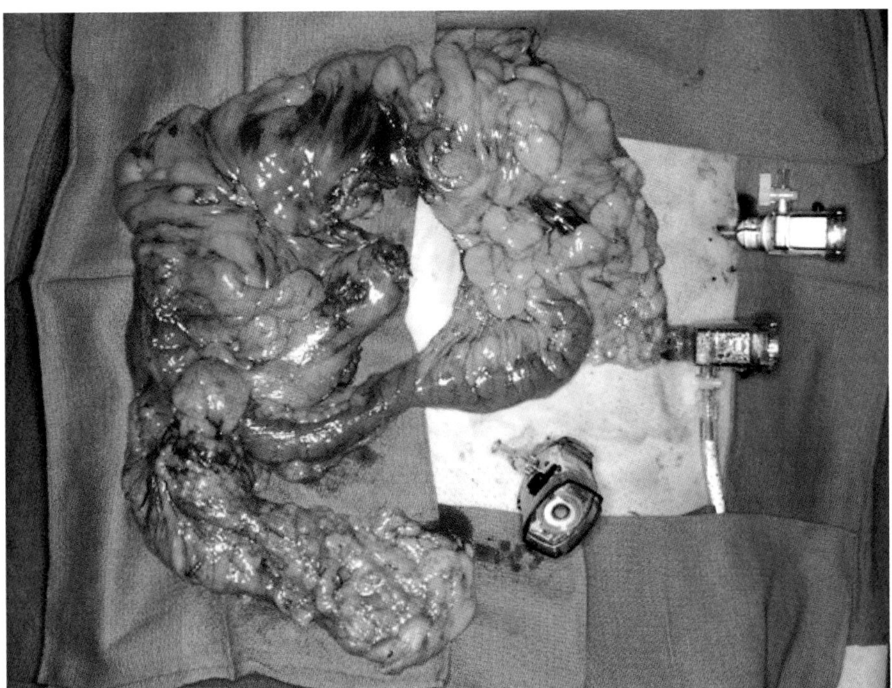

Fig. 48-10. The right colon is exteriorized from the distal ileum to the mid-transverse colon.

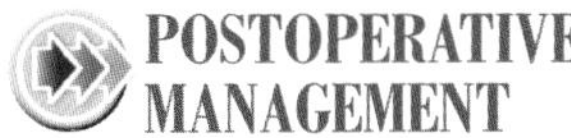

POSTOPERATIVE MANAGEMENT

On completion of the operation the orogastric tube is removed, and the patient returns to the ward with intravenous fluids, a urinary catheter, and patient-controlled analgesia (PCA). On postoperative day 1 the patient is allowed clear fluids, provided he/she is not nauseated and the abdomen not distended, and is encouraged to ambulate. If liquids are tolerated, a low-fiber diet is commenced on postoperative day 2, intravenous fluid replacement is stopped, analgesia is converted to oral medication, the urinary catheter is removed, and mobilization of the patient increased. By postoperative day 3 the patient may be discharged if he/she is comfortable, tolerating the diet, and passing gas. Patients who do not tolerate diet advancement at this rate are not pushed to start eating unduly, and the withdrawal of intravenous fluid and PCA are governed by resolution of the patient's ileus.

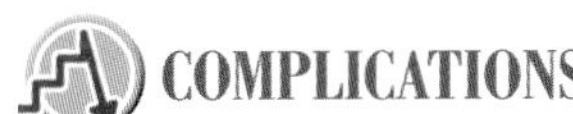

COMPLICATIONS

The risks of developing complications such as wound infection, hemorrhage, or anastomotic dehiscence are similar in laparoscopic and open colectomy. However it is important when performing laparoscopic resection that one adheres to traditional surgical principles such as ensuring adequate colon and particularly splenic flexure mobilization to prevent tension when performing left-sided anastomosis. Smaller incisions do not justify shortcuts.

Complications unique to laparoscopic colectomy are "off-screen" injuries and inadvertent small bowel damage. Off-screen injuries occur when instruments are not visible on screen, such as when they are introduced into the abdominal cavity or when hot cautery scissors are moved out of the field of view. These injuries can be minimized by insisting that everything is performed under direct vision. Small intestinal injuries such as serosal tears may occur when the bowel is being moved from the operative field with graspers. The risk is minimized by utilizing gravity to move the small intestine and helping by gently pushing the bowel, rather than grasping. If intraabdominal complications are suspected in the postoperative period, standard imaging techniques such as CT scan and contrast enema should be employed. Laparoscopy may be of use to treat some complications by creating a stoma, washing out the abdominal cavity, or controlling a bleeding vessel, but a negative finding at laparoscopy does not preclude the possibility of a missed injury. If sufficient doubt exists, conversion to laparotomy may be required.

SELECTED READING

The American Society of Colon and Rectal Surgeons approved statement: laparoscopic colectomy for curable cancer. *Dis Colon Rectum* 2004;47(8):A1.

The Colon Cancer Laparoscopic Open Resection Study Group – (COLOR). Laparoscopic surgery versus open surgery for colon cancer: short term outcomes of a randomized trial. *Lancet Oncol* 2005;6: 477–484.

Fleshman JW, Nelson H, Peters WR, et al. Early results of laparoscopic surgery for colorectal cancer: retrospective analysis of 372 patients treated by Clinical Outcomes of Surgical Therapy (COST) Study Group. *Dis Colon Rectum* 1996;39:S53–S58.

Guillou PJ, Quirke P, Thorpe H, et al. Short-term endpoints of conventional versus laparoscopic-assisted surgery in patients with colorectal cancer (MRC CLASICC trial): multicentre, randomised controlled trial. *Lancet* 2005;365:1718–1726.

Johnstone PAS, Rohde DC, Swartz SE, et al. Port site recurrences after laparoscopic and thoracoscopic procedures in malignancy. *J Clin Oncol* 1996;14:1950–1956.

Kuhry E, Bonjer HJ, Haglind E, et al. COLOR Study Group. Impact of hospital case volume on short-term outcome after laparoscopic operation for colonic cancer. *Surg Endosc* 2005;19:687–892.

Lacy AM, Garcia-Valdecasas JC, Delgado S, et al. Laparoscopy-assisted colectomy versus open colectomy for treatment of non-metastatic colon cancer: a randomised trial. *Lancet* 2002;359:2224–2229.

Nelson H. The Clinical Outcomes of Surgical Therapy Study Group. A comparison of laparoscopically assisted and open colectomy for colon cancer. NEJM 2004;350:2050–2059.

Reza MM, Blasco JA, Andradas E, et al. Systematic review of laparoscopic versus open surgery for colorectal cancer. *Br J Surg* 2006;93:921–928.

Veldkamp R, Gholghesaei M, Bonjer HJ, et al. European Association of Endoscopic Surgery (EAES). Laparoscopic resection of colon cancer. Consensus of the European Association of Endoscopic Surgery. *Surg Endosc* 2004; 18:1163–1185.

Young-Fadok TM, Fanelli Rd, Price R, et al. Laparoscopic resection of curable colon and rectal cancer: An evidence-based review. *Surg Endosc* 2007;21:1063–1068.

COMMENTARY

Drs. Lawes and Young-Fadok have written an authoritative chapter on laparoscopic colectomy. For many years, general surgeons were awaiting the results of prospective randomized trials to justify the performance of laparoscopic resections for colon cancer. These trials have now been published and have the power to show equivalency of the laparoscopic and open approaches to colectomy in regards to morbidity and cancer-related survival. Several other studies have suggested that laparoscopic operations result in shorter hospital stays and decreased period of ileus. Furthermore, the laparoscopic approach may be associated with less immunosuppression and may ultimately be proven to be superior in terms of long-term cancer survival.

The indications for laparoscopic colectomy are essentially identical to those for open colectomy. The experience of the surgeon is critical in determining whether a curative resection should be performed laparoscopically. Position statements from several surgical societies have suggested that a minimum of 20 cases be done before a surgeon begins a program of laparoscopic resections for colon cancer. Surgeons performing laparoscopic colectomies should be prepared to perform intraoperative colonoscopy to localize lesions if the exact site of tumor cannot be identified intraoperatively. To facilitate the laparoscopic approach, many surgeons have employed preoperative tattooing of the lesion using India ink.

The authors advocate a very standardized and reproducible approach for patient positioning and port placement for all laparoscopic colorectal procedures. This systematic approach facilitates performance of the procedures by trainees and improves teamwork among allied health personnel. The authors have separated colonic resections into those performed for the left colon, the right colon, and the transverse colon. Each of these procedures is divided into distinct steps that can be followed in a logical fashion. The steps are illustrated well with cartoons and intraoperative photographs. Many different methods can now be used for mobilization of the colon and division of the vasculature. Mobilization can be performed sharply, while using harmonic shears, or by cautery administered via scissors or hook devices. Blood vessels can be divided using harmonic energy or bipolar cautery, clips, or stapling devices. Each surgeon will arrive at a comfort zone with his or her own techniques and be able to apply them to the specific patient. At our institution, all distal anastomoses are checked for leaks prior to finishing the case. This is usually done by inserting an endoscope transanally and insufflating the anastomosis under water. Any bubbles emanating from the anastomosis should result in additional sutures being placed with a recheck, and consideration should be given to performing a diverting proximal loop ilesotomy.

Postoperatively, most patients can be "fast tracked" with discharge on the 2nd to 4th postoperative day. Nasogastric tubes are generally avoided and oral liquids are started regardless of whether flatus has been passed. One of the side effects of the increased scrutiny paid to laparoscopy has been a reevaluation of postoperative care following traditional "open" surgery. Many of the dogmas that were held in the "good old days" (use of nasogastric tubes, awaiting flatus prior to oral feeds, hospitalization until after a bowel movement, etc.) have been debunked. Surgeons involved in laparoscopic colectomy are sure to learn a few new tips and tricks from this chapter.

NJS

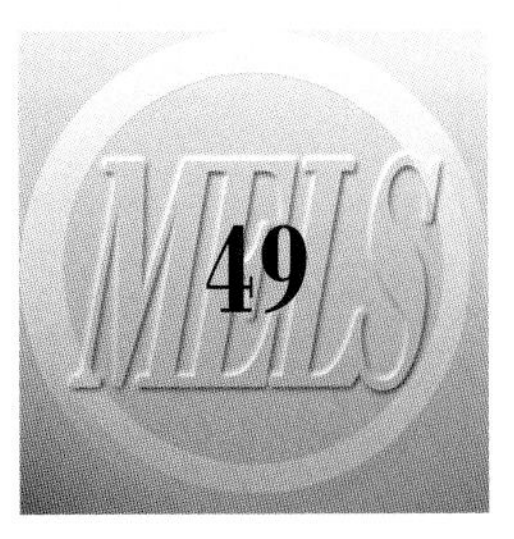

Laparoscopic Resection for Carcinoma of the Rectum

BASHAR SAFAR AND STEVEN D. WEXNER

INTRODUCTION

Colorectal cancer is the third most common cancer and the third leading cause of cancer-related mortality in the United States. An estimated 41,420 new rectal cancers were projected for 2007 according to the American Cancer Society. Rectal cancer is a highly treatable and often curable disease when localized. Surgery is the primary treatment, and results are curative in approximately 45% of all patients. Ernest Miles transformed rectal cancer surgery at the turn of the 20th century when he introduced the abdominoperineal approach to rectal cancer, as opposed to a pure perineal approach that was practiced during that time. He managed to significantly reduce the local recurrence rate, but this success came at the price of a high morbidity and mortality rate. In 1978, Heald emphasized the importance of the complete excision of the lymphovascular fatty tissue surrounding the rectum under direct vision, in a procedure now known as total mesorectal excision or TME. This technique resulted in significantly reduced local recurrence rates and has been adopted and accepted throughout the world as the procedure of choice for surgical treatment of rectal cancer.

Since the introduction of laparoscopic surgery in the early 1990s, most digestive tract procedures have been successfully attempted and confirmed to be safe and feasible. One issue that remained to be answered was the oncologic adequacy of these procedures in cancers of the gastrointestinal tract. This question was definitively answered in the case of colon cancer by several prospective controlled multi-institutional randomized trials; however no such trials have yet been completed for rectal carcinoma. Rectal cancer resection is further complicated by the relatively more aggressive characteristics of the tumor and by the fact that TME is a more challenging procedure than colon resection, due to the anatomy of the pelvis and the pattern of lymphatic distribution. The two fundamentals of performing laparoscopic surgery for gastrointestinal malignancies are adequate training and sufficient experience. These issues are of vital importance in rectal cancer surgery, where even in open procedures the surgeon's volume and training have been shown to be independent risk factors in local recurrence and survival. Moreover, a risk–benefit ratio needs to be established when attempting such an endeavor; any compromise to the long-term onclogical quality of the operation is unacceptable even if it provides certain short-term advantages.

Laparoscopic surgery for rectal cancer should only be performed by adequately trained surgeons with considerable expertise in laparoscopy who have a significant interest in colorectal surgery. Multiple reports have confirmed the safety of the procedure; nonetheless, most data reported must be considered to be preliminary and medium-term results at best. A prospective multi-institutional clinical trial attempting to address this issue is awaited in the U.S.

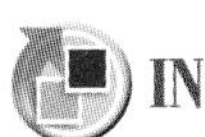

INDICATIONS

The indications for surgery in rectal cancer are the same whether approached via a laparoscopic technique or by laparotomy. There is evidence that laparoscopic TME (LTME) results in less blood loss, a quicker return to normal diet, less pain, decreased narcotic use, and less immune response. However, it seems likely that LTME is associated with longer operative times and higher costs (Table 49-1).

Factors that influence the decision as to whether a laparoscopic approach should be attempted include body mass index (BMI), multiple previous abdominal operations, a history of extensive lysis of adhesions, and peritonitis, all of which increase the procedure complexity and result in a higher incidence complications and conversions. Large bulky tumors that show poor response to preoperative chemoradiation and have potentially invaded local structures are not well suited for the laparoscopic approach due to the difficulty in performing the dissection and the large incision needed for extraction of the specimen.

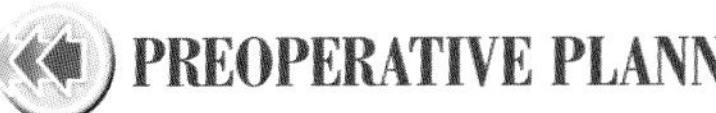

PREOPERATIVE PLANNING

The initial evaluation includes a complete history and physical exam, laboratory studies including a complete blood count, chemistries, liver function tests, and CEA level, computed tomography (CT) of the abdomen and pelvis, chest X-ray, and full colonoscopy with biopsies. Clinical assessment should include a careful, thorough digital rectal examination assessing the specific factors that influence further decision-making, including tumor mobility, involvement of the sphincters, distance from the anal verge, and fixation to adjacent organs. The location of the tumor either in relation to rectal valves or as distance from the anal verge or dentate line must be accurately

TABLE 49-1. COMPARISON OF OPEN AND LAPAROSCOPIC RESECTIONS FOR RECTAL CANCER

Author (year)	Lap/Open (n)	Morbidity (%)	OR time (minutes)	EBL (mL)	LOS (days)
Fleshman (1999)	42/152	55/50	278/209	NR	7/12
Zhou (2004)	82/89	6.1/12.4	120/106	20/92	8.1/13.3
Leung (2004)	203/200	19.8/22.5	190/144	169/238	8.2/8.7
Breukink (2005)	41/41	27/51	200/180	250/1000	12/19
Law (2006)	98/167	25/29	200/127	200/250	7/8
Braga (2007)	83/85	28.9/40	262/209	213/396	10/13.6

Lap, laparoscopic; OR, operating room; EBL, estimated blood loss; LOS, length of hospital stay; NR, no results.

Diseases of the Small and Large Bowel

TABLE 49-2. MORBIDITY AND MORTALITY AFTER LAPAROSCOPIC RECTAL RESECTION

Author (year)	Patients (n)	Procedure (%)	Morbidity (%)	Mortality (%)
Fleshman (1999)	42	APR (100)	55	0
Leroy (2004)	102	AR (84.7)	27	2
		APR (13.3)		
Leung (2004)	203	AR (100)	25	2.5
Barlehner (2004)	194	AR (91)	20	0
		APR (8)		
Scheidbach (2004)	520	AR (64)	33	1.5
		APR (36)		1.6
Dulucq (2005)	218	LAR (65)	22	1
		AR (35)		
Tsang (2006)	105	LAR (100)	25	0
Kim (2006)	312	AR (85)	21.5	0.3
		APR (14)		
Law (2006)	98	AR (100)	25	1.0
Braga (2007)	83	AR (91)	29	1.2
		APR (9)		

AP, ablative procedure; APR, abdominoperineal resection; LAR, low anterior resection.

documented. A careful search for distant metastases must be done; identification of systemic disease significantly changes the operative planning from a potentially curative procedure to a palliative one.

The goal of the initial evaluation is to stratify the patients into one of two groups: locoregional disease (Stages I to III) or systemic disease (Stage IV). Patients with locoregional disease are further stratified depending on degree of penetration of the tumor through the bowel wall (T) and the presence or absence of nodal involvement (N). Both endorectal ultrasound (EUS) and magnetic resonance imaging (MRI) with pelvic or endorectal coil have been employed to provide information regarding the T stage of the tumor as well as the lymph node status (N). EUS is more widely utilized in the U.S., with an accuracy approaching 95% in assessing the T stage in experienced centers; however EUS is less accurate in assessing lymph node status (up to 74% accuracy).

Accurate locoregional staging can influence therapy by helping to determine which patients may be candidates for local excision rather than more extensive surgery, patients who are eligible for a restorative procedure (low anterior resection) vs. an ablative procedure, and patients who may be candidates for combined modality treatment (CMT), including preoperative chemotherapy and radiation therapy. Patients with full-thickness tumors (T3) and/or node-positive disease are at high risk for local and systemic relapse. Most trials of preoperative or postoperative CMT have shown a decrease in the local recurrence rate but no definite effect on survival. Neoadjuvant therapy is associated with less treatment toxicity and a better chance of sphincter preservation; a 6-week course of radiation 5040 Gy combined with infusional 5-FU is the preferred method in the U.S.

A multidisciplinary approach has transformed cancer care in recent years. Rectal cancer treatment is highly individualized; multiple factors are taken into account when management decisions are undertaken. The algorithm must follow the same pathway for the laparoscopic approach that it would for an open one. Ultimately it is the surgeon's responsibility to discuss with the patient the various types of procedures available and which type of operation the patient would benefit from the most. Table 49-3 outlines the preoperative evaluation summary.

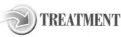

TABLE 49-3. PREOPERATIVE EVALUATION SUMMARY

Preoperative assessment	Locoregional staging	Systemic staging
Complete H&P	Digital rectal exam	CEA
CBC, CMP	Colonoscopy	CT abdomen and pelvis
+/− Manometry	EUS vs. MRI	PET scan
Stoma therapist		Chest X-ray

H&P, history and physical; CEA, carcinoembryonic antigen; CBC, complete blood count; CMP, comprehensive metabolic profile; CT, computed tomography; EUS, endorectal ultrasound; MRI, magnetic resonance imaging; PET, positron emission tomography.

TREATMENT

Surgical approaches for rectal cancer can be divided into local and radical. The local procedures include transanal (transanal excision, transanal endoscopic surgery, or TEM) and posterior (Kraske and York-Mason) procedures. The local procedures are usually reserved for well-differentiated, localized tumors in a select group of patients and will not be discussed any further in this chapter.

Radical procedures include low anterior resection (LAR) and abdominoperineal resection (APR). Both of these procedures may be performed utilizing either open or laparoscopic techniques. The initial approach to both procedures is identical, with an emphasis on total mesorectal excision, ensuring adequate radial and distal margins. Multiple reports have emerged in the last few years confirming the feasibility and safety of both procedures laparoscopically performed.

With the advent of improved preoperative staging, neoadjuvant therapy and surgical techniques, the use of APR has significantly decreased. APR is now reserved for the few patients with direct tumor invasion into the sphincter complex, when there is technical inability to obtain an adequate distal margin, or for patients with baseline sphincter dysfunction and incontinence.

SURGICAL TECHNIQUE

Preparation

Every patient considered for a proctetomy needs a full cardiac, pulmonary, and renal evaluation. A preoperative consultation with a stoma therapist must also be obtained, as the likelihood of acquiring a stoma either for diversion or permanently is high; we therefore emphasize the importance of bilateral preoperative marking in all patients. This allows the patient to be acquainted with the stoma appliance and reduces postoperative anxiety.

Full mechanical bowel preparation is a controversial topic, however it remains the standard of care in the U.S.; it allows easier laparoscopic handling of the bowel as well as intraoperative endoscopy. All patients are instructed to have a mechanical bowel preparation the day before surgery. Patients are admitted on the day of surgery and are given prophylactic subcutaneous heparin as well as intravenous antibiotics on call to the operating room; in addition, a pneumatic compression device should be routinely used.

Patient Positioning

The patient is placed in the modified lithotomy position using Allen stirrups with both arms tucked and well padded to avoid any injury, especially at bony prominences (Fig. 49-1). The patient is secured to the operating table with particular attention to the shoulders to prevent the patient from slipping with extreme position changes that may be needed to perform the procedure. The hips must be flexed no more than 15 degrees to avoid interference with the surgeon's hand movements during the procedure. We routinely place ureteric catheters in the radiated pelvis for laparoscopic pelvic dissection; these catheters can facilitate the identification of the ureters and help prevent ureteral injury. Digital rectal examination is performed to assess the tumor or scar and confirm the level and relation to the sphincters; this evaluation is particularly important if neoadjuvant therapy was administered in order to assess the tumor response. Rectal irrigation using betadine is optional; the abdomen and the perineum are prepped and draped in the usual manner.

The abdominal cavity is entered using the open Hasson technique above or below the umbilicus, depending on the distance from the pubis. Pneumoperitoneum up to 15 mmHg is created, using a 30-degree telescope. A careful exploration of the entire abdominal cavity is undertaken, including the liver and all peritoneal surfaces, to exclude tumor dissemination.

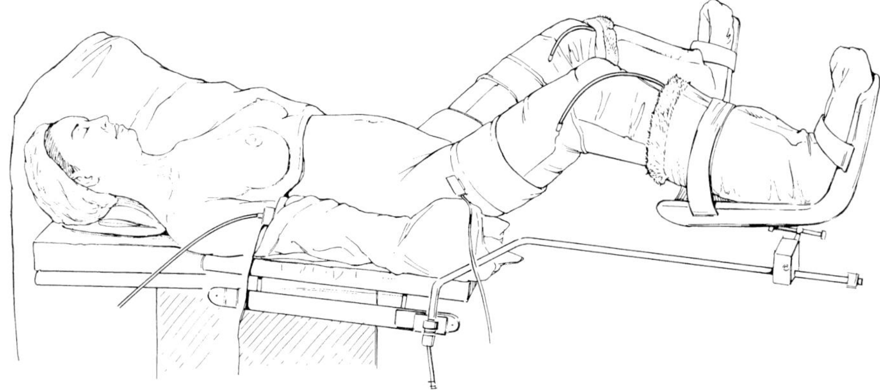

Fig. 49-1. The patient is placed in positionable stirrups and the arms padded and tucked.

Trocar Placement and Laparoscopic Equipment

The team consists of the operating surgeon, first assistant, camera assistant, and a scrub technician. Two monitors are employed; one positioned in line with the surgeon's vision over the patient's left leg and other is placed over the right shoulder or in a convenient position for the first assistant. The surgeon and camera assistant stand on the right side while the first assistant stands to the left of the surgeon. The scrub technician with the Mayo table is usually positioned below the right leg of the patient (Fig. 49-2). The equipment needed to

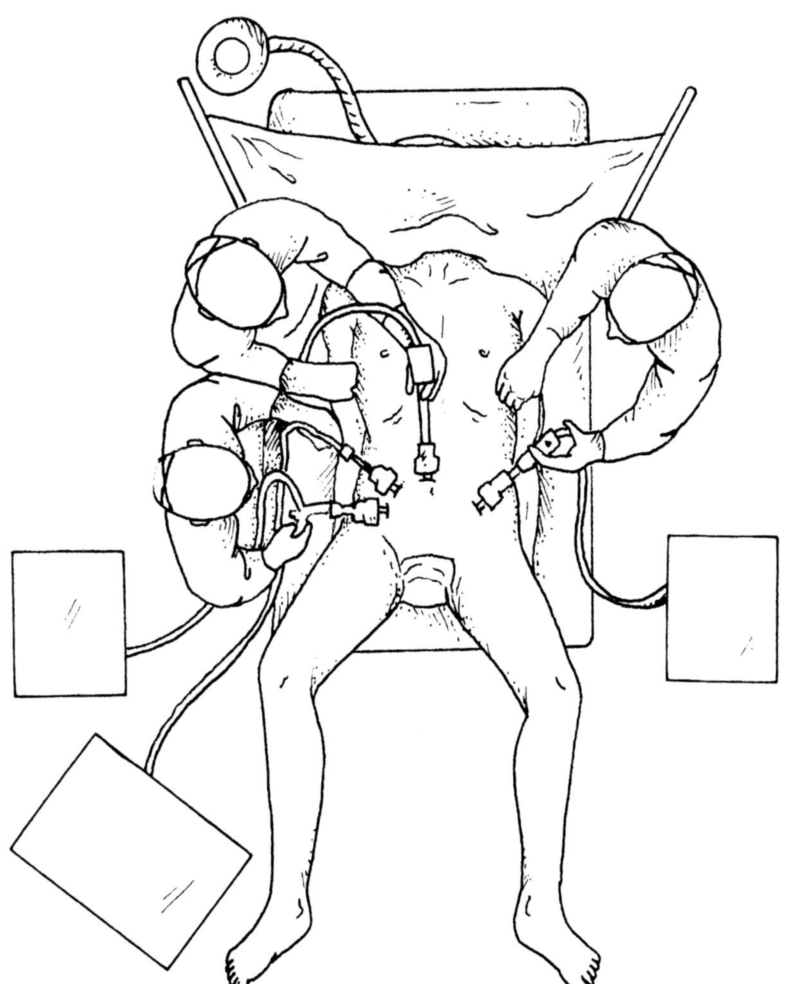

Fig. 49-2. Typical room setup for laparoscopic rectal surgery.

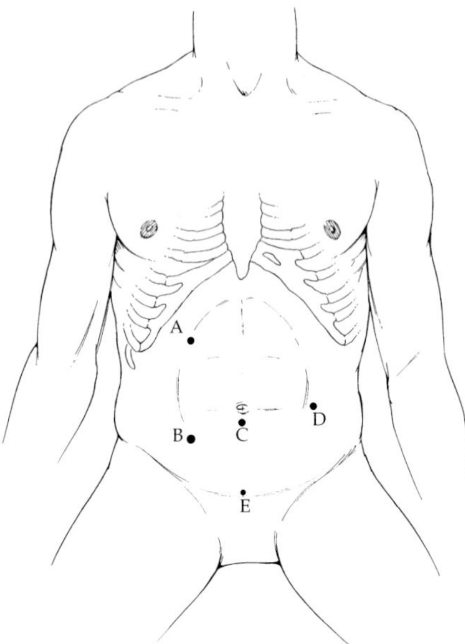

Fig. 49-3. Typical port placement for laparoscopic rectal resections.

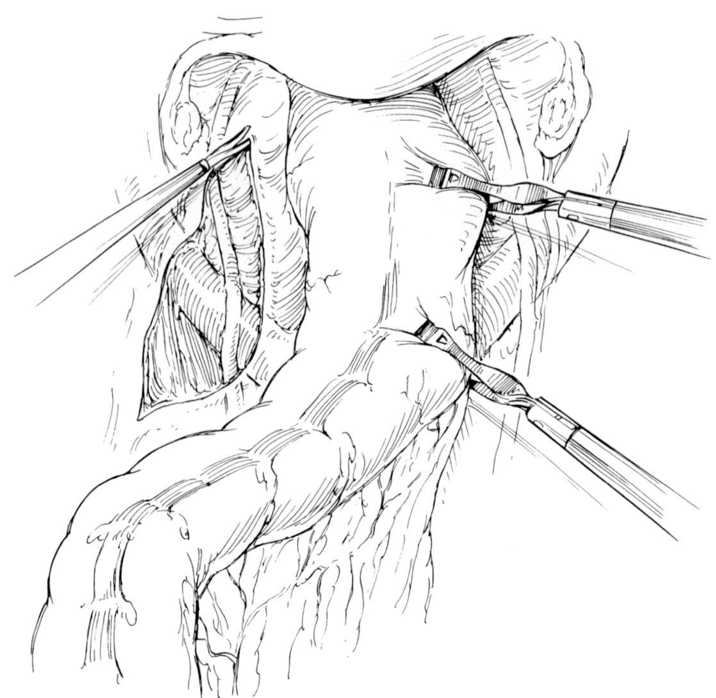

Fig. 49-4. The line of Toldt of the left colon is divided and blunt dissection is used to sweep the colon medially and expose the ureter.

perform the procedure includes three 10- to 12-mm trocars, nontraumatic bowel graspers (we prefer to use laparoscopic 10-mm Babcock bowel clamps), a 30-mm endoscopic articulating linear cutting stapler, a wound protector, and a laparoscopic dissecting device such as the HARMONIC SCALPEL (Ethicon Endo-Surgery; Cincinnati, OH), the laparoscopic LigaSure sealing device (Valleylab; Boulder, CO), or the EnSeal (SurgRx; Redwood City, CA).

Once the procedure is deemed feasible, the other trocars are inserted: two trocars on the right side lateral to the rectus muscle avoiding the inferior epigastric vessels, one in the right lower quadrant, and the other in the right middle or upper quadrant. An additional trocar may be subsequently inserted based on the procedure selected and the patient's anatomy; thus the position may be the left lower quadrant (site of stoma creation) for APR or suprapubic (extraction site) in LAR. It is important to adhere to the laparoscopic triangulation principle and not place the trocars too close to each other, which might prevent the surgeon from having free mobility of his or her arm. We use 10- to 12-mm trocars for all the access ports as we feel that this allows for the flexibility and interchangeability frequently required in these cases (Fig. 49-3).

Mobilization of the Colon

The patient is positioned in steep Trendelenburg with the left side up to allow gravity to move the small bowel and omentum away from the operating field. The sigmoid and descending colon are mobilized utilizing the lateral-to-medial approach. The sigmoid colon is grasped with a Babcock grasper and retracted medially with the left hand, taking care to avoid handling the tumor and not using the locking function of the grasper in order to avoid bowel injury. The white line of Toldt is identified and dissection is undertaken with the right hand using the ultrasonic coagulating shears in the avascular plane between the mesocolon and posterior peritoneum. The colon is progressively mobilized medially until the ureter is identified crossing the iliac vessels (Fig. 49-4). Proximal dissection is performed by incising the line of Toldt and sweeping the mesocolon off of the Gerota fascia.

The splenic flexure is then mobilized, either with the surgeon standing between the patient's legs or remaining on the patient's right side. The patient is then placed in the reverse-Trendelenburg position. Starting to the right of the middle colic vessels, the omentum is dissected from the colon and the lesser sac is entered. The dissection is then extended towards the spleen using the harmonic scalpel to free all of the attachments of the spleen to the colon (Fig. 49-5).

Once the splenic flexure has been fully mobilized, the mesenteric vessels are dissected, which may require an extra trocar. The colon is retracted laterally, allowing for the medial dissection to be undertaken. The extra trocar may be placed either in the left lower quadrant or suprapubically, depending on the anticipated procedure. With the colon retracted laterally, a window is created in the base of the mesocolon at the level of the sacral promontory. Careful dissection in the avascular plane should help identify the left ureter and create a window in the mesentery, which can be followed cephalad until the inferior mesenteric artery is reached (Fig. 49-6). The artery should be isolated and divided using an endoscopic linear cutting stapler with a vascular cartridge. The inferior mesenteric artery should be divided 1 cm distal to its origin from the aorta, avoiding the sympathetic nerves and allowing further intervention should any doubt arise regarding hemostasis (Fig. 49-7, page 494). The division can be proximal or distal to the colic artery. It is crucial to visualize the ureter while closing the stapler to avoid entrapping it in the jaws of the stapler. Once the artery is divided, attention is turned to the inferior mesenteric vein, which can be identified at the ligament of Treitz, lateral to the fourth portion of the duodenum and near the inferior border of the pancreas. The vein is divided using a vascular cartridge with the endoscopic linear stapler. Additional hemostasis can be achieved

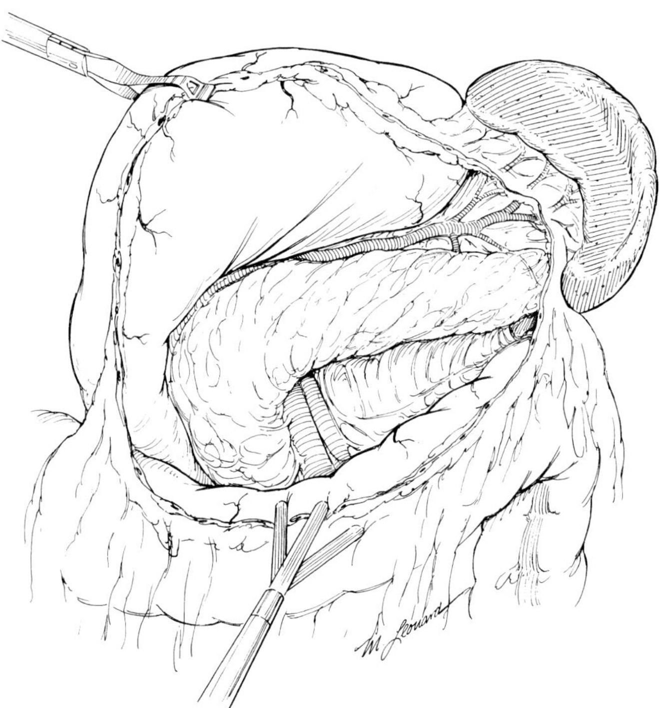

Fig. 49-5. The splenic flexure is mobilized with the ultrasonic shears while the assistant provides traction.

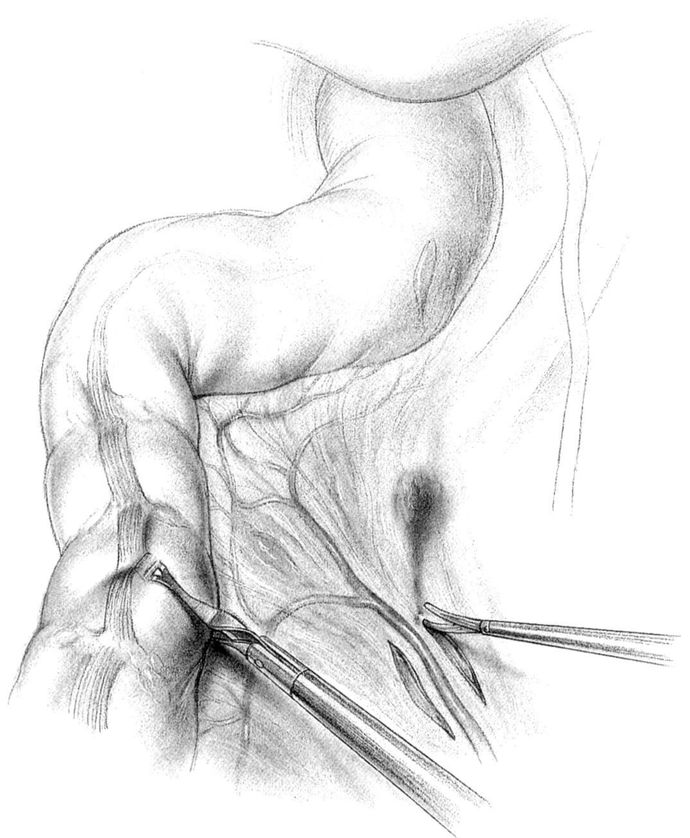

Fig. 49-6. From the medial approach, windows are made on either side of the inferior mesenteric artery and blunt sweeping will once again expose the ureter.

using laparoscopic endoloop or clips if needed. The inferior mesenteric vein is routinely divided as it affords the colon more mobility, allowing for a tension-free and well vascularized anastomosis.

THE PROCTECTOMY

Dissection is undertaken in the avascular areolar plane surrounding the mesorectum between the parietal and visceral facial planes of the pelvis. We start the dissection posteriorly using the ultrasonic shears in a plane anterior to the hypogastric and autonomic nerves and then continue to the lateral stalks, leaving the anterior dissection as the final step (Fig. 49-8, page 494). The utility of the extra port is again emphasized for this stage of the procedure as the extra grasper may help retract the rectum towards the anterior abdominal wall while the surgeon develops the posterior plane as far as needed; alternatively a suture can be placed through the sigmoid colon fixing it to the anterior abdominal wall if further retraction is required. The posterior plane can be developed as far as the levator muscles, if deemed necessary. In females the uterus may need to be anteriorly retracted to facilitate exposure; this can be done by securing the uterus to the anterior abdominal wall with a straight needle or using a laparoscopic retractor to reflect it out of the way (Fig. 49-9, page 495). The peritoneum of the rectovaginal or rectovescical pouch is incised; this should allow the avascular plane and Denonvilliers fascia to be identified. The fascia is divided and the rectum is freed anteriorly as far as necessary (Fig. 49-10, page 495).

At this stage of the operation, the rectum has been circumferentially mobilized and the surgeon must decide whether a restorative resection or a sphincter-sacrificing procedure is to be performed. The proximal dissection is performed in an identical fashion irrespective of which procedure is chosen.

Multiple hybrid procedures have been described which involve a combination of laparoscopic mobilization and open proctectomy including hand-assisted techniques. Mobilization of the colon and the splenic flexure is performed laparoscopically and the proctectomy done through a Pfannenstiel or lower midline incision; in a conventional manner. We do not advocate utilizing these techniques and adhere to the laparoscopic approach whenever possible as the laparoscope provides a magnified view of the pelvis, improving visualization for TME and allowing a precise dissection as opposed to blunt manual dissection.

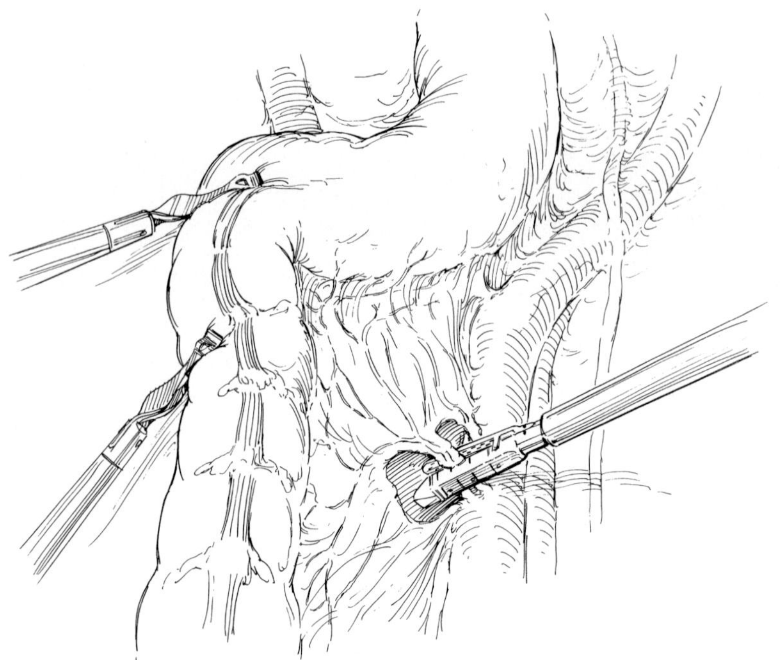

Fig. 49-7. The inferior mesenteric artery is divided with a vascular stapler.

Low Anterior Resection

In the case of a low anterior resection, the distal extent of the dissection depends upon the level of the tumor. A 5-cm mesorectal distal margin is recommended for high and middle rectal cancers, whereas a 1- to 2-cm mucosal margin is deemed adequate in low cancers. The level of transection can be identified by gently clamping the rectum with an atraumatic bowel clamp and performing a sigmoidoscopy. This evaluation ensures that the required margin is not being compromised by the lack of tactile feedback. It also prevents too large a dissection of the middle and lower rectum in upper rectal cancers. Once the level of transaction is determined, the harmonic scalpel can be used to divide the mesorectum; care must be taken to avoid undercutting the mesentery during this part of the procedure and the mesorectum must be divided at the same level as the rectal transection. If the tumor is in the lower third of the rectum, the entire mesorectum must be excised.

Transecting the rectum at the predetermined level can be challenging; we prefer using an endoscopic articulating linear 30-mm stapler with a 3.5-mm cartridge to perform this maneuver. The stapler is introduced through the right lower quadrant port and the rectum is retracted to the left. The stapler is then articulated so that the line of transection is at a right angle to the rectum (Fig. 49-11, page 496). This results in a transverse straight staple line lying in the coronal plane. Two or more staple loads are frequently needed to complete the transection. Again, care must be taken to avoid injury to the ureter and iliac vessels on the left while closing the jaws of the stapler. An alternative method has also been described whereby the suprapubic port is utilized to insert the stapler and the rectum is retracted cephalad with a grasper inserted through the right upper quadrant port. The stapler is then applied in an anterior–posterior direction, leaving the rectal stump with a staple line that lies in the sagittal plane.

After transecting the rectum, the rectal stump should be examined with a finger as well as endoscopically with an air leak test. For the latter, the pelvis is filled with saline and air is insufflated into the stump as flexible endoscopy is performed. Any evidence of a leak warrants careful search for a defect at the staple line and may require further intervention, including completely revising the anastamosis by restapling lower in the rectum if the length allows or performing a mucosectomy and handsewn coloanal anastomosis, if possible. The descending/sigmoid colon, which should be completely mobile, is brought down to the pelvis and the proximal margin of transaction is determined and marked with two endoscopic clips for future identification.

The extraction site is created next. A suprapubic port is inserted two fingerbreadths above the symphysis pubis unless it was created earlier to aid in the dissection. A laparoscopic Babcock is inserted and the transected end of the bowel is grasped across the staple line; the ratchet is locked fully to avoid dislodgement. The skin incision around the port is enlarged to accommodate the width of the specimen. Using the port as a guide, the incision is extended into the abdominal cavity on either side of the port and then a wound protector is inserted around the port. The port is extracted through the wound along

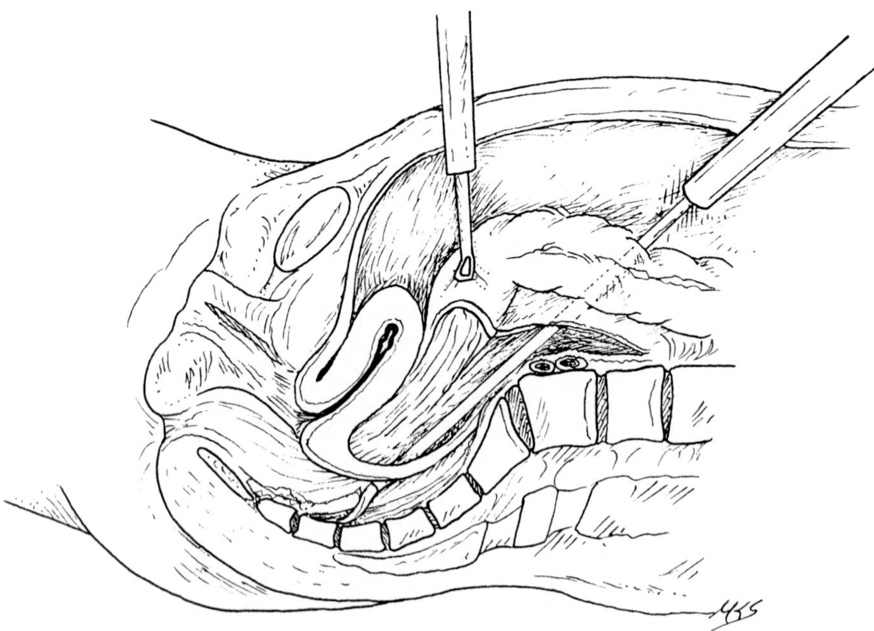

Fig. 49-8. Posterior dissection is continued down the sacral hollow until the levator muscles are reached.

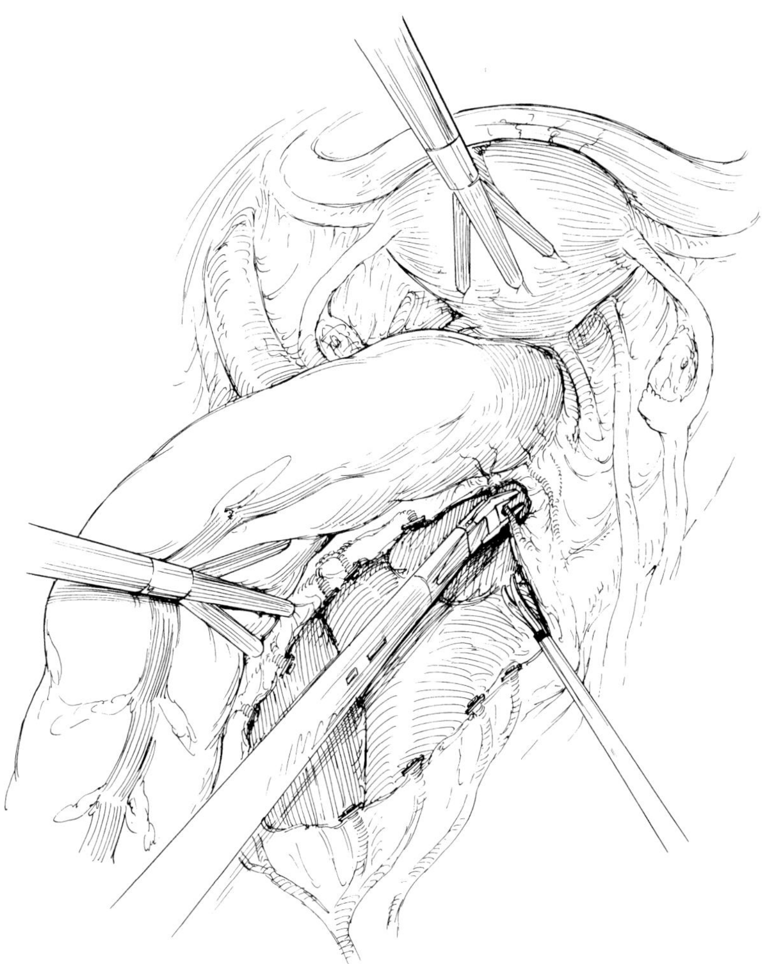

Fig. 49-9. In females, it is necessary to retract the uterus anteriorly with sutures or an atraumatic retractor.

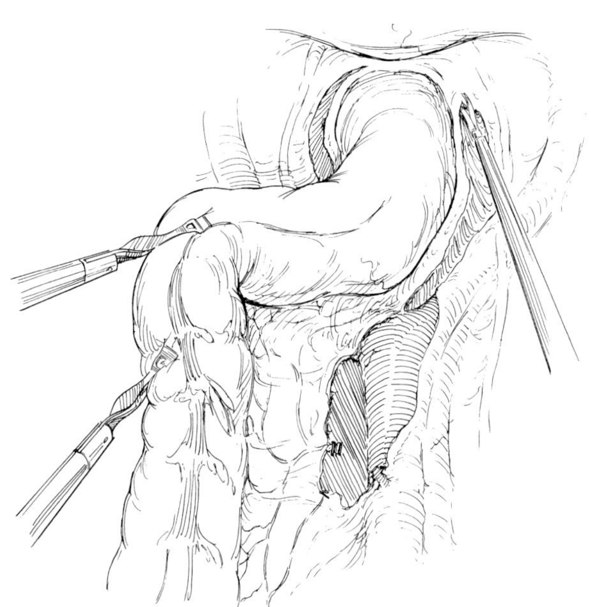

Fig. 49-10. Following the posterior dissection, the lateral and anterior peritoneum is incised and the Denonvilliers fascia exposed.

with the grasper and the bowel. The bowel is pulled out until the endoscopic clips placed earlier in the procedure to mark the location of transection are identified and a proximal bowel clamp is applied; the bowel along with the mesentery is divided.

Bowel continuity can be restored utilizing a variety of methods depending on the length of the rectal stump and the surgeon's preference. We prefer performing a double-stapled end-to-end anastomosis for high lesions and creating a colonic J-pouch for coloanal or low anastomoses within 5 cm from the anal verge.

Double stapled end-to-end anastomosis proceeds by placing a purse-string suture around the cut edge of the colon using 2-0 polypropylene. A 33-mm circular anvil is inserted, the purse-string suture is secured around it, and the bowel is prepared for the anastomosis by clearing the mesentery and the appendices epiploicae off the anvil. If a colonic J-pouch is to be performed, then the distal colon is folded on itself in a J configuration, creating a pouch that is 5 to 6 cm in length. The pouch is created using a linear stapler; the anvil is introduced through the colotomy and a purse-string suture is performed as described earlier around the colotomy at the apex of the pouch. The bowel is carefully returned to the abdominal cavity, the incision is closed with a running polydioxanone suture (PDS), and pneumoperitoneum is reestablished. The anastomosis is then performed under direct vision. The circular stapler shaft is introduced through the anus after gentle dilatation and guided into the desired location with the endoscopic Babcock clamp. We prefer to deploy the stapler at or near the staple line. The anvil shaft is guided with an endoscopic anvil grasper introduced through the right lower quadrant into the stapler (Fig. 49-12, page 496). Care must be taken to ensure that the bowel mesentery is not twisted and no additional tissue has been trapped in the stapler while closing. The mesenteric edge is traced from the origin of the middle colic artery to the free edge of the bowel. Once the stapler is deployed, it should be very gently withdrawn and the two "donuts" inspected. The pelvis is again filled with saline, the proximal bowel clamped with an atraumatic grasper, and the anastomotic integrity is verified by direct vision through sigmoidoscope and by air leak test (Fig. 49-13, page 497).

An alternative technique for low-lying tumors requiring a hand-sewn colonic J-pouch coloanal anastamosis has been described. After completion of laparoscopic total mesorectal excision, the surgeon turns

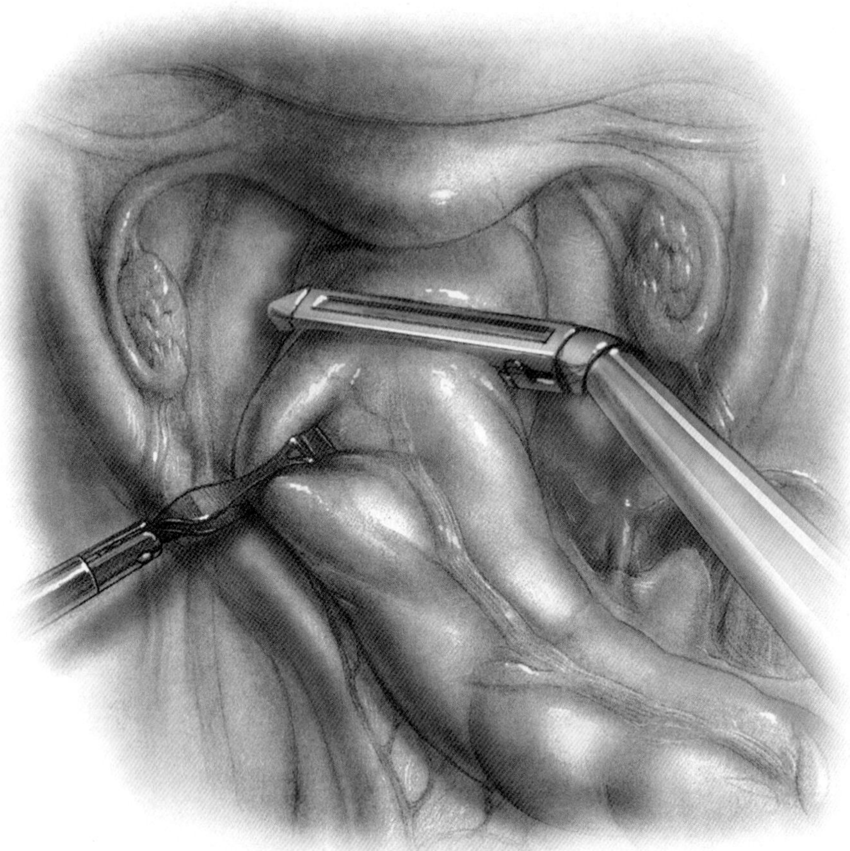

Fig. 49-11. Articulating endoscopic staplers with short loads are used to divide the rectum transversely.

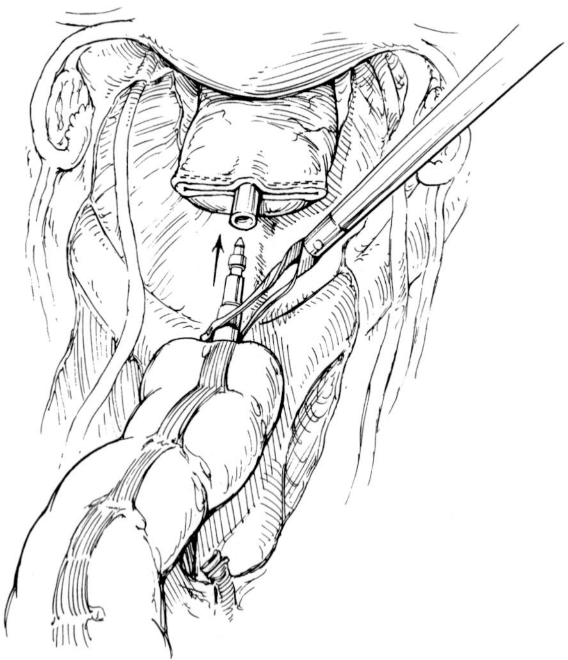

Fig. 49-12. The anvil of the circular stapler is grasped with a Babcock and firmly docked with the stapler itself.

his or her attention to the perineal aspect of the procedure; no extraction site is needed. The anus is effaced with a Lone Star Retractor (Lone Star Medical Products, Inc.; Trumbull, CT). A circumferential full-thickness incision is created at the dentate line and the peritoneal cavity is entered. A wound protector is placed and the rectum, along with the colon, is delivered through the anus. The colon is transected extracorporeally at the predetermined location marked by the endoclips. A colonic J-pouch is constructed extracorporeally and a hand-sewn pouch-anal anastomosis is performed (Fig. 49-14). The abdomen is insufflated and a diverting loop ileostomy is created. This technique is limited to small tumors and to a highly select group of patients.

A loop ileostomy and drains should be used liberally. All patients with coloanal anastomosis, colonic J-pouch, and anastomosis within 5 cm of the anal verge receive a diverting loop ileostomy and drain placement. Other factors that lower our threshold to divert and drain include preoperative chemoradiation, immunosuppresion, questionable anastomotic integrity, and diabetes.

Abdominoperineal Resection

The abdominal portion of the procedure proceeds in the same fashion as described earlier for low anterior resection. A TME is performed and the dissection is carried down to the levators circumferentially. The transection site in the proximal colon is chosen and the bowel is divided using the endoscopic linear stapler with a GI cartridge. A left lower quadrant port is inserted where the stoma site has been marked unless it was created earlier to aid in the dissection. A laparoscopic Babcock is inserted and the transected end of the bowel is grasped across the staple line; the ratchet is locked fully to avoid dislodgment.

Perineal Portion

The perineum is exposed using a lone star retractor and the anus is closed with a heavy purse string suture. A circumferential perineal incision is made and dissection is undertaken using electrocautery in the ischiorectal fossa to expose the levator ani muscle and the anococcygeal ligament (Fig. 49-15, page 498). The anococcygeal ligament is incised and the pelvis is entered. An index finger is introduced through this defect to guide the lateral division of the levator (Fig. 49-16, page 498). The specimen is exteriorized through the posterior

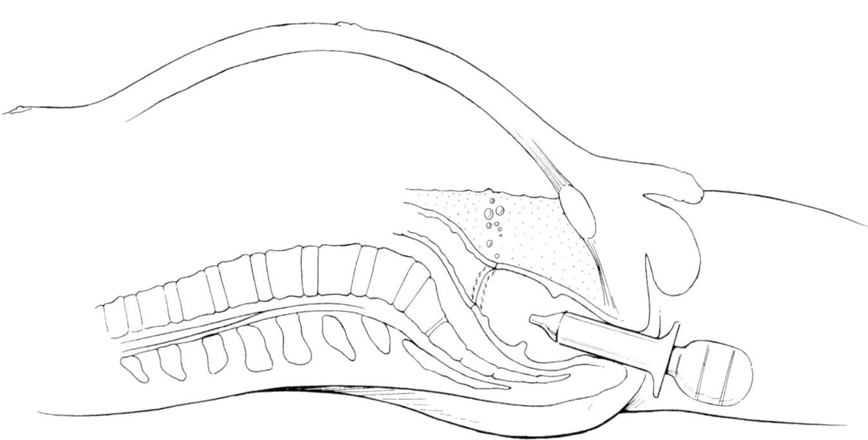

Fig. 49-13. Low anastomoses are tested by filling the pelvis with saline and insufflating air into the rectum to look for bubbles.

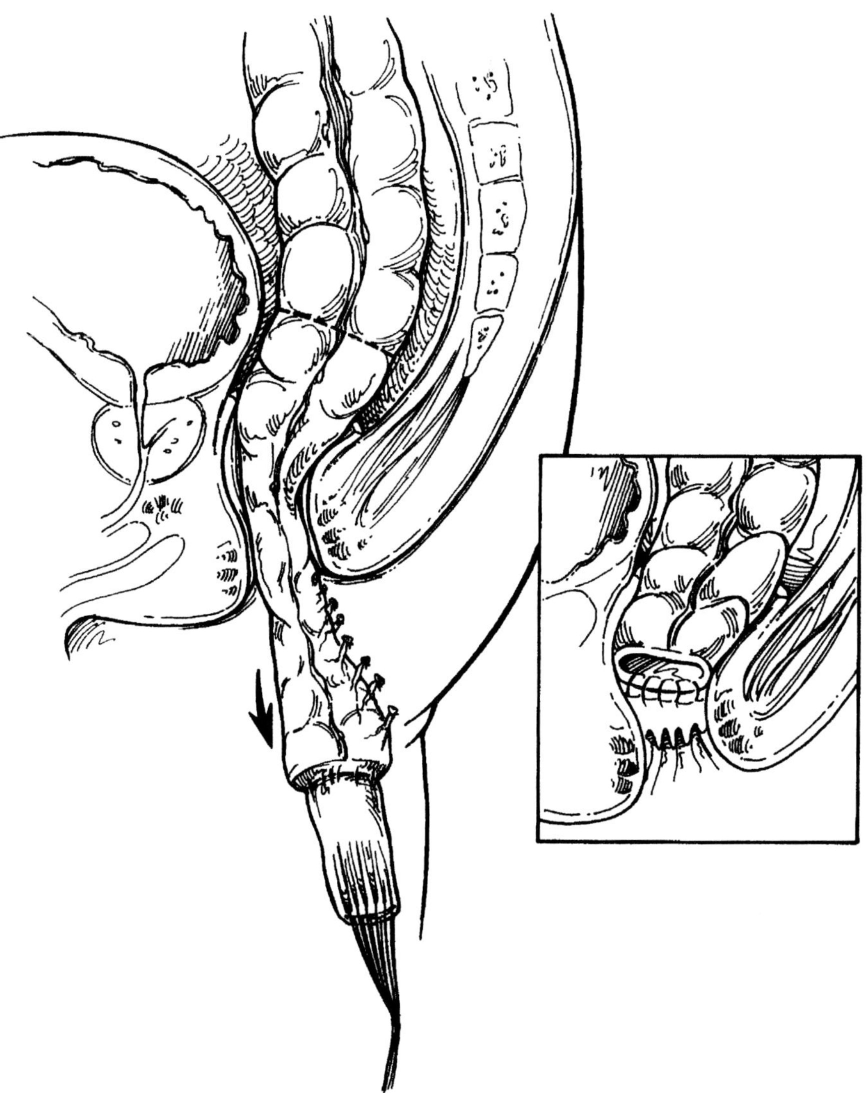

Fig. 49-14. Ultra-low resections are possible by performing an anal mucosectomy and a subsequent hand-sewn coloanal anastamosis.

defect and the anterior portion of the procedure is completed taking care to avoid injury to the urethra in males or the vagina in females. The perineal defect is closed in layers and the abdomen is re-insufflated. Careful inspection is performed ensuring adequate hemostasis. A drain is left in the pelvis from the right lower quadrant incision.

A circular incision is made around the left lower quadrant trocar and the colostomy aperture is created. The defect in the fascia should be no more than two fingerbreadths wide; the trocar is pulled out along with the Babcock and the end of the bowel. The abdomen is re-insufflated and verified for meticulous hemostasis after which an eversion technique is used to mature the end colostomy.

We routinely close all trocar defects using a figure-eight absorbable suture to avoid hernia formation.

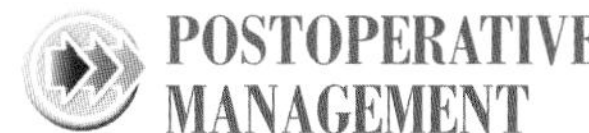

POSTOPERATIVE MANAGEMENT

The nasogastric tube and the ureteral stents are removed at the conclusion of the procedure. After stabilization in the recovery room, the patient is transferred to a regular floor bed and is allowed a clear diet on the evening of the procedure. The diet is then advanced as tolerated, starting on postoperative day 1. The patient is encouraged to ambulate early and is given a patient-controlled analgesia (PCA) pump for pain relief. The urinary catheters are kept for 3 to 5 days postoperatively and reinserted in cases of urinary retention; post-void residual volume measurement can aid in early identification. The pelvic drain is removed on postoperative day 3, unless the effluent is worrisome for a leak. The enterostomal therapist initiates stoma care early in the postoperative period.

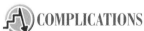

COMPLICATIONS

Complications associated with laparoscopic rectal cancer include all complications associated with conventional surgery with the addition of a unique set of complications related to the laparoscopic approach. Postoperative complications, including anastomotic leak, autonomic nerve damage, and wound complications, are similar in both techniques and will not be discussed further in this chapter (Tables 49-1 and 49-2).

Conversion to an open technique at any stage of the procedure should not be viewed as a complication but rather as the

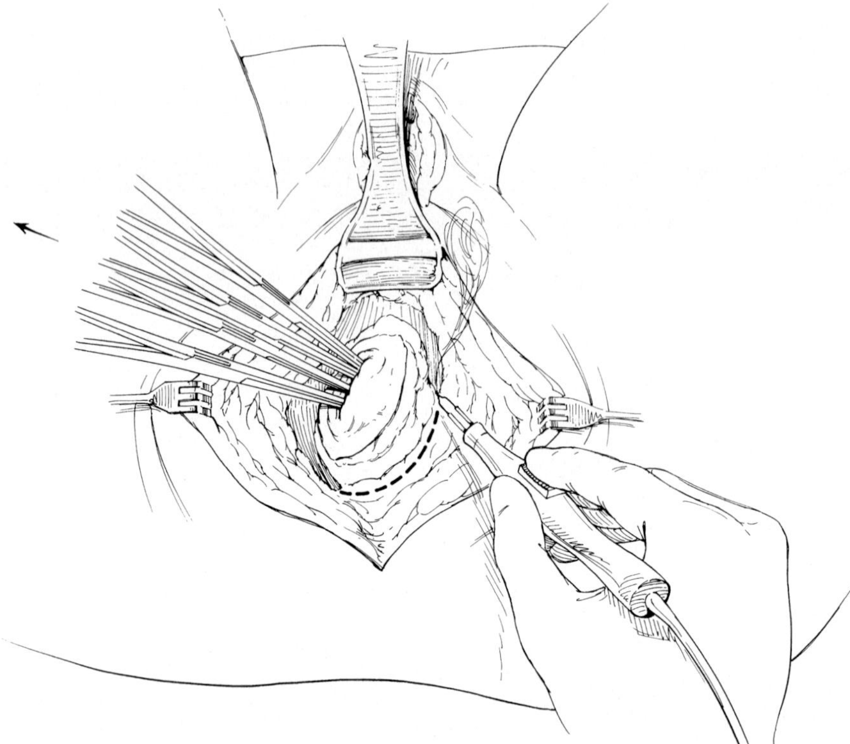

Fig. 49-15. Cautery is used to circumferentially excise around the anus.

application of astute clinical judgment. There are two types of conversions: reactive and preemptive. Preemptive conversions are initiated early in the procedure when there is evidence, including severe adhesions, coagulopathy, unclear anatomy, and dilated bowel, that it may be unsafe or unwise to proceed with laparoscopy; preemptive conversion in such cases has been shown to decrease morbidity. Reactive conversions are initiated secondary to an event, such as bleeding or visceral injury, and are associated with a much higher morbidity and mortality. Therefore, whenever possible, preemptive rather than reactive conversion should be employed.

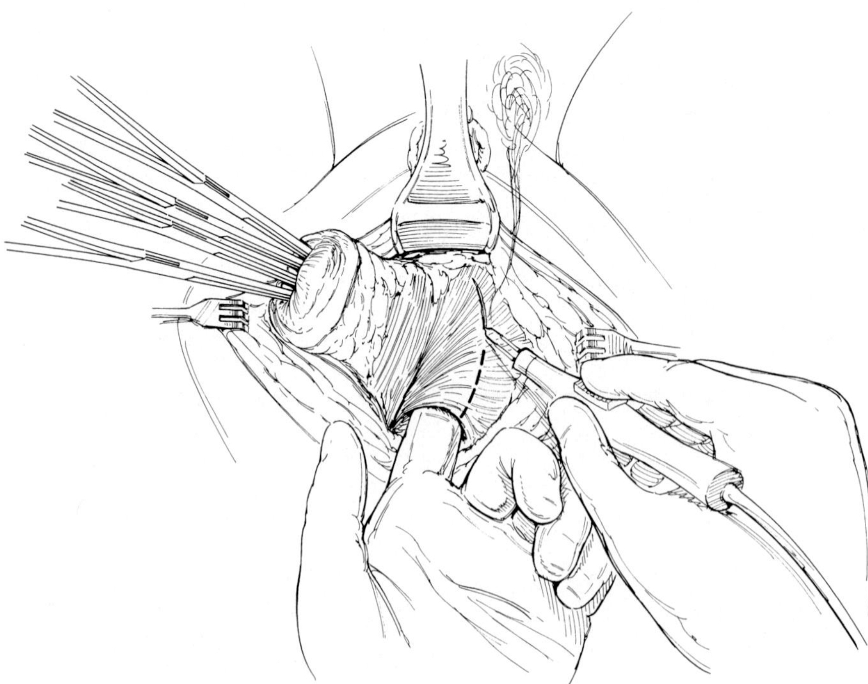

Fig. 49-16. The abdomen is entered posteriorly and the levators divided over the surgeon's finger.

CONCLUSION

Laparoscopic resection for rectal cancer is an exciting new field that remains under much scrutiny. It provides measurable postoperative outcome improvements in the short term; however insufficient level-one data are available regarding oncologic outcomes. The adoption of laparoscopic proctectomy has been slow, mostly due to the complexity of the procedure and the lack of adequate training for many surgeons. Only surgeons with extensive experience in performing laparoscopic colorectal operations and proficient in total mesorectal excision for cancer should be attempting these complex procedures. In addition, just like in conventional surgery, laparoscopic rectal resections should be limited to surgeons with high volumes performing these procedures in high-volume institutions. The learning curve for these procedures is steep, with a minimum of 20 cases needed to overcome this obstacle. We have described our preferred methodology for performing these procedures; readers must be aware that many variations are available and surgeons should acquaint themselves with these modifications and choose their own preferred approach.

SUGGESTED READING

Barlehner E, Benhidjeb T, Andres S, et al. Laparoscopic resection for rectal cancer: Outcomes in 194 patients and review of the literature. *Surg Endosc* 2005;19:757–766.

Fleshman JW, Wexner SD, Anvari M, et al. Laparoscopic vs. open abdominoperineal resection for cancer. *Dis Colon Rectum* 1999;42:930–939.

Leung KL, Kwok SPY, Lam SDW, et al. Laparoscopic resection of rectosigmoid carcinoma: Prospective randomized trial. *Lancet* 2004,363:1187–1192.

Person B, Vivas DA, Wexner SD. Totally laparoscopic low anterior resection with transperineal handsewn colonic J-pouch anal anastomosis for low rectal cancer. *Surg Endosc* 2006;20:700–702.

Pikarsky AJ, Rosenthal R, Weiss EG, et al. Laparoscopic total mesorectal excision. *Surg Endosc* 2002;16:558–562.

Weiss E, Wexner S. Laparoscopic segmental colectomies, anterior resection, and abdominoperineal resection. In: The Sages Manual: Fundamentals of Laparoscopy and Endoscopy. Scott-Conner CEH, ed. New York: Springer, 1999:290–295.

COMMENTARY

One of the last gastrointestinal surgical procedures to begin conversion to laparoscopic approaches has been surgery for rectal cancer. Reasons for that are multifactorial and include the relatively small numbers of the cancer, the aggressive nature of the cancer and its history of significantly higher local failure rates, the technical difficulty of operating low in the pelvis, and the perception that it would be impossible to reproduce the total mesenteric excision (TME) laparoscopically. TME is in fact a perfect case in point. First described by Heald in 1978 and supported over the years with reams of superior outcomes data, it wasn't until more than 20 years later that the approach became the recognized oncologic standard. Changes are slow to be accepted in the world of rectal surgery.

Laparoscopic resection of the rectum for cancer has been greatly facilitated by definitive evidence that TME can be replicated, by the equivalent outcomes of laparoscopic colon cancer surgery, and by technology developments such as the development of improved stapling devices: articulating, flexible, or curved. Some would also list hand ports, for hand-assisted surgery. I remain unconvinced that this is a true advance, aside from the fact that it may offer some psychological reassurance to surgeons in their learning curve period. It seems to compromise the less-is-more premise of minimally invasive surgery; LeRoy has referred to it as "laparoscopic-assisted open surgery." Still, it is a popular modality and has at least introduced a generation of surgeons to the benefits of laparoscopy. Our own institution uses the hand ports for a step-down approach to conversion. If the procedure is not progressing satisfactorily, or there is indication for emergent conversion for bleeding or other occurrences, we will make a 7- to 10-mm incision, rapidly place a hand port, and try to use a hand to control the situation. If this does not succeed, full conversion is performed.

Drs. Safar and Wexner gives many technical pearls for surgeons who perform rectal excisions. I particularly like the suggestion to plot the distal resection using intraoperative endoscopy. This offers a useful alternative to the open tactile input for margins. Also, achieving a good transverse staple rectal division is an important consideration for a secure anastomosis. The authors recommend the use of several firings of an articulating 30-mm endoscopic stapler. Another alternative is the use of the newer curved TA stapler inserted through the specimen removal site. Regardless, the main thing is to test the security of the anastomosis before considering the procedure finished.

LLS

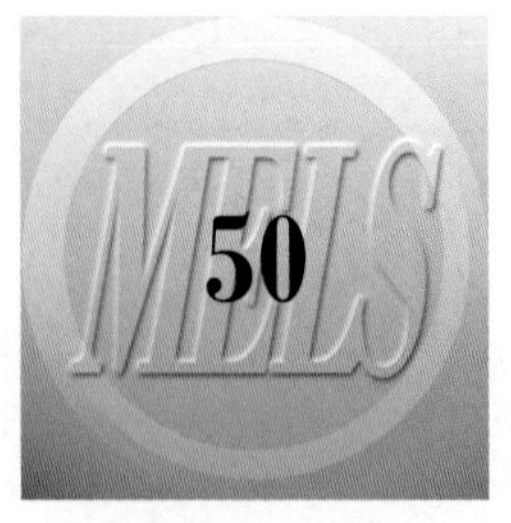

Laparoscopic Enterostomies

JAMES W. FLESHMAN

INTRODUCTION

An operation to primarily construct an intestinal stoma without intestinal resection is usually performed when a fecal diversion proximal to an intestinal fistula (temporary or permanent) or decompression of an obstructed intestine is necessary. The construction of an intestinal stoma plays a role in the management of a wide variety of colorectal and anal diseases, such as anastomotic leak after colorectal anastomosis, Crohn anal disease, obstructing cancer, or severe diverticulitis. The intestinal stoma can be performed as an end ostomy with divided limbs or as a loop with both ends present at the stoma site. Selection of each of these depends on the overriding need for decompression (loop stoma with both ends open) or diversion (end stoma with the distal end closed).

Open laparotomy has been used to accomplish diversion or decompression for many years. Numerous techniques for the construction of emergency or elective ostomies have been described. Mobilization of the ileum or colon is often necessary to bring the intestine out of the abdomen as a stoma. Minimally invasive techniques are now being described to avoid laparotomy. The trephine technique is used to deliver the ileum or colon through the stoma site incision without laparotomy. This technique prohibits adequate inspection of the abdominal cavity. An accurate identification of the proximal and distal intestinal segment of the ostomy is essential to prevent twisting of the stoma or maturation of the wrong segments of the ostomy. Mobilization of the intestinal segment to reach the stoma site without tension may also be difficult when using the left or sigmoid colon for a trephine stoma. Use of laparoscopic techniques may eliminate these disadvantages of a minilaprotomy approach and retain the "minimal access" advantages.

The first laparoscopic colon operation was performed in 1991. Since then, indications for laparoscopic surgery were quickly expanded to a wide variety of colorectal diseases. Laparoscopic colorectal surgery has been reported to have some advantages over open laparotomy (e.g., less pain, shorter time of hospitalization, fewer wound complications, quicker recovery), but it has the same rate of intraabdominal complications.

Laparoscopic stoma construction has been reported in small series of patients having mixed problems with good outcomes and the same advantages shown for laparoscopic techniques used in other disease processes: less pain, low risk of wound infection, short recovery time, low incidence of conversion, and low rate of complications. The use of laparoscopic stoma usually allows earlier initiation of chemotherapy and radiation therapy in obstructing rectal cancers and earlier feeding in patients with non-resectable complicated diverticulitis. Laparoscopic ostomy construction is usually technically feasible with only minimal intestinal mobilization and manipulation of mesentery. The literature does not contain any controlled randomized study comparing laparoscopic and open ostomy construction and less invasive (such as trephine or percutaneous) techniques. An initially overlooked advantage of laparoscopic ostomy is the lack of adhesions at the time of construction. Subsequent take down of the ostomy is made much easier by the absence of adhesions.

The procedure is normally easy for surgeons with laparoscopic colorectal experience. The advantages of using laparoscopic stoma construction are that the laparotomy incision and all of its consequences are avoided. The only sizeable incision is made at the ostomy site. Laparoscopic techniques theoretically cause fewer adhesions and allow more rapid return of intestinal function. This can allow earlier feeding in an already compromised patient and facilitate earlier self-care of the ostomy because pain is reduced. Lack of adhesion formation may also allow earlier ostomy closure if the reason for diversion or decompression has resolved (e.g., diverting loop ileostomy for small colorectal anastomotic leak that resolves with diversion of fecal stream for 2 weeks). The shorter recovery time after a palliative procedure is important for patients with advanced colorectal or anal cancer. As a result, neoadjuvant chemoradiation before definitive operation or palliative chemotherapy might be started earlier. It is usually necessary to wait at least a month after laparotomy. In most cases, treatment can be started within 1 to 2 weeks after laparoscopic ostomy construction.

The clinician's learning curve for laparoscopic colectomy is estimated between 20 to 50 cases. The complexity of laparoscopic colorectal surgery involves expertise with mobilization of more than one intestinal segment, familiarity with new anatomic perspectives through the laparoscope's lens, and the use of single-faceted, rudimentary laparoscopic instruments. However, laparoscopic stoma formation is a relatively easy procedure requiring minimal intestinal mobilization and almost no mesentery manipulation or vascular division. A rigid straight laparoscope is usually adequate. No expensive instruments are needed to complete the surgery and no special energy sources, access ports, or stapling devices are required. For these reasons, it can be used as one of the first procedures for surgeons with no experience in laparoscopic colorectal surgery.

The basic requirements for performing laparoscopic ostomy construction are knowledge of general principles of ostomy construction and an operating room laparoscopic procedure team of nurses and technicians familiar with equipment and room setup.

General Principles of Ostomy Construction

It is essential to involve the enterostomal therapist in the care of the patient at the onset of planning construction of an ostomy. Education regarding stoma function, lifestyle changes, coping methods, support groups (e.g., the local chapter of the United Ostomy Association) plays a large role in the rapid recovery of the ostomate, whether the stoma is constructed by open methods or laparoscopically.

Patient interview and education is done preoperatively by an enterostomal therapy nurse if at all possible (even in emergency situations). The potential stoma sites are chosen and marked with the patient sitting, standing, and dressed. The site should ideally be free of incisions, sutures, drains, rods, bony prominences, scars, and waistline and skin folds because each may form defects in the abdominal contours that may result in pouch leakage. Depending on the type of stoma (i.e., colostomy, ileostomy) the quadrant will be chosen, but as a principle the site should always be the middle of the rectus sheath on the apex of the supra or infraumbilical fat fold. Some exceptions are made in obese patients, young children, and patients with a barrel-shaped abdomen. It is generally important to mark these stomas in the upper quadrants so that the patient is able to see and, therefore, care for the stoma independently.

In the operating room, in the emergency setting when a preoperatively selected site is not marked, the site can be selected relative to the umbilicus on the infra- or supraumbilical fat fold in the center of the rectus muscle in the appropriate quadrant. Although this may result in a poorly positioned ostomy on occasion, the stoma usually can be pouched and skin issues managed.

Clear pouches are applied in the early postoperative period for better observation of mucosal vascularity. A flexible adhesive base on a one-piece sizable system is selected that will be cut to the size of the patient's stoma. Presized or two-piece "snap-on" systems are not recommended in the operating room because postoperative mucosal edema may occur that could result in stoma laceration and bleeding. A properly fitted and applied pouching system is essential for patient comfort and confidence in the immediate postoperative period. While the site is painful, limited pressure should be applied, thus eliminating the use of snap-on two-piece appliances.

After the mucosal edema has disappeared, the actual size of the stoma is determined using a measuring guide, and pre-cut faceplates can be ordered. Convex pouching systems are generally not used because application of pressure to the newly sutured mucocutaneous junction may result in separation. Many pouching systems have integrated skin barriers. The appliance must fully protect the skin around an ileostomy because of the alkalinity and enzymatic activity of the stoma effluent. The ileostomy must protrude 2 to 3 cm, with a close fit of the stoma to the edge of the appliance adhesive faceplate essential (Fig. 50-1A). Conversely, a colostomy does not place the skin surrounding the stoma at risk for erosion and damage. A larger opening that is less precisely matched to the ostomy is adequate.

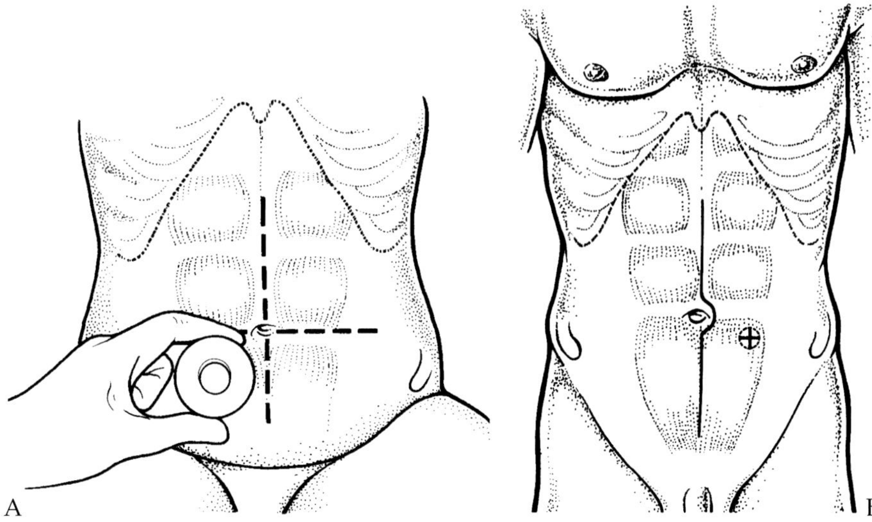

Fig. 50-1. Stomas sites. **A.** Ileostomy. **B.** Colostomy.

Diet

In most patients, except those with obstructing tumor, a nasogastric tube is not used. If the procedure is completed early in the day, most patients are able to tolerate some liquids the same evening; otherwise, introduction of liquids is delayed until the next morning. The diet is started with liquids and is advanced according to the patient's tolerance. Standard dietary precautions for ileostomates should be followed by the dietary service in the hospital and taught by the enterostomal therapist. There are no restrictions in diet for patients after sigmoid colostomy construction. Stool softeners and laxatives are still necessary for patients with a history of constipation.

Restrictions

The daily output of an ileostomy is approximately 500 to 800 mL, with variation from person to person. The amount of water lost through an ileostomy is higher than the amount of water normally contained in feces. Thus, patients need to be aware of the volume of their output and adjust liquid intake or use of antidiarrheal medications accordingly. Undigested fiber and any other food that may obstruct the ileostomy output should be avoided. High osmotic load liquids, usually resulting from sugar content, should be avoided unless the use is intended to cause diarrhea to overcome partial blockage at the new edematous stoma.

Pure Laparoscopic Ostomy Construction

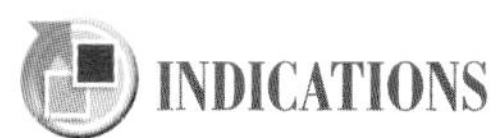

INDICATIONS

Indications for laparoscopic stoma construction are the same as for open techniques. These include all situations in which the fecal stream must be diverted. Surgical options include loop ileostomy and loop or loop-end colostomy. Selection of an ileostomy or colostomy depends on the indication for the procedure and surgeon preference. Indications for laparoscopic ostomy in colorectal practice are listed in Table 50-1, page 502.

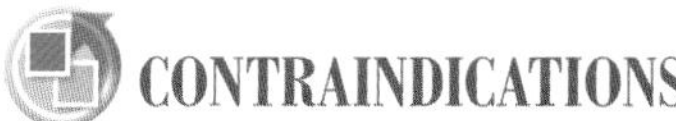

CONTRAINDICATIONS

Contraindications for laparoscopic stoma construction are the same as for other laparoscopic colorectal procedures. The presence of a known coagulopathy with ongoing bleeding, medical intolerance of anesthesia, and known severe adhesions are absolute contraindications for laparoscopic procedures. It is very difficult to explore, irrigate, drain, and debride the abdominal cavity completely in patients with fecal or purulent peritonitis through the laparoscopic approach. However, there are reports in the literature using laparoscopic approaches to

TABLE 50-1. INDICATIONS FOR PURE LAPAROSCOPIC ENTEROSTOMIES

Ileostomy
Anastomotic leak at colorectal, ileoanal anastomosis
Obstructing or advanced rectosigmoid cancer before neoadjuvant therapy
Rectal Crohn disease with multiple abscesses or fistulae
Sigmoid phlegmon due to diverticulitis or perforated cancer
Ileocolic phlegmon secondary to Crohn disease
Colostomy
Obstructing or advanced rectosigmoid cancer before neoadjuvant therapy
Advanced anal cancer before neoadjuvant therapy
Nonresectable diverticulitis
Rectal trauma
Fournier's disease
Anal incontinence
Failed anal sphincter repair or sliding flap repair of fistula

TABLE 50-2. CONTRAINDICATIONS FOR LAPAROSCOPIC ENTEROSTOMIES

Absolute
Uncorrectable bleeding or dyscrasia
Extensive previous surgery with known severe adhesions
Relative
Colonic perforation and free peritonitis
Inflammatory bowel disease with friable bowel wall
Morbid obesity
Large abdominal aortic aneurysm

these problems with good outcome. The absolute and relative contraindications are listed in Table 50-2.

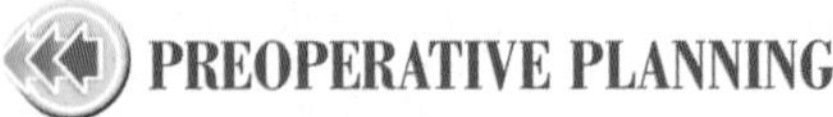

PREOPERATIVE PLANNING

The attendant benefits and risks of laparoscopic stoma construction should be discussed with the patient and informed consent obtained, followed by the administration of appropriate antibiotics as indicated perioperatively. The stoma site should be marked by an enterostomal therapist and educational material provided. Mechanical preparation by repeated rectal enemas should be attempted before colostomy construction, it at all possible.

SURGICAL TECHNIQUE

Operation Room and Patient Positioning

The patient is placed in a modified lithotomy position, for colostomy, with the buttocks near the lower edge of the operating table and the legs in stirrups (either Allen or Lloyd-Davies) (Fig. 50-2). For ileostomy, the supine position is used. The patient is fixed in position using a beanbag attached with Velcro strips to the table. All patients are submitted to general anesthesia. The surgeon and camera operator are positioned on the side opposite the involved segment of intestine (Fig. 50-3). The assistant is positioned opposite to the surgeon or between the patient's legs. The flexible or angled laparoscope is inserted through an umbilical port or through the ostomy site if possible. The critical feature of performing any laparoscopic ostomy includes limiting the number of trocars by utilizing the ostomy site as a trocar site while making every effort to ensure that the correct end of the bowel is matured as the functioning stoma. This can be accomplished by using anatomic landmarks, delivering the distal limb until tethering occurs in the proper direction, or inserting a flexible scope down the distal limb to document connection to the distal part of the bowel. If a secondary port is needed, a 5-mm trocar is place in the opposite side of the abdomen or at the suprapubic position.

Ileostomy

Access to the abdominal cavity is achieved by either a closed or open technique at the stoma site. The disc of skin is excised at the previously marked stoma site, the skin and fat are removed, the rectus muscle sheath is opened vertically over 3 cm, the muscles are separated in the direction of its fibers, and the trocar is inserted through a 1-cm incision in the posterior rectus sheath. After the pneumoperitoneum is established, a laparoscopic camera (flexible is preferred) is inserted through the trocar at the stoma site (Fig. 50-4). The abdominal cavity is carefully inspected. The second trocar is usually placed at the umbilicus when the camera

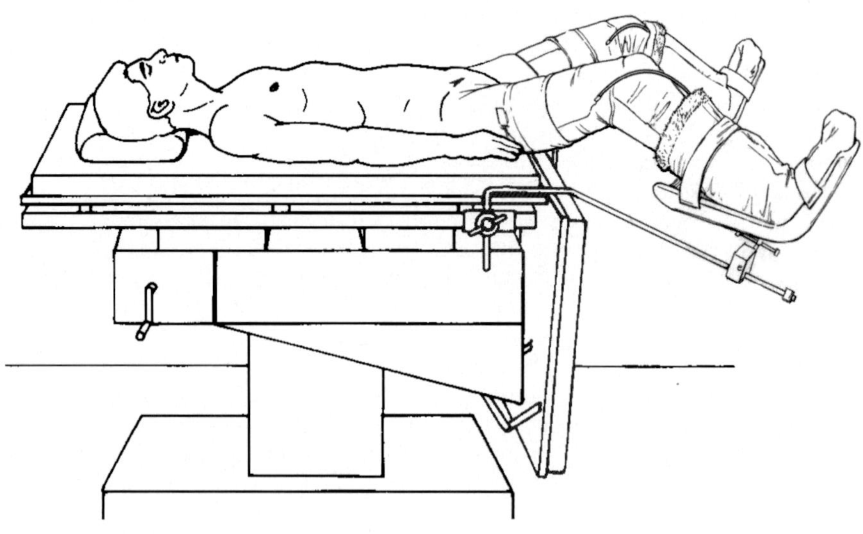

Fig. 50-2. Patient position.

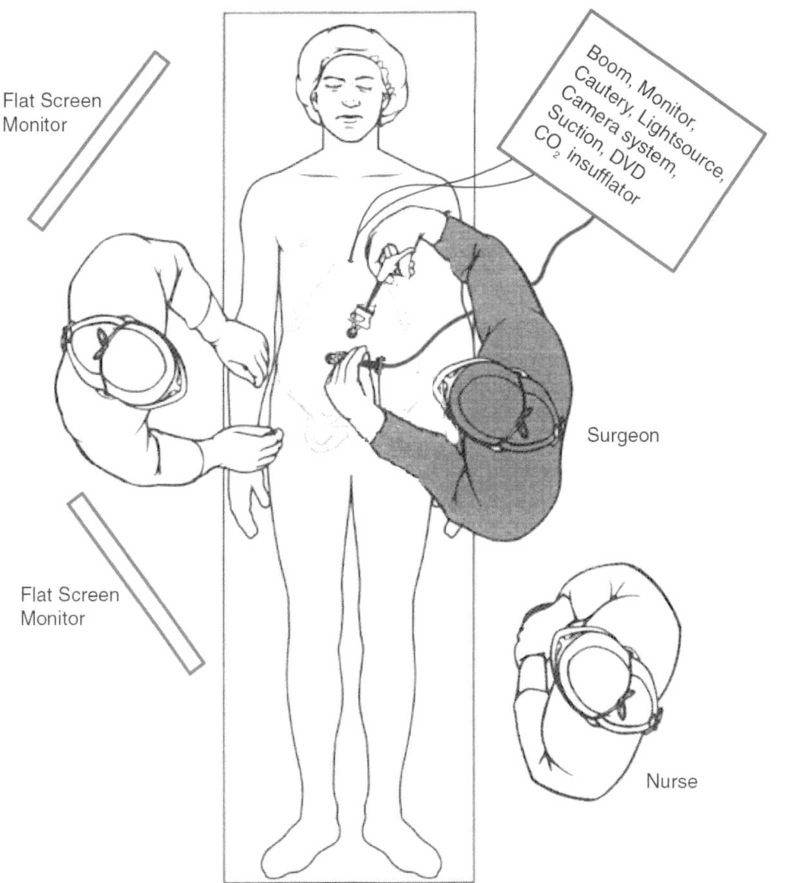

Fig. 50-3. Position of the equipment and personnel for ileostomy.

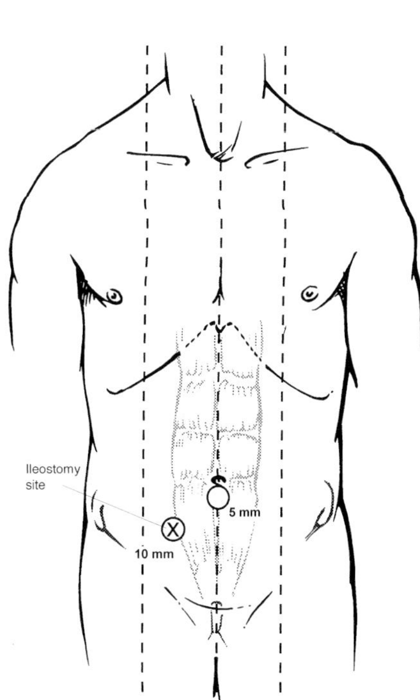

Fig. 50-4. Trocar placement for ileostomy.

is in the stoma site. Alternatively, if a 5-mm camera is available, the camera can be placed through the 5-mm umbilical trocar. The terminal ileum is grasped 20 cm proximal to the ileocecal valve with an atraumatic 5-mm grasper (Fig. 50-5, page 504). Intestinal mobility and capacity to reach the abdominal wall without tension are tested. Additional mobilization at the base of the right colon and small-bowel mesentery along the pelvic brim will guarantee free movement of the ileum to the abdominal wall. This is critical in the obese patient to prevent tethering, retraction, and ischemia. Placing the patient in Trendelenburg position and airplaning the table to the left will help expose the retroperitoneal attachments of the cecum and terminal ileum. The correct position and identification of proximal and distal limbs are confirmed and then the loop of bowel is kept close to the abdominal wall and the grasper fixed on the abdominal surface to prevent rotation. Additional 5-mm trocars and working instruments can be added as needed to accomplish mobilization. The posterior sheath is opened to the maximum diameter of the ostomy site using the trocar as a guide. The ileum is delivered through the ostomy site as the pneumoperitoneum is deflated, still grasped by the 5-mm grasper and oriented in the appropriate anatomic position. The grasper is exchanged to a regular Babcock clamp to pull the bowel as a knuckle through the abdominal wall opening. The trocars are removed and only the site away from the ostomy site containing a 10-mm port (if used) is closed at the fascia level. The ileostomy is matured as a 2.5-cm spigot. The ileostomy is incised 80% around the circumference of the bowel at the skin level on the distal limb of the bowel. The full-thickness bowel-to-subcuticular-layer sutures at the skin fix the so called "mucus fistula" in the inferior part of the stoma opening. The proximal bowel is then everted (i.e., folded back on itself) using full thickness sutures placed through the cut edge of the intestine, then a seromuscular suture 5-cm proximal, and finally a subcuticular suture in the skin in matched position around the bowel circumference and ostomy opening (Fig. 50-6, page 504). A rod is only used if the bowel is under tension (e.g., in an obese patient), in which case the rod is passed through the mesentery at the midpoint of the knuckle of the bowel to suspend the intestine above the skin level.

Colostomy

Operating room personnel are positioned as shown in Figure 50-7, page 505. A working trocar is inserted through the ostomy site in the left lower quadrant (Fig. 50-8A, page 505). The circle of skin is incised at the previously marked stoma site, the skin and fat are removed, and the anterior rectus muscle sheath is opened. The rectus muscle fibers are then split and the trocar inserted through a 1-cm incision in the posterior sheath. The camera port is inserted at the umbilicus under direct vision through the stoma site trocar. A 5-mm camera is helpful if available and a flexible tip scope is preferable. The abdominal cavity is carefully inspected under the 15-mmHg pneumoperitoneum. An additional 5-mm trocar is placed at the suprapubic site where the scissor is inserted. Other 5-mm trocars can be inserted as needed for dissection. Another 5-mm port inserted at the right lower quadrant is usually most helpful. The table is placed in the Trendelenburg position and airplaned to the right. The sigmoid is identified and retracted medially with the laparoscopic atraumatic clamp inserted through the stoma site. The lateral and pelvic peritoneal attachments are

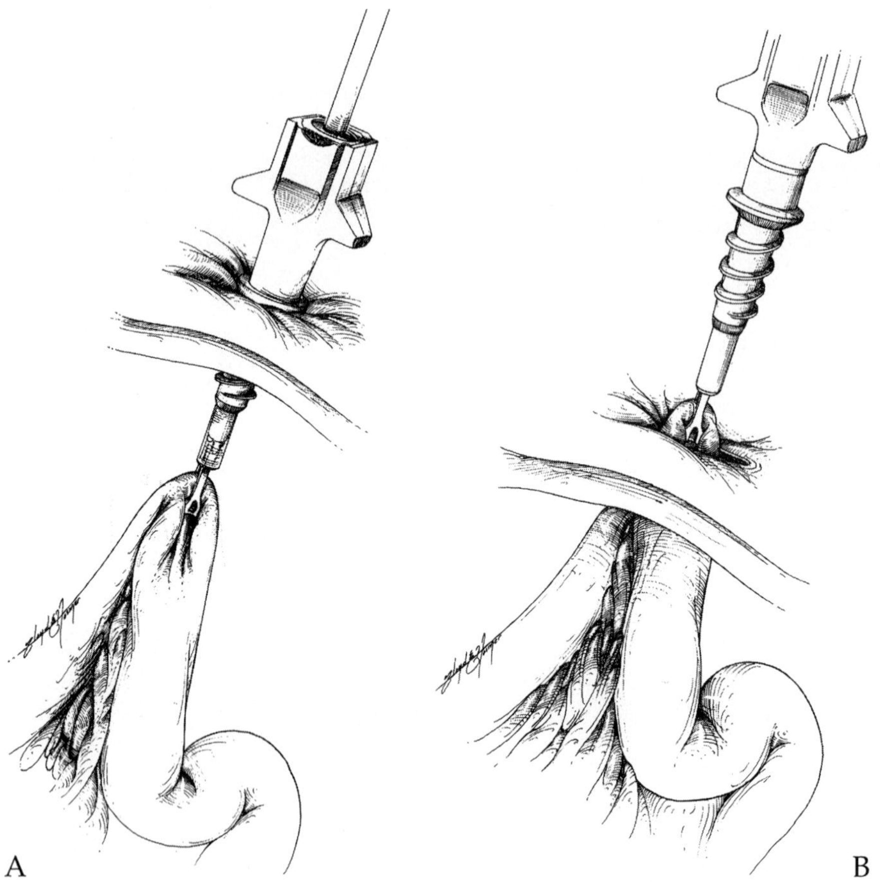

Fig. 50-5. Ileostomy technique. **A.** The ileum is grasped with a Babcock clamp. **B.** The clamp is used to pull the bowel through the abdominal wall.

sharply incised using sharp scissor dissection via the suprapubic working port. The sigmoid and descending colons are mobilized along the white line of Toldt in the avascular plane between the colon, its mesentery, and the retroperitoneal structures and should produce little if any blood loss. The ureter should be identified and visualized crossing the iliac artery (Fig. 50-9, page 506). If mobility is still an issue, the splenic flexure can be mobilized from the lateral abdominal wall, the tip of the spleen, and tail of the pancreas. The inferior mesenteric vessels are divided only in the most unusual circumstances where mobility is limited, such as obesity and inflammation. The inferior mesenteric artery can be divided at its origin without compromising blood supply in most instances due to rich collaterals from proximal and distal. The apex point of the sigmoid or left colon is grasped and held close to the abdominal wall testing the mobility and capacity to reach the stoma site without tension. The proximal and distal limb orientations are made by direct vision and, taking care to not twist the colon, the grasper is pulled straight up to the stoma site. The posterior rectus sheath is opened to deliver the colon easily. Releasing the pneumoperitoneum should allow the bowel to easily pass through the stoma site. The trocars are removed, any 10- to 12-mm port site is closed with sutures, and

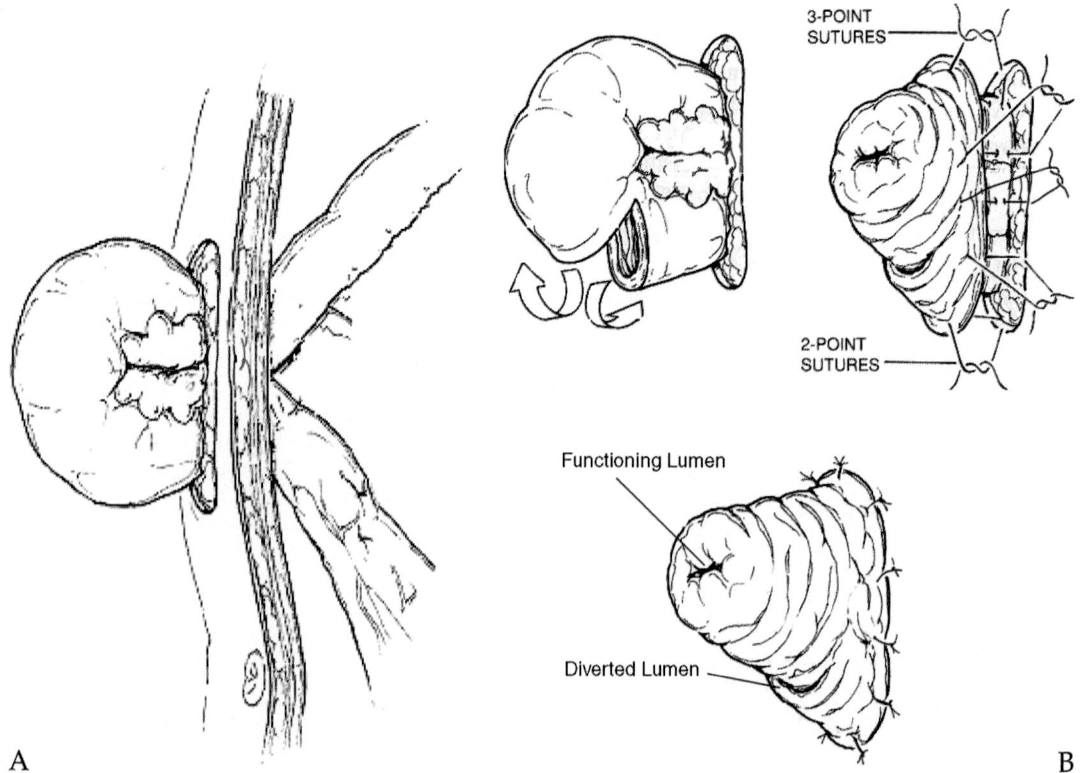

Fig. 50-6. Construction of a loop ileostomy.

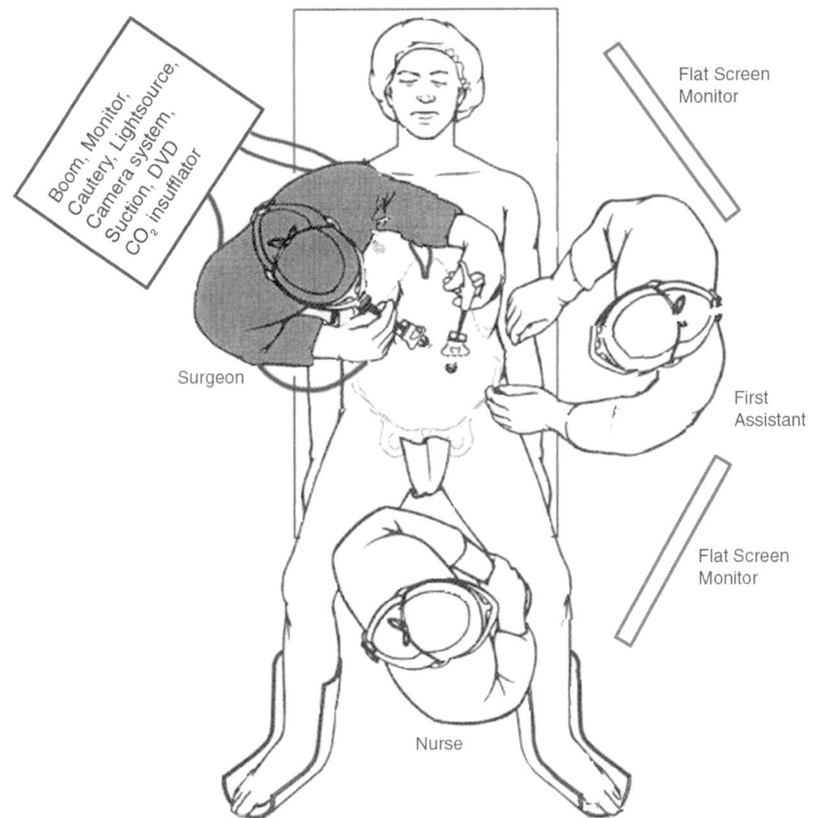

Fig. 50-7. Position of the equipment and personnel for colostomy.

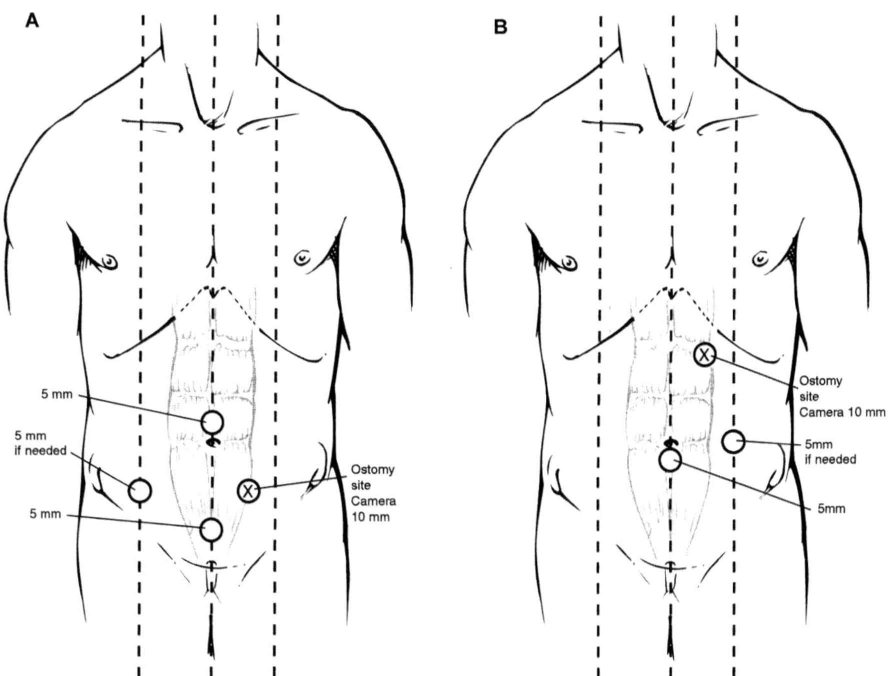

Fig. 50-8. Trocar placements of colostomy. **A.** Sigmoid colostomy. **B.** Transverse colostomy.

the skin is closed with staples. The sigmoid colon is divided at the skin level in the inferior aspect of the ostomy site with the GIA stapler. The corner of the staple line of the distal colon is secured with a single suture subcutaneously or subfascially. In patients with obstructing rectal lesions the corner of the staple line of the distal colon is opened and matured as a mucus fistula in the lower portion of the ostomy site. The opening is limited to 5-mm to act only as a blow hole. The proximal limb is matured at the skin with absorbable full-thickness sutures through bowel and skin, covering the distal limb or bridging to the mucus fistula in the lower part of the ostomy site (Fig. 50-10, page 506). The appliance is then placed.

Special Considerations for Ostomies after Bowel Resection

Several issues that influence the outcome of the patient must be considered during construction of a laparoscopic ostomy. The abdominal wall opening must be adequate to preserve blood supply to the everted stoma or subcutaneous portion of the colostomy. The tendency is to use a trocar site incision that has been only slightly enlarged. This results in an ischemic stoma to the level of the fascia and requires revision. In an obese patient, blood supply to the entire loop of bowel may be tenuous because of tension, volume of tissue at the level of the fascial opening, or compression of an already bulky mesentery. In these circumstances, it is reasonable to perform a divided loop-end colostomy/ileostomy, which leaves the stapled closed distal limb within the abdominal cavity and delivers only the proximal functioning end through the fascia. Thus, less tissue is brought through the abdominal wall opening.

By suspending the loop of intestine from the abdominal wall without fixation, there is a theoretic risk of volvulus at the stoma site. The surgeon must be aware of this possibility in the postoperative period. For example, in the patient undergoing a laparoscopic total proctocolectomy and pouch, the ileostomy is placed approximately 20 to 30 cm proximal to the pelvic pouch. The forces of nature (i.e., gravity) tend to drag all bowel loops to the pelvis. This may result in a loop of bowel becoming wrapped around both sides of the suspended loop of ileum and causing a twist or partial obstruction. It is important to replace the bowel in the abdominal cavity to avoid this if at all possible and remember that postoperative obstruction may not always be caused by adhesions.

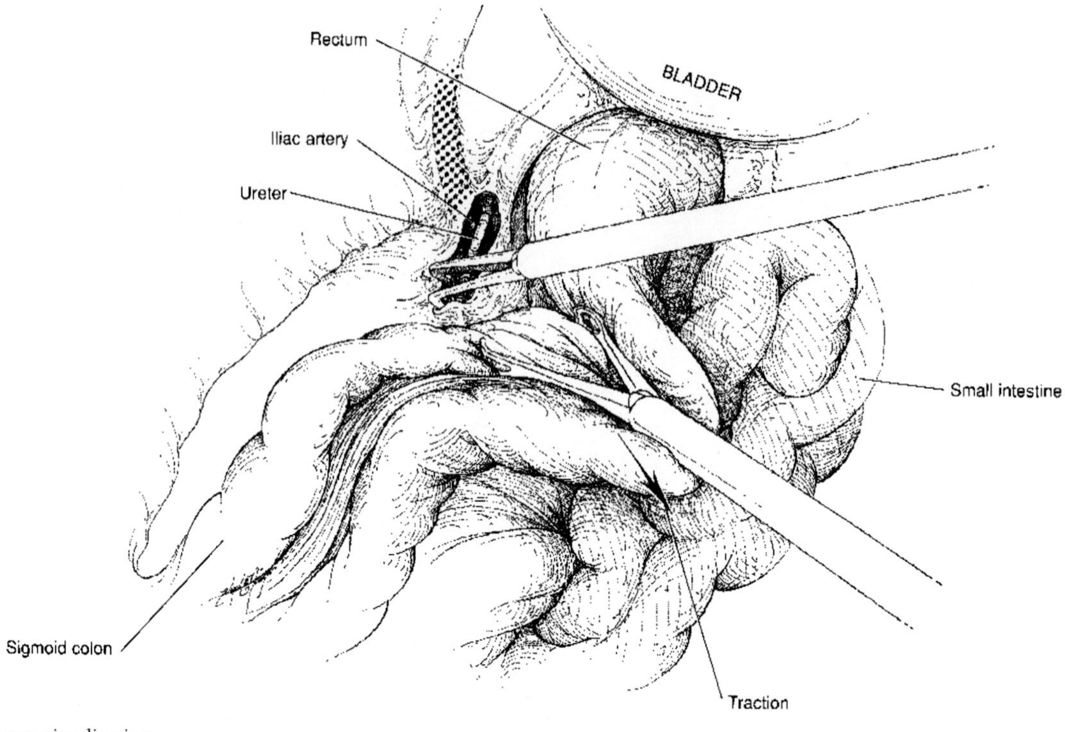

Fig. 50-9. Ureter visualization.

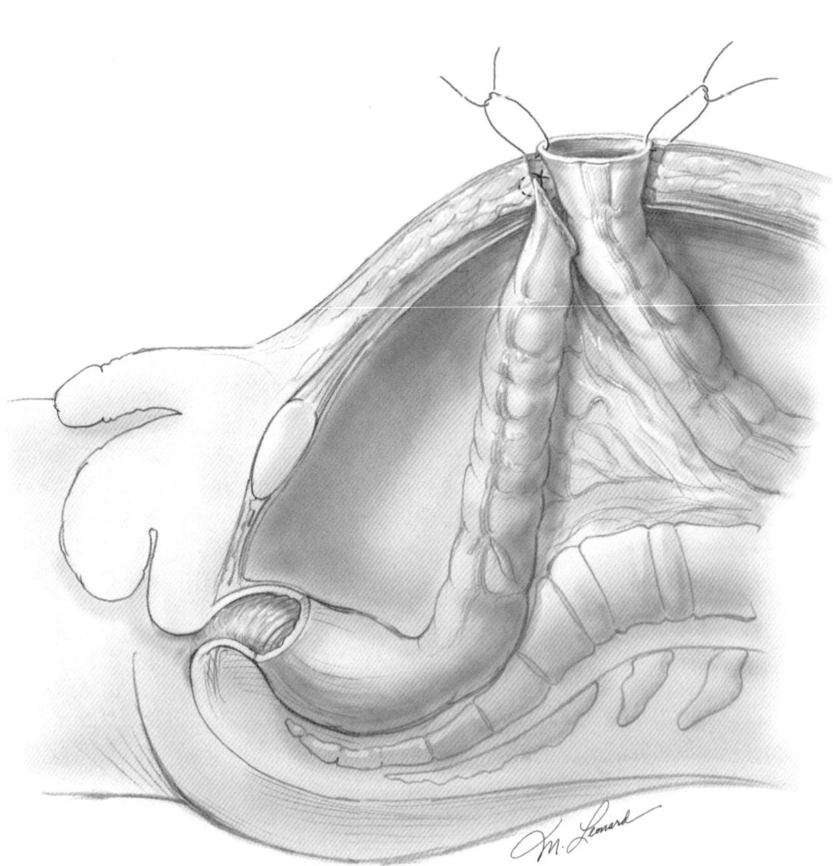

Fig. 50-10. Colostomy.

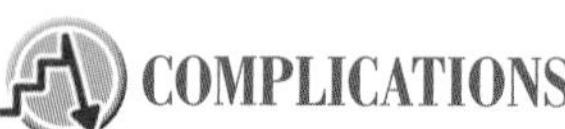

COMPLICATIONS

Potential complications of laparoscopic stoma are usually related to surgical actions. Care is needed during the procedure to prevent these postoperative problems. A patent vascular supply is essential. Mobilization of a larger portion of the colon than the area of stoma is necessary to avoid tension, maintain blood supply, and consequently prevent retraction and ischemia-related complications. As previously mentioned, the size of the fascial opening must be large enough to permit the intestinal segment to pass through freely but not so large that a hernia develops. Placement of the ostomy through the rectus muscle has been shown to reduce herniation and prolapse of the stoma. Preoperative or intraoperative site selection is critical to provide a good base for appliance adherence to avoid skin breakdown.

Intraoperative Complications

Potential intraoperative complications include those associated with any laparoscopic procedure, such as injury cased by insufflation needle or trocar to bowel or vessels, air embolism, arrhythmias, CO_2 intolerance, and subcutaneous emphysema. Another group of potential complications include those specific to laparoscopic colorectal surgery. The familiarity with anatomy visualized through the camera is necessary for perfect identification of anatomic structures. Visualization of ureter, iliac vessels, mesenteric vessels, and correct position of distal and proximal intestinal limbs are necessary to avoid iatrogenic injuries. The immediate recognition of any potential injury must be clarified and promptly treated. Failure to recognize a collateral injury to any of the aforementioned structures is even worse than the injury itself. It is important to avoid retraction or grasping out of the field of view, and care must be taken to show the entire surface of the energy source of the dissecting instrument. During the construction of ileostomy, mobilization of terminal ileum is not necessary in most patients. However, when it has to be done, identifying the right ureter is important but not critical during the dissection. Mobilization of the left colon to allow the sigmoid to reach the anterior abdominal wall without tension is necessary in most circumstances when a left-sided colostomy is formed, even for a sigmoid colostomy, unless it is extremely redundant. Identification of the left ureter as it crosses the iliac vessels is absolutely necessary to avoid injury during dissection.

Postoperative Complications

Possible complications in the postoperative period are the same as traditional stoma construction. The complications are also similar between colostomies and ileostomies. The most frequent complications are ischemia, stoma retraction, prolapse, wound infection, bleeding, and parastomal hernia.

Laparoscopic Ostomy Closure

The only comment to be made regarding ostomy closure is to remind surgeons who construct end colostomies during emergency open Hartmann resection of the rectosigmoid that the first operation is the opportune occasion to make a laparoscopic colostomy closure easy. Mobilization of the splenic flexure to lengthen the left colon mesentery and allow stretch to the pelvis is helpful. Resection of the entire sigmoid colon down to soft rectum (well into the pelvis if need be) is essential, so that no resection of constricted diverticular-affected sigmoid is needed to perform a double stapled end-to-end anastomosis between the rectal stump and left colon. Finally, use of adhesion barrier (such as Seprafilm, Genzyme; Cambridge, MA) is extremely helpful to reduce or prevent adhesions along the left gutter and in the pelvis over the rectal stump.

SUGGESTED READING

Fleshman JW, Fry RD, Birnbaum EH, et al. Laparoscopic-assisted and minilaparotomy approaches to colorectal diseases are similar in early outcomes. *Dis Colon Rectum* 1996; 39:15–22.

Fuhrman GM, Ota DM. Laparoscopic intestinal stomas. *Dis Colon Rectum* 1994;37:444–449.

Hollyoak MA, Lumley J, Stitz RW. Laparoscopic stoma formation for faecal incontinence. *Br J Surg* 1998;85:226–228.

Oliveira L, Reissman P, Nogueras J, et al. Laparoscopic creation of stomas. *Surg Endosc* 1997;11:19–23.

Senapati A, Phillips RKS. The trephine colostomy: a permanent left iliac fossa end colostomy without recourse to laparotomy. *Ann R Coll Surg Engl* 1991;3:305–306.

Swain BT, Ellis CN. Laparoscopy-assisted loop ileostomy: an acceptable option for temporary fecal diversion after anorectal surgery. *Dis Colon Rectum* 2002;45:705–707.

Wexner SD, Reissman P, Pfeifer J, et al. Laparoscopic colorectal surgery: analysis of 140 cases. *Surg Endosc* 1996;10:133–136.

Williams NS, Nasmyth DG, Jones D, et al. Defunctioning stomas; a prospective controlled trial comparing loop ileostomy with loop transverse colostomy. *Br J Surg* 1986; 73:566–570.

Young CJ, Eyers AA, Solomon MJ. Defunctioning of the anorectum: historical controlled study of laparoscopic vs open procedures. *Dis Colon Rectum* 1998;41: 190–194.

COMMENTARY

Recent prospective randomized trials have demonstrated the superiority of laparoscopic colon resections to open colectomies over the short term and have shown equivalent long-term survival rates for cancer operations. As a result, more general surgeons are taking on laparoscopic colectomies and ascending the learning curve for these difficult procedures. Using laparoscopic techniques to perform ileostomies and colostomies represent a good opportunity for the surgeon to become familiar with many of the basic technical skills involved in laparoscopic colon operations with generally lower technical difficulties and risk. The author draws on an extensive experience with both laparoscopic and open intestinal and colonic procedures. He rightfully emphasizes the preoperative considerations that must be appreciated to maximize the quality of life of the patient undergoing enterostomy creation. This is particularly true in planning the appropriate type of ostomy and its precise location on the abdominal wall. It can be quite discouraging to perform a technically perfect operation but be left with a patient whose lifestyle is markedly impaired due to an improperly located ostomy or major morbidity associated with skin problems. Additionally, the importance of maintaining adequate blood supply, minimizing tension on the bowel, and optimizing the size of the fascial and skin incisions are clearly explained.

Surgeons performing laparoscopic intestinal surgery should keep several caveats in mind. Visualization of the ureters should be undertaken whenever the right colon or left colon is mobilized. Second, the bowel wall should be handled with care using atraumatic instruments; seromuscular tears with occult perforation can occur quite easily. Third, many of the patients requiring creation of stomas will have had prior abdominal operations, and adhesions will need to be managed. Appropriate gentle traction and counter traction to expose the appropriate plane is the most important tenet. Sharp dissection of any adhesions near the wall of the intestine needs to be performed to avoid thermal injury to the underlying bowel wall. If a serosal tear does occur, it should probably be oversewn unless so clearly superficial that the muscularis is not visible.

Although Dr. Fleshman has clearly illustrated many fine points in the technical performance of enterostomy, surgeons would be wise to involve enterostomal therapists in the postoperative management of their patients. These individuals can manage stomas that may have technical issues seemingly trivial to the surgeon but that are a major inconvenience to the patient. The work of these allied professionals has the capability of markedly simplifying the surgical care required following creation of enterostomies.

NJS

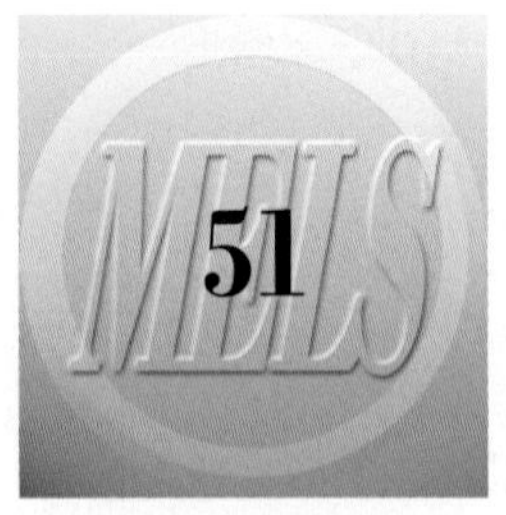

Minimally Invasive Approaches to Anorectal Disorders

JAMES F. FITZGERALD AND LEE E. SMITH

INTRODUCTION

Over the past several years, three minimally invasive techniques have emerged in the treatment of anorectal disease: transanal endoscopic microsurgery (TEM), the procedure for prolapse and hemorrhoids (PPH), and Doppler-guided hemorrhoidal artery ligation (HAL). As these surgeries become more common, surgeons not specializing in this field may be called upon to evaluate and treat patients who have undergone these procedures; an understanding of the procedures and their potential complications is therefore essential. This chapter will discuss the indications, preoperative evaluation, and complications of these procedures, with the necessary equipment, the technique used, and the postoperative care for each procedure outlined.

Transanal Endoscopic Microsurgery

Transanal endoscopic microsurgery is one of the first minimally invasive surgical techniques devised. Developed in 1982 by Gerhard Buess, the technique has been widely accepted in Europe and many parts of the world. However, because it has a very specific indication and requires expensive equipment and special training, TEM is only just gaining widespread acceptance in the United States.

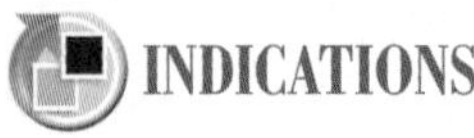

INDICATIONS

Tumors in the middle to upper rectum are acceptable for TEM. For lesions in the distal third of the rectum, it can be difficult to maintain operative exposure using TEM. Fortunately, these lesions can usually be approached under direct vision with standard anal instrument sets. Using the longer TEM scope, lesions as high up as 24 cm can be excised and sutured closed.

Generally any benign adenoma within the rectum and rectosigmoid can be excised using this technique; size is not a deterrent. Other benign tumors such as lipomas and carcinoids are also appropriate. Other rectal procedures, such as prolapse resections and stricturoplasties, have been described but are not widely practiced. Select small, superficial carcinomas may be eligible if they are less than 3 cm in size and moveable, which suggests that the tumor is confined to the rectal wall. Rectal ultrasound should be performed to verify the depth of penetration of suspected or confirmed cancers. While Stage 1 cancers are appropriate for transanal excision, the final pathology should be reviewed. If the lesion is more advanced, or if there are adverse prognostic features such as poor differentiation or lymphovascular invasion, a more extensive resection with removal of the lymphatic bed should be considered. If the ultrasound suggests a Stage 2 or higher lesion, radical resection of the rectum should be performed as the initial surgery unless there are mitigating circumstances that prevent laparotomy or laparoscopy.

Transanal endoscopic microsurgery also has been useful to remove the site of lesions previously excised with a colonoscope that are found on pathology to be a carcinoma with a close or involved margin. The site of such an excision should be tattooed as soon as the pathology reveals the need for additional surgery so that it will not heal and be lost to easy visualization.

Finally, TEM may have a palliative role in those patients in whom general anesthesia or a laparotomy is not acceptable, usually due to medical conditions or extensive cancer. The TEM will remove the primary tumor, but distant sites and nodes are not included in the specimen. Palliative resection must be carefully explained to the patient.

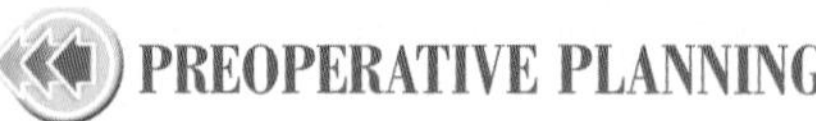

PREOPERATIVE PLANNING

During the initial preoperative evaluation, the tumor is assessed for its distance from the anal verge and its orientation in the rectum. If the lesion is in the distal half of the rectum, it can generally be palpated and mobility can be assessed. A hard site with fixation or tethering to the rectal sidewall suggests a carcinoma. In female patients, the relationship to the vagina can also be determined.

A rigid sigmoidoscopy is performed to verify the mobility of the tumor, to look for visual cues that might denote carcinoma such as ulceration, and to measure the distance from the anal verge. The apex of the tumor should be assessed to determine whether the apical margin can be visualized and controlled for excision and closure. It is not possible to do TEM when the lumen becomes narrower than the scope, when there is not a straight approach, or when the distal rectum contains a stenosis. In general, these findings will relegate the patient to an abdominal procedure.

Colonoscopy is essential to verify that there are no other colorectal tumors. If the lesion is a carcinoma, rectal ultrasound is utilized to identify the depth of penetration and lymph node status, and a computed tomography (CT) scan or a positron emission tomogram (PET) scan is performed to define possible metastases. In addition, a baseline carcinoembryonic antigen (CEA) measurement should be obtained.

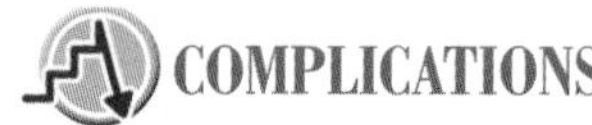

COMPLICATIONS

The patient must be informed of the potential for cure and the risks and complications of TEM. The patient must understand that a carcinoma is found, additional therapy or even a salvage surgery may be advisable. When surgery is indicated, it should be performed at least 6 weeks after full-thickness excision to allow the bowel wall to heal, but is quite successful if it is applied at that time.

The most important complications to discuss are perforation into the peritoneal cavity and, in females, perforation into the vagina. Such perforations require careful closure and may even require an ostomy, although this is rarely the case. Closure can be performed by suturing transanally but could also be done by laparoscopy or by laparotomy.

The 4-cm proctoscope rarely causes a sphincter injury. Generally the sphincter recovers in a period of a few months;

rarely it loses resting tone on a permanent basis. This is much more common in patients with a preexisting problem or with previous sphincter reconstituting surgery.

Urinary retention can be a problem for males with enlarged prostates. The operating proctoscope lying on the prostate sometimes results in some swelling and thereafter urinary retention.

Bleeding is seldom a problem in the follow-up period. Generally electrocoagulation at the time of surgery and suture closure minimizes subsequent bleeding. If bleeding does occur, it generally happens 5 to 10 days after surgery. It can usually be controlled endoscopically or by repeat TEM with suture ligation. Infection of the excision area can occur, but is usually only manifested to the patient as a low-grade fever and malaise. Broad-spectrum antibiotics treat this problem and re-intervention is seldom needed.

The follow-up must be agreed upon with the patient before undertaking TEM. If an adenoma is found, there is only a very small recurrence rate. If it is a carcinoma, early detection of a recurrence permits salvage surgery. In general, a repeat sigmoidoscopy at 3 months is recommended following TEM for any reason, with repeat colonoscopy depending on standard recommendations, which vary by indication.

A complete bowel preparation, including mechanical and antibiotics, is performed, because laparotomy may be necessary.

INSTRUMENTS

The equipment used for this technique was designed by Gerhard Buess and is produced by the Richard Wolf Company in Germany. The operating proctoscopes are 12 cm and 20 cm in length and 4 cm in diameter. The scopes may be fitted with one of two faceplates. First, there is a clear window faceplate for use in situating the scope over the tumor and locking the scope in position. Second, the operating faceplate has several ports for introduction of instruments. The system is made gastight by silastic sleeves attached to the ports and caps that fit on the ends of the sleeves. These caps are solid-faced or contain a small hole to permit introduction of the instruments.

A special arm is attached to the operating table rail and then fastens to the operating proctoscope to hold the scope in a fixed position. This arm is double-ball jointed and can be locked by the tightening of a single knob (Fig. 51-1). There is a binocular microscope with an attachment to connect it to a monitor. This microscope provides a 2.5× magnification and provides a three-dimensional image. Alternately, there is an adapter for a standard 25-degree 10-mm laparoscope that broadcasts to standard laparoscopic video screens. The operating instruments include a needle-knife cautery, forceps, scissors, needle holders, injection needle tip, and a clip applier.

The needle-knife has an angled, pointed tip for use with either cutting or coagulation currents. The tips of the forceps and the scissors are angled either right or left. There are two types of needle holders: one that is angled and another that is straight at the tip. The angled tip is often preferred because it provides a better needle sweep during closures. A needle-tipped instrument is available for the injection of a dilute epinephrine solution for hemostasis or a dye for tattooing. The clip applier is used to crimp silver clips onto sutures. This avoids the need for intracorporeal knots. The suction probe is used frequently to remove blood, liquid stool, and smoke and is typically left in situ the entire case. This suction probe is double-angled so that the assistant can keep it out of the way of the operating surgeon (Fig. 51-2, page 510).

Laparoscopic instruments may be used in special circumstances in place of some of the TEM instruments. The knife, the forceps, and a suction probe are electrified so that electrocautery can be readily used for hemostasis. A special CO_2 insufflation unit is used to control both insufflation and suction in a controlled, balanced way (Fig. 51-3, page 511).

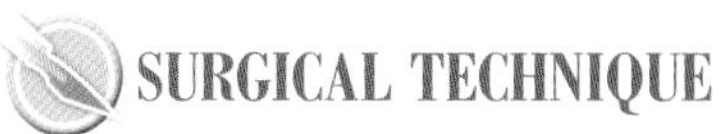

SURGICAL TECHNIQUE

The day before surgery, the patient has a mechanical and oral antibiotic preparation. Just prior to surgery, intravenous antibiotics are given. The rectum is irrigated with a solution of Betadine diluted with an equal amount of water through a urinary catheter with a 30-cc balloon. A urinary catheter is inserted into the bladder. Compression stockings are placed on the legs to aid in the prevention of deep venous thrombosis.

The patient is positioned with the center of the tumor directly down toward the tabletop. This is necessary because the scope is best fixed so that the surgeon is looking down at the tumor. Thus, the patient's position will typically be rotated depending upon the site of the tumor (Fig. 51-4, page 511). If the tumor is lateral, the patient will need be on his or her side with the legs extended onto a surgical arm board. The anus must extend off of the bottom of the table for access with the proctoscope. If the tumor is anterior, the patient is placed prone and the legs are separated and supported to gain access to the perineum. The easiest position is for the patient with a posterior tumor, in which case a standard high lithotomy position is used. The patient is then placed on a beanbag and the body and legs are taped to the table; thus the table can be

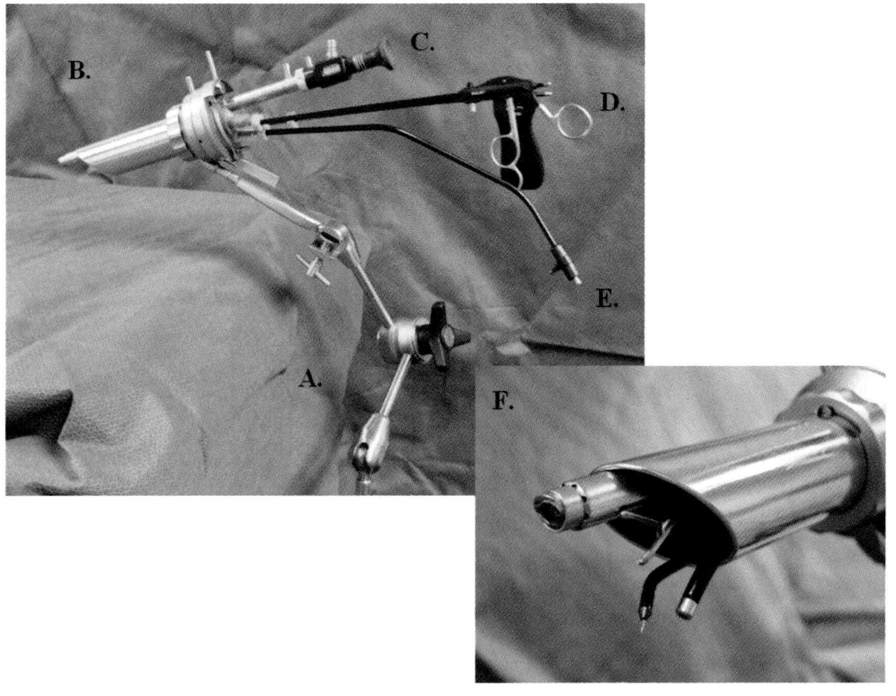

Fig. 51-1. Transanal endoscopic microsurgery unit assembled. **A.** Arm. **B.** Proctoscope. **C.** Microscope. **D.** Instruments. **E.** Suction. **F.** Closeup of proctoscope with instruments.

Diseases of the Small and Large Bowel

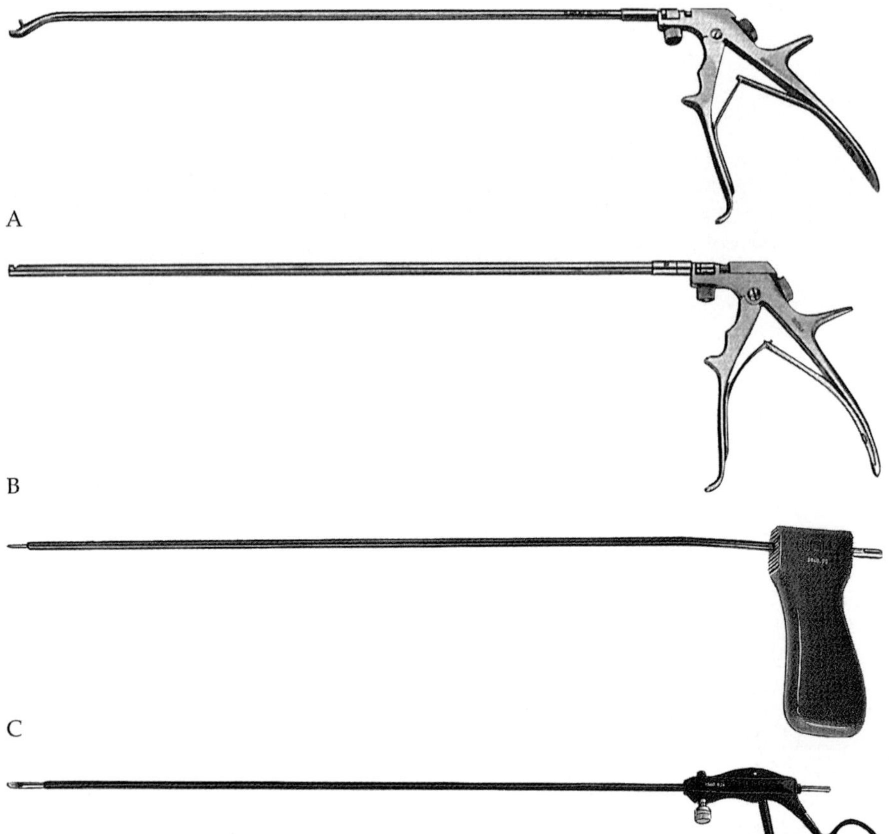

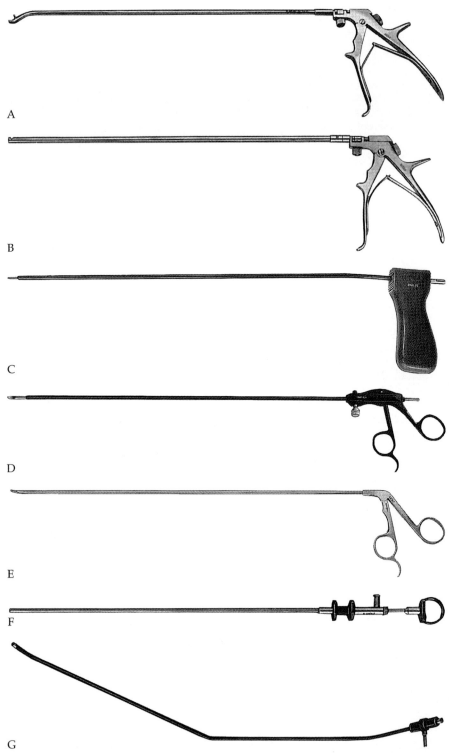

Fig. 51-2. Unique, laparoscopic-like instruments for transanal endoscopic microsurgery. **A.** Needle holder. **B.** Clip applier. **C.** Electric knife. **D.** Forceps. **E.** Scissors. **F.** Injection needle. **G.** Suction probe.

rotated to adjust the field of surgery if there is a margin that is out of the field in one direction or the other. An anal block of bupivacaine with epinephrine relaxes the sphincter and contributes to hemostasis. General anesthesia is usually employed, but regional anesthesia also can be used for small lesions.

The sphincter is gently dilated. The well-lubricated operating proctoscope with a clear window faceplate is introduced with its obturator and carefully situated over the center of the tumor. The Martin arm is used to fix the scope in place. The Martin arm is valuable because the tightening knob is released and tightened frequently, as the scope tip must be moved around the intraluminal field frequently. Generally the procedure is carried out from the right to the left of the field, whether one is marking, cutting, or sewing.

The first step in the surgical procedure is to outline the tumor with a 1-cm margin. The three-dimensional image provided by the microscope is valuable in making certain that the entire tumor is enclosed within the outline. The outline is created using the electrocautery current through the needle-knife to create eschar dots. After the outline is made, the dotted margins are cut down upon to the level desired. If the tumor is benign by all criteria, dissection down to the submucosal plane is possible, although many do a full-thickness excision for all lesions (Fig. 51-5, page 512). Suspected cancerous lesions require a full-thickness excision with an effort to remove contiguous fat for lymph node assessment. The tumor is undercut through the perirectal fat plane, again working from the right toward the left. A helpful tip is to make the left border greater than 1 cm in order to provide a tumor-free area that can be grasped more easily to better avoid manipulating the tumor. After the tumor is undercut and bleeding controlled, the specimen is removed. The specimen is subsequently pinned out on a board and placed in formalin; the flat specimen provided permits perpendicular cuts for better pathological evaluation. The wound is closed using 3-0 PDS (polydiaxanone) suture. The sutures are prepared in 6-cm lengths, with a silver clip on the tip to serve as a knot. Again, the suture line is run working from right to left. Then another silver clip is applied to the suture to hold the suture line taut (Fig. 51-6, page 512).

If the peritoneal cavity is entered, the perforation must be closed securely. Closure via intrarectal suturing techniques is usually adequate. If there is concern about the integrity of the closure, the site may be approached for closure by laparoscopy.

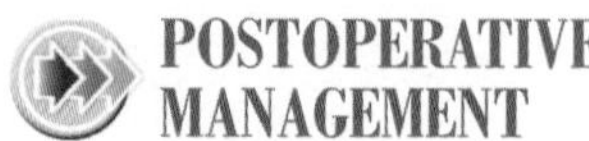

POSTOPERATIVE MANAGEMENT

Most procedures can be performed in an outpatient setting. Patients may require admission for observation if there are bleeding problems or when there is perforation into the abdominal cavity. Social considerations including geographic distance from the hospital may also warrant admission. Oral antibiotics are continued for 48 hours. Pain medicine is prescribed. Most patients have little or no pain because the rectum is not innervated with pain neurons. A regular diet can be taken the next day and the patient should be discharged with stool softeners. A return to work can be in a few days, when fatigue is overcome.

The patient is followed up at 3-month intervals for the first year. If the lesion is a carcinoma, the follow-up is extended to 6-month intervals up to 5 years. The primary follow-up is aimed at detection of local recurrence by digital examination and proctoscopy. Colonoscopy at 2- to 3-year intervals is recommended to survey for new neoplasms. If a recurrence is detected early, salvage surgery is often successful.

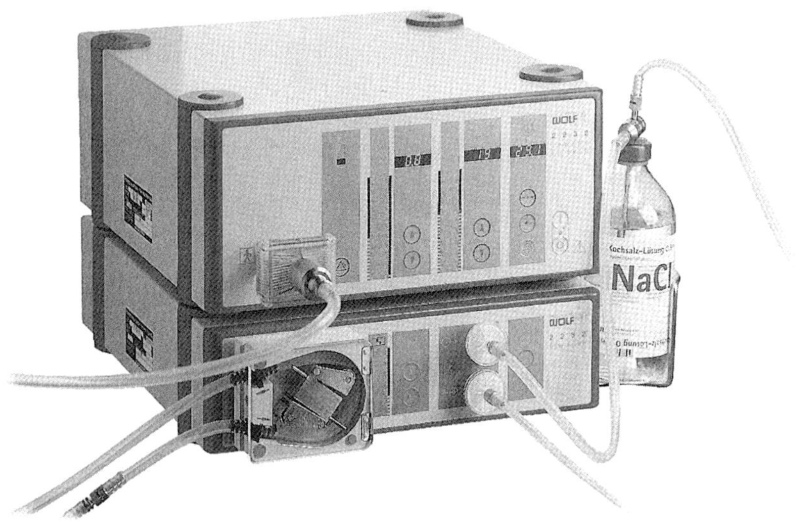

Fig. 51-3. The insufflator unit controls both CO_2 insufflation and suction.

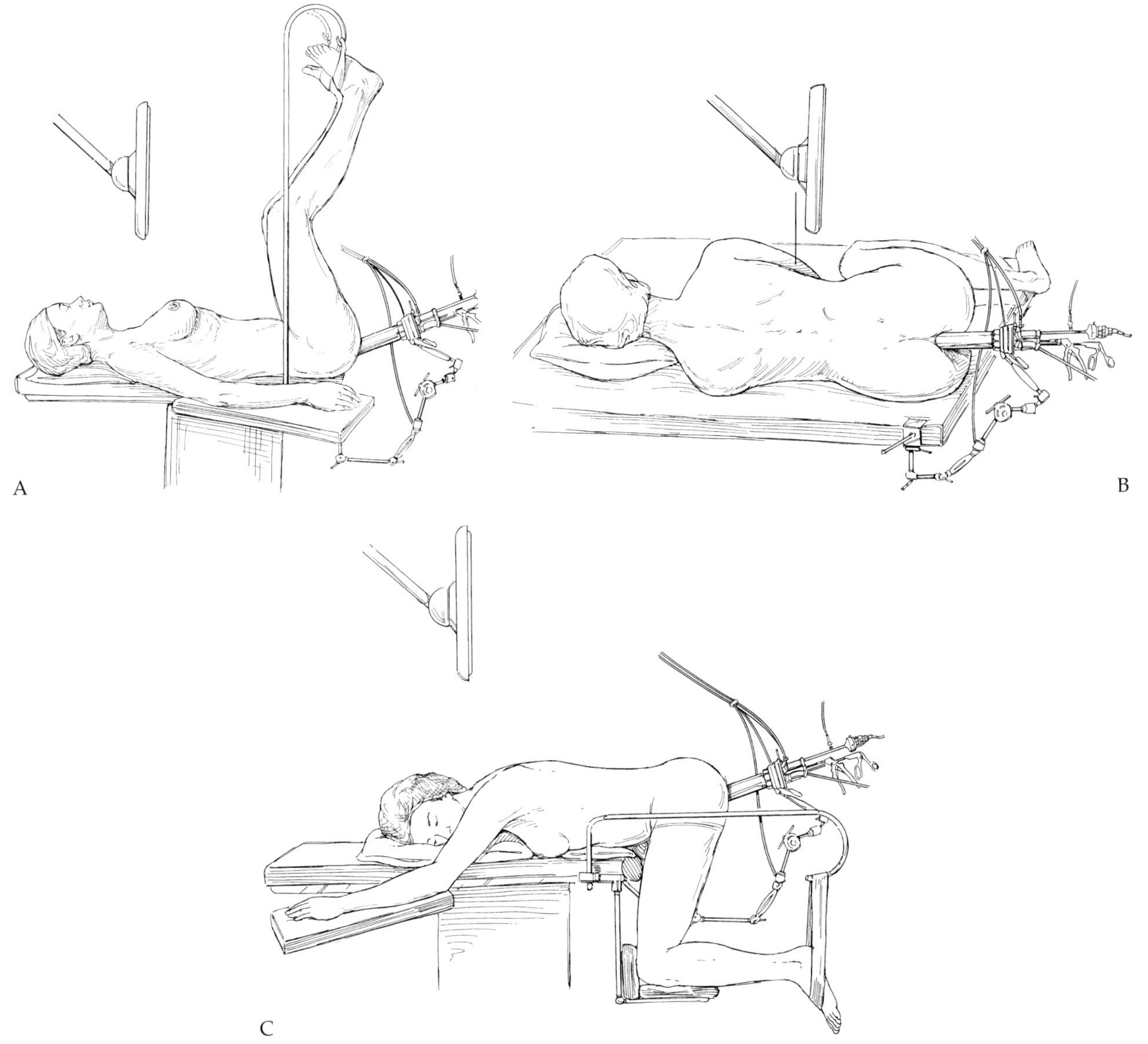

A

B

C

Fig. 51-4. Patient positioning varies depending on tumor location. **A.** The tumor is posterior. **B.** The tumor is lateral. **C.** The tumor is anterior.

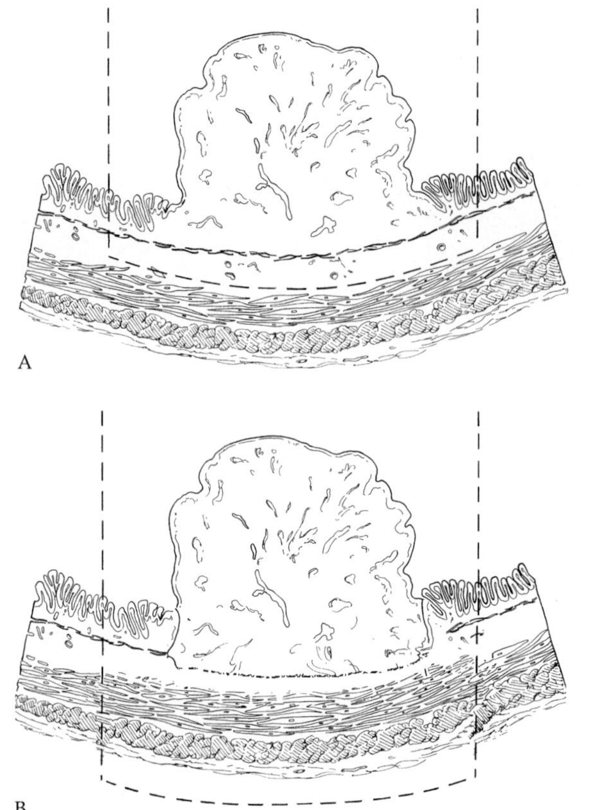

Fig. 51-5. Transanal endoscopic microsurgery allows both (A) precise submucosal resections and, more commonly, (B) full-thickness resections often including perirectal fat.

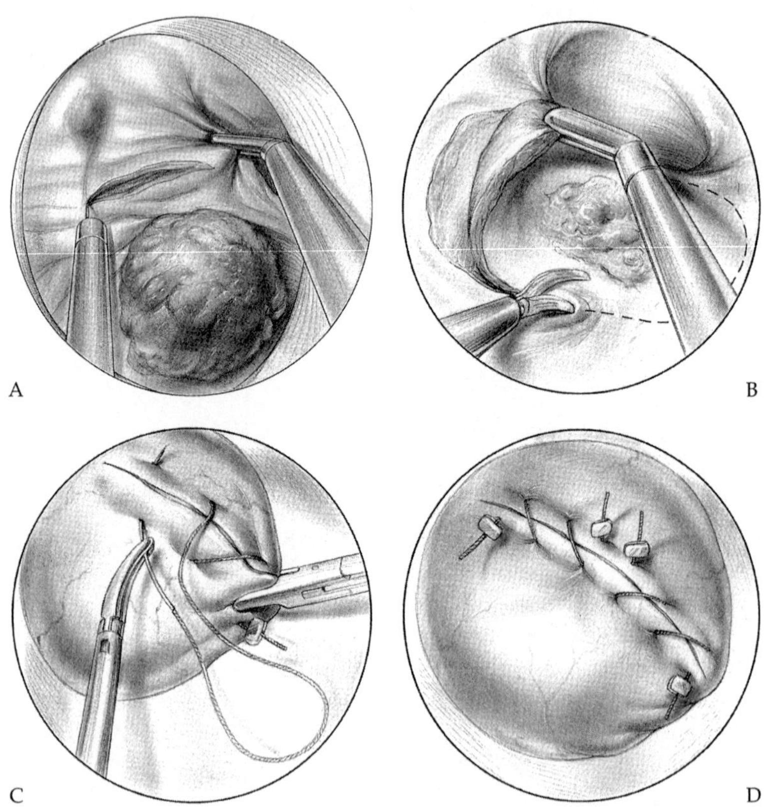

Fig. 51-6. A. Outlining the resection margin. B. Resection of the tumor. C, D. Suture closure of the defect with clips applied.

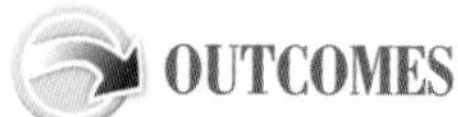

OUTCOMES

The role of TEM in the surgical treatment of rectal neoplasms continues to evolve. There is general agreement on its value for benign disease. Recurrence rates following TEM excision of adenomas are generally less than 5%, and close follow-up is advised.

The use of TEM to treat rectal cancer is more controversial. Winde et al. performed the only randomized controlled trial of TEM vs. anterior resection for Stage 1 (T1) lesions. Although the study size was small, no difference was detected out to 4 years. A recent study by Borschitz et al. stratified patients with T1 lesions who had undergone TEM resection into two groups based upon histological features. Patients with a complete resection and favorable pathology had a 6% recurrence rate, compared to 20% of patients with unfavorable histology. They concluded that complete excision of low-risk T1 lesions compares favorably with radical surgery. Another study by Stipa et al. showed an 8.6% recurrence rate for T1 lesions, but good long-term outcomes following salvage surgery. However, recent evidence suggests that the recurrence rate following local excision of favorable T1 lesions is higher than previously believed and may be as high as 29%, although this study included standard transrectal excision as well as TEM. Patients need to be advised of these concerns, and close observation is essential until the factors controlling recurrence are better understood.

Data on patients treated with adjuvant chemoradiation and TEM is limited, but appears promising. Further advances in preoperative evaluation of tumor biology and lymph node status are needed to more appropriately select patients for TEM.

Procedure for Prolapse and Hemorrhoids

The procedure for prolapse and hemorrhoids (PPH), commonly referred to as the stapled hemorrhoidectomy, uses a modified circular stapler to excise a ring of anal mucosa. This theoretically disrupts the hemorrhoidal vessels and tacks the prolapsing tissue up in the anal canal.

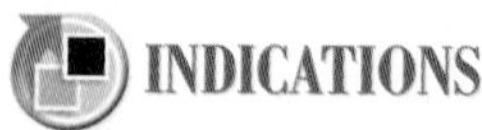

INDICATIONS

Patients with symptomatic grade II or III hemorrhoids are candidates for this procedure. Because the suture line is placed proximal to the dentate line, the procedure is felt to produce less pain and a shorter recovery than a standard hemorrhoidectomy. While it does not remove external skin tags, it may reduce their size. Alternately they can be removed separately during the same operation.

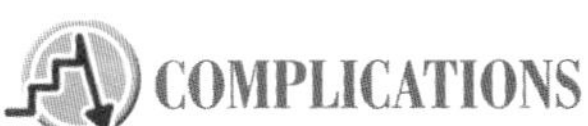

PREOPERATIVE PLANNING

A detailed history should be taken to ascertain the exact symptoms that the patient has been experiencing and ensure that they are related to hemorrhoidal disease. The initial preoperative examination involves a complete anorectal exam including anoscopy. This should be done to evaluate the hemorrhoids and to look for other perianal pathology, including rectal prolapse, fissures, condylomas, and carcinomas that may mimic the symptoms of hemorrhoids. In addition, patients with bleeding should have a screening colonoscopy.

COMPLICATIONS

Before undergoing this procedure, patients need to understand the various options for treating hemorrhoids. First-line treatment generally involves modifying bowel habits and diet to improve symptoms. This is generally done using fiber supplements, increasing water consumption, and limiting the duration of time patients spend on the toilet. For early hemorrhoidal disease, this is often all that is required. The next step in treatment involves office-based procedures designed to reduce hemorrhoidal tissue and create scarring in the anal mucosa. These include rubber band ligation, chemical sclerosis, or photodynamic therapy. Surgery is generally reserved for more severe and chronic disease.

Complications from hemorrhoid surgery include bleeding, urinary retention, infection, anal stenosis, and injury to the sphincter muscles. Infection is relatively uncommon. With close attention to proper surgical techniques, the incidence of anal stenosis and sphincter injury should be minimal.

Proper placement of the staple line during the PPH is essential. If the staples are placed too low, the patient will have immediate and significant pain. Staple lines placed too high result in a recurrence of the hemorrhoids.

Other rare complications of the PPH include pelvic sepsis, rectovaginal fistulas, fissures, and chronic pain. While the incidence of these complications appears to be low, they can be extremely debilitating for the patient and perplexing for the surgeon. Chronic anorectal pain after this procedure can be extremely difficult to treat. Anti-inflammatory suppositories, oral and topical nifedipine, and staple line removal have all been tried with varying degrees of success.

INSTRUMENTS

The PPH kit comes prepackaged with a hemorrhoidal circular stapler, a clear plastic circular anal dilator with an obturator, and a plastic anoscope. The tissue is excised using a modified 33-mm circular stapler with the anvil permanently attached. A 2-0 polypropylene suture on a 30-mm curved needle is used for the purse-string. 2-0 Vicryl sutures secure the anal dilator and contribute to hemostasis.

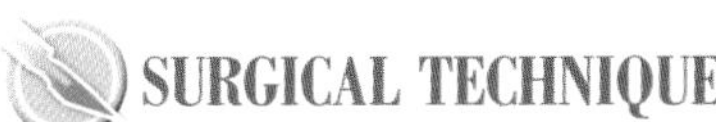

SURGICAL TECHNIQUE

Two Fleet enemas are given prior to surgery. The patient is placed in the prone jackknife or lithotomy position, depending upon surgeon preference. A mixture of 1% lidocaine mixed with 0.5% Marcaine with epinephrine is used to achieve local anesthesia and muscle relaxation. A digital rectal exam is performed to gently dilate the sphincters. The circular anal dilator with the obturator is inserted into the anal canal. The obturator is removed. The perianal skin should be slowly pushed back until the dentate line is in the middle of the clear plastic dilator. The dilator is then secured in position using two interrupted 2-0 Vicryl sutures.

The plastic anoscope is then placed through the clear plastic dilator. A 2-0 polypropylene suture is then used to place a circumferential purse-string approximately 2 to 3 cm proximal to the dentate line (Fig. 51-7). The suture should be placed in the mucosal layer only. Once this has been achieved, the anoscope is removed. With gentle tension on the purse-string suture, the circular stapling device is introduced into the anal canal. A slight pop is felt when the device is in position, with the purse-string between the two limbs of the stapler. The purse-string is tied around the stapler, and the two ends of the purse-string are brought up through two holes in the shaft of the stapling device. Again, gentle pressure is applied to the purse-strings, and the stapler is closed (Fig. 51-8). After approximately 30 seconds, the stapler is fired, and the device removed.

The staple line should be carefully examined for hemostasis (Fig. 51-9). Bleeding can generally be controlled using suture ligation and electrocautery. In female patients, a vaginal exam should be performed at each step in the procedure to ensure that the vaginal wall will not be included in the purse-string or staple line.

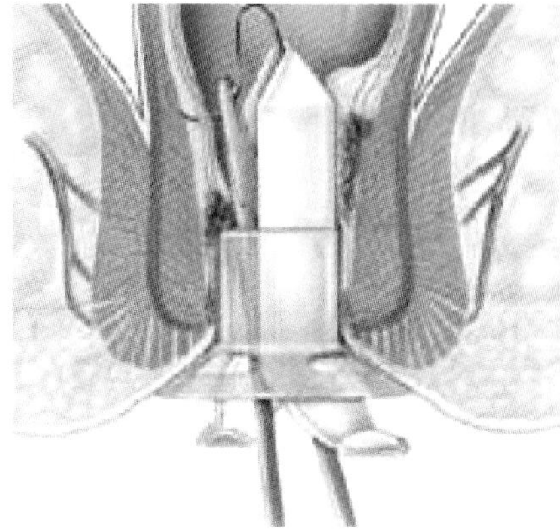

Fig. 51-7. The operating anoscope is inserted through the clear plastic dilator and a purse-string is placed 2 to 3 cm above the dentate line.

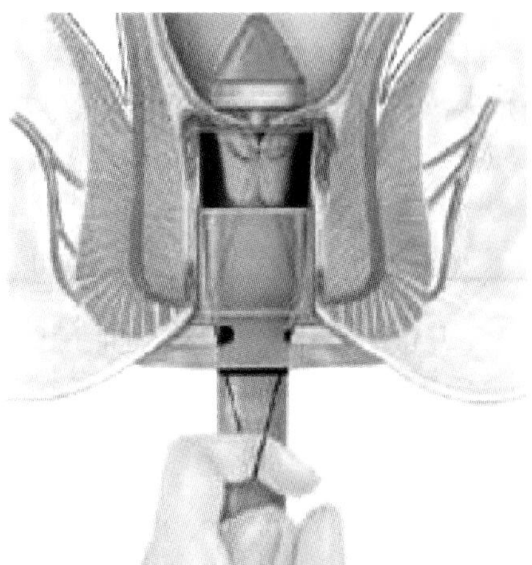

Fig. 51-8. The stapler is introduced through the dilator, and gentle retraction is held on the purse-string suture.

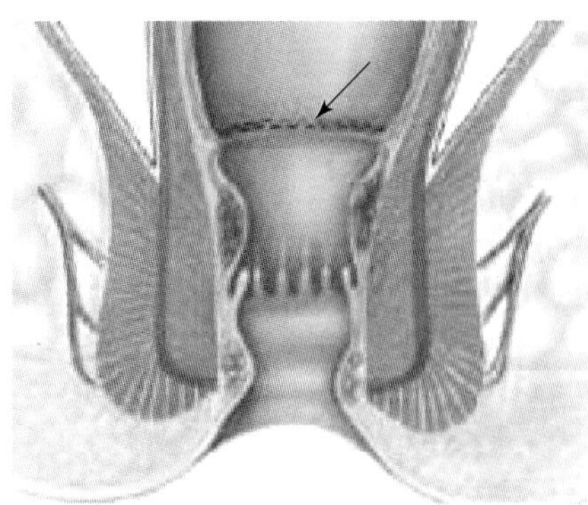

Fig. 51-9. The procedure for prolapse and hemerrhoids (PPH) works by resecting redundant mucosa, pexying the prolapsing hemorrhoids, and dividing the feeding vessels. The arrow marks the circumferential staple line.

POSTOPERATIVE MANAGEMENT

Most procedures can be performed in an outpatient setting. Admission may be required for pain control or urinary retention. However, pain can usually be controlled in the outpatient setting using oral medications. Stool softeners and warm baths are recommended.

OUTCOMES

The majority of studies confirm that PPH is safe and effective in treating patients with grade I or III hemorrhoidal disease. In a prospective, randomized multicenter trial, 134 patients were randomized to an open procedure or a stapled hemorrhoidectomy. Patients in the PPH group had a shorter recovery and less pain. At 2 years, there was no difference in the resolution of symptoms or complications.

The procedure has been compared to open hemorrhoidectomies using both the harmonic scalpel and the LigaSure device. Chung et al. conducted a study of 88 patients with grade III hemorrhoids. The patients were randomized into either an open hemorrhoidectomy using the harmonic scalpel or a PPH. Patients in the PPH group had reduced pain, shorter length of stay, and an earlier resumption of work than those in the harmonic scalpel group. In another prospective randomized trial, Kraemer et al. compared the PPH with the LigaSure device. They found no difference in postoperative pain scores, patient satisfaction, or self assessment of activity. However, a second randomized study by Basdanis et al. in patients with grade III or IV hemorrhoids found that the LigaSure device resulted in more pain but fewer bleeding complications than the stapled hemorrhoidectomy.

While the incidence of complications appears to be low, they can be quite devastating. Pelvic sepsis, rectovaginal fistulas, fissures, strictures, incontinence, and persistent perianal pain have all been reported. Although the exact numbers continue to be debated, these problems can be a difficult challenge for even the most experienced colorectal surgeons.

Hemorrhoid Artery Ligation

Hemorrhoid artery ligation utilizes a specially designed Doppler ultrasound device placed in the anal canal to identify the location of the terminal hemorrhoidal arteries. The arteries can then be suture ligated, disrupting blood flow to the hemorrhoidal tissue (Fig. 51-10). In addition, a mucopexy can be performed, lifting the hemorrhoidal tissue more proximal in the anal canal. Like the PPH, the procedure is promoted as having less pain and shorter recovery.

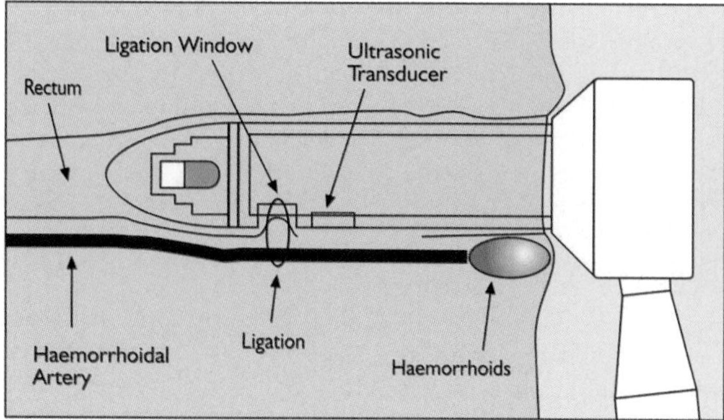

Fig. 51-10. The hemorrhoidal feeding arteries are identified using Doppler guidance and suture-ligated, disrupting blood flow to the hemorrhoidal tissue.

INDICATIONS

Hemorrhoidal artery ligation has been performed in patients with grades I through IV hemorrhoidal disease. As with any hemorrhoid operation, a detailed history should be taken to ensure the symptoms are related to hemorrhoids. The preoperative evaluation is otherwise the same as for the PPH.

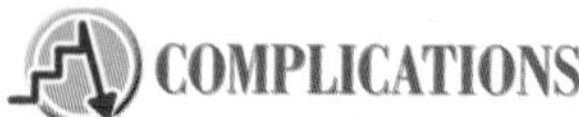

COMPLICATIONS

Theoretically, any of the complications related to hemorrhoid surgery can occur with this procedure. Based on early studies, however, the incidence of postoperative bleeding, urinary retention, persisting pain, incontinence, and fecal impaction is extremely low. A small percentage (1% to 5%) of patients develops anal fissures, thrombosed external hemorrhoids, or pain lasting more than 48 hours.

INSTRUMENTS

The Doppler probe is made of clear plastic and has a transducer buried in the side wall of the cylinder. The probe connects to the handpiece, which is attached to the Doppler ultrasound machine. A reusable sleeve is placed over the probe. Both the probe and the sleeve have a side window through which the ligation is performed. Rotating the sleeve clockwise about the probe creates a larger window through which the mucopexy can be performed. The device is illuminated. A long needle holder and knot pusher are needed to place the sutures (Fig. 51-11). Approximately four to six 2-0 Vicryl sutures are generally used during the procedure.

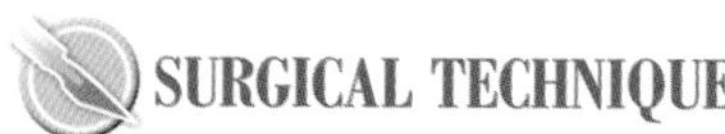

SURGICAL TECHNIQUE

Two Fleet enemas are generally given prior to the procedure. The patient may be placed in lithotomy, left lateral decubitus, or prone jackknife position, based upon the surgeon's preference. The machine is assembled by connecting the probe to the handpiece and sliding the sleeve over the transducer.

After careful anorectal examination, the device is inserted into the anal canal. The Doppler head is positioned approximately 2 cm proximal to the dentate line. The device is rotated around the anal canal to identify the hemorrhoidal arteries. Once the vessels have been identified, a 2-0 Vicryl figure-eight suture is placed through the side window proximal to the vessel. The absence of the Doppler signal distal to the sutures confirms the vessel has been appropriately ligated. The procedure is repeated around the entire circumference of the anal canal. Generally, there are six vessels identified.

Once all of the vessels have been identified and ligated, the surgeon may opt to perform a mucopexy. The sleeve is rotated about the probe. A 2-0 Vicryl suture is placed at the apex of the hemorrhoids and run distal. At the base of the internal hemorrhoids, proximal to the dentate line, the last stitch is used to pexy the hemorrhoids up in the anal canal. At the completion of the case, a careful examination is performed to ensure proper positioning of the suture and adequate hemostasis.

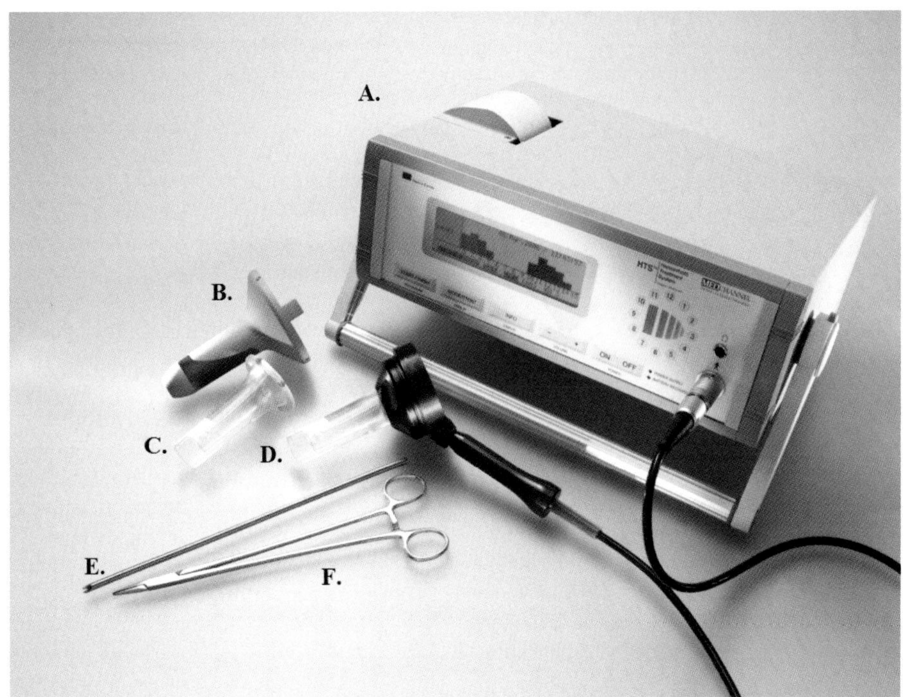

Fig. 51-11. Equipment for hemorrhoidal artery ligation. **A.** Doppler machine. **B.** Reusable probe sleeve. **C.** Doppler probe. **D.** Assembled handpiece. **E.** Knot pusher. **F.** Needle driver.

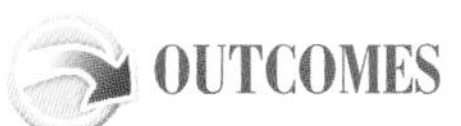

OUTCOMES

Several studies have been performed showing that this technique is safe and effective in the treatment of hemorrhoids. Bursics et al. randomized 60 patients to undergo either closed hemorrhoidectomy or hemorrhoid artery ligation. Patients undergoing hemorrhoid artery ligation needed significantly less pain medication, had a shorter hospital stay, and returned more quickly to their normal daily activity. At 1 year, the results were comparable to closed hemorrhoidectomy. A larger study of 308 patients demonstrated the procedure can be safely performed for grades II, III, and IV hemorrhoids. Complications included residual protrusion (15%), bleeding (4.8%), thrombosis (2.9%), defecation pain (1.6%), fissure (1.3%), and urinary retention (1.3%).

FUTURE DEVELOPMENTS

The role of minimally invasive techniques in the treatment of anorectal disease continues to evolve. Transanal endoscopic microsurgery will continue to benefit from advances in laparoscopic equipment and improvements in laparoscopic techniques. As the technique continues to be refined and increases in popularity, it will need to be studied more extensively to better elucidate its place in the treatment of rectal cancer.

Both PPH and Doppler hemorrhoidal artery ligation are promising techniques designed to improve patient comfort while effectively treating hemorrhoidal disease. As experience grows, the safety and efficacy of these procedures will need to be compared to rubber band ligation and surgical hemorrhoidectomy.

Two minimally invasive procedures for patients with incontinence who fail or are not eligible for more conventional therapies are being investigated: the Secca procedure and sacral nerve stimulation. The Secca procedure delivers radiofrequency energy to the anorectal junction. While the exact mechanism is not fully understood, the heat generated by this device is believed to induce tissue contraction and remodeling of the wall of the anal canal. Short-term follow-up has demonstrated an improvement in patient symptoms. While this procedure has been approved by the Food and Drug Administration (FDA), the company making the device has gone bankrupt and is no longer manufacturing the product. The use of the technique may have a resurgence if these financial issues can be resolved. The second procedure, sacral nerve stimulation, uses a small device implanted beneath the skin to send mild electrical pulses to the sacral nerves. The FDA has approved the device for patients with urinary incontinence and is currently examining its use in patients with fecal incontinence.

As with any new procedure, the long-term outcomes need to be investigated further and tested against more traditional techniques. However, advances in technology and increased patient demand will continue to drive surgeons to explore less-invasive options in the care of their patients.

SUGGESTED READING

Basdanis G, Papadopoulos VN, Michalopoulos A, et al. Randomized clinical trial of stapled hemorrhoidectomy vs. open with LigaSure for prolapsed piles. *Surg Endosc* 2005;19(2): 235–239.

Borschitz T, Heintz A, Junginger T. The influence of histopathologic criteria on the long-term prognosis of locally excised pT1 rectal carcinomas: results of local excision (transanal endoscopic microsurgery) and immediate reoperation. *Dis Colon Rectum* 2006; 49:1492–1506.

Buess G, Thiess R, Gunther M, et al. Endoscopic operative procedure for the removal of rectal polyps. *Coloproctology* 1984;6:254.

Bursics A, Morvay K, Kupcsulik P, et al. Comparison of early and 1-year follow-up results of conventional hemorrhoidectomy and hemorrhoid artery ligation: a randomized study. *Int J Colorectal Dis* 2004;19:176–180.

Chung CC, Cheung HY, Chan ES, et al. Stapled hemorrhoidopexy vs. harmonic scalpel hemorrhoidectomy: a randomized trial. *Dis Colon Rectum* 2005;48(6):1213–1219.

Kraemer M, Parulava T, Roblick M, et al. Prospective, randomized study: proximate PPH stapler vs. LigaSure for hemorrhoidal surgery. *Dis Colon Rectum* 2005;48(8):1517–1522.

Scheyer M, Antonietti E, Rollinger G, et al. Doppler-guided hemorrhoidal artery ligation. *Am J Surg* 2006;191(1):89–93.

Stipa F, Burza A, Lucandri G, et al. Outcomes for early rectal cancer managed with transanal endoscopic microsurgery: a 5-year follow-up study. *Surg Endosc* 2006;20(4):541–545.

Winde G, Nottberg H, Keller R, et al. Surgical cure for early rectal carcinomas (T1): transanal endoscopic microsurgery vs. anterior resection. *Dis Colon Rectum* 1996;39: 969–976.

COMMENTARY

Proctology often receives little attention or credit in the gastrointestinal surgery field. Painful, unpleasant, and largely considered to be a "minor" surgery, it seldom attracts much thought or attention; until, that is, you are the one who needs it. It is however, an important area of surgery and one that has undergone a pretty substantial evolution in technique over the last decade or two. While hemorrhoids may not be a life-or-death condition, they can be disabling for the patient. Until recently, hemorrhoid surgery was based on 18th-century techniques and widely considered to be almost as bad as the original condition, obviously leaving room for improvement. The two new procedures described by Drs. FitzGerlad and Smith are ingenious reworkings of the whole hemorrhoid treatment approach; rather than mass excision of the sensitive anorectal junction they depend on focal interruption of feeding vessels and minimal tissue excision. In other words, they achieve minimally invasive credentials by altering the treatment based on a rethinking of the pathologic process. The obvious benefit to the patient is less pain and a quicker recovery. These procedures have had a slow but constant adoption by surgeons. The slowness is from the commendable insistence by the equipment manufacturers that surgeons receive fairly extensive training before being allowed to use the instrumentation. This approach may be a model for adoption of other new technology dependent surgeries.

Transanal endoscopic microsurgery is a different story. A truly minimally invasive surgery, it has the intention and capability of sparing patients truly morbid interventions ranging from multiple piecemeal resections all the way to abdominal perineal resections. The capabilities of TEM are truly remarkable; full-thickness excisions of lesions as high as 24 cm, precise closure of even intraabdominal excisions, stricturoplasties, fistula repair, and sleeve resections have all been described. It is a mystery why, more than 20 years after its introduction, it still is not widely available to patients. There is no doubt that it is a technically demanding procedure, however we have found that the learning curve is fairly short for most surgeons familiar with laparoscopic techniques. It is definitely worthwhile for any major surgery centers to start a TEM program; it acts as an important adjunct to comprehensive colorectal cancer care as well as a regional draw for the program. The patient benefits for this approach, particularly for benign lesions that would otherwise require a major resection, can not be understated. Its role as a definitive cancer treatment for early malignancies is also currently receiving close scrutiny. If it becomes a proven modality for T1 and T2 cancers, it would herald a new era for rectal surgery as significant as the introduction of breast conservation surgery was to masectomy. Finally, in the new era of natural orifice transluminal endoscopic surgery (NOTES), TEM may well serve as a proven platform for the introduction of flexible endoscopes and specimen retrieval.

LLS

Abdomen and Abdominal Wall

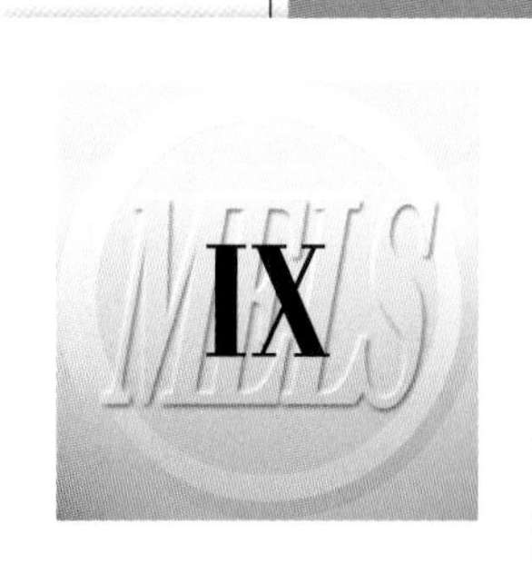

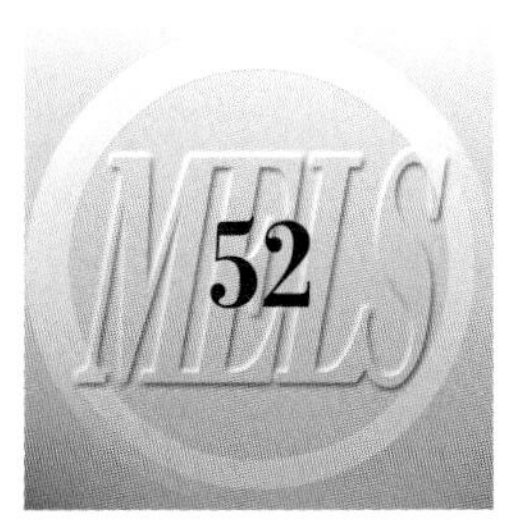

Exploratory Laparoscopy and Lysis of Adhesions

ALFRED TRANG AND BARRY SALKY

INTRODUCTION

Laparoscopic surgery has revolutionized the approach to surgical patients who present with unclear diagnosis for abdominal complaints. These patients typically complain of subacute abdominal pain or have chronic partial obstructive symptoms. In the past, surgeons would order numerous lab and imaging studies to determine the cause of a patient's symptoms when they were unsure of the diagnosis. Sometimes, these tests would fail to reveal an etiology of the symptoms, leaving doctors and patients perplexed and frustrated. Many times, these patients have seen many different specialists with no relief. The morbidity of a laparotomy for diagnostic purposes does not seem justified for a patient who does not have a clear indication for surgery. Despite the advancement in imaging modalities, there remains one superior method of ruling out abdominal surgical pathology, that is, by taking a direct look inside. Laparoscopy provides a less invasive means to directly evaluate the abdomen with minimal morbidity.

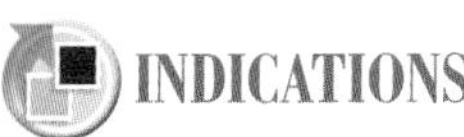

INDICATIONS

Exploratory laparoscopy can be used as a staging tool for cancer. There are times when the findings during staging laparoscopy have changed the operative plan. For example, the presence of peritoneal implants is very difficult to detect on any preoperative imaging modality. Confirming the presence of implants could spare the patient a potentially morbid resection without any benefit of increased survival and allow the surgeon to pursue a palliative approach to patient care. Laparoscopy allows the surgeon to detect occult pathology such as metastatic implants with minimal morbidity. In addition, node sampling can also be performed, which could lead to optimal timing of surgery after neoadjuvant chemotherapy has been administered, thus changing the multimodality treatment of the patient.

There is also an increasing role for exploratory laparoscopy in the bariatric surgery population. Patients who have undergone gastric bypass surgery may develop internal hernias that cause intermittent bowel obstructions after they have lost a considerable amount of weight. These patients rarely develop a complete obstruction but experience episodes of crampy abdominal pain and partial obstruction, likely due to small bowel loops intermittently sliding in and out of these hernia defects. Exploratory laparoscopy allows the surgeon to diagnose and close the mesenteric defects that lead to these types of hernias.

One of the most frustrating clinical scenarios for surgeons is the patient who presents with chronic abdominal pain. Often, these patients have had prior abdominal surgeries and have been told that their symptoms may be due to adhesions. Performing a laparotomy to remove scar tissue seems counterintuitive, because the surgery will lead to more scar tissue. Laparoscopy provides a method of diagnosing whether or not adhesions may be the cause of the patient's symptoms. Up to 5% of diagnostic laparoscopies detect pathology other than adhesions as the cause of chronic pain. Occult hernias and abnormal appendices have been reported.

When adhesions are suspected as the etiology of pain, adhesiolysis can be performed with little trauma to the tissues, minimizing further adhesion formation. There is debate in the literature over the true benefit of adhesiolysis for chronic abdominal pain versus the placebo effect of a diagnostic laparoscopy. The majority of reported studies are biased and retrospective. Regardless, the majority of patients report relief of their symptoms and an improved quality of life.

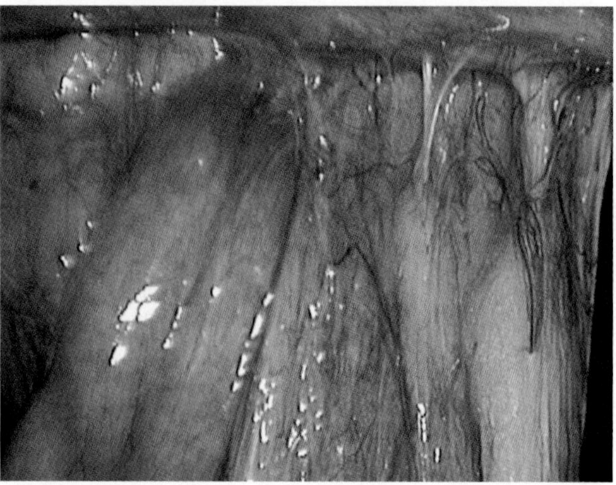

Fig. 52-1. Dense adhesion and bowel stuck to the anterior abdominal wall.

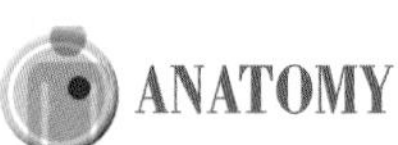

ANATOMY

Postoperative adhesions are caused by trauma, ischemia, infection, and foreign bodies. Initially, fibrin-rich exudate forms in response to intraabdominal injury. Normally these early adhesions are lysed by fibrinolytic activity of plasminogen activation. However, in the presence of traumatized peritoneal surfaces, there is a decrease in plasminogen activation. Trauma to the peritoneal surfaces, ischemia to the tissues, and the presence of foreign bodies all decrease the impact of plasminogen activity. The fibrinous adhesions persist and become organized by neovascularization and fibroblast infiltration to form a fibrous adhesion. Different types of adhesions may form: fine-filmy, dense vascularized, or thick cohesive. Unfortunately, it is impossible to predict which adhesions will eventually lead to clinical symptoms in the future.

Adhesions may also develop without surgery. Inflammatory processes such as infiltrating carcinoma, pelvic inflammatory disease, cholecystitis, and diverticulitis can lead to adhesion formation although the exact incidence is unknown as the majority of them do not cause symptoms. Patients who have been treated with pelvic radiation for malignancy are also susceptible to scar formation.

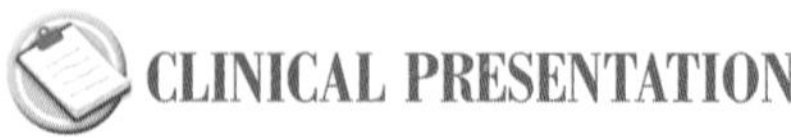

CLINICAL PRESENTATION

Bowel obstruction secondary to adhesions accounts for 12% to 17% of hospital admissions following abdominal operations. These adhesions cause a kink or twist in the bowel, leading to obstruction (Fig. 52-1). Patients may present with partial or complete bowel obstructions. Those who do not show signs of bowel ischemia or sepsis may be managed nonoperatively with nasogastric decompression and fluid resuscitation. Eventually 2% to 5% of patients fail to resolve, requiring exploration and adhesiolysis; up to one-third of them will require another operation later in life due to adhesion-related complications.

Midgut and hindgut operations are responsible for the majority of adhesion-associated bowel obstructions, followed by gynecologic operations and foregut procedures. This preponderance of lower abdominal procedures causing small bowel obstruction is presumed to be due to the bowel being more mobile in the pelvis and tethered in the upper abdomen.

Although difficult to diagnose preoperatively, pain secondary to adhesions has been described in the literature. This pain is described as chronic in nature and difficult to associate with an activity or pathologic process. These patients with chronic abdominal pain will have seen many specialists and have undergone numerous tests yet have an undetermined etiology. Many times, the surgeon is unsure whether or not adhesiolysis will resolve the patient's symptoms. It is only after the operation and the patient's pain is resolved that it can be assumed that the pain was due to adhesions. Unfortunately, it is impossible to predict which patients will have a favorable outcome.

Laparotomy vs. Laparoscopy

As technology improves and techniques are refined, the standard of care is being modified. Although laparotomy and adhesiolysis remains the standard of care for treatment of small bowel obstruction due to scar tissue, an increasing number are being treated laparoscopically. There are many reasons for this evolution. The incidence of ventral hernia ranges between 11% and 20% after laparotomy incisions and increases with each subsequent incision. This compares unfavorably with the 0.02% to 2.4% incidence of port site hernias. The other inherent benefits of laparoscopy, namely decreased wound infection rates, postoperative ileus, and postoperative pain and a shorter length of hospital stay, make the laparoscopic approach very beneficial. Up to one-third of patients may require repeat laparotomy for recurrent small bowel obstruction from intraabdominal adhesions. With each operation, more scar tissue is formed, increasing the likelihood of further complications. Laparoscopy has been shown to cause less adhesion formation when compared to open surgery. The long-term clinical outcome of this finding has yet to be determined.

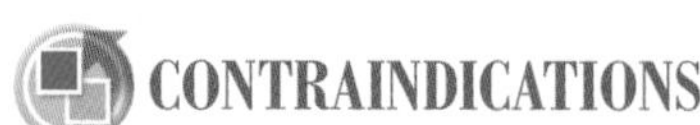

CONTRAINDICATIONS

With all the benefits of laparoscopic adhesiolysis, why should laparotomy still be performed? Unfortunately, there are surgeon, patient, and technical limitations to laparoscopic adhesiolysis. Contraindications include: (1) massive abdominal distension that precludes visualization and establishment of a working space; (2) the presence of peritonitis with the need for bowel resection and handling in a highly inflamed environment; (3) hemodynamic instability; (4) severe comorbid heart and lung disease that preclude the use of pneumoperitoneum; and finally (5) the surgeon's comfort level with the procedure. Many surgeons are not adequately trained to handle a dilated bowel with laparoscopic instruments. Others feel that the risk of enterotomy outweighs the benefits of laparoscopy. Predictors of successful outcomes after laparoscopic adhesiolysis have been reported to include surgeon training in advanced laparoscopic techniques, the degree of bowel dilation, and whether or not the obstruction was partial or complete.

PREOPERATIVE PLANNING

Patients who present with bowel obstruction requiring surgical intervention must be evaluated on an individual basis to determine if laparoscopy should be attempted. A thorough history and physical exam will provide valuable information as to whether a laparoscopic exploration can be safely performed. Patients who are completely obstructed and have a history of multiple prior open abdominal operations may be better served with an exploratory laparotomy. Laparoscopy requires enough space in the peritoneal cavity after insufflation to visualize and manipulate bowel. Proximal obstructions tend to have a lesser degree of dilated intestine compared to distal obstructions. This is also the case when comparing partial versus complete obstructions. Extremely dilated intestines may prevent adequate laparoscopic visualization.

There are times when a computed tomography (CT) scan of the abdomen and pelvis may aid in the decision on whether or not to attempt laparoscopic adhesiolysis. The CT scan could delineate a transition point in the bowel suggestive of the point of obstruction. This type of obstruction can be more amenable to a laparoscopic approach. In addition, the degree of dilation and thickness of the bowel on imaging could provide an impression of anticipated problems with handling the bowel with laparoscopic instruments and preventing serosal tears or enterotomies. In patients who have had prior surgeries, a CT scan might also guide the surgeon to the optimal location for obtaining access to the peritoneal cavity. Loops of intestine adherent to a particular area of the abdominal wall, which would be wise to avoid on initial approach, can be seen on CT scan.

Access to the Abdominal Cavity

There is considerable debate over the "open" versus "closed" technique for access to the abdominal cavity. Hasson described the original "open" technique in 1971 and has recently reported his 29-year experience: only 1 of 5284 patients (0.02%) who underwent open laparoscopic access experienced an inadvertent injury to the small bowel, which was repaired without adverse outcome. There were no major vascular injuries or mortalities in his series. Other retrospective reviews indicate that the risk of visceral and vascular injury was decreased by the open technique. General opinion is that the open approach is safer because of the decreased incidence of major vascular injuries but that it does not always prevent all visceral injuries. As a result of this ongoing debate, different access trocars have been developed for safer and more efficient access to the peritoneal cavity.

The classical open technique uses a Hasson trocar, a blunt-nose trocar that is held to the fascia with anchoring sutures. Several optical-access trocars on the market allow for direct visualization of the layers of the abdominal wall during placement. The tips of the trocars have clear ends through which a 0-degree laparoscope is placed. The surgeon is then able to watch as the trocar traverses the visible tissue planes. Although advertised as safer, optical-access trocars have been implicated in several serious complications according to the Food and Drug Administration's Medical Device Reporting Program and the Manufacturer and User Facility Device Experience (MAUDE) databases. These have included major vascular injuries, bowel perforations, liver lacerations, significant bleeding from port sites, and even patient deaths.

Certain clinical scenarios make access to the abdominal cavity even more difficult. Patients with multiple prior abdominal surgeries are more likely to have adhesions and bowel adherent to their anterior abdominal wall. Also, a virgin abdomen does not guarantee the absence of adhesions. Patients may have spontaneous adhesions from bouts of infection (diverticulitis, chronic cholecystitis, and pelvic inflammatory disease), inflammation (Crohn disease or ulcerative colitis) or from radiation to the abdomen.

It is recommended that the initial access site be made away from any previous scars to avoid underlying adhesions. Reviewing old operative reports can provide clues as to which part of the abdomen to avoid. In addition, as mentioned before, a CT scan may show areas of dense bowel loops that would be preferably avoided.

Once the initial trocar is placed, one must decide the number, size, and position of the other trocars needed to perform an adequate lysis of adhesions. This will depend on the anatomy inside the peritoneal cavity and the amount of adhesions. Many times, some adhesiolysis must be performed before other trocars can be placed. Initial trocars should be placed as laterally as possible. This aids in adhesiolysis of bowel that may be stuck to the anterior abdominal wall. If the trocar is placed too far medially, the proper angle to lyse scar adherent to a midline incision is difficult to attain. The ports should also be placed so that the small bowel may be run from ligament of Treitz to ileocecal valve and vice versa.

Choice of Instruments

Tactile feedback is diminished in laparoscopic surgery. A three-dimensional image is shown on a two-dimensional screen, limiting the depth of perception. Therefore, it is important to use a 30- or 45-degree laparoscope when performing adhesiolysis (Fig. 52-2, page 520). The angled scope enables the surgeon to look around corners to make sure there are no bowel loops stuck behind a dense adhesion before cutting it. It is also useful for looking up into abdominal wall hernias with incarcerated bowel.

Complications can occur with the improper selection of instruments. Atraumatic graspers should be used at all times when handling intestine. Even graspers that are advertised as atraumatic may cause injury to small bowel, especially in the setting of a dilated or inflamed bowel. Laparoscopic scissors should be kept sharpened with rounded tips to allow for gentle dissection without the worry of causing inadvertent injuries or enterotomies (Fig. 52-3, page 520). If the choice to use electrically energized instruments is made, the shafts should be isolated to prevent unwanted conduction of current to adjacent structures. Electrocautery can be attached to scissors or ultrasonic dissection can be used to lyse dense adhesions or those that might bleed (Fig. 52-4, page 520).

SURGICAL TECHNIQUE

The same general principles that guide safe exploratory laparotomy and adhesiolysis should be applied to the laparoscopic approach. This starts with proper visualization of all the structures within the abdominal cavity, paying attention to areas of distorted anatomy. During open

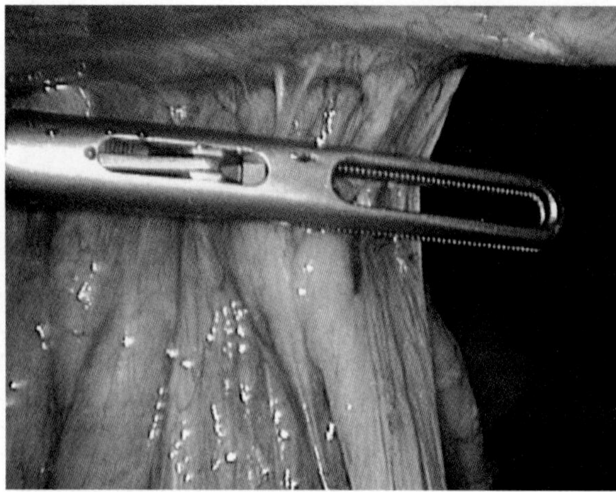

Fig. 52-2. Using the 30-degree laparoscope and blunt retraction to look around a corner.

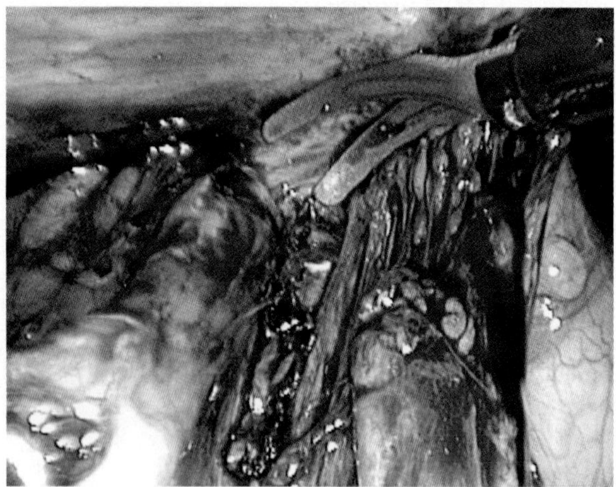

Fig. 52-3. Sharp adhesiolysis with round-tip scissors.

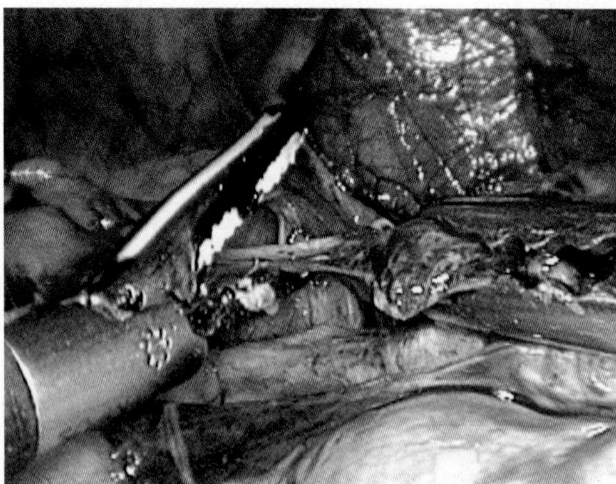

Fig. 52-4. The ultrasonic division of dense adhesive band, making sure there is no adjacent bowel affected.

adhesiolysis, surgeons have the ability to rub tissue between their fingers to either break up an adhesion or to determine if it can be divided sharply. This tactile advantage is lacking in laparoscopy. Therefore, we must more diligently apply the other principles of safe surgery: traction and countertraction as well as looking at the structures from many different views to fully define the anatomy.

Initially, adhesions to the anterior abdominal wall are divided. This should be attempted through the most lateral ports in order to gain the proper angle. On occasion, the laparoscopic instrument will not reach an adhesion due to patient body habitus or the presence of a large ventral hernia. Gentle firm pressure may be applied from outside the abdominal wall in the posterior direction. This will bring the target area closer to the instruments. Often gravity is sufficient to provide adequate traction in order to lyse adhesions from the anterior abdominal wall. One main rule always applies: if you can see through it, you can cut it. The difficulty occurs when dense scar tissue either resembles bowel or masks a segment of bowel that is lying directly behind it. Whether by changing the camera angle or by moving the tissue itself, it is important to visualize the scar from all angles. If nothing of significance is there, one feels much more at ease cutting the scar. If there is a piece of bowel directly behind, more care should be taken.

Laparoscopic adhesiolysis can be performed safely as long as dissection is maintained in the proper avascular planes. This reduces any bleeding that could diminish visualization as well as distort tissue planes. Occasionally, despite meticulous dissection and firm but gentle traction, the anatomy will remain unclear. The scar may be too dense or resemble bowel. In this case, there are certain maneuvers that may be attempted.

Changing the working perspective can sometimes reveal new tissue planes. If taking down adhesions from the left side becomes too difficult, try approaching it from the right side. If this does not work, switch to a different area altogether and work for a while before coming back at a later time. It is amazing how new tissue planes appear when you take a second look. On the rare occasion that the anatomy is still distorted, stick to certain principles: It is better to remove a piece of peritoneal lining that is stuck to the bowel than to injure the bowel itself. Some surgeons feel that no electrical cautery or ultrasonic device should be used in this situation. Sharp dissection with scissors is wise as the risk for bowel injury with electrical cautery or ultrasonic device is great.

Lastly, how much adhesiolysis is enough? The answer depends on the clinical scenario. If laparoscopy is performed for obstructive symptoms, then adhesiolysis should be performed until the point of obstruction is determined and corrected. This can include taking down all of the scar tissue from the anterior abdominal wall in order to fully inspect the small bowel. Once the point of obstruction is fixed, the bowel should be "run" from the ligament of Treitz to the ileocecal valve to ensure no other areas of obstruction remain. This also provides an opportunity to inspect the bowel for potential sites of inadvertent injury. Interloop adhesions generally do not cause obstruction and should be left alone.

Laparoscopic adhesiolysis for chronic pain symptoms presents a more challenging situation. Some clinicians refute the utility of this indication for adhesiolysis, citing the placebo effect of a diagnostic laparoscopy. It would be reasonable to limit adhesiolysis to areas of reported pain as the data is inconclusive on this matter.

One potential method of trying to determine which adhesion is causing pain is to perform the procedure under local anesthesia with anesthesia on standby. By pulling on adhesions with the patient awake, it is possible to localize the adhesion causing the pain. The insufflation gas should be changed to nitrous oxide instead of carbon dioxide, as the latter forms carbonic acid with the fluid in the abdomen. This can be irritative to the peritoneum under local anesthesia.

Despite advancements with the laparoscopic approach, it should be emphasized that, as with all laparoscopic procedures, the surgeon should not be hesitant to convert to an open procedure should the situation warrant. As more surgeons attempt this approach, the success of laparoscopic adhesiolysis has been reported in several cases and multiple series (Table 52-1). Although the long-term data are still accumulating, the success rate has been reported between 46% and 87%, with a conversion rate ranging between 6.7% and 43%. The incidence of intraoperative enterotomy ranged from 3% to 17.6%.

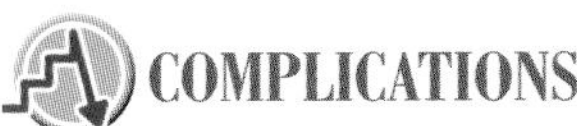

COMPLICATIONS

Complications can occur with any surgical procedure. Unfortunately, they are further magnified when they occur during a new, more advanced procedure compared to the standard of care. As mentioned previously, injuries can occur as access is being gained to the abdominal cavity. Even the Hasson approach does not prevent such injuries all the time. It is prudent to look around the abdomen through the laparoscope to assess potential initial injury, especially the area directly under the initial incision, before putting in any more trocars.

Bleeding complications can occur either at the port site or in the abdomen. Some adhesions are well vascularized and will bleed if cut or torn. Meticulous hemostasis should be attained with ultrasonic device or electrocautery. Adhesions that are stuck to the liver or spleen can tear the capsule with excessive traction and cause significant bleeding. Bleeding can usually be stopped with gentle pressure or other hemostatic agents. If bleeding is profuse, conversion to an open procedure may be warranted.

The most feared complication after adhesiolysis, whether the procedure is done open or laparoscopic, is a missed bowel injury. These patients present a few days later usually in septic shock with high mortality. Ideally, there would be no bowel injuries, but if they do occur, the next best thing would be to recognize and repair them at the time of injury. Tears and perforations can occur by direct or indirect means. Direct injuries occur when sharp instruments inadvertently cut or penetrate tissue. They can also occur with electric burn or heat from the ultrasonic dissector. This type of injury is more likely to manifest in the delayed septic patient. Indirect injures can result from improper selection or use of instruments, causing disproportionate tension on tissues. Dilated or inflamed bowel is especially prone to this type of injury. The tenuous bowel wall easily tears when excessive shearing forces are applied. Indirect injuries can also occur when improperly insulated energy devices lead to stray energy burns. These injuries occur outside of the visual field and only present days later.

Certain practice guidelines should be followed to decrease the likelihood of missed injuries. The entire bowel should be carefully examined at the end of the procedure. Any injury that occurs during adhesiolysis should be repaired promptly to minimize the degree of contamination. The decision to repair primarily versus resection should be clinically based on the mechanism and degree of injury. Electrical cautery and ultrasonic injuries tend to extend beyond the visible blanched area and

TABLE 52-1. RESULTS OF LAPAROSCOPIC ADHESIOLYSIS AS REPORTED IN SEVERAL SERIES

Series/year	N	Operative time (min)	Conversion (%)	Bowel injury (%)	Length of stay (days)	Follow-up (months)	Reoperation (%)	Mortality (%)
Pekmezci et al., 2002	15	99	6.7	6.7	4	17.2	0	0
Levard et al., 2001	308	NR	40.9	8.4	4	1.6	4.5	2.2
Sato et al., 2001	17	105	17.6	17.6	10.4	61.7	5.8	0
Suter et al., 2000	83	NR	43	15.6	5.9	NR	9	2.4
Al-Mulhim et al., 2002	19	58	32	NR	5	27	0	0
Chosidow et al., 2000	134	71.7	16	3	5.03	NR	NR	0
Strickland et al., 1999	40	68	32.5	10	3.6	22	5	0
Leon et al., 1998	40	108	35	7.5	2.9	12	17.5	0
Bailey et al., 1998	65	64	21.5	NR	3	NR	10.8	1.8
Navez et al., 1998	69	77	40	9	6.6	46	2.9	2.9
Ibrahim et al., 1996	33	NR	15	9.1	NR	NR	3	3
Overall (range)		58–208	6.7–43	3–17.6	2.9–18	1.6–61.7	0–17.5	0–3

NR, not recorded.

will more likely require resection. Depending on surgeon experience and comfort level, this can be attempted laparoscopically or done as an open procedure.

Enterotomies that occur during laparoscopic adhesiolysis are often treated differently based on the amount of spillage and contamination. An enterotomy on a decompressed and relatively healthy bowel segment usually can be controlled and repaired laparoscopically, as the amount of spillage is minimal. This approach might not be optimal for a dilated bowel segment enterotomy, which results in a much greater amount of enteric content spillage. Whenever the amount of spillage that occurs before the surgeon gains control of the hole, the enterotomy should be held closed with a grasper while the procedure is converted to open. The repair can then be performed and the abdomen adequately irrigated of all the enteric spillage. Otherwise, the patient is susceptible to severe chemical peritonitis and eventual sepsis.

CONCLUSIONS

Exploratory laparoscopy has provided surgeons with another tool to diagnose and treat patients. Findings on diagnostic laparoscopy can alter treatment plans and improve the quality of patient care. Common surgical problems such as small bowel obstructions and intractable abdominal pain due to adhesions can thus be treated with minimal morbidity.

Intraadbominal adhesions are often associated with significant morbidity and mortality. Laparoscopic adhesiolysis can be safely performed by well-trained laparoscopic surgeons. As more procedures are being performed, the data suggest that the properly selected patient would benefit greatly from this approach compared to the standard laparotomy. The advanced laparoscopic surgeon should learn proper technique and sound principles so that they may be applied to adhesions encountered during all types of laparoscopic procedures.

SUGGESTED READING

Amaral JF, Chrostek, C. Depth of thermal injury: ultrasonically activated scalpel versus electrosurgery. *Surg Endosc* 1995;9:226.

Bemelman WA, et al. Efficacy of establishment of pneumoperitoneum with the Veress needle, Hasson trocar, and modified blunt nose trocar: a randomized study. *J Laparosc Adv Surg Tech* 2000;10:325–330.

Bhoyrul S, Vierra MA, Nezhat CR, et al. Trocar injuries in laparoscopic surgery. *J Am Coll Surg* 2001;192:677–683.

Catarci M, Carlini M, Gentileschi P, et al. Major and minor injuries during the creation of pneumoperitoneum. A mutlicenter study on 12,919 cases. *Surg Endosc* 2001;15: 566–569.

Fevang BS, Fevang J, Lie SA, et al. Long-term prognosis after operation for adhesive small bowel obstruction. *Ann Surg* 2004;240: 193–201.

Miller G, Boman J, Shrier I, et al. Natural history of patients with adhesive small bowel obstruction. *Brit J Surg* 2000;87: 1240–1247.

Salky BA, Edye MB. The role of laparoscopy in the diagnosis and treatment of abdominal pain syndromes. *Surg Endosc* 1998;12: 911–914.

Salky BA. Diagnostic laparoscopy. *Surg Laparosc Endosc* 1993; vol. 3, No. 2:132–134.

Swank DJ, Swank-Bordewijk SC, Hop WC, et al. Laparoscopic adhesiolysis in patients with chronic abdominal pain. *Curr Opin Obstet Gynecol* 2004;16:313–318.

Szomstein S, Lo Menzo E. Laparoscopic lysis of adhesions. *World J Surg* 2006;30:535–540.

COMMENTARY

Exploratory laparoscopy can be considered to be the most basic of laparoscopic operations. In its simplest form, a single port and scope are all that are required to examine the peritoneal cavity. Often the surgeon opts to add other trocars and instruments in order to facilitate exposure and manipulation of intraperitoneal organs. Despite the relatively basic nature of exploratory laparoscopy, injuries and complications can occur. Gaining safe access to the peritoneal cavity is essential in all laparoscopic procedures. Additionally, the physiologic responses to pneumoperitoneum can range from the unnoticeable to cardiovascular collapse and sudden death.

Laparoscopic lysis of adhesions is commonly performed as a part of many operations. This procedure can range from simply cutting or sweeping aside a few bands of tissue to hours of tedious and dangerous dissection. The authors point out the dangers associated with the use of cautery and other energy sources during lysis of adhesions. A balanced representation of this debate must include the view that the use of energy sources during adhesiolysis can allow the surgeon to maintain excellent hemostasis and subsequently better visualization, which can in turn enhance one's ability to avoid injuries. Blunt sweeping of adhesions can effectively clear an area but often leaves raw surfaces that can continue oozing after the surgeon moves to dissect another area. When many raw surfaces are exposed and oozing persists, it can be difficult to maintain adequate visualization to make safe progress.

Bowel obstruction was at one time considered to be an absolute contraindication to laparoscopy. The thoughts related to this topic evolved through a phase where it was considered to be a relative contraindication to where bowel obstruction is now considered to be a good indication for a laparoscopic approach in selected patients. Surgeons must be mindful that there is a higher risk of bowel injury and perforation in this setting and that the size of the working space can be compromised by dilated loops of bowel. Gentle manipulation of dilated bowel and the use of atraumatic instrumentation are strongly encouraged in this situation.

WSE

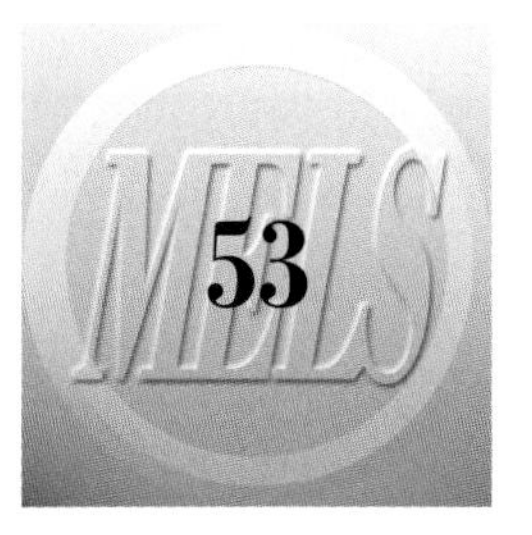

Laparoscopic Inguinal Hernia Repair

EDWARD L. FELIX

INTRODUCTION

Inguinal hernioplasty has undergone a gradual evolution over the last 100 years. In the beginning, surgeons like Edoardo Bassini, William Halsted, and Chester McVay championed new understandings of hernia anatomy and fresh approaches to dissection and repair of the inguinal floor. In the 1970s surgeons began to incorporate prosthetic materials into their repairs to eliminate tension and to decrease recurrence. Later Nyhus, Stoppa, and Wantz further changed the direction of inguinal hernioplasty by applying prostheses to the posterior wall of the groin. The evolution reached its current level in 1990 shortly after the introduction of laparoscopic cholecystectomy, when the laparoscopic approach to inguinal hernia repair was introduced.

The introduction of video laparoscopy and the development of new laparoscopic instruments and skills offered the potential to take the posterior approach to inguinal hernioplasty one step further and make it less invasive and disruptive to patients. Early laparoscopic surgeons tried to replicate established posterior techniques rather than attempt to satisfy the concepts that had originally made these approaches so successful. Because these surgeons failed to adequately dissect and repair the entire floor of the groin, recurrence rates of the early laparoscopic repairs were quite high. Once it was accepted that any laparoscopic repair had to mimic the established gold standard of open posterior mesh repair, recurrence rates decreased to less than 2% in most series.

Initially, most laparoscopic surgeons used a transabdominal preperitoneal (TAPP) approach to access the posterior floor of the groin. Surgeons were familiar with intraperitoneal laparoscopy, and the anatomy of the groin viewed via this approach was relatively intuitive and easy to learn (Fig. 53-1). Some early investigators failed to understand the need for placing the prosthetic material in the preperitoneal space, outside the peritoneal cavity. They utilized an intraperitoneal "on-lay" technique (IPOM), which resulted in the mesh being in direct contact with intraperitoneal contents and, in many cases, the staples used to fasten the mesh blindly placed into the pelvic floor. This approach, however, was abandoned for the most part because of high recurrence and complication rates. The TAPP approach soon became the standard for laparoscopic hernia repair and many studies were published demonstrating recurrence rates of less than 1%. When complications such as internal hernias from inadequate closure of the peritoneum and injury to viscera from trocars and needles placed in the peritoneal cavity were reported, a totally extraperitoneal approach (TEP) was developed and subsequently adopted by many laparoscopic surgeons. This approach required the surgeon to laparoscopically expose the extraperitoneal space without entering the peritoneal cavity. Although the TAPP approach had a history of success, the TEP approach potentially offered several advantages and slowly gained popularity. The approach had the potential to eliminate complications related to violating the peritoneal cavity and to reduce operative times, especially for bilateral hernia repairs.

Initially, the dissection of the extraperitoneal space in the TEP approach tended to be difficult, confusing, and therefore hard to learn. With the advent of balloon dissectors, this exposure became simpler. Complications related to the TAPP technique were almost completely eliminated by the TEP approach, operative times were reduced, and recurrence rates remained low. Simultaneous with the increased popularity of the TEP approach, however, were modifications in the TAPP approach that have made outcomes with both approaches comparable. Current thinking is that both approaches are acceptable, with special circumstances when one laparoscopic technique is preferred over the other or

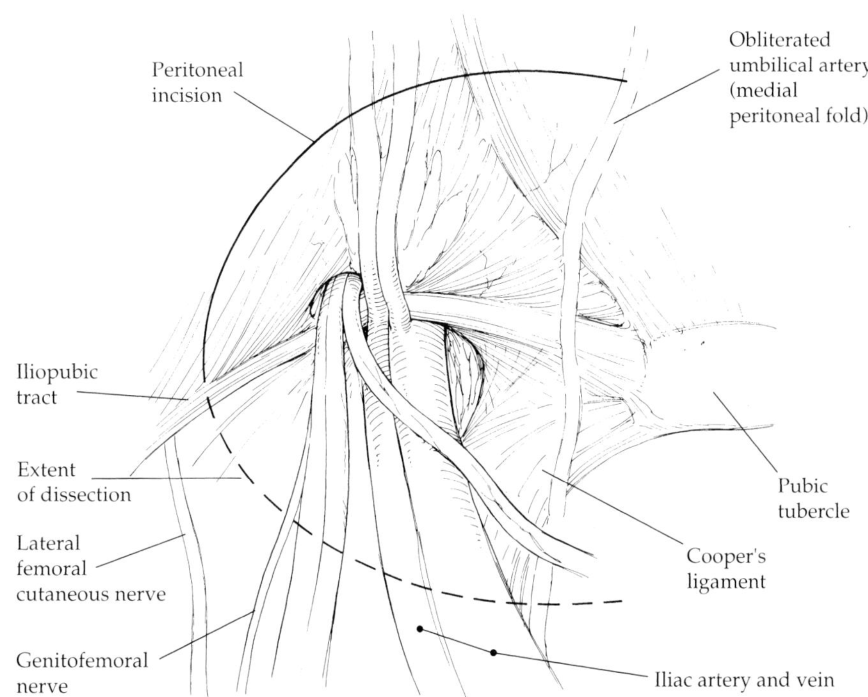

Fig. 53-1. Peritoneal incision in a left-sided transabdominal preperitoneal (TAPP) hernia repair.

where even an open anterior repair will better serve the patient.

CHOICE OF APPROACH

When a surgeon evaluates a patient for inguinal hernia repair, it is ideal that he or she is experienced in the conventional anterior approach, as well as both the TAPP and the TEP laparoscopic approaches. This allows the selection of an operation that best fits the patient's overall condition, as well as the particular hernia being treated. In general, patients who are not candidates for general anesthesia should have an open anterior hernioplasty under local anesthesia. Several centers have also reported successful results with local or regional anesthesia for the TEP approach. It has been our experience, however, that a small but significant percentage of these patients will become anxious if carbon dioxide (CO_2) enters the peritoneal cavity, requiring the urgent induction of general anesthesia. Therefore, laparoscopic repair should be reserved for patients who would be candidates for general anesthesia, even if a local or regional anesthetic technique is initially used. An absolute contraindication to laparoscopic hernioplasty is the presence of infection. Neither the TAPP nor the TEP approach should be used in the face of local or systemic infection because of the risk of mesh infection.

The choice of laparoscopic approach depends on the surgeon's level of experience, the type of hernia present, and the patient's history. The TEP approach is now favored by most laparoscopic surgeons for most patients because it avoids entering the peritoneal cavity. It is therefore less likely to have intraoperative complications and is often performed more quickly than the TAPP approach because it does not require peritoneal closure after mesh placement. There are, however, a few exceptions. If the patient has an incarcerated hernia, a TAPP approach is usually preferred. The TAPP procedure permits an accurate analysis of the contents of the hernia sac and of the viability of the incarcerated structures, as well as a safe and usually easy reduction of the contents. With incarceration, use of a balloon dissector to develop the extraperitoneal space for a TEP repair may lead to a large tear in the peritoneum or even an injury to incarcerated omentum, bowel, or bladder. Although there are reports of good results with the TEP approach for incarcerated hernias by using manual dissection rather than a balloon dissector, in most surgeons' hands the TEP approach should be avoided if the hernia cannot be reduced after the induction of anesthesia.

In women with abdominal pain, the etiology may be in question. If the surgeon has to differentiate between a groin hernia and other possible causes of the patient's symptoms, such as endometriosis, the surgeon should perform a diagnostic laparoscopy and then a TAPP repair, if indicated. For women in whom the diagnosis is certain, the TEP technique can still be utilized. The presence of a Pfannenstiel incision is common in many of these patients because of a previous cesarean section or pelvic surgery, but does not usually contraindicate the TEP dissection.

There are some abdominal incisions, operations, or treatments that may preclude adequate or safe dissection of the extraperitoneal space. Radical prostatectomy or pelvic irradiation will prevent the surgeon from separating the peritoneum from the abdominal musculature. Balloon dissection of the extraperitoneal space in these cases can actually result in a large rent in the peritoneum or injury to the bladder. A lower abdominal incision crossing the rectus sheath can also obstruct the safe passage of the balloon dissector. Forcing the dissector through the obstruction will tear the peritoneum and possibly injure an intraabdominal organ adherent to the preperitoneum. A transverse incision is not an absolute contraindication to the use of the TEP approach, but if resistance is experienced while passing the dissector, the procedure should be converted to a TAPP approach. A lower abdominal midline incision is almost never a problem when the TEP approach is used. The dissector will simply slide to the pubis parallel to the old incision. The midline peritoneum will usually separate from the abdominal wall when the balloon is inflated or can be dissected manually after the trocars are placed. If bilateral repairs are planned there is a small chance that a previous midline incision may hinder the surgeon's ability to dissect the opposite side at the same sitting and this should be discussed with the patient preoperatively.

Recurrent hernias are ideally suited for laparoscopic repair. The unobstructed view of the usually virgin posterior wall allows complete identification of the sites of recurrence and repair of the entire posterior floor. The decision as to which approach to use, TAPP or TEP, depends on the surgeon's expertise and preference. The dissection of an adherent recurrent indirect sac can be difficult with the TEP technique and requires more skill than in a primary hernioplasty. With experience, the difference in difficulty disappears and allows the surgeon to choose which hernioplasty he or she will use on the basis of other factors. Recurrent laparoscopic hernias are usually best handled by the TAPP approach although some have reported results using the TEP technique. Dissection of the extraperitoneal space after a previous laparoscopic repair with mesh is quite challenging and has a potentially high incidence of complications no matter what approach is used.

Large scrotal hernias are similar to recurrent hernias in that the dissection of the indirect sac can be quite difficult with the TEP technique. Such sacs however, can be dissected off the cord and reduced with patience and precise dissecting techniques. To avoid problems, surgeons should use the TAPP approach until they have mastered some of the special maneuvers required to deal with the long scrotal sac.

The age of a patient can influence the type of hernioplasty chosen. In general, laparoscopic hernioplasty is reserved for adults or fully developed adolescents. Some surgeons have suggested that laparoscopic repairs should be limited to working younger adults and avoided in the elderly. It is our experience that patients of all ages benefit from the laparoscopic approach. More than 400 patients greater than 65 years of age have undergone a successful laparoscopic hernioplasty in our center during a 15-year period. Their rapid recovery and early return to normal activity testify to the value of laparoscopic repair for older patients. It is therefore not indicated to restrict the laparoscopic approach by age, but rather to use other criteria already discussed.

PREOPERATIVE PLANNING

A full history and physical examination are essential in every patient to rule out medical problems that might preclude the laparoscopic approach or favor one laparoscopic technique over another. Before the operation, each patient should be informed of the possibility that the TEP approach might be converted to either a TAPP or open repair. In addition, it is important to review the major and minor complications that can be seen with the different hernioplasties. If patients are prepared for the possible sequelae of the repair, they will be better able to deal with them. This is especially true of minor problems, such as seromas, CO_2 or bruising in the scrotum, transient neuralgia, and hematomas.

Patients receive one dose of a prophylactic antibiotic, usually a first-generation cephalosporin, just before going into the operating room. All patients should void to completely empty their bladders immediately before the procedure and thereby avoid the need for an indwelling catheter.

Anesthesia

For laparoscopic hernioplasty, general anesthesia is preferred for most patients. In a few ideal instances, regional or even local anesthesia may be possible with a TEP approach with a well-experienced anesthesiologist and confidant surgeon, but the surgeon must be prepared to convert to general anesthesia if CO_2 enters the peritoneal cavity and causes the patient to become anxious. Because of the low CO_2 pressures used and the limited space present in thin or muscular patients, complete relaxation of the abdominal rectus muscles is important. With the patient under general anesthesia, if the abdominal wall begins to regain its tone, the surgeon will become aware of it before any of the anesthesiologist's monitors become alerted. If the operative field begins to collapse, the anesthesiologist should deepen the level of relaxation to increase the available visual space.

At the end of the procedure, anesthesia should be reversed in a manner that avoids bucking on the endotracheal tube, which can place a tremendous strain on the posterior floor of the groin. In our center when performing TEP repairs, use of a laryngeal mask airway has markedly improved the reversal procedure. It essentially eliminates the endotracheal tube and its irritation. The anesthesiologist maintains control of the airway, but the postoperative sore throat and irritation are eliminated, as well as the extreme abdominal contractions so often seen with reversal of the endotracheal anesthetic.

Operating Room Setup and Patient Positioning

Laparoscopic hernias are easily performed with just the surgeon and a single assistant, who can also be the scrub nurse. The monitor and video equipment should be placed at the foot of the operating bed at the patient's midline or slightly toward the side of the hernia. The surgeon stands opposite the hernia for TEP repairs. If there are bilateral hernias, the surgeon should start by standing opposite the larger or more complicated side and reverse sides when the second repair is begun. For TAPP repairs the surgeon usually stands on the patient's right side for all repairs. The scrub nurse or assistant stands opposite the surgeon and holds the camera and passes the instruments. A Mayo stand should be placed over the legs so that both the surgeon and the nurse can handle the instruments. It is important both arms of the patient be carefully tucked to the sides to allow enough room for the surgeon and assistant to work comfortably. The operating table can be flat or in a slight head-down position. A steep Trendelenburg position is not typically required.

Equipment

Minimizing costs is an important element of any high-volume surgical procedure such as a laparoscopic hernia repair. Reusable unipolar scissors and a bipolar coagulator should be set up on the field, as well as two atraumatic graspers. A 5-mm clip applier may be occasionally needed and should be available. A suction/irrigator is rarely used but can be set up if required. A 6 × 6-inch (15.24 × 15.24-cm) sheet of polypropylene mesh is used for each hernia. Several mesh options are now available, including 3DMax mesh (Bard/Davol Inc.; Cranston, RI), a large preformed mesh that can be used with or without the use of a fixation device. A fixation device (stapler or screw tacker) to anchor the mesh is used by many surgeons but is not necessary and can cause pain. In some patients, endoloops are required to ligate the hernia sac or close a tear in the peritoneum. A 0-degree laparoscope can be used, but a 25- or 30-degree lens may work better as long as the surgeon and assistant are accustomed to operating with an angled scope.

Some open instruments are necessary, such as a no. 11 blade and Kelly or Mayo clamps to dissect the fat and muscle at the umbilicus. Hasson-type S-retractors facilitate this dissection and preperitoneal exposure. A Hasson-type blunt trocar is used at the umbilicus, and two 5-mm or one 5- and one 10-mm trocar are used for the instruments. The extraperitoneal space can be dissected using a balloon dissector or with blunt dissection using insufflation and the laparoscope if the surgeon is experienced and so inclined. For TAPP repairs three trocars are required: a 10-mm camera port and two 5-mm ports for dissection.

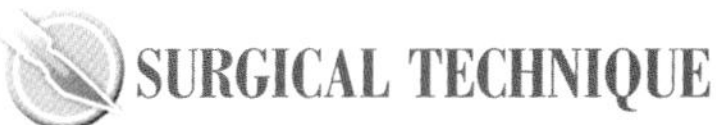

SURGICAL TECHNIQUE

Totally Extraperitoneal (TEP) Approach

Access

The TEP repair begins with a horizontal skin incision just below the umbilicus that extends from the midline 2 cm laterally toward the side of the dominant hernia (Fig. 53-2, page 526). It is important to stay off the midline to avoid entering the peritoneal cavity, as that is where the anterior and posterior rectus sheaths merge. The side of the dominant hernia is chosen because the balloon dissector will dissect more completely on the side of the midline on which it is placed, making subsequent exposure simpler.

After the incision is made, the subcutaneous fat is carefully spread with a clamp to avoid bleeding from small vessels, which would obscure identification of the anterior rectus sheath. Two S-retractors are placed in the wound and used as dissectors to expose the white fibers of the fascia. The fascia is incised laterally with a no. 11 blade, and the rectus muscle is exposed. The S-retractor is placed under the muscle, the muscle is swept laterally, and the posterior rectus sheath is visualized (Fig. 53-2B); the space behind the muscle is dilated with a finger. At this point, the surgeon is ready to dissect the extraperitoneal space.

Dissection of the Extraperitoneal Space

The balloon dissector can simplify the dissection of the extraperitoneal space. Dissection can also be performed manually, without a dissector, but may be more difficult and time-consuming for the inexperienced surgeon. Manual dissection is performed by initiating insufflation through the umbilical port. The laparoscope is inserted and used to sweep down the areolar connective tissue with a horizontal back and forth motion. This is done until the symphysis is exposed and there is enough space for placement of secondary ports.

Because the posterior rectus sheath ends at the Douglas line, any instrument passed on top of the sheath will automatically fall into the extraperitoneal space (Fig. 53-3, page 526). The dissecting balloon is therefore inserted behind the rectus muscle with its tip on the posterior rectus sheath. Aimed slightly upward, it is gently passed downward, on top of the sheath, toward the pubis until the bone is palpated with the dissector. If resistance is

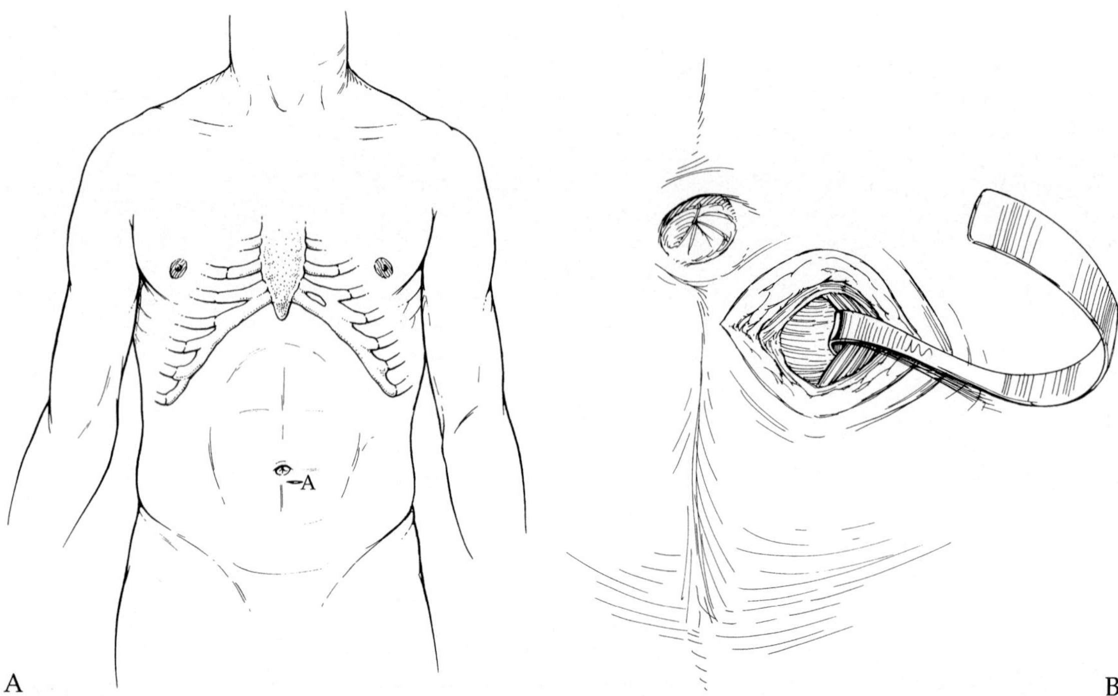

Fig. 53-2. A. The initial 1-inch incision is just off the midline below the umbilicus. **B.** An S-retractor holds up the anterior rectus fascia and muscle for insertion of the balloon dissector.

encountered, the balloon dissector should not be forced into the space because it could break into the peritoneal cavity. A second attempt to pass the instrument may be tried after dilating the space with a finger and will usually be successful. If such access fails, the procedure can be converted to the TAPP approach.

Once the bone is felt, the balloon portion of the dissector can be inflated. With the laparoscope inside the balloon, the progress of the dissection can be followed directly on the monitor. After a maximum of 40 compressions of the bulb, the space will be adequately expanded. If the bowel is visualized during inflation of the balloon, the balloon dissection should be stopped immediately. The methods available to complete the hernioplasty laparoscopically at that point will be discussed later (see "Intraoperative Complications"). After successful dissection of the extraperitoneal space, the balloon dissector is deflated by releasing the air valve and is removed.

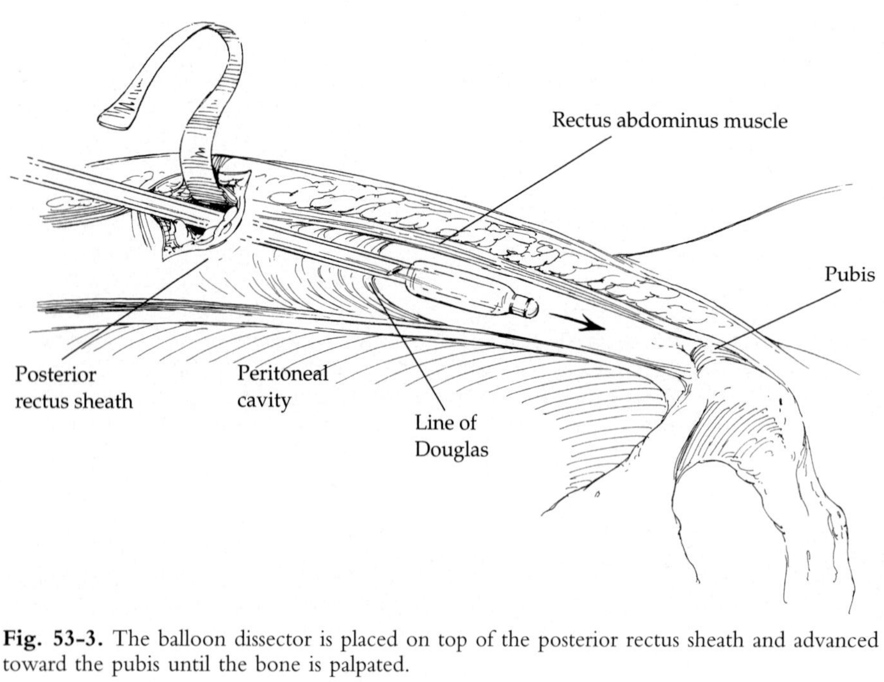

Once again, the S-retractor is placed under the rectus muscle, and the muscle is retracted upward to create a tunnel. This will ensure that when the blunt Hasson trocar is placed, it will be positioned on top of the posterior fascia and behind the muscle. Next, the Hasson trocar is secured in the tunnel, and the extraperitoneal space is insufflated with CO_2 to a maximum of 12 mmHg. The laparoscope is inserted, and the dissected extraperitoneal space is examined.

At this stage, the surgeon will be looking down the rectus sheath, which opens into the dissected extraperitoneal space. If this tunnel is very short, it will not interfere with placement of the other trocars or with the hernia exposure, but if it is very long, the available space will be limited and vision will be impaired. If the tunnel is long or the posterior rectus sheath extends to the pelvis, it must be dissected with an endoscopic scissors after all trocars are in place. A special Hasson trocar equipped with a balloon tip may

Rectus abdominus muscle
Pubis
Posterior rectus sheath
Peritoneal cavity
Line of Douglas

Fig. 53-3. The balloon dissector is placed on top of the posterior rectus sheath and advanced toward the pubis until the bone is palpated.

also be used to retract the posterior fascia. This can open up the exposure and may facilitate the procedure.

Trocar Placement

Subsequent trocars can be placed either laterally or in the midline. A midline placement minimizes the chance of an intraperitoneal insertion. A 10-mm Hasson trocar is placed just below the umbilicus for the camera, one 5-mm trocar in the middle, and another 5-mm trocar 4 to 5 cm above the pubis. The upper instrument trocar should be as close to the subumbilical camera trocar as possible to leave space between the lowest trocar and the pubis. The inferior trocar is positioned approximately three fingerbreadths below the middle trocar, which is enough space between trocars to prevent instrument sword-fighting and still have the lowest trocar above the level of the mesh (Fig. 53-4). The penetration of both instrument trocars should be watched carefully to prevent lacerating a branch of the inferior epigastric vessel if placed laterally or overshooting into the peritoneal cavity when placed medially. The trocars should be anchored at the skin level with paper tapes to prevent them from slipping in and out during instrument manipulation.

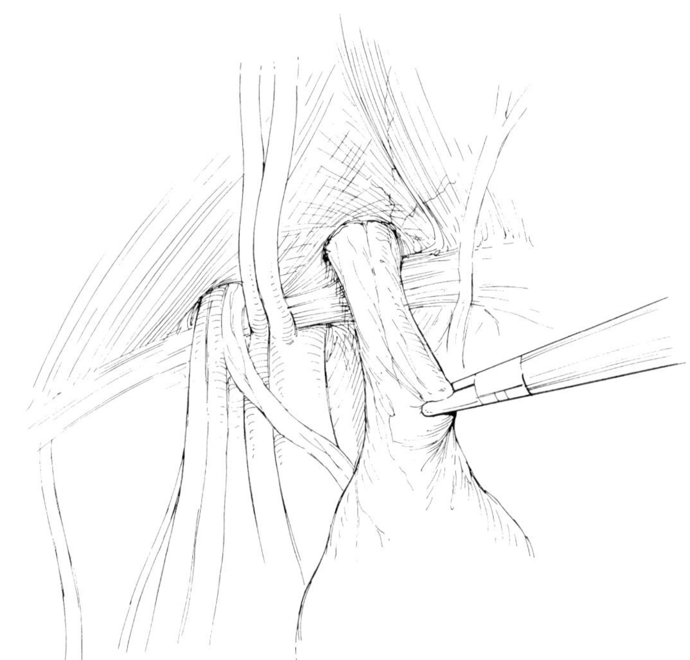

Fig. 53-5. A direct sac is reduced by gentle traction on the peritoneum with countertraction on the transversalis fascia.

Dissection of the Inguinal Floor

Dissection of the posterior aspect of the abdominal wall begins by sweeping off any tissue remaining on the pubis to expose the Cooper ligament. If a direct hernia is present, it is hopefully completely reduced at this point. If it is not, it can usually be reduced with gentle traction on the peritoneal attachments within the defect (Fig. 53-5). On the occasion that the hernia contents are not completely reduced by the balloon dissector, or with gentle traction, the fascial defect can be incised on the superior aspect to release the incarcerated hernia. After the direct sac is reduced, it should not be ligated because the bladder may be involved with the medial aspect of the sac and ligation could result in a bladder injury.

After dissection of the direct floor, the femoral area should always be examined. The iliac vein will be visible just lateral to the Cooper ligament, unless there is an incarcerated femoral hernia. In this situation, the vein will be under the incarcerated hernia contents. The surgeon must carefully reduce these hernias, taking care not to tear small vessels present in the canal. If the hernia is adherent within the canal, an incision in the medial superior edge of the femoral ring should release the hernia (Fig. 53-6, page 528).

The dissection of the lateral floor begins with identification of the inferior epigastric vessels on the anterior wall of the dissection. Care must be taken to avoid dissecting between the vessel and rectus muscle because this will complicate subsequent mesh placement and will cause more bleeding from avulsed muscle

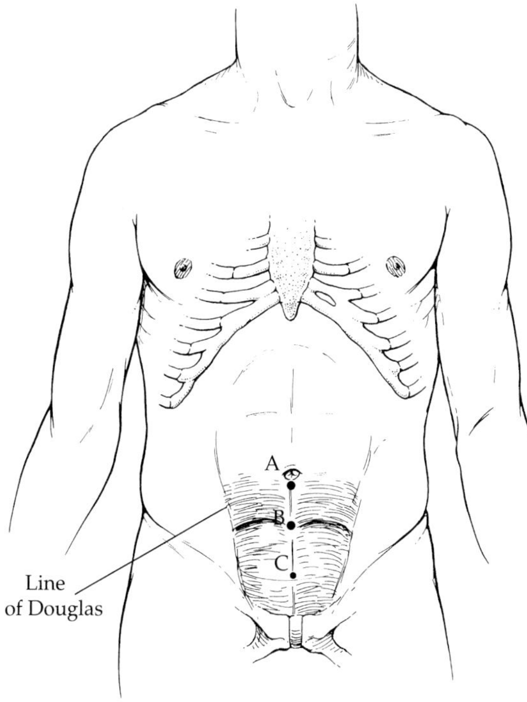

Fig. 53-4. The second trocar is positioned at approximately the Line of Douglas, and the third trocar is positioned three fingerbreadths below. **A.** A 10-mm Hasson (camera) port. **B.** A 5- or 10-mm port. **C.** A 5-mm port.

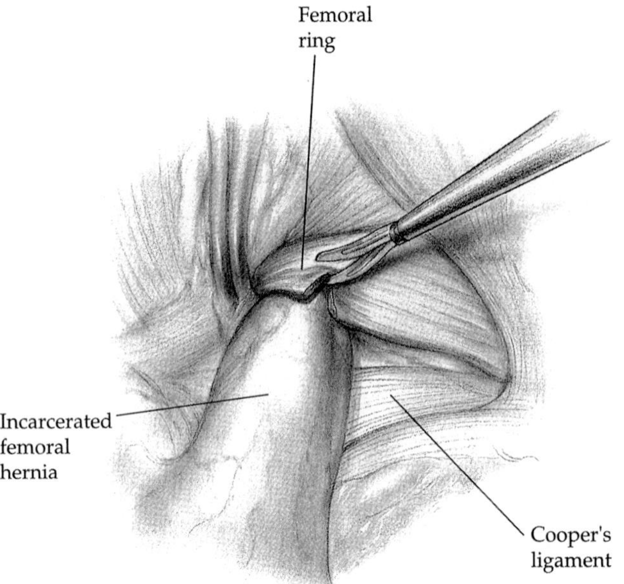

Fig. 53-6. If an incarcerated femoral hernia cannot be reduced, an incision in the supermedial aspect of the ring will release the contents.

branches (Fig. 53-7). All loose connective tissue and fat are swept off the posterior abdominal wall just lateral to the vessels and the peritoneum pushed posteriorly. This will fully expose the inguinal cord (Fig. 53-8). If there is a lipoma of the cord within the canal, it will be lateral to the cord and covering it. The lipoma should always be pulled out of the internal ring and left in the retroperitoneum behind the operative field (Fig. 53-8). Not doing so will often result in a palpable mass in the inguinal canal—much to the distress of the patient. The lateral femoral cutaneous and femoral branch of the genitofemoral nerve lie directly under this lipoma; therefore cautery should be avoided in this dissection (Fig. 53-10, page 530).

The cord should be skeletonized with careful dissection. Once the cord structures are visualized, the peritoneum of an indirect sac will be identified. (If there is no indirect hernia, the peritoneal edge will be found set well back from the internal ring.) The edge of the peritoneum is grasped with an atraumatic grasper and lifted off the testicular vessels. It should be pulled as far cephalad as possible, so that the mesh that will be placed over the posterior floor will be covered by the peritoneum when the CO_2 is evacuated. The peritoneum must also be dissected off the vas deferens, as originally described by Stoppa in the open posterior repair, to once again prevent the peritoneum from lifting the mesh on the medial aspect when de-insufflation is performed.

If there is an indirect hernia, the peritoneal sac will be encountered anterior and lateral to the cord structures as the tissue is dissected off the lateral abdominal wall. A short or small sac can usually be delivered out of the internal ring by stripping it off of the anterior surface of the testicular vessels and vas deferens. With both hands in a hand-over-hand technique, the entire sac can be dissected back until an adequate space is achieved for the placement of the mesh. It is essential that the peritoneum be dissected back completely cephalad to the inferior edge of the mesh. If the peritoneum or any of its filamentous attachments to the canal are left under the mesh, a door is left open for an early recurrence.

When the indirect sac is very long, descending deep into the scrotum, the dissection of the entire sac may be difficult and potentially traumatic. If the progress of this dissection is too slow or difficult, the superior lateral edge of the peritoneum can be opened. From this point, the rest of the sac can be safely transected if one remembers that the testicular vessels and the vas deferens are sometimes quite adherent to the undersurface of the hernia sack. The vas deferens will be on the medial side, and the testicular vessels will be on the lateral side. To avoid injury, both the structures should be identified before the inferior peritoneal surface is cut (Fig. 53-11, page 530). After the proximal sac is completely separated from the distal sac, it can be dissected off the cord structures and ligated with an endoloop. An alternative technique is to circumferentially dissect the sac and pass a ligature around it. Care must be taken not to include any of the elements of the cord and to reduce the peritoneal contents before tying this suture. In general, the first technique is safer and less likely to cause complications; however, it does allow CO_2 to escape into the peritoneal cavity, which can compromise visualization. If intraperitoneal CO_2 causes the peritoneum to balloon into the operative field, obscuring the exposure, a Veress needle can be placed intraperitoneally to decompress

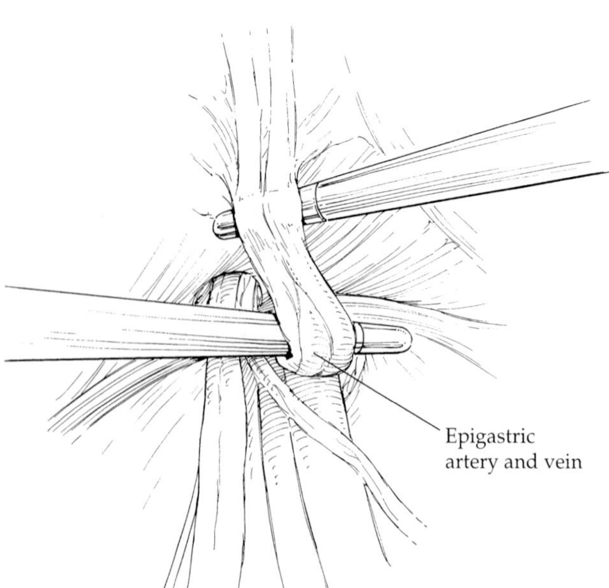

Fig. 53-7. Care must be taken to not dissect above the superficial epigastric vessels, as this can lead to bleeding and mesh placement problems.

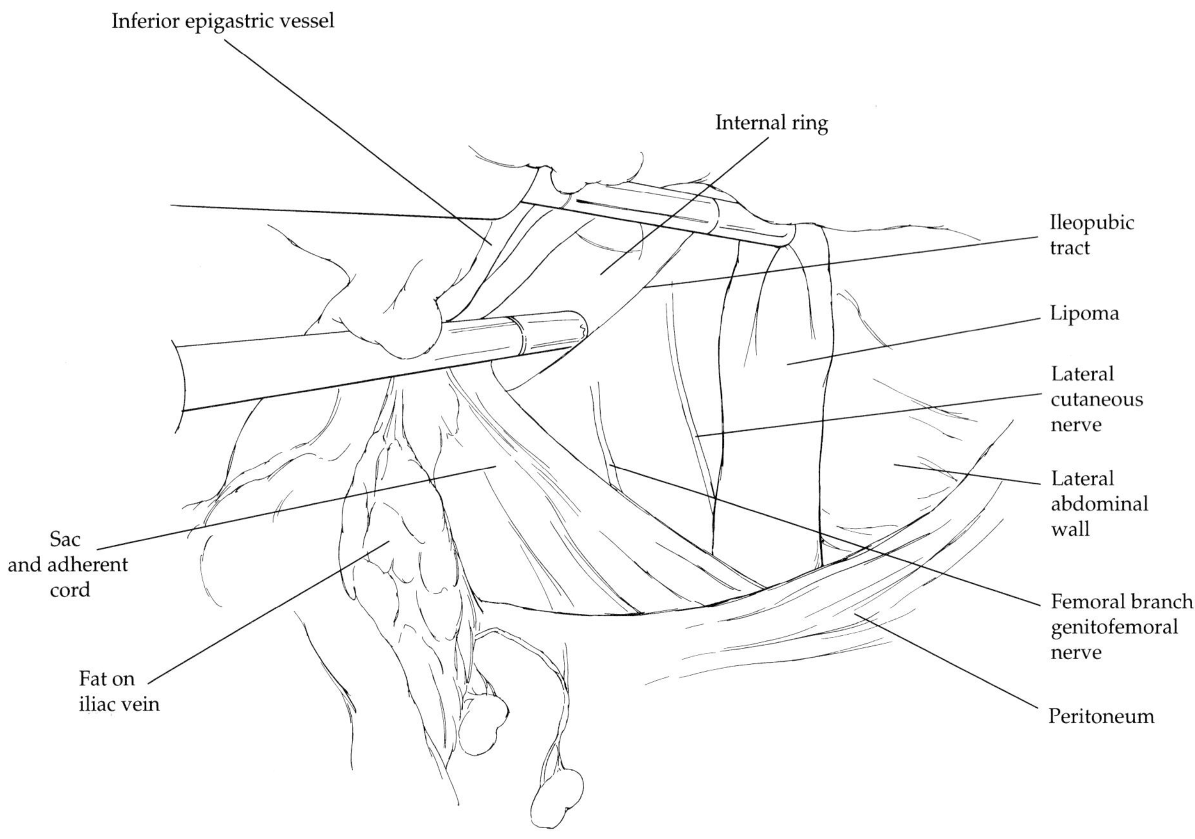

Fig. 53-8. The cord is dissected free and identified.

the abdominal cavity. Usually, however, this is unnecessary, and the surgeon only needs to dissect the peritoneum further back to allow gravity to hold it out of the field of vision. Sometimes in fact, it is better to wait until the mesh is in place before ligating the indirect sac, thus leaving the peritoneal pressure in equilibrium with the extraperitoneal space. However, at the end of the procedure, the indirect sac and any other tears in the peritoneum must be closed to prevent later internal herniation or adhesions to the mesh. If a small hole is made in the peritoneum during dissection, it can be found and completely ligated later in the procedure. If the surgeon sees quivering of the peritoneal surface during dissection, this typically means that CO_2 has entered the peritoneal cavity. Such holes should be identified and ligated with an endoloop.

It is important to remember that one cannot always tell whether there is an indirect component to a hernia until the lateral dissection is completed. Unlike the TAPP approach, in which an indirect hernia is immediately obvious, the indirect sac cannot be identified in the TEP approach until the cord is completely dissected. In essence, the entire posterior floor needs to be dissected in every patient (Fig. 53-12, page 531). Even when there is an obvious direct or femoral hernia, up to 30% of patients will have an indirect component that must be uncovered.

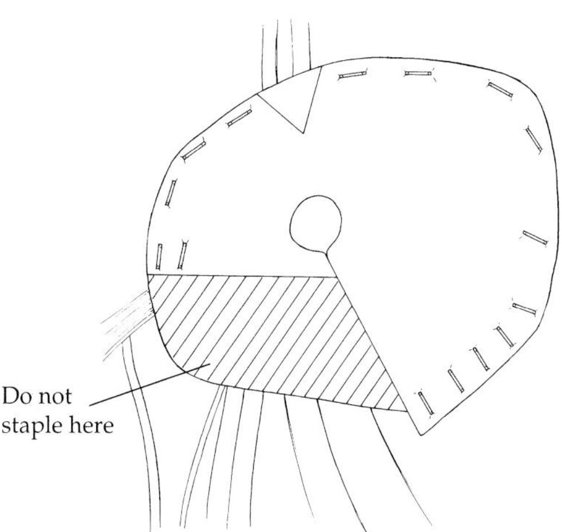

Fig. 53-9. Safe areas for placement of mesh anchors. (Note designated area where anchors cannot be placed.)

Transabdominal Preperitoneal (TAPP) Approach

Incisions and Trocar Placement

The TAPP repair begins with a skin incision within or just below the umbilicus, identical to that used to begin a laparoscopic cholecystectomy. Insufflation is performed using a Veress needle or

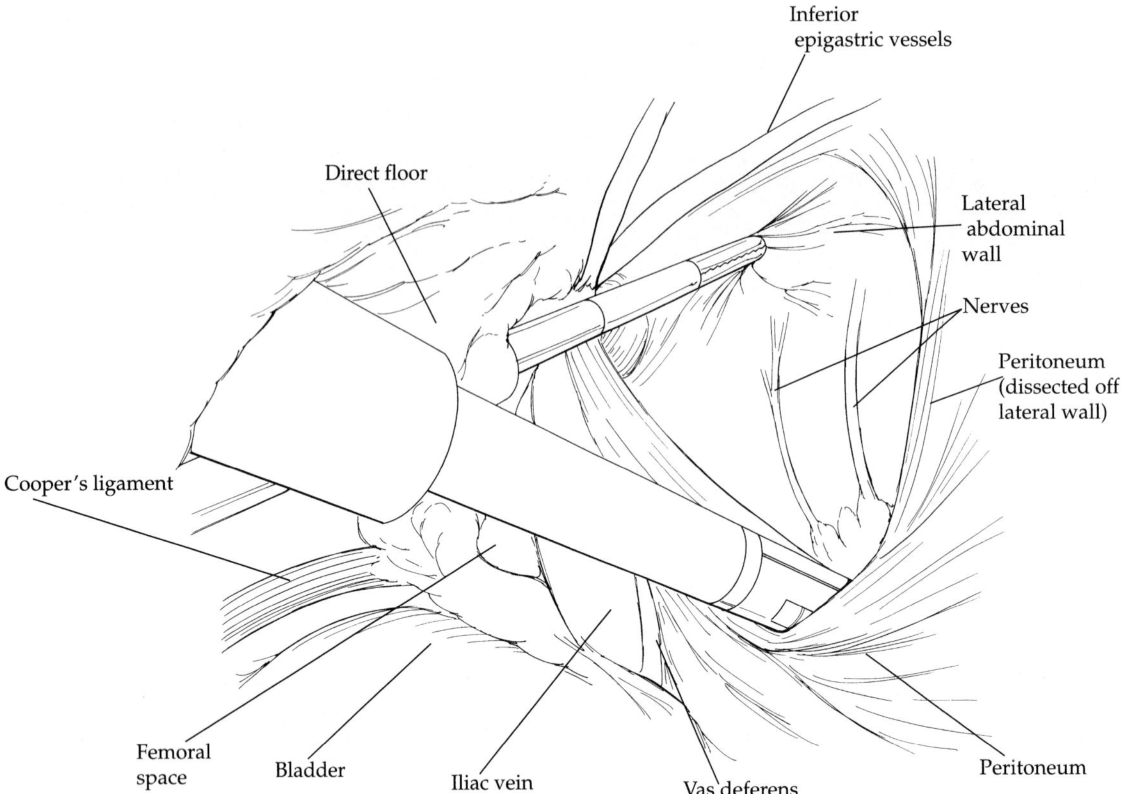

Fig. 53-10. The completed preperitoneal dissection exposing the cord, bony structures, and the lateral nerves.

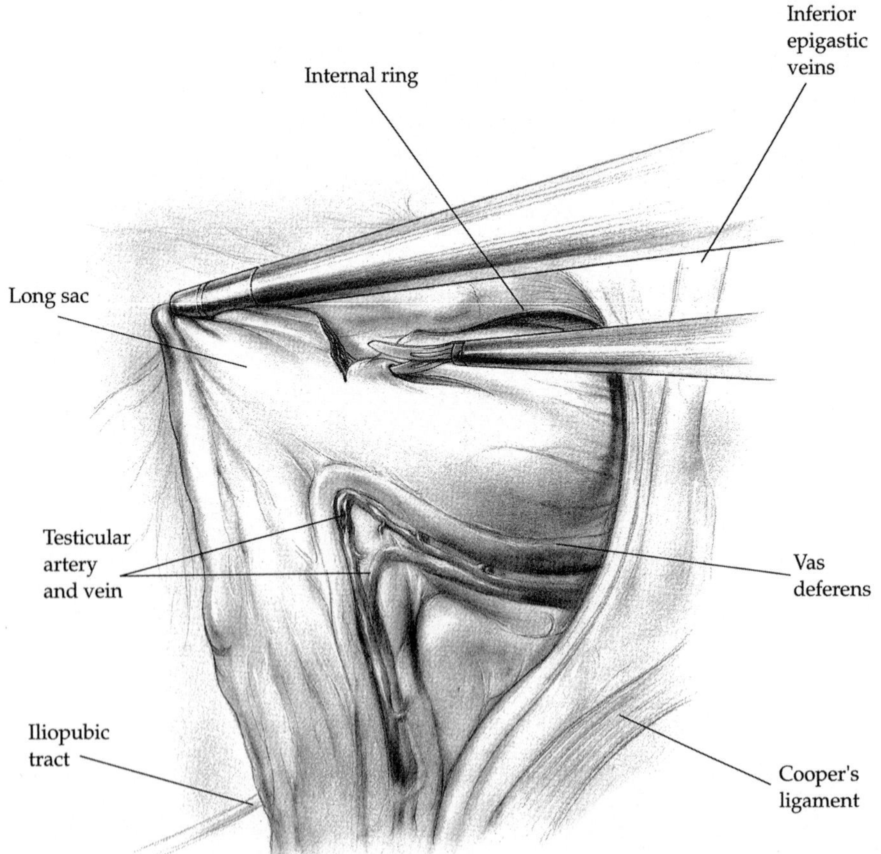

Fig. 53-11. When the sac cannot be easily reduced, it is transected and dissected off the cord structures.

Hasson technique. A 10-mm trocar is placed and the peritoneal cavity viewed with a 10-mm 30-degree endoscope. The two lateral 5-mm trocars are placed at the level of the umbilicus lateral to the transilluminated inferior epigastric vessels on each side. If a 10-mm lateral trocar is used, this incision will have to be sutured at the end of the procedure. For TAP procedures the assistant stands opposite the surgeon and if an additional nurse is available he or she may stand on either side (Fig. 53-13, page 532).

Dissection of the Posterior Floor

The surgeon should always examine the anatomy of the pelvic floor (Fig. 53-14, page 533) before proceeding with the dissection of the extraperitoneal space. Using an endoscopic scissors, the extraperitoneal space is opened by making a small incision lateral to and well above the indirect defect. The incision is continued in a medial direction above the direct space (see Fig. 53-1). The peritoneum is dissected off the abdominal wall with downward sweeping motions, reducing the direct and indirect peritoneal sacs when possible. The peritoneum must be dissected cephalad far enough to allow the peritoneum to be positioned on top of the mesh after the peritoneum is closed.

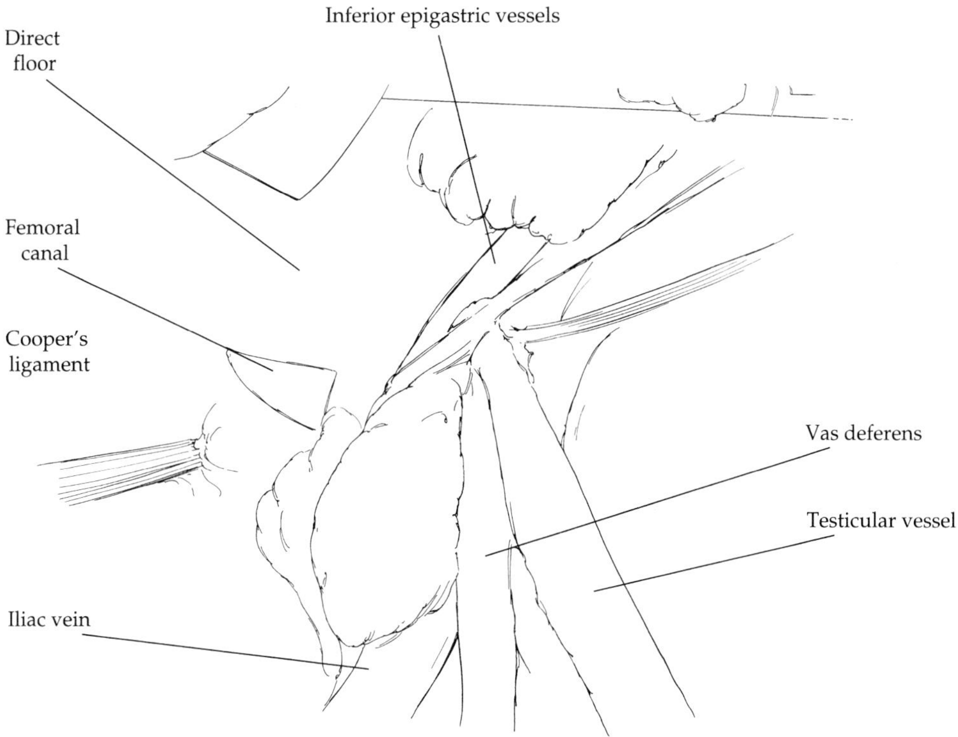

Fig. 53-12. The completed dissection of the posterior wall of the groin exposes all three potential hernia sites.

After the peritoneal flaps are developed, the dissection of the pelvic floor and hernias is identical to that described in the TEP section.

Mesh

After the dissection of all three potential hernia sites, the mesh repair is performed. Whether for a TEP or TAPP repair, an oversized 6 × 6-inch (15.24 × 15.24-cm) sheet of nonabsorbable mesh is cut to fit the pelvic floor. The medial half is cut wider than the lateral so that it drapes over the Cooper ligament when it is placed in the pelvis. The overall shape can be reminiscent of a map of Australia (Fig. 53-15, page 534). To differentiate the medial from the lateral side of the mesh when it is positioned laparoscopically, a stitch can be placed at the bottom of the medial side of the mesh before it is placed in the extraperitoneal space. The suture marker will make subsequent orientation of the mesh much simpler.

To decrease the morbidity of laparoscopic repairs, alternative meshes have been developed. A contoured mesh that does not require fixation was introduced after the publication of a cadaver study demonstrating that in approximately 15% of patients the posterior nerves of the groin (the ilioinguinal and iliohypogastric nerves) are at risk of injury from even proper posterior fixation of mesh. During a 5-year period, this type of mesh has demonstrated the same low recurrence rate seen with a flat sheet of mesh and fixation. Shaped mesh should be marked for orientation on the medial inferior edge, and a right or left mesh is used as appropriate. In an attempt to decrease shrinkage and create a softer, less reactive mesh some surgeons have chosen to use a polyester mesh and have also eliminated fixation. Most recently, surgeons have reported preliminary results of a series of repairs using a biological mesh that becomes a scaffold for the patient's own collagen and is eventually absorbed. Early recurrence rates with both types of these meshes has been promising, but only long-term follow-up will determine which mesh is most appropriate for laparoscopic hernioplasty.

Placing the mesh in the extraperitoneal space does not require any special instruments. The mesh is simply grasped with a 5-mm instrument and pushed into the extraperitoneal space through the 10-mm camera port. The laparoscope is then replaced, and the mesh is gently pushed into the pelvis with the scope. After the mesh is fully inside the extraperitoneal compartment, it is positioned using two graspers until the marking stitch is in place below the Cooper ligament. Using a two-handed technique, the smaller end of the mesh is placed over the indirect area and the larger end is placed over the direct and femoral areas. The mesh must cover all three potential hernia sites in every patient (Fig. 53-16, page 534). When the mesh is smoothed out, it overlaps the pubic bone and crosses the midline. If the patient has bilateral hernias, the mesh from each side will most likely overlap in the midline. It is important to examine the mesh carefully to eliminate any wrinkles or folds before it is anchored in place. It is also essential to note the location of the inferior epigastric vessels and the iliopubic tract, as well as any aberrant obturator vessels, to prevent complications when the mesh is fixed to the abdominal wall.

As discussed earlier, the peritoneum and any lipomas of the cord must be reduced well below the inferior edge of the mesh before the mesh is fixed in place. In some patients, a large sac or lipoma can be placed on top of the mesh after the mesh is anchored and before the CO_2 is evacuated. Alternatively, if the mesh appears to be too large, a portion of it can be cut away with endoscopic scissors and removed through one of the ports. This

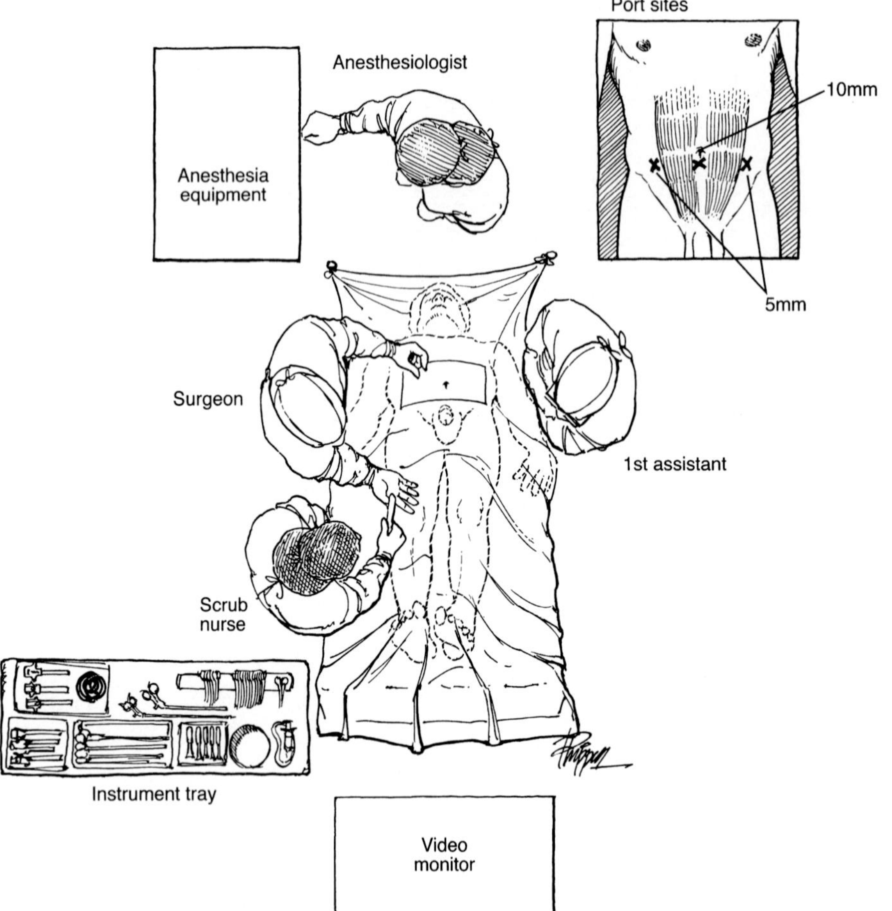

Fig. 53-13. Operating room setup and trocar placement for a transabdominal preperitoneal (TAPP) hernioplasty.

prevents the mesh from being lifted off the pelvic wall by the peritoneal edge when the CO_2 is released.

Occasionally, the mesh placed over the posterior floor will be discovered to be too small to adequately cover it because of the unusually large size of the patient or the hernia defect. When this happens, a second piece of mesh can be added in a patchwork fashion to complete the repair. When there is a very large direct hernia, one should not hesitate to add an additional mesh running in a longitudinal direction extending well above the defect and below the pubic bone. This can also be done to add coverage to an incidentally discovered large femoral hernia.

In a small number of patients, the testicular vessels will not lie comfortably against the pelvic floor. Instead, they seem to run across the extraperitoneal space like a clothesline, actually suspending the mesh above the floor. This is more common in very thin patients or those with recurrent open hernias. In these situations, to prevent a recurrence under the mesh into the internal ring, a double-buttress repair as originally described for the TAPP hernioplasty can be used. In this technique, a smaller 2.5 × 4-inch (6.35 × 10.16-cm) mesh with a slit in the lower third for the cord is used to secure the indirect defect. The slit is placed around the cord and reapproximated over Cooper ligament. A second mesh exactly like that previously described for the single-layer repair is placed over this smaller one. The second mesh prevents recurrence through the slit and completes the repair of the direct and femoral areas (Fig. 53-17, page 535).

Anchoring the Mesh

Anchoring the mesh to the posterior wall of the groin is performed by the majority of laparoscopic surgeons. Fixing the mesh ensures that it will remain where the surgeon first placed it long after the operation. In general, such fixation is safe in most patients. Because the nerves at risk for injury are typically below the iliopubic tract, injury or entrapment of the genitofemoral, lateral femoral cutaneous, or femoral nerve can therefore be avoided by placing all mesh anchors into or above the iliopubic tract (Fig. 53-9). As stated previously, however, in a small percentage of patients the nerves are above the iliopubic tract and can be compromised by fixation. This is why many surgeons now use approaches that do not require fixation, including the use of a contoured mesh and the preperitoneal approach. We now prefer this approach in most patients and use fixation only in selected situations, such as in patients with multiple recurrences or in whom the direct floor is almost entirely absent.

When placing fixation one must identify the landmarks. The iliopubic tract is recognized as a white fibrous band running transversely at the lower edge of the internal ring. In some patients, it is obvious, whereas in others it is subtle and barely visible. Identification is confirmed by placing one hand on the abdominal wall and pressing a laparoscopic grasper against the wall so the tip is felt with the opposite hand. If the surgeon cannot feel the instrument, it is below the iliopubic tract and in an area where the nerves are at risk for injury. This same maneuver is performed when the staples or fixation tacks are being placed. No anchors should be placed unless the anchoring device can be felt with the opposite hand. In addition, with the opposite hand on the abdominal wall, the stapler achieves a more perpendicular angle, which improves its reliability. However, the surgeon should not press so hard as to force the staple deeply into the wall, possibly injuring a more superficial nerve such as the ilioinguinal nerve.

The first anchors are placed through the mesh into the Cooper ligament. This stabilizes the mesh and allows the surgeon to fan the mesh out in a lateral direction, taking out any wrinkles or folds. The next staples or tacks are placed into the transversalis fascia medial to the inferior epigastric vessels. The mesh is again smoothed out in a lateral direction, with care taken that the peritoneum and lipoma of the cord are well back from the edge of the mesh. Before the lateral fixation is completed, the mesh can be trimmed or further dissection of the sac or lipoma can be performed. The lateral anchors are

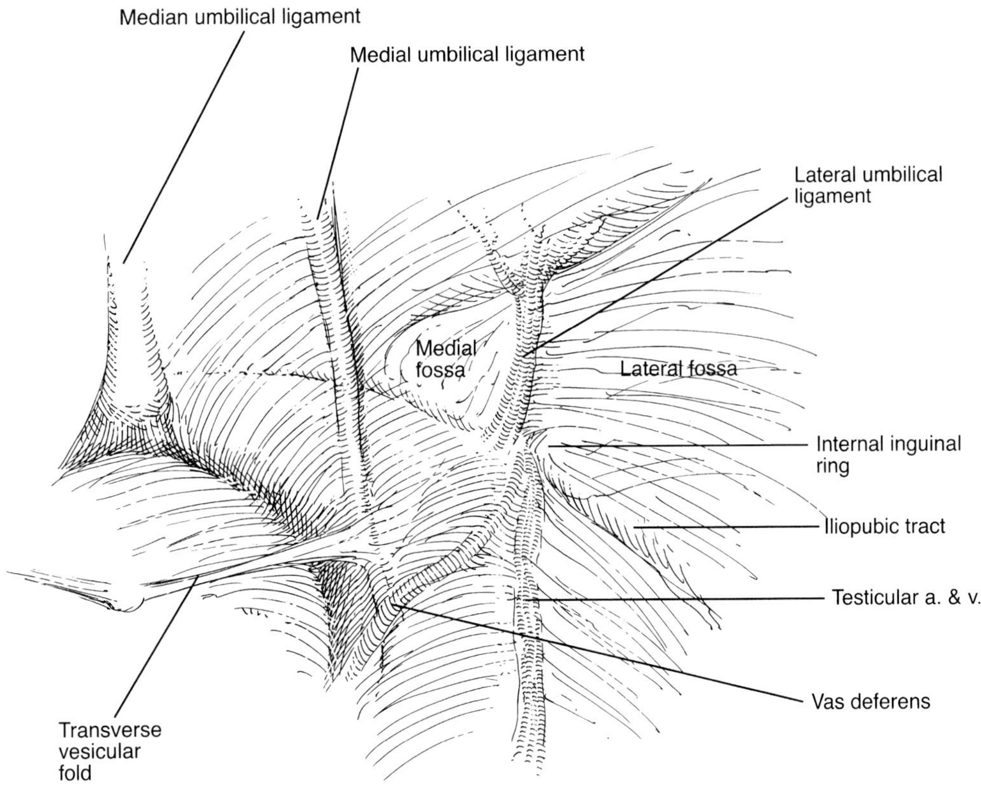

Fig. 53-14. Laparoscopic view and anatomy of right lower abdominal wall.

inserted by using the bimanual technique to prevent any damage to the neural structures below the iliopubic tract. The final mesh anchor is placed into the Cooper ligament just medial to the iliac vein (Fig. 53-18, page 535). Its purpose is to remove any slack in the lower mesh edge that would otherwise allow a recurrence from under the polypropylene patch. It is mandatory to feel the pubic bone when placing this final fixation to avoid inadvertent laceration of the iliac vessels. If aberrant obturator vessels are present coursing over the pubis, they must be avoided or serious bleeding will result.

There is no minimum number of staples or tacks that should be used to hold the mesh in place. Their purpose is not to give strength to the repair but to hold the mesh smoothly against the posterior wall until the body's own inflammatory response takes over in a few days. The surgeon should resist placing unnecessary anchors, especially in the lateral aspect of the mesh. Many surgeons, in fact, no longer use any fixation of the mesh, particularly for the TEP repair. When the mesh is completely stabilized, the extraperitoneal space is examined for possible bleeding and, if necessary, irrigated to clear any residual blood.

When using a TAPP technique, the peritoneum must be completely closed to prevent internal hernias and exposure of the mesh to viscera. Closure is best performed with a running baseball stitch. Closure with clips is usually inadequate and tacks may injure underlying nerves. In TEP repairs formal closure of the peritoneum is unnecessary, but careful evacuation of the gas is required as described below.

Wound Closures

Closing any 10-mm trocar sites is essential to prevent the development of incisional hernias. Usually, a simple figure-eight absorbable suture will do the job. A full-thickness closure of the umbilical incision is important in TAPP repairs. Before closing any ports in the TEP approach, the position of the mesh is evaluated, and the CO_2 is slowly evacuated through the 5-mm port. The peritoneum must come to rest on top of the mesh to hold it in place. If the peritoneum is seen to be lifting the edge of the polypropylene patch, further manipulation should be performed until the mesh is properly covered by the peritoneum. The 5-mm ports are removed and wounds closed. The camera port is closed after evacuating any CO_2 trapped in the peritoneal cavity. This can be done by holding up the abdominal wall with a clamp on the fascia and puncturing the posterior fascia and peritoneum with a Veress needle. After the abdominal cavity is deflated, the anterior rectus sheath is sutured closed. Bupivacaine is injected at each of the incisions to aid in early pain control.

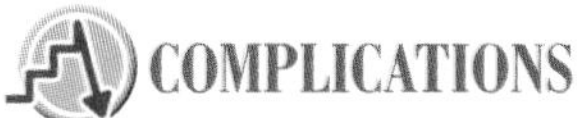

COMPLICATIONS

Intraoperative Complications

There are three complications of balloon dissection that may cause problems for the surgeon early in the procedure: dissection above the inferior epigastric vessels, bleeding, and tearing of the peritoneum. Any of the differently shaped balloons can drop the inferior epigastric vessels off of the posterior abdominal wall, but balloons that fan out laterally

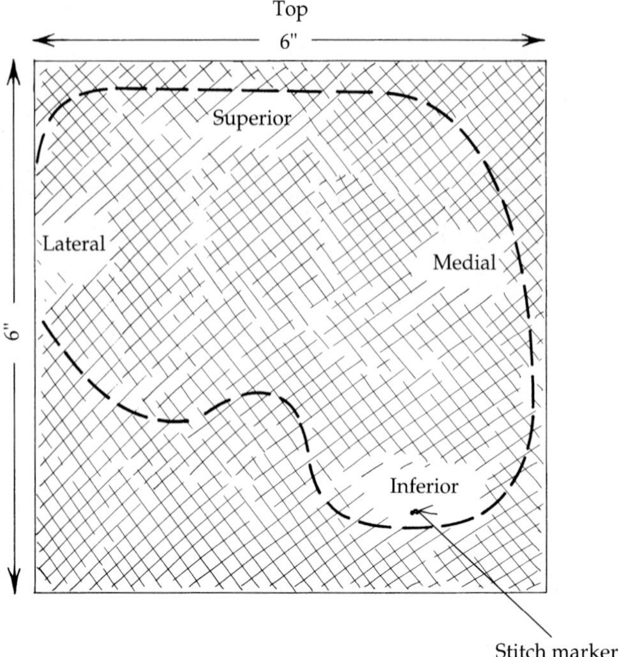

Fig. 53-15. The polypropylene mesh, cut from a 6 × 6-inch (15.24 × 15.24-cm) sheet, is made large enough to cover the entire floor of the groin.

are more likely to cause the problem. If the vessels are off the wall, they will interfere with further dissection. They should be ligated with clips or endoloops or cauterized with bipolar current before further dissection of the floor. Bleeding can occur if small vessels are torn from the inferior epigastric or pelvic vessels. If this happens, it is a matter of locating the bleeding site and controlling it with cautery or clips. Irrigation is required if the bleeding has been brisk. Tears in the peritoneum are the most difficult problem to handle. Avoiding the TEP approach in patients with an incarcerated hernias, a history of pelvic irradiation, or a radical prostatectomy will reduce the incidence of significant peritoneal tears. When tears do occur, the surgeon can switch to a TAPP approach or proceed with the TEP technique, just making sure to close the rent at the end of the procedure. Endoloops are usually sufficient and much easier than suturing such defects in the peritoneum. Venting the gas from the peritoneum during the case is usually unnecessary, but placing the patient in steep Trendelenburg position can help.

Bleeding during dissection of the posterior wall is usually minor and will stop spontaneously. If it does not stop, careful isolation of the bleeding point and coagulation or clipping of the individual bleeder is indicated. Mass coagulation must be avoided to prevent inadvertent injury to the cord structures or groin nerves. Severe hemorrhage can develop from dissection around the iliac vein. If bleeding develops from a tear in a small branch of the vein or the vein itself, it must be controlled promptly and CO_2 embolus prevented by compression of the bleeding site. Open exploration will be required if the surgeon cannot rapidly gain control laparoscopically.

Injury to major vessels and viscera has been reported after conventional laparoscopic procedures including TAPP hernia repairs. These complications fortunately are now rare because surgeons have an increased familiarity with proper access techniques. Bleeding from lateral trocar placement can be avoided by being aware of the position of the inferior epigastric vessels. If it does occur, the vessels can be secured with a full-thickness suture placed with a suture passer.

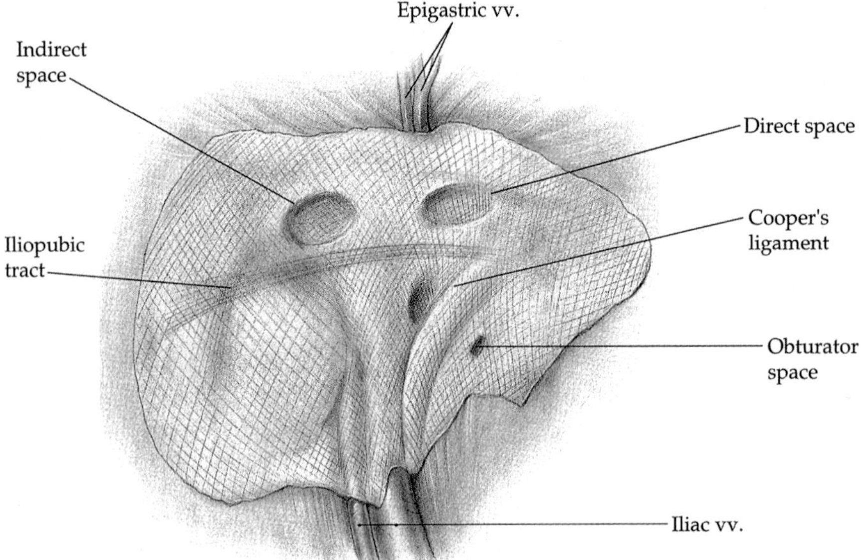

Fig. 53-16. The polypropylene mesh covers the entire area of potential groin hernias, with the wider half placed over the Cooper ligament. vv, vessels.

Postoperative Complications

Unfortunately, complications occur with every hernioplasty technique, but some are peculiar to the laparoscopic approach. Seromas are the most common problem, but they usually resolve spontaneously or rarely with aspiration. Injuries to the femoral branch of the genitofemoral nerve, the lateral femoral cutaneous nerve, and the femoral nerve are more serious potential complications of the laparoscopic approach (Fig. 53-19, page 536). These injuries can be avoided in all but rare instances if the proper techniques of anchoring the mesh are followed; namely, staying above the iliopubic tract or by avoiding fixation entirely.

Small-bowel obstruction has been reported by several authors after the TAPP approach, but only rarely after a TEP

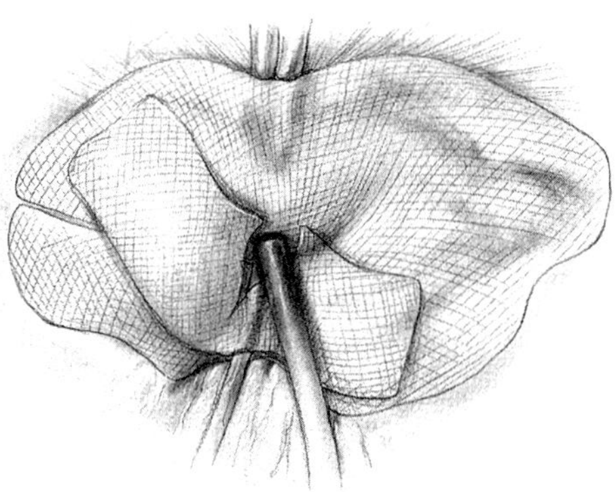

Fig. 53-17. When the cord structures appear to suspend the mesh off the pelvic floor, a second piece of mesh with an upwards slit is placed behind the cord.

repair. The key to preventing this complication is the repair of tears or holes in the peritoneum created during dissection and meticulous closure of the peritoneum in TAPP repairs.

Recurrence after laparoscopic hernioplasty is rare when the techniques that are used follow the principles outlined in this chapter. Many hernia centers have demonstrated that the TEP and TAPP repairs are effective approaches to inguinal hernia repair. If the surgeon, however, is not meticulous in the dissection and repair of the entire posterior floor, early recurrence will be more common than after technically simpler open repairs (Table 53-1, page 536). This fact is borne out in a recent Veterans Affairs (VA) multicenter study in which laparoscopic outcomes were significantly worse than after open repairs, except when performed by more experienced surgeons.

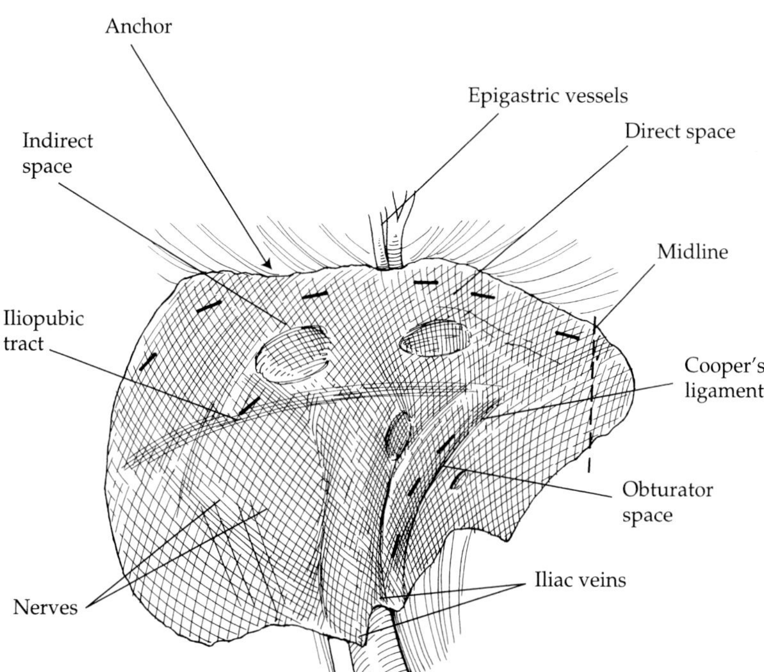

Fig. 53-18. Staples or tacks anchor the mesh to the transversalis fascia above the iliopubic tract medial and lateral to the inferior epigastric vessels, as well as into the Cooper ligament (left groin).

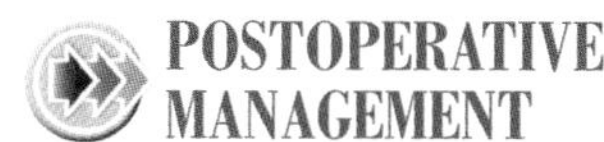

POSTOPERATIVE MANAGEMENT

Activity after TEP and TAPP laparoscopic repairs is not restricted. Patients are told to resume all activities and work as soon as they feel able. The average return to normal activity is less than 1 week. Return to work depends on patient motivation and varies from 1 to 2 weeks. To avoid anxiety, patients should be forewarned about the possibility of CO_2 becoming trapped in the scrotum, seroma formation, and discoloration of the scrotum and penis developing a few days after the operation. Wearing supportive underwear and use of anti-inflammatory drugs are extremely helpful in alleviating early postoperative discomfort. If a seroma develops, usually reassurance and time are all that is needed. When patients are symptomatic or the fluid collection is large, aspiration is indicated. There does not seem to be an association between seroma formation and later development of a hydrocele, which is seen in approximately 0.5% of hernioplasties.

OUTCOMES

Since the introduction of laparoscopic hernioplasty 15 years ago, laparoscopic techniques, equipment, and results have improved dramatically. Utilizing both TAPP and TEP repairs, centers worldwide have demonstrated that, with experience and laparoscopic expertise, laparoscopic hernioplasty can be performed efficiently with a recurrence rate of less than 1% and with less immediate postoperative and long-term pain. The surgeon, however, must use judgment in choosing which hernioplasty is best for each patient and each hernia in order to achieve the lowest recurrence rate with the least morbidity.

Our own center has had experience with more than 3000 laparoscopic repairs during this 15-year period. Our approach has evolved as described in this chapter, and recurrence rates have remained well below 1%. The laparoscopic approach has fulfilled its original promises, but the technique remains a difficult one and should be reserved for surgeons willing to take the time to master the advanced laparoscopic skills required.

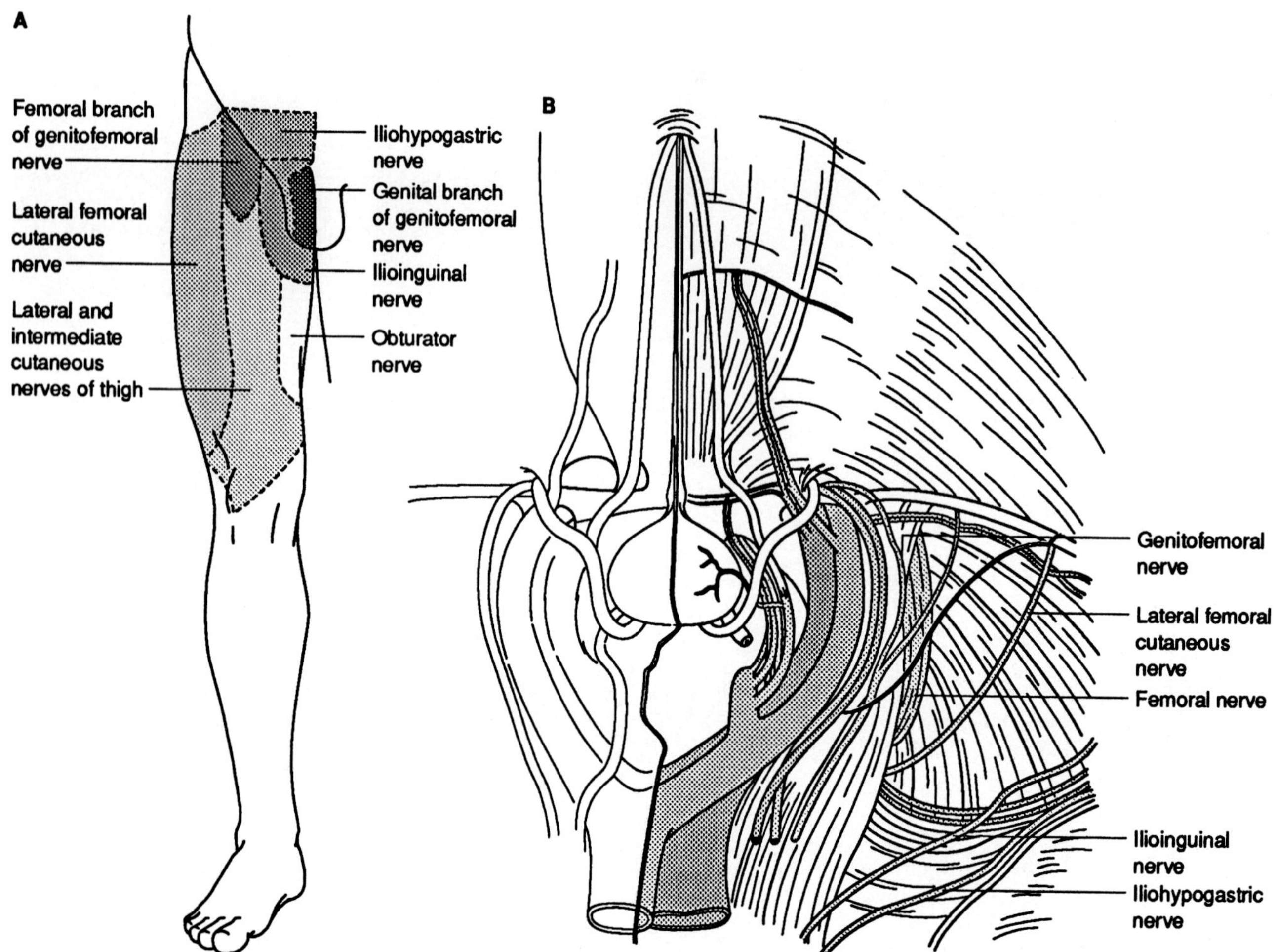

Fig. 53-19. A. Location and distribution of sensory nerves of the pelvis that are at risk of injury during a laparoscopic hernia repair. **B.** Location of these nerves in the preperitoneal space.

TABLE 53-1. EFFECT OF LEARNING CURVE ON RECURRENCE AND COMPLICATIONS FOR LAPAROSCOPIC HERNIOPLASTY

Authors	Technique	Patients/number of repairs	Total recurrence (%)	Recurrence rate in learning curve (%)	Recurrence rate after learning curve (%)	Total comp. rate (%)	Comp. in learning curve (%)
Leibel et al.	TAPP	2225/2700	1.03	NS	NS	4.60	7.8 (1–50)
Felix et al.	TEP and TAPP	1087/1423	0.40	NS	NS	2.70	5.6 (1–46)
Sayad et al.	TEP	724/958	2.20	NS	NS	4.10	NS
Kapiris et al.	TAPP	3017/3530	0.62	5 (1–375)*	0.16 (376–3205)*	3.68	NS
Shultz et al.	TAPP	1952/2500	1.04	2.2 (1–500)*	0.3 (501–1500)*	3.56	13.0 (1–20)
Ramshaw et al.	TEP and TAPP	955/1224	2.60	2.0 (1–300)*	0.3 (301–1224)*	13.6	10.0 (1–30)

Comp., complication; NS, not studied.
*Case numbers in the series authors used to define "in" and "after" learning curve.

SUGGESTED READING

Andersson B, Hallen M, Leveau P, et al. Laparoscopic extraperitoneal inguinal hernia repair versus open mesh repair: a prospective randomized controlled trial. *Surgery* 2003;133: 464–472.

Felix EL. A unified approach to recurrent laparoscopic hernia repairs *Surg Endosc* 2001;15:9.

Felix EL, Michas CA, Gonzalez M. Laparoscopic hernioplasty: why does it work? *Surg Endosc* 1997;11:36–41.

Felix EL, Scott S, Crafton B, et al. A multicenter study: causes of recurrence after laparoscopic hernioplasty. *Surg Endosc* 1998;12: 226–231.

Khajanchee YS, Urbach DR, Swanstrom LL, et al. Outcomes of laparoscopic herniorrhaphy without fixation of the mesh to the abdominal wall. *Surg Endosc* 2001;15:1102–1107.

Lal P, Kajla RK, Chander J, et al. Randomized controlled study of laparoscopic total extraperitoneal versus open Lichtenstein inguinal hernia repair. *Surg Endosc* 2003;17: 850–856.

Lau H, Patil G, Yuen W. Day-case endoscopic totally extraperitoneal inguinal hernioplasty versus open Lichtenstein hernioplasty for unilateral primary inguinal hernia in males. *Surg Endosc* 2006;20:76–81.

Leibl B, Schmidt J, Daubler P, et al. A single institution's experience with transperitoneal laparoscopic hernia repair. *Am J Surg* 1998; 175 6:446–452.

Neumayer L, Giobbie-Hurder A, Jonasson U, et al. Veterans Affairs Cooperative Studies Program 456 Investigators (2004) Open mesh versus laparoscopic mesh repair of inguinal hernia. *N England J Med* 350: 1819–1827.

Puri V, Felix E, Fitzgibbons R. Laparoscopic vs conventional tension free inguinal herniorrhaphy: 2005 Society of American Gastrointestinal Endoscopic Surgeons (SAGES) annual meeting. *Surg Endosc* 2006:1809–1816.

Rosenberger R, Loeweneck H, Meyer G. The cutaneous nerves encountered during laparoscopic repair of inguinal: new anatomical findings for the surgeon. *Surg Endosc* 2000; 8:731–735.

Schneider BE, Castillo JM, Villegas L, et al. Laparoscopic totally extraperitoneal versus Lichtenstein herniorrhaphy: cost comparison at teaching hospitals. *Surg Laparosc Endosc Percutan Tech* 2003;13:261–267.

Swanstrom LL. Laparoscopic hernia repairs: the importance of cost as an outcomes measurement at the century's end. *Surg Clin N Am* 2000;80:1341–1351.

COMMENTARY

Inguinal hernia repair is the most common general surgery procedure in North America and one of the oldest practiced reconstructive operations known. Changes in this bread-and-butter surgery are slowly accepted and require much data, persuasion, and encouragement. As Dr. Felix has commented, laparoscopic hernia repairs have been around for almost 20 years and yet they only account for 15% of the total number of repairs done. Why is this? Is it a poor repair? The answer, as the author points out, is definitely no; laparoscopic repairs are well documented to have excellent outcomes—both low failure rates and less patient trauma. This translates to less postoperative pain and a quicker recovery. So, why the poor adoption rate? Laparoscopic hernia repairs are often criticized as being too expensive, and they certainly can be. Surgeons interested in performing laparoscopic hernia repairs should take care to operate in a cost-effective fashion when it comes to such a high-volume operation. The elimination of unneeded devices or instruments is important, as is the minimization of the use of disposables. If this is done, we have found that laparoscopic hernia procedures cost almost the same as open (hospital charges are another matter, of course). Perhaps a larger issue is the difficulty in learning both the TEP and TAPP approaches. As pointed out by the author, the learning curve is quite long and, as such, discouraging to many surgeons. This becomes a self-fulfilling prophecy as there are few expert practitioners available to teach the next generation of residents and fellows, who are then faced with the burden of struggling through a long learning curve on their own. Many give up for a surgery that just doesn't seem to be worth it. This is a shame, because laparoscopic herniorrhaphy is an elegant and potentially mechanically advantaged way to treat hernias. Certainly few would deny that the literature supports the laparoscopic approach *at least* for certain indications: namely bilateral and recurrent disease. Perhaps it is time to include laparoscopic approaches to inguinal hernias as a part of a mandatory core curriculum for surgery residents so that training in this useful approach will begin early and allow skills to build gradually over 5 years.

Practitioners of laparoscopic herniorrhaphy continue to divide into camps between the TAPP and TEP repairs. This is probably a spurious argument; as Dr. Felix points out, the laparoscopic herniorrhaphist should master both the TAPP and TEP as there are ideal indications for each approach. Certainly, it is not infrequent that a TEP approach needs to be converted to a TAPP due to failure to access the preperitoneal space or loss of exposure due to a hole in the peritoneum. Likewise it has been shown that TEP can be faster and safer, particularly in cases where the patient has had previous lower abdominal surgery, obviating as it does the need for adhesiolysis. In short, practicing only one approach for all hernia repairs is counterintuitive and probably unfair to the patient—surgeons should be masters of all and selective in their application.

LLS

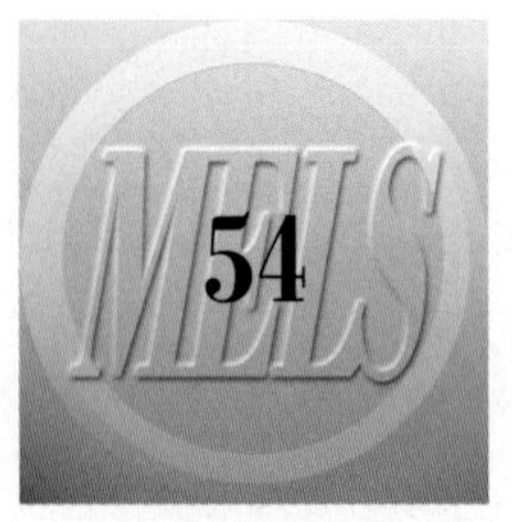

Laparoscopic Incisional and Ventral Hernia Repair

BRUCE RAMSHAW AND SHARON BACHMAN

INTRODUCTION

In the past few years, thousands of laparoscopic ventral hernia repairs have been reported, including one study reviewing 850 cases. A large, multicenter Veterans Affairs (VA) trial comparing laparoscopic and open ventral hernia repair was terminated at an early safety review, due to the significant reduction in wound complications in the laparoscopic group. The many reports of excellent clinical results in addition to the sound principles of the repair have made laparoscopic ventral hernia repair one of the fastest growing minimally invasive techniques in the past ten years.

The ventral hernia repair is based on the principles of the Rives-Stoppa open retrorectus tension-free mesh repair, in which the plane between the rectus muscle and the posterior fascia is dissected widely. Mesh is then placed posteriorly and fixed to healthy abdominal wall fascia using full-thickness permanent sutures. The laparoscopic approach differs, however, with mesh placement in the intraabdominal cavity rather than in the retrorectus plane. Laparoscopic ventral hernia repair allows for clear visualization of the abdominal wall, wide mesh coverage beyond the defect, and secure fixation to healthy abdominal wall fascia, ensuring a successful repair.

The intraabdominal location of mesh may lead to a possible mechanical advantage; similar to the placement of a patch inside a punctured tire, the intraabdominal pressure may help to push the mesh against the abdominal wall. A generous mesh overlap may also relieve some of the pressure off of the area around the defect, allowing for medialization of the fascial edges of the defect.

This chapter will review the indications, contraindications, appropriate patient selection, technique, and postoperative care for laparoscopic ventral hernia repair. Particular attention will be paid to the avoidance and management of complications.

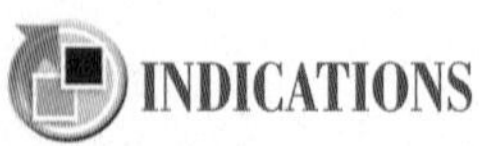

INDICATIONS

The appropriateness of mesh hernia repair in children is being debated; this chapter will focus on the technique for patients beyond puberty. Based on published studies, it is apparent that tension-free mesh repair for ventral hernias excels in terms of low rates of recurrence, even for the smallest primary hernia. Essentially any ventral hernia that can be repaired using an open tension-free mesh repair may potentially be repaired laparoscopically. Patient selection is of critical importance for this procedure, during the surgeon's learning curve. Certain patient groups can minimize the potential for complications even when performed early in a surgeon's experience, such as a primary or first-time recurrent umbilical hernia in patients without previous abdominal surgeries. However, this same technique in a patient with many previous abdominal operations, especially in patients with previous intraabdominal placement of polypropylene mesh, can be a significant challenge for even the most skilled laparoscopic surgeon. Bleeding, enterotomy, and other intraabdominal organ injuries can be relatively common in patients with severe intraabdominal adhesions. Of course, this is the case regardless of the approach—open or laparoscopic.

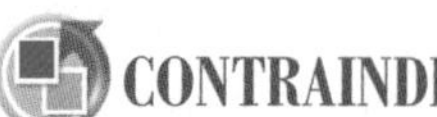

CONTRAINDICATIONS

As mentioned, essentially all adult ventral hernias may be approached laparoscopically. However, depending on the surgeon's experience, relative contraindications may include active wound infection, loss of abdominal domain, a history of severe abdominal adhesions, and/or previous intraabdominal mesh placement. In patients with acute infection or at a high risk of bacterial contamination, alternatives to standard prosthetic mesh placement include laparoscopic placement of a biologic mesh or the use of a non-mesh repair, such as the components separation technique. Although rare given the current safety of general anesthesia, patients with significant cardiopulmonary disease or other medical problems may not be candidates for general anesthesia and therefore are not candidates for a laparoscopic repair. Hernias in these patients may be most appropriately managed nonoperatively, with abdominal binders and activity restrictions, to avoid the unnecessary risks of surgery.

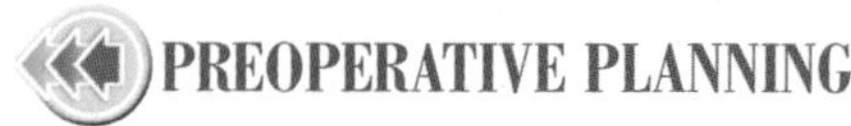

PREOPERATIVE PLANNING

In preparation for laparoscopic ventral hernia repair, preoperative patient education is imperative, especially in patients with complex and/or large hernias. It should be stressed that the laparoscopic ventral hernia repair combines the benefits of minimal recurrence and minimal wound complications. Yet, postoperative pain may be significant and often requires a hospital stay for pain management, except following repair of the smallest hernias.

Other important patient education topics include the expectation of postoperative seroma formation, extra incisions for suture fixation, and the potential for bowel injury as well as its management. The last point is especially important in patients with multiple previous abdominal surgeries, multiple previous ventral hernia repairs (especially with mesh), and very large defects. These patients should be prepared preoperatively for the possibility of delayed mesh placement at a second surgery, should a bowel injury occur or be suspected. The management of these patients may be aided by preoperative CT scan to evaluate anatomy and preoperative bowel preparation for decompression.

For patients with suspected loss of abdominal domain, additional discussion should include the increased likelihood of multiple operations, conversion to open operation, prolonged recovery, and even the possibility of death. There are several considerations that can be discussed preoperatively. The first option is no surgery (conservative management with binders). Operative strategies include placement of an intraabdominal port for chronic pneumoperitoneum with several weeks of injection of air to attempt to expand the true abdominal cavity, followed by delayed mesh placement (open or laparoscopic) after regaining some domain. One of the separation of components procedures may be considered for open repairs. If open abdominal-wall reconstruction is required,

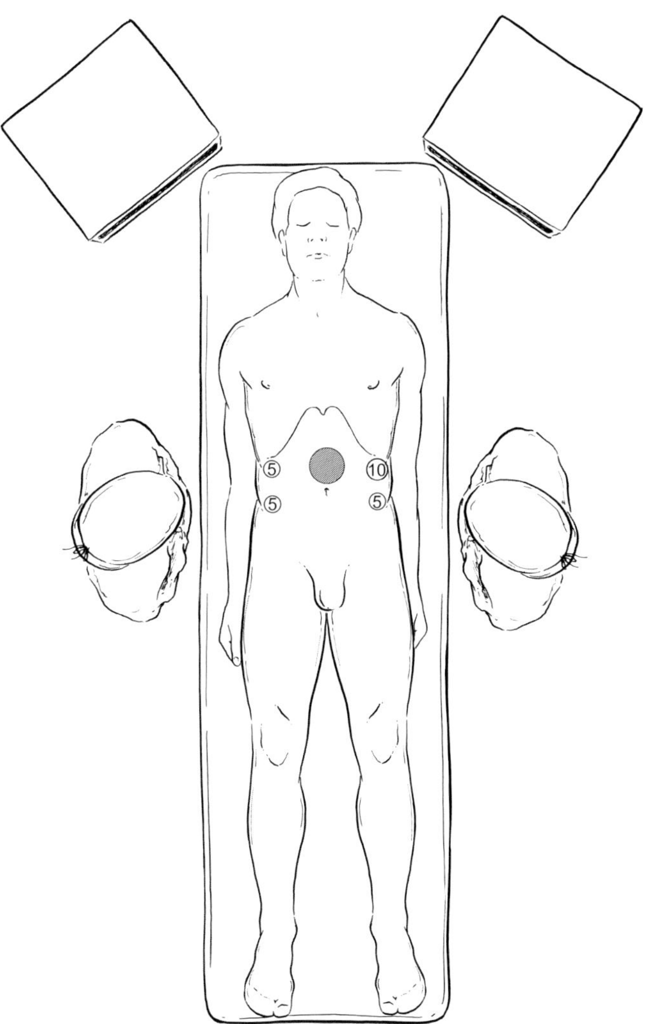

Fig. 54-1. Standard trocar placement and operating room setup for laparoscopic ventral hernia repair. Three 5-mm sites and one 10-mm site are depicted.

wound complications are common and frequently will require additional operative procedures to manage them.

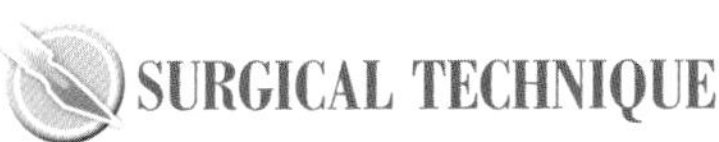

SURGICAL TECHNIQUE

Positioning and Preparation

The patient is generally placed in the supine position with arms tucked at the side or on armboards, depending on the size and location of the defect. Many hernias, especially larger ones, require the surgeon to move about the operating table during the procedure. In most situations, having the patient's arms tucked allows for more flexibility in handling instruments.

As opposed to most laparoscopic procedures, the surgeon, trocar, and monitor positions for a laparoscopic ventral hernia repair can be quite variable. For most long midline hernias, the initial access would be lateral, with additional trocars on the contralateral side (Fig. 54-1). Monitors would be required on each side of the patient, either toward the head or the foot depending on the location and extent of the midline defect. For upper abdominal hernias, the monitors should be at the head of the bed, similar to placement for laparoscopic cholecystectomy. For lower abdominal hernias, the monitor is placed at the foot of the bed, similar to placement for a laparoscopic inguinal hernia repair. For a ventral hernia away from the midline, such as a spigelian hernia or an ostomy site hernia, the surgeon stands on the side of the patient opposite the hernia, and the monitor is placed on the same side as the hernia (opposite the surgeon). The surgeon should make the operating room staff aware of this variability to avoid the potential for incorrect room setup. (See specific hernias at the end of the chapter.)

Preoperative antibiotics against skin flora are typically administered, as well as an orogastric tube for gastric decompression and a Foley catheter for bladder decompression. Sequential compression devices are utilized for deep vein thrombosis prophylaxis. The patient is shaved, prepped, and draped widely to allow for the lateral placement of ports. Using an Ioban drape helps to avoid mesh-to-skin contact.

Access and Port Placement

The initial access port is usually a 10-mm trocar. The decision to use a Veress needle or open technique for trocar placement should be based on the surgeon's experience. If a closed technique is chosen, an optical trocar is recommended. Another safe method of entry utilizes blunt digital dissection. Because most of these patients have had previous abdominal surgery, accessing the abdomen away from previous incisions minimizes the risk of intraabdominal injury. Two relatively safe areas for access include the subxiphoid midline, where the left lateral lobe of the liver usually protects other intraabdominal organs, and subcostal off the tip of the 11th rib at the anterior axillary line, where the presence of preperitoneal fat or intraabdominal adhesions is rare.

Once safe access is achieved, the laparoscope is inserted and the abdominal cavity is explored. An angled scope is used to better view the anterior abdominal wall, where much of the procedure is performed. Typically, two to four 5-mm trocars are used as secondary ports. One or two are placed on the same side of the abdomen as the scope for initial adhesiolysis, if necessary. Trocars are placed laterally as far from the hernia defect as possible to avoid covering them with mesh during the repair. Having both 10-mm and 5-mm laparoscopes available maximizes the surgeon's options for visibility by allowing either scope to be placed through any port.

Lysis of Adhesions

The lysis of adhesions is frequently the most difficult and dangerous portion of this operation. Bleeding and injury to bowel or other organs may occur, especially in patients with multiple previous surgeries or previously placed intraabdominal mesh. Typically, a plane is developed between the abdominal wall and the adherent abdominal contents to allow for safe, gentle, blunt and cold, sharp dissection (Fig. 54-2, page 540). If no plane is discernable, abdominal wall is sacrificed to protect the bowel. Energy sources, including ultrasonic dissection devices, should be used only if bowel or other organs are clearly not adjacent or adherent to the abdominal

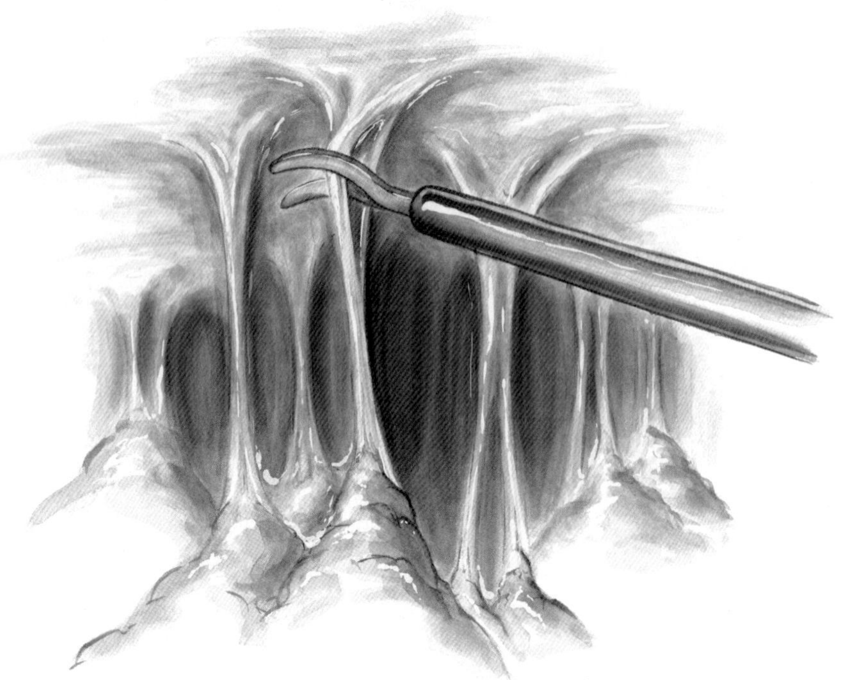

Fig. 54-2. Beginning adhesiolysis from the free edge of an adhesion helps identify any potential loops of bowel adhered to the anterior abdominal wall.

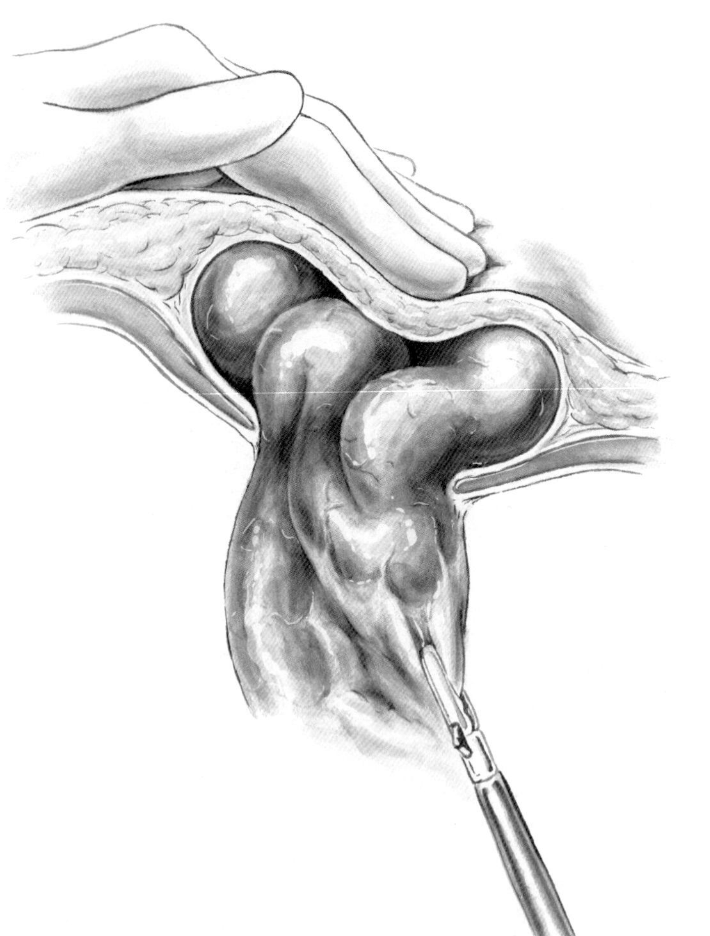

Fig. 54-3. Applying manual pressure on the hernia will help reduce incarcerated bowel and ease the lysis of adhesions of bowel to the abdominal wall in the defect.

wall. Delayed bowel injury can occur with the use of electrocautery or scissors or following ultrasonic dissectors, scissors, or grasper retraction. Thermal injury may occur and not be identified during initial dissection. Bleeding may be controlled with pressure, clips, or cautery after all nearby viscera has been cleared away.

When operating for recurrent incisional hernias, lysis of adhesions can be complicated by the previous repair. If bowel is eroded, or ingrown, into previously placed mesh, the mesh and any attached abdominal wall is transected and left on the bowel. However, if there are signs of bowel obstruction or if in the surgeon's judgment the mesh should not be left on the bowel, a bowel resection may be necessary. In this situation, a conversion to an open or laparoscopic assisted approach may be appropriate. It may be necessary to delay mesh placement, based on the surgeon's judgment.

Reduction of Hernia Contents

In most patients, hernia contents can be reduced safely with gentle traction using atraumatic laparoscopic graspers. External manual compression on the hernia will assist with safe reduction (Fig. 54-3). If bowel is incarcerated or is even possibly included within a mass of incarcerated contents, care should be taken to avoid excessive tension with graspers to minimize the risk of bowel injury. For incarcerated omentum, the main risk during reduction is bleeding. The use of energy sources, clips, sutures, or endoloops may be required if bleeding occurs. In rare cases when incarcerated contents are not reducible, sharp division of the fascial edge of the defect will facilitate reduction. As in open surgery, the viability of reduced contents should be assessed. An open incision centered over the incarcerated hernia contents is an option if contents are not reducible. Laparoscopic repair can proceed after closure of the incision, or this may facilitate bowel resection if necessary.

Preparation of the Anterior Abdominal Wall

For centrally located hernias, no additional dissection is necessary prior to mesh placement. However, hernias located above, below, or lateral to the midabdominal wall may require additional dissection to expose the posterior abdominal wall and prevent possible lead points for re-herniation. Division of the falciform or median umbilical ligament or the exposure of Cooper ligament may be necessary. This is typically performed with cautery or ultrasonic dissection due to vasculature running within these ligaments.

Hernia Evaluation

Once the entire defect is exposed and adequate dissection of the abdominal wall allowing for wide mesh coverage is achieved, the defect is measured. Accurate measurement of the hernia defect can be difficult, especially in obese patients, due to the differential of the abdominal circumference at the skin and at the peritoneum. A piece of mesh measured and cut to size outside the abdomen would typically be larger than necessary when placed inside the abdomen and fixed to the peritoneum. Various tips are provided that may help to accurately measure the size of the defect at the peritoneal level. First, the abdomen can be deflated to minimize the difference in external and internal circumference of the abdominal wall. Spinal needles are also helpful when placed perpendicular to the abdominal wall at the edges of the defect. Measurement of the distance between the spinal needles during desufflation of the abdomen increases accuracy. The hernia defect can also be measured directly, using a suture or laparoscopic instrument or by cutting a plastic ruler lengthwise and placing it inside the abdominal cavity.

In the presence of multiple defects, the maximum distance between all defects is typically measured, and one piece of mesh is used to cover all defects. Occasionally, defects are separated by long distances of healthy abdominal wall and use of two separate pieces of mesh may be more appropriate, based on the surgeon's judgment. For incisional hernia repair, it is recommended that the entire previous incision be covered with mesh unless adhesiolysis in this area would significantly increase the risks of the procedure.

Mesh Preparation

The mesh should be placed on the desufflated abdomen and, using the marked outline of the hernia, fashioned to allow for coverage beyond the edges of the defect by at least 4 to 5 cm in all directions. Once the appropriate size of mesh is cut, it is marked for orientation (top/bottom, etc.) and the planned location of the preplaced sutures. Markings on the skin or Ioban drape help to plan the site of externalization of the cardinal stay sutures. Typically, four sutures are initially placed in the mesh. Too many sutures would make it difficult to find the appropriate suture inside the abdominal cavity, and too few sutures would not provide enough mesh fixation to simplify tack placement for additional fixation. Permanent sutures are used; Goretex sutures offer strength and a lack of memory that allows for ease of placement, but must be handled carefully to prevent fracturing. Prolene sutures are inexpensive and strong, but the memory may make handling them difficult intraabdomially.

Mesh Placement

After securing sutures at the cardinal points of the mesh and marking the mesh and abdomen, the mesh is rolled up and, depending on its size, inserted through either the 10-mm trocar or the wound itself. A 5-mm grasper placed through a trocar on the opposite side of the patient can be used to grasp the mesh through the 10-mm wound and pull it into the abdomen. In order to visualize mesh placement, a 5-mm laparoscope in a third trocar may be utilized.

Mesh Fixation

The mesh is then unrolled and the proper orientation is verified (Fig. 54-4A, page 542). The sutures are brought out through small incisions in the skin using a suture-passing instrument to grasp each arm of the suture in a separate pass. Local anesthesia is injected prior to inserting the suture passer. The angle of the suture passer is slightly different with each pass, allowing the needle to enter the abdominal wall through the same skin incision but exit the peritoneal surface of the abdominal wall approximately 1 cm away from the first suture arm (Fig. 54-4B and C). The sutures are not tied down until all four have been placed and lifted to demonstrate the appropriate tautness of the mesh. If a suture is in an unacceptable position, it is pulled back into the abdominal cavity and brought out through another more appropriate skin incision. Once the mesh is confirmed to be in an appropriate position, the sutures are gently tied down, approximating the anterior fascia and up to 1 cm of full-thickness abdominal wall to the mesh (Fig. 54-4D).

The edge of the mesh is then fixed to the abdominal wall with tacks or other point-fixation devices at approximately 1-cm intervals (Fig. 54-4E, page 543). Although the constructs may not provide long-term fixation, they stretch the mesh taut for additional suture fixation and help to prevent internal herniation between the mesh and the abdominal wall. The point-fixation device must typically be inserted into trocars opposite the mesh edge being tacked. Pressure is applied to the abdominal wall using the nondominant hand to approximate the edge of the mesh to the device at a 90-degree angle, ensuring appropriate tack placement (Fig. 54-4F). A tack that is not fired perpendicular to the abdominal wall may not be flush with the mesh. If a construct is only partially penetrating the mesh or falls into the abdominal cavity, it is removed if possible to avoid potential injury. Tacking one quadrant of the mesh at a time, and moving to the opposing quadrant rather than continuing down the length of the mesh, will help prevent migration of the mesh to one side of the abdomen.

After the mesh is appropriately taut, additional full-thickness abdominal wall suture fixation may minimize the likelihood of recurrence (Fig. 54-4G). Most experts recommend that sutures be placed at 3 to 5 cm intervals. Small defects or "Swiss cheese" types of hernia defects with most of the mesh approximating healthy abdominal wall might require less additional suturing, at intervals of 5 to 8 cm. Large defects with less mesh approximated to the abdominal wall relative to the defect will require more sutures at 3- to 5-cm intervals to minimize the risk of recurrence.

The mesh should tent tautly over the defect at the conclusion of the procedure (Fig. 54-4H). This ensures the mesh will follow the curve of the abdominal wall when the abdomen is desufflated, without wrinkling or enventrating out into the defect (Fig. 54-4I).

Closure

After complete fixation of the mesh, the abdominal cavity should be explored for active bleeding or other injuries. The fascia of the 10-mm incision may be closed laparoscopically, utilizing the suture passer, or in an open fashion. Alternatively, in patients felt to be at high risk for trocar herniation, the mesh can be used to cover the 10-mm incision. The CO_2 is pushed out of the abdominal cavity, and subcuticular sutures are used to close the skin of all trocar wounds. Sutures or skin adhesives are used to close suture incision sites, and steristrips and dry dressings are applied to all wounds. Prior to dressing the suture-site wounds, a hemostat or other thin instrument should be used to elevate the skin of these incisions in at least two directions. This will help to prevent the skin dimpling that can occur from the fixation sutures entrapping subcutaneous tissue.

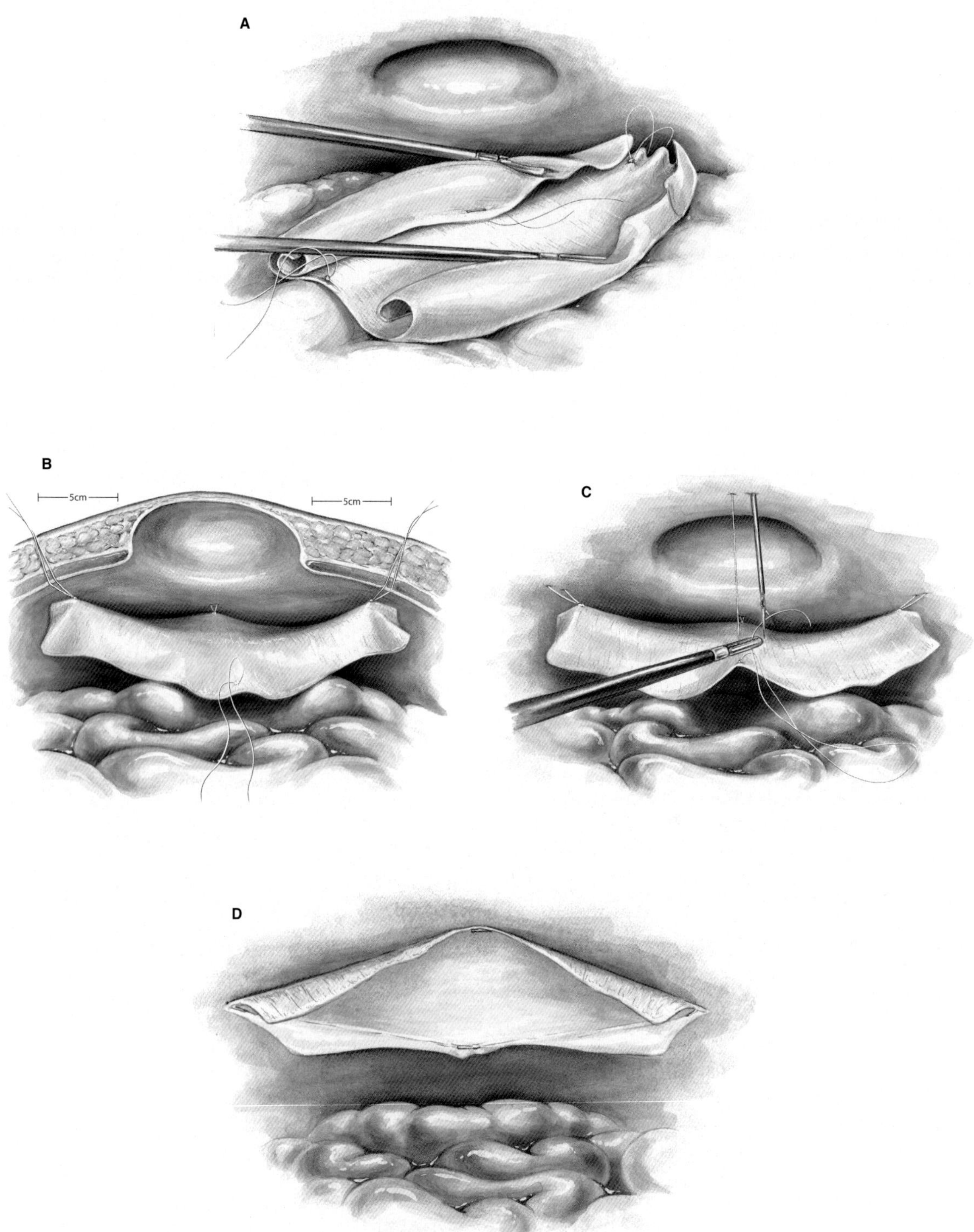

Fig. 54-4. A. Mesh is oriented in the peritoneal cavity and then unrolled. Stabilizing the center of the mesh with one grasper and unfurling one side at a time works well. **B.** Sutures are preplaced 1 cm in from the mesh edge. The mesh is seen extending at least 5 cm beyond the edges of the hernia defect. The two legs of the suture are brought out of the same skin incision but enter at two different sites intraabdominally, with at least 1 cm of fascia between the legs. **C.** Sutures are clamped but not tied until all four cardinal sutures have been externalized, allowing for adjustments in the placement of the transfascial sutures if necessary. Alternating between pulling the sutures tight and allowing slack helps allow for precise suture placement. **D.** All four cardinal fixation sutures have been gently tied, and the mesh has the appropriate diamond shape, demonstrating tautness. **E.** The point-fixation device should be introduced from ports on the side of the abdomen opposite the area to be fixed. Ideally, the camera is on the same side as the device. Fixing one quadrant at a time and alternating between opposite quadrants helps prevent inadvertent shifting of the mesh across the abdomen. **F.** Proper seating of the fixation device is accomplished by placing external pressure on the abdominal wall with the palm or fingers of the hand not using the fixation device. The abdominal wall should be pushed onto the tip of the device at a 90-degree angle. **G.** After placing fixation constructs at 1-cm intervals, additional transabdominal fixation sutures are placed 3 to 5 cm apart. One end of the suture is placed in the suture passer and introduced into the abdomen. The suture passer is then reintroduced at a slightly different angle to pull the suture end out. **H.** At completion of the repair, the mesh is stretched taut across the defect. **I.** At desufflation, the mesh will relax slightly, following the curve of the abdominal wall, but will not become loose enough to wrinkle or eventrate into the defect.

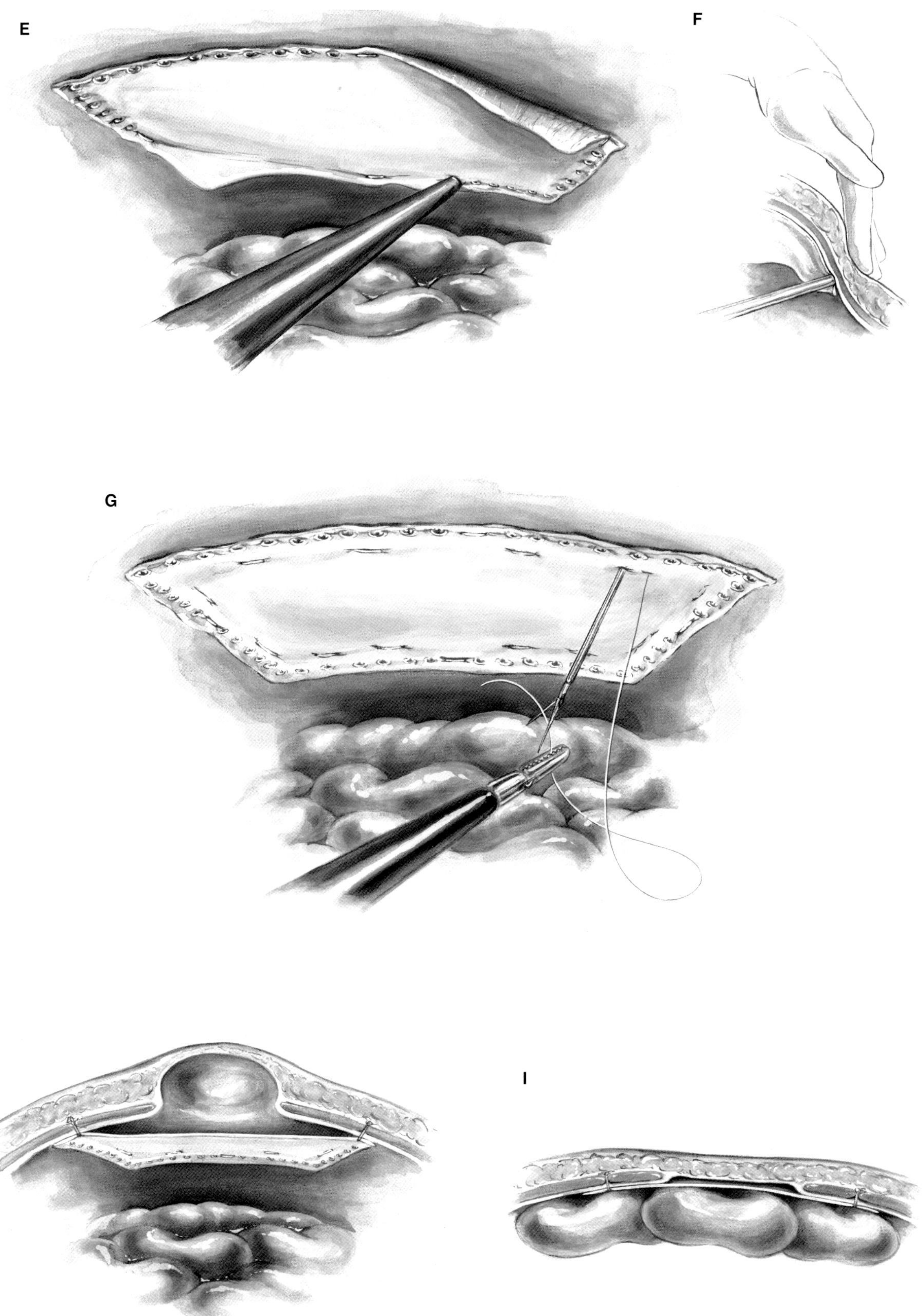

Fig. 54-4. Continued

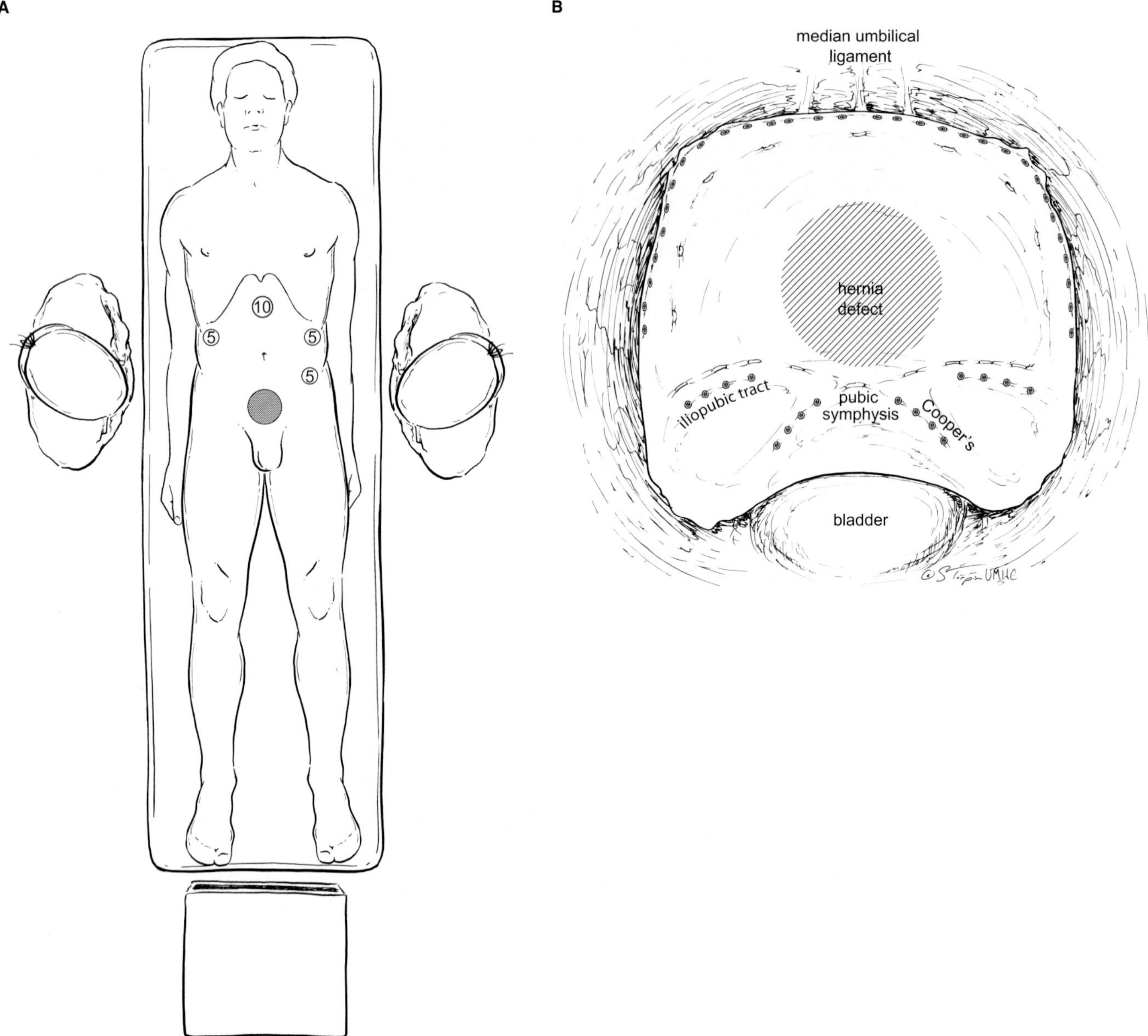

Fig. 54-5. A. Trocar and operating room positioning for hernias below the umbilicus. **B.** Example of a completed suprapubic hernia repair. Note the extension of mesh below the pubic symphysis and Cooper ligament and the extra fixation along the iliopubic tract.

VARIATIONS OF HERNIA TYPES

Suprapubic Hernias

Suprapubic hernias require additional mesh coverage inferiorly into the pelvis to avoid increased potential for recurrence when the mesh is fixed only to the pubis (Fig. 54-5B). For repair of small suprapubic hernias, the initial 10-mm trocar can be placed in the upper midline. The peritoneum is divided and dissected off the rectus muscles bilaterally down to the pubis. The peritoneum and bladder are then displaced posteriorly and inferiorly, exposing the Cooper ligament bilaterally. An extra 6 to 10 cm of mesh are placed into the pelvis and fixed permanently to the Cooper ligament bilaterally. Inferolaterally, standard full-thickness abdominal wall suture fixation may be performed at or just superior to the inguinal ligament bilaterally.

Lumbar/Flank Hernias

The patient is placed in the lateral position for lateral abdominal wall hernias (Fig. 54-6A). These hernias may occur primarily or, more commonly, following flank incisions for nephrectomy or iliac crest bone harvest. The peritoneum is incised and reflected posterior and medial to stay in the plane between the retroperitoneal organs and the paraspinal musculature. After adequate dissection, mesh is fixed with full-thickness sutures to the paraspinous muscles between the costal margin and the iliac crest (Fig. 54-6B). Inferiomedially, the mesh may be fixed to the ipsilateral Cooper ligament and, with sutures, superior to the inguinal ligament. Alternately, the mesh is fixed to the iliac crest with sutures passed through drilled holes or with bone anchors. Standard fixation techniques are used for the medial and superior edges of the mesh. For flank hernias that are near the costal margin, mesh may be placed up to the diaphragm

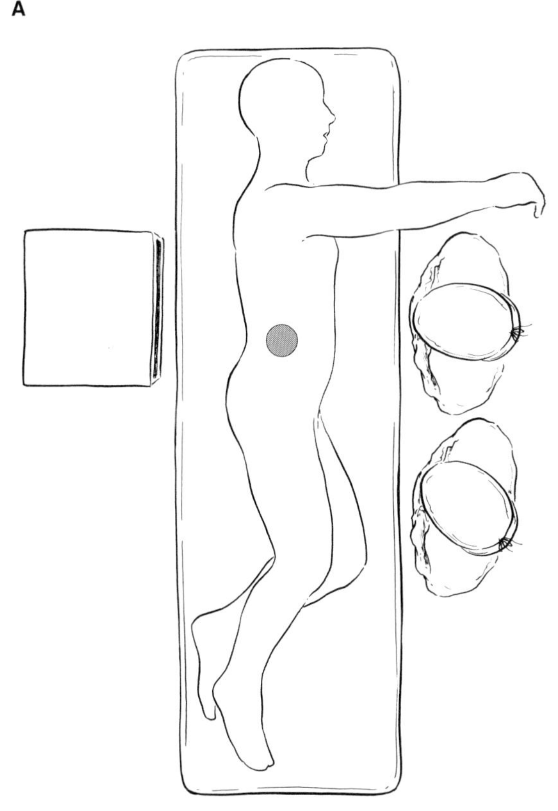

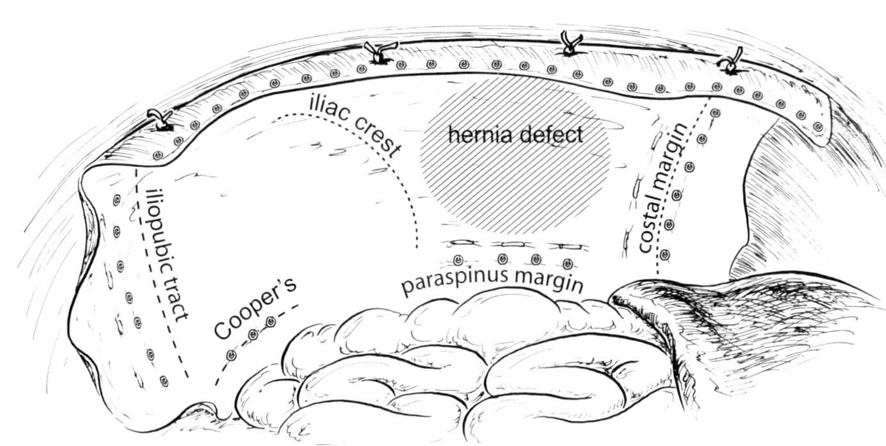

Fig. 54-6. A. Patient positioning and operating room setup for repair of flank hernias. **B.** Retaining orientation to bony structures can be difficult during repair of flank hernias. This schematic demonstrates these relationships when the patient is in the lateral position, as well as the sites of point and suture fixation.

with point fixation to the ribs and suture fixation at the costal margin.

Subxiphoid Hernia

Subxiphoid incisional hernias are frequently seen in patients with previous mediastinal chest tubes following coronary artery bypass graft or other cardiac surgery. In small subxiphoid hernias, the umbilicus may be used for the initial 10-mm trocar. As with most upper abdominal hernias, the falciform ligament should be divided to allow for mesh coverage flush with the anterior abdominal wall. Sutures are placed on either side of the xiphoid process with 4 to 6 cm of mesh extending superior to the sutures, providing adequate overlap superior to the defect (Fig. 54-7B, page 546). Fixation of the mesh to the anterior abdominal wall superior to the xiphoid process can be accomplished with tacks and/or sutures, taking care to avoid mesh fixation into the diaphragm, especially in the vicinity of the heart. Tacking along the posterior surface of a rib can aid fixation. Additional sutures are placed immediately below the coastal margin bilaterally. Standard fixation techniques are utilized for the inferior and lateral edges of the mesh.

Parastomal Hernia

Parastomal hernias can be repaired laparoscopically with minimal change in the described technique. Careful attention should be paid to dissecting the hernia sac away from the colon. Without cutting a slit in the mesh, the hernia is covered and the limb of bowel is brought out of the edge of the mesh (Fig. 54-8B and C, page 547). Sutures are used to fix the mesh at either side of the bowel to prevent internal hernias. An alternate technique described by LeBlanc uses two pieces of mesh with slits in opposite directions, designed to minimize the risk of recurrence through the mesh slit.

VARIATIONS IN TECHNIQUE

No Sutures

Some surgeons have advocated laparoscopic mesh placement without suture fixation. Reasons to avoid the use of suture fixation include the potential for bleeding caused by the suture-passing instrument and the potential for postoperative pain caused by the suture. Carbajo has described a "double-crown" technique in which two circumferential rows of tacks are placed to provide fixation. Published results show low recurrence rates; however, suture fixation was actually used in selected patients. Other surgeons propose that sutures are unnecessary with certain types of polypropylene mesh because of excellent ingrowth into the abdominal wall. However, many cases of mesh migration and contraction of various types of mesh are seen clinically, and the fact that the mesh is being fixed to the mobile peritoneum, not directly to the fascia, would argue for the use of suture fixation regardless of the type of mesh used.

Choice of Mesh

The optimal mesh for laparoscopic ventral hernia repair placement requires a mesh with two unique characteristics. The side of the mesh toward the abdominal wall is usually placed directly on the peritoneum and ideally will incorporate through the peritoneum and preperitoneal fat into the abdominal wall fascia with significant strength to minimize migration and therefore

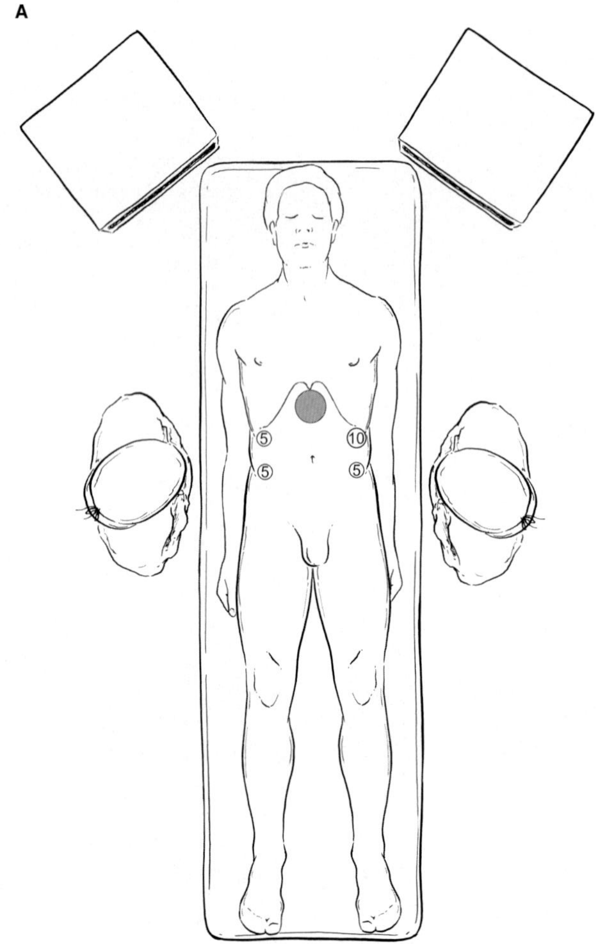

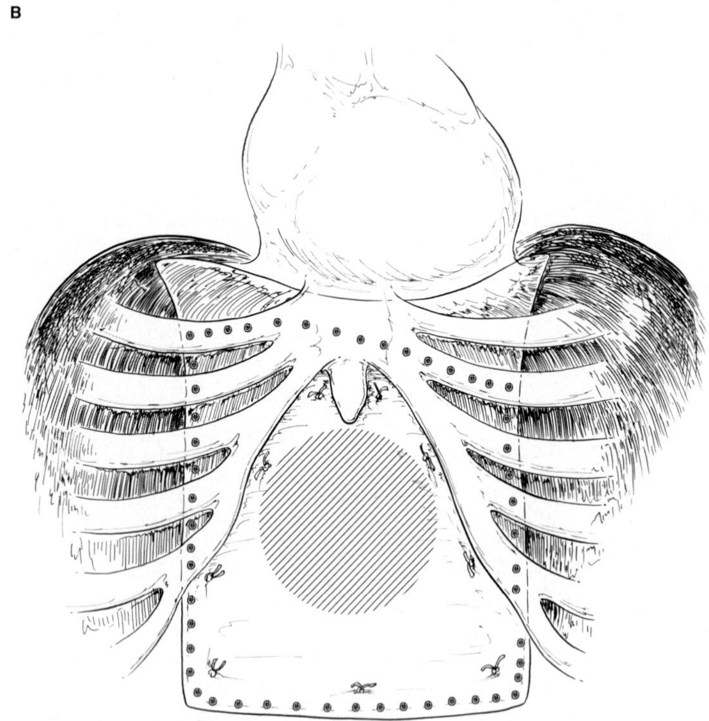

Fig. 54-7. A. Patient positioning and operating room setup for repair of subxiphoid hernias. In small hernias the umbilicus can be used for the 10-mm port site. **B.** Extra mesh is allowed to extend superiorly towards the dome of the diaphragm. The first fixation sutures are placed on either side of the xiphoid process. Superior tack fixation is performed following the posterior rib surface, with the location of the pericardium well in mind.

recurrence. On the visceral side, the mesh will ideally minimize adherence of the abdominal contents and, most importantly, prevent the ingrowth of any adherent organ to help eliminate long-term complications. These opposing characteristics make it difficult to create the ideal mesh.

Although not ideal, there are numerous meshes currently available that are appropriate for intraabdominal placement. Expanded poly-tetraflouoro-ethylene (ePTFE) solid mesh has been used for over a decade in this situation, and the significant advantage of this type of mesh is the lack of ingrowth on the side placed toward the abdominal cavity. However, there is also less ingrowth on the abdominal wall side, necessitating secure fixation. There are many clinical publications documenting the use of this mesh with good outcomes.

A variety of "composite" mesh materials have been developed to promote ingrowth into the abdominal wall and prevent adhesions and/or ingrowth of the abdominal viscera. These products consist of a macroporous mesh that allows for collagen ingrowth on the abdominal wall side and some form of barrier on the visceral side. Polypropylene (hydrophobic) and polyester (hydrophilic) meshes are the most common in this category. The barriers include a thin layer of ePTFE or an absorbable anti-adhesion film. A number of these films have been developed, including products that are collagen-based or utilize oxidized regenerated cellulose.

The common assumption that mesh remains inert when placed in vivo is being challenged, and a focus on materials that are "lightweight" is another trend in modern mesh. (Working in collaboration with biomaterials engineers, our materials- characterization lab has shown that essentially all hernia meshes, especially heavyweight polypropylene, undergo chemical changes caused by oxidation in the body. These reactions result in degradation of mesh and physical changes that may cause significant contraction and can make mesh stiff and brittle.) These lightweight meshes are still several times stronger than the native abdominal wall, but reduce the total load of foreign body that may stimulate a chronic inflammatory reaction. Mesh made with other polymers that are more hydrophilic than polypropylene, such as polyester, and mesh with coatings on lightweight polypropylene are also being used.

The number of biologic mesh materials available is multiplying rapidly and eventually may come to play a role in primary laparoscopic ventral hernia repair. Currently, the most common indication for biologic mesh is a hernia repair in an infected or

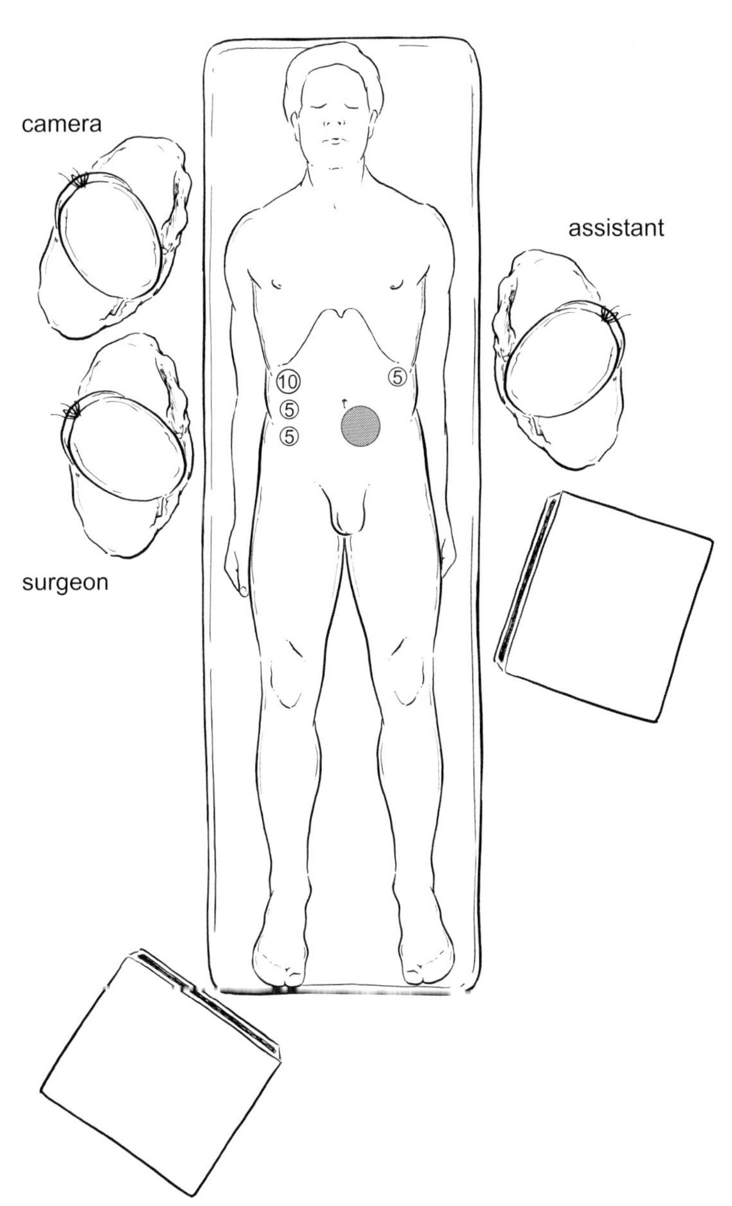

contaminated operative field due to previously placed mesh that has become infected, or after an enterotomy. The clinical data available to evaluate the biologic mesh is growing, but does not yet support the primary use of these materials at this time, especially when cost is considered.

INTRAOPERATIVE PITFALLS

Adhesions

The potential for increased difficulty and danger due to severe dense adhesions has been mentioned. For the surgeon without significant laparoscopic experience, the best way to avoid complications associated with difficult adhesiolysis is to select patients unlikely to have complex adhesions.

Bleeding during adhesiolysis should be isolated and controlled with clips or endoloops or possibly with thermal energy when bowel or other organs are not near the site of bleeding. Bleeding that cannot be controlled laparoscopically requires conversion to an open procedure.

As in open surgery, enterotomy during laparoscopic adhesiolysis is likely to occur at some point in a surgeon's experience. When encountering an enterotomy, surgeons must use their best judgment given their experience and their patient's situation. Conversion to an open procedure is always an option and should not be considered a failure. Alternately, a small incision may be created to allow for repair of the enterotomy. Following abdominal wall closure, the procedure may proceed as a laparoscopic-assisted repair. For the experienced laparoscopic surgeon, a laparoscopic repair of the enterotomy utilizing laparoscopic suturing techniques may be appropriate.

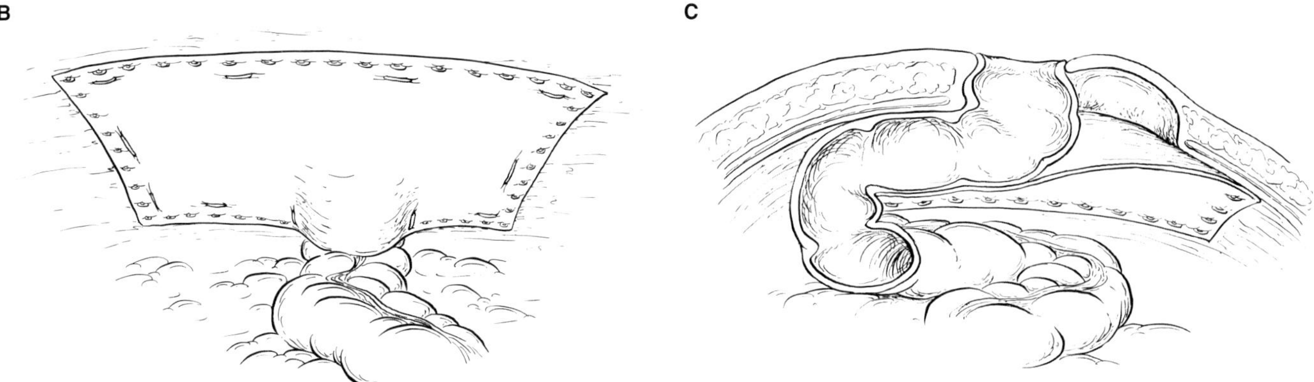

Fig. 54-8. A. Patient positioning and operating room setup for repair of parastomal hernias. The patient should be well secured, as the table may be rotated into a steep lateral position. **B.** Finished view after mesh placement for the Sugarbaker (nonslit) technique for repair of parastomal hernias. Note the two fixation sutures on either side of the bowel. **C.** Cutaway view demonstrating the course of the bowel prior to emerging from the edge of the mesh.

The decision whether or not to place mesh following an enterotomy also requires good judgment. The size of the enterotomy, degree of spillage, and the portion of the bowel injured all play a role in the decision. One option is to repair the injury and complete the adhesiolysis but to delay mesh placement. The patient is admitted to the hospital for observation and for antibiotics and returned to the operating room for laparoscopic mesh placement 2 to 6 days later. Placing a biologic mesh at the time of enterotomy repair is another option.

Suture-Site Bleeding

The suture-passing instrument used to secure the mesh can cause bleeding in the abdominal wall (notoriously at the epigastric vessels). Direct pressure and/or tying the suture will usually stop this abdominal wall bleeding. If bleeding persists, additional sutures above and below the site of bleeding will usually control the bleeding.

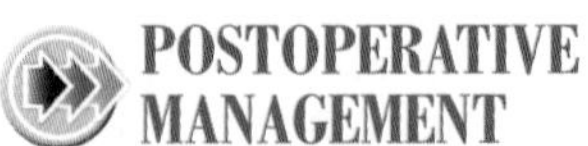

POSTOPERATIVE MANAGEMENT

Patients are given clear liquids postoperatively and advanced to a regular diet as tolerated. Early ambulation is encouraged, and return to normal activities is limited only by the patient's degree of pain and discomfort. Patients with repair of relatively small ventral hernias often go home the day of surgery, whereas those with repair of larger ventral hernias require a hospital stay.

For large ventral hernia repairs, adequate pain control will almost always require intravenous (IV) narcotics such as patient-controlled analgesia devices (PCAs). Placing an epidural preoperatively in patients with large hernias may provide equivalent or better pain control during the most painful immediate post-op period. During the early postoperative period, pulmonary toilet with frequent use of incentive spirometry is encouraged and sequential compression devices (SCDs) are frequently maintained until the patient is ambulating. Patients who are ambulating well, tolerating a diet, and able to control pain with oral analgesics alone are discharged from the hospital.

Abdominal binders can provide patients with support of their abdominal wall, which may reduce some discomfort due to movement. Additionally, the gentle compression may help reduce, although not eliminate, postoperative seromas.

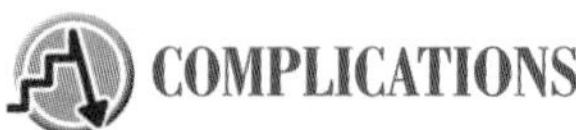

COMPLICATIONS

Ileus

Patients requiring extensive adhesiolysis or those with very large defects are at risk for a postoperative ileus. Most patients with an ileus will require intravenous hydration and, possibly, suppositories or oral cathartics for return of bowel function. A nasogastric tube may be required for severe ileus. Internal herniation between the mesh and the abdominal wall is a rare complication that presents with symptoms similar to acute bowel obstruction and can occur if fixation devices fail. This may be mistaken for a severe ileus, and a persistent ileus may warrant follow-up with imaging.

Seroma

The presence of a seroma is common, especially after repair of a large hernia defect. Because fluid will naturally fill the empty space created by reducing hernia contents in laparoscopic ventral hernia repair, essentially all patients will have a seroma unless the space is obliterated. In general, seromas are not considered a complication. Most seromas resolve without therapy and rarely produce symptoms. It is important to explain to the patient that the "bulge" is not a recurrent hernia. Seromas are usually significantly improved within 6 to 8 weeks after surgery, although very large seromas can take several months to resolve. Rarely, a symptomatic or persistent seroma is aspirated. A sterile technique is essential to avoid secondary mesh infection.

Most surgeons would not attempt to drain a seroma within the first 2 to 3 months. If a symptomatic seroma recurs after 2 to 4 aspiration attempts, additional radiographic evaluation or reoperation should be considered. Although fibrin glue, cauterization of the hernia sac and other attempts have been used to decrease seroma rates, none have been uniformly adopted. Encouraging the patient to wear a binder with or without a bulky dressing to compress the empty space is the most common strategy used by surgeons to decrease seroma formation.

In rare cases, patients develop a "mesh allergy," where the peritoneum actively secretes fluid in response to the presence of mesh. These seromas are typically below the mesh and may require surgery to drain the seroma or to remove the offending mesh.

Suture Site Pain

After the initial pain of the procedure resolves, it is not uncommon for patients to experience pain at one or more of the suture sites. Typically, this pain will resolve with time and conservative therapy. For severe or persistent suture site pain, an injection of a combination of short- and long-acting local anesthetic usually leads to resolution of the pain. Occasionally, repeat injections are required for permanent pain relief. Suture site pain can present or recur up to several months after the operation, usually due to increased activity. It is very rare to need to remove a suture for pain control.

Bleeding

Significant postoperative bleeding is rare because brisk bleeding is usually visualized during the procedure. In the largest study to date, Fewer than 2% of patients required blood transfusions in the postoperative period. This could be a result of intraabdominal bleeding from raw surfaces after extensive adhesiolysis, omental bleeding, or abdominal wall bleeding from injury to inferior epigastric vessels or muscular branches. This type of bleeding is almost always self-limiting, and reoperation rarely results in identification of a specific source of active bleeding. The patient will often experience significant bruising in the pelvis and/or flanks as the hematoma resolves. As with all patients, suspected postoperative bleeding in a patient who is hemodynamically unstable requires aggressive intervention for diagnosis and definitive treatment.

Missed or Delayed Bowel Injury

A missed or delayed bowel injury should be suspected in a patient who has worsening abdominal pain and tenderness and begins to show signs of sepsis, such as elevated temperature and white blood cell count, tachycardia, and decreasing urine output and blood pressure during the first few days after surgery. Other potential causes of the patient's worsening condition should be evaluated. An intraabdominal source must be considered, especially in patients who required extensive adhesiolysis. Close monitoring and radiographic evaluation, including a CT scan, may be appropriate in stable patients, although the decision to reoperate should be made in a relatively short period of time, depending on the results of resuscitation, diagnostic testing, and close monitoring. A missed or delayed enterotomy and the resulting intraabdominal sepsis can be fatal even when diagnosed and repaired in a timely fashion.

Recurrence

The recurrence rate for this procedure is excellent compared to published results for a variety of open ventral hernia repairs. In the largest series of laparoscopic hernia repair, the recurrence rate was less than 5% and included cases performed during each surgeon's learning curve. The range of recurrence rates in the surgical literature for laparoscopic ventral hernia repair is from 1.1% to 17.7%. Theoretically, the repair should have no recurrence if the basic principles of clear visualization, wide coverage, and secure fixation are adhered to. The common causes of recurrence are technical: a missed hernia from lack of visualization of the entire abdominal wall, inadequate mesh coverage leading to mesh eventration out of the defect, and inadequate mesh fixation resulting in failure to cover the defect at one edge of the mesh or migration of a portion or all of the mesh. We have also experienced another mechanism of recurrence due to lack of secure fixation. In giant ventral hernias, it is often necessary to sew multiple pieces of mesh together to achieve adequate coverage. During laparoscopic reoperation for a recurrent ventral hernia, we found that the suture used to sew two pieces of mesh together had broken. We now use interrupted sutures in addition to running permanent sutures when multiple pieces of mesh are required.

Acknowledgment

The authors thank Stacy Turpin for contributing the illustrations to this chapter.

CONCLUSION

The laparoscopic approach for ventral hernia repair has achieved widespread acceptance based on excellent clinical results, especially when compared to traditional open techniques. A low combined recurrence and wound complication rate differentiates it from most open repairs. As with other advanced laparoscopic procedures, safe adoption of the technique requires appropriate training and patient selection. As we continue to gain experience with this procedure and with further advances in equipment and mesh, our hope is that clinical results will continue to improve.

SUGGESTED READING

Carbajo MA, del Olma JC, Blanco JI, et al. Laparoscopic approach to incisional hernia. Lessons learned from 270 patients over 8 years. *Surg Endosc* 2003;17:118–122.

Constanza MJ, Heniford BT, Arca MJ, et al. Laparoscopic repair of recurrent ventral hernias. *Am Surg* 1998;64:1121–1127.

Costello CR, Bachman SL, Ramshaw BJ, et al. Materials characterization of explanted polypropylene hernia meshes. *J Biomed Mater Res Part B: Appl Biomater* 2007;83:44–49.

DeMaria EJ, Moss JM, Sugerman HJ. Laparoscopic intraperitoneal polytetraflouoroethylene (PTFE) prosthetic patch repair of ventral hernia. Prospective comparison to open prefascial polypropylene mesh repair. *Surg Endosc* 2000;14:326–329.

Heniford BT, Park A, Ramshaw BJ, et al. Laparoscopic repair of ventral hernias: nine years' experience with 850 consecutive hernias. *Ann Surg* 2003;238:391–400.

Klosterhalfen B, Junge K, Klinge U. The lightweight and large porous mesh concept for hernia repair. *Expert Rev Med Devices* 2005; 2(1):1–15.

Koehler RH, Voeller G. Recurrences in laparoscopic incisional hernia repairs: a personal series and review of the literature. *JSLS* 1999; 3:293–304.

LeBlanc KA. Incisional hernia repair; laparoscopic techniques. *World J Surg* 2005;29: 1073–1079.

LeBlanc KA. Laparoscopic incisional and ventral hernia repair: complications—how to avoid and handle. *Hernia* 2004;8:323–331.

Perrone JM, Soper NJ, Eagon JC, et al. Perioperative outcomes and complications of laparoscopic ventral hernia repair. *Surgery* 2005; 138:708–716.

Ramshaw BJ, Esartia P, Schwab JL, et al. Comparison of laparoscopic and open ventral hernias. *Am Surg* 1999;65:827–832.

Toy FK, Bailey RW, Carey S, et al. Prospective, multicenter study of laparoscopic ventral hernioplasty. Preliminary results. *Surg Endosc* 1998;12:955–959.

COMMENTARY

Laparoscopic ventral hernia repair is a procedure for which the concept seems remarkably simple yet the technical challenges and potential for complications are daunting. In more complex patients the surgeon can encounter a morbidly obese individual who has undergone more than 20 abdominal operations. Multiple attempts at abdominal wall repair with a variety of prosthetic materials are a frequent part of the patient history. Longstanding large hernias could have led to loss of domain, and the multiple medical diseases present can make wound healing less than optimal. The surgeon who approaches this patient must be adept at extensive adhesiolysis, possess the ability to dissect bowel from old mesh, and be prepared to stage the procedures and possibly utilize chronic pneumoperitoneum to overcome loss of domain issues.

Few, if any, surgeons have mastered this field as has been done by one of the authors, Bruce Ramshaw. Dr. Ramshaw provides our readers with a basic understanding of the issues related to the repair of more routine ventral hernias. He then provides readers with pearls from his vast experience and expertise in dealing with difficult patients. Both authors are true experts in materials used for hernia repair. Their groundbreaking work in materials characterization and the development of biologic and synthetic hernia repair materials has been widely recognized.

The surgeon who chooses to repair ventral hernias on an infrequent basis should develop a strong appreciation for the potential for life-threatening complications. Missed bowel injuries can lead to sepsis and death. Additionally, attempts to limit the use of energy sources during adhesiolysis in an attempt to avoid bowel injury can lead to bleeding and hemodynamic instability. Furthermore, one can perform a safe and seemingly effective procedure and then have the patient reappear with hernia recurrence. Rarely during the repair of ventral hernias will anything be done to address the underlying problems that led to the development of a hernia. The patient, therefore, remains at high risk to develop new hernias or recurrent hernias.

The authors have provided us with the current state of care for the laparoscopic repair of ventral hernias. These same authors will be the first to state that tremendous opportunities exist for improvements in our techniques, the understanding of hernia formation, and materials used to repair these defects.

WSE

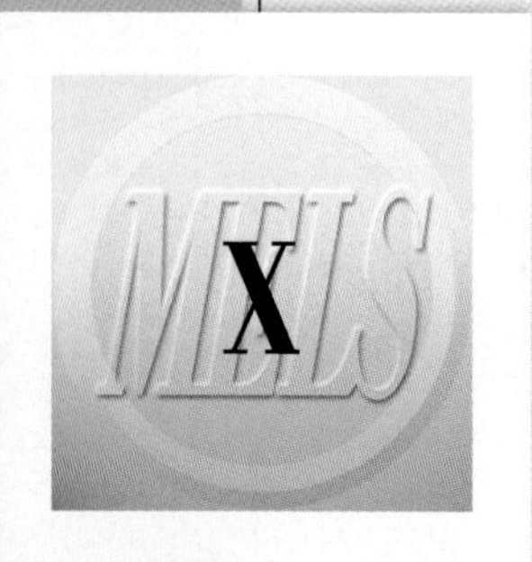

X Thoracic Surgery

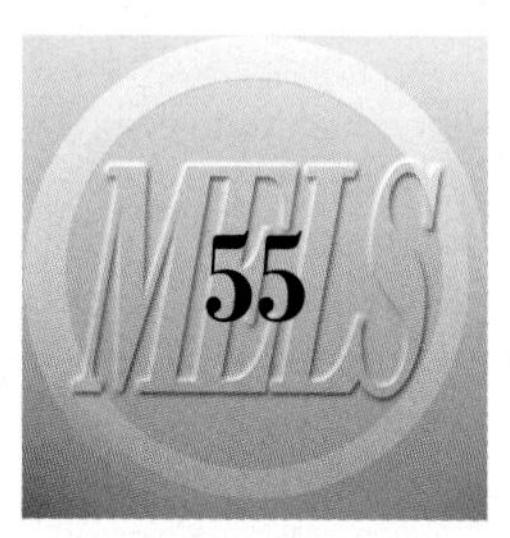

55 Thoracoscopic Surgery of the Mediastinum and Esophagus

GORDON BUDUHAN AND RICHARD J. FINLEY

INTRODUCTION

The growth of video-assisted thoracic surgery (VATS) over the past several years has given the thoracic surgeon an alternate approach in the management of diseases of the mediastinum. Thoracoscopy for mediastinal disease offers the potential advantages of smaller incisions, decreased pain and analgesic requirements, and a shortened hospital stay compared with conventional open thoracotomy or sternotomy approaches. Visualization within the mediastinum with the aid of the angled thoracoscope is often superior to open techniques, where exposure is limited by the rigid bony thorax. Virtually all diseases of the mediastinum may be approached with a VATS approach, depending on the expertise of the treating surgeon in minimally invasive surgery (Table 55-1).

Thoracoscopy

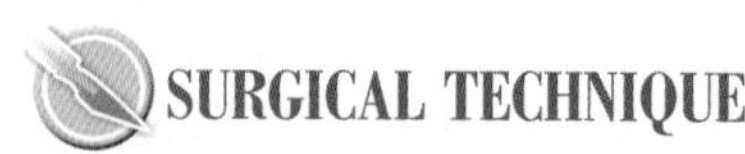

SURGICAL TECHNIQUE

General anesthesia with endotracheal intubation using a double-lumen tube is used to allow single-lung ventilation on the nonoperative side and deflation of the ipsilateral lung. For shorter cases, the use of a regular endotracheal tube with either intermittent apnea or low-pressure (8 mmHg) carbon dioxide (CO_2) insufflation may provide reasonable exposure of the mediastinum. Although positioning of the patient ultimately depends upon the precise location of the target area, our general preference is to place the patient in lateral decubitus position with the bed flexed to open up the intercostal spaces for port placement (Fig. 55-1).

TABLE 55-1. COMMON LESIONS OF THE MEDIASTINUM AND ESOPHAGUS

Mediastinum			
Anterior	**Middle**	**Posterior**	**Esophagus**
Thymoma, myasthenia gravis, thymic cyst	Lymphoma	Neurogenic tumors: nerve sheath, paraganglioma, neurofibroma	Leiomyoma
Lymphoma	Bronchogenic cysts	Lymphoma	Diverticula
Germ cell tumors	Pericardial cysts	Neuroenteric cyst	Duplication cysts
Thyroid: substernal extension, ectopic	Granuloma		Carcinoma
Parathyroid adenoma	Hamartoma		

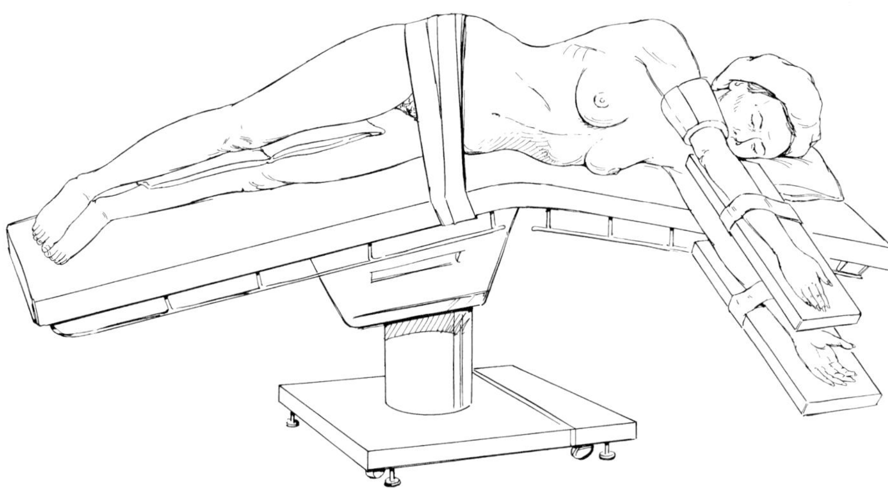

Fig. 55-1. A typical lateral decubitus patient placement for most thoracoscopic approaches to the mediastinum.

Optimal port placement is one of the most important technical factors for any minimally invasive operation. In general, three trocars are placed to "triangulate" the target area with the apex being the approximate field of dissection (Fig. 55-2). Careful preoperative study of available imaging is necessary in order to decide where to place the necessary ports. Another variation is to use two 5-mm trocars and one 12-mm trocar, which will accommodate the 5-mm 30-degree angled thoracoscope and two working ports. The 12-mm port incision allows passage of a thoracoscopic stapler if necessary, facilitates extraction of specimens, and may be used as the site for chest tube insertion at the conclusion of the operation. During the operation, several general principles may be noted:

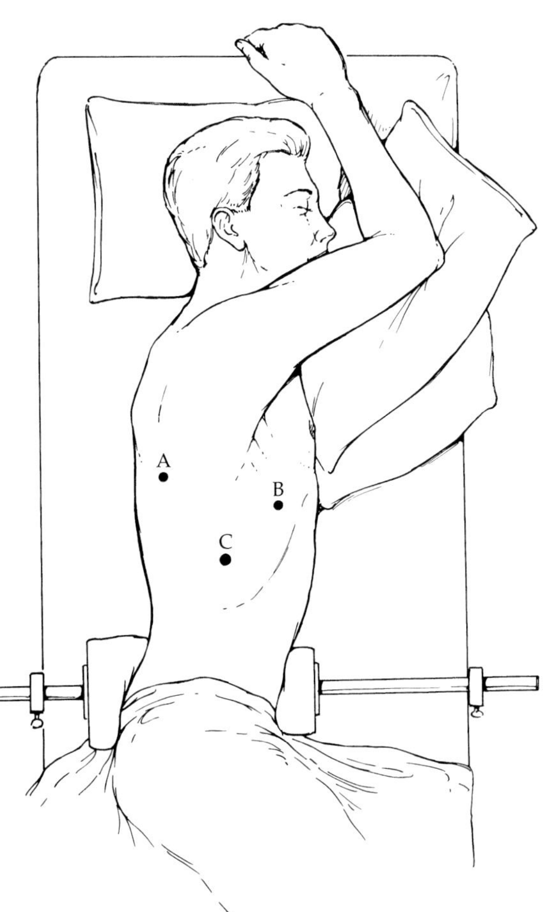

Fig. 55-2. Port positioning using triangulation. Ports A and B point are cephalad at the apex of an imaginary triangle. Port C is used for the thoracoscope. The instruments and camera can be moved at different ports to facilitate different parts of the procedure.

1. Precise port placement is necessary to facilitate both exposure and ease of dissection. It is important that instruments approach the target area in a perpendicular manner. Imprecise placement of the trocars leads to excessive levering of the instruments against the ribs, which greatly contributes to postoperative incisional pain. If initial port placement is suboptimal, additional port(s) should be placed under direct vision. Once port site incisions are made, instruments may be inserted directly through the incisions without trocars to minimize levering and allow use of larger instruments (e.g., staplers, scissors).
2. For thoracoscopy, the patient is usually placed in lateral decubitus position with the body held in place with sandbags or a deflatable beanbag and the bed flexed to open up the space between the costal margin and iliac crest. The reverse-Trendelenburg position allows the diaphragm to fall back and expose the operative field. Exposure can be further facilitated by angling the operating table appropriately. For anterior and middle mediastinal masses, the patient may be placed in the lateral decubitus supine position, tilting the patient slightly dorsally (that is, patient's back towards the floor) to allow the ipsilateral lung to fall away (Fig. 55-3, page 552). Similarly, in VATS for posterior mediastinal masses and esophageal diseases the patient is placed in lateral decubitus prone position and rotated ventrally (chest rotated toward floor) to achieve optimal exposure of the target area. Note that securing the patient on the bed (beanbags, tape) is essential to prevent inadvertent slippage during bed manipulation.
3. Skin incisions for ports should be just large enough to allow passage of the port. Excessively large incisions may allow the trocars to become dislodged when instruments are withdrawn.
4. All instruments entering the thorax should be visualized upon entry and exit to avoid inadvertent injury to vital structures.

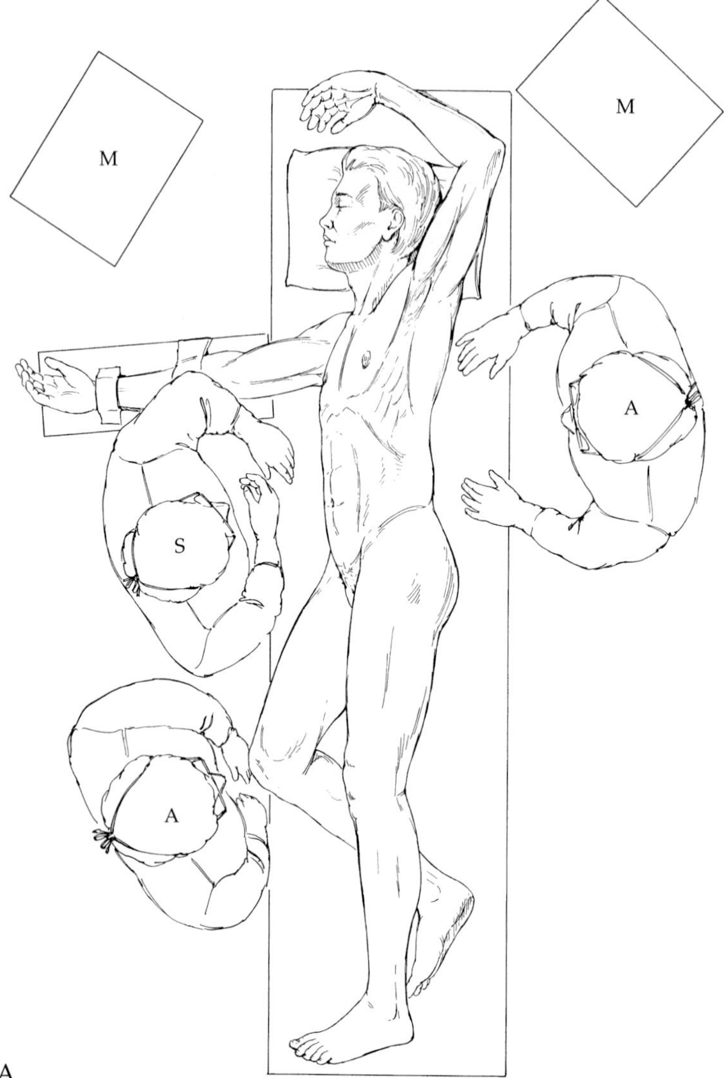

Fig. 55-3. Sometimes the lateral decubitus supine position, with the patient rolled slightly backwards, is advantageous. S, surgeon; A, assistant; M, monitor.

5. As in all minimally invasive cases, optimal visualization is essential. Common technical problems such as camera lens fogging can usually be minimized by use of an anti-fog solution applied to the lens or by simply warming the instrument with warm saline prior to insertion.
6. Extraction of specimens: Larger specimens are best extracted through a port site placed in the anterior aspect of the intercostal space, which is larger than the posterior aspect. The excised tissue should be placed in a bag to facilitate removal and to prevent port site seeding in cases of malignancy. Small benign specimens may be extracted without a bag, but it is helpful to withdraw the instrument until the specimen is partially or fully shielded by the 12-mm trocar, which is then removed along with the lesion.

MEDIASTINAL MASSES–ANTERIOR

The anterior mediastinum is bound superiorly by the thoracic inlet, inferiorly by the diaphragm, anteriorly from the sternum to the anterior pericardium, and laterally by the phrenic nerves. The most common anterior mediastinal masses are listed in Table 55-1, with thymomas being the most frequent. The four **Ts** of anterior mediastinal masses are **t**hymoma, **t**eratoma or germ cell tumor, "**t**errible" lymphoma, and **t**hyroid; one must keep a broad differential in mind when working up any mediastinal mass. Often these lesions are found incidentally, frequently during workup of local (pain, dyspnea, stridor) or constitutional symptoms (fever, night sweats). In the setting of mediastinal lymphadenopathy, the thoracic surgeon is called upon to make a definitive histologic diagnosis after an exhaustive workup—including image-guided needle biopsy—remains equivocal (Fig. 55-4).

While diagnosis and staging of mediastinal masses are the more common VATS procedures for the anterior mediastinum, thoracoscopy may also play a therapeutic role in management. While the treatment of malignant mediastinal germ cell tumors is usually nonoperative, a residual nonseminomatous germ cell tumor mass following treatment with combination chemotherapy may require resection.

Thymectomy for myaesthenia gravis (MG) may also be approached thoracoscopically. Although there is some debate regarding the ability of achieving a complete resection with a VATS thymectomy, centers with considerable experience in VATS have reported equivalent results compared with transsternal or transcervical approaches. Masaoka stage 1 thymomas may also be completely resected via VATS, although this approach remains controversial. Transsternal thymectomy is the standard approach for suspected thymomas.

A thyroid goiter or malignancy may extend substernally and cause compression of the trachea. Rarely, an ectopic intrathoracic thyroid tumor may develop separate from the cervical thyroid. Most intrathoracic thyroid goiters or malignancies can usually be excised through the neck. If the intrathoracic tumor cannot be safely dissected through the neck, a VATS approach may be used to mobilize the thoracic component.

Parathyroid adenomas may be found in ectopic locations within the chest in 1% to 2% of patients with primary hyperparathyroidism and are a common cause of

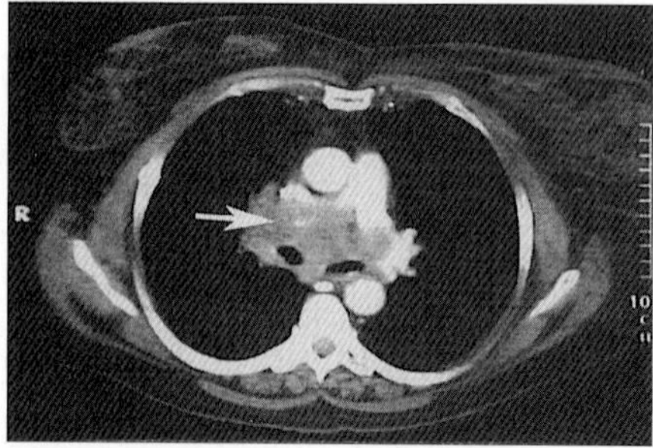

Fig. 55-4. The arrow points to an extensive mediastinal lymphadenopathy. Following thoracoscopic biopsy, a diagnosis of small-cell lung cancer was made.

persistent hypercalcemia following neck exploration. The most common intrathoracic parathyroid is an inferior gland that had descended within the thyrothymic ligament or thymus, although cases of parathyroid adenomas in the subaortic and pretracheal regions have been noted. Imaging studies, including ultrasound, computed tomography (CT) scan, and technetium–99m sestamibi scintigraphy, are essential to diagnosis and in planning the operative approach to excision of mediastinal parathyroid glands. The use of intraoperative parathyroid hormone (PTH) assays has been well described for excision of cervical parathyroid adenomas. Similar techniques may be utilized in VATS exploration and the excision of mediastinal parathyroid adenomas to guide resection and confirm complete removal of the offending gland.

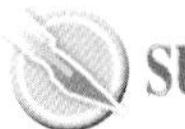

SURGICAL TECHNIQUE

Careful study of the available imaging is essential when planning the operative approach to a VATS biopsy or resection of an anterior mediastinal mass. Depending on its location, a right- or left-sided approach may be utilized. Our own preference to access a midline anterior mediastinal mass is through the right hemithorax, as the heart does not obscure exploration and the superior vena cava and innominate vein are easily identified and serve as landmarks. A standard VATS setup is used, with the patient in the lateral decubitus supine position and one-lung ventilation with a double-lumen tube. Trocars are placed in the posterior axillary line in the third to sixth interspaces, triangulating them with the target lesion as the apex. Diagnostic biopsies by VATS may be preceded by needle aspiration of the lesion to avoid injuring vital structures. Diagnostic specimens are sent for frozen section before concluding the procedure to ensure that a confirmatory histological diagnosis is obtained. A chest tube is placed if there has been extensive dissection within the mediastinum or if there is concern for iatrogenic lung injury.

VATS THYMECTOMY

The positioning and trocar placement are identical to the technique described above. A right- or left-sided approach may be used, depending on the particular location and orientation of the target lesion. After general exploration with the 30-degree thoracoscope, the first structure identified is the phrenic nerve, which runs along the lateral surface of the pericardium. Dissection of the thymus gland off the pericardium is begun anterior to the phrenic nerve at its inferior pole (Fig. 55-5). Continuing this plane cephalad, the thymus is elevated off the pericardium. One or more thymic veins will be encountered draining from the innominate vein, which are doubly ligated with endoclips (Fig. 55-6, page 554). Anterior mobilization of the thymus off the sternum is then performed after incising the mediastinal pleura. Arterial branches of the internal mammary and inferior thyroid arteries supplying the superior poles of the thymus are ligated with clips. Mobilization of the superior poles may be technically difficult as the uppermost limit lies at the base of the neck. One option is to also use a transcervical incision in order to fully dissect out the upper poles of the thymus. Care must be taken when mobilizing the upper poles in order to avoid inadvertent avulsion of the inferior thyroid veins, which lie just posterior to the thymus. During dissection of the gland, it is important to stay extracapsular and to incorporate a wide margin of perithymic tissue so as not to leave behind residual gland. The thymus can be extracted through one of the trocar sites after placing it in an endoscopic bag. A chest tube is optional. Results following thoracoscopic thymectomy for myasthenia gravis are comparable to transsternal and transcervical techniques, with comparable remission rates and decreased need for medication. There has been debate regarding the adequacy of resection margins for VATS thymectomy for thymoma. However, in specialized centers, extent of resection has been shown to be equal for both open and thoracoscopic approaches. In addition, at the time of writing there have been no reports of thymoma recurrence following VATS thymectomy in the literature. However, as previously stated, transsternal thymectomy is the preferred approach for thymomas. A further role for VATS may be in re-exploration of patients who have had a previous transsternal thymectomy but have persistent MG symptoms, obviating the need for and morbidity of a redo sternotomy.

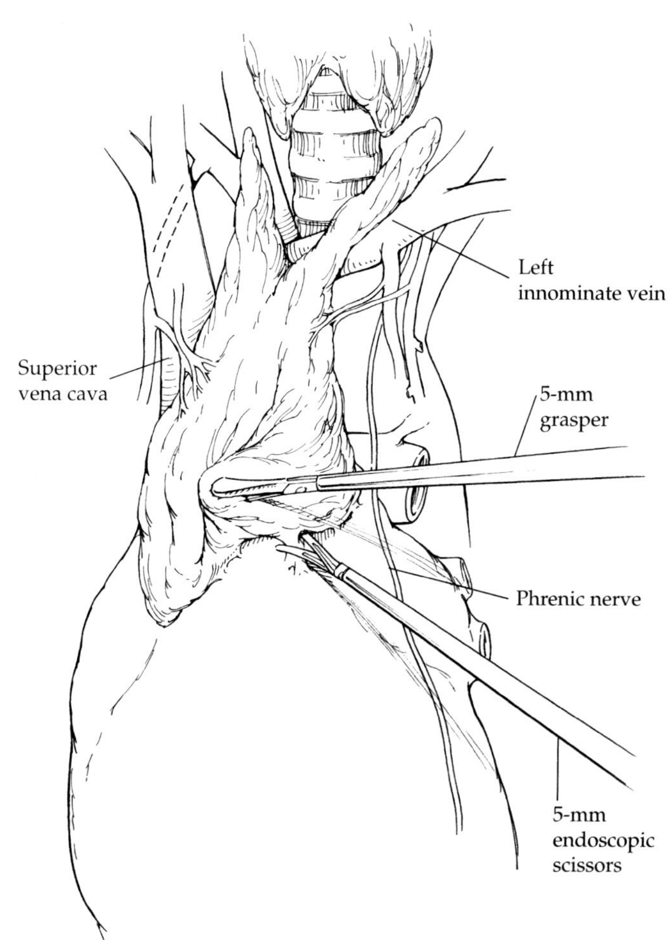

Fig. 55-5. The inferior poles of the thymus are carefully dissected anterior to the phrenic nerve.

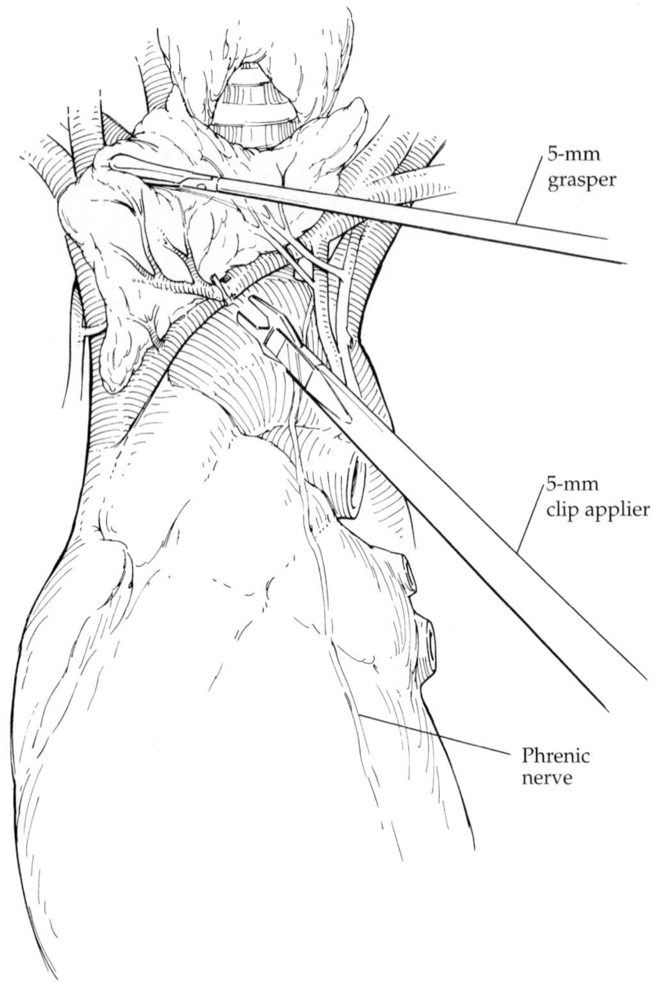

Fig. 55-6. The thymic vein branches are identified, ligated, and divided.

VATS RESECTION–MEDIASTINAL THYROID AND PARATHYROID

With caudal growth of a substernal thyroid there is glandular tissue in both the cervical area and within the mediastinum. In a combined cervical-VATS excision, the patient is positioned with the neck extended and the ipsilateral arm abducted with the bed rotated 15 degrees. After dissection of the cervical thyroid through the neck incision, the lung is collapsed using CO_2 insufflation and the intrathoracic thyroid is visualized with a camera in the fifth intercostal space, anterior axillary line. Dissection is carried out through 5-mm ports placed in the second and fifth intercostal spaces, midclavicular line. During mobilization within the anterosuperior mediastinum, care is taken to identify key adjacent structures such as the phrenic and vagus nerves and innominate vein. The vascular supply of the tumor is identified, ligated, and divided. A complete en bloc excision of an intrathoracic thyroid should be attempted, particularly if there is concern for malignancy.

The operative positioning and instrument setup for mediastinal parathyroid excision is similar to that used for a VATS thymectomy. Mediastinal parathyroid adenomas are often embedded within the thymus and are often difficult to visualize; thus, careful study of the preoperative imaging is essential. Use of intraoperative PTH rapid assays can be helpful in localization, as a "step up" in PTH level is noted when the venous catheter passes the region of the adenoma. Other centers have described using radioguided techniques with a gamma probe following injection with radiolabeled colloid to help localize the adenoma. Once the gland is located, it is carefully dissected away from surrounding structures. Small blood vessels are clipped and divided. Often, a discrete gland is not definitively visualized and a wide resection of mediastinal fatty tissue including thymic tissue and mediastinal pleura is taken in the approximate location of the gland judging from the imaging studies. Confirmation of removal of the adenoma can be done by frozen section or by noting a greater than 50% decrease in PTH level from preoperative baseline 5 minutes following excision.

MEDIASTINAL MASSES–MIDDLE

The middle mediastinal compartment is bound laterally by the left and right pleural cavities, anteriorly and posteriorly by the pericardium, superiorly by the thoracic inlet, and inferiorly by the diaphragm (see Table 55-1). Indications for thoracoscopy in the middle mediastinum may be diagnostic and/or therapeutic. In the presence of mediastinal lymphadenopathy, VATS exploration and biopsy may be required for histologic confirmation and staging of a malignancy such as lung cancer or lymphoma (see Fig. 55-4). Resection of foregut duplication cysts, most commonly bronchogenic, is indicated for symptoms of dysphagia or dyspnea from compression of adjacent viscera, infection, increasing cyst size, bleeding, and for diagnostic confirmation. Thoracoscopic pericardial window is a good treatment option for large symptomatic or recurrent pericardial effusions, especially if there is associated pulmonary or pleural pathology or if pericardial tissue is required for diagnosis.

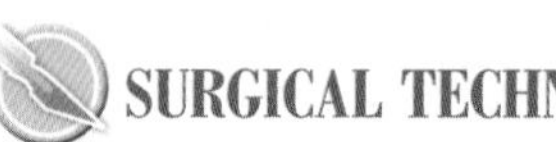

SURGICAL TECHNIQUE

The standard VATS setup is identical to that described for anterior mediastinum above. A right- or left-sided approach may be used depending on the particular location and orientation of the target lesion. Trocar placement again depends on the level of the lesion. In general, if the mass is more posterior within the mediastinum, the corresponding trocars are placed further anteriorly on the lateral chest wall to achieve optimal instrument angulation and maneuverability. Prior to beginning any dissection in the middle mediastinum, it is essential to identify the course of the phrenic nerve. The mediastinal pleura overlying the mass is incised and dissection is performed with sharp and blunt dissection with careful hemostasis. Mediastinal lymph nodes may be biopsied or excised. Aspiration of the node with a long spinal needle and syringe is useful to prevent inadvertent vessel injury. For foregut duplication cysts, complete excision is preferred, but usually the cyst has a common wall with the tracheobronchial tree or esophagus. Therefore, if the cyst wall is densely adherent to adjacent vital structures, partial excision with fulguration of the inner wall is acceptable. Placing the specimen in an endoscopic bag facilitates extraction without fear of cyst rupture and is necessary if there is suspicion of malignancy. Enlarging or symptomatic pericardial cysts may be removed in the same manner, again taking care to identify and preserve the ipsilateral phrenic nerve. The lower lobe may need to be mobilized and retracted away from the surgical field after incising the inferior pulmonary ligament. For pericardial effusions, great care is taken to avoid the phrenic nerve as the pericardium is incised after tenting it up with grasping forceps. The initial incision is made anterior and parallel to the phrenic nerve and extended from the level of the superior pulmonary vein to the diaphragm. A blunt suction catheter may be used to gently break up loculations within the pericardial sac and drain the effusion. The pericardial "window" is completed by extending the incision medially and excising the free margin (Fig. 55-7). Low-level cautery is used and care is taken to protect the heart from injury. After the pericardial flap has been excised and the effusion adequately drained, a drainage catheter is placed within the pericardial space and brought out through a port site.

A chest tube is usually placed in the pleural space after ensuring adequate hemostasis.

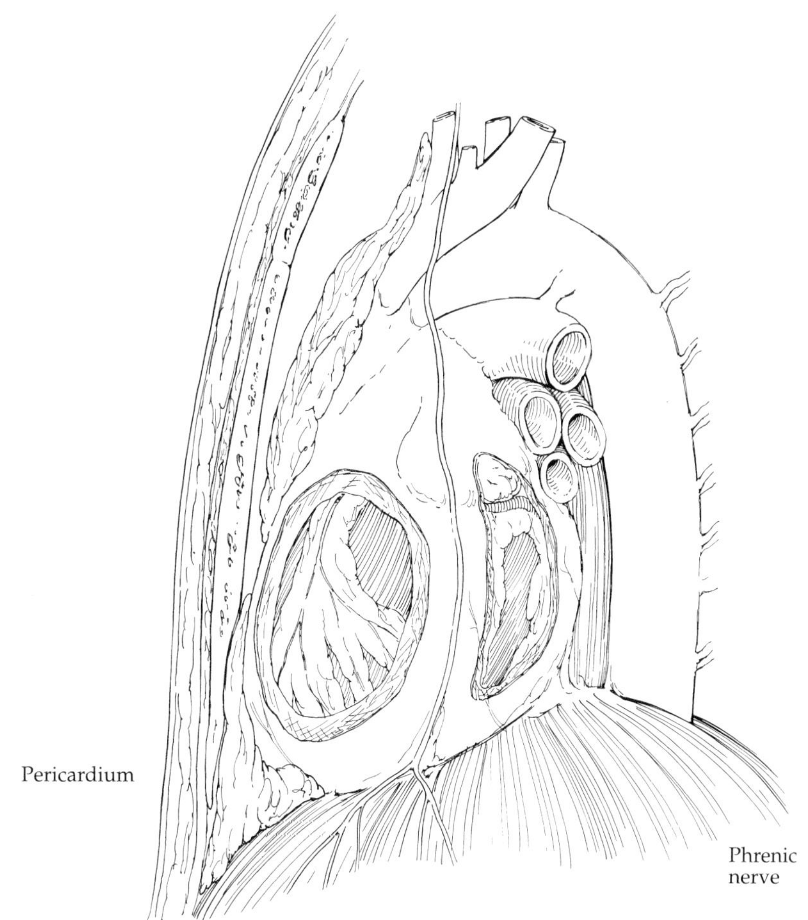

Fig. 55-7. A completed pericardial window, preserving the phrenic nerve.

MEDIASTINAL MASSES–POSTERIOR

The most common lesions encountered in the posterior mediastinum are benign neurogenic tumors of the sympathetic chain or peripheral nerve sheath (Fig. 55-8). Symptomatic lesions or concern for malignancy are indications for resection. Proper imaging is essential to define the extent of the tumor and its relationship with the spinal cord. A combined neurosurgical and thoracic team approach may be necessary for dumbbell tumors with intraspinal extension.

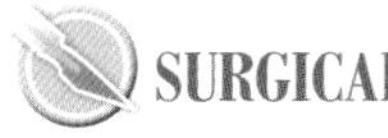

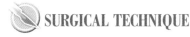

SURGICAL TECHNIQUE

A similar operative setup of the thoracoscopic instruments is used for resection of lesions of the posterior mediastinum, with the patient in lateral decubitus prone position and on one-lung ventilation. Triangulation of the two working instruments on either side of the camera port will facilitate tumor dissection. The overlying pleura is incised and the plane between the mass and surrounding pleura is dissected out. Study of preoperative CT and magnetic resonance imaging (MRI) will help to define the vascular supply. Exiting nerves and vessels are clipped and divided. If the tumor lies close to the origin of the ipsilateral brachial plexus or sympathetic chain, care should be taken to try to preserve these structures. The excised specimen is placed in a bag and extracted through the anterior working port incision, which is extended. A chest tube is placed after ensuring adequate hemostasis.

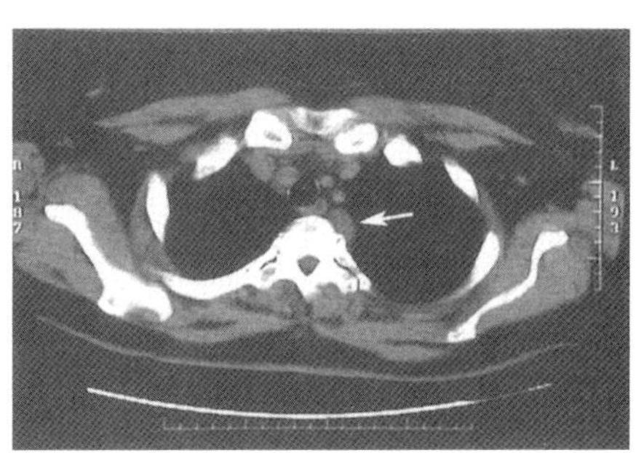

Fig. 55-8. A benign neurogenic tumor (arrow) in the posterior mediastinum.

Esophageal Disorders

THORACOSCOPIC MYOTOMY–ACHALASIA

Achalasia is the most common primary motility disorder of the esophagus, typified by persistent dysphagia and regurgitation to both solids and liquids. Contrast swallow may show the classic "bird's beak" deformity of a dilated esophagus narrowing down to the noncompliant gastroesophageal junction. The classical manometric features of failure of relaxation of the lower esophageal sphincter (LES) to deglutition, hypertensive LES, aperistalsis of the esophageal body, and elevated intraluminal esophageal pressure confirm the diagnosis of achalasia. A distinct subtype of achalasia, characterized by simultaneous esophageal contractions in association with LES non-relaxation, is known as vigorous achalasia. While numerous studies have confirmed the effectiveness of the Heller myotomy for the treatment of achalasia, the indications for thoracoscopic myotomy in this setting are less clear. Laparoscopic Heller myotomy is the preferred approach for achalasia, with several studies citing superior results compared to thoracoscopic myotomy in terms of increased relief of dysphagia and decreased incidence of postoperative reflux, operative time, and length of stay. The limitations of the thoracoscopic approach in the treatment of achalasia include inadequate exposure to the gastroesophageal junction leading to inadequate distal extent of myotomy as well as higher technical difficulty in creating a fundoplication. Nevertheless, a thoracoscopic approach may be indicated if a laparoscopic myotomy cannot be performed, such as in the case of severe obesity, dense intraabdominal adhesions from previous laparotomy, or redo myotomy. The vigorous achalasia subtype may be better approached thoracoscopically, where the myotomy should be extended to the most proximal peristaltic abnormality on the manometry study. In experienced hands, thoracoscopic myotomy can provide adequate relief of dysphagia with minimal morbidity.

SURGICAL TECHNIQUE

Following induction with general anesthesia and double-lumen endotracheal intubation, flexible esophagoscopy is performed and the tip of the scope left just proximal to the gastroesophageal junction. The reasons for leaving the scope within the esophageal lumen are threefold. First, the scope may be used to push the distal esophagus up into the left chest to facilitate dissection. Second, the scope acts as a guide to judge the extent of myotomy. Third, air insufflation via the scope is used to detect a mucosal perforation following myotomy.

The patient is positioned in right lateral decubitus position with the bed flexed. With the left lung collapsed, five trocars are placed:

1. An 11-mm port at the seventh intercostal space, anterior axillary line for insertion of the 30-degree thoracoscope
2. An 11-mm port at eighth or ninth midaxillary intercostal space for retraction of the left crus and the dome of the diaphragm
3. An 11-mm port in the tenth intercostal space, posterior axillary line for the thoracoscope
4. A 5-mm working port in tenth intercostal space, anterior to the previously described port
5. A 5-mm working port at eighth intercostal space, posterior axillary line

After identification and incision of the inferior pulmonary ligament with hook electrocautery, the left lung is displaced anteriorly and superiorly, exposing the lower thoracic esophagus (Fig. 55-9). Care must be taken to avoid injury to the descending thoracic aorta, just lateral to the esophagus. Manipulation of the endoscope may facilitate identification of the esophagus. The mediastinal pleura overlying the esophagus is incised with cautery in a caudal direction from the level of the inferior pulmonary vein superiorly to the diaphragmatic crus inferiorly. Periesophageal fatty tissue is cleared off to expose the left lateral wall of the esophagus, taking care not to injure the anterior or posterior vagal trunks. The distal esophagus is exposed by incising the diaphragmatic reflection of the mediastinal pleura in an anterior-to-posterior direction. This maneuver is key to achieving sufficient exposure of the distal muscular fibers of the esophagus and gastric cardia. The esophagomyotomy is carefully performed using either hook cautery or curved Metzenbaum scissors (Fig. 55-10). The proper submucosal dissection plane is developed and the myotomy extended caudally. Blunt dissection is used to sweep the muscle 180 degrees off the mucosa. The most inferior extent of the myotomy is usually 1 to 2 cm distal to the gastric cardia. Extreme care must be taken not to perforate the mucosa, as the submucosa and muscular layers of the esophagus may be fused together. The position of the endoscope within the esophagus and stomach serves as a useful guide to gauge the limit of the myotomy. Following completion of the

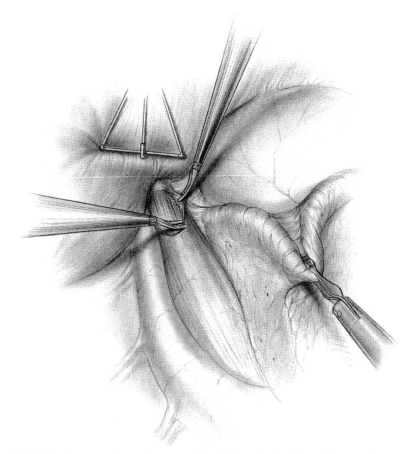

Fig. 55-9. The lower esophagus is exposed by dividing the inferior pulmonary ligament and retracting the lung cephalad.

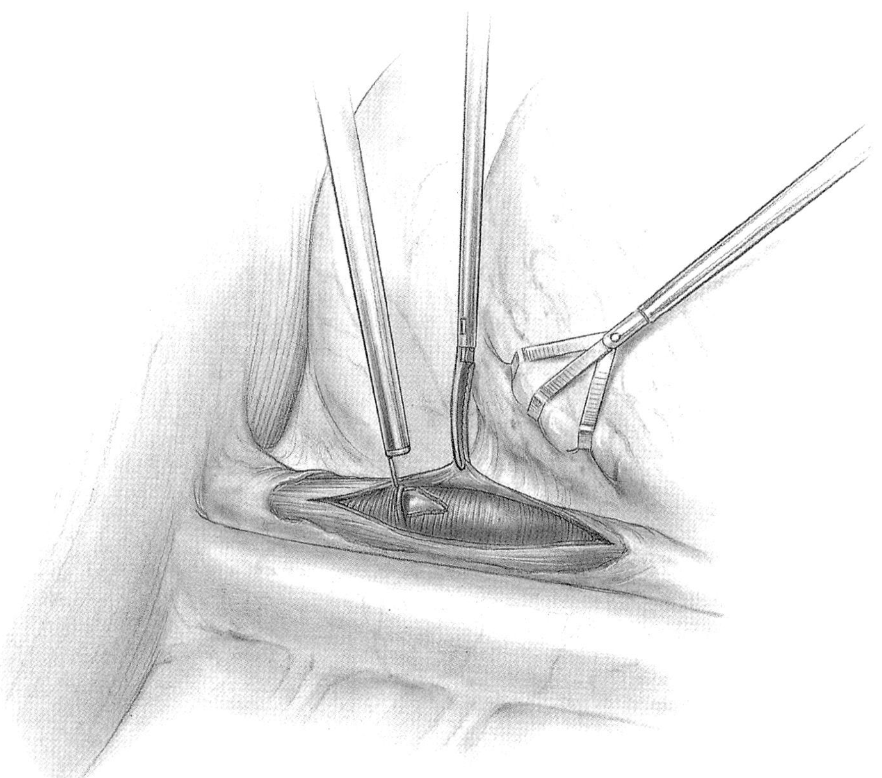

Fig. 55-10. A hook cautery or endoscopic scissor is used to divide longitudinal and circular muscle fibers.

myotomy, it is tested for leaks by gentle air insufflation through the endoscope after submerging the thoracic esophagus in saline. A small mucosal perforation may be repaired thoracoscopically using carefully placed interrupted absorbable sutures approximating the mucosa. An antireflux procedure is not typically performed. Following irrigation of the hemithorax, a chest tube is placed through one of the port incisions. A nasogastric tube is placed into the stomach and removed on the first postoperative day and a clear fluid diet is given.

OUTCOMES

Results for thoracoscopic myotomy in the treatment of achalasia have generally shown higher recurrence of dysphagia, up to 38%, compared with laparoscopic myotomy in most series. In our institution, we prefer a laparoscopic approach, citing shorter operative time, decreased length of hospitalization, and more durable alleviation of symptoms. Thoracoscopic myotomy for achalasia however, remains a viable option if a transabdominal approach is contraindicated.

THORACOSCOPIC LONG MYOTOMY–FOR SPASTIC ESOPHAGEAL MOTILITY DISORDERS

Diffuse esophageal spasm (DES) and nutcracker esophagus (NE) are uncommon primary esophageal motility disorders with distinct manometric features. Typical symptoms include dysphagia and chest pain. Diffuse esophageal spasm is characterized by frequent, repetitive high-amplitude esophageal contractions occurring simultaneously without peristaltic coordination. Nutcracker esophagus is also characterized by abnormally high-amplitude (>180 mmHg) esophageal contractions, but in the setting of normal coordinated peristalsis (Fig. 55-11, page 558). In the past, extended or "long" myotomy was indicated for NE and DES refractory to medical therapy. More recent evidence has shown that DES may be effectively treated with laparoscopic myotomy, similar to achalasia. Indeed, DES may exist on a continuum in the spectrum of motility disorders characterized by the progressive loss of peristalsis, with achalasia being the most severe form. In contrast, refractory NE is usually an indication for long myotomy of the thoracic esophagus, although variable success in relief of symptoms is reported. Several points may be made related to the treatment of these disorders.

1. It is most important to rule out a primary diagnosis of gastroesophageal reflux disease (GERD) using ambulatory pH studies. Motility abnormalities may be secondary to acid reflux, and the approach to treatment in such cases would be to treat the primary reflux disorder. Conversely, coexisting reflux symptoms in the setting of a primary motility disorder such as NE or DES necessitating surgery may benefit from an antireflux procedure such as a partial fundoplication in addition to a short myotomy.
2. In cases of primary NE, the manometry study should be carefully evaluated to determine the extent of esophageal myotomy.

SURGICAL TECHNIQUE

The operative approach to long myotomy is similar to that described for thoracoscopic myotomy for achalasia previously, with the patient placed in right lateral decubitus prone position under single-lung ventilation. The key difference in technique is the need for sufficient exposure of the thoracic esophagus in order to perform an adequate myotomy. After division of the inferior pulmonary ligament, the left lung is retracted anteriorly to expose the esophagus. Again, the preoperative placement of an esophagoscope or nasogastric tube facilitates identification of the esophagus. The myotomy is extended distally to the GE junction and may be extended further distally onto the stomach, especially if manometry demonstrates an abnormally high LES pressure. Proximally, the myotomy is extended to the level of the aortic arch in DES and up to the level of the most proximal peristaltic abnormality as determined by manometry in cases of NE (Fig. 55-12, page 559). Again, care is taken to adequately dissect the muscle layers from the underlying mucosa and achieve complete division of all muscle bands over the entire length of the myotomy. Typically, an antireflux procedure is not performed if the patient did not have a preoperative diagnosis of GERD. If an antireflux procedure is deemed necessary, a partial wrap

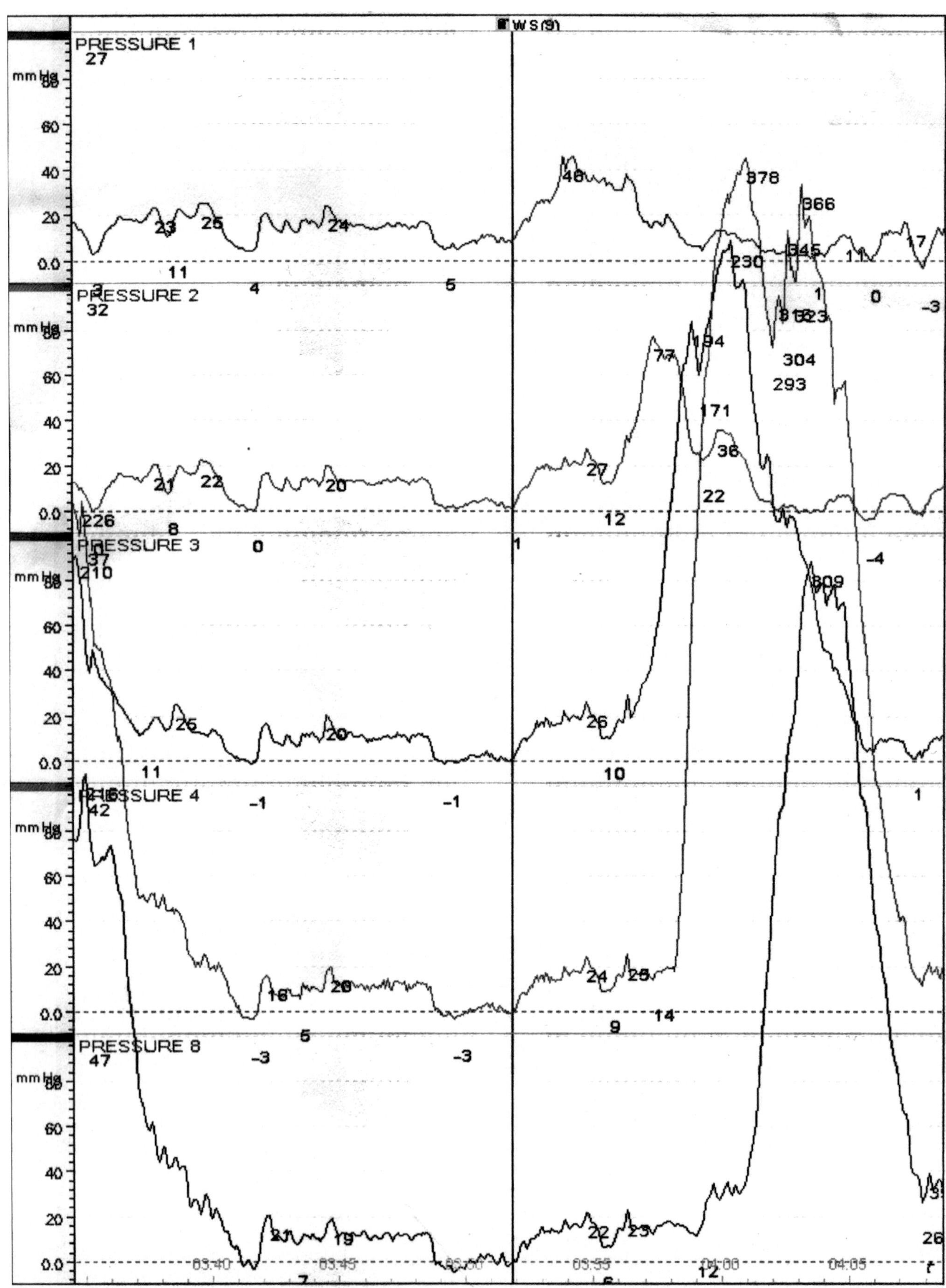

Fig. 55-11. A motility tracing typical for nutcracker esophagus showing high-pressure peristaltic contractions. DES, diffuse esophageal spasm.

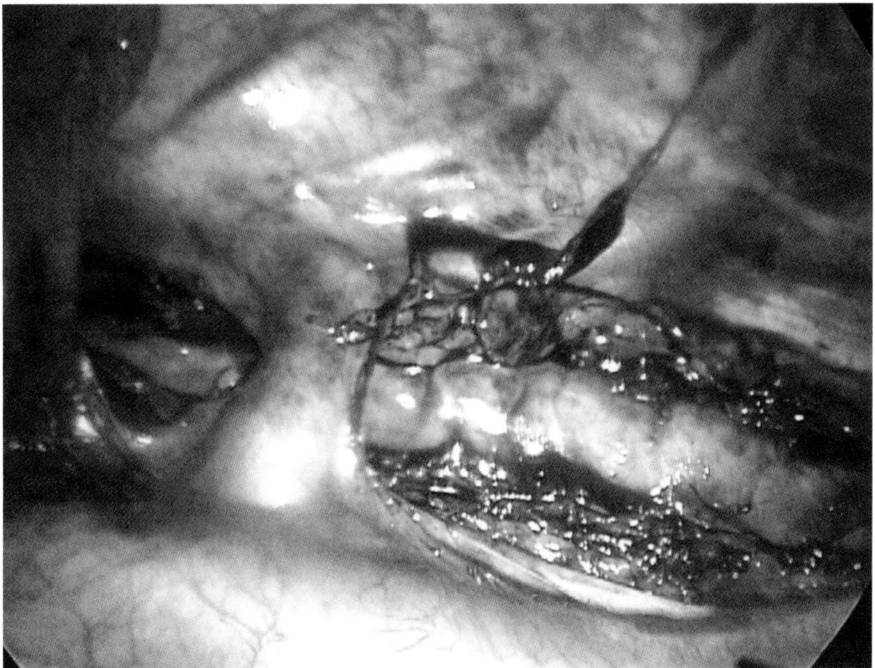

Fig. 55-12. A completed long thoracic myotomy extending from the stomach to the thoracic inlet.

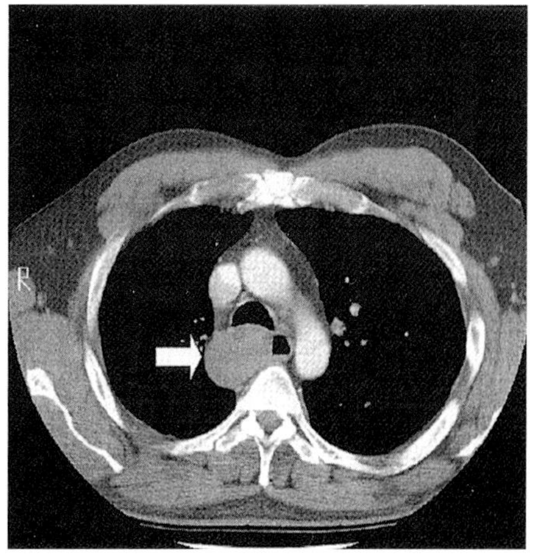

Fig. 55-13. A computed tomography (CT) scan clearly shows the homogeneous solid mass (arrow) of the esophageal wall consistent with a stromal tumor or leiomyoma.

such as a Dor (90-degree) or a Belsey (270-degree) may be constructed, securing the gastric fundus to the cut distal edges of the esophageal muscle.

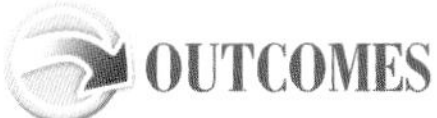

OUTCOMES

Controversy surrounds the surgical approach for the treatment of DES and NE, as outcomes have been mixed. A recent review by Patti et al. of the results following thoracoscopic myotomy demonstrated relief of dysphagia in 80% of patients with DES and in 60% with NE, but relief of chest pain in only 65% and 40%, respectively. In addition, superior relief of dysphagia was demonstrated following laparoscopic myotomy for the treatment of both DES and NE (86% and 83%, respectively). DES may present in association with a hypertensive non-relaxing LES, and in these cases a laparoscopic myotomy alone may be sufficient to relieve dysphagia. In cases where the primary pathologic dysmotility is in the proximal thoracic esophagus, a thoracoscopic approach is necessary to perform an adequate extended myotomy. For cases of NE, in general, surgery should only be considered primarily for symptoms of severe refractory dysphagia. Treatments aimed at relieving symptoms of chest pain have been disappointing, and surgery is less likely to be successful.

ESOPHAGEAL TUMORS–BENIGN

Benign tumors of the esophagus are relatively rare and usually arise from the submucosa. The most common submucosal esophageal tumors are leiomyomas, comprising 75% of all benign esophageal lesions. Leiomyomas typically originate in the lower two-thirds of the esophagus, owing to the abundance of smooth muscle at this location. Diagnosis is made on barium swallow, which will demonstrate the typical smooth, well-circumscribed submucosal mass that moves freely with swallowing, with normal overlying mucosa. Biopsy is not necessary to confirm histology and may increase the risk of mucosal perforation during enucleation, as explained later. Double-contrast CT or endoscopic ultrasound shows the extent of involvement of the esophageal wall, which is important for planning the approach to enucleation of the lesion (Fig. 55-13). Leiomyomas are slow-growing and have minimal risk of malignant degeneration. In spite of these characteristics, surgical removal is recommended for symptomatic lesions and those that are larger than 5 cm. Asymptomatic leiomyomas found incidentally may be followed but in general all should be eventually resected to confirm the diagnosis and prevent future development of symptoms.

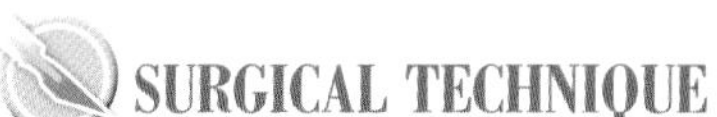

SURGICAL TECHNIQUE

Surgical enucleation is the procedure of choice for removal of esophageal leiomyomas. As most of these lesions arise from the distal esophagus, a left-sided thoracoscopic approach generally allows optimal exposure. Proximal and midlevel tumors above the level of the carina are better accessed through the right side. If a proximal tumor appears on CT scan to encompass the left side of the esophagus, a right-sided thoracoscopic approach with rotation of the esophagus for enucleation is still necessary as the aortic arch prevents safe excision of these proximal leiomyomas from the left side. After induction and positioning of the patient in lateral decubitus prone position, two working ports are placed on either side of the camera port, which is placed at the fourth intercostal space near the scapula tip for distal tumors and in the seventh intercostal space for more proximal lesions. An extra port is optional to aid in retraction of the lung or diaphragm. As for other thoracoscopic esophageal procedures, intraoperative placement of an esophagoscope helps to identify the esophagus within the hemithorax. Endoscopic visualization of the tumor with transillumination may also assist in identifying smaller tumors. The mediastinal pleura is incised directly over the identified mass. The esophagus may be encircled with a Penrose drain to assist in retraction, especially for large or circumferential lesions. The longitudinal esophageal muscle is split with scissors or hook electrocautery in the direction of its fibers directly over the tumor (Fig. 55-14). Care is taken to identify and preserve the vagal nerves. Once split, the esophageal muscle layer enveloping the leiomyoma is bluntly dissected off the mass by finding the anatomic plane and extending it circumferentially. The tumor may then be gently grasped with Babcock forceps and retracted away from the esophagus. The adherent mucosa is then carefully dissected off the mass, taking great care not to perforate this layer. Inflammation from previous endoscopic biopsy may make the mucosal dissection especially difficult. Insufflation with the previously placed esophagoscope helps to confirm the integrity of the mucosa, and any disruption may be repaired with absorbable sutures. The superficial esophageal muscle layer is reapproximated over the mucosa following removal of the tumor (Fig. 55-15). Rarely, extensive circumferential tumors may necessitate short segment esophagectomy and end-to-end anastomosis. Should such a resection be necessary, conversion to thoracotomy is advised unless the operator has sufficient experience in thoracoscopic esophageal resection. Otherwise, following successful enucleation of the tumor, the pleura is irrigated and a chest tube is left in place following the procedure and may be removed the following day. Recurrent leiomyoma following enucleation is rare. Postoperative stricture formation is uncommon and may be managed with endoscopic dilatation.

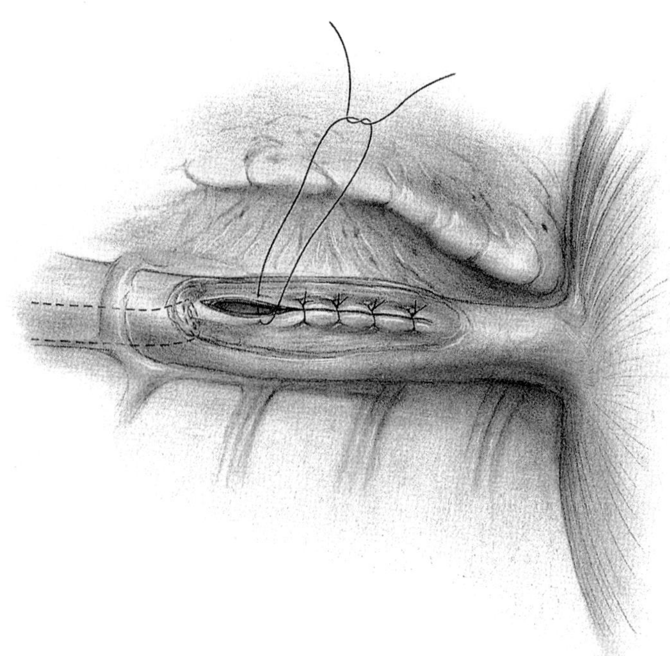

Fig. 55-15. The superficial muscles of the myotomy are loosely reapproximated to prevent late diverticulization.

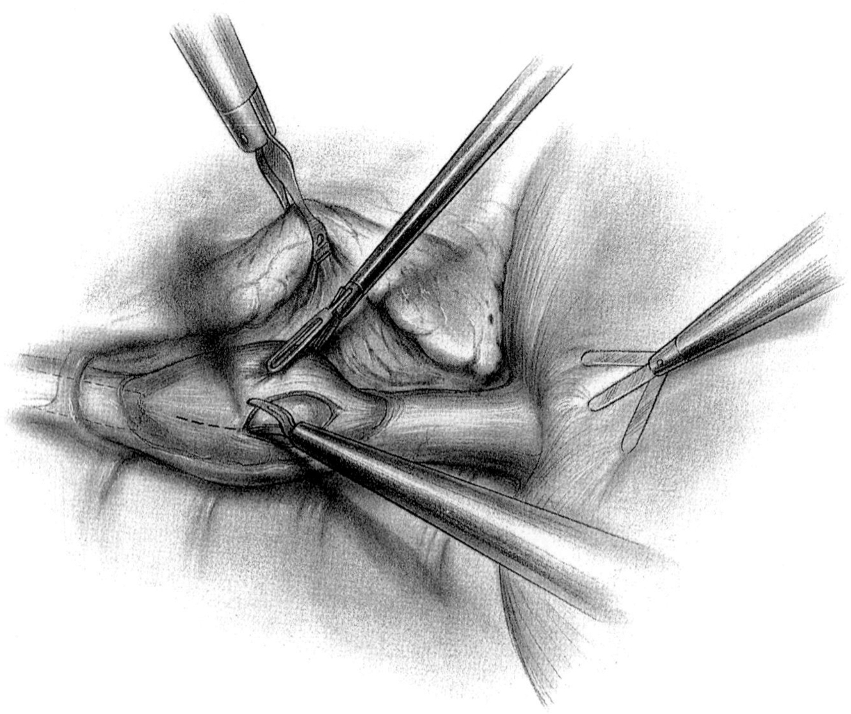

Fig. 55-14. Endoscopic scissors are used to split the muscle layers overlying the tumor.

ESOPHAGEAL TUMORS–MALIGNANT

Surgical resection of malignant neoplasms of the esophagus remains the only potentially curative treatment option. Unfortunately, many patients present at an advanced stage with disseminated metastases or local tumor invasion into vital structures, precluding surgery. For those patients with localized disease, the traditional open esophagectomy—whether performed via combined right thoracotomy and laparotomy (Ivor Lewis), transhiatal, or left thoracoabdominal approach—is associated with considerable morbidity. With the refinement of thoracoscopic surgery, various applications have been developed to minimize the morbidity in the surgical management of esophageal cancer. Diagnostic thoracoscopy may be used to first rule out invasive or metastatic disease and assess gross resectability of bulky tumors. Minimally invasive esophagectomy has been described using laparoscopy or combined thoracoscopy and laparoscopy. It should be noted that minimally invasive esophagectomy is a technically demanding operation requiring advanced skills in minimally invasive surgery as well as in esophageal resection. Patients selected for minimally invasive esophagectomy should have resectable tumors based on diagnostic imaging without evidence of distant or nodal metastases. Patients with

Barrett high-grade dysplasia are ideal candidates for minimally invasive esophagectomy. The steps in the combined VATS and laparoscopic esophagectomy as previously developed and described by Luketich et al. at the University of Pittsburgh Medical Center are outlined below.

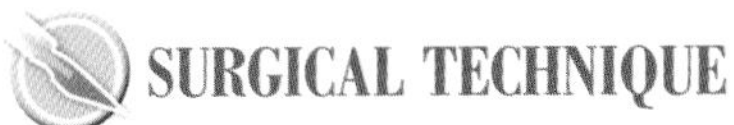

SURGICAL TECHNIQUE

Minimally Invasive Esophagectomy

Right Thoracoscopy

With the patient in left lateral decubitus, one port is placed for the camera and two to three additional ports for dissection and retraction. The esophagus is exposed by incising the inferior pulmonary ligament and retracting the lung anterior and cephalad. The overlying mediastinal pleura is incised over the esophagus and mobilized with blunt and sharp dissection. Preoperative placement of a nasogastric tube facilitates esophageal dissection. A wide lateral margin is obtained to include paraesophageal nodal tissue (Fig. 55-16). Dissection is extended to the level of the azygous vein, which is divided with a vascular stapler. Any feeding vessels and lymphatics are divided with clips, ultrasonic shears, or coagulating shears. Following complete mobilization of the esophagus, the ports are removed and a chest tube is placed.

Laparoscopy

With the patient placed supine, abdominal ports are placed identical to the setup for fundoplication (see Chapter 10). With the left lobe of the liver retracted using a self-retaining retractor, the gastrohepatic ligament is divided up to the hiatus. Lymphoareolar tissue within the lesser curve is swept toward the stomach for later removal with the specimen. The greater curve of the stomach along with the greater omentum is separated from the transverse colon, taking care to preserve the right gastroepiploic vessels. As the dissection is carried cephalad along the greater curve, we prefer using a vascular stapler to divide the left gastroepiploic and short gastric vessels. The left gastric artery and vein are identified and divided with a vascular stapler close to the celiac axis. A pyloromyotomy is created to prevent delayed gastric emptying. The duodenum is not routinely mobilized. At the level of the hiatus, a rim of crural tissue is dissected circumferentially for neoplasms of the distal esophagus. The gastric tube is then made by dividing the stomach using multiple firings of an Autosuture ENDO GIA stapler, beginning at the distal aspect of the lesser curve and extended superiorly to the fundus, preserving the right gastric artery. The distal thoracic esophagus and proximal stomach should now be free. The gastric tube is then sutured to the previously divided proximal stomach in order to deliver both the specimen and conduit up to the neck. A laparoscopic jejunostomy is then placed for postoperative feeding and secured to the abdominal wall.

Cervical

The cervical phase of the esophageal mobilization is generally identical to that described for transhiatal esophagectomy (see Chapter 20). The main difference with the minimally invasive approach is that the esophageal specimen must be extracted through the cervical incision. Once the cervical esophagus has been fully mobilized and divided, the specimen and attached gastric conduit are carefully delivered into the neck wound. The delivery is guided by laparoscopy to maintain proper orientation of the conduit. The specimen is removed from the operative field. The cervical esophagogastric anastomosis may be performed using handsewn or stapled technique. Our own preference is the side-to-side stapled anastomosis as described in Chapter 20. A Penrose drain is left in the neck to alert the surgeon of postoperative anastomotic leak (Fig. 55-17).

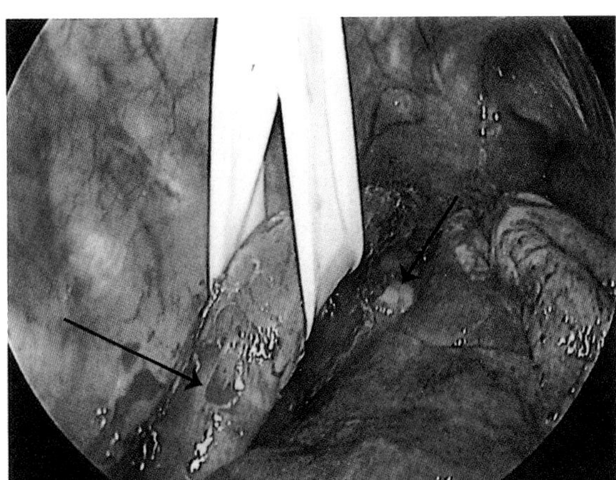

Fig. 55-16. Complete thoracoscopic mobilization, with mediastinal nodes left attached to the esophagus (long arrow). Transected azygos vein also shown (shorter arrow).

CONCLUSION

While minimally invasive esophagectomy represents a major advance in thoracic surgery, the longer operative time, steep learning curve, and questionable benefit compared with traditional open techniques have limited its application to a small number of centers with clinical expertise in advanced minimally invasive foregut surgery. Nevertheless, as minimally invasive techniques continue to become more widespread among current and future thoracic surgeons, acceptance of potentially less morbid procedures will continue to grow. Further studies are needed to demonstrate any significant advantages of minimally invasive esophagectomy over open techniques.

SUGGESTED READING

Champion JK, Delisle N, Hunt T. Comparison of thoracoscopic and laparoscopic esophagomyotomy and fundoplication for primary motility disorders. *Eur J Cardiothor Surg* (Suppl 1)1999;S34–S36.

Cheng YJ, Kao EL, Chou SH. Video-thoracoscopic resection of stage 2 thymoma: prospective comparison of the results between thoracoscopy and open methods. *Chest* 2005;128:3010–3012.

de Hoyos A, Litle VR, Luketich JD. Minimally invasive esophagectomy. *Surg Clin N Am* 2005;85:631–647.

Filipi CJ, Hinder, RA. Thoracoscopic myotomy—a surgical technique for achalasia, diffuse esophageal spasm and "nutcracker esophagus." *Surg Endosc* 1994;8:921–926.

Kitami A, Suzuki T, Usuda R, et al. Diagnostic and therapeutic thoracoscopy for mediastinal disease. *Ann Thorac Cardiovasc Surg* 2004;10: 14–18.

Patt MG, Gorodner MV, Galvani C, et al. Spectrum of esophageal motility disorders—implications of diagnosis and treatment. *Arch Surg* 2005;140:442–445.

Rammaciato G, Mercantini P, Amodio PM, et al. The laparoscopic approach with anti-reflux surgery is superior to the

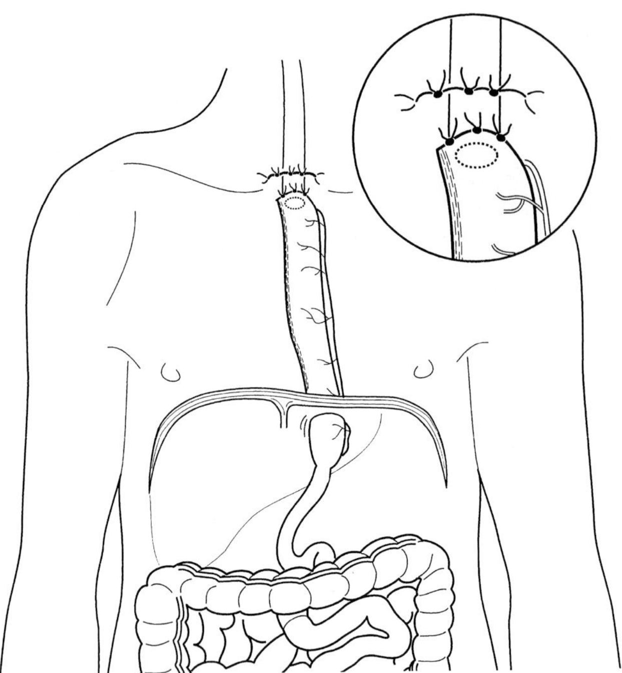

Fig. 55-17. The final result after esophagectomy with cervical anastamosis.

thoracoscopic approach for the treatment of esophageal achalasia—experience of a single surgical unit. *Surg Endosc* 2002;16: 1431–1437.

Ruckert JC, Gellert K, Muller JM. Operative technique for thoracoscopic thymectomy. *Surg Endosc* 1999;13:943–946.

Stewart KC, Finley RJ, Clifton JC, et al. Thoracoscopic versus laparoscopic modified Heller myotomy for achalasia: efficacy and safety in 87 patients. *J Am Coll Surg* 1999; 89:164–170.

Von Rahden BHA, Stein HJ, Feussner H, et al. Enucleation of submucosal tumors of the esophagus—minimally invasive vs. open approach. *Surg Endosc* 2004;18:914–920.

Wagner AJ, Cortes RA, Strober J, et al. Long term follow-up after thymectomy for myasthenia gravis: thoracoscopic vs. open. *J Ped Surg* 2006;41:50–54.

Weigel TL, Murphy J, Kabbani L, et al. Radioguided thoracoscopic mediastinal parathyroidectomy with intraoperative parathyroid testing. *Ann Thorac Surg* 2005; 80:1262–1265.

COMMENTARY

Drs. Finley and Buduhan give us a fairly comprehensive survey of mediastinal pathology and the thoracoscopic approaches to their treatment. They demonstrate that no portions of the mediastinum (anterior, posterior, or middle) are out of reach to the thoracoscopist. I would like to emphasize several of the technical point that they discuss in passing:

- Thoracoscopic approaches to the mediastinum have been somewhat eclipsed over the last several years by the popularity of transhiatal laparoscopy. This is due to the lingering feeling that transthoracic access is morbid and by the fact that it has been primarily abdominal surgeons who pioneered and mastered advanced laparoscopic techniques. This group may have felt somewhat out of their comfort zone in utilizing transthoracic approaches. This is unfortunate as thoracoscopy provides an excellent view of all of the mediastinal structures, permitting wide resections of various lesions and avoiding the awkwardness of tight, transhiatal approaches and the morbidity of a thoracotomy.
- A very interesting evolution in thoracoscopy has been the flexibility or variations of access. Patient position has varied from traditional lateral decubitus positions with traditional VATS to innovative access with lateral supine or lateral prone positions as illustrated by the authors. The use of prone positioning, as described by others, is a truly novel approach, only applicable to endoscopic surgery. It provides a great view of the posterior and medial compartments of the mediastinum with fewer ports, as retraction of the lung is performed by gravity.
- Another advance that has made thoracoscopy more appealing has been the realization that a mini-thoracotomy, as is common with VATS, is not really needed for thoracoscopy. Briefly mentioned by the authors, another approach is the use of positive pressure capnothorax or the use of standard laparoscopic valved ports with carbon dioxide insufflation. This obviates the need for dual-lumen endotracheal intubation, which simplifies the anesthesia of these patients tremendously. We have found the visualization to be excellent with this technique.

- Flexible endoscopy, a useful adjunct in any mediastinal procedure, is particularly useful in thoracoscopy and should be mandatory in esophageal procedures. Without the ability to palpate the structures of the mediastinum, it is easy to become disoriented and dissect in the wrong area. The transillumination of the endoscope provides instant orientation and the real-time ability to detect injuries to the esophagus.
- Finally, we agree with the authors that spastic esophageal motility disorders should rarely come to surgery and then only after a comprehensive workup and exhaustion of all medical alternatives. Particularly when dealing with noncardiac chest pain and DES or nutcracker esophagus, we advocate a trial treatment of endoscopic Botox injections before committing to an irreversible long myotomy.

Thoracoscopic mediastinal access is an important modality for both the thoracic and the upper GI surgeon. Mastering the "tricks" of access and dissection allows a minimally invasive approach to a wide spectrum of uncommon but morbid diseases.

LLS

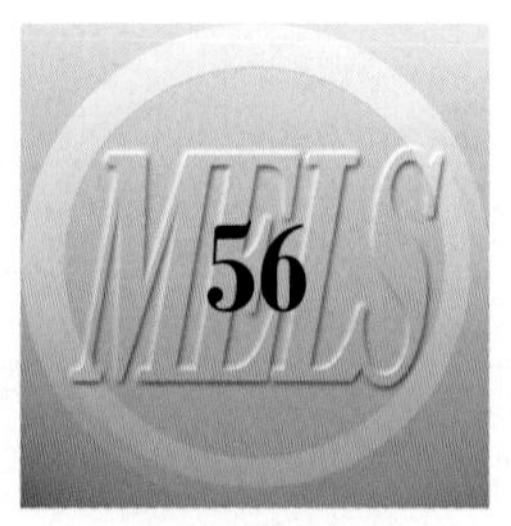

Video-Assisted Thoracoscopic Surgery (VATS) for the General Surgeon

ALBERTO DE HOYOS, MATTHEW BLUM, AND RODNEY LANDRENEAU

INTRODUCTION

The field of body cavity endoscopic surgery became common practice in gynecology and general surgery in the 1970s and 1980s. Thoracic surgeons however, did not apply this technique widely until after the development of laparoscopic equipment and procedures such as cholecystectomy and appendectomy were commonly performed. In the last two decades thoracoscopy has expanded from a simple, pleural diagnostic procedure to an intervention through which many other thoracic procedures can be performed, as depicted in Table 56-1. It is important to emphasize that the operations performed through video-assisted thoracic surgery (VATS) are not new. Identical procedures to those performed with open thoracotomy can be replicated with minimally invasive techniques. The benefits of VATS are depicted in Table 56-2. As experience has accumulated with VATS, open thoracotomy is becoming less common in many surgical practices. This chapter describes the use of thoracoscopic techniques that may be useful for the practicing general surgeon with some experience in minimally invasive surgery; advanced techniques such as lobectomy and robotic thoracic surgery are out of the scope of this chapter. Surgery of the mediastinum and esophagus is covered in Chapter 55.

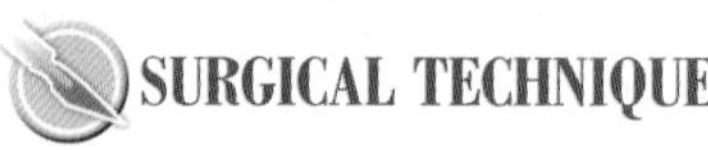

SURGICAL TECHNIQUE

Patient Positioning

Patients are usually placed in full lateral decubitus position with all pressure points well padded to prevent tissue and nerve injury. The use of a beanbag is optional, but the patient should be safely secured to the table. The hips are placed below the break point of the table to allow opening of the intercostal spaces as the table is angulated. The contralateral leg is gently flexed while the ipsilateral leg is maintained extended. The ipsilateral arm should rest in a natural position to avoid hyperextension and to prevent injury to the brachial plexus. The thorax is prepared and draped as for open thoracotomy should this arise. Patient positioning for hyperhidrosis is somewhat different, as will be described later.

TABLE 56-1. INDICATIONS FOR VATS

Diagnostic
Lung biopsy
Interstitial lung disease
Indeterminate pulmonary nodule
Biopsy of mediastinal lymph nodes
Biopsy of mediastinal mass
Biopsy of pleural-based lesions
Pleural biopsy and drainage of effusion
Therapeutic
Lung
Lobectomy for lung cancer
Sublobar resection (segmentectomy, wedge) for lung cancer
Placement of brachytherapy mesh for sublobar resection for lung cancer
Resection of blebs for recurrent pneumothorax
Lung-volume reduction surgery
Pleura and Pericardium
Drainage of large pleural effusion (benign or malignant)
Pleurodesis (pleurectomy, mechanical, chemical)
Drainage of large pericardial effusion (subclinical or clinical tamponade)
Drainage of empyema and decortication of the lung
Drainage of retained hemothorax
Mediastinum
Excision of small mediastinal masses or cysts
Thymectomy for myasthenia gravis
Sympathectomy for hyperhidrosis
Ligation of the thoracic duct for chylothorax
Esophageal
Resection of leiomyomata
Resection of enteric cysts
Esophagomyotomy
Esophagectomy

VATS, video-assisted thoracoscopic surgery.

Anesthetic Considerations

All patients require monitoring of the EKG, continuous pulse oxymetry, and CO_2 capnometry. An arterial line is utilized selectively in patients in poorer condition or for prolonged procedures. For most VATS procedures single-lung ventilation is required in order to facilitate manipulation of the lung and instruments within the limited pleural space.

Lung isolation may be achieved through a double-lumen tube (DLT) or single-lumen tube (SLT) with a bronchial blocker. Patients with pneumonia and parapneumonic empyema require DLT to ensure strict lung isolation and to prevent soiling of the dependent normal lung with purulent secretions. Malposition (migration) or mucous plugging of the endotracheal tube is the usual cause of significant intraoperative hypoxemia. The anesthesia and surgical teams must be prepared to immediately suction secretions from the ventilated lung and to perform bronchoscopic examination of the bronchial blocker or DLT to correct any potential misplacement. When significant hypoxemia persists despite confirmation of correct tube positioning, brief periods of bilateral lung re-expansion and continuous positive airway pressure for the ipsilateral lung during the single-lung ventilation usually correct the hypoxemia. Alternatively, patients may tolerate better brief periods of bilateral lung ventilation alternating with periods of apnea of up to 2 to 3 minutes,

TABLE 56-2. THE BENEFITS OF VATS

Reduced acute pain
Reduced use of intravenous narcotics
Reduced need for epidural catheters
Reduced length of hospitalization
Reduced time to return to regular activities
Reduced impact on immune system
Reduced overall cost

VATS, video-assisted thoracoscopic surgery.

during which the procedure can be performed in steps. On occasion, lung collapse is aided with gentle CO_2 insufflation to 8 to 10 mmHg. This requires special ports to maintain pressurization of the thoracic cavity, as is performed in laparoscopy.

Pain Control

Thoracic incisions are more painful and less well tolerated than abdominal incisions. Complications of poorly controlled incisional pain include splinting, poor pulmonary hygiene, atelectasis, and pneumonia. Most patients undergoing VATS do not require epidural catheter for pain control. Common clinical practice includes the use of intraoperative nerve blocks with 0.25% to 0.5% bupivicaine (1 to 3 cc into each intercostal space), nonsteroidal anti-inflammatory drugs (ketorolac), subcutaneous placement of catheters (pain pump) and patient-controlled analgesia with narcotics. In patients undergoing pleurectomy and pleurodesis for recurrent pleural effusion or pneumothorax, an option is to utilize an epidural catheter and avoid the use of nonsteroidal anti-inflammatory drugs, as they may interfere with the desired inflammatory reaction necessary for pleurodesis.

Instrumentation and General Approach to Thoracoscopy

The basic concepts of VATS are summarized in Table 56-3. Most VATS procedures can be performed using two to four 5-mm to 12-mm ports and reusable standard or thoracoscopic sponge holders, lung graspers, tissue forceps, scissors, and disposable endoscopic staplers. If standard open instruments are used, it is important to select instruments that have the proper mechanism to open widely when inserted through thoracoscopic ports. In some cases disposable endoscopic kittners (Ethicon Endo-Surgery, Inc.; Cincinnati, OH or U.S. Surgical; Norwalk, CT) are useful for manipulation of the lung.

For most cases the surgeon stands in front of the patient, and the assistant and scrub nurse opposite the surgeon. Monitors should be placed on both sides of the patient for optimal visualization.

The 10-mm, 30-degree angled telescope is preferred in our practice for the vast majority of VATS procedures. This telescope allows great visibility and the ability to reach areas difficult to access with the 0-degree telescope. For simple pleural procedures such as drainage of effusions and pleural biopsies, the 10-mm, 0-degree operating thoracoscope is preferred. This thoracoscope has a 5-mm biopsy channel that can accommodate most 5-mm endoscopic instruments. This feature allows single intercostal access for many pleural-related problems. On occasion, a 5-mm 30-degree telescope can be utilized, although the quality of the image is not as clear as the one obtained with the 10-mm telescope.

Endoscopic stapling devices are safe, quick, and convenient and can reliably divide pulmonary parenchyma and vessels while maintaining excellent hemostasis and pneumostasis. Commonly available models include the Ethicon (Ethicon Endo-Surgery, Inc.; Cincinnati, OH) and ENDO-GIA (U.S. Surgical; Norwalk, CT). A variety of staple sizes and stapler lengths is now available. For division of pulmonary parenchyma such as for wedge biopsy for diffuse infiltrates or pulmonary nodule, the blue load is preferred (cartridge length 45 to 60 mm, staple size 3.5 mm). For large wedges or segmental resection of thick lung tissue, the green load is preferred (cartridge length 45 to 60 mm, staple size 4.8 mm). In select cases, such as the resection of blebs or bullae, buttressing material with permanent or absorbable material is recommended to reinforce the staple line and prevent prolonged air leaks.

Proper selection of patients is vital for successful surgical results. Suggested guidelines for indications and contraindications for VATS are listed in Tables 56-1 and 56-4 respectively. A careful preoperative review of the chest roentgenogram and the computed tomography (CT) scan is vital to formulate the plan for the initial and subsequent intercostal access for the thoracoscope and surgical instruments. For instance, in a VATS lung biopsy for diffuse bilateral interstitial pulmonary disease, a right-sided approach is favored. Because of the trilobar anatomy of the right lung,

TABLE 56-3. BASIC CONCEPTS OF VATS

1. Work together with your anesthesiologist to ensure adequate lung isolation.
2. Place ports for thoracoscope and instruments at a distance across the chest cavity from the target lesion to achieve a panoramic view of the operative field, optimize working space, and avoid instrument crowding and fencing.
3. Conceptualize the three-dimensional location of target lesion based on examination of the CT scan to "triangulate" the lesion.
4. Keep the thoracoscope and instruments in the same 180-degree arc to maintain the same videoendoscopic perspective and avoid "mirror imaging."
5. Keep ports anterior to the posterior axillary line, if possible, where the intercostal spaces are wider.
6. Utilize both hands to manipulate the instruments in coordinated fashion.
7. Minimize the use of electrocautery to avoid smoke and the need to suction (the lung will reexpand). The suction-irrigation device is very helpful to maintain a clean field and to control suctioning.
8. Become familiar with the required thoracoscopes, instrumentation and choice of staplers.
9. Ensure good hemostasis and pneumostasis.
10. Understand that conversion to thoracotomy is not a failure but an appropriate option when the performance of VATS is limited by availability of equipment, technical difficulty, or clinical condition of the patient.

VATS, video-assisted thoracoscopic surgery.

TABLE 56-4. CONTRAINDICATIONS FOR VATS

Considered contraindications
Dense pleural symphysis
Inability to tolerate single-lung ventilation
Pulmonary hilar mass
Deeply located pulmonary nodules
Pulmonary lesion invading the mediastinum or chest wall
Large pulmonary lesions (>5 cm)
Inability to achieve ipsilateral pulmonary atelectasis
Inadequate visualization of the target lesion
Inadequate instrumentation
Not considered contraindications
Neoadjuvant chemotherapy or radiotherapy
Lesions abutting mediastinum, chest wall, or diaphragm
Ventilator dependency
Prior thoracotomy

VATS, video-assisted thoracoscopic surgery.

there are simply more lung "edges" available for obtaining a stapled lung biopsy.

The operation begins with the selection of an appropriate initial intercostal site of access for exploratory thoracoscopy. This skin incision is made directly over the intercostal space to be entered, as opposed to the traditional subcutaneous tunnel made for simple chest tubes. This allows for a full 360-degree arc of mobility of the port and reduces the incidence of postoperative neuritis secondary to excessive pressure due to improper port placement. Careful introduction of a finger or a small, curved pointed clamp (Kelly or Crile) through the intercostal muscles and pleura is made, avoiding the intercostal vessels and nerve along the inferior edge of the more cephalad rib. Direct digital exploration of the initial access intercostal site, rather than blind trocar placement into the chest, is used to identify the presence of local pleural adhesions and to confirm atelectasis of the lung. Pleural adhesions to the lung can impede the introduction of instruments and potentially result in pulmonary parenchymal injury. Flimsy focal adhesions can be divided with blunt finger dissection. More extensive pleural adhesions in the location of the proposed initial access site may require alternative access to perform the VATS procedure. On occasion, if extensive pleural adhesions are present, a second incision in the vicinity of the initial incision may facilitate creation of a pleural space by working simultaneously with two fingers until they reach each other, creating enough space for introduction of the thoracoscope. This will facilitate adequate selection of the other ports for completion of the procedure. On rare occasion, convertion to thoracotomy is required due to complete symphysis of the pleural space.

Strategic positioning of the thoracoscopic camera and endoscopic instruments is vital to the success and efficiency of the procedure. In general, the initial thoracoscopic incision is placed on the sixth or seventh intercostal space in the mid- to anterior axillary line. This initial thoracoscopic location usually provides a clear view of the mediastinum, all pleural surfaces, and the pulmonary parenchyma. Carbon dioxide insufflation is rarely used for VATS as it requires a closed chest to maintain pressurization, which would in turn limit the use of standard instruments. Occasionally, CO_2 may be utilized at the beginning of the procedure to facilitate and expedite collapse of the lung, particularly in the presence of adhesions.

The visibility of the entire thoracic cavity obtained through VATS contrasts favorably with the direct view obtained thorough a limited axillary, inframammary or lateral mini thoracotomy. Following the initial exploration of the pleural cavity, additional intercostal access sites are selected as required and placed under direct thoracoscopic vision. The specific locations for these additional ports are determined by the site of the primary pathology and the procedure to be performed, but in general the ports are placed across the ipsilateral pleural cavity to allow for some "working room" between the port sites and the lesion. It is also very useful to conceptualize the three-dimensional location of the target lesion within the thorax and to then place the port access sites to "triangulate" the lesion, as depicted in Figure 56-1. With proper port placement and by keeping adequate distance between the ports, any crossing over or "fencing" of the instruments can be avoided. Furthermore, the instruments and the thoracoscopic camera must be oriented so that they all are being utilized to face the target pathology from the same direction; otherwise, difficulties in instrument manipulation will occur because of "mirror imaging" when the instruments are directed toward the thoracoscopic camera. Once the camera is introduced into the thoracic cavity and all additional ports placed, the trocar for the camera can be slid out of the chest wall onto the thoracoscope to optimize the range of motion and minimize pressure on the intercostal nerve. Most other thoracoscopic instruments, including staplers, do not require the use of trocars. Specimens containing malignant lesions should be retrieved in endoscopic bags to avoid implantation of tumor in the access incisions. In most cases, a single 20 to 28F intercostal drain is required and directed posteriorly and apically taking care to avoid the fissure.

VATS FOR THE DIAGNOSIS OF INTERSTITIAL LUNG DISEASE

Interstitial lung disease (ILD) includes more than 100 specific entities. Surgical biopsy is frequently necessary to establish the diagnosis, direct the most appropriate

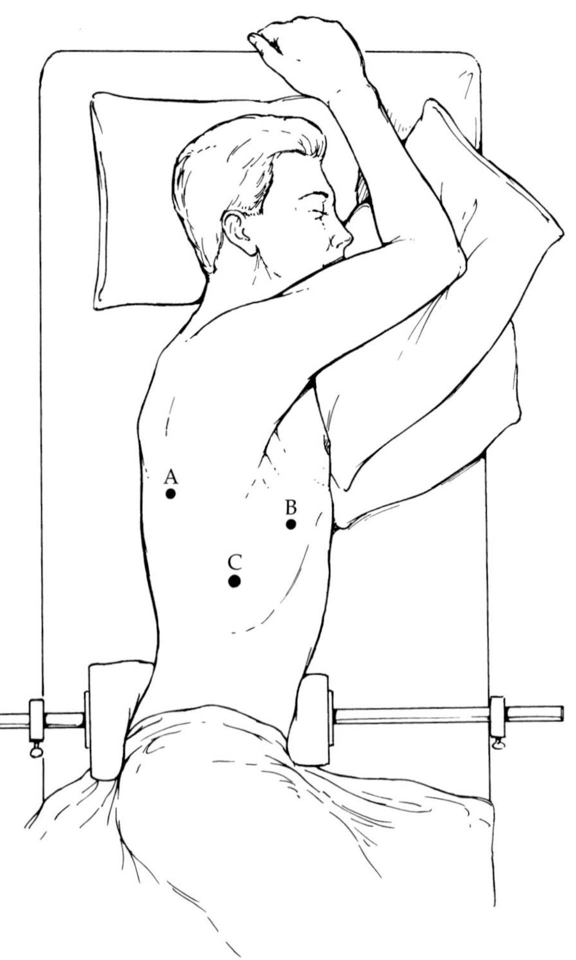

Fig. 56-1. Port placement. The usual sites of intercostal access utilized to accomplish video-assisted thoracic surgical exploration and wedge resection of the lung.

therapy, and estimate the prognosis. Preoperative assessment of the patient should include a discussion regarding potential complications such as prolonged air leak and the inability to arrive to a specific diagnosis despite extensive pathologic examination of the biopsy specimen. Not every patient with ILD warrants a lung biopsy.

Lung biopsy for ILD can be accomplished by a small limited anterior thoracotomy or by VATS. The ability to visualize the entire pleural cavity and sample remote areas of the lung, in addition to decreased early postoperative pain and early discharge, are attractive factors in favor of VATS.

VATS has been criticized because of the greater overall cost compared to thoracotomy, but our experience conflicts with this report. The liberal use of reusable instruments in VATS and the reduced overall length of hospitalization in turn reduce the overall cost of VATS. Less time missed from work in the postoperative period adds to the cost-effectiveness of VATS, compared with open procedures.

An open lung biopsy is recommended in the presence of contraindications for VATS, such as patient inability to tolerate single-lung ventilation or intraoperative findings of extensive pleuropulmonary adhesions. Other potential contraindications include pulmonary hypertension and uncorrected coagulopathy.

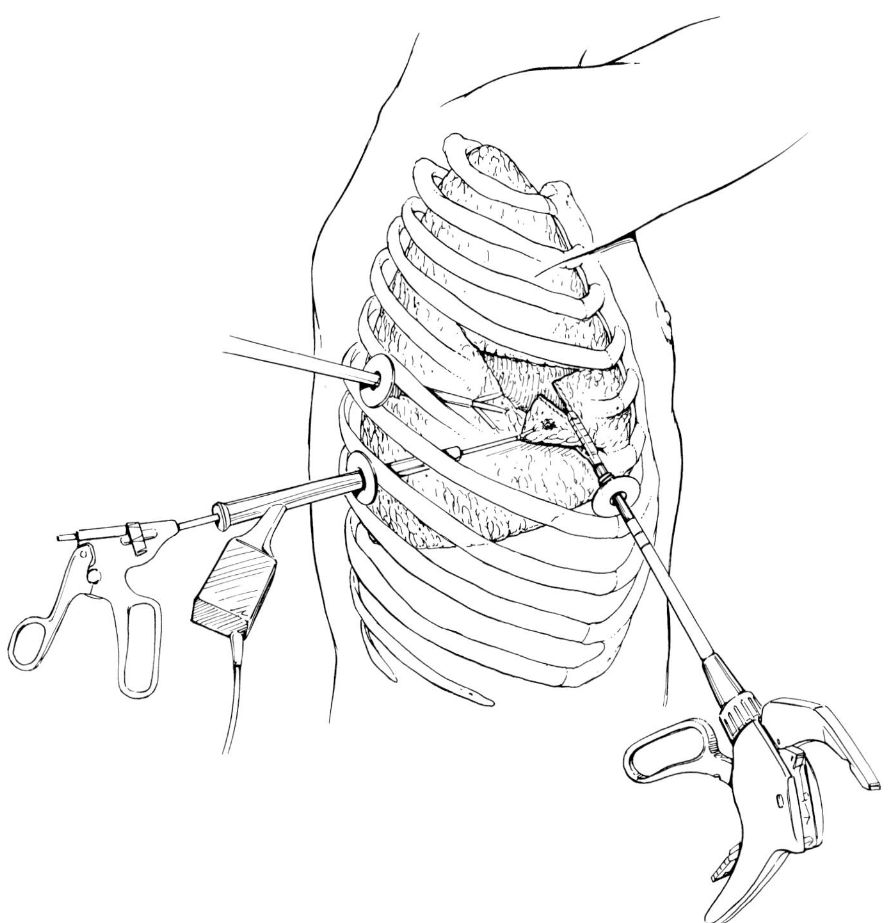

Fig. 56-2. The usual three intercostal access sites utilized for excisional biopsy via VATS. Note that the video camera, the grasper, and the stapler are within the same 180-degree arc.

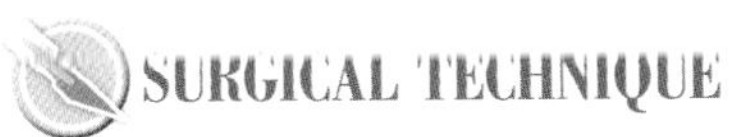

SURGICAL TECHNIQUE

Access incisions for biopsy for ILD are placed anterior to the posterior axillary line. The thoracoscope is placed at the seventh intercostal space in the anterior to midaxillary line. Operating instruments and the stapling device are introduced through intercostal access at the fourth or fifth interspace on the anterior axillary line or sixth to eighth interspace just anterior to the posterior axillary line. This intercostal access arrangement allows ideal thoracoscopic visualization of the entire lung surface for appropriate selection of biopsy sites. The free edges of the lobes along the fissures and the superior and basilar segments of the lower lobes are relatively easy sites for biopsy (Fig. 56-2). Similarly, the apical segments of the upper lobes or lateral segments of the lingual or middle lobe are also readily accessible with VATS. This orientation also facilitates alignment of the stapling device along the fissures. The flat surfaces of the lung should be avoided. Buttressing of the staple line may be helpful for patients considered at high risk for air leak, such as those requiring positive pressure ventilation or high dose corticosteroids and patients with emphysematous lungs. In general, two to three biopsy specimens are resected from different lobes to ensure representative sampling of the ILD. To perform the biopsy, the selected edge of the lung is held with a grasping instrument and one or more firings of the stapler are applied. Multiple firings of the stapler may be needed to complete the excision. Roticulation of the stapler may be required in order to avoid the "banana" effect, where a long narrow specimen is obtained.

Following removal of the specimen, the lung is partially expanded and the staple line inspected for hemostasis and air leak. Most staple lines are hemostatic and pneumostatic, but if an air leak is identified, a commercially available product such as DuraSeal or Tisseal can be utilized in an attempt to control the air leak. Intercostal nerve blocks are applied and a small single chest tube (16 to 28F) is introduced through one of the inferior intercostal incisions and positioned under thoracoscopic guidance toward a posterior and apical direction avoiding the fissure. The other intercostal incisions are closed in layers. The chest tube can be removed when drainage is minimal (<150 to 200 cc per day) and the air leak has resolved. Early chest tube removal after 90 minutes in the recovery room was evaluated in a prospective, nonrandomized study with 59 patients. Among those patients, 26 underwent VATS for ILD and 33 underwent resection of lung nodules. Results from this study showed it to be a safe and cost-effective practice if strict criteria for this strategy are met, as depicted in Table 56-5, page 568). Patients managed with this strategy had a shorter hospitalization compared with the traditional approach.

VATS EXCISIONAL BIOPSY OF INDETERMINATE PULMONARY NODULES

Diagnostic Assessment

With the recent widespread use of CT scans, a larger number of patients is found to have one or more small lung nodular

TABLE 56-5. CLINICAL CRITERIA FOR EARLY REMOVAL OF CHEST TUBES AFTER A VATS WEDGE BIOPSY OF THE LUNG

Peripherally located disease
Absence of extensive adhesions or dissection
Absence of visceral pleural disruption
No obvious air leak during and at conclusion of the operation
Complete expansion of the lung on postoperative chest roentgenogram
Drainage <50 mL/hour
Extubation before chest tube removal
Absence of an air leak in the recovery room

VATS, video-assisted thoracoscopic surgery.

opacities. The consulting surgeon needs to have a clear understanding of the differential diagnosis, evaluation, and treatment options to propose a rational management algorithm. A solitary pulmonary nodule (SPN) is defined as a single ovoid or spherical lesion, up to 3 cm in diameter, completely surrounded by lung without associated atelectasis or adenopathy. Lesions larger than 3 cm are almost always malignant and are referred to as masses; prompt diagnosis and resection is the preferred strategy. The differential diagnosis of SPN includes neoplastic, infectious, inflammatory, vascular, traumatic, and congenital lesions. Other benign etiologies for lung nodules are hamartoma, rheumatoid nodules, intrapulmonary lymph nodes, plasma cell granulomas, histoplasmosis, granulomas, and nodular sarcoidosis. Previous CT scans, chest radiographs, and other pertinent imaging studies should be obtained for comparison whenever possible, as they may serve to demonstrate either stability or interval growth of the nodule in question. After completing an initial clinical and radiographic assessment, clinicians will be able to classify solitary pulmonary nodules into one of three categories: benign, malignant, or indeterminate. Between 70% and 75% of nodules that remain indeterminate will ultimately be identified as malignant.

The malignant potential of peripheral noncalcified pulmonary lesions depends primarily on the patient's age, the lesion size, the degree of tobacco smoke exposure, the pattern of nodule growth and calcification, and a history of previous malignancy.

Until now, it has been accepted standard practice to regard all noncalcified pulmonary nodules as potentially malignant lesions that require close monitoring until proved stable over a period of 2 years. This approach was adopted prior to the widespread use of CT and was based on the observation that a substantial proportion of noncalcified nodules that were detected at chest radiography turned out to be lung cancers. These nodules were almost all larger than 5 mm in diameter and most were in the 1 to 3 cm range.

Since the introduction of helical CT in the early 1990s and multidetector row CT in the late 1990s, the detection of focal rounded pulmonary opacities or nodules as small as 1 to 2 mm in diameter has become routine. In fact, the majority of smokers who undergo thin-section CT have been found to have small lung nodules, most of which are smaller than 7 mm in diameter. However, the clinical importance of these extremely small nodules differs substantially from that of larger nodules detected on chest radiographs in that the vast majority of the small nodules are benign.

It has been clearly demonstrated that there is a positive relationship of lesion size to likelihood of malignancy. For nodules less than 3 mm in diameter, the incidence of malignancy is less than 0.2%, whereas the risk of malignancy for nodules 4 to 7 mm in diameter is 0.9%. This risk increases to 18% for nodules 8 to 20 mm and to 50% for those larger than 20 mm.

Until recently, serial CT scans were recommended at 3, 6, 12, 18, and 24 months for all low-probability indeterminate nodules regardless of size. The rationale for this approach was that some of these nodules would turn out to be cancers and that early intervention would provide an opportunity for cure. The downside of this policy includes potential morbidity and mortality from resection for benign nodules and other false-positive findings, poor utilization of resources, increased health care costs, unnecessary patient anxiety, and increased radiation burden.

Current recommendations for follow-up and management of nodules smaller than 8 mm in diameter detected incidentally at nonscreening CT are depicted in Table 56-4. A low-dose, thin-section, unenhanced technique should be used, with limited longitudinal coverage, when follow-up of a lung nodule is the only indication for the CT examination. Because at least 99% of all nodules 4 mm or smaller are benign and such small opacities are extremely common on thin-section CT scans, we do not recommend follow-up scans in every case except in high-risk patients. In the case of nodules larger than 8 mm, additional options such as contrast-enhanced CT, positron emission tomography (PET),

TABLE 56-6. RECOMMENDATIONS FOR CT SCAN FOR PULMONARY NODULES DETECTED INCIDENTALLY AT NONSCREENING CT

Nodule size (mm)[*]	Low-risk patient[†]	High-risk patient[‡]
<4	No follow-up needed[§]	Follow-up CT at 12 mo; if unchanged, no further follow-up[¶]
4–6	Follow-up CT at 12 mo; if unchanged, no further follow-up[¶]	Initial follow-up CT at 6–12 mo then at 18–24 mo if no change[¶]
6–8	Initial follow-up CT at 6–12 mo then at 18–24 mo if no change	Initial follow-up CT at 3–6 mo then at 9–12 and 24 mo if no change
>8	Follow-up CT at 3, 9, and 24 mo, dynamic contrast-enhanced CT, PET, and/or biopsy	Same as for low-risk patient

CT, computed tomography.
[*]Average of length and width of newly detected indeterminate nodule in persons 35 years of age or older
[†]Minimal or absent history of smoking and other known risk factors
[‡]History of smoking or other known risk factors
[§]The risk of malignancy in this category is substantially less (<1%) than that in a baseline CT scan of an asymptomatic smoker
[¶]Nonsolid (ground-glass) or partly solid nodules may require longer follow-up to exclude indolent adenocarcinoma

percutaneous needle biopsy, and thoracoscopic resection can be considered.

Management decisions should not be made on nodule size alone. While any calcification in a small nodule favors a benign etiology, central, laminar, or dense diffuse patterns of calcification are reliable evidence of benignancy. Fat content suggests a hamartoma or occasionally a lipoid granuloma or lipoma. Solid versus nonsolid appearance, speculation, or other characteristics influence the likelihood of malignancy. Longer follow-up intervals are appropriate for nonsolid (ground glass opacities) and very small opacities. For instance, even if malignant, a nonsolid nodule that is smaller than 6 mm will probably not grow perceptibly in much less than 12 months. In addition, obtaining an accurate measurement of growth in subcentimeter nodules is problematic.

Several recent studies support the use of screening CT for the early detection of lung cancer in high-risk patients. The International Early Lung Cancer Action Program (I-ELCAP) investigators recently reported their experience on survival of patients with Stage I lung cancer detected on CT screening. Among participants with clinical Stage I cancer who underwent surgical resection within 1 month after diagnosis, the 10-year estimated survival rate was 92%, suggesting that screening CT is effective in detecting early lung cancer likely to be cured by surgical resection.

Positron emission tomography (PET) scanning is becoming more commonly used to differentiate benign from malignant nodules (Fig. 56-3). An estimated sensitivity of 96.8% and specificity of 77.8% for identifying malignant processes have been reported in a recent meta-analysis of 40 studies; however, little information exists about 18F-fluorodeoxyglucose (FDG)-PET performance for nodules less than 1 cm in diameter. False negative results can occur in lesions smaller than 1 cm because a critical mass of metabolically active malignant cells is required for PET diagnosis. False negative results are also observed in bronchoalveolar carcinomas with ground glass opacity and carcinoid tumors. False positive results can be expected with active inflammatory processes such as granulomatous lesions (as a result of histoplasmosis or tuberculosis, for example), pneumonia, abscess, aspergillosis, and sarcoidosis. In these cases the FDG uptake has been attributed to granulocyte and/or macrophage activity.

Positron emission tomography should be included as part of the workup of an SPN if clinical decision-making will be changed by its findings. PET is not only useful in visualizing the nodule, but it can also change patient management by detecting unsuspected nodal and metastatic disease. Because of its high negative predictive value, PET excludes malignancy correctly in the vast majority of cases. In these patients, excisional biopsy can be avoided and follow-up CT scan is advised. A prospective study of 87 patients examined whether FDG uptake could differentiate malignant from benign nodules. The investigators found that when a mean standardized uptake value (SUV) of greater than or equal to 2.5 was used for detecting malignancy, the sensitivity, specificity, and accuracy were 97%, 82%, and 92% respectively. In a recent study PET and CT were used for 5 years in a screening trial in heavy smokers. PET sensitivity was 90% in nodules greater than 7 mm in diameter and correctly identified eight of nine prevalence cancers and ten of eleven incidence cancers. PET is not recommended for lesions less than 7 mm in diameter.

A cost-effectiveness study of alternative management strategies for patients with SPN utilizing 40 possible clinical combinations of five diagnostic interventions (CT, FDG-PET, transthoracic needle biopsy, surgery, and watchful waiting) demonstrated that PET should be used selectively when pretest probability of malignancy and CT findings are discordant or in patients with intermediate to high pretest probability who are at high risk for surgical complications.

Invasive Staging

The sensitivity of bronchoscopy for diagnosis of malignancy in a solitary pulmonary nodule varies from 20% to 80%. The sensitivity increases with size, from 10% in nodules less than 1.5 cm to up to 60% for nodules 2.0 to 3.0 cm. When a bronchus is leading to the lesion on CT scan, 70% of the cases are diagnosed as malignant. More recently, ultra-thin bronchoscopy and navigational bronchoscopy have been utilized successfully to reach peripherally located nodules, which are out of reach from conventional bronchoscopy utilizing fluoroscopy.

Transthoracic needle aspiration biopsy identifies peripheral pulmonary lesions as malignant in up to 95% of cases; however, the false negative rate is 3% to 29%. Complication rates are higher than those for bronchoscopy, with an incidence of pneumothorax of up to 30%. Unfortunately, less than 15% of patients with specific benign diagnoses (such as infectious organisms, hamartoma, or pulmonary infarct) have a final confirmation of the etiology, and many of these "benign" lesions will ultimately be found to be malignant at subsequent surgical excision. In fact, the nonspecific "benign" percutaneous biopsy results in a 60% false negative rate when surgical excision was later carried out. The relative accuracy, complication rate, and effect on subsequent clinical management of patients with peripheral *indeterminate* pulmonary nodules approached with an initial VATS excisional biopsy are superior to those of an initial percutaneous biopsy approach. Caution, however, should be exercised to avoid resection of many benign nodules, exposing patients to unnecessary risk and expense.

A percutaneous CT-guided biopsy approach, is however, appropriate in selected instances. It is certainly a reasonable diagnostic approach for obviously unresectable pulmonary lesions for which primary radiotherapy, chemotherapy, or ablative techniques (radiofrequency ablation, radiosurgery ablation) are being considered. Percutaneous biopsy is also acceptable for patients with severe physiologic impairment who are not candidates for any surgical intervention, including VATS as a compromised wedge resection. Finally, it

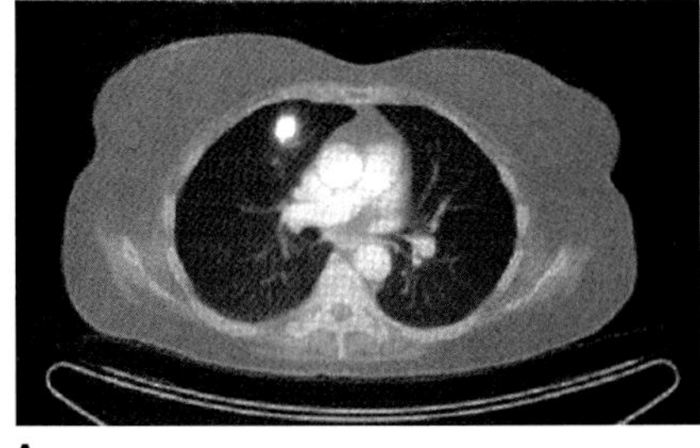

A

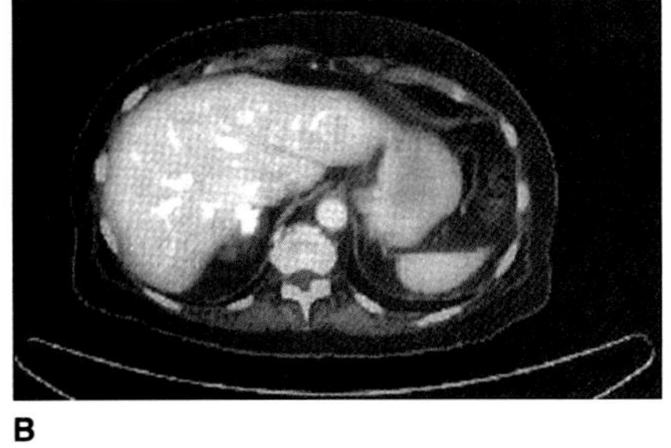

B

Fig. 56-3. Integrated PET-CT scan for lung cancer staging. **A.** The lung nodule demonstrates increased FDG uptake. **B.** Metastatic disease of the adrenal gland demonstrated by whole-body PET-CT scan. PET-CT, positron emission tomography-computed tomography; FDG, fluorodeoxyglucose.

is acceptable to perform percutaneous biopsy in deep seated lesions not amenable for VATS resection prior to embarking on formal resection for lung cancer (lobectomy).

VATS FOR THE DIAGNOSIS OF A PULMONARY NODULE

The significant limitation of the "nonsurgical" techniques to establish the final diagnosis of a pulmonary nodule has led many physicians to move directly to surgical excisional biopsy as the primary diagnostic modality in patients who can withstand thoracic surgical exploration and resection. The VATS approach is an attractive minimally invasive surgical alternative to open thoracotomy for the surgical management of *indeterminate* pulmonary nodules. The ability to identify and accurately diagnose peripheral pulmonary nodules with thoracoscopic excisional biopsy approaches 97% in selected candidates. Criteria for thoracoscopic biopsy of pulmonary nodules are depicted in Table 56-7.

Thoracoscopic biopsy of indeterminate pulmonary nodules provides definitive diagnosis and eliminates the need for follow-up and serial CT scans required for assessment of potential growth and malignancy. Also, there is a potential therapeutic benefit through a compromise nonanatomic wedge resection of subcentemiter peripheral lung cancers in patients with impaired cardiopulmonary reserve that otherwise would not have been considered for lobectomy. Nonetheless, patients should be evaluated preoperatively to rule out significant compromise of cardiopulmonary function that might worsen even with a small amount of lung resection. Patients with severe pulmonary hypertension are particularly at risk. It is important, however, to minimize the number of unnecessary procedures for benign diagnoses by applying the current understanding of the role of CT and PET for diagnosis and follow-up of patients with SPN.

TABLE 56-7. CRITERIA FOR THORACOSCOPIC EXCISIONAL BIOPSY OF SOLITARY PULMONARY NODULES

Size less than 3 cm in diameter
Indeterminate etiology after appropriate workup
Location in the outer third of the lung
Absence of endobronchial extension
Ability to tolerate general anesthesia with one-lung ventilation

It should be emphasized that VATS wedge resection, when done for primary malignant lung nodules, should be followed by formal resection (segmentectomy or lobectomy) in the same setting. Therefore, nodules that have the possibility of being lung cancer should not be biopsied unless the surgeon is prepared to proceed with a definitive resection at that setting.

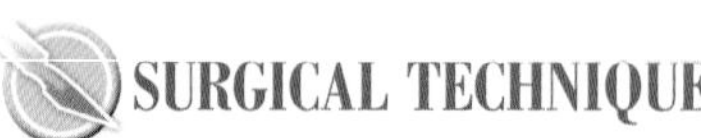

SURGICAL TECHNIQUE

The basic techniques for VATS excisional biopsy of peripheral pulmonary nodules are similar to those used for thoracoscopic wedge resection biopsy for ILD. Some important differences relate to the strategies for lesion localization and intercostal access for instrumentation to approach the lesion in question from the best angle. Port placement is based on careful examination of the CT scan to estimate the location of the nodule in relation to landmarks such as the apex of the lung, tip of the scapula, carina, fissures, pulmonary veins and diaphragm. The camera is usually inserted in the anterior axillary line at the seventh or eighth interspace to provide a panoramic view of the entire pleural cavity. It is helpful to have a port placed near the estimated location of the nodule to introduce a finger and palpate nonvisible lesions with minimal lung manipulation. Careful examination of the surface of the lung in the region of the suspected lesion identified by CT will often reveal local visceral pleural scarring or puckering. Nodular lesions are easier to identify with a completely atelectatic lung. Once the nodule has been located, strategic placement of other intercostal access is crucial to adequately position the endoscopic tools for wedge resection. In general, a three-port technique can be utilized to accommodate the camera, grasper, and stapler. In the case of potentially malignant nodules that may require a formal lung cancer operation such as segmentectomy or lobectomy, planning should include the placement of a 4- to 5-cm access incision to perform the procedure.

With the nodule clearly identified, the stapling device can usually be positioned beneath it when the lesion is located near an edge of the lung or when the lesion is small (<2 cm in diameter) and in a subpleural location. For patients undergoing diagnostic wedge biopsy prior to proceeding to VATS lobectomy for lung cancer, margins are not crucial as a formal cancer operation will follow. In patients with poor pulmonary reserve in whom a compromise wedge resection is being performed as the cancer operation, efforts should be made to achieve a 2- to 4-cm margin to ensure complete resection. The specimen should be retrieved from the thoracic cavity in a bag to prevent seeding of the soft tissues of the chest wall.

In patients for whom VATS is not ideal, generally due to a deep location in the lung parenchyma, several techniques have been described for localization of pulmonary nodules. These techniques include careful preoperative assessment of the CT scan, preoperative injection of methylene blue, and wire needle localization or injection of radiolabeled albumin for intraoperative localization with a gamma counter. Ultrasonography has also been utilized, although with limited success.

The rate of local recurrence after sublobar resection for lung cancer is greater than following lobectomy. Aiming to improve local control and to avoid the potential morbidity and radiation treatment planning difficulties associated with "postage stamp" local radiotherapy, the use of radioactive iodine (^{125}I) brachytherapy in conjunction with sublobar resection of Stage I non-small cell lung cancer has been explored. This technique can be applied thoracoscopically or after thoracotomy. It consists of preparing and positioning a permanent implant of ^{125}I seeds sewn within a polyglycolic sheet of absorbable hernia mesh (Fig. 56-4). A uniform distribution of the radioactive seeds is greatly facilitated by the use of an absorbable suture product in which the seeds are imbedded at 1-cm intervals. A significant reduction in local recurrence was observed among these patients (2%), compared with a similar cohort of patients treated earlier with sublobar resection alone (19%).

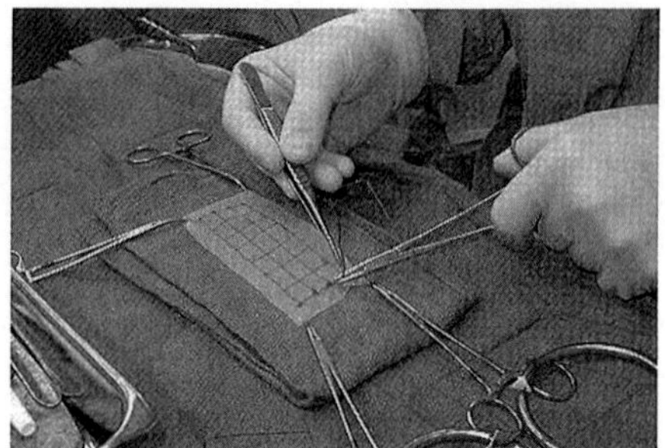

Fig. 56-4. Configuration of the absorbable Vicryl suture ^{125}I seeds utilized to deliver brachytherapy following VATS sublobar resection.

VATS PULMONARY METASTASECTOMY

Pulmonary metastasectomy is indicated in selected patients with favorable tumor etiologies. Selected patients with indeterminate pulmonary nodules and a history of malignancy also benefit from metastasectomy, as the presence of metastases will provide prognostic information and indicate further therapy.

Patients with metastatic disease who do not receive treatment have a median survival of less than 10 months and a 5-year survival of less than 5%. In patients with colorectal carcinoma metastatic to the lung, however, the 5-year survival after pulmonary metastasectomy ranges from 21% to 62%. The number of pulmonary metastases, serum carcinoembryonic antigen level, and thoracic lymph node metastases were identified as prognosis-related criteria. Selected patients with metastatic melanoma are also candidates for pulmonary metastasectomy.

Several techniques have been described for the surgical management of lung metastases, including VATS, sternotomy, and thoracotomy. Chosing the best technique is based on the potential pain-related morbidity, preservation of the pulmonary function, and capability of complete palpation of the lung.

The resistance that many surgeons have regarding a VATS approach to metastatic disease is that some foci will be missed due to the restricted palpation of the lung. In a prospective study designed to compare the values of CT scan, VATS exploration, and open thoracotomy in the management of pulmonary metastases, analysis of early results with 18 patients revealed a 56% failure rate of CT and VATS to detect all lesions.

In a small study of patients with three or fewer metastases (diameters <3 cm in CT scan) located in the periphery of the lung in which a confirmatory thoracotomy was performed and the thoracoscopic resection of solitary metastasis was considered feasible, the 2-year follow-up of these patients suggests that VATS resection of solitary pulmonary metastasis is associated with the same survival rate as resection by thoracotomy.

Candidate lesions for pulmonary metastasectomy are similar to those described for VATS resection of indeterminate pulmonary nodules. The VATS approach is a valid alternative to thoracotomy for the resection of limited metastatic disease (fewer than three nodules) identified as small, peripheral nodules on helical CT scan. Generous wedge biopsies with 1- to 2-cm margins are adequate for the resection of metastases. Repeated procedures are indicated in some patients with favorable response to prior operations and well-controlled primary tumors. In patients with lung metastases not considered for VATS resection due to the number and size of the lesions or compromised segmental boundaries and with high risk of incomplete resection, an open thoracotomy or sternotomy should be performed. Palpation of the lung through small thoracotomies could minimize the need for conversion to full, open thoracotomy in selected patients.

PLEURAL DISEASE

The indications for thoracoscopy for pleural disease have expanded greatly in the last decade. Thoracoscopy is ideally suited for biopsy of the pleura and drainage of pleural effusions with or without pleurodesis for benign and malignant effusions, pleurodesis and blebectomy for recurrent pneumothorax, debridement and decortication for empyema, evacuation of retained hemothorax, chylothorax, and biopsy of pleural based masses. The basic technique for all of these procedures is relatively standard and can be achieved with two to three port incisions, a 5- or 10-mm 30-degree angled telescope, and basic instrumentation.

The preoperative evaluation for pleural disease is straightforward. A thorough history and physical examination should be performed. Imaging studies usually include a chest roentgenogram and CT with or without contrast. A CT scan will clearly demonstrate the amount of effusion, areas of consolidation or atelectasis, pneumonthorax and blebs, and pleural-based masses and it can also demonstrate pleural thickening, fluid loculations or evidence of trapped lung. Percutaneous interventional procedures are often performed initially for diagnostic and therapeutic purposes. The indication to proceed with thoracoscopy is made on an individual basis, taking into consideration the clinical situation and results of prior investigations or interventions.

RECURRENT BENIGN AND MALIGNANT PLEURAL EFFUSION

Most patients with moderate to large benign pleural effusions can be treated medically or with one or more thoracenteses for diagnosis and symptomatic relief of their dyspnea. On occasion, recurrent benign pleural effusion may require thoracoscopy for pleural biopsy, drainage of effusion, and pleurodesis in an attempt to avoid further recurrences and prevent trapped lung. For malignant effusions, thoracoscopy may be performed to confirm the diagnosis of suspected malignancy if the diagnosis has not been established by prior thoracentesis and to perform pleurectomy, pleural abrasion, and chemical pleurodesis. In patients with large pleural effusions, we prefer to drain the effusion with a small-bore catheter such as a pigtail the day prior to the operative procedure to prevent re-expansion pulmonary edema.

SURGICAL TECHNIQUE

The procedure is best performed with the patient in full lateral decubitus position to allow access to the entire pleural cavity. If the effusion is free-flowing, the initial access incision is placed at the level of the seventh intercostal space in the mid- to anterior axillary line. A general exploration of the thoracic cavity is performed. One or two additional 5-mm ports are then placed for the instruments. One is placed in the fourth or fifth intercostal space anterior axillary line and the other just below the tip of the scapula or slightly lower. If the lung is partially adhered to the parietal pleura, the placement of these ports may need to be altered as necessary. In the absence of multiloculated fluid collections, no attempt is made to free the lung from the chest wall. Attention is directed at assessing the tumor burden in the pleural cavity. If the diagnosis of malignant effusion has not been made prior to the procedure, the biopsy of pleural nodules can be performed to confirm the diagnosis on a frozen section. The appearance of the parietal pleura leaves little doubt of the diagnosis when it is studded with malignant nodules. The lung is then examined and assessed for its pliability and probability to fully expand and completely obliterate the pleural cavity. If the lung is trapped and there is little possibility of complete obliteration of the pleural cavity and pleural apposition, pleurodesis is contraindicated and a pleurex catheter should be considered. This can be easily placed under direct thoracoscopic vision and directed at the desired location. There is no role for decortication in malignant pleural effusion. For benign effusions, a partial pleurectomy and pleural abrasion are performed to aid in pleurodesis.

The agent of choice for chemical pleurodesis for malignant effusions continues to be a matter of debate. Options include sterile talc, bleomycin, and doxycycline. In our practice we prefer sterile talc 5 to 10 grams insufflated into the thoracic cavity taking care to evenly cover the entire surface of the lung and chest wall. If bleomycin or doxycycline is utilized, the chest tubes should remain either elevated or clamped for 4 to 6 hours after the procedure to prevent their immediate evacuation from the thoracic cavity. Chest drains are usually left on suction for at least 2 days to allow time for initial pleural adhesion. If fluid drainage persists, the chest drains are left until the output decreases to less than 200 mL/day (usually 2 to 4 days).

EMPYEMA

Thoracic empyema is the collection of pus or infected pleural effusion within the pleural space. It can involve the entire pleural space or it can be loculated. Empyema is usually secondary to an underlying infectious process in the lung, such as pneumonia or abscess (parapneumonic empyema), or as a complication of operative procedures in the chest. Other causes of empyema include trauma, esophageal perforation, descending infections from the neck, infection of the chest wall, spine, or mediastinal lymph nodes, or transdiaphragmatic extension of a subphrenic abscess. The causative agent may be anaerobic, aerobic, or mixed pathogens. Mortality from empyema ranges from 1% to 19%; prognosis is worse in the elderly and in patients with underlying cardiac, renal, and pulmonary conditions or with hospital-acquired or culture-positive empyema. Diagnosis is usually made on clinical grounds, radiographic signs, and demonstration of infected fluid on thoracentesis. Findings indicating the presence of empyema include a pH less than 7.0, positive gram stain or culture, and frank pus on the aspiration of pleural fluid. Empyema is usually classified into exudative, fibrinopurulent, or organizing stages depending on the characteristics of the infectious process in the chest cavity. These stages represent a continuum, and there are no sharply defined boundaries. Once the diagnosis of empyema is established, it is necessary to determine whether the collection is free or loculated. Imaging studies helpful in evaluation of patients with empyema include chest roentgenograms, CT scan, and ultrasonography. Computed tomography and ultrasonography are highly sensitive in demonstrating the presence of septa, membranes, and loculations.

Treatment of empyema requires antibiotics and drainage of the pleural space. Drainage procedures vary from simple interventions such as chest tube thoracostomy to invasive operations such as open thoracotomy depending on the size of the effusion, condition of the patient, and stage of the empyema. Other treatment modalities include pleural irrigation, fibrinolytics, and thoracoscopy. Recent literature does not support the routine use of fibrinolytic agents in the treatment of empyema. Thoracoscopic debridement of the pleural space offers an opportunity to provide early intervention to diminish the risk of potential complications such as trapped lung requiring formal decortication. VATS is particularly effective during the exudative and fibrinopurulent stages of empyema. Thorough empyemolysis can be achieved with complete breakdown of all loculations and drainage of the gelatinous exudates restricting lung expansion. The goals of the operation are to (1) remove as much of the infected material as possible, (2) achieve a unilocular pleural space and adequate drainage, and (3) achieve full expansion of the lung and obliteration of the pleural cavity. On occasion, a formal thoracotomy is required to decorticate a trapped lung, and one should not hesitate to proceed if indicated. Lung encasement with a fibrotic peel is the most frequent cause for conversion.

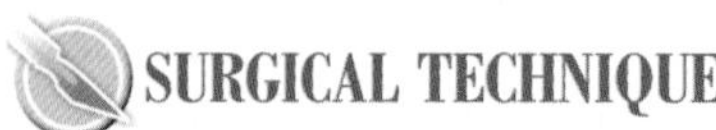

SURGICAL TECHNIQUE

Access port placement is somewhat variable, depending on the area of the chest cavity most involved. Compared to the general strategies in trocar placement for most VATS procedures, the approach to a localized or loculated pleural inflammatory process such as an empyema is reversed. Because of the inflammatory reaction that results in degrees of pleural symphysis, there is a greater risk of injury to the lung when the empyema pocket is approached from across the pleural cavity. Instead, the initial trocar should be inserted toward the central portion of the fluid collection from a dependent approach and the empyema is drained first, thus lessening the risk of lung injury. Following drainage and decompression of the empyema pocket, the other trocars can be placed to facilitate completion of the procedure. The entire pleural cavity needs to be explored, including the fissures of the lung and the subpulmonic space, to avoid leaving undrained infected fluid collections. Once the scope and a suction cannula are placed, gentle manipulation of the lung is performed to avoid lacerations. If access to the pleural space is limited due to adhesions, a finger, the telescope, the suction device, or an endoscopic kittner can be used as blunt probes to take down adhesions and create more working space. During this maneuver, the instrument is kept next to the chest wall as a sweeping motion is performed to avoid trauma to the lung. Breaking down the adhesions allows the lung to collapse and improves visualization. Once enough space has been created, additional ports are placed under direct visualization.

Thick gelatinous material is removed with a ring forceps or a large-bore suction cannula. Irrigation of the pleural cavity with warm saline may expedite this maneuver. A blunt grasper is used to grasp exudative or fibrous peels from the surface of the lung and chest wall, stripping as much as possible. This is performed in a systematic fashion to address all areas of the lung, taking care to avoid a deep plane of dissection with resultant injury to the lung. It is however, not necessary to remove every piece of peel as long as complete lung expansion can be achieved, as doing so will result in creation of multiple lung lacerations and air leaks. Removal of the peel is facilitated in the open procedure by partially inflating the lung. This, however, is not practical during VATS. Once the goals of the operation are achieved, one or more chest tubes are placed in strategic locations to provide optimal drainage. On occasion, large Jackson-Pratt drains are helpful to access localized pockets not easily drained by chest tubes. Gentle manual ventilation of both lungs is performed to expand all areas of atelectatic lung. Most patients can be extubated at the end of the procedure. Postoperative pleural irrigation is rarely indicated but can be performed by instilling 500 to 1000 cc of saline in the pleural cavity through a special chest tube adaptor. The chest tubes are clamped to allow the fluid to dwell for 1 hour and then are connected to suction. The cycle can be repeated every 4 to 6 hours for 2 to 3 days. Depending on the severity of the process, chest tubes can be removed after a few days or are converted to empyema tubes. A repeat CT scan of the chest may need to be performed if there is any concern regarding undrained fluid collections, which can be drained successfully with percutaneous catheters. The use of postoperative fibrinolytics has not been formally investigated.

PNEUMOTHORAX

Spontaneous pneumothorax is a disease with an estimated incidence of 4 to 9 per 100,000 patients per year with a 5:1 male predominance. Its management differs depending upon its etiology, duration, number of previous occurrences, and patient occupation, lifestyle, and general health. The risk of recurrence is between 20% and 40% after the first episode and rises to 60% after a second episode.

Primary spontaneous pneumothorax (PSP) occurs due to the rupture of blebs in the absence of other pulmonary pathology. It typically affects patients between the ages of 25 and 30 years who are tall, thin and who often have a history of smoking. Blebs are blister-like areas (<1 cm) composed of visceral pleura and located in the surface of the lung, particularly at the apex of the upper lobes and superior segment of the lower lobes. These blebs have no epithelial lining. The precise etiology for their formation is unknown, but there is increased incidence in asthmatics and smokers.

Pain is the most common symptom, followed by dyspnea. Rarely, hemorrhage may occur from a torn vascular adhesion. A tension pneumothorax may result from a ball-valve effect creating hemodynamic instability.

Secondary spontaneous pneumothorax (SSP) usually occurs in patients 50 to 65 years old with underlying pulmonary parenchymal conditions. The most common etiology is rupture of a bulla. Bullae are larger then blebs (>2.5 cm) and are most common in patients with emphysema. Because of their underlying pulmonary condition, these patients do not tolerate their pneumothoraces as well as younger patients with PSP. Other predisposing conditions include necrotic peripheral malignancies, infection, interstitial lung disease, lymphangiomyomatosis, endometriosis, and *Pneumocystis jirovecii* pneumonia. Catamenial pneumothorax occurs during menstruation as a result of endometrial implants, affecting the right hemithorax in 90% of cases.

Diagnosis is suspected clinically and confirmed on a chest roentgenogram. The size of the pneumothorax may be estimated on plain films, but the result is highly inaccurate. For patients suspected of having SSP, CT scan may be cost-effective in identifying other target areas for possible resection not easily identified on plain films.

The general goals of treatment are the same for PSP and SSP and include the elimination of the source of the air leak, complete lung re-expansion, and the minimization of the risk of recurrence. Options for the management of pneumothorax include simple aspiration, chest tube thoracostomy, and thoracoscopy, or open thoracotomy. For patients with a small (<20%) pneumothorax and minimal symptoms, observation with a repeat chest X-ray may be advisable. Patients with larger or more symptomatic pneumothorax are initially treated with a chest tube to evacuate the pneumothorax and re-expand the lung. Indications for operative intervention include recurrence of pneumothorax, prolonged air leaks (>3 days), associated hemothorax, large cystic areas, and patient occupation or lifestyle (such as pilots, scuba divers, and patients living in remote areas or with no access to immediate medical care).

Video-assisted thoracic surgery has become the preferred approach to treat PSP or SSP. Alternatively, a limited axillary thoracotomy through the third or fourth intercostal space may be performed. VATS offers far greater visualization of the entire pleural cavity and the ability to reach areas in the lower lobes. If pleurectomy is anticipated, an epidural catheter may be beneficial for optimal postoperative pain control.

SURGICAL TECHNIQUE

Most VATS procedures for pneumothorax require two to three port incisions and single-lung ventilation with a DLT or a SLT and a bronchial blocker. The initial incision is usually placed at the midaxillary line, seventh intercostal space. With the scope in the thoracic cavity, two additional 5- to 10-mm incisions are placed in higher interspaces for instruments and staplers. All incisions are placed anterior to the posterior axillary line. Trocars are not necessary in the majority of situations. A grasper is used to gently mobilize the lung and identify all areas affected with blebs or bullae. Areas of adhesions are gently taken down if necessary to gain access to the blebs or bullae. The preferred method for their excision is to utilize a mechanical stapler, taking care to apply the stapler in the adjacent preserved lung parenchyma and avoiding the blebs or bullae. Reinforcement buttressing material is available and recommended for patients with severe emphysema but not for otherwise healthy lungs. Additional maneuvers to prevent recurrences of pneumothorax include partial pleurectomy, mechanical abrasion of the pleura with a sponge or electrocautery scratch pad, and chemical pleurodesis. Particular attention should be placed at avoiding a deep plane of dissection during pleurectomy to prevent stripping intercostal neurovascular structures and bleeding. Pleurectomy is easily performed from the apex to the mid chest (fifth intercostal space). The remaining pleura can be mechanically abraded with a sponge or scratch pad. Troublesome bleeding can be easily controlled with argon plasma coagulation.

Chemical pleurodesis for recurrent pneumothorax can be achieved with doxycycline, 500 to 1000 mg. The chest tubes should be clamped or elevated for 4 to 6 hours to allow sufficient dwelling time. Every effort should be made to see that the patient leaves the operating room without air leaks. Postoperatively, the chest tubes are kept on suction for 48 to 72 hours and removed when drainage is less than 200 to 300 cc per day. Particular attention should be directed at avoiding air entry into the thoracic cavity during removal of the chest tubes, which will result in pneumothorax and failure of pleurodesis. For the same reason, anti-inflammatory medications such as ketorolac and other non steroidal antiinflammatory drugs should be avoided for pain control, as they may interfere with the inflammatory reaction necessary to cause pleurodesis.

For patients who are not candidates for VATS, a bedside pleurodesis may be attempted. Our preference is to use talc slurry (5 g diluted in 100 cc of normal saline). If doxicycline is utilized, patients should be premedicated with intravenous narcotics and a mild sedative to abrogate the intense pain associated with its instillation in the pleural space. In any case, this procedure does not address the origin of the problem, and recurrence is high.

HYPERHIDROSIS

Hyperhidrosis is a pathologic condition characterized by excessive sweating for normal thermoregulation with an extraordinary low palmar temperature. The excessive sweating may occur in any part of the body, but the most troublesome manifestations occur in the hands, arms, face, and axillae. Patients range in age from teens to people in their 30s. Hyperhidrosis is not a life-threatening condition but it markedly impedes the patient's social life and professional activities. Most patients referred for thoracic sympathectomy for hyperhidrosis have already failed medical therapy.

In the past, approaches used for thoracic sympathectomy included the cervical or supraclavicular, transaxillary, dorsal, and transthoracic routes. These approaches caused excessive morbidity and were not commonly performed. Thoracoscopic sympathectomy offers many advantages, including improved visualization, reduced pain and morbidity, and better results compared to open approaches. Other indications for thoracic sympathectomy include causalgia or dystrophic reflex, Raynaud disease, and other vascular disorders of the upper extremities.

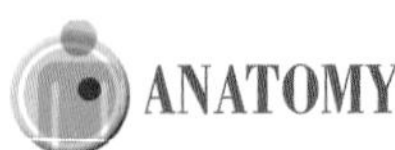

ANATOMY

Surgeons performing sympathectomy for palmar hiperhidrosis should become very familiar with the anatomy of the thoracic sympathetic chain and its variations. The thoracic sympathetic ganglia rest under the pleura against the heads of the ribs. The first thoracic ganglion is usually fused with the lower cervical ganglion to form the stellate ganglion. The next ganglion, which rests on the head of the second rib, is the second thoracic ganglion. Each of the thoracic ganglia corresponds numerically to the number of the rib. Adjacent ganglia are connected via the sympathetic trunk. In some cases, one or more accessory sympathetic fibers, known as Kuntz fibers, are found lateral to the thoracic sympathetic chain. Kuntz fibers communicate with the sympathetic system and should be treated at the same time. Undivided accessory fibers have been postulated as cause of inadequate operation or recurrence of symptoms.

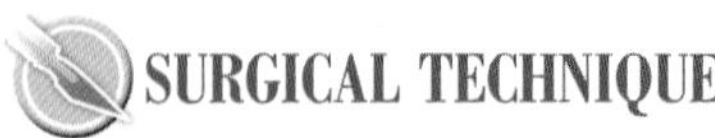

SURGICAL TECHNIQUE

There are several thoracoscopic approaches for thoracic sympathectomy for hyperhidrosis. The procedure can be performed under local anesthesia or intubated with or without split-lung ventilation and CO_2 insufflation. Techniques ranging from one to three ports have been described. The procedure can be performed in the lateral decubitus position or supine for access to both hemithoraces without need to reposition the patient. The instruments required for the different approaches are very similar to the conventional thoracoscopic instruments. A 3-, 5-, or 10-mm videothoracoscope is utilized. Our preferred method is to utilize two or three 5-mm ports placed around the breast with the patient in the supine position and the arms suspended for unimpeded access to both hemithoraces. A single-lumen tube and CO_2 insufflation to 6 to 8 mmHg is utilized. We do not routinely employ split-lung ventilation.

The first trocar is placed at the level of the nipple and lateral to the breast tissue. A 5-mm incision is made and the soft tissues gently dissected. High-flow CO_2 is then connected to the Veress needle introduced over a universal introducer. The high-flow CO_2 insufflation helps push the lung away as the pleura is punctured, creating a place for the safe introduction of the trocar. The 5-mm scope is then introduced, and the CO_2 pressure is kept at approximately 6 to 8 mmHg. This effectively collapses the lung and pushes it posteriorly, making access to the paraspinal region easier. One or two additional 5-mm ports are placed, one for the standard electrocautery instrument (hook or scissors) or harmonic hook and the other for a grasper if necessary. The advantage of the harmonic hook over standard electocautery instruments is that less smoke, which can interfere with visualization, is produced. These two additional ports are placed at the submammary fold midclavicular line and two intercostal spaces higher than the camera port at the anterior axillary line.

The first step in performing a thoracic sympathectomy is the correct identification of the ganglia to be resected. The uppermost rib seen on the back side is usually the second rib. The second rib has an intercostal muscle on its upper side, whereas the first rib does not; this helps in differentiating these two ribs. If in doubt, confirmation of the second rib can be made by introducing a needle at the second intercostal space midclavicular line (at the level of the angle of Louis). Thoracoscopically the needle will be clearly seen, and the second rib can be traced to the spine. The sympathetic chain can be seen under the translucent parietal pleura as a thin, whitish cord.

With the second rib clearly identified, the parietal pleura is opened longitudinally over the sympathetic nerve from the second to the third or fourth ribs. Small vessels in the proximity can be cauterized or avoided. A small flap of pleura is created and the nerve dissected. For palmar hyperhidrosis the second thoracic ganglia is excised. If the patient has coexistent palmar and axillary hyperhidrosis, the second and third thoracic ganglia are excised. We prefer to divide and excise the nerve tissue and cauterize the corresponding ribs and adjacent tissue to coagulate potential Kuntz fibers, although this is controversial. Alternative procedures include applying clips to the chain and cauterization of the chain without excision. Once hemostasis is achieved, a 5F pigtail catheter is introduced through the submammary incision. The lung is reinflated and the incisions closed in layers. The procedure is repeated in the opposite hemithorax and the pigtails are removed several hours later. The patient is discharged home the same or the next day.

PERICARDIAL WINDOW

Surgical indications for pericardial disease include two large categories of patients: those with pericardial effusions with or without tamponade and those with chronic constrictive pericarditis. In this section we will describe our approach for management of pericardial effusions requiring surgical intervention. Pericardial effusions can result from acute, subacute, or chronic processes. Most pericardial effusions can be treated medically or with percutaneous interventions. Recurrent effusions or malignant effusions may require surgical drainage. The selection of the appropriate therapy is related to the nature of the underlying disease process. General indications for surgical intervention include clinical or subclinical (echocardiographic) tamponade, failure to control the underlying disease process with medical therapy or percutaneous techniques, the need for histologic documentation of the etiology, and associated pleural effusions.

Two general approaches are widely employed for drainage of pericardial effusions: the subxiphoid pericardial window and the thoracoscopic pericardial window. Thoracoscopy offers the advantage of greater visibility and exposure of the pericardium, as it allows resection of a greater portion of the pericardium, and the ability to simultaneously examine and drain the pleural space. Patients considered for thoracoscopic management of pericardial effusion must be able to tolerate general anesthesia and split-lung ventilation. Preoperative and intraoperative transesophageal echocardiography is recommended to estimate the amount of fluid present, its location, and its effect on myocardial and hemodynamic function. High-risk patients may not tolerate general anesthesia and split-lung ventilation and are therefore better candidates for the subxiphoid approach.

We prefer to approach the pericardium from the right hemithorax. The right chest cavity normally provides a greater space, better exposure, and easier manipulation of instruments to perform a larger pericardial resection. A large pericardial effusion may take a significant portion of the left pleural space, limiting the exposure and the ability to perform the procedure safely. The presence of an associated pleural effusion or lung abnormality may influence the choice of approach.

SURGICAL TECHNIQUE

The patient is positioned in full lateral decubitus. If there is any concern of intraoperative hemodynamic instability, a roll is placed under the hemithorax and the patient placed 45 degrees off center to allow quick access to perform a subxiphoid approach. A single-lumen tube with a bronchial blocker or a double-lumen tube is employed for split-lung ventilation. Pacing-defibrillation patches are placed prophylactically in the event of intraoperative supraventricular or ventricular arrhythmia. The surgeon stands in the back of the patient, facilitating the approach to the anteriorly located pericardium. The initial 10-mm incision is placed at the seventh intercostal space in the anterior axillary line. The hemithorax is explored with a 30-degree telescope. Two additional 5-mm incisions are made, one at the seventh intercostal space mid- to posterior axillary line and the other just anterior to the tip of the scapula. The lung is retracted posteriorly and the distended pericardium exposed. The phrenic nerve is clearly identified and thoracoscopic forceps are used to grasp the pericardium anterior to the nerve. Thoracoscopic electrocautery scissors are utilized to open the pericardium, taking care to avoid contact with the myocardium to avoid inducing a potentially fatal ventricular fibrillation. Once a small opening is made, a suction cannula can be introduced to collect fluid for chemical analysis and cytology. This prevents mixing of the fluid with pleural fluid if the pericardial effusion is allowed to drain freely into the thoracic cavity. With the pericardium decompressed, a generous portion of the pericardium covering the right atrium can be safely excised with electrocautery scissors to ensure hemostasis. The specimen is then submitted for pathologic and microbiologic examinations as necessary. If the echocardiogram reveals a posterior effusion, the pericardium posterior to the phrenic nerve can also be excised, taking care to avoid injury to the inferior pulmonary vein. On the right side, exposure to the posterior pericardium is facilitated by mobilizing the esophagus circumferentially after retracting the lung anteriorly. This dissection is better performed with a harmonic scalpel. If the diaphragm interferes with adequate access, a retracting endostitch is placed in the dome of the diaphragm and brought out under the lower ribs, as performed for minimally invasive esophagectomy, to improve the exposure. This maneuver provides unimpeded access to the posterolateral pericardium. A generous resection of the pericardium can then be performed taking care to avoid injury to the inferior pulmonary vein and the phrenic nerve. Intraoperative transesophageal echo confirms adequate drainage of the pericardial effusion. One or two 10-mm Jackson-Pratt drains are then placed in the pericardial space and a chest tube positioned behind the lung for drainage of any pleural effusion. Most patients are extubated immediately in the operating room and transferred to a monitor ward for 24 hours. Drains are usually removed after 5 days. We do not recommend the use of sclerosing agents, even for malignant pericardial effusions.

CHYLOTHORAX

A chylothorax is an uncommon condition that arises from a broad range of conditions, including malignancy, trauma, operative procedures, and congenital abnormalities. The diagnosis of chylothorax is suspected by the excessive drainage of milky fluid from the chest cavity and confirmed by a triglyceride level greater than 110 mg/dL. The optimal management of chylothorax requires a detailed knowledge of anatomy, pathophysiology, and available treatment options. These options include thoracic duct ligation (open or thoracoscopic), pleurodesis, pleuroperitoneal shunt, and percutaneous embolization of the cysterna and thoracic duct.

The initial management of chylothorax requires complete drainage of the pleural cavity, full expansion of the lung, fluid repletion, nutritional support, and reduction of lymph flow (by administering octreotide). For patients in whom conservative measures fail, percutaneous or surgical intervention is required. Postsurgical chylothorax, particularly after esophagectomy, requires early intervention as the injury usually involves the main thoracic duct and is unlikely to respond to medical management. Smaller leaks from tributary channels, in contrast, may respond to nonoperative measures. The timing and type of intervention depend on the underlying cause and condition of the patient. The smaller the daily volume of chyle loss, the longer conservative measures can be considered. However, daily fluid losses greater than 500 to 1000 cc suggest that spontaneous cessation is unlikely and intervention should be considered within a week of diagnosis. Early surgical management should be avoided in patients who are in poor overall medical condition caused by other underlying medical causes and in those with nonsurgically induced chylothorax. These patients may benefit from interventional coiling embolization of the thoracic duct. This modality is becoming an effective alternative for any cause of chylothorax where a localized leak can be demonstrated radiographically, including post-esophagectomy patients. At our institution, percutaneous embolization of the cysterna chyle and thoracic duct is the procedure of choice for chylothorax requiring an intervention. Those patients that fail are considered for surgical approach.

SURGICAL TECHNIQUE

Chylothorax in either the right or left chest is surgically treated with thoracic duct ligation at the level of the diaphragmatic hiatus through the right hemithorax. General anesthesia and isolated left lung ventilation are used. Port placement is very similar to the placement employed for dissection of the esophagus during esophagectomy. The camera port is placed in the midaxillary line in the sixth or seventh intercostal space. Two additional 5- to 10-mm ports are placed, one just below the tip of the scapula and the other as low as possible along the same line. An additional 10-mm port is placed at the anterior axillary line lateral to the nipple for a fan retractor. The target area is the supradiaphragmatic region in the posterior mediastinum between the azygos vein and the aorta. To improve access and exposure to this area, a diaphragmatic retraction stitch is placed in the dome of the diaphragm and brought out as low as possible at the level of the posterior axillary line. This maneuver will retract the diaphragm several centimeters caudally, allowing unimpeded access to the target area above the diaphragm, just as it is done in the open procedure. The chylothorax and all loculations are drained. A peel of fibrinous membranes may need to be removed to allow full lung reexpansion. The pulmonary ligament is divided and the lung retracted cephalad and anteriorly with a fan retractor placed at the level of the fifth intercostal space anterior axillary line. The parietal pleura adjacent to the azygos vein is opened. If the site of the leak can be identified, the duct is controlled with clips or suture ligature.

Care is taken to avoid skeletonizing the duct. Clips should be applied with extreme caution to avoid lacerating the duct and creating additional injury. It should be remembered that the duct is a very fragile structure and easy to tear.

Whether or not the actual site of leak is identified, circumferential dissection around the tissue in between the aorta and azygos vein is also performed and the entire thickness of this tissue is encircled with a suture ligature. It is not necessary to divide the duct in between suture ligatures. The site of repair is observed for several minutes to ensure that the lymph leak has been effectively controlled. Fibrin glue or bioglue can be applied with a thoracoscopic catheter to cover this area, although its effectiveness remains unproven. Mechanical or chemical pleurodesis is usually not required but is recommended by some as an adjunct to operative repair. With the entire pleural space drained, one or two chest tubes are placed. The patient receives nothing by mouth for 2 days and then is started on low fat diet. If there is no increase in the chest tube output, the diet is advanced to regular. The chest tubes can then be removed. One should not hesitate to convert the procedure to an open one if difficulty is encountered in achieving the goals of safe and reliable ligation of the duct.

RETAINED HEMOTHORAX

A retained hemothorax, either traumatic, postsurgical, or spontaneous can be drained successfully with thoracoscopy. Initial management for hemothorax is simple chest tube insertion, utilizing one or two large-bore (32 to 36F) drains. If the hemithorax is not completely evacuated, VATS with two or three ports can be employed. Port placement is similar to that for pleural effusions. A retained clot can be removed with a rigid large-bore suction cannula or ring forceps. Warm saline solution or water may help break down the clots and facilitate their extraction. Once the clot is removed, a detailed inspection of the entire thoracic cavity is performed to identify potential bleeding sites. If the bleeding is originating from a peripheral lung laceration, a generous wedge biopsy is performed with the stapler to control the bleeding. Other sites of bleeding may be controlled with direct suture, clips or pressure with a sponge stick, and hemostatic agents such as oxidized cellulose and thrombin. Electrocautery and argon plasma coagulation are also useful alternatives. On rare occasion, a small thoracotomy might need to be performed to a troublesome bleeding site.

SUGGESTED READING

Bunyaviroch T, Coleman E. Pet evaluation of lung cancer. *J Nuc Med* 2006;46:451–469.

Chen DL, Dehdashti F. Advances in positron emission tomographic imaging of lung cancer. *Proc Am Thorac Soc* 2005;2:541–544.

Cho DG, Cho KD, Jo MS. Thoracoscopic direct suture repair of thoracic duct injury after thoracoscopic mediastinal surgery. *Surg Laparosc Endosc Percutan Tech* 2007;1:60–61.

Dresler CM, Olak J, Herndon JE, et al. Phase III intergroup study of talc poudrage vs talc slurry sclerosis for malignant pleural effusion. *Chest* 2005;3:909–915.

Georghiou GP, Stamler A, Sharoni E, et al. Video-assisted thoracoscopic pericardial window for diagnosis and management of pericardial effusions. *Ann Thor Surg* 2005;2:607–610.

Henschke CI, Yankelevitz DF, Naidich DP, et al. CT screening for lung cancer: suspiciousness of nodules according to size and baseline scans. *Radiology* 2004;231:164–168.

Hyland MJ, Ashrafi AS, Crepeau A, et al. Is video-assisted thoracoscopic surgery superior to limited axillary thoracotomy in the management of spontaneous pneumothorax? *Can Resp J* 2001;8:339–343.

The International Early Lung Cancer Action Program Investigators. Survival of patients with Stage I lung cancer detected on CT screening. *N Eng J Med* 2006;355:1763–1771.

Landreneau RJ, Mack MJ, Hazelrigg SR. Video-assisted thoracic surgery: basic technical concepts and intercostal approach strategies. *Ann Thorac Surg* 1992;54:800–807.

MacMahon H, Austin JH, Gamsu G. Guidelines for the management of small pulmonary nodules detected on CT scans: a statement from the Fleischner society. *Radiology* 2005;237:395–400.

Petersen RP, Hanish SI, Haney JC, et al. Improved survival with pulmonary metastasectomy: an analysis of 1720 patients with pulmonary metastatic melanoma. *J Thorac Cardiovasc Surg* 2007;133:104–110.

Pfannschmidt J, Muley T, Hoffmann H, et al. Prognostic factors and survival after complete resection of pulmonary metastases from colorectal carcinoma: experience in 167 patients. *J Thorac Cardiovasc Surg* 2003;126:732–739.

Roviaro GC, Varoli F, Vergani C, et al. State of the art in thoracoscopic surgery: a personal experience of 2000 videothoracoscopic procedures and an overview of the literature. *Surg Endosc* 2002;16:881–892.

Stefani A, Natali P, Casali C, et al. Talc poudrage versus talc slurry in the treatment of malignant pleural effusion. A prospective comparative study. *Eur J Cardiothorac Surg* 2006;6:827–832.

Weiner-Muran HT. The solitary pulmonary nodule. *Radiology* 2006;239:34–49.

COMMENTARY

In this chapter, the authors give a broad overview of the primary indications for video-assisted thoracoscopic surgery (VATS) that a general surgeon in practice may encounter. These indications range from diagnostic biopsies of chest structures to therapeutic procedures involving the lung, pleura, or pericardium. They carefully describe the general concepts of VATS, including patient positioning, control of the airway, instrumentation, and port placement. As opposed to video-assisted surgery of the abdominal cavity, in most instances a pneumothorax is not induced using carbon dioxide gas under pressure; rather, the lung is collapsed by the use of single-lung ventilation. The port positions are more limited due to the presence of the ribs, but standard instruments can be used with or without access ports because of the lack of concern regarding the escape of pneumoperitoneum. Similar to laparoscopy, however, the port position should be chosen carefully to allow triangulation of the operative field.

General surgeons preparing to perform VATS should have a background in thoracotomy in order to be familiar with the anatomy and indications for surgery. As with laparoscopy, conversion to thoracotomy may be necessary and should not be considered a "failure." Using VATS procedures, many common abnormalities of the pleura often managed by general surgeons (such as pneumothorax, hemothorax, or empyema) can be managed under direct visualization and without the morbidity of a full thoracotomy incision. Advances in VATS technology and increasing experience have now extended the indications for this technique to many procedures formerly requiring thoracotomy.

NJS

Miscellaneous Procedures

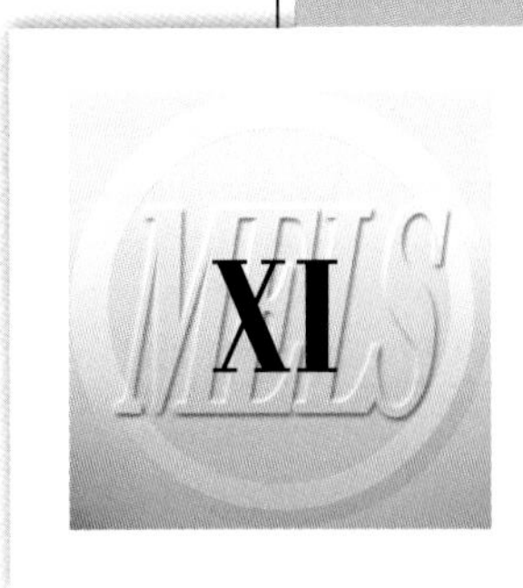

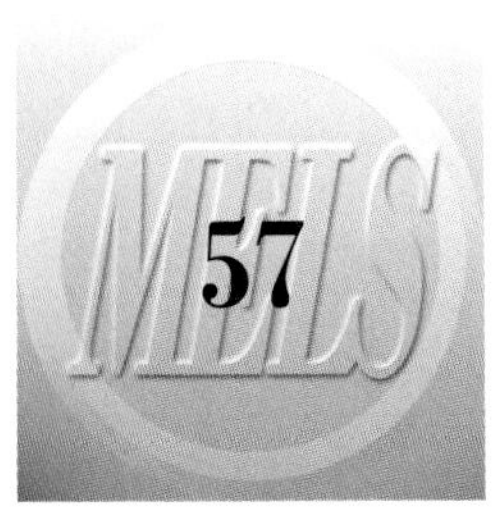

Laparoscopic Approaches to Vascular Disease

RALF KOLVENBACH AND
CATHERINE CAGIANNOS

INTRODUCTION

The initial enthusiasm given to endovascular techniques of safely excluding abdominal aortic aneurysms (AAA) has markedly diminished, due to the significant late failure rates, persistent risk of aneurysm rupture, and costs. With today's improvements in minimally invasive technology, laparoscopic techniques can be a durable alternative to endovascular repair. In fact, the outcome of laparoscopic AAA resection or aortoiliac bypass can be expected to be similar to that of an open transperitoneal tube graft repair, the gold standard, of treatment, because the conventional operation is simply replicated laparoscopically.

There are currently two rapidly evolving laparoscopic techniques for abdominal vascular surgery: total laparoscopic aortic surgery and laparoscopy to treat failing aortic endografts (hybrid techniques).

Total Laparoscopic Procedures

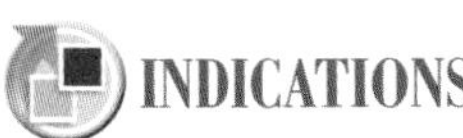

INDICATIONS

Total laparoscopic aortic procedures can be performed in patients with occlusive disease as well as for those with AAAs. A defining principle of a total laparoscopic operation is that the anastomosis is performed with laparoscopic needle holders under pneumoperitoneum.

Total laparoscopic aortic surgery in patients with aortic occlusive disease can routinely be performed in the majority of patients. Since the description of the first total laparoscopic aortic bypass procedures, the technique has been further refined and can now be used in patients with aortic aneurysms.

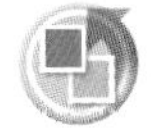

CONTRAINDICATIONS

Patients with previous aortoiliac surgery, a hostile abdomen, inflammatory aneurysms, or any aortic aneurysms requiring suprarenal cross-clamping are not candidates for a totally laparoscopic approach. In cases of aortic occlusive disease we exclude patients with a proximal "porcelain" aorta, which does not permit safe cross-clamping of the aorta.

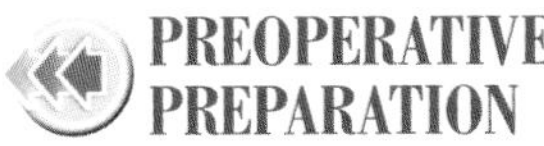

PREOPERATIVE PREPARATION

All patients receive the standard preoperative examination required for any major aortic surgery. If indicated, coronary angiography is performed, as well as pulmonary function tests. We routinely administer a standard bowel prep the day before surgery to facilitate exposure. Standard invasive monitoring lines are placed immediately before surgery, and a dose of a first-generation cephalosporin is given 30 minutes before the procedure.

Patient Positioning and Initial Exposure

These procedures are best done in designated minimally invasive operating suites with adequate monitor placement to enable the entire team to observe the case. During the whole procedure all three surgeons will be standing on the right side of the patient. The patient is placed on the operating table on a vacuum bag, which will help to keep the patient in position during the procedure. Securing the patient to the operating table is important as the table will be tilted to the right as much as 70 degrees. Six or seven laparoscopic ports are used, depending on the size of the patient (Fig. 57-1).

The left hemicolon including the splenic flexure, is mobilized medially (Fig. 57-2). In many patients there are intraabdominal adhesions that should be taken down to avoid a postoperative ileus. The technique of medial mobilization to separate the abdominal contents from the retroperitoneal space was originally described by Dion. The line of Tolt is used as a landmark when incising the lateral attachments of the sigmoid colon. Incomplete mobilization of the splenic flexure can cause lacerations of the spleen during retraction, particularly in cases with adhesions from previous surgery. In most of our patients we prefer a left hemicolic retrorenal approach

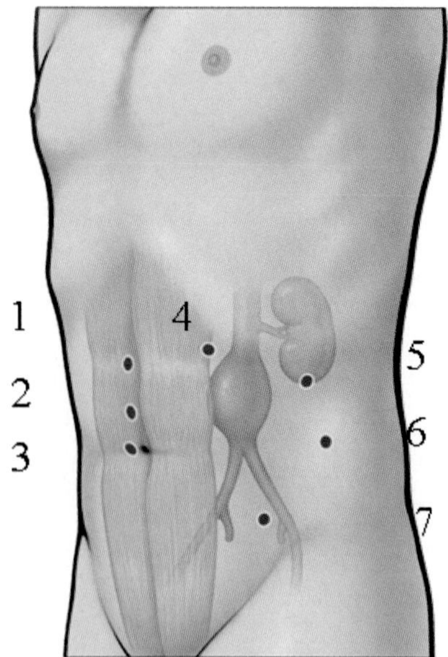

Fig. 57-1. Port placement for a total laparoscopic procedure. Ports 1 to 3: needle holders and graspers; Port 4: aortic crossclamp; Port 5: camera port and table-mounted retractor; Port 7: iliac clamp and suction device.

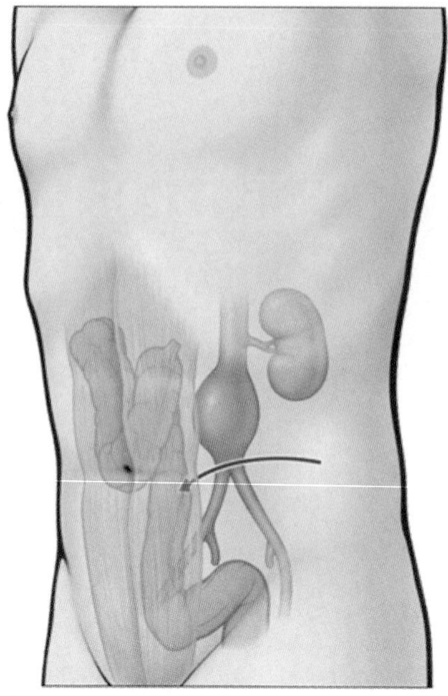

Fig. 57-2. Schematic drawing of transperitoneal left retrocolic approach.

with medial en bloc mobilization of the left kidney and the ureter; this permits expeditious exposure of the aorta, even in obese patients. We try to avoid any separate dissection of the ureter, which is only left laterally when necessary. In most cases any mobilization of the ureter can be avoided. Even in obese patients, only one laparoscopic retractor is generally required to maintain aortic exposure. This approach can also be used for medial visceral rotation to obtain access to the suprarenal aorta.

Laparoscopic exposure of the aorta is initiated at the level of the neck of the aneurysm. The left renal vein is one of the first structures seen when dissection is started. The laparoscopic camera stays in port 2 most of the time during exposure of the aorta. Especially in patients with occlusive disease only the anastomosis site proximal to the origin of the inferior mesenteric artery is dissected. This exposure technique avoids damage of the lumbrosacral nerves adjacent to the aortic bifurcation. During retroperitoneal dissection, the first assistant holds the camera and also helps to put the tissue on tension with a grasping clamp (Fig. 57-1).

Lumbar arteries are controlled extraluminally from the left side using a laparoscopic clip applier. After the left-sided lumbar arteries are clipped and divided, the adjacent right-side lumbar arteries can be clipped. When the sac of the aneurysm is incised and collapsed, most lumbar arteries can be expeditiously identified medially and laterally of the aorta and occluded with a clip. Lumbar arteries that are still bleeding after incision of the sac of the aneurysm will be controlled from the lumen with laparoscopic sutures, which can be secured with a titanium clip to save time. Hernia staplers have also been used to stop bleeding from lumbar arteries.

Aortoiliac Aneurysms

In large iliac or aortoiliac aneurysms, a hybrid procedure is used to obtain proximal and distal control, combining endovascular and laparoscopic techniques. This hybrid procedure consists of transfemoral balloon occlusion of the right common iliac artery after insertion of an 8F hemostatic sheath. The left common iliac artery is occluded from within the aneurysm by balloon catheters introduced through an 8F hemostatic sheath inserted directly through the abdominal wall. Three endovascular balloons are used, on average, in each case. One endovascular balloon is used for occlusion of the hypogastric artery from within, and a second is often needed for the external iliac. If the distal anastomosis is performed with the iliac bifurcation, this anastomosis can be sutured laparoscopically. In cases with hypogastric artery aneurysms, coil embolization is performed, followed by staple occlusion of the common iliac and the proximal external iliac artery with a subsequent distal anastomosis to the external iliac artery, which can be performed through a small inguinal incision. Using this technique, no distal clamps are required. Only the infrarenal aorta is clamped, using a laparoscopic aortic clamp (Karl Storz; Tuttlingen, Germany).

Controlling Bleeding from Lumbar Arteries

Lumbar arteries are controlled extraluminally from the right side before crossclamping or opening the aneurism. Lumbar arteries that are still bleeding after incision of the aneurysm sac are stitched with pledgeted laparoscopic sutures and secured with a titanium clip.

When the sac of the aneurysm is incised and collapsed, most lumbar arteries can expeditiously be identified medially and laterally of the aorta and occluded with a clip.

Clamping

A deployable aortic clamp is used to occlude the iliac arteries. Using this novel device, only the port for the proximal aortic clamp is obstructed with an instrument. Alternatively, two laparoscopic clamps are inserted through ports in the lower abdomen to occlude the iliac arteries. A laparoscopic aortic clamp is placed through a port in the upper abdomen. Easy access at all times is mandatory for the proximal aortic clamp.

A suction/irrigation device is connected with a cell-saving machine and a large-bore 10-mm suction device (Karl Storz; Tuttlingen, Germany) is used to evacuate the thrombus material and any kind of debris. At the end of the procedure we routinely place a closed suction drain into the retroperitoneum.

Laparoscopic Anastomosis

Laparoscopic dissection and suturing is performed with the surgeon standing on the patient's right side (Fig. 57-3). In patients with a bifurcated graft, the right limb of the graft is tunnelled first to the right groin to achieve a certain degree of stabilization of the prosthesis. Alternatively the first assistant has to stabilize the graft with a grasping clamp. Tunneling to the left groin is performed later to avoid gas loss from the left-sided retroperitoneum. In patients with an end-to-end anastomosis, the aorta is completely transected. transection is carefully performed under laparoscopic visualization with a 30-degree angled laparoscope to avoid any injury to lumbar arteries or veins. The scissors are introduced with the surgeon's left hand through port 1 to guarantee a right angle and to avoid any oblique transection of the aorta, which can make suturing of the left hemi circumference much more difficult, as it only leaves a small posterior aortic wall. In patients with an end-to-side anastomosis, an aortotomy is performed and the anastomosis is started posteriorly with a 10-cm 3-0 Prolene suture. A second suture is taken anteriorly, and both are tied together intracorporeally. A laparoscopic nerve hook is useful to put the suture line on tension. Time can also be saved by using two 3-0 Prolene sutures with a pledget fixed at the end as originally described by Coggia. The first assistant can follow the suture with an atraumatic DeBakey clamp from Storz, which has been shown in the lab to not cause breakage of Prolene sutures. The assistant also keeps the operating field free of blood with the suction device. While the anastomosis is performed, the camera is in the left upper abdomen.

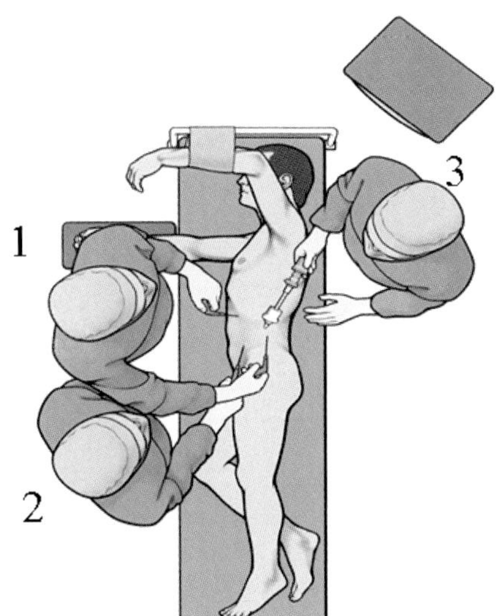

Fig. 57-3. The operating surgeon (1) and first assistant stand (2) on the right side of the patient; the second assistant (3) stands on the patient's left.

Partial or Complete Conversion

Reasons for conversion to a minilaparotomy should be planned before surgery. According to our self-established guidelines, they include an aortic cross-clamping time of more than 2 hours and a total operating time exceeding 4 hours. In these cases, we convert to a laparoscopic hand-assist procedure (HALS), where the anastomosis is performed under pneumoperitoneum but with the nondominant hand of the surgeon inserted into the abdomen to provide exposure and assist with the anastomosis. Other reasons for conversion are extensive adhesions, excessive calcification, and uncontrollable blood loss. When severe calcification does not permit safe clamping of the iliac artery, a balloon catheter can be inserted through a laparoscopic port to block the vessel intraluminally.

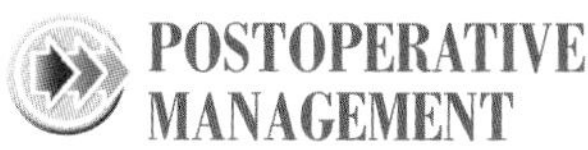

POSTOPERATIVE MANAGEMENT

The nasogastric tube is removed in the operating room together with the endotracheal tube. All patients are permitted to drink on the evening of the day of the operation. Solid food is routinely given on the first postoperative day. The retroperitoneal drain is removed on the first postoperative day, and mobilization can be started the same day.

Hybrid Techniques

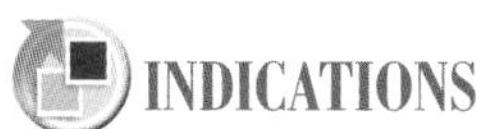

INDICATIONS

Endoleaks, endotension, and graft migration are the major problems of endovascular abdominal aortic aneurysm (AAA) exclusion (EVAR). There is an increasing number of patients with endotension and aneurysms that increase in diameter without any evidence of patent lumbar arteries or a patent inferior mesenteric artery (IMA). Endovascular coiling of patent lumbar arteries or of the IMA is cumbersome, often requiring several treatment sessions by experienced radiologists. Traditionally, the only option for these endograft issues was an open surgery for repair. This was problematic as these operations are difficult secondary to periaortic inflammation and the patient population receiving stents were often considered too ill for surgery. These problems have led investigators and clinicians to explore the use of laparoscopy as a hybrid procedure, which is less invasive than open surgery and more definitive and cost-effective than endovascular "patch-up" jobs. Several hybrid procedures have been described (Table 57-1).

TABLE 57-1. HYBRID PROCEDURES COMBINING LAPAROSCOPY WITH ENDOVASCULAR TECHNIQUES

Laparoscopic treatment options for patients with endografts
• Clipping of the IMA and of lumbar arteries to treat type II leaks
• Thrombus removal
• Tight closure of the sac of the aneurysm
• Fixation of the endograft to the aortic neck
• Banding of the aorta to prevent neck dilatation

IMA, inferior mesenteric artery.

Miscellaneous Procedures

Laparoscopic techniques can be used to treat patients with type II endoleaks after EVAR. Lumbar arteries as well as the IMA can be easily accessed and occluded with laparoscopic clips. An even greater advantage is the ability to further alter the external aneurism from the outside in order to stabilize and prolong the life of the endoprosthesis. The thrombus can be removed laparoscopically, which permits wrapping of the endograft in a way similar to a Creech procedure. Considering that thrombus is not an inert substance but a place for macrophages generating free oxygen radicals that can further weaken the aortic wall, the removal of thrombus material, as is routinely done in open surgery, can potentially enhance graft incorporation. Using special suturing techniques the endoprosthesis can actively be attached to the aortic wall preventing graft migration. This can be combined with a banding procedure to enlarge the landing zone and prevent neck dilatation (Fig. 57-4).

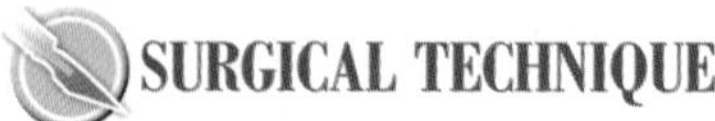

SURGICAL TECHNIQUE

A pneumoperitoneum is established and the abdomen is inspected. If possible, a transperitoneal left retrocolic access is chosen. When an endograft has been in place for several months there is quite often a dense inflammatory retroperitoneal reaction. In very rare cases under these circumstances a totally transperitoneal approach must be chosen.

The left hemicolon is mobilized medially as described above and as originally published by Dion. The origin of the inferior mesenteric artery (IMA) is identified and the artery is divided between clips. When clips are too small to safely occlude the IMA, a vascular stapler is used. This will facilitate further mobilization of the aorta. The aneurysm and the aortic neck are identified and dissected free to enable proximal control. As many lumbar arteries as accessible are clipped on the left side of the aorta. Because access to the right-side lumbar arteries is often very difficult because of the inflammatory changes, we now prefer a more direct approach: stitching lumbar arteries from inside like in open surgery.

Laparoscopic Remodeling of the Aorta after EVAR

The principal laparoscopic steps outlined above are performed without clamping the aorta, as this would damage the endograft. Instead, an aortic balloon occlusion catheter is introduced transfemorally from the groin through a hemostatic sheath and advanced proximally under fluoroscopic guidance. This balloon is inflated before the sac of the aneurysm is incised to stabilize the graft inside the aorta. Dislodgement of the endograft when taking out the thrombus is impossible when the balloon is inflated. This is performed after systemic heparinization of the patient and with adequate monitoring of the patient's blood pressure.

With the surgeon standing on the right side of the patient, the sac of the aneurysm is incised and opened with laparoscopic scissors in a H-shaped configuration (Fig. 57-5). The graft is inspected using the magnification of the 30-degree endoscope to exclude any damage of the fabric or stents. Laparoscopic graspers and a 10-mm suction-irrigation device are used to remove the thrombus material. Patent lumbar arteries are stitched with a Vicryl suture blocked with a pledget at the end. With a laparoscopic running suture (2-0 Prolene), the sac of the aneurysm is overlapped, wrapping the aorta tightly around the endograft. In addition to these measures we like to place a band around the neck of the aneurysm to prevent neck dilatation. This requires careful circumferential dissection of the proximal aorta. Using a curved grasping instrument originally designed for laparoscopic fundoplication, a self-made band of PTFE is wrapped around the aortic neck (Fig. 57-6). The band is put on tension and secured with several interrupted Prolene sutures. When this can be successfully accomplished, there is probably no need for

- Clipping of lumbar arteries
- Clipping of the inferior mesenteric artery
- Thrombus removal
- Tight closure of the sac of the AAA
- Banding of the neck
- Suture fixation of the endograft

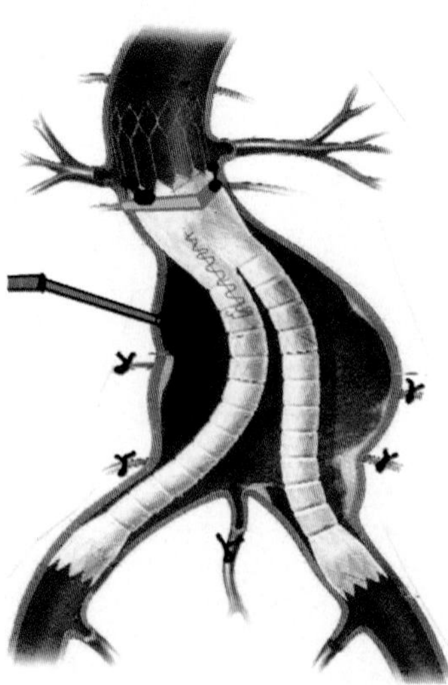

Fig. 57-4. Adjunctive measures that can be performed laparoscopically after endografting. AAA, abdominal aortic aneurysm.

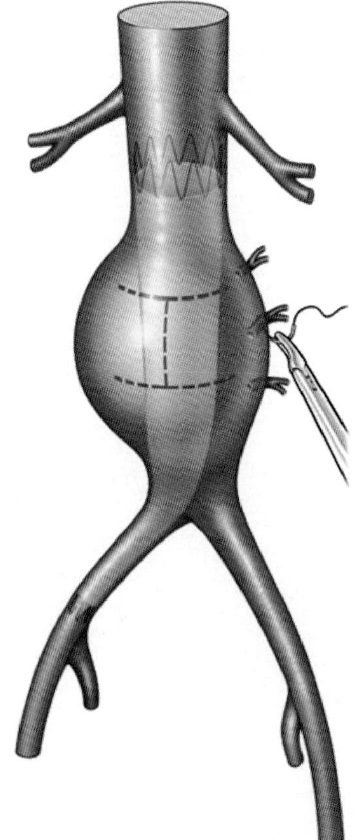

Fig. 57-5. An H-shaped incision of the sac of the aneurysm to remove thrombus and to stitch lumbar arteries.

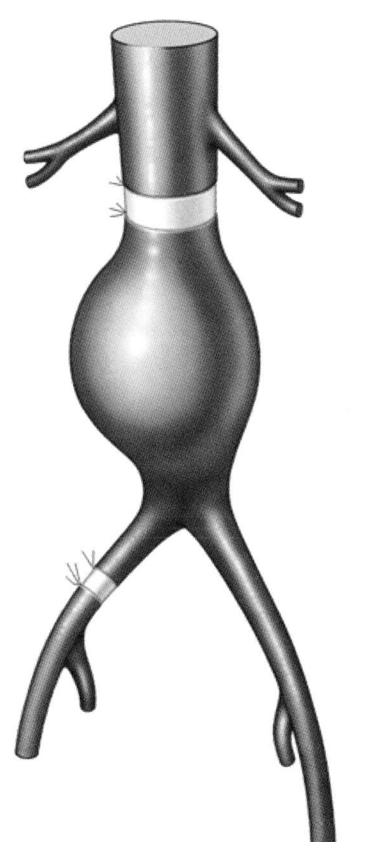

Fig. 57-6. Proximal and distal banding of the landing zone, which laparoscopically can be increased.

placing additional sutures to prevent migration. When it is felt that sutures are needed to stabilize the proximal endograft, fluoroscopy should be used to identify the bare wires of the stent and the part of the graft where the interrupted stitches will incorporate the fabric of the endograft's body.

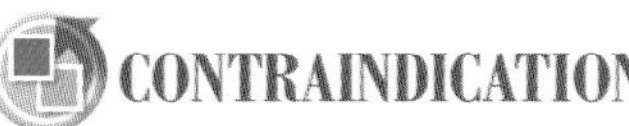

CONTRAINDICATIONS

The technique described should not be used in cases with extensive graft migration, even with the balloon catheter in place, as free rupture would be possible. Another contraindication is patients with hostile abdomen where laparoscopic exposure of the retroperitoneum can not be accomplished. We have used this technique in combination with endovascular repair techniques such as the placement of extension cuffs or angioplasty as well as graft limb thrombectomy.

Our experience with laparoscopic techniques as part of a hybrid approach to treat patients with AAA has demonstrated that we now have the operative technique and the instrumentation to improve the long-term performance of endografts or to salvage failing grafts, reducing the need for conversion to open surgery and saving money by avoiding multiple attempts at correction with expensive endoprostheses.

SUGGESTED READING

Coggia M, Bourriez A, Javerliat I, et al. Totally laparoscopic aortobifemoral bypass: a new and simplified approach. *Eur J Vasc Endovasc Surg* 2002 Sep;24(3):274–275.

Dion YM, Gracia CR, El Kadi, H. Totally laparoscopic abdominal aortic aneurysm repair. *J Vasc Surg* 2001;33:181–185.

Dion YM, Thaveau F, Fearn S. Current modifications to totally laparoscopic "apron technique." *J Vasc Surg* 2003;38: 403–406.

Kolvenbach R, Ceshire N, Pinter L, et al. Laparoscopy-assisted aneurysm resection as a minimal invasive alternative in patients unsuitable for endovascular surgery. *J Vasc Surg* 2001;34:216–221.

Kolvenbach R, Da Silva L, Schwierz E, et al. Video assisted aortic surgery. *J Am Coll Surg* 2000;190:451–457.

Kolvenbach R, Ferrari M, Shifrin EG. Laparoscopic assisted aortic surgery. A review. *J Cardiovasc Surg (Torino)* 2006 Oct;47(5): 547–556.

Kolvenbach R, Pinter L, Raghunandan M, et al. Laparoscopic remodeling of abdominal aortic aneurysms after endovascular exclusion: a technical description. *J Vasc Surg* 2002;36: 1267–1270.

Kolvenbach R, Puerschel A, Fajer S, et al. Total laparoscopic aortic surgery versus minimal access techniques: review of more than 600 patients. *Vascular* 2006;14(4): 186–192.

Veith F. et al. Nature and significance of endoleaks and endotension: Summary of opinions expressed at an international conference. *J Vasc Surg* 2002;35:1029–1035.

Wassiljew S, Kolvenbach R, Puerschel A, et al. Total laparoscopic iliac artery aneurysm repair using endoscopic techniques and endovascular balloon occlusion. *Eur J Vasc Endovasc Surg* 2006;32(3): 270–272.

Wisselink W, Cuesta AM, Berends FJ, et al. Retroperitoneal endoscopic ligation of lumbar and inferior mesenteric arteries as a treatment of persistent endoleak after endoluminal aortic aneurysm repair. *J Vasc Surg* 2000; 31:1240–1244.

COMMENTARY

Drs. Kolvenbach and Cagiannos are true pioneers in the application of minimally invasive techniques to intraabdominal aortic surgery. They describe their large experience with the laparoscopic equivalent of open repair of aneurisms and aortic occlusive disease. The latter indication is now widely treated in Europe with laparoscopic access—either with hand-port assistance or totally laparoscopically as is described here. Many surgeons prefer the use of the hand port in this surgery as it provides a margin of safety if rapid proximal control is needed and provides a port to allow standard direct vision anastomosis for the proximal graft. As has happened, however, in many other hand-assisted laparoscopic procedures, once the surgeon has experience and achieves comfort with the laparoscope, the hand port is abandoned–or, as described by Dr. Kolvenbach, is reserved as a fallback if progress can't be made laparoscopically.

The description of the use of laparoscopy to salvage failing endografts is yet another indication of this group's creative quest for the least invasive and most effective treatment of abdominal vascular disease. Stented endografts seemed to be the ideal minimally invasive solution to AAA. However, this early promise has not been totally borne out. Stenting remains an extremely expensive procedure, typically more than an open aneurismectomy. More worrisome is the risk of late rupture due to endoleaks, distal migration of the grafts as aneurism morphology changes, and the gradual deterioration

(continued)

of the grafts due to stent fracture and material tears. These problems have mandated that patients with stent grafts have to have lifelong surveillance and repeated interventions to keep the prosthesis patched and functioning. This further adds to the cost and inconvenience of this option. The possibility, therefore, of using laparoscopy to treat early problems such as endoleaks or late problems such as migration is truly exciting. It may be that Dr. Kolvenbach's investigations point the way to a future primary surgery where laparoscopy and interventional radiology work together to permanently implant and fix in place a durable endoprosthesis that will ensure the patient a cost-effective and permanent repair of their aneurism.

LLS

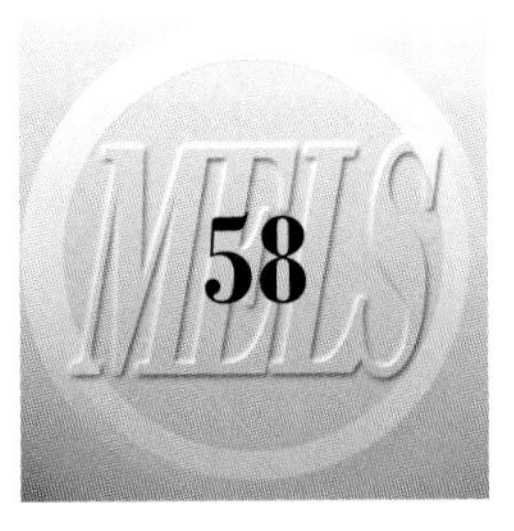

Pediatric Laparoscopy and Endoscopy

STEVEN S. ROTHENBERG

INTRODUCTION

While minimally invasive surgical techniques have been embraced by general surgeons over the last 20 years, pediatric surgeons have been reluctant to use these techniques, especially in infants and small children. The initial resistance to minimally invasive surgery (MIS) was justified by comments stating that the procedures took too long, that they were too difficult to perform in small patients, and that the benefits of decreased surgical trauma, shorter hospitalization, and an earlier return to normal activity were not significant in the pediatric and especially the neonatal population. Some pediatric surgeons who did try to embrace this new technology had their initial enthusiasm dampened by a lack of experience and appropriately sized instrumentation for children. However, over the last decade, an increasing number of reports have documented the safety and efficacy of such procedures as minimally invasive appendectomy, fundoplication, and splenectomy in the pediatric population, showing the same benefits as in the adult population. There has also been a large push in the development of neonatal- and pediatric-specific procedures such as pyloromyotomy for pyloric stenosis, colon pull-through for Hirschsprung disease and imperforate anus, repair of intestinal atresias, and advanced thoracoscopic procedures in neonates and children. Many of these developments came about not only because of the advanced skills that come with experience but with the development of pediatric-specific instrumentation to facilitate these procedures. Because of the limited scope of this chapter, discussion will be limited to the most common and pediatric-specific procedures.

GENERAL PRINCIPLES

It is worth mentioning just a few basic principles. In general the approach to pediatric MIS is the same as in adults. Because the patients are smaller, they are often moved to the edge of the table to achieve the most ergonomic position. In infants, a number of the procedures such as pyloromyotomy and pull-through are performed with the patient crosswise on the table, giving the surgeon equal access to the head and foot of the patient while keeping the patient closer to the anesthesiologist during the case. In the case of a Nissen fundoplication, the patient is moved towards the foot of the table, which leaves a fairly long gap between the head of the table and the head of the patient. Pneumoperitoneum is achieved in the same manner as in adults, and the decision to use a closed Veress needle technique or an open Hasson technique is purely surgeon-dependent. Many have felt that insufflation pressures need to be less in infants and children, but there is no physiologic data to support this point. An increase in end-tidal CO_2 may develop with insufflation but this can be remedied by increasing the minute ventilation. Hypotension and other physiologic effects have not been shown to be significant in most cases. In neonates a starting pressure of 10 to 12 mmHg is acceptable, and most patients, even those with cardiac anomalies, will tolerate a pressure of 12 to 15 mmHg. Laparoscopy in most children can be performed at a standard pressure of 15 mmHg. However, in neonates who weigh less than 5 kg some insufflators are not sensitive enough to detect the rapid changes in pressure in the small peritoneal cavities of these patients. This may result in overinsufflation, which can cause physiologic changes. Therefore the surgeon must be sure to have an appropriate insufflator and to start out at flows of only $\frac{1}{2}$ to 1 liter/minute.

In thoracoscopic procedures CO_2 insufflation is routinely used, as are valved trocars, because most pediatric patients cannot accommodate a double-lumen endotracheal tube. In most cases, single-lung ventilation is obtained by mainstem intubation of the contralateral side. Occasionally bronchial blockers may be used but these are often difficult to position. The slight tension pneumothorax created by the CO_2 helps provide complete collapse in most cases, creating an adequate working environment.

The other major difference is instrumentation. In patients weighing less than 10 kg and certainly those less than 5 kg, the surgeon should have available instruments with shafts that are shorter (18 to 20 cm) in length and smaller (2.5 to 3 mm) in diameter. These instruments improve the ergonomics and allow the surgeon to perform fine dissection and suturing in a relatively confined space. Smaller scopes (3- and 4-mm) of shorter (20-cm) lengths are also important. With these scopes, however, light retrieval can be compromised; therefore a good light source and digital camera are imperative.

Using these modifications of standard adult instruments, equipment, and techniques, almost every pediatric surgical procedure has now been accomplished using MIS techniques (Table 58-1, page 584).

PYLOROMYOTOMY FOR PYLORIC STENOSIS

Laparoscopic pyloromyotomy was probably the first truly pediatric laparoscopic procedure. Many felt that a laparoscopic approach added little advantage over a standard right upper quadrant or supraumbilical incision, but the ease and quickness of the procedure along with the superior cosmetic result has made it one of the most commonly adopted MIS procedures.

CLINICAL PRESENTATION

In most cases, the infant is 4 to 6 weeks of age and presents with a history of projectile vomiting. The diagnosis is generally confirmed with ultrasound, which shows the thickened pyloric wall. The infant is taken to the operating room after his or her electrolytes and hydration status have been corrected.

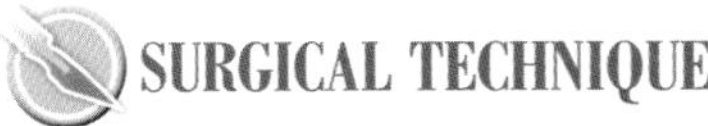

SURGICAL TECHNIQUE

After induction the infant is placed crossways on the table. This allows the surgeon and assistant to stand at the infant's feet without moving the patient all the way to the foot of the table. The abdomen is accessed

TABLE 58-1. CURRENT TECHNIQUES IN PEDIATRIC ENDOSCOPIC SURGERY

Thoracoscopy	Laparoscopy	Ileocolectomy
Division of tracheoesophageal fistula	Gastrostomy	Colectomy
Esophageal atresia repair	Fundoplication	Pull-through for Hirschsprung disease
Patent duct arteriosus (PDA) ligation	Pyloromyotomy	Pull-through for anorectal malformation
Resection of mediastinal mass	Repair of duodenal atresia	Cloacal repair
Debridement of empyema	Repair of malrotation	Splenectomy
Lung biopsy	Roux-en-Y jejunostomy	Adrenalectomy
Lobectomy	Resection of Meckel diverticulum	Pancreatectomy
Diaphragmatic plication	Repair of intestinal atresia	Resection of nesidioblastosis
Repair of diaphragmatic hernia	Release of small-bowel obstruction	Ovarian cystectomy
Difficult central venous access	Liver biopsy	Oophorectomy
Thymectomy	Cholecystectomy	Evaluation for ambiguous genitalia
Resection of mediastinal mass	Resection of choledochal cyst	Fowler-Stevens orchiopexy
Resection of neurogenic tumor	Portoenterostomy for biliary atresia	Inguinal hernia repair
Aortopexy for tracheomalacia	Reduction of intussusception	Laparoscopic-assisted inguinal hernia repair
	Appendectomy	Ventral hernia repair

through an umbilical incision, and a 3- or 4-mm 30-degree lens is introduced through an appropriate-sized trocar. Two small stab wounds are then made in the right mid-quadrant and in the mid-epigastrium to the left of the falciform ligament, at approximately the liver edge. A 3-mm atraumatic grasper (Babcock or bowel clamp) is placed through the mid-quadrant incision to grasp the duodenum, just distal to the pylorus. A retractable arthroscopy blade is placed through the epigastric incision. Once in, the blade is advanced 2 to 3 mm past the shield, and a longitudinal myotomy is made extending from just proximal to the duodenum to the proximal edge of the pylorus. A deep, straight initial cut should be made. The blade is then retracted back into the sheath, and the blunt sheath is used to deepen and widen the myotomy (Fig. 58-1). At this point the surgeon has two options. The first is to grab the upper muscle rim with the Babcock clamp and retract the lower muscle rim using the blunt sheath. The surgeon can visualize the muscle fibers splitting and can tell when the myotomy is complete by the bulging mucosa and the ability of the upper and lower muscle rims to slide tangentially to each other. The other option is to remove the arthroscopic blade and insert a laparoscopic pyloromyotomy spreader. This is a double-action instrument that spreads between the muscle rims achieving the same effect (Fig. 58-2). The spreader may need to be repositioned along the myotomy to achieve an adequate disruption of the muscle fibers. If a mucosal perforation is noted it should be sutured closed, the pylorus rotated 90 degrees, and another myotomy made.

Postoperatively feeds are started 1 to 2 hours after surgery and volumes are rapidly increased. Most patients are discharged in under 24 hours.

LAPAROSCOPIC FUNDOPLICATION AND GASTROSTOMY BUTTON

Esophageal-gastric fundoplication is one of the most common procedures performed by pediatrics surgeons today. A recent report of over 7,000 cases from seven major U.S. institutions concluded that fundoplication was a safe and effective procedure in the pediatric population but failed to make any mention of a laparoscopic approach.

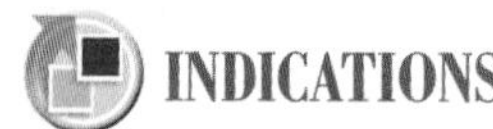

INDICATIONS

Indications for antireflux procedures in children include respiratory compromise, neurologic impairment, failure to thrive, and esophagitis and stricture formation. An increasing incidence of Barrett esophagitis is also being documented in children.

A

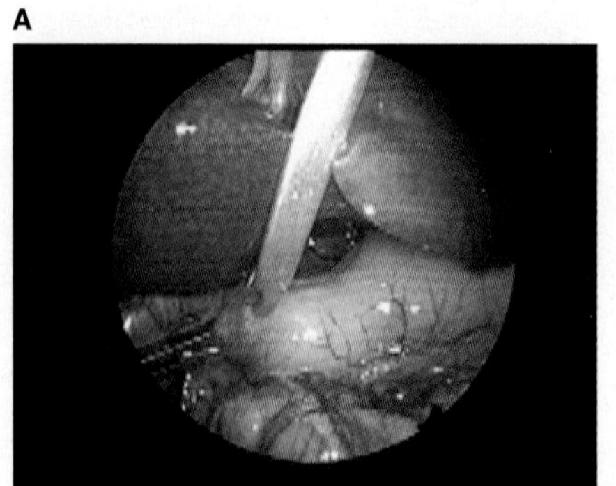

B

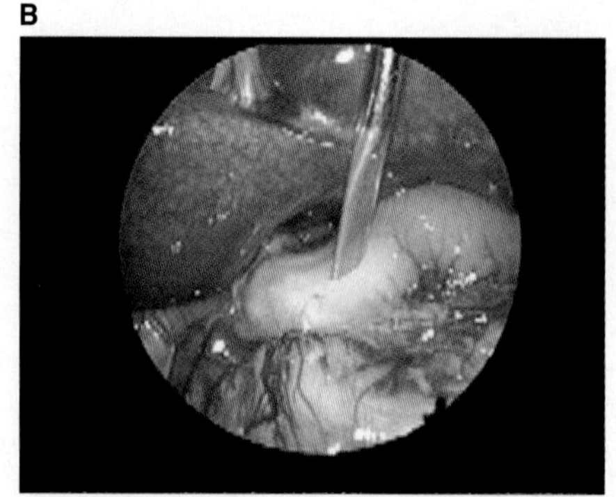

C

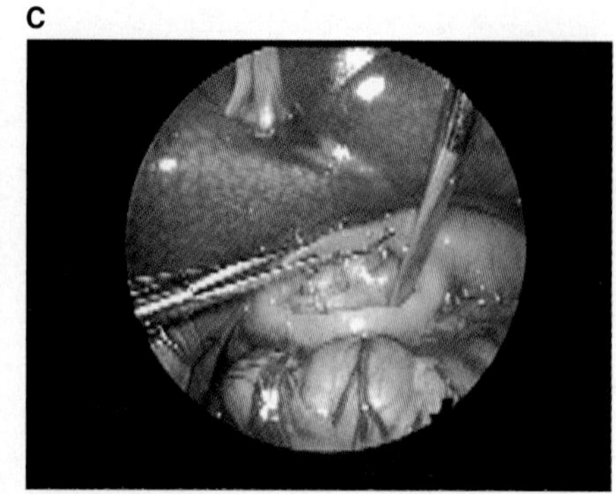

Fig. 58-1. A. The pylorus is stabilized by grasping the duodenum as the sheathed arthrotomy blade is inserted. **B.** A longitudinal incision is made along the length of the pylorus and the blunt sheath is used to deepen and widen the cut. **C.** The muscle fibers are spread using the grasper and blunt sheath.

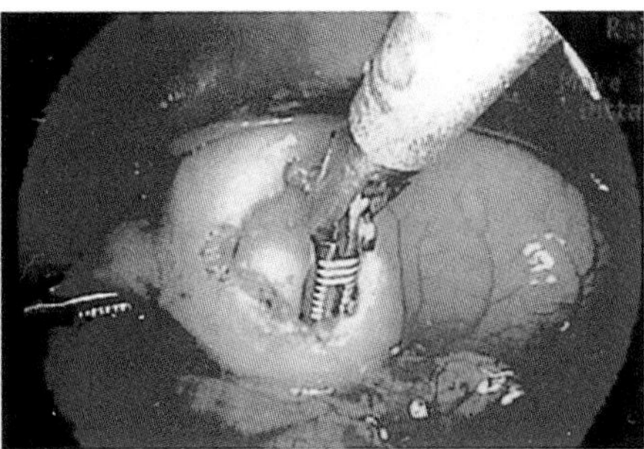

Fig. 58-2. The muscle layers are gently spread along the length of the pylorus, with care taken to avoid injury to the underlying mucosa.

Another common association has been the placement of a gastrostomy tube for feeding and a significantly increased risk of gastroesophageal reflux (GER); 10% to 50% of these patients will eventually require fundoplications. Recent studies have also indicated that GER plays an important role in respiratory problems, including the development of apnea and bradycardia, sudden death spells, recurrent lung infections, and even reactive airway disease. All of these factors have resulted in a large increase in the number of these procedures performed.

Laparoscopic fundoplications have routinely been done in infants and children for 15 years; a number of large series shows excellent results and recurrence rates at 10-year follow-up better than that achieved with traditional open surgery. There is also a striking decrease in morbidity, especially in terms of pulmonary complications and the incidence of postoperative bowel obstructions.

SURGICAL TECHNIQUE

The most commonly performed procedure is the Nissen fundoplication. In most instances this is done through a five-port technique (Fig. 58-3), with trocars being placed in the umbilicus (camera port), the right and left mid-quadrants (working ports), the right mid- or upper-quadrant (liver retractor), and the left upper-quadrant (stomach retractor and gastrostomy tube site). The positioning of the retracting ports high in the abdomen limits any instrument dueling. The abdomen is insufflated through the infraumbilical ring incision using a Veress needle and a closed technique. If there was a previous incision in this area, an alternate site is chosen to avoid adhesions. Insufflation pressures between 10 and 15 mmHg are chosen depending on the size and respiratory status of the patient. Oxygen saturation and end-tidal CO_2 should be monitored in each case.

Instrumentation and trocars are 5-mm or 3-mm in size, depending on the size of the patient. A standard length 5-mm 30-degree scope or a short wide-angle 4-mm 30-degree scope is chosen, also based on patient size.

The left lobe of the liver is retracted superiorly to expose the gastroesophageal (GE) junction. This is accomplished in most cases by using a locking Babcock clamp placed through the right upper quadrant incision, which is just to the right of the falciform ligament at the liver edge. The shaft of the clamp hooks the falciform, helping to elevate the liver, and the clamp is used to grasp the diaphragm above the esophageal hiatus, thus allowing the shaft of the instrument to act as a self-retaining retractor. In some cases with an extremely large liver it is necessary to place a snake or fan retractor. The esophagogastric and phrenoesophageal ligaments are then divided and the right and left diaphragmatic crus are identified and cleared. The short gastric vessels are divided using hook cautery in patients under 10 kg or one of the 5-mm sealing/dividing instruments that are routinely used in larger patients, making sure that the stomach is mobilized adequately to perform a tension-free wrap. A retroesophageal window is then developed, taking care not to injure the posterior vagus nerve. An adequate length of intraabdominal esophagus is then mobilized to allow for an adequate wrap. All posterior attachments to the stomach are

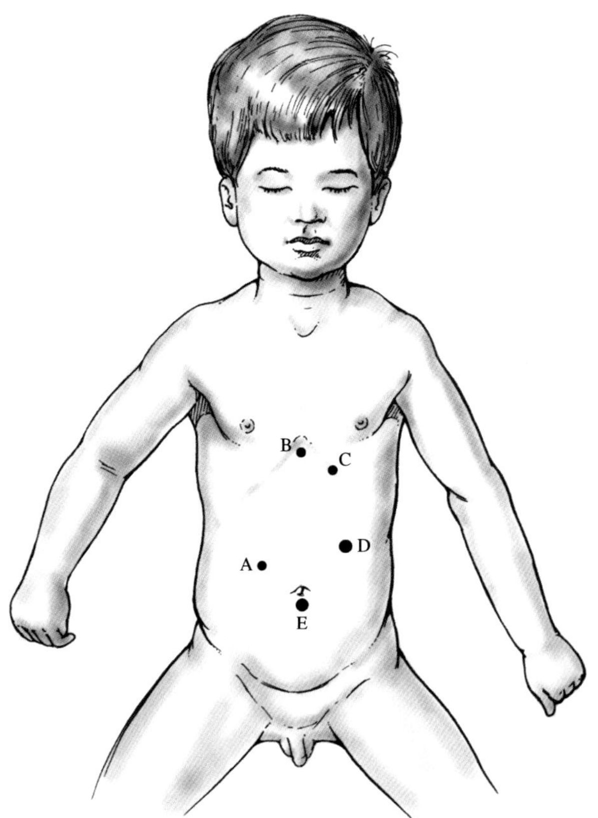

Fig. 58-3. Trocar positioning in a pediatric Nissen fundoplication.

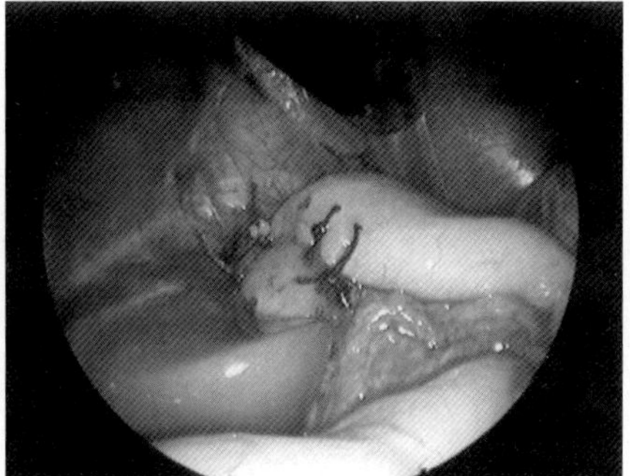

Fig. 58-4. A completed wrap.

divided at this time. A crural repair is performed in all cases, using a braided nonabsorbable suture. The wrap is formed around an intraesophageal stent, the size dependent on the size of the patient. The wraps are made 1.5 to 3 cm in length and consist of two to three sutures going from stomach, to the anterior wall of the esophagus, and to the retroesophageal portion of the stomach. The junction of the two parts of the fundus should lie at approximately 11 o'clock to prevent tension on or torsion of the esophagus (Fig. 58-4). This decreases the incidence of dysphagia. The first stitch can also include the anterior diaphragmatic rim; some choose to place collar stitches between the wrap and crus.

If the patient is a poor eater or has primary aspiration, a gastrostomy button is placed. In infants and smaller children this is most easily accomplished by bringing the stomach up through the left upper quadrant trocar site (Fig. 58-5). The button is secured with a purse-string suture, and the stomach is tacked to the anterior abdominal with two stay sutures, all placed through the trocar site. Another method is to use a Seldinger technique with a guidewire and dilators as depicted in Figures 58-6, 58-7, and 58-8.

Liquids are started 2 hours postoperatively, and most patients are discharged on the first postoperative day and maintained on a soft diet for approximately 1 week. Patients with gastric buttons are left to gravity overnight, and feeds are started the next morning.

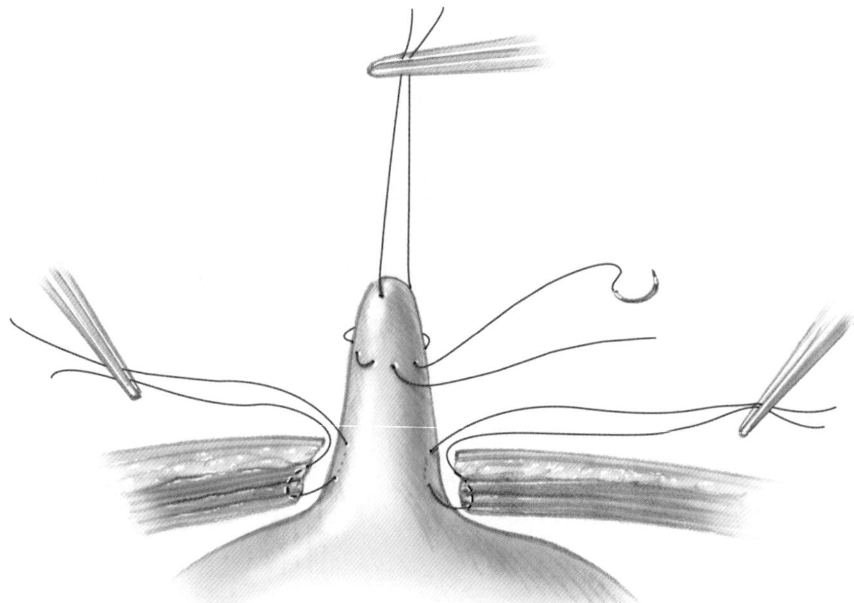

Fig. 58-5. The stomach is brought up through left upper quadrant trocar site to place a gastrotomy button.

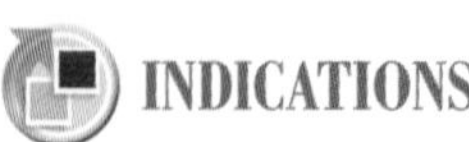

INDICATIONS

INTESTINAL ATRESIA REPAIR

Many intestinal stenoses or atresias can be managed laparoscopically. The proximal atresias are more amenable because the distal bowel is decompressed, allowing for a large intraperitoneal working space. The most commonly performed laparoscopic repair in infants is for duodenal atresia, with many variations including complete and partial obstruction. This can occur secondary to a failure of recanalization, a partial stenosis, or an annular pancreas. More distal atresias are usually secondary to some sort of ischemic event. Patients with complete obstruction present early in life with feeding intolerance and recurrent vomiting. Many cases are now diagnosed in utero. The classic double bubble can be seen on prenatal ultrasound or postnatal kidney-ureter-bladder film (KUB). This condition may present later in life as reflux and failure to thrive if the obstruction is not complete.

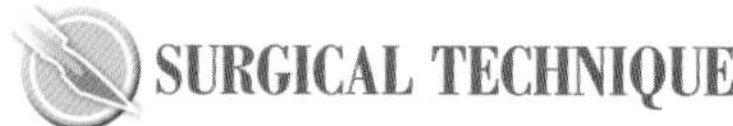

SURGICAL TECHNIQUE

For the repair, standard 3-mm neonatal laparoscopic instruments and trocars are used. The patient is placed supine at the end of the table, and the surgeon stands at the patient's feet. The abdomen is insufflated through an umbilical ring incision, and the first port is placed here. Two other ports are placed in the right lower

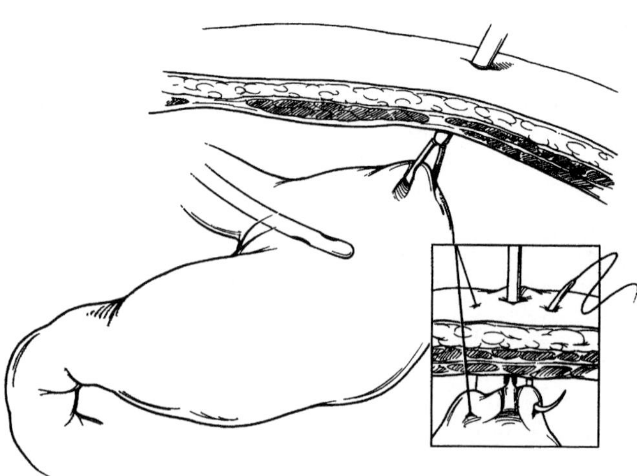

Fig. 58-6. After the site for gastrostomy is carefully chosen, a grasper is used to hold the stomach and U-sutures are placed through the abdominal wall, through the stomach, and back through the abdominal wall (inset).

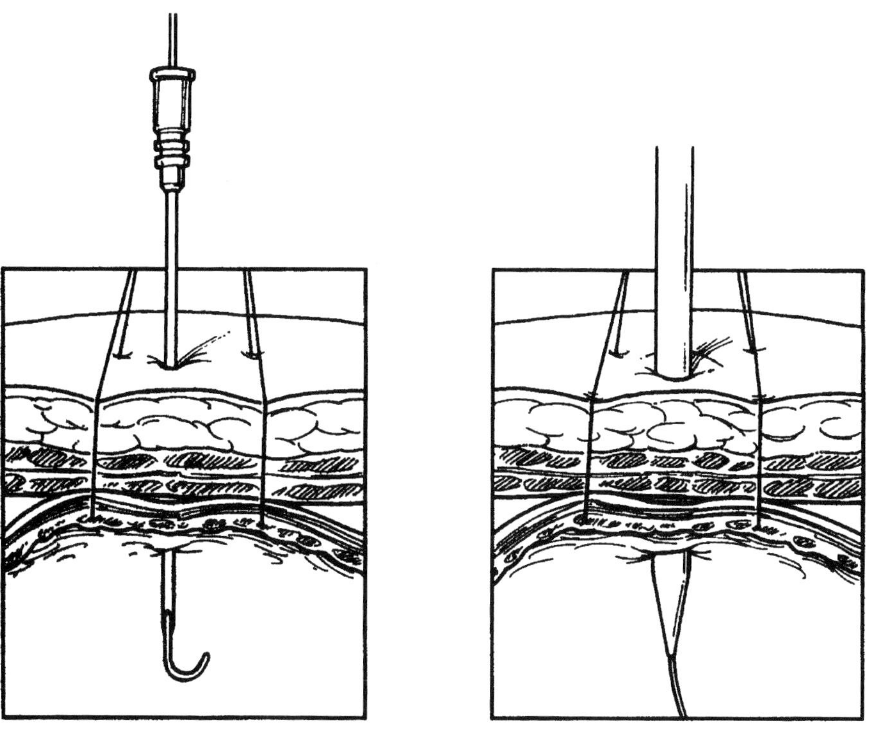

Fig. 58-7. While traction to the U-sutures is applied and the stomach insufflated via an orogastric tube, the stomach is accessed with an 18-gauge needle (left) followed by a wire (right).

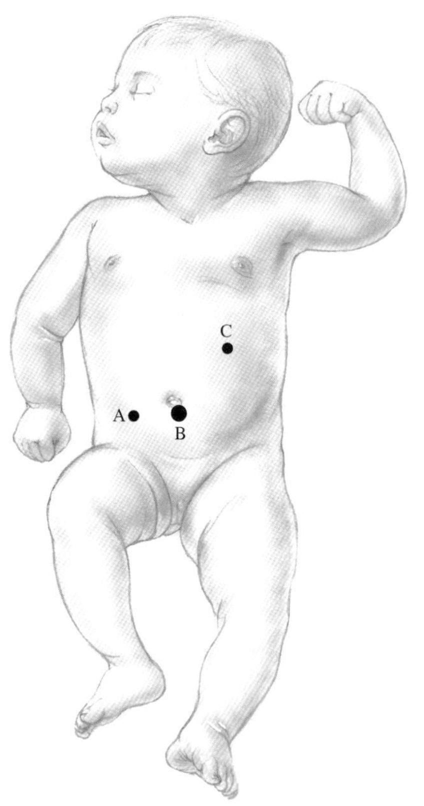

Fig. 58-9. Trocar placement for duodenal atresia repair.

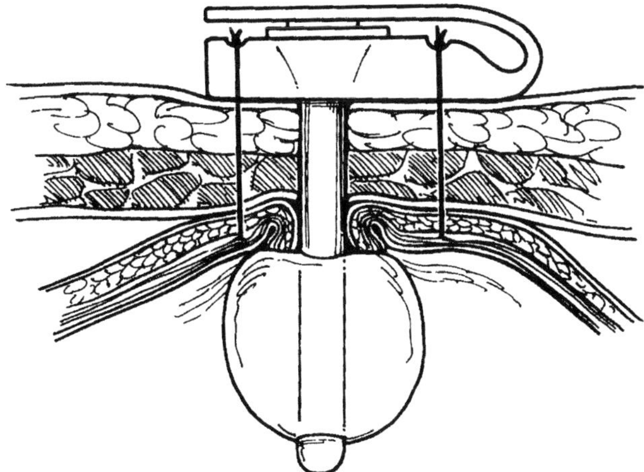

Fig. 58-8. The balloon on the button gastrostomy is insufflated, and the U-sutures are secured around the gastrostomy. These sutures are removed in 48 hours to prevent abdominal wall necrosis. The stomach is insufflated via the gastrostomy to check proper placement as it is visualized with the laparoscope.

quadrant and left mid quadrant, respectively (Fig. 58-9). Because of the decompressed nature of the distal bowel, there is generally abundant intraabdominal space and excellent visualization of the C-loop of the duodenum. The duodenum is Kocherized, and the site of the obstruction is usually easily visible. Proximal and distal duodenotomies are made, transverse in the dilated upper pouch and longitudinal in the smaller distal segment, and a standard diamond anastomosis is performed using 4-0 absorbable sutures. Care must be taken to avoid injury to the ampulla of Vater, which is often close to the distal enterotomy. Stay sutures are placed at each corner to set up the anastomosis, and then first the back wall and then the front wall are sewn with a running suture (Fig. 58-10). The distal bowel should then be run to look for evidence of other, distal atretic segments. In the cases where a web is suspected, a longitudinal duodenotomy is made across the area of apparent transition. The web is identified, partially resected, and a transverse closure is performed with running suture.

Other intestinal atresias can also be diagnosed and treated laparoscopically. However, because of the distended loops of bowel and the large size discrepancy between the proximal and distal segment, it is often best to exteriorize the atresia through an extended umbilical ring incision and perform the repair extracorporeally.

Postoperatively a nasogastric tube is left in until daily volumes diminish and the bile staining clears. Most of the neonates have started feeds within 5 days, which is

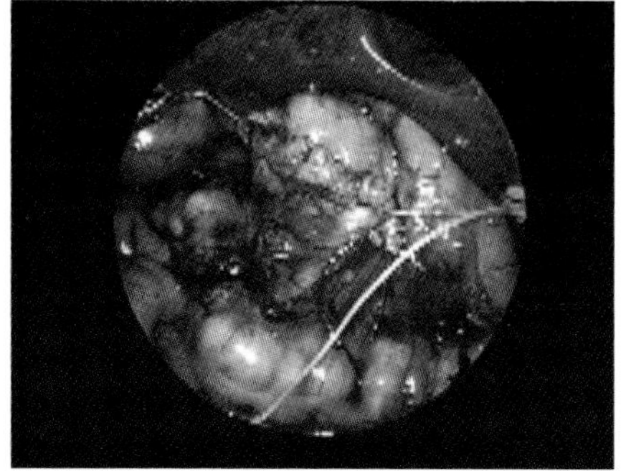

Fig. 58-10. A duodenal anastomosis.

a much quicker return to bowel function than noted with the standard open repair.

INTESTINAL MALROTATION (LADD PROCEDURE)

Intestinal malrotation is another condition that can present as a partial proximal bowel obstruction or, in cases of volvulus, a surgical emergency.

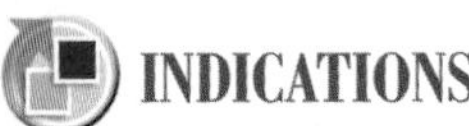

INDICATIONS

Generally the diagnosis of malrotation is made by contrast study. The upper GI shows an incomplete or abnormal C-loop, and barium enema may show the cecum to be floating, not positioned in the right lower quadrant. If the diagnosis is not clear a Doppler ultrasound can be helpful to determine the orientation of the superior mesenteric artery and vein. Once the diagnosis is made the patient is explored in a fashion similar to that for duodenal atresia. In some cases, laparoscopy is necessary to make or rule out the diagnosis.

The duodenum is examined and a search made for the ligament of Trietz. If the ligament of Trietz is present but the cecum is not fixed, this is an incomplete rotation but not a malrotation, and no intervention is necessary.

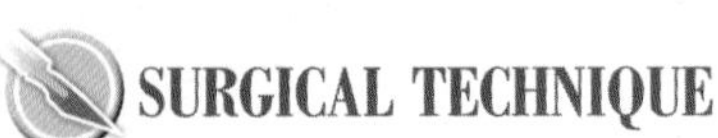

SURGICAL TECHNIQUE

If the diagnosis of malrotation is confirmed, the adhesions overlying the malpositioned duodenum (Ladd bands) are divided (Fig. 58-11). These are often draped over the duodenum and extend to the right colon, causing external compression and partial obstruction. Once these bands are divided, the duodenum is mobilized and straightened so that it lies in the right gutter. The bowel is then run from proximal to distal, untwisting the bowel and dividing any congenital adhesions. During this process the small bowel mesentery is widened. Once the colon is reached it is positioned along the patient's left gutter and an appendectomy is performed. In infants it is often easiest to bring the appendix up through the umbilical incision to ligate and divide it extracorporeally.

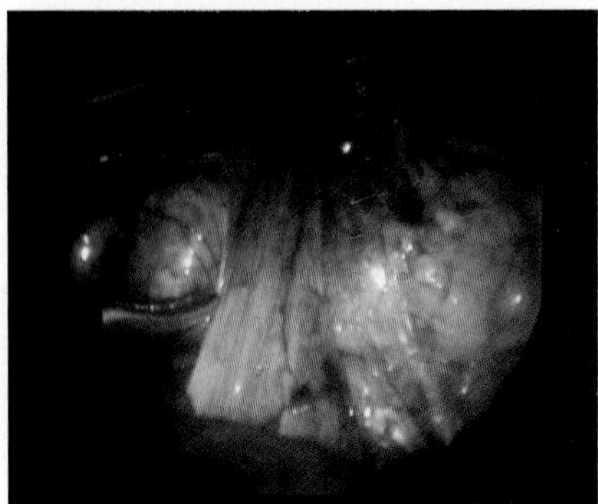

Fig. 58-11. Division of Ladd bands.

HIRSCHSPRUNG DISEASE

One of the most dramatic changes in pediatric surgical practice over the last 10 years has been the shift from staged open procedures to minimally invasive primary procedures for the correction of Hirschsprung disease. The most popular and widely used minimally invasive technique is the laparoscopic-assisted endorectal pull-through or its derivative, the transanal endorectal pull-through. The laparoscopic-assisted technique has the advantage of obtaining a biopsy to document normal ganglional cells above the transition zone prior to the irreversible step of the endorectal dissection. Additionally, the endorectal dissection and subsequent pull-through are much easier after division of the sigmoid mesocolon laparoscopically. Traction on the internal and external sphincters is minimized by this preliminary intraabdominal dissection, particularly in infants and children over 6 months of age. When the aganglionic segment extends beyond the splenic flexure, biopsies can be taken and the pull-through procedure delayed until permanent section assessment has been completed to accurately determine the best level for the pull-through.

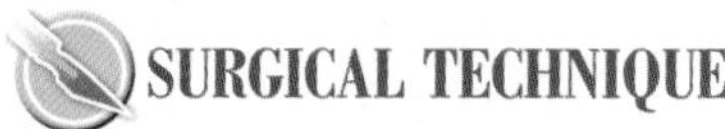

SURGICAL TECHNIQUE

The laparoscopic endorectal pull-through is begun by the placement of three trocars: in the umbilicus, in the right upper quadrant subcostally, and in the right lower quadrant in the anterior axillary line. Biopsies are obtained above the level of the anticipated transition zone. The surgeon should delay any further dissection until these biopsies confirm the presence of normal ganglion cells. Once the pathologist has confirmed the presence of ganglion cells and, in some centers, normal acetylcholinesterase activity, the mesocolon is divided adjacent to the colon along the entire length of aganglionic bowel. In longer aganglionic segments, a pedicle can be developed by continuing the division of the mesocolon medial to the marginal artery, which will allow an anastomosis without tension between the neorectum and the anus (Fig. 58-12). Once an adequate colon pedicle has been developed, the transanal endorectal dissection is begun. Six retraction sutures are placed in the perineum. A circumferential incision is made in the distal rectal mucosa 3 to 5 mm above the dentate line. Fine traction sutures are placed on the rectal mucosa. The rectal mucosa is separated from the circular smooth muscle using a needle-tip electrocautery and blunt

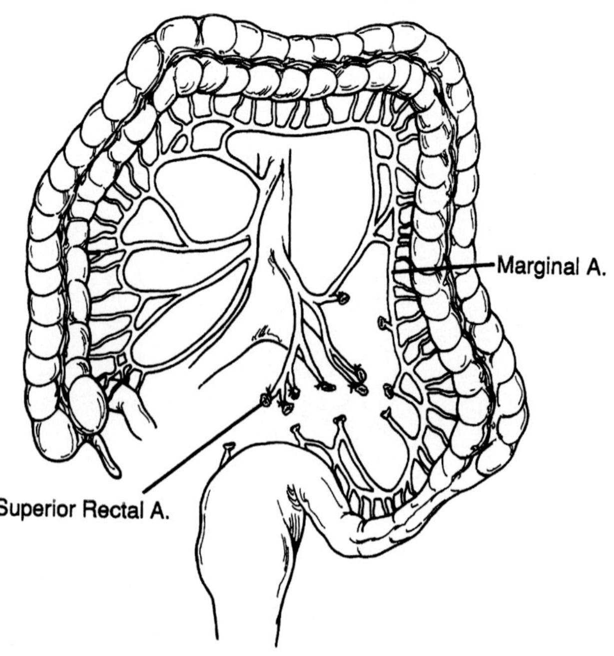

Fig. 58-12. The laparoscopic division of the sigmoid mesentery facilitates mobilization to make the endorectal pull-through easier.

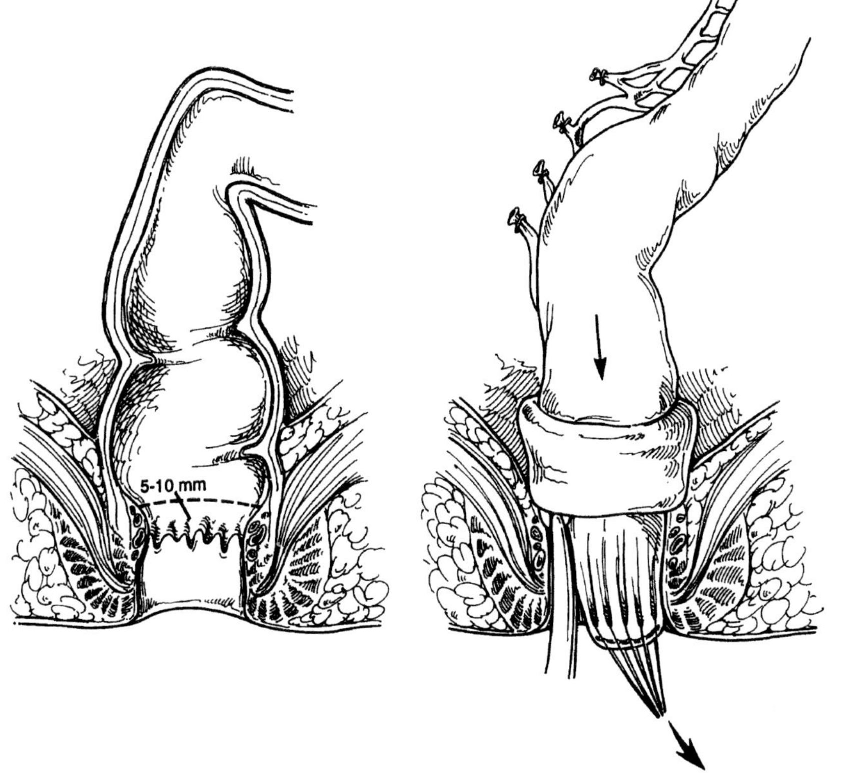

Fig. 58-13. The rectal mucosa is divided just above the dentate line, and a submucosal plane is developed. This prevents injury to the sphincter complex and pelvic nerves.

dissection (Fig. 58-13). The mucosa is cored out for a distance of 4 or 5 cm. At this point, the muscular cuff turns inside out and can be brought out through the anus. The peritoneal cavity is entered, and the dissection is carried out circumferentially, releasing the colon from the rectal cuff. The bowel is pulled down to a point above the documented transition zone. The colon is amputated at this point and secured with a single-layer anastomosis to the rectal mucosa located just above the dentate line (Fig. 58-14, page 590). The pull-through segment is visualized laparoscopically to make certain that no twists have developed. Also, the potential for internal herniation is avoided in patients with a long pedicle by securing the mesentery of the neorectum to the posterior peritoneum. The trocars are removed and the pneumoperitoneum evacuated.

POSTOPERATIVE MANAGEMENT

These patients usually stool within 24 hours and can then be placed on a regular diet. Most are discharged within 3 days of the operative procedure. The complications of this technique are similar to the open endorectal technique. Enterocolitis remains the primary complication. Splitting the posterior wall of the endorectal cuff prior to performing the anastomosis seems to reduce the incidence of enterocolitis (Fig. 58-15, page 591) Additionally, resecting 10 to 20 cm of bowel above the transition zone and leveling the pull-through anastomosis at a point where the acetylcholinesterase activity is determined to be normal may also help diminish the problem of chronic enterocolitis in these patients.

HIGH ANORECTAL MALFORMATIONS

Surgical repair of high anorectal malformations has resulted in fecal incontinence in the majority of patients. A laparoscopic-assisted pull-through for high anorectal malformations allows for the performance of a procedure similar to perineal operations for low anorectal malformations. Unfortunately, the underdevelopment of both the external and internal sphincters in patients with high anorectal malformations makes the achievement of continence problematic no matter what surgical procedure is performed. Patients with high anorectal malformations are diverted with a distal descending colon colostomy and proximal sigmoid colon mucous fistula. At the time of the initial colostomy formation, it is critical to leave as much slack in the sigmoid colon as possible to facilitate the subsequent pull-through of the high anorectal malformation without tethering of the colon by the attachment of the mucous fistula to the abdominal wall.

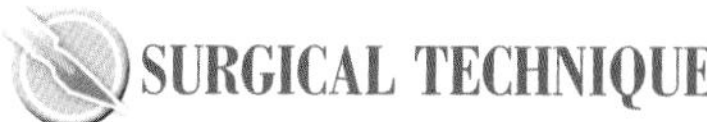

SURGICAL TECHNIQUE

The pull-through operation is begun by placing three trocars in the right upper quadrant. A suture is passed through the abdominal wall, through the bladder near the bladder neck, and back up through the abdominal wall to better expose the bladder neck and prostate during the laparoscopic dissection. The dissection of the fistula is begun at the peritoneal reflection. Great care is taken not to injure the sigmoid mesocolon, which could compromise the blood supply to the distal rectum. Additionally, the dissection is carried out right on the muscular wall of the rectum and fistula to avoid injury to the seminal vesicles, the prostate, the urethra, and the nervi crigentes. The dissection should be performed first posteriorly and then laterally on both sides and lastly anteriorly. In this way, the muscular wall of the rectourethral fistula can be better visualized, further aiding in the effort to avoid injury to important pelvic structures. Once the fistula has been dissected down to its junction with the urethra, the fistula is divided sharply about 5 mm proximal to the urethra. A loop ligature is applied to the fistula on the urethral side, snugging down the ligature directly adjacent to the catheterized urethra. A strobe light in the urethra also aids in the dissection of the distal fistula and accurate placement of the loop ligature. Once the fistula has been divided, a minimal amount of dissection is made to help visualize the levator muscles on the pelvic floor from above. Great care should be taken to avoid injury to the branches of the pudendal nerve, which innervates the levator mechanism primarily on its cephalic surface.

The legs are lifted and the perineal dissection begun. Electrical stimulation is used to identify the center of the external sphincter muscles (Fig. 58-16, page 591). These muscles are oval in orientation. A 1-cm incision is made in the skin over the central portion of the external sphincter muscles (Fig. 58-17, page 591). A plane is bluntly developed inside the external

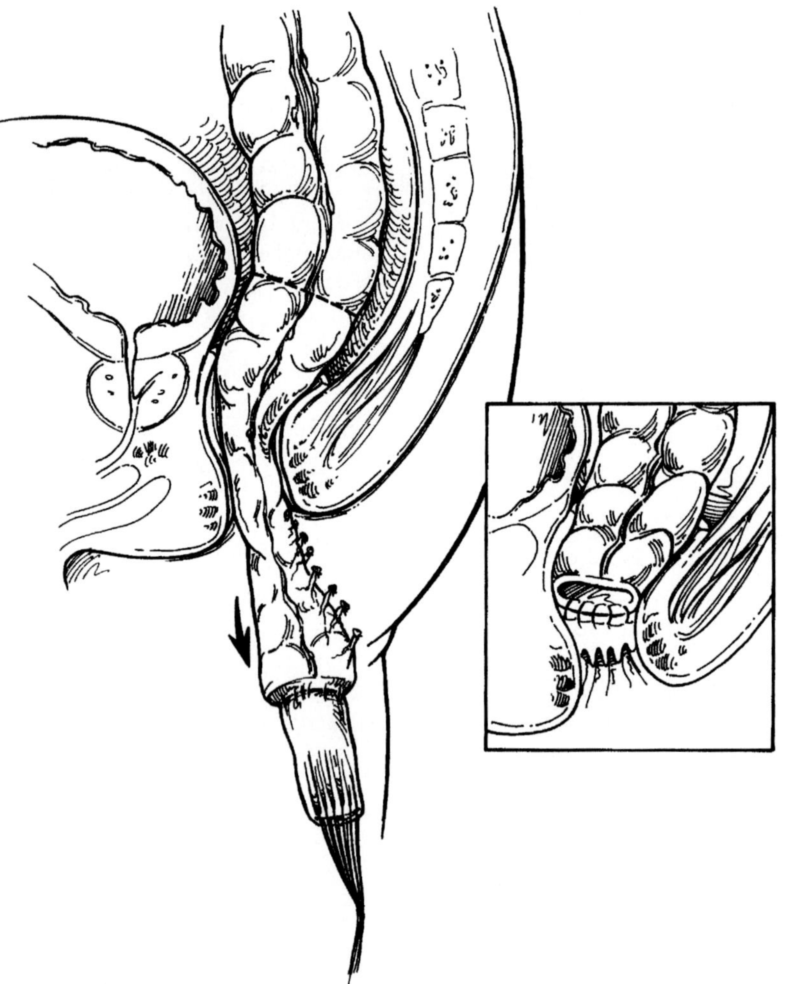

Fig. 58-14. The submucosal plane is converted to a full-thickness plane higher in the pelvis. The aganglionic colon is then pulled through and resected, and the ganglionic colon that remains is anastomosed to the anal cuff (inset).

sphincter complex and carried up for a distance of 2 cm. A Veress needle covered by an expandable sheath is then applied to the perineum through the recently developed plane inside the sphincter complex and passed under laparoscopic surveillance through the midline inside the visible puborectalis muscle. The Veress needle is removed from the expansile sleeve, and 5- and 10-mm trocars are applied through the expansile sleeve to dilate the tract. A 12-mm sleeve is passed through this expansile sleeve in larger infants. A laparoscopic Alice clamp is passed through this trocar and the fistula grasped (Fig. 58-18, page 592). The fistula is brought into the 12-mm trocar, but no effort is made to pull it through the trocar. The fistula and rectum are trailed behind the trocar as it is pulled down and out onto the perineum. The fistula is attached to the perineal skin using interrupted absorbable suture. The rectum is grasped transabdominally and pulled upward to deepen the anal dimple and lengthen the skin-lined anal canal. The rectum should be secured to the presacral fascia in this tethered position to preserve the deepened anal dimple (Fig. 58-19, page 592). The pneumoperitoneum is evacuated and the trocar sites closed. The anus should be dilated beginning 2 to 3 weeks postoperatively. Once adequate dilatation has been achieved over a 6- to 12-week period, the colostomy can be closed.

Adequate long-term assessment of continence has not yet been determined in patients operated on by the laparoscopic technique. However, reliable indicators of potential continence such as the presence of an anorectal reflex and improved compliance of the rectum have been noted in increased numbers in patients treated by laparoscopic-assisted pull-through when compared with the posterior sagittal anorectoplasty.

Thoracoscopic Procedures

EMPYEMA

In the past, empyema in children was treated with antibiotics, prolonged chest tube drainage, and, if this failed, open thoracotomy for debridement. This was often associated with long hospitalizations and significant morbidity due to the delayed interventions. With the expanded use of endoscopic techniques, thoracoscopy has been increasingly used in the treatment of empyema and often applied much earlier in the course of disease. The minimal morbidity associated with this procedure makes it ideal for the treatment of empyema in children. It has resulted in much shorter hospitalizations and a quicker resolution of respiratory symptoms.

PREOPERATIVE PLANNING

The preoperative workup consists of primarily a chest X-ray and computed tomography (CT) scan. Once the diagnosis of empyema is confirmed the child is prepared for surgery. After induction of general anesthesia a mainstem intubation of the contralateral bronchus is performed. This helps keep the lung collapsed during the procedure as the peel and effusion are removed.

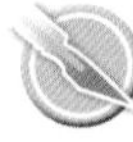

SURGICAL TECHNIQUE

The patient is placed in a lateral decubitus position with the affected side up (Fig. 58-20, page 592). An axillary roll and appropriate protective padding are used and the patient is secured with tape or straps. In an older child, support can be provided by a beanbag. The upper arm is extended upward and outward and secured in position. If the patient does not tolerate this position because of persistent desaturation, he or she may be placed more supine. Also if the patient does not tolerate single-lung ventilation a standard tracheal intubation is acceptable.

As the surgeon will need to access the entire chest cavity, he or she may stand on either side of the patient. The surgical assistant is usually positioned on the other side of the table to hold the camera. Two monitors are used, with one placed on each side of the patient at the level of the patient's chest near the shoulders to allow unobstructed views by the surgeon and assistant. A Veress needle is placed just anterior to the midaxillary line

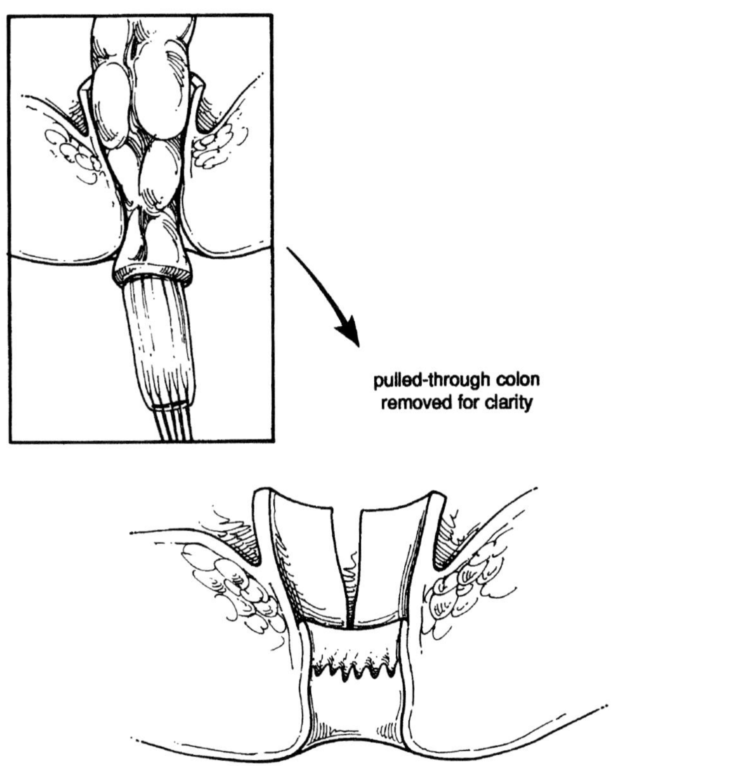

Fig. 58-15. The muscular cuff that remains is divided posteriorly. This may help prevent enterocolitis following pull-through.

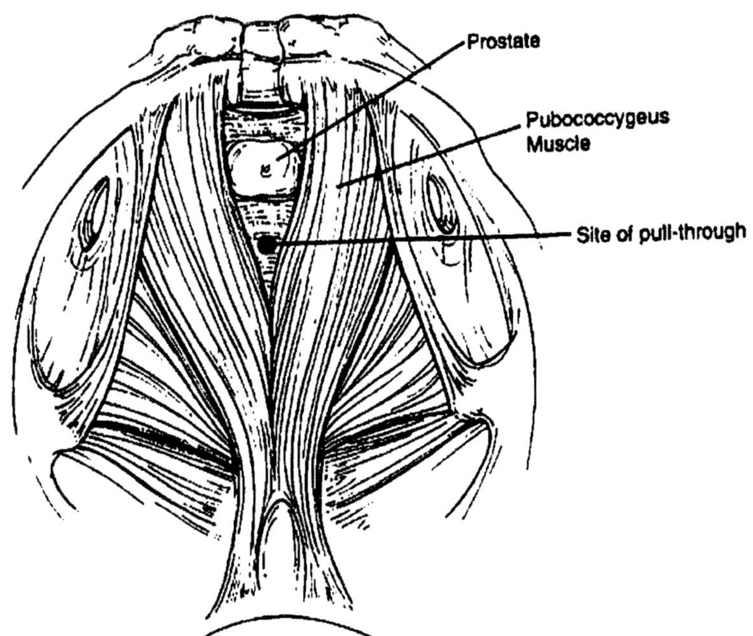

Fig. 58-16. A central location situated between the pubococcygeus muscle and the anatomic location of the sphincter complex becomes the eventual site of pull-through of the high rectal fistula.

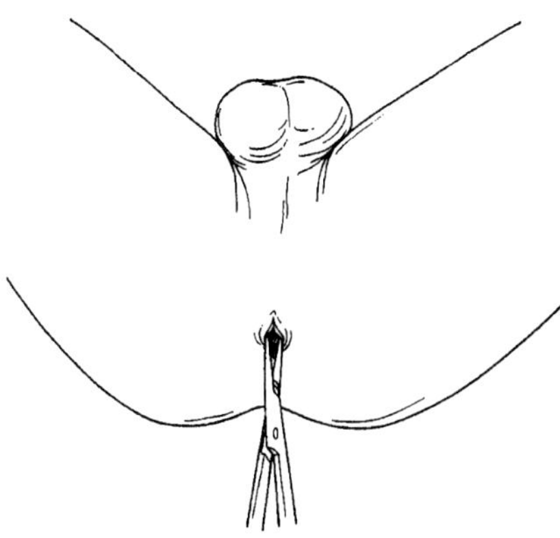

Fig. 58-17. Electrical stimulation identifies the proper site for the sphincter complex externally. An incision is made over this site and blunt dissection starts to create a tract. Progressively dilating, radially expanding trocars are then passed through this site into the pelvis under laparoscopic visualization.

at approximately the fourth or fifth intercostal space after infiltrating the site with local anesthetic and making a small transverse incision. Alternatively, an open approach may be used for placement of the first trocar. If there is an identified site on ultrasound or CT with a large fluid pocket close to one of the proposed port sites, this should be chosen as the point of entry. Insufflation with low-flow CO_2 to a pressure of 4 to 5 mmHg may help collapse the lung and improve visualization as the fibrinous adhesions are taken down. A 5-mm trocar is then placed and the 30-degree scope is introduced.

The endoscope can be used to bluntly take down adhesions and break up loculations, in order to allow for placement of the second trocar under thoracoscopic vision. This second 5-mm port is placed more posteriorly and inferiorly at approximately the sixth intercostal space along the posterior axillary line.

A suction-irrigator is introduced to aspirate the free pleural fluid and to further break down loculations with blunt dissection. A sample of the fluid can be collected at this time with a trap. A grasping forceps can then be used to peel off and remove the fibrinous debris through the trocar (Fig. 58-21, page 593). A bowel clamp works well for this purpose.

The scope and operating instrument can be interchanged from one port site to another to ensure that all of the pleural surfaces are reached. A systematic approach within the chest also helps ensure that no surface is left untouched.

Once the lung has been completely freed, all of the pleural fluid drained, and most of the fibrinous peel removed, the thoracic cavity is irrigated with warm normal saline that is subsequently aspirated out. The suction-irrigator is removed and the pneumothorax dissipated. The lung is allowed to expand fully with the help of positive pressure breaths from the anesthetist. Once full expansion is confirmed, the lower trocar is removed and a chest tube, appropriate to the child's size, is placed and positioned posteroinferiorly under thoracoscopic vision and secured in

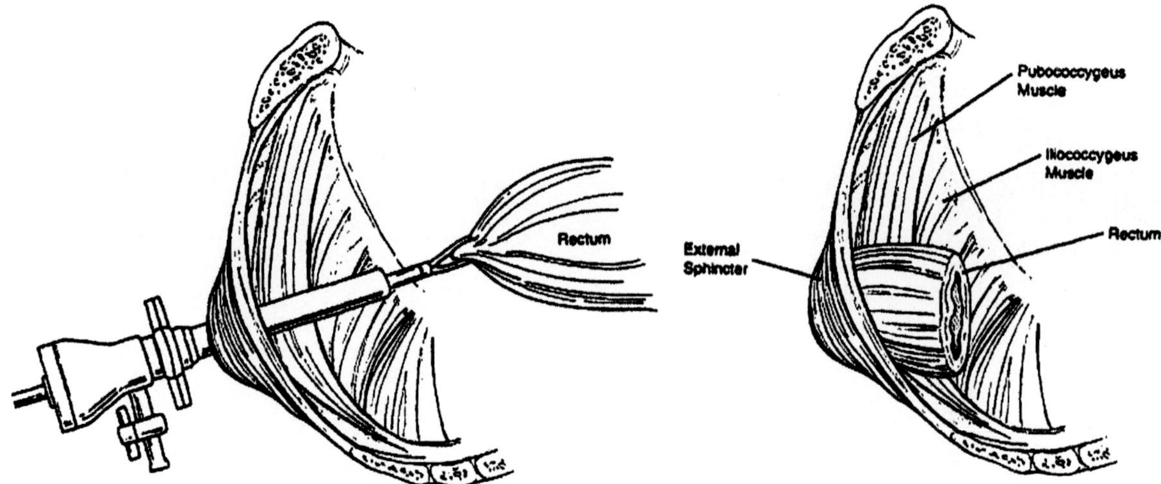

Fig. 58-18. The rectal fistula is grasped through the perineal trocar and pulled down to the perineum, where it is anastomosed.

place. The scope and remaining trocar are removed. This site is closed in two layers. The chest tube is attached to a Pleurovac and appropriate dressings are placed.

The chest tube is initially left to suction at −10 to −20 cm H_2O pressure. Once drainage becomes minimal, there is no evidence of an air leak, and the child is improving, the chest tube can be removed, usually after a trial of underwater seal. This is usually by the 3rd or 4th postoperative day. The patient is usually discharged on antibiotics after he or she has been afebrile for 48 hours.

MEDIASTINAL MASS RESECTION

Traditional approaches to the evaluation and treatment of mediastinal masses have included mediastinoscopy, anterior thoracotomy, sternotomy, and standard posterolateral thoracotomy. All of these procedures can be associated with significant surgical morbidity and recovery time. Over the last decade, thoracoscopy or video-assisted thoracic surgery (VATS) has been utilized to perform increasingly complex diagnostic and therapeutic procedures in the chest. The greater exposure and diminished morbidity now makes this the preferred method for diagnosis and resection of congenital and mediastinal masses. The most common lesions in the posterior mediastinum are foregut duplications, bronchogenic cyst, and neurogenic tumors such as neuroblastoma. The most common anterior masses are teratoma, thymoma, and lymphoma. Preoperative evaluation of these children includes chest X-ray, CT scan, magnetic resonance imaging (MRI), and barium upper GI tract contrast study.

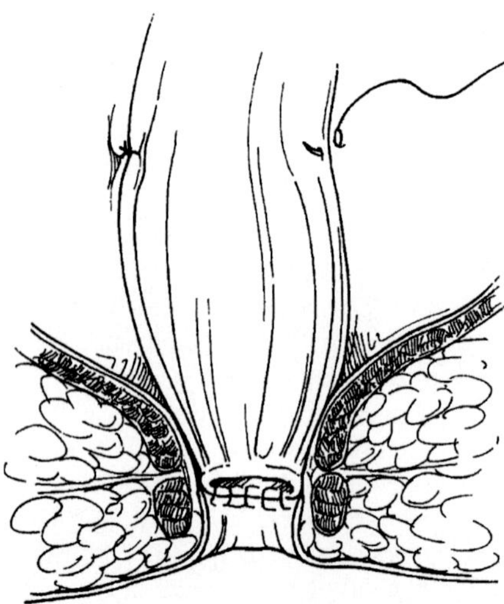

Fig. 58-19. The rectal fistula is secured under mild tension to the presacral fascia to recreate the anal dimple and prevent prolapse.

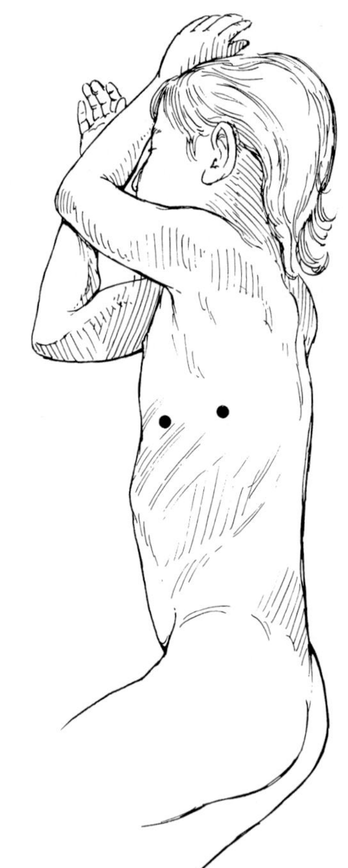

Fig. 58-20. Trocar positioning to allow maximal access to the entire thoracic cavity through a limited number of ports. One port is usually 10 mm to allow for adequate removal of the fibrous peel.

SURGICAL TECHNIQUE

Patients with an anterior mediastinal mass are positioned in a modified supine position with the affected side elevated slightly, 10 to 20 degrees (Fig. 58-22A). Patients with posterior masses are positioned in a modified prone position with a similar degree of elevation (Fig. 58-22B). Single-lung ventilation is obtained in most patients by performing a mainstem intubation of the contralateral side. All cases are started by inserting a Veress needle in the mid-axillary line and initiating a low-pressure, low-flow of CO_2 (at a pressure limit of 3 to 4 mmHg) to help collapse the lung. Three or four ports are placed between the anterior and posterior axillary lines; valved ports are used in all cases to help maintain a slight tension pneumothorax and thus aid thoracoscopic visualization. A nasogastric tube, esophageal bougie, or flexible gastroscope should be placed to help identify the esophagus in cases of posterior masses. A

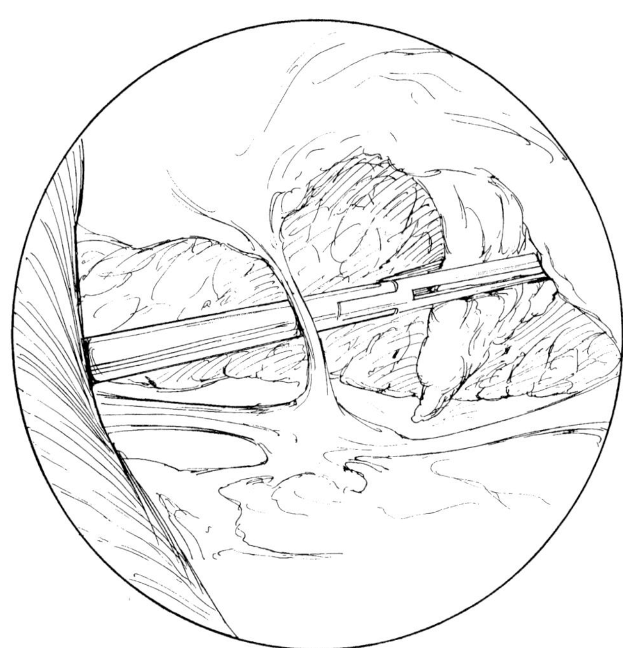

Fig. 58-21. A blunt grasper used to strip the fibrous peel off the parietal and visceral pleura.

combination of 3- and 5-mm instruments with cautery, ultrasonic dissector, or LigaSure are used to perform the procedures. Dissection is performed circumferentially, mobilizing the lesion towards its stalk. In the case of foregut duplication, this is relatively narrow and there is generally not an intraluminal connection to the esophagus (Fig. 58-23, page 594). Neural tumors may have a more broad-based attachment. Once resected, all solid masses should be placed in an endoscopic specimen bag prior to removal from the chest cavity to eliminate any risk of tumor spread or port site recurrence. Once the lesion is removed, the collapsed lung is re-expanded with a drain placed to water seal. If no air leak is apparent the drain is removed prior to extubation in the operating room, which eliminates the source of greatest postoperative pain. Most patients not requiring other therapy are discharged within 24 hours following surgery.

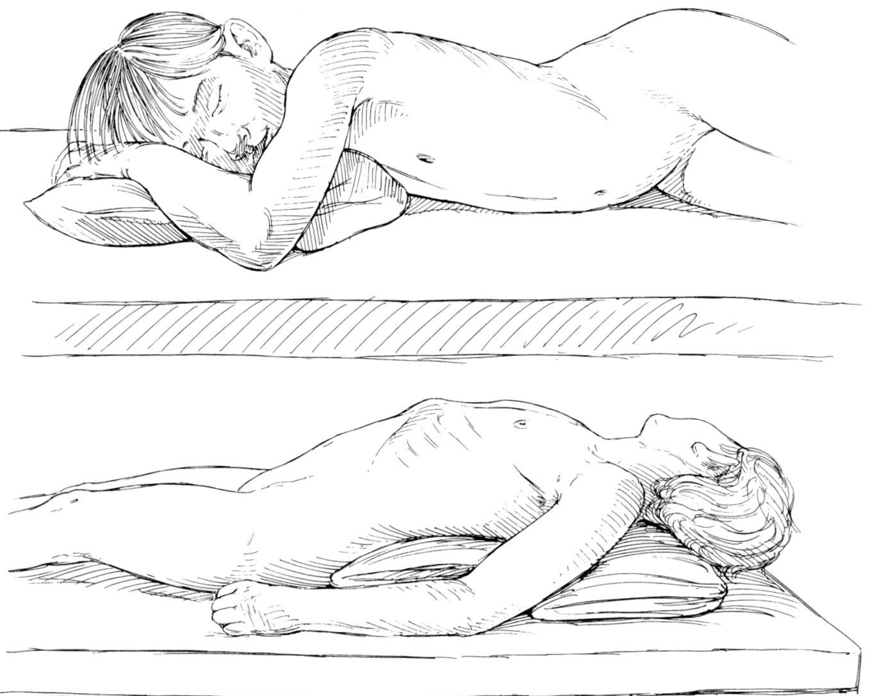

Fig. 58-22. Patient positioning: **(A)** modified supine and **(B)** modified prone. The position selected depends on the type and location of their pleural-based processes.

ESOPHAGEAL ATRESIA REPAIR

Esophageal atresia (EA) with or without a tracheoesophageal fistula (TEF) is one of the rarer congenital anomalies, occurring once for every 5000 births.

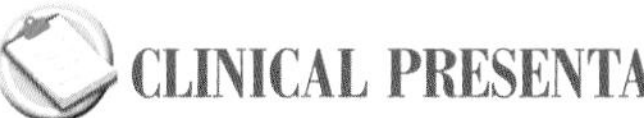

CLINICAL PRESENTATION

Traditionally these patients have presented shortly after birth because of respiratory distress or an inability to pass an orogastric tube or to tolerate feeds. The condition maybe associated with other major congenital anomalies (VATER syndrome) or may be an isolated defect. Improvements in maternal-fetal ultrasound have resulted in prenatal diagnosis in a number of cases. This allows the surgeon to plan for delivery and eventual surgery. Patients with a TEF require relatively emergent surgical intervention to prevent aspiration of gastric acid and over-distension of the intestines. Those with pure atresia can be dealt with in a more leisurely fashion as long the infant's oral secretions are controlled by continuous or intermittent suction.

In 2000 the first successful repair of an esophageal atresia with TEF in a newborn using a completely thoracoscopic approach was performed, and the operation has now become the standard in many major pediatric centers across the world. The greatest advantage of this technique is the avoidance of the major morbidity associated a formal thoracotomy in a neonate.

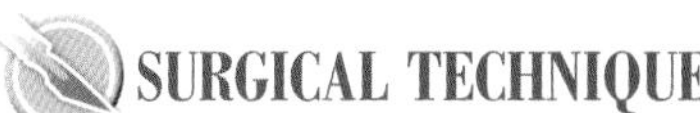

SURGICAL TECHNIQUE

The procedure is performed under general endotracheal anesthesia, but low peak pressures should be used until the fistula is ligated to prevent over-distension of the abdomen. Local anesthetic (0.25% Marcaine) is inserted at the trocar sites. Initially attempts were made to obtain a left mainstem intubation. However this can be difficult and time-consuming in a compromised newborn. We now perform the procedure with just a standard tracheal intubation, as excellent right lung

A

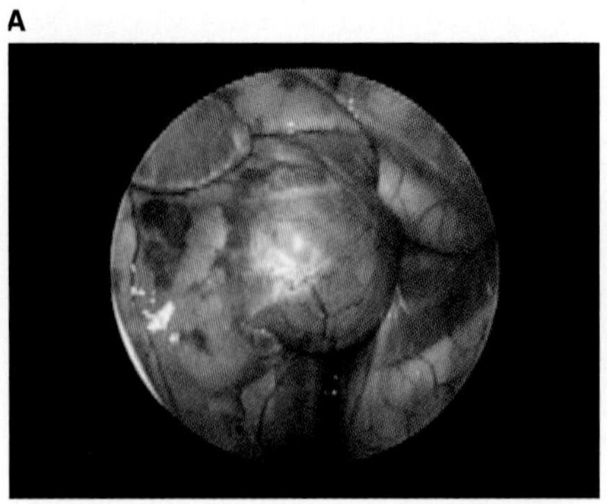

B

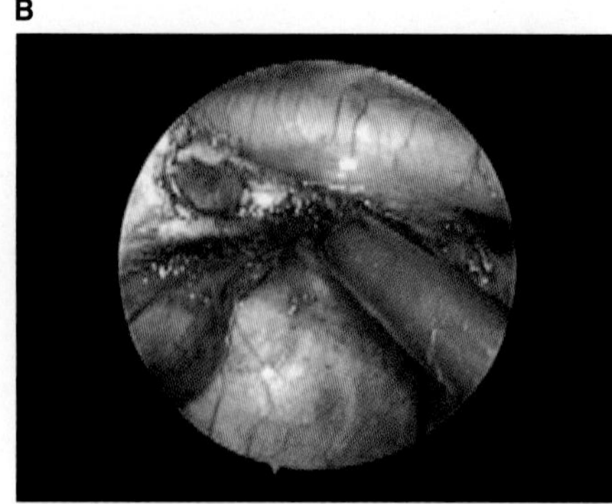

Fig. 58-23. A. Esophageal duplication. **B.** Division of the esophageal stalk.

collapse in newborns can be achieved with CO_2 insufflation alone. Wasting even minutes trying to place a bronchial blocker or other manipulations can compromise the eventual success of a thoracoscopic approach.

Once the endotracheal tube is secured, the patient is placed in a modified prone position with the right side elevated approximately 30 to 45 degrees (Fig. 58-22B). If there is a right sided aortic arch, the left side is approached. This positioning gives the surgeon access to the area between the anterior and posterior axillary lines for trocar placement while allowing gravity to retract the lung away from the posterior mediastinum, giving excellent exposure of the fistula and esophageal segments without the need of an extra trocar for a lung retractor. Generally small rolls are sufficient to provide stabilization for positioning or a small beanbag can be used.

The surgeon and the assistant stand at the patient's front and the monitor placed at the patient's back. Because of the fine manipulation necessary the surgeon and the assistant should position themselves so that they are in the most ergonomic and comfortable position.

Port placement is extremely important because of the small chest cavity and the intricate nature of the dissection and reconstruction. The procedure can be performed with three ports but occasionally a fourth port is necessary to retract the lung.

The initial 3- to 5-mm port is placed in the fifth intercostal space at approximately the posterior axillary line. This is the camera port and gives excellent visualization of the posterior mediastinum in the area of the fistula and eventual anastomosis. As mentioned, a 30-degree lens is used to allow the surgeon to "look down" at the instruments and avoid "dueling" (Fig. 58-24).

The two instrument ports are placed in the mid-axillary line one to two interspaces above and below the camera port. The upper port is 5 mm to allow for a clip applier and suture. The lower port is 3 mm in size. Ideally, these ports are placed so that the instrument tips will approximate a right angle (90 degrees) at the level of the fistula. This positioning will facilitate suturing the anastomosis.

Once the chest has been insufflated and the lung collapsed, the surgeon must identify the fistula. In most case the fistula is attached to the membranous portion of the trachea just above the carina. This level is usually demarcated by the azygus vein. After the azygus is identified it should be mobilized for a short segment using a curved dissector or scissors. The vein is then cauterized and divided. It is often easiest to do this with a small hook cautery, although bipolar cautery or other sealing devices can be used. Ties or clips are generally not necessary and could interfere with the dissection of the fistula.

With the vein divided, the lower esophageal segment is identified and followed proximally to the fistula. Because of the magnification afforded by the thoracoscopic approach it is easy to visualize

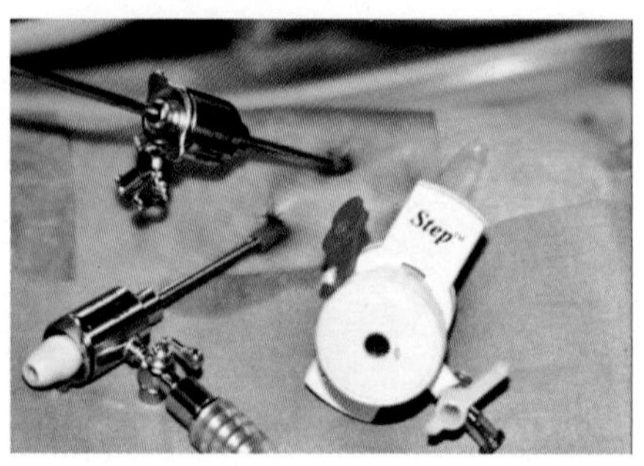

Fig. 58-24. Port placement for a tracheoesophageal fistula (TEF).

exactly where the fistula enters the back wall of the trachea. A 5-mm endoclip can then be applied safely (Fig. 58-25). Care should be taken to avoid the vagus nerve. The fistula can then be safely divided with scissors. The distal segment may retract, making it difficult to visualize; in that case it may be preferable to wait until the upper pouch is dissected out before completely dividing the fistula.

Attention is now turned to the thoracic inlet. The anesthesiologist places pressure on the nasogastric (NG) tube to help identify the upper pouch. The pleura overlying the pouch is incised sharply and the pouch is mobilized with blunt and sharp dissection. In some cases it is helpful to place a stay suture in the tip of the pouch to aid in applying traction. The plane between the esophagus and trachea can be easily seen, and the two should be separated by sharp dissection. Mobilization of the upper pouch is carried on up into the thoracic inlet.

Once adequate mobilization is achieved the distal tip of the pouch is resected. This should be an adequate section so that there is a sufficient opening to prevent later stricture formation. With the two ends mobilized, the anastomosis is performed using

A

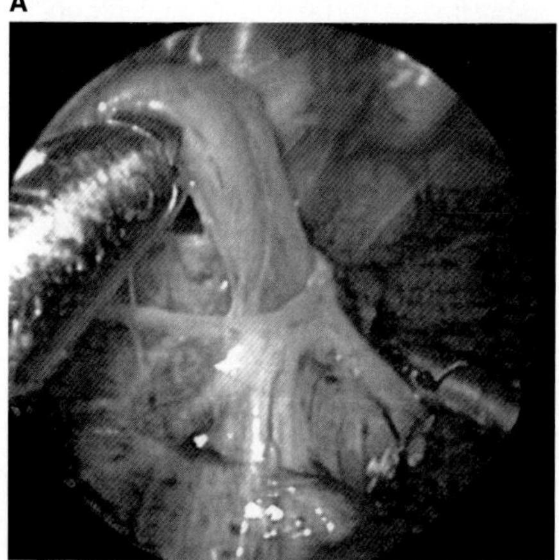

B

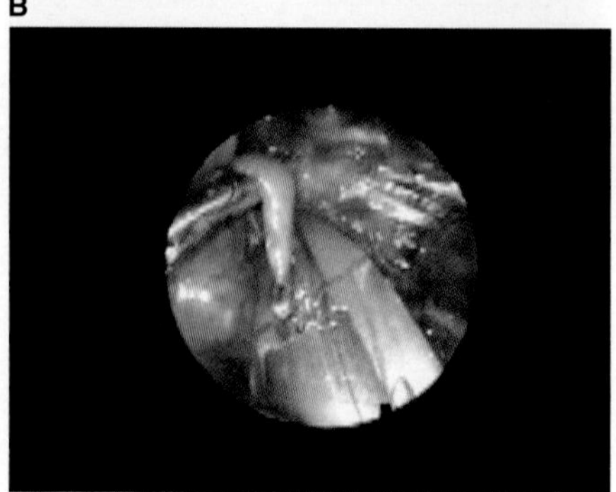

Fig. 58-25. A. Isolating a fistula for clip application. **B.** Applying the clip to the fistula.

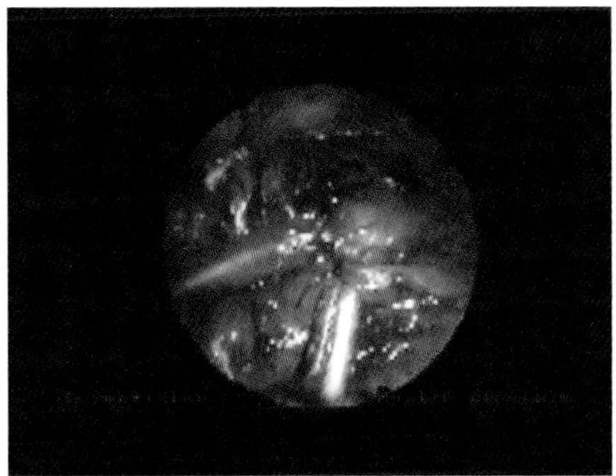

Fig. 58-26. A completed repair of an esophageal atresia.

A

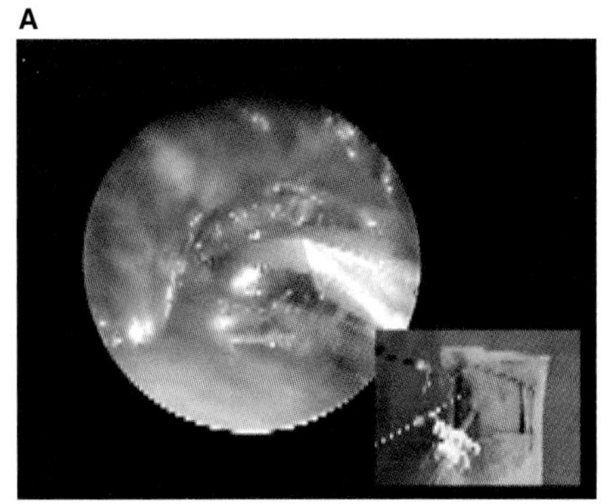

B

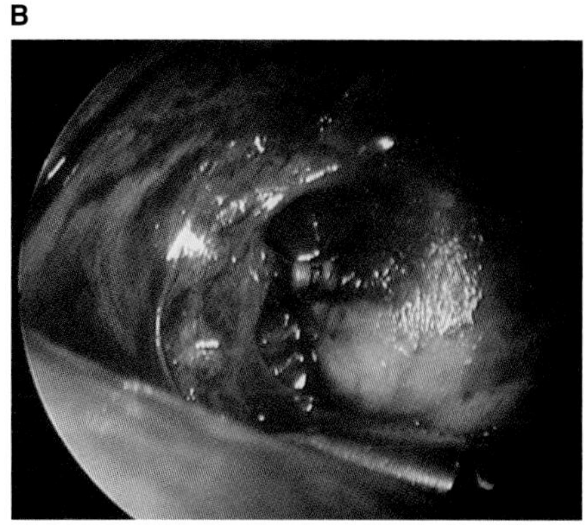

Fig. 58-27. A. Applying a clip to patent ductus arteriosus. **B.** A completed ligation with the clip in place.

a 4-0 or 5-0 monofilament absorbable suture on a small taper needle. The sutures are placed one at a time in an interrupted fashion. The back wall is placed first (3 to 5 sutures) with the knots intraluminal. The NG tube is then passed under direct vision into the lower pouch and on into the stomach. The anterior wall is then completed, with the NG tube acting as a guide to prevent incorporation of the posterior wall and ensuring patency of the anastomosis (Fig. 58-26). Adequate bites should be placed to prevent the sutures from tearing out; just as in the open procedure, it is important to include mucosa with all bites. The anastomosis generally requires only eight to nine sutures.

Once the anastomosis is completed a chest tube is then placed through the lower trocar site and the tip is placed near the anastomosis (under direct vision with the endoscope). The other ports are removed and the sites are closed with absorbable suture.

Generally the patient is left NPO (nil per os, or nothing by mouth) for 4 to 5 days, and then an esophagogram is obtained to check for any leaks. If none are found, oral feeds are started and the chest tube is removed.

PATENT DUCTUS ARTERIOSUS AND VASCULAR RINGS

Closure of a persistent patent duct arteriosus (PDA) has traditionally been performed through a standard posterolateral thoracotomy incision with either suture ligation or vascular clip closure. Over the last 15 years an increasing experience with intravascular occlusive devices such as coils and plugs has been seen but often this procedure is limited by the size of the patient and the diameter of the ductus. Thoracoscopic closure offers an alternative to these two techniques and affords many of the same benefits as seen in other thoracoscopic procedures.

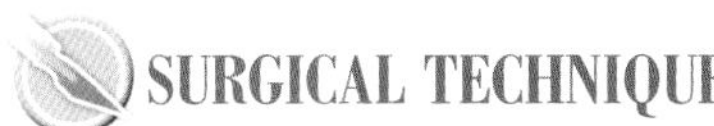

SURGICAL TECHNIQUE

The procedure is performed with the patient in a modified prone position with the left side elevated approximately 30 degrees. Two 3-mm ports and one 5-mm port are used to perform the surgery. A right mainstem intubation is obtained and the collapsed left lung is retracted anteriorly by gravity exposing the ductus. The pleura overlying the ductus is dissected, starting in the middle of the aorta, and then retracted medially. This exposes the ductus and pulls the vagus nerve out of the field of dissection. The endoscope provides excellent visualization of the ductus and the recurrent laryngeal nerve, which should help prevent injury to this structure. A 5-mm endoscopic clip can then be safely applied to the ductus, thereby occluding flow (Fig 58-27). In some cases it is necessary to use a larger clip or to perform a suture ligation. In these cases the 5-mm port is removed and a standard hemoclip can be placed through a widened trocar incision. In general a chest tube is not necessary postoperatively. Most patients admitted for this operation are discharged the next day.

The same approach is used for vascular rings that constrict the trachea or esophagus. Most require the ligation and division of the ligamentum arteriosum. In this case the ligament is dissected out, ligated in continuity, and divided. In most cases there is not persistent blood flow through the ligament, but the surgeon should not count on that.

SUGGESTED READING

Avansino JR, Goldman B, Sawin RS, et al. Primary operative versus nonoperative therapy for pediatric empyema: a meta-analysis. *Pediatrics* 2005;115:1652–1659.

Bax NM, Van der Zee DC. Laparoscopic treatment of intestinal malrotation in children. *Surg Endosc* 1998;12:1314–1316.

Georgeson KE, Inge TA, Albanese C. Laparoscopically assisted anorectal pull-through for high imperforate anus—a new technique. *J Pediatr Surg* 2000;35:927–930.

Georgeson KE, Jona JZ, Rothenberg SS, et al. Primary laparoscopic assisted endorectal colon pull-through for Hirschsprung's Disease—a new gold standard. *Ann Surg* 1999;229: 678–683.

Holcomb GW, Rothenberg SS, et al. Thoracoscopic repair of esophageal atresia and tracheoesophageal fistula: a multi-institutional analysis. *Am J of Surg* 2005;242:1–9.

Laborde F, Folligut T, Batisse A, et al. Video-assisted thoracoscopic surgical interruption: the technique of choice for patent ductus arteriosus. Routine experience in 230 pediatric cases. *J Cardiovasc Surg* 1995;110:1681–1684.

Levitt MA, Rothenberg SS, Tantoco JG, et al. Complication avoidance in miniature access pyloromyotomy. *Ped Endosurg Innov Techniques* 2003;7:291–296.

Partrick DA, Rothenberg SS. Thoracoscopic resection of mediastinal masses in infants and children: an evolution of technique and results. *J Ped Surg* 2001;36:1165–1167.

Rothenberg SS. First decades experienced with laparoscopic fundoplication in infants and children. *J Pediatr Surg* 2005;40:142–147.

Rothenberg SS. Laparoscopic duodeno-duodenostomy for duodenal obstruction in infants and children. *J Ped Surg* 2002;37: 1088–1089.

Rothenberg SS. Thoracoscopy in infants and children. *Semin Pediatr Surg* 1998;7:213–219.

Rothenberg SS, Bealer J, Chang J. Primary laparoscopic gastrostomy button for feeding tubes. *Surg Endosc* 1999;13:995–997.

COMMENTARY

Dr. Rothenberg has written a chapter covering the spectrum of minimally invasive surgery in the pediatric population. This summary is complete and well illustrated, discussing many thoracoscopic and laparoscopic operations currently being performed in newborns, infants, and children. Many general surgeons perform pediatric surgery as part of their practice, particularly in older children and adolescents. Furthermore, it is not uncommon for pediatric surgeons to ask for general surgeons experienced in laparoscopy to assist them in a pediatric case. Thus, this chapter has broad relevance despite its restrictive title.

Laparoscopic operations in small individuals entail some difficulties unique to the patient population. Positioning of the patient on the operating table involves different considerations related to the target organ and size of the individual. Intraabdominal pressures can and should probably be limited to levels lower than those traditionally used in the adult population. Smaller ports and shorter instruments are also commonly used. Thankfully, the number of small diameter instruments has increased markedly over the past few years as a result of the evolution and maturation of pediatric laparoscopic surgery. Despite the well-publicized trend towards obesity in childhood, most pediatric patients have less intraabdominal fat than their adult counterparts, which usually simplifies the dissection necessary in a given case. However, the tissues themselves are often more delicate, so the surgeon must exert care to minimize undue tissue trauma.

Laparoscopic surgery was initially not embraced by pediatric surgeons. During the last few years, as instrumentation has improved and become more widely disseminated, an increasing number of pediatric surgeons have conquered the laparoscopic learning curve. We are fortunate to have Dr. Rothenberg, one of the early adopters and acknowledged experts in the field, share his technical experience.

NJS

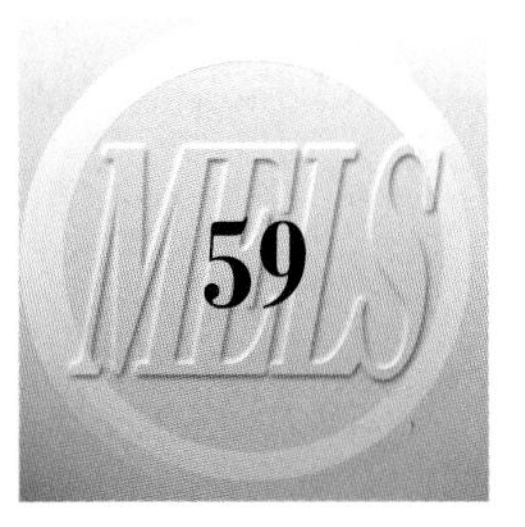

Diaphragm and Gastric Pacing

RAYMOND P. ONDERS

INTRODUCTION

Functional electrical stimulation (FES), a rapidly expanding area of medicine, no longer involves only cardiac applications. There are presently two laparoscopic applications of FES: gastric pacing (Enterra; Medtronic; Minneapolis, MI) and diaphragm motor point pacing (NeuRx RA/4; Synapse Biomedical; Oberlin, OH). To understand these procedures one has to understand the basics of electrical engineering and humanitarian use of devices. In the United States these two applications are only being used under a Food and Drug Administration (FDA) Humanitarian Device Exemption (HDE) of a Humanitarian Use Device (HUD). HUDs are medical devices approved by the FDA for the treatment of medical conditions affecting fewer than 4000 patients per year. In granting HDE approval for a HUD, the FDA mainly looks at the safety and probable benefit rather than a statistically significant demonstration of efficacy that is required of a pre-market application used for complete FDA approval. Federal regulations regarding HDEs state that each hospital's Institutional Review Board (IRB) must consider the use of this type of device at their hospital even though its use may not be in formal research studies.

A basic FES unit involves stimulating electrodes, an anode, a pulse generator, and a programmer. The types of electrodes that can be implanted are variable. There are electrodes that are only used to map or assess nerve function, electrodes that are placed near muscle motor points, or electrodes that are placed in contact with nerves. Electrodes that are placed in contact with nerves are many times called cuff electrodes. Electrodes have a non-insulated area to transfer the electrical impulse to the target. The connecting lead between the exposed electrode and the pulse generator needs to have a low resistance and be insulated, flexible, and capable of transferring current. Depending on where the electrode needs to be placed, an appropriate implant instrument needs to be used, such as the one used for diaphragm pacing. All electrical systems need an anode, or ground electrode, which can be the pulse generator if implanted. The pulse generator is one of the key aspects of functional electrical stimulation, commonly referred to in surgery as the "pacemaker" or "stimulator." This contains the battery to store the charge as well as the hardware and software that allow it to be programmable to give the stimulus with different rates, amplitude, frequency, and pulse width. If the pulse generator is implanted, it is commonly referred to as an IPG (implanted pulse generator). All pulse generators have an external programmer that will allow the clinician to assess the system and program the stimulation parameters the patients will receive.

Diaphragm Pacing

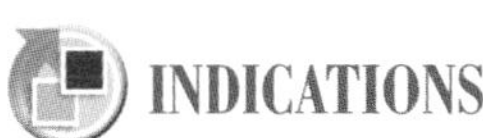

INDICATIONS

The diaphragm pacing stimulation (DPS) system was designed to replace or delay the need for patients requiring long-term positive pressure mechanical ventilation via tracheostomies. The use of ventilators, although lifesaving, leads to a myriad of complications: difficulty with speech, increased secretions and need for suctioning, loss of sense of smell, constant noise, difficulty with transfers, inability to find living facilities or nursing care, and an annual cost that approaches $200,000. In addition, the use of mechanical ventilation greatly decreases life expectancy, primarily due to respiratory infections that result from the inherently poor posterior lobe ventilation the devices provide. Diaphragm pacing provides natural negative pressure ventilation and overcomes many of these issues.

The initial clinical indications for phrenic nerve or diaphragm pacing have been cervical spinal cord injuries and congenital central hypoventilation syndromes (CCHS or Ondine curse). Although both of these conditions manifest in the individual's inability to independently breathe, spinal cord injury involves the disruption of the signal pathway from the respiratory center in the brain to the respiratory nerves (primarily the phrenic nerves), whereas central hypoventilation syndromes generally involve a decreased respiratory drive. In the latter case, the signal from the respiratory center to the phrenic nerves is not generated or sent, although the conduction pathway to deliver the signal is intact. CCHS is a rare diagnosis affecting 1 in 50,000 live births with presentation as newborns. Once the syndrome is identified by evidence of hypoventilation during sleep, these children will require nighttime positive pressure ventilation for the rest of their lives unless they are able to undergo DPS to control nighttime ventilation.

Of 11,000 new SCI injuries each year in the U.S., slightly more than one-half are affected by quadriplegia, with only 4% requiring long-term mechanical ventilation. In a prospective worldwide trial in this group, a total of 50 (37 male) patients were implanted, with failure in only one patient due to a false positive phrenic nerve study. There was no perioperative mortality. There were no operative time differences between sites. Average age was 36 years (range of 18 to 74 years), and the average time from injury to implantation was 5.6 years (ranging from .3 to 27 years). Ninety-eight percent of the patients had DPS-stimulated tidal volumes above 5 to 7 cc/kg for 4 or more continuous hours, with 50% utilizing DPS for continuous 24-hour ventilation. During the over 75 cumulative years of follow-up there have been three unrelated deaths (1 sepsis, 2 cardiac). In analyzing 10 patients with preexisting cardiac pacemakers, there was no cardiac or device-to-device interaction. Age and time from injury directly affects conditioning time to achieve ventilation with DPS, with younger and more recently injured patients weaning from ventilators more quickly. In a long-term analysis of patient satisfaction (24 patients), over 60% report less secretions, over 95% report greater freedom and independence, 100% would recommend

DPS to others, and no patients stopped utilization. This multicenter trial has shown that DPS implantation is safe and easily reproducible and that it can provide natural diaphragm ventilation. Most important is the patients' perception of improved quality of life DPS provided.

Another area where DPS is increasingly used is in patients with amyotrophic lateral sclerosis (ALS or Lou Gehrig disease), where the major cause of mortality is respiratory insufficiency as patients lose 3% to 5% of their motor neurons monthly, leading to respiratory muscle weakness. In this group of patients, the goal is to delay the need for mechanical ventilation, rather than replacing it, by implanting the DPS and stimulating the muscle to maintain diaphragm strength prior to the end-stage weakness. The results to date show that patients can be safely implanted, even when feeding tubes are placed at the same time. Experience has shown that DPS can improve diaphragm excursion with diaphragm stimulation compared to the patient's maximal voluntary effort. The procedure significantly increases muscle thickness when assessed with ultrasound ($p = 0.02$). After conditioning the diaphragm with the DPS, preliminary results show an average rate of decline in FVC of 0.9% per month from the preimplantation decline of 2.4% a month, which extrapolates to an additional 24 months of ventilator-free survival. Additional findings include: DPS can convert fast-twitch glycolytic (IIb) to functional slow-twitch (I) oxidative muscle fibers; DPS improves posterior lobe lung ventilation; DPS increases lung compliance, leading to decreased effort in breathing; and patients have started utilizing DPS to improve nighttime ventilation. It has been found that ALS patients develop central hypoventilation that can be overcome with night DPS use. The DPS system can be safely implanted and utilized in ALS patients, with a documented decrease in the decline of respiratory failure leading to increased survival. A multicenter pivotal trial is now enrolling patients and collecting data to further identify the optimal patient and time for implantation. The ability to specifically target and improve diaphragm function with the DPS system will increase therapeutic options in ALS patients.

Because muscle motor point electrodes can be removed and used for short periods of times, further investigations are being done to assess the use of temporary DPS for patients in intensive care units (ICUs). Over 100,000 tracheostomies are done yearly in the U.S. because of a failure to wean from ventilators; DPS may have a role in these patients. Table 59-1 outlines how DPS could help these patients. Subsequent studies have led to less invasive methods of application, including the possibility of natural orifice transluminal endoscopic surgery (NOTES) techniques, so that, for example, the pacing wires can be placed at the bedside for patients in the ICU at the time of their percutaneous endoscopic gastrostomy (PEG) tube placement.

TABLE 59-1. PRIMARY AND SECONDARY EFFECTS OF DIAPHRAGM PACING IN PATIENTS IN THE ICU

Primary effects	Secondary effects
Diaphragm strengthening	Maintenance of slow-twitch oxidative muscle fibers Decreased weaning time and length of stay
Reduction in airway pressure	Decreased barotrauma Improved alveolar ventilation
Posterior lobe ventilation	Decreased atelectasis Pneumonia risk reduction
Maintenance of negative chest pressure	Improved venous return Increased cardiac output Reduced third spacing

PREOPERATIVE PLANNING

For the DPS device to be effective, the phrenic nerve must be able to provide conduction pathways through to the muscle. Therefore, the lower motor neurons in the spinal cord and the phrenic nerve must be intact. If a phrenic nerve has been completely severed or injured, the diaphragm cannot be paced. Prior to implanting, an assessment of phrenic nerve function should be performed. In patients with ALS or CCHS, fluoroscopy of the diaphragm should be done to see that volitional diaphragm movement is intact (commonly referred to as a sniff test). The ALS patients should also be stabilized from a respiratory standpoint so that they can tolerate the general anesthesia. If they have low pulmonary function, they should be trained to tolerate noninvasive positive pressure ventilation (NIPPV) or bi-level positive pressure ventilation (BiPaP) preoperatively.

For SCI patients, their trauma history has to be consistent with intact motor neurons in cervical segments 3 to 5 with no phrenic nerve injuries. If the history is questionable, then phrenic nerve function should be assessed both by measurements of phrenic nerve conduction times and by fluoroscopic evaluation of diaphragm movement during phrenic nerve stimulation.

Because the diaphragm has to be stimulated during the operation, no neuromuscular blocking or paralyzing agents can be used by the anesthesiologist. The overall strategy is to use rapid reversible short-acting analgesic and amnestic agents such as remifentanil, sevoflurane, and propofol. At the end of each procedure the DPS system is also utilized to increase the respiratory system compliance by decreasing posterior lobe atelectasis. If an ALS patient was on NIPPV preoperatively, he or she should bring it and the mask for postoperative use.

SURGICAL TECHNIQUE

The DPS procedure, which takes about 1.5 hours, is described in four phases: exposure, mapping, implantation, and routing. The exposure consists of the setup for the standard four-port laparoscopy to visualize the diaphragm. Because these patients are not paralyzed, the use of preemptive local anesthetics in the skin and abdominal muscles at the planned trocar sites helps to decrease abdominal muscle spasms. The initial port is placed in the midline supraumbilical so that adequate visualization of the diaphragm can be obtained; this can be a 5- or 10-mm port depending on the laparoscope choice. A zero-degree laparoscope is usually adequate, although an angled one can be used. Two lateral subcostal 5-mm ports are placed for the mapping probe for each side and these are used initially to completely

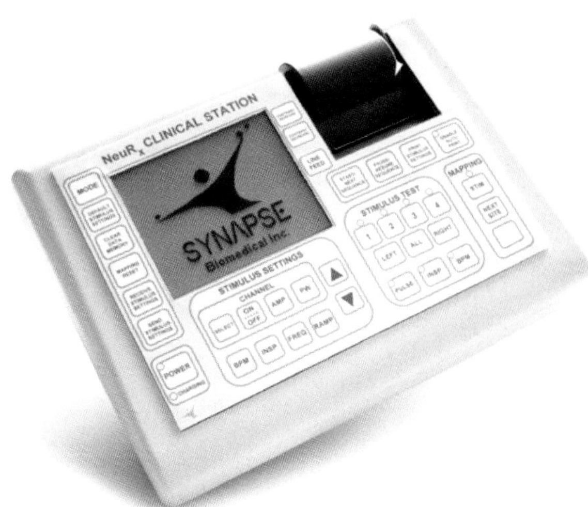

Fig. 59-1. Clinical station for diaphragm pacing used intraoperatively to map the diaphragm and record intraabdominal pressures during stimulation and postoperatively to program the patient's stimulator.

divide the falciform ligament, which allows easier visualization of the medial aspect of the right diaphragm and easier exit of the pacing electrodes through a 12-mm epigastric port. The epigastric port is used for the diaphragm implant instrument. An additional grounding patch is placed on the patient and attached to the clinical station (Fig. 59-1). From one of the secondary trocar insufflation ports, pressure tubing is attached and handed off the sterile field to connect to the pressure sensor of the clinical station.

Mapping involves finding the point on the abdominal side of the diaphragm where stimulation causes the greatest diaphragm excursion. The mapping instrument has flexible tubing inside a rigid cannula that connects to the operating room suction. The working part of the mapping instrument has a circular electrode that can be stimulated when temporarily attached to the diaphragm by the suction (Fig. 59-2). Its flexibility allows an unimpeded diaphragm contraction. The vacuum line is controlled by a tubing clamp. Placement and movement of the suction tip is best done with a two-handed procedure. The tip of the probe is pulled out from the metal cannula after insertion into the abdomen to provide slack in the tubing. The tip is grasped with a non-racheted dissector and small movements along the surface are made to move test locations. The other hand manipulates the back of the metal cannula, pushing in or withdrawing tubing as needed with a gentle slack in the tube (Fig. 59-3, page 600). Stimulation is applied in either a twitch or burst mode from the clinical station through a connecting cable. Mapping allows qualitative and quantitative data to be obtained. Quantitatively, changes in abdominal pressures are measured. Qualitatively, observation of the diaphragm contraction is performed. The stronger the stimulated contraction, the closer the mapping probe is to the motor point of the diaphragm. During mapping the entire diaphragm is assessed in a grid pattern to be sure the point of maximal contraction is not missed. The magnitude of the abdominal pressure change to the applied stimuli is recorded for each location. The primary electrode site is identified at the location of maximal pressure change in each hemi-diaphragm. A secondary electrode site is identified as either a backup to the primary site or at a location in each hemi-diaphragm that recruits another region (e.g., anterior, lateral, or posterior) of the diaphragm at a similar magnitude. The nerve does not travel with the vessels in the diaphragm so the motor point is not related to the visible vascular bundles. On the right diaphragm the motor point is just lateral to the central tendon; on the left diaphragm the motor point tends to be much more lateral because the phrenic nerve travels on the lateral aspect of the pericardium and enters the diaphragm more laterally. In later-stage ALS patients, the diaphragm will be weaker because of the decreased motor units from loss of motor neurons. In these patients a burst or train of stimulation is needed to see diaphragm contraction and finalize the site for electrode implantation. Repeated burst stimulations can tire out the ALS diaphragm as it is composed of mostly type IIb muscle fibers, so bursts are used infrequently. At times the abdominal insufflation pressure even has to be decreased because the diaphragm is too weak to overcome normal abdominal insufflation pressure. Once the optimal response sites are identified a temporary surgical marking pen is used to place a mark at the target implant sites. Further mapping may be done around the mark to confirm that the marks are at the optimal locations.

Once the primary and secondary electrode sites are identified in each hemi-diaphragm, the implantation phase begins. Since every diaphragm is at a slightly different angle, the approach to the

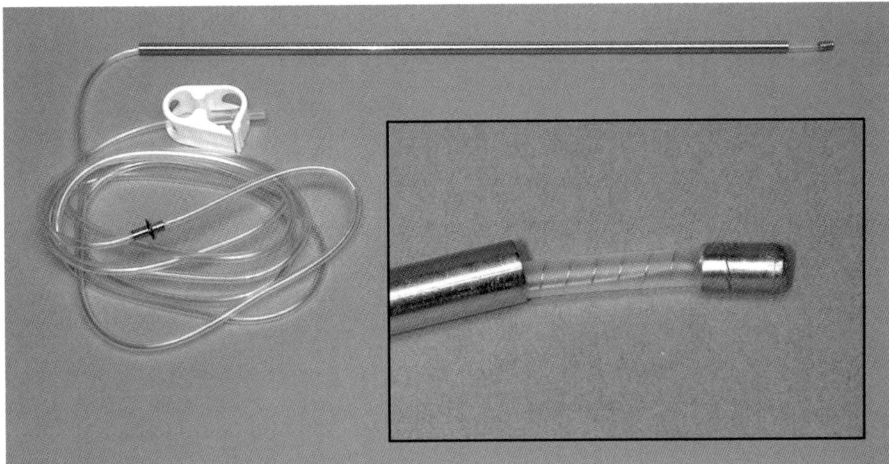

Fig. 59-2. A laparoscopic mapping probe. This has a suction port attached to the operating room vacuum so that the contact electrode at its tip can be noninvasively attached to the surface of the muscle. It receives a stimulus from the clinical station.

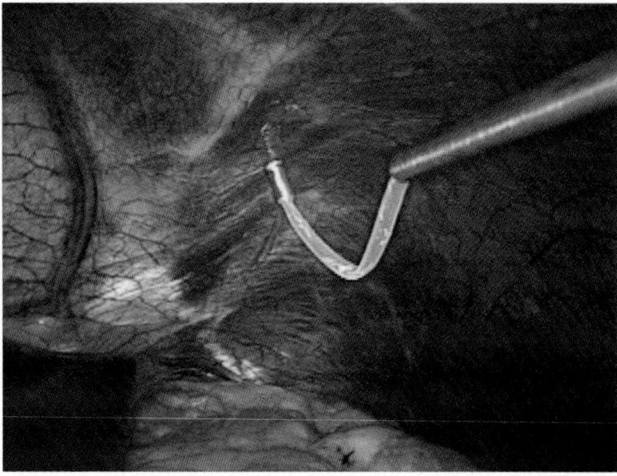

Fig. 59-3. A mapping probe being used on patient's left diaphragm; note the gentle slack of the vacuum tubing.

marked implant sites is first tested with an empty implant instrument (Fig. 59-4). The angle of approach and any torques on the instrument are identified. The epimysium of the diaphragm is also opened, at the site of insertion, with the empty needle. This allows for an easier entry of the loaded instrument. The electrode is loaded down the lumen of the implant instrument with only the hooked tip of the electrode and one piece of the blue polypropylene barb extending out of the needle. The entire skirt of the barb should be inside the needle. The instrument is inserted into the trocar with the needle closed. The inferior electrode should be placed first so that the lead is not interfering with the placement of the next electrode. The needle should approach the diaphragm orthogonally to the direction of the muscle fibers, when possible, to allow for the barbs to catch into the fibers easier. When withdrawing the needle, slight counterpressure on the diaphragm surface with a dissector at the tip of the needle will also allow the barbs to release from the needle and catch on the muscle fibers (Fig. 59-5). As the needle is withdrawn from the diaphragm, care is taken to not over-extend the needle and cause a capnothorax, which is air tracking from the abdominal cavity to the pleural cavity along the needle. This is seen in up to 50% of cases of very weak and thin diaphragms this may at times be unavoidable. The electrode is then tested to assure the desired response to twitch stimuli is achieved and the procedure is repeated for the remaining electrodes. If the response is not adequate when tested the electrode may be withdrawn by gently pulling on it and another implanted. A second electrode is implanted at the previously marked site during mapping (Fig. 59-6). Once all four electrodes are implanted, they are brought out through the epigastric port, keeping the right and left side separated. Excess electrode length is kept in the abdomen on top of the liver.

The electrodes will be tunneled subcutaneously to an area in the upper chest at a site deemed appropriate by the surgeon and patient's caregivers. Each wire is tunneled separately, with the right electrodes inferior to the left electrodes. A ground electrode will be placed subcutaneously in the upper chest through a separate percutaneous exit site. The electrodes are then retested to make sure that all of the connections have been made properly. An electrocardiogram (EKG) strip is recorded with all four electrodes active to be sure there is no capture of the cardiac rhythm. A chest X-ray will be obtained to be sure no intraabdominal air has tracked with the needle to the chest cavity causing a capnothorax. If a capnothorax is observed on chest X-ray, it is treated by initially giving much larger breaths via the patient's tracheostomy and repeating the chest X-ray. If the capnothorax is still present, then it is aspirated by a method most familiar to the implanting surgeon: either with a small pediatric chest tube or a thoracentisis needle. At this time if the patient needs a gastrostomy a standard percutaneous endoscopic technique can be done and the wires are once again checked. The port incisions are then closed and the patient is transferred to recovery. In the recovery room or later that day the patient's wires are placed in a block to allow for connection to the stimulator (Fig. 59-7, page 602).

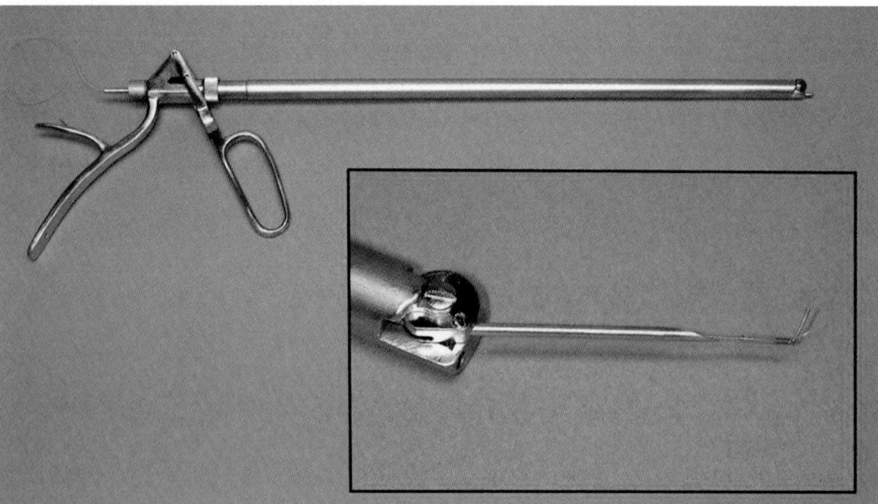

Fig. 59-4. A laparoscopic electrode implant tool. The electrode is carried in a hypodermic needle that is enclosed in the instrument for insertion into the abdominal cavity. The trigger rotates the needle outward to allow the surgeon control over the angle of insertion into the tissue.

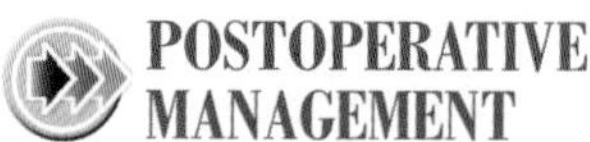

POSTOPERATIVE MANAGEMENT

After the surgery, patients are placed in the hospital in an observational status and are able to eat a regular diet for dinner and have no activity restrictions. SCI patients are placed on their usual mechanical ventilator settings until conditioning of their diaphragm is begun. ALS and CCHS patients need to be monitored for hypoventilation perioperatively as both have lost

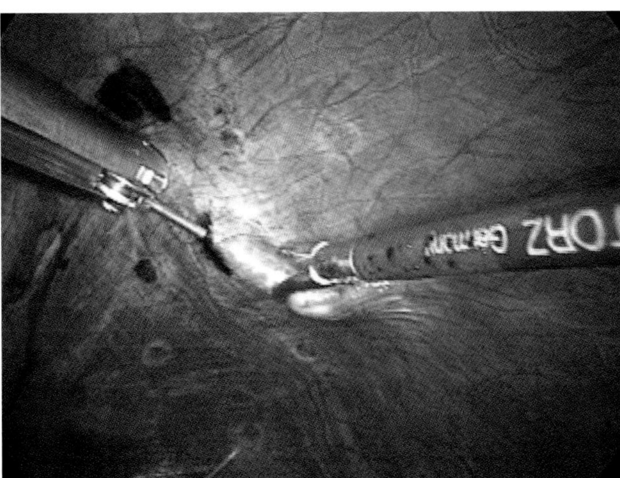

Fig. 59-5. A laparoscopic implant device with the needle housing the electrode being placed in the diaphragm muscle. Countertraction is applied with another laparoscopic instrument to help to deploy the electrode, which has a small barb, into the diaphragm muscles.

some central control of respiration that can be affected by sedation. ALS patients are placed on their NIPPV in the recovery room if they were on it beforehand.

Characterization of electrodes and system evaluation is done when the patient is stable post-implantation. Electrode evaluation is performed by adjusting individual stimulus parameters (amplitude, pulse width, rate, and frequency) so that a comfortable level of stimulation can be identified for the diaphragm conditioning sessions. The DPS will be set to provide a tidal volume that provides 15% above the basal needs (5 to 7 cc/kg) and that the SCI patient can easily tolerate and, for ALS patients, the highest setting that causes no discomfort. The settings will always be below 25 mA for amplitude, below 20 Hz for frequency, and below 200 us for pulse width.

ALS patients begin conditioning for their diaphragm by pacing five 30-minute sessions a day. If patients are having daytime or nighttime episodes of hypoventilation (identified through night polysomnography or hypercarbia on arterial blood gas analysis), the amount of DPS time can be increased and then used at night. Continuous positive airway pressure (CPAP) or NIPPV may still be needed to maintain an upper airway and can be used in conjunction with DPS.

A weaning program for SCI patients is then begun in which the DPS is turned on and the ventilator is turned off. The patients' tidal volume is checked initially with a Wright spirometer and then every 5 minutes. They are placed back on the ventilator when they feel uncomfortable or if their tidal volumes start dropping because of diaphragm fatigue. Initially patients may only tolerate 15 minutes of diaphragm pacing. Due to disuse atrophy and the conversion of muscle fibers to fast-fatigueable type during periods of inactivity, patients who have long-standing and significant respiratory paralysis will require conditioning of the diaphragm muscle in order to sustain ventilation. The diaphragm can recover quite rapidly from training so that patients and their caregiver can repeat a session every hour. The length of time it takes to tolerate DPS for greater than 4 continuous hours depends on the amount of time the patient and caregivers devote to this process.

Because the abdominal muscles of spinal cord-injured patients are also paralyzed, the diaphragm muscles will not elongate up into the chest after contraction. This can lead to smaller tidal volumes and respiratory distress. This effect is alleviated to a large extent by use of a snug-fitting abdominal binder that maintains intraabdominal pressure.

After full-time pacing is achieved throughout the day, pacing can be extended to sleep for SCI patients. During sleep, however, upper airway obstruction can occur with paced breaths. To prevent this, the tracheostomy should be capped with a valve such as the Passy-Muir device, which allows airflow through the tracheostomy.

With any respiratory support device, adequate monitoring needs to be maintained. Pacemaker function should be monitored on routine basis and SCI patients will need to have backup ventilation in case of failure of the electrodes. It is important to note that reductions in inspired volume can occur despite a normal functioning pacemaker system. Retained secretions, for example, may cause an increase in airway resistance and lead to the development of atelectasis with secondary reductions in lung compliance. Inspired volumes will be reduced as a consequence of these mechanical derangements. Fortunately, removal of airway secretions results in prompt improvement in volume generation.

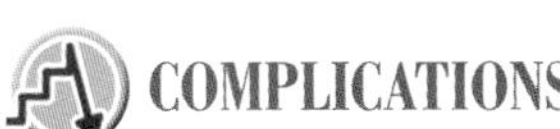

COMPLICATIONS

The groups of patients undergoing DPS implantation are at an inherent risk for problems given the comorbidities of their disease process. ALS patients have a terminal disease; the goal is to increase their quality of life by delaying their need for tracheostomy ventilation. The most common problem intraoperatively is a capnothorax,

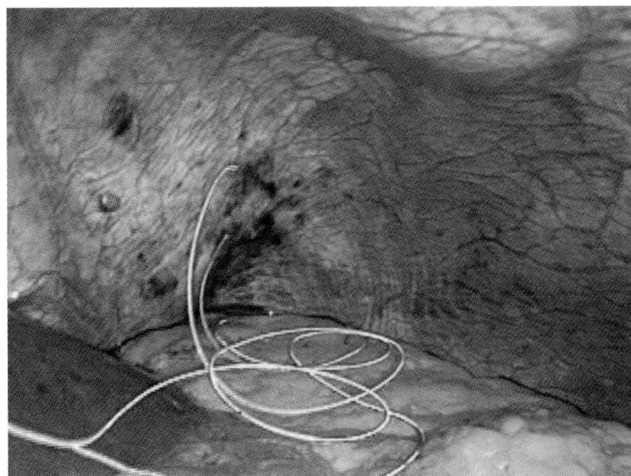

Fig. 59-6. Two electrodes have been implanted on the left diaphragm and exit the abdomen through the epigastric port.

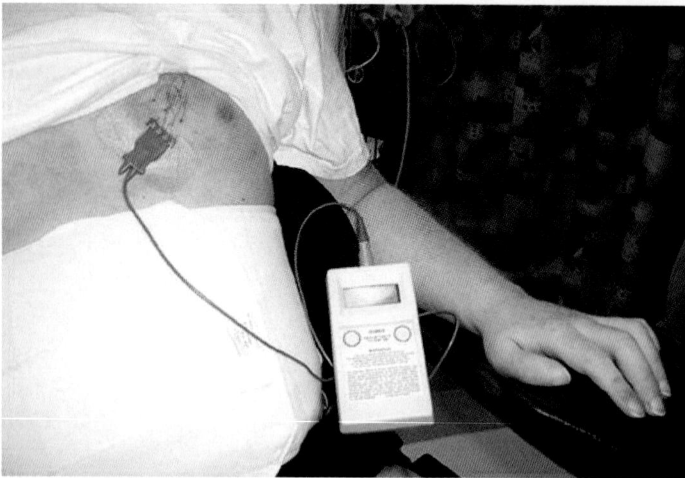

Fig. 59-7. The percutaneous electrodes are attached to a connector block in which the external stimulator can be attached. Note the spinal cord injured patient utilizing an abdominal binder with the DPS system. DPS = diagram pacing stimulation.

TABLE 59-2. INCLUSION CRITERIA FOR GASTRIC ELECTRICAL STIMULATION (GES)

Gastroparesis for longer than one year
Delayed gastric emptying; more than 60% retention at 2 hours and more than 10% at 4 hours
A condition that is refractory or intolerant to at least two drug classes
More than seven vomiting episodes per week
Stable medical therapy for at least 1 month prior to implantation
Stable nutritional support for 1 month prior to implantation

which occurs from intraabdominal air tracking to the chest cavity from the needle being placed in the thin diaphragm of these patients. This occurs up to 50% of the time and can easily be managed by watchful waiting as the carbon dioxide is absorbed readily or easily aspirated via a thoracentesis catheter. An overall 3% wound infection rate is most likely due to the simultaneous gastrostomy tube placement. No electrodes have needed to be removed or replaced, and no electrodes, to date, have stopped functioning. The possibility of phrenic nerve injury is minimal in that the electrodes do not come in direct contact with the nerves.

Gastric Pacing

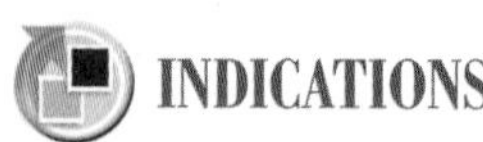

INDICATIONS

Gastroparesis, defined as delayed gastric emptying in the absence of mechanical obstruction, affects more than 1.5 million Americans with approximately 100,000 suffering from a severe form. Causes for gastroparesis include idiopathic, diabetic, and post-foregut surgery. Patients present with nausea, vomiting, abdominal pain, bloating, early satiety, malnutrition, and weight loss. Treatment options for gastroparesis are limited and include medical therapy, operative therapy, and nutritional support. Treatment including dietary and behavioral modifications and drug therapy are often used as the first line of treatment, and may alleviate symptoms in patients with mild to moderate disease. Prokinetic agents used include cisapride, domperidone, erythromycin, and metoclopramide, although only the last two are available in the U.S. Even with a multidisciplinary approach, treatment is often challenging and medical therapy may only offer temporary or partial relief. In cases of severe disorder, nutritional support and more aggressive medical treatment may be indicated. Invasive interventions are reserved for patients with severe disease, including nutritional deficiencies, refractory symptoms despite medical treatment, and frequent emergency room visits or hospitalizations. These treatments include enteral nutritional support (such as a jejunostomy), endoscopic injections of botulinum toxin in the pylorus, pyloroplasty or pyloromyotomy, partial or total gastric resection, and gastric electrical stimulation (GES).

Various methods of GES have been studied with the most widely applied method being used the high-frequency short-pulse low-energy method. A number of studies have shown that this short-pulse GES demonstrates significant antiemetic effect but only modest improvement in gastric emptying. However, symptom improvement does not rely solely on improved gastric emptying, and the quality of life improvement with GES has been significant. This has been shown in both a randomized, double-blind, placebo-controlled study and in a crossover study. In a publication by Forster, GES patients showed improvements in body mass index, hemoglobin A1C levels (in diabetic patients), quality of life, and number of hospital admissions. GES can easily be performed laparoscopically and it is a relatively safe treatment option for patients with refractory gastroparesis that results in improvement in gastrointestinal and quality of life symptoms and a reduction of drug therapy. The primary inclusion criteria for placement of a gastric stimulator are listed on Table 59-2.

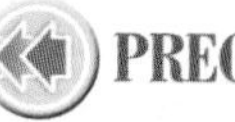

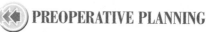

PREOPERATIVE PLANNING

The diagnosis and the severity of gastroparesis should not only be based upon symptoms, but also documented with delayed gastric emptying (radio labeled solid meal) and the absence of a mechanical obstruction. A patient's nutritional status should be optimized if possible prior to surgery. A frank discussion should also be undertaken with patients so that it is understood that GES will not cure all of their symptoms. Most successful GES patients indicate while they still suffer from gastrointestinal symptoms after undergoing the procedure, the symptoms are less severe and less frequent. The location of the planned implanted neurostimulator should also be discussed with the patient and care must be taken to place it in an area away from any future planned feeding tubes. The location also should be in a cosmetically acceptable position away from bony structures and possible areas of friction with abdominal clothing. If the patient has had a significant number of upper abdominal operations, consideration should be given to an open procedure because the GES device will be implanted and an enterotomy may require delay of implantation. Patients are given intravenous antibiotics prior to surgery.

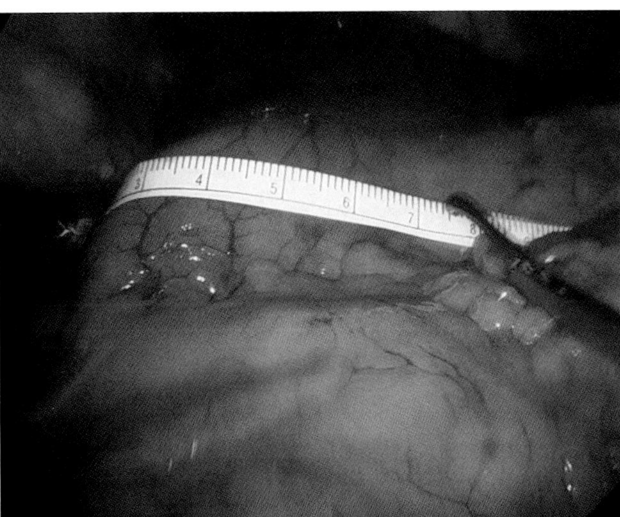

Fig. 59-8. Measuring to determine the site for electrode implantation. This should be 10-cm proximal to the pylorus.

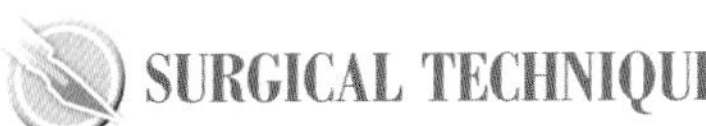

SURGICAL TECHNIQUE

Standard laparoscopic access is performed away from any previous or present feeding tubes and, if necessary, an adhesiolysis may be performed to identify the anterior gastric wall. All previous gastrostomies should be taken down, preferably with a stapler to decrease the possibility of contamination. The liver is retracted cranially and the stomach is marked 10-cm proximal to the pylorus on the greater curvature (Fig. 59-8). The conducting end of the electrode is attached to a monofilament, which is in turn attached to a straight needle. This needle is pushed tangentially through the muscular wall of the stomach without entering the gastric lumen (Fig. 59-9). This should be confirmed with intraoperative esophagogastroduodenoscopy (EGD). If any part of the needle is seen in the lumen, the needle should be removed and replaced prior to pulling the electrode into position. The monofilament is then used to pull the electrode into the stomach wall (Fig. 59-10, page 604). The electrodes are secured to the serosa of the stomach using silk sutures proximally and a plastic disc with two clips on the monofilament suture distally. Clips are also used over the monofilament to hold the disk in position. A second electrode is implanted 1-cm parallel to the first electrode and secured to the gastric wall in a similar fashion (Fig. 59-11, page 604). The leads are extracted through the fascia at the planned location of the pulse generator where a subcutaneous pocket is made. There should be enough slack on the electrode lead to minimize stress, tension, and the possibility that patient movement could dislodge it (Fig. 59-12, page 604). Excess wire should be wrapped around the neurostimulator, and the connector pins and leads should have bodily fluids wiped off before they are connected. The etched identification side should face outward and away from muscle tissue to minimize the possibility of skeletal muscle stimulation, which may be perceived by the patient as twitching or burning. The external programmer device sets the gastric stimulator in a standard configuration and the electrode impedance and gastric wall conductance is tested to verify correct placement of electrodes.

Once the pocket for the stimulator is closed, the placement of a simultaneous feeding jejunostomy can be considered. Feeding jejunostomies are used if the patient has been dependent on parenteral nutrition or is markedly malnourished.

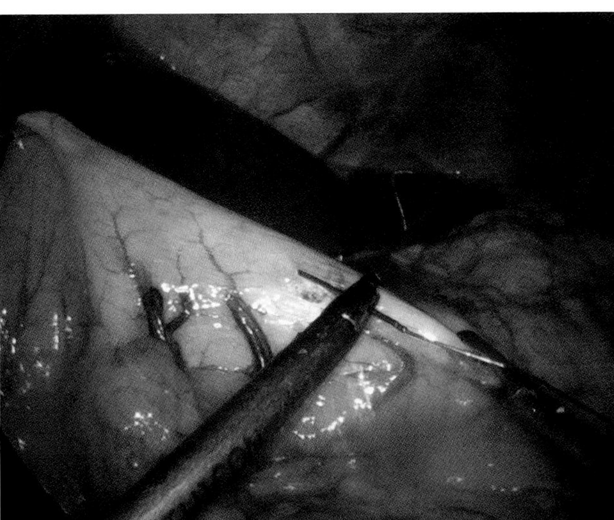

Fig. 59-9. The introducer needle is placed in the gastric wall and confirmation of not violating the gastric lumen should be made with intraoperative flexible endoscopy.

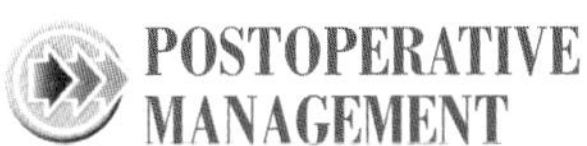

POSTOPERATIVE MANAGEMENT

The pulse generator is initially programmed to standardized settings of a frequency of 14 Hz, amplitude of 5 mA, and a pulse width of 300 ms and set to cycle on for 0.1 second and off for 5 seconds, resulting in 12 pulse doublets per minute. This is considered high-frequency and low-energy GES. Because of their comorbidities, these patients may spend several days in the hospital managing both their diabetes and their nausea. It is imperative to have a team aspect in managing these complicated patients, including endocrinology, gastroenterology, and chronic pain management, because many patients have chronic pain associated with their gastroparesis.

In the long-term, these patients may experience that their overall gastric emptying does not improve but their symptoms do. In addition, the improvement may not be instantaneous and in fact may not appear for several months. Nausea and vomiting symptoms improve more than postprandial fullness, bloating, and early satiety. The average days of hospitalization for these patients decreases significantly but still averages a little over two weeks a year.

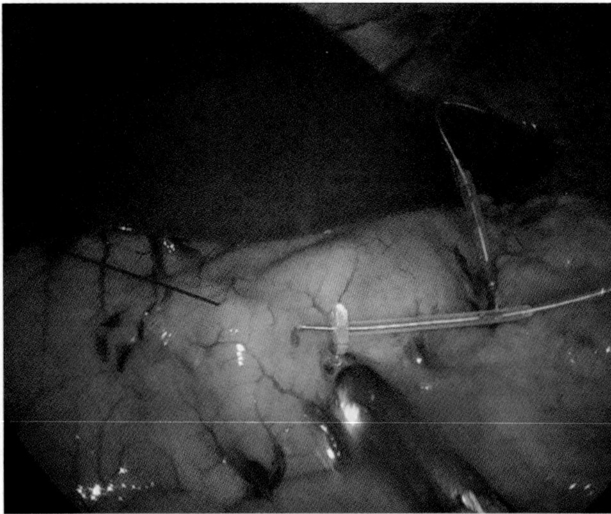

Fig. 59-10. Pulling the electrode into the gastric seromuscular layer.

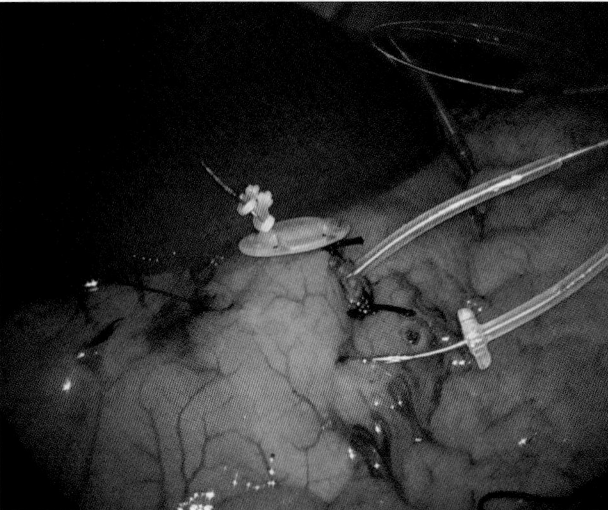

Fig. 59-11. The first electrode is visualized with the proximal end sutured and the distal end having a plastic disc and clips. The second electrode is being inserted parallel to the first one.

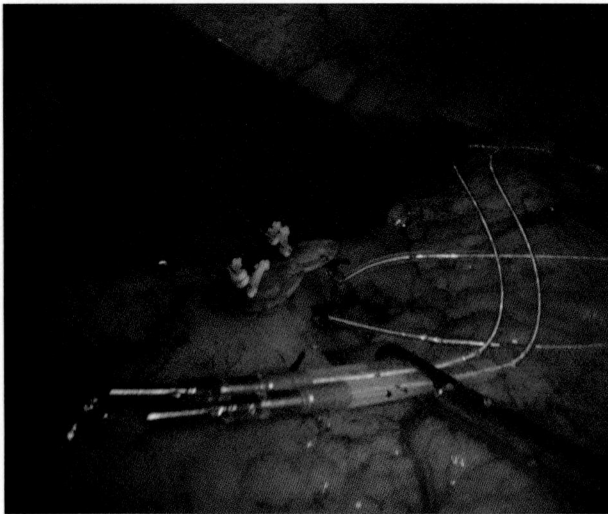

Fig. 59-12. Both electrodes are in place and the ends will be brought to the location of the implanted stimulator.

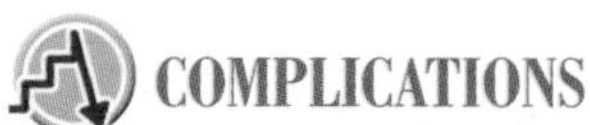

COMPLICATIONS

The laparoscopic implantation of the GES, historically done in an open fashion, has not had any significant reported rates of conversion to a laparotomy. The major postoperative complication as with any implantable foreign body is infection. This most commonly involves infection of the hardware, but case reports have described electrode erosion into the stomach, electrode dislodgment, electrode malposition, abdominal pain, and small bowel volvulus around the electrodes. Of the 51 patients enrolled in the two studies submitted to the FDA, four patients had side effects that resulted in the surgical removal of the implant system. Three patients had implants that became infected or eroded through the skin, and in one patient the lead perforated the stomach wall. In another patient, the neurostimulator migrated under the skin and was re-anchored surgically, but not removed. Forster removed only four out of 55 GES devices in the largest series with the longest follow-up to date. In the experience presented by Abell only two out of 33 GES devices were removed due to infection.

Electrode erosions into the gastric lumen may present with an increase of electrode impedance and worsening symptoms of gastroparesis. If erosion is suspected the initial and simplest test is an abdominal X-ray. In the best case, the electrode and the clip used to secure it to the gastric wall should be closely approximated on X-ray. The next and best study is probably an EGD to document an intraluminal position of the electrodes. Eroded electrodes need to be removed; this can be performed laparoscopically. Any fibrous capsules that have developed around the electrodes need to be opened up so the electrodes can be detached from the gastric wall by pulling alone. Intraoperative endoscopy allows for the assessment of gastric perforation; if this occurs closure can be performed with either sewing or stapling. When electrode erosion occurs, the stimulator usually needs to be removed because of contamination.

The optimal timing of stimulator and electrode reimplantation is unknown. With minimal gastric wall inflammation or infection, immediate replacement of the electrodes appears reasonable as long as the stimulator is not infected. The inflammation induced by the electrode erosion and infection can distort the gastric wall, making electrode reimplantation at the manufacturer's recommended site of 10-cm from the pylorus difficult, thereby risking suboptimal positioning of the electrodes. In that case allowing inflammation to resolve and attempting reimplantation at a later time is warranted.

SUGGESTED READING

Abell T, Lou J, Tabbaa M, et al. Gastric electrical stimulation for gastroparesis improves nutritional parameters at short, intermediate, and long-term follow-up. *J Parenter Enteral Nutr* 2003;27(4):277–281.

Abell T, McCallum R, Hocking M, et al. Gastric electrical stimulation for medically refractory gastroparesis. *Gastroenterology* 2003; 125(2):421–428.

Abell TL, Van Cutsem E, Abrahamsson H, et al. Gastric electrical stimulation in intractable symptomatic gastroparesis. *Digestion* 2002;66(4):204–212.

Forster J, Sarosiek I, Delcore R, et al. Gastric pacing is a new surgical treatment for gastroparesis. *Am J Surg* 2001;182(6):676–681.

Forster J, Sarosiek I, Lin Z, et al. Further experience with gastric stimulation to treat drug refractory gastroparesis. *Am J Surg* 2003; 186(6):690–695.

Lin Z, Forster J, Sarosiek I, McCallum RW. Treatment of gastroparesis with electrical stimulation. *Dig Dis Sci* 2003;48(5):837–848.

Liu RC, Sabnis AA, Chand B. Erosion of gastric electrical stimulator electrodes: evaluation, management and laparoscopic techniques. *Surg Laparosc Endosc Percutan Tech* 2007;17(5):438–441.

Mason RJ, Lipham J, Eckerling G, et al. Gastric electrical stimulation: an alternative surgical therapy for patients with gastroparesis. *Arch Surg* 2005;140(9):841–846.

Onders R, Marks J, Schilz R, et al. Diaphragm pacing with natural orifice transvisceral endoscopic surgery (NOTES): Potential for difficult to wean intensive care unit (ICU) patients. *Surg Endosc* 2007;21:475–479.

Onders RP, Aiyar H, Mortimer JT. Characterization of the human diaphragm muscle with respect to the phrenic nerve motor points for diaphragmatic pacing. *Am Surg* 2004;70:241–247.

Onders RP, Elmo MJ, Ignagni AR. Diaphragm pacing stimulation system for tetraplegia in individuals injured during childhood or adolescence. *J Spinal Cord Med* 2007;30:25–29.

Onders RP, Ignagni AI, Aiyer H, et al. Mapping the phrenic nerve motor point: the key to a successful laparoscopic diaphragm pacing system in the first human series. *Surgery* 2004; 136:819–826.

Onders RP, Ignagni AI, DeMarco AF, et al. The learning curve of investigational surgery: lessons learned from the first series of laparoscopic diaphragm pacing for chronic ventilator dependence. *Surg Endosc* 2005;19: 633–637.

COMMENTARY

This chapter by Dr. Onders addresses one of the most futuristic topics covered in this book. Diaphragm and gastric pacing are not brand-new concepts, but the procedures range from a few accepted operations to the investigational and the experimental. The author is truly one of very few international experts in the arena of diaphragm pacing. Anecdotal reports of patient successes are exciting and prompt great expectations for the results of studies involving large patient cohorts.

Attention to methodical mapping and adherence to proven technical steps increase the likelihood of a successful outcome. Education and training, mentoring and proctoring, and credentialing will be of vital importance as this field further develops and these techniques and technologies are applied by increasing numbers of surgeons worldwide.

WSE

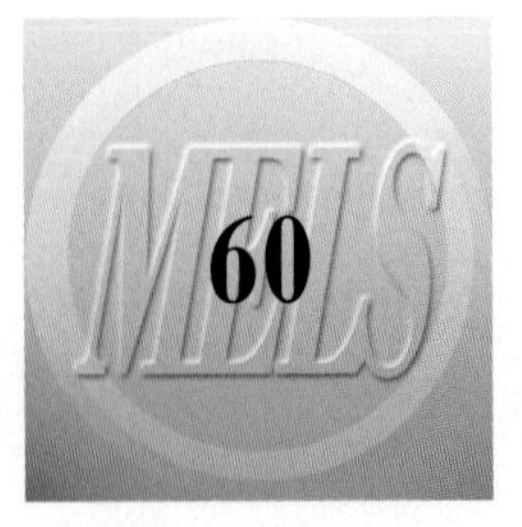

Laparoscopy and Endoscopy in Organ Transplant

ROBERT A. CATANIA AND ADRIAN E. PARK

INTRODUCTION

Organ transplantation continues to be a major indication for surgical intervention; as of this writing, the United Network for Organ Sharing (UNOS) has 94,683 people on waiting lists for organ transplant in the United States. From January through September 2006 there were 22,016 transplants performed, and organs were procured from 16,878 deceased and 5,138 living donors in that same time period. The role of laparoscopy and endoscopy continues to expand in the field of transplantation, with minimally invasive techniques now being used both diagnostically and therapeutically.

Role of Endoscopy and Laparoscopy

Prior to transplantation or living organ donation, all patients are required to undergo age appropriate cancer screening; thus upper endoscopy and colonoscopy play an important role in the initial evaluation of both live organ donors and transplant recipients. Flexible endoscopy is also used in the postoperative period and provides an excellent window for the diagnosis of rejection following intestinal and pancreatic transplant and gastrointestinal graft versus host disease after bone marrow transplantation. Advanced endoscopic procedures, including endoscopic ultrasound, endoscopic retrograde cholangiopancreatography (ERCP), and stent placement, are crucial for the diagnosis and management of biliary complications following liver transplant. The laparoscopic management of post-kidney transplant lymphoceles is well described, as is the biopsy of transplanted organs that are not amenable to percutaneous biopsy.

PANCREAS TRANSPLANT

Laparoscopic organ harvest is the most common minimally invasive transplant operation; it has been described for kidney, liver, and pancreas procurement. That being said, live donation of pancreatic tissue for transplant remains a rare operation. Since 1990, 5,048 pancreas transplants and 13,294 combined kidney/pancreas transplants have been performed in the United States, for a combined total of over 18,000 pancreatic transplants, of which only 61 live donor harvests occurred. Several reasons underlie the paucity of live donor pancreatectomy cases. Chief among them is the fact that it remains unclear how much pancreas must be harvested to ensure an adequately functional graft. At the same time the donor cannot be deprived of so large a portion of his or her pancreas that endocrine or exocrine insufficiency is a potential result. Furthermore, because pancreatic transplantation is currently not considered a life-saving procedure, the "burden of proof" is even greater upon transplant surgeons to ensure the safety and long-term health of the donor.

Thus, pancreas transplant is currently the least common indication for live donor harvest. Despite these small numbers, laparoscopic donor distal pancreatectomy has been described, and a case series of five successful hand-assisted laparoscopic procedures has been published by the transplant team from the University of Minnesota. In that series, two of the donors underwent simultaneous left donor nephrectomy as well. None of the donors developed complications related to the procedure, suggesting that live donor pancreatectomy and combined donor pancreatectomy/nephrectomy can be performed safely and with minimal morbidity to the donor. The technique is similar to that for distal pancreatectomy (Fig. 60-1), which is described in Chapter 39.

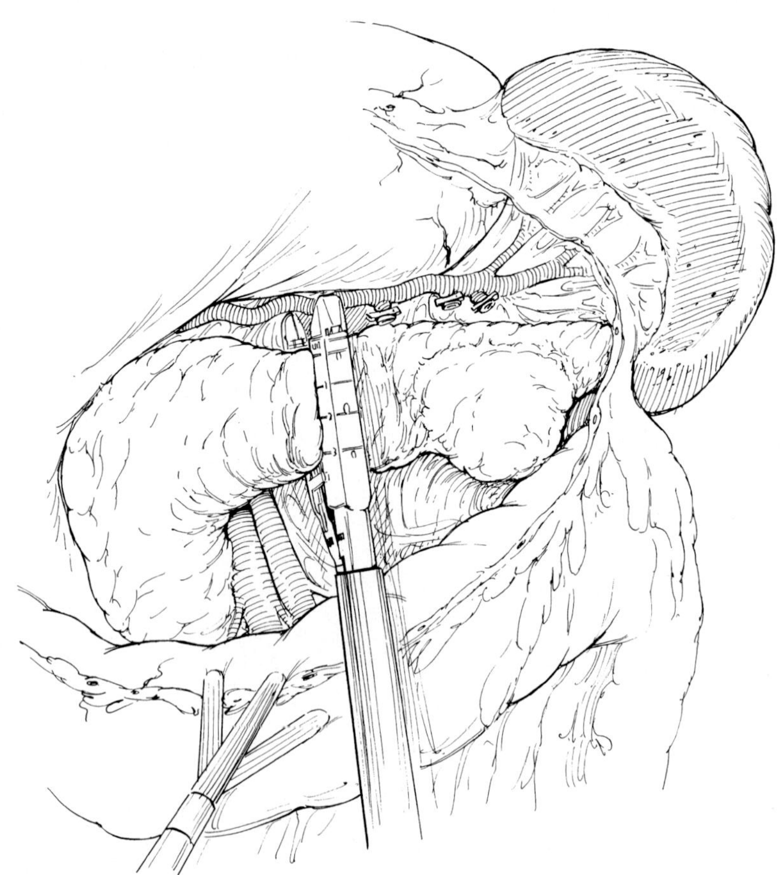

Fig. 60-1. Laparoscopic resection of the distal pancreas for islet cell harvest.

LIVER TRANSPLANT

Live donor hepatectomies are much more common than pancreatectomies, with 3,233 cases performed in the United States since January 1990. Despite this larger number, living donor transplants still account for only 4% of the total number of liver transplants performed in that time period. Considering the dramatic increase in kidney donation following the development of laparoscopic donor nephrectomy, several groups are working to establish a minimally invasive technique for liver harvest. Laparoscopic donor hepatic lobectomy has been well described in both the sheep and pig model; however, only individual case reports of human procedures have been published from groups in the United States. The European experience with laparoscopic liver donation has been larger, with a series of 15 cases reported in France. In Japan, video-assisted live donor hepatic lobectomies performed through 12-cm excisions have also been reported.

LAPAROSCOPIC DONOR NEPHRECTOMY

Of all the roles played by laparoscopy and endoscopy in transplantation surgery, by far the most prevalent procedure currently performed is laparoscopic donor nephrectomy (LDN). The technique was pioneered at Johns Hopkins Hospital and The University of Maryland in Baltimore, Maryland after being first described by Ratner in 1995. Live donor nephrectomy, initially seen as a mechanism to expand the pool of available donors, was quickly found to be superior to cadaveric donation in terms of both graft and recipient survival. Kaplan-Meier graft survival rates for transplants performed from 1997 to 2004 demonstrate that kidney graft survival rates at 1, 3, and 5 years are all significantly better following live donor transplant, with survivals of 95%, 87.9%, and 79.7% for live donor graft survival versus 89%, 77.8%, and 66.5% for cadaveric donors. The same can be said for recipient survival, with living donor recipient survival of 97.9%, 94.3%, and 90.2% versus 94.5%, 88.3%, and 82.0% in patients who received cadaveric transplants.

Laparoscopic donor nephrectomy was developed to further reduce barriers to living donation and offers several advantages over open nephrectomy to the kidney donor, including less postoperative pain, shorter hospitalization, and a quicker return to activity. In addition, LDN has been shown to have an equivalent complication rate to open donor nephrectomy (ODN), although the pattern of complications differs between the two procedures. As expected, LDN results in fewer wound and pulmonary complications relative to ODN, while mechanical and vascular complications appear to be more common with the laparoscopic technique. When comparing LDN with ODN, there was initial concern that the pneumoperitoneum would have a detrimental effect on intraoperative kidney perfusion and thus post-transplant graft function. Early studies supported the hypothesis that delayed graft function would be more prevalent following LDN, but subsequent refinements in technique have resulted in equivalent graft survival and function. Current reviews of LDN versus ODN graft outcome demonstrate equivalence in the need for postoperative dialysis, early and late recipient serum creatinine levels, 1-year creatinine clearance, 1-year rejection rates, and graft and patient survival up to 3 years post-transplant. Given that for transplant recipients both graft and patient survival is known to be improved following transplant with a live donor organ, LDN has clear benefits for both the donor and recipient.

Of the 16,481 kidneys transplanted in the United States in 2005, 6,568 (40%) were harvested from living donors. Prior to the advent of LDN, less than 30% of transplanted kidneys were obtained from a living donor. The most common technique for living donor harvesting in 2005 was a laparoscopic, hand-assisted nephrectomy (3,839 cases), followed by totally laparoscopic nephrectomy (1700), with ODN accounting for 953 cases (Figs. 60-2 and 60-3).

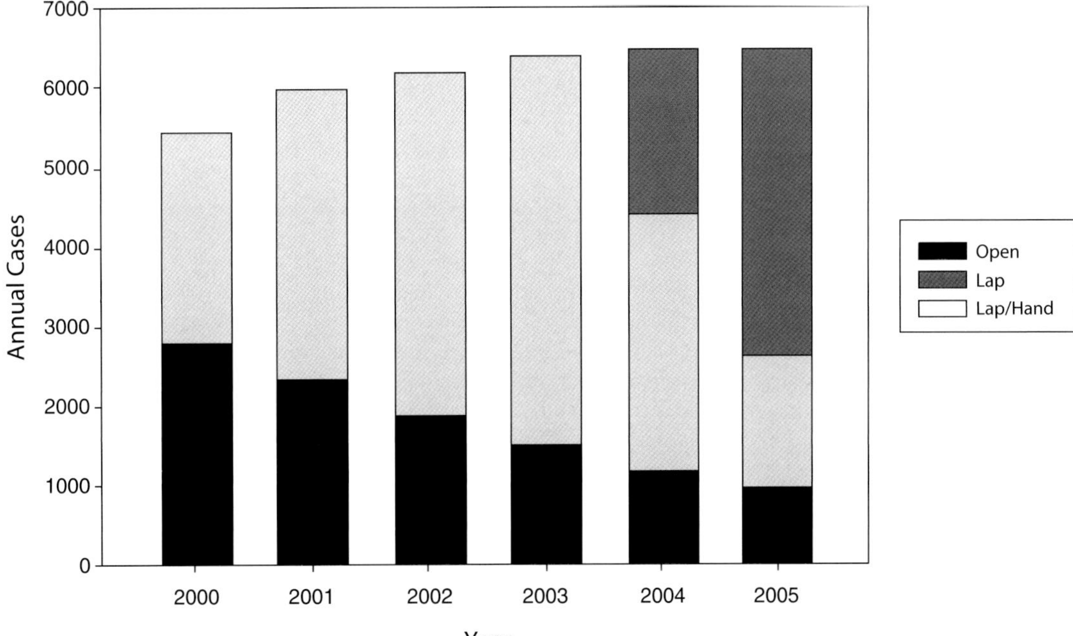

Fig. 60-2. Live donor nephrectomy case volume by type of procedure.

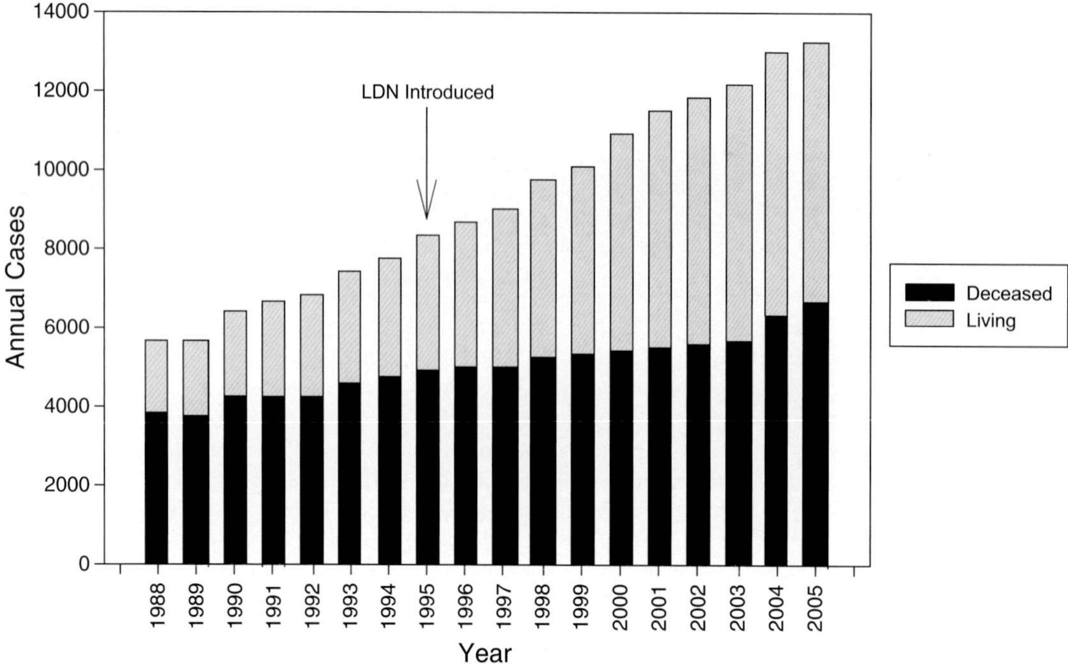

Fig. 60-3. Number of individuals acting as kidney donors by year. LDN, live donor nephrectomy.

Laparoscopic nephrectomy is currently utilized in 85% of all living donor nephrectomies performed, a proportion that continues to grow year after year. It is fair to say that LDN, which provides benefit to both the kidney transplant donor and recipient, has become the preferred method for donor nephrectomy.

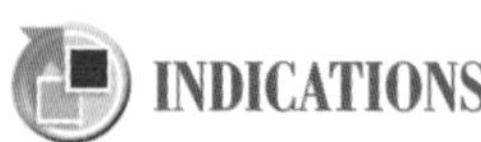 INDICATIONS

The indication for donor nephrectomy is the altruistic desire to improve the life of a less fortunate individual. Historically, living donors were recruited from the family of a patient with renal failure, with the belief that transplanting organs between histocompatable family members would yield optimal graft function and survival. Experience has shown that living donor transplants yield superior results to cadaveric transplants even when the donor is not human leukocyte antigen (HLA)-identical. This finding has opened the door to transplants between genetically unrelated individuals. Typically, unrelated donors are spouses, friends, or individuals related to the recipient by other close bonds, such as coworkers or church members. Unrelated, nondirected donations by anonymous donors have also been performed. Prior to donation, it must be confirmed that no coercion or undue pressure has been placed on the donor, and the option to withdraw from the process should be made clearly available to the donor during the evaluation.

Once an individual has expressed the desire to become an organ donor, an extensive medical and psychological workup is initiated. At the University of Maryland, blood type compatibility between donor and recipient is first determined. If compatible, the donor next undergoes a battery of tests, including serum chemistries, complete blood count, coagulation profile, liver function testing, urinalysis, urine culture, 24-hour creatinine clearance, chest radiograph, electrocardiogram (ECG), and serology testing. Potential female donors require serum human chorionic gonadotropin (HCG) testing. Next, a computed tomography (CT) angiogram of the kidneys is obtained to determine renal vascular and collecting system anatomy. A complete history and physical examination is performed by the surgical team, and, if health issues are identified, further medical consultation may be requested. All age-appropriate cancer screening tests are obtained prior to transplant, as is a stress test in patients over age 50. Patients with communicable diseases, morbid obesity, diabetes, coronary artery disease, or kidney disorders are excluded from the donation process. A psychological evaluation is performed to ensure the patient is competent and under no duress to serve as an organ donor. Additionally, every patient who has volunteered to serve as an organ donor undergoes an extensive informed consent discussion. Finally, a cross match is performed to verify there are no preformed antibodies to donor-specific antigens that would result in early transplant failure. At our institution, the case is then reviewed by a multidisciplinary board consisting of a transplant surgeon, donor surgeon, nephrologist, psychologist, and transplant nurse/coordinator. If no outstanding issues are identified, the transplant is scheduled.

 PREOPERATIVE PLANNING

Donor renal anatomy is the most important technical consideration when planning a donor nephrectomy; the importance of preoperative imaging can not be overstated. Various imaging protocols are employed at the nation's transplant centers, including digital angiography, magnetic resonance angiography (MRA), and computerized tomographic angiography (CTA). Our center performs standard three-dimensional (3-D) CTA to determine renal arterial, venous, and ureteral anatomy. We have developed a unique protocol using commercially available software that allows the data to be manipulated to create a 3-D reconstruction of the kidney that can be rotated around any axis. By creating a virtual mesh structure

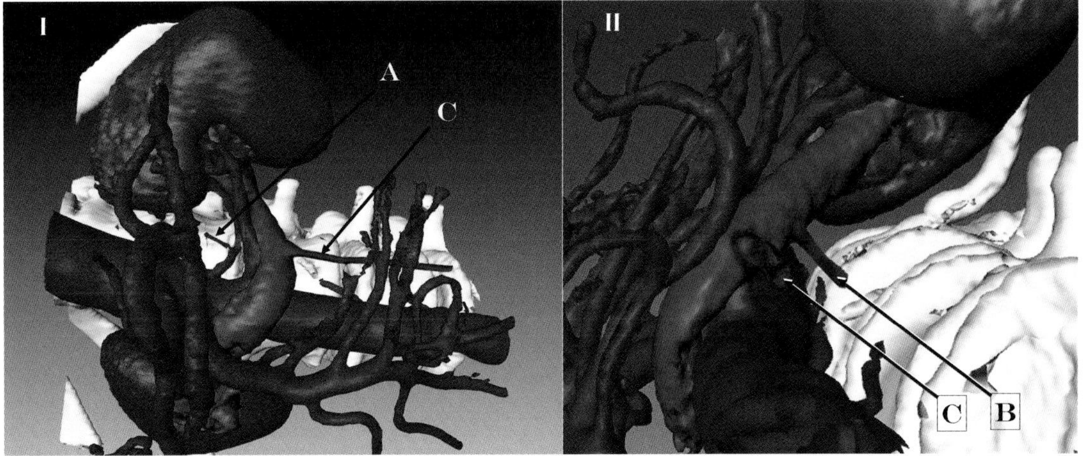

Fig. 60-4. Preoperative 3-D reconstruction. The renal anatomy is reconstructed in such a fashion as to assist in the interpretation of operative findings. In particular, view I shows the 3-D imaging in the operative plane of view. One can appreciate the adrenal vein (A) in this view; however, it is not visible in the inferior view (view II). In the inferior view, one can appreciate the lumbar vein (B), but not the adrenal artery. In both instances the gonadal vein (C) remains recognizable though in alternate orientations. Note that typically the small mesenteric artery (SMA) and its branches would be rotated out of view with the patient in the lateral decubitus position.

around the different densities in the CT scan, it is possible to virtually navigate through the actual patient anatomy and easily establish landmarks to facilitate spatial orientation for surgical planning. This allows examination in exquisite detail of the configuration of the renal vasculature, including the gonadal, lumbar, and adrenal vessels, permitting them to be viewed as they will appear at the time of surgery (Fig. 60-4).

LEFT NEPHRECTOMY

As a rule, the left kidney is removed during donor nephrectomy, unless there is a distinct benefit to the donor for a right-sided harvest, because of the longer length of the left renal vein. Anatomic variants such as multiple renal vessels or collecting systems are considered for transplant depending upon the degree of anomaly. A discussion between the transplant and donor (harvest) surgeon as to the acceptability of a kidney for transplant is essential in these situations; it typically occurs at the multidisciplinary transplant conference.

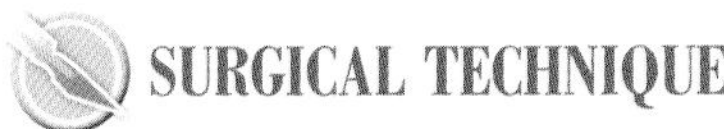

SURGICAL TECHNIQUE

Patient Positioning and Preparation

Pneumatic compression devices are placed on the legs and a dose of preoperative antibiotic is administered. After the patient has been anesthetized and intubated, a Foley catheter is placed. While the patient is still in the supine position, the kidney extraction site is marked. A 6-cm Pfannenstiel incision is utilized for the extraction, and we mark several proposed incision sites, with the lowest being 3 cm cephelad of the pubic tubercle. The next marking is 2 cm cephelad to the first, and the next is again 2 cm cephelad. This gives us several options for the incision once the patient has been turned to the right decubitus position (Fig. 60-5, page 610). While the patient is positioned, the anesthetist is instructed to volume-load the patient to maintain adequate renal perfusion once pneumoperitoneum is established. During positioning, the patient's lumbar region is centered over the table break and the patient is then turned onto his or her right side and an axillary roll placed. A pneumatic beanbag can obstruct the surgical field; thus rolls of sheets are used to stabilize the patient on his or her side. The table is then flexed and the kidney rest extended. Once positioned, the patient is prepped anteriorly and posteriorly from the mid-chest to below the pubic tubercle.

Trocar Placement

A Veress needle is placed in the left upper quadrant and used to establish pneumoperitoneum to 15 mmHg with carbon dioxide. A 5-mm optical trocar is then placed in the left lower quadrant just lateral to the midclavicular line at the level of the umbilicus. An additional 5-mm trocar is placed in the upper abdomen along the same line, and a 12-mm trocar is placed several centimeters below the costal margin in the anterior axillary line. When necessary for retraction or to maintain exposure, an additional 5-mm trocar can be placed in the posterior axillary line several centimeters inferior to the costal margin (Fig. 60-5). A 30-degree, 5-mm scope is used to provide the image for the procedure and is placed though the periumbilical port. The surgeon's left hand is used to provide exposure with an atraumatic grasper, and the right hand is used to dissect with ultrasonic shears.

Exposure of the Left Kidney

The patient is placed in reverse-Trendelenburg position, and the splenic flexure of the colon is mobilized inferiorly and medially. This dissection is carried caudad along the peritoneal reflection of the left colon to the sigmoid. The splenophrenic ligament is then divided to allow the spleen to rotate medially. The splenic hilum and tail of the pancreas are rotated medially to expose the superior pole of the kidney. Maintaining spacial orientation allows dissection through this bloodless plane, referred to as "the valley of the adrenal" (Fig. 60-6, page 610). Once entered, blunt dissection is sufficient to separate the abdominal and retroperitoneal organs anterior to the kidney and great vessels in a maneuver analogous to a medial visceral rotation. Inferiorly, blunt dissection and ultrasonic power are utilized to elevate the colonic mesentery until the descending colon has been mobilized to the midline, thus exposing the infrarenal aorta. Superiorly, care must be taken to prevent injury to the diaphragm at the upper limits of the dissection. At all times attention to staying in the proper plane prevents entry into the Gerota

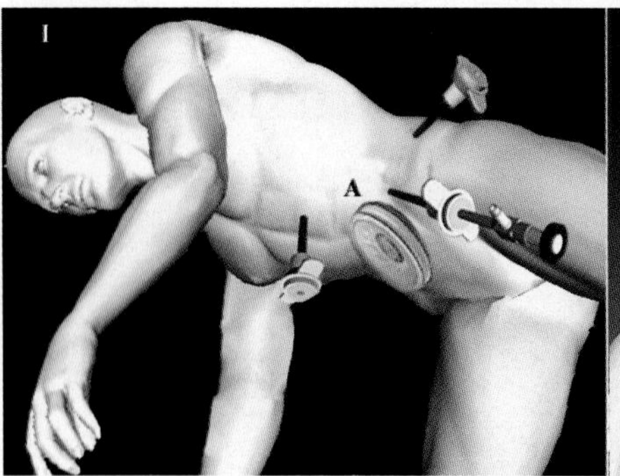

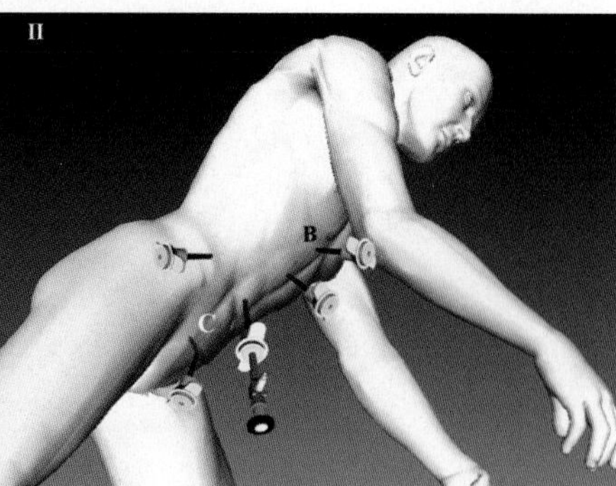

Fig. 60-5. Trocar placement for laparoscopic donor nephrectomy: Shown in view I (left lateral decubitis position) is a hand port (A) for hand-assisted technique. The hand port may be placed via a periumbilical or Pfannenstiel incision, initial to the procedure, during the procedure, or just prior to extraction. Both view I and view II (right lateral decubitis position) show standard port positioning for donor nephrectomy, with 5-mm ports used as sites for the camera and left-hand instrument while the right-hand site port is 12 mm to accommodate the laparoscopic stapler. In view II, a right donor nephrectomy requires the placement of an additional subxiphoid port for liver retraction (B). In both views an 18-mm port is placed through the Pfannenstiel incision to introduce the extraction bag once the donor kidney has been fully mobilized. Preoperative marking for possible Pfannenstiel incision and extraction sites may be performed (C).

fascia during the mobilization of the spleen, pancreas, and colon. In places, the difference of one cell layer can turn a straightforward blunt dissection into a difficult and bloody field. Once the colon, pancreas, and spleen have been rotated, the gonadal vessels and ureter should be exposed from the renal hilum to the level of the iliac vessels. Tracing the gonadal vein cephelad will then allow identification of the inferior border of the renal vein at its junction with this vessel.

Exposure of the Renal Vessels and Mobilization of the Kidney

Once the Gerota fascia has been exposed and the gonadal vessels identified, dissection is commenced along the inferior border of the renal vein. Sharp and blunt dissection are utilized to identify the junction of the renal vein with the gonadal, adrenal, and, if present, lumbar veins. The use of preoperative 3-D CT angiography provides a road map for this portion of the dissection and also allows preoperative determination of the relationship of the renal vein and artery. After identifying the branches of the renal vein, these vessels are dissected for several centimeters and divided between 5-mm surgical clips (Fig. 60-7). A right-angle clip applier is used for this purpose; care is taken to ensure that these clips will not interfere with the application of the stapling device that will subsequently be utilized to divide the renal vein. Once the vein has been circumferentially mobilized, it may be gently retracted to expose the renal artery. Now that the vascular supply to the left kidney has been isolated, the organ itself may be mobilized from within the Gerota fascia. The dissection is initially carried cephelad from the superior margin of the renal vein in the plane between the kidney and the adrenal gland. Care must be taken not to cause troublesome bleeding in this location; the ultrasonic dissector is helpful in this regard. A significant amount of perinephric fat may be encountered, particularly in men, which requires meticulous dissection to avoid injury to the kidney or adrenal gland.

After separating the kidney and the adrenal gland, mobilization continues along the anterior and medial surfaces of the kidney. By reserving the lateral dissection for the end of the procedure, the kidney remains suspended, allowing good visualization of the organ with minimal need for additional retraction. As the lateral attachments are divided, allowing access to the posterior surface of the organ, it is sometimes necessary to place a fourth trocar to maintain exposure. Posterior dissection requires rotating the organ anteromedially, which can compromise the vascular pedicle by torsion; thus the kidney should be returned to its normal anatomic position from time to time to prevent the development of warm ischemia during dissection. Once the kidney is nearly freed, a 12.5-gram intravenous bolus of mannitol is administered to promote diuresis. Retraction of the renal vein with a blunt dissector exposes the renal artery, which is typically surrounded by lymphatic tissue and highly vascular fatty tissue, which may be dense at times. Dissection along this vessel is carried to its junction with the aorta to provide the transplant team with the greatest possible length for subsequent anastomosis. Once again, the use of preoperative imaging is helpful in defining the branching pattern of the renal artery. Complete dissection of the renal artery may require rotation of the kidney medially along its vascular pedicle to completely free the posterior aspect of the vessel from the surrounding connective tissue under direct visualization. Again, care must be taken not to impede vascular flow to the organ for any length of time.

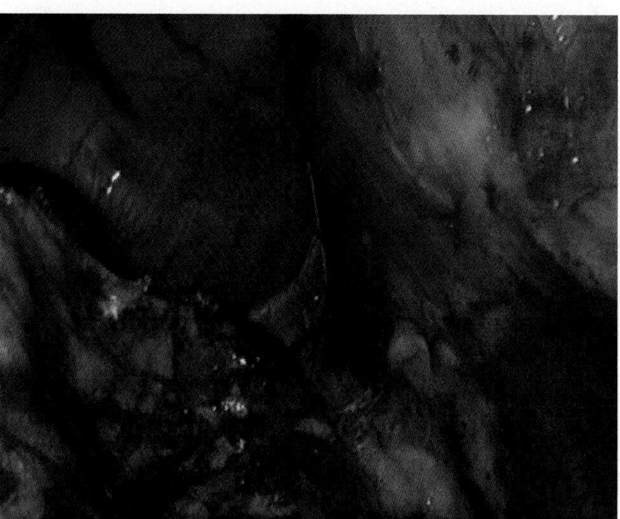

Fig. 60-6. The valley of the adrenal. The pancreas and spleen are mobilized medially by dissecting along the medial border of the left kidney without entering the Gerota fascia.

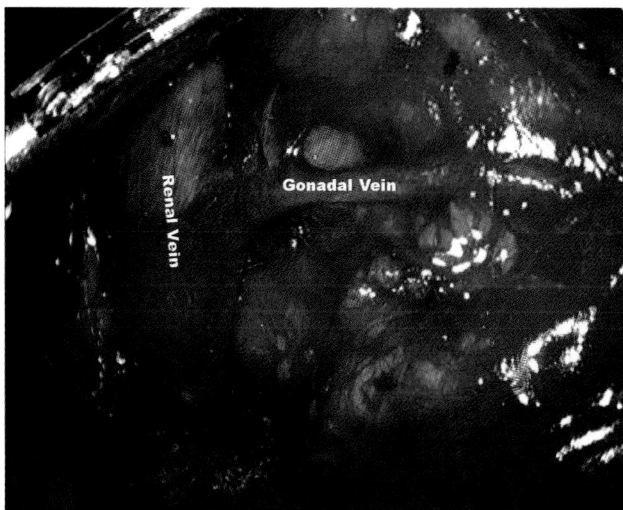

Fig. 60-7. The exposed gonadal vein. The kidney remains suspended from the retroperitoneum and can be gently rotated laterally with the left-hand retractor. After identification of the gonadal vein, it can be traced cephalad to its junction with the left renal vein.

Division of the Ureter and Renal Vasculature

The ureter and gonadal vessels, which have been previously exposed, are now dissected en bloc along their course in the retroperitoneum. An additional dose of mannitol is administered at this time. This dissection is carried out from the renal hilum to the pelvic inlet using ultrasonic shears and is best accomplished by elevating the structures off of the psoas muscle in a pedicle consisting of vessels, ureter, and intervening fat and lymphatics. An earlier laparoscopic practice in which the ureter was skeletonized and isolated separately from the gonadal vessels should be avoided as it resulted in unacceptable rates of recipient ureteral complications. Once the necessary length of ureter has been mobilized, the extraction site is prepared for the rapid removal of the kidney. The previously marked incision sites are inspected and the appropriate one is chosen. The incision should be made as low as possible, but the best working position should not be sacrificed for cosmesis. A 6-cm transverse incision is performed and dissection is carried down to the anterior abdominal fascia. In obese patients it is particularly important to identify the midline, as any pannus may alter skin landmarks. The fascia is divided transversely and superior and inferior fascial flaps are developed so that the midline is widely exposed. A blunt 18-mm trocar is placed between the rectus muscles under direct visualization. This port will be utilized to introduce the 15-mm specimen retrieval bag once the hilar vessels are divided. Before firing the stapler a final equipment check is conducted to ensure that the necessary equipment, including staplers, reloads, and extraction bag, is available and on the instrument table. Warm ischemia time begins immediately upon dividing the renal artery, and there is no time to search for missing supplies once the stapler has been applied. Most centers have established a routine in which warm ischemia time can be limited to 120 seconds or less by using a well-practiced surgical team including surgeon, first assist, scrub nurse, and circulator. Immediately prior to stapling, a 5000-unit bolus of heparin is administered; after a 4-minute circulation time, a 45-mm articulating endoscopic GIA stapler (2.5-mm staple) is passed through the subcostal port and used to divide the ureteral pedicle at the level of the iliac vessels (Fig. 60-8). If an adequate angle cannot be obtained to preserve ureteral length, the 18-mm extraction port can alternately be used for passage of the stapler.

Once the ureteral pedicle is free, the stapler is then applied to the renal artery. A 2.0-mm staple is used for this firing, and the stapler is applied directly alongside of the aorta to preserve arterial length (Fig. 60-9, page 612). In the case of multiple arteries, repeated firings may be required. Care must be taken during this maneuver to avoid incorporating the sidewall of the aorta, which can result in significant bleeding or narrowing of the vessel. After dividing the artery, the vein is divided in a similar fashion. The stapler is applied to the vein where it crosses the aorta, again maximizing length for the transplant surgeon. Once the vessels have been divided and the kidney is free in the abdomen, a rapid inspection of the surgical staple lines occurs.

Specimen Extraction

Immediately upon dividing the renal vein, the specimen extraction bag is inserted through the 18-mm trocar located in the Pfannenstiel incision. The anesthesiologist is notified to administer a fully reversing dose of protamine sulfate as soon as the renal vein is divided. Once the kidney is placed in the specimen bag, the rectus muscles are bluntly separated in

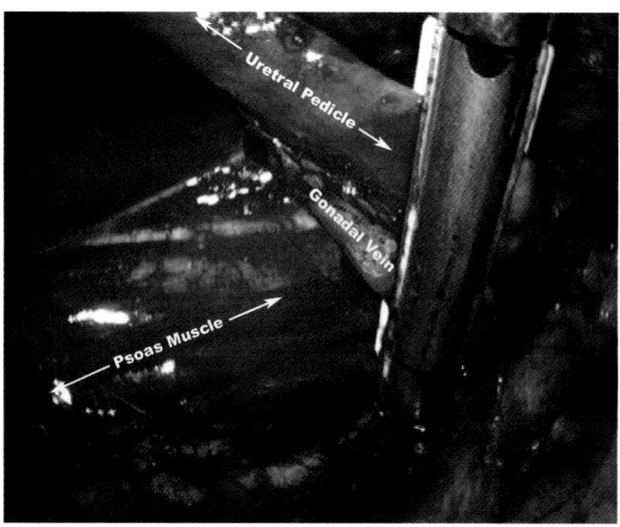

Fig. 60-8. Dividing the ureteral pedicle. The ureteral pedicle including the gonadal vessels is dissected off the psoas muscle using blunt dissection and ultrasonic energy. The pedicle is then divided where it enters the pelvis with a vascular load of the endoscopic stapler.

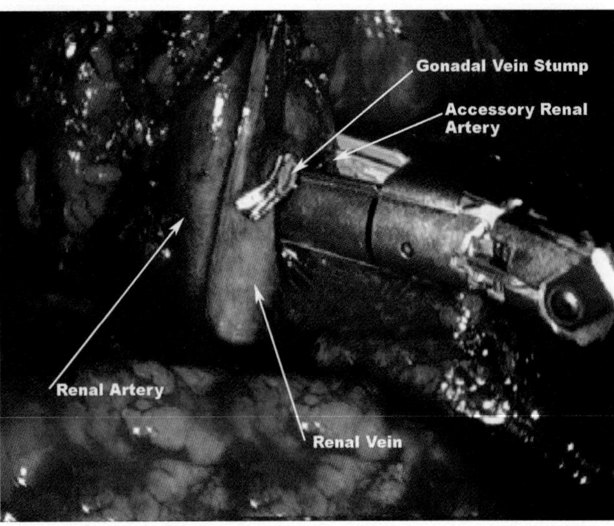

Fig. 60-9. Division of the renal artery (vein intact). The stapler is placed across the renal artery and cinched up against the aorta prior to dividing the vessel. Warm ischemia time begins upon closing the stapler. The vein is then divided in a similar manner.

the midline and the kidney extracted. Pneumoperitoneum is lost as the specimen is extracted; due to the length of the fascial incision required to accommodate the kidney, it is not easy to rapidly reestablish pneumoperitoneum to allow laparoscopic visualization of the kidney bed. Thus, hemostasis of the staple lines and kidney bed must be ensured prior to extraction. Once removed, the specimen is placed on ice and transported to the recipient operating theater, where it is prepared for implantation.

Fascial closure is quickly achieved with a running polydioxanone suture so that reinsufflation can be achieved and the kidney bed is irrigated and further inspected for hemostasis. Particular attention is paid to the vascular staple lines and surgical clips. Rarely will a topical thromobotic agent such as SURGICEL be required to control oozing from the vascular staple lines. Once hemostasis has been ensured and any residual blood or clot irrigated from the abdomen, the trocars are removed under direct visualization. The 12-mm trocar site is closed at the fascial level with polyglactin suture and all skin incisions are closed with subcuticular poliglecaprone suture. Steri-Strips are applied and the patient is returned to the supine position.

Right Kidney Considerations

Several technical considerations make a laparoscopic right-sided donor nephrectomy significantly more difficult than a left-sided procedure. For this reason, absolute comfort with a left-sided procedure is essential prior to considering a right donor nephrectomy. There should be a distinct advantage to the donor in maintaining the left kidney, and vascular or collecting system anomalies of the left kidney should not be the sole determinant in choosing a right-sided donor nephrectomy. If a significant kidney size discrepancy exists in the donor, the smaller of the two organs should be chosen for donation.

Port placement requires modification to allow for the placement of a liver retractor, as is demonstrated in Figure 60-5. To medially rotate the liver sufficiently, the right triangular ligament is divided with an ultrasonic dissector. After the liver has been mobilized, the hepatic flexure is taken down and the duodenum Kocherized to expose the Gerota fascia and the inferior vena cava. Bothersome bleeding from tributaries of the renal vein can occur during this mobilization; the use of ultrasonic energy can aid in maintaining a bloodless field. Once the renal vein has been identified, blunt dissection is used to clear its anterior surface and its length is assessed. Posterior dissection of the vein is necessary to expose the renal artery, and short lumbar veins crossing the artery are easily avulsed during this phase of the operation. Careful division of the lumbar, adrenal, and gonadal veins is then performed between surgical clips. Placement of these clips should be performed in such a manner as to prevent their interference with the vascular stapler that will be used to divide the renal vein. Suture ligation or ultrasonic energy may be necessary to control very short vessels if clips can not be utilized.

Division of the posterior and lateral attachments of the kidney allows it to be rotated anteromedially, facilitating dissection behind the vena cava to maximize the length of the arterial cuff. The isolation of the ureter may then be performed as previously described. When dividing the right renal artery, rotating the kidney medially prior to application of the stapler will allow additional length to be achieved. Division of the short renal vein requires the tight application of the stapler along the vena cava, and care must be taken to position the stapler parallel to the great vessel to avoid compromising its lumen. If insufficient length of vein is available, a small subcostal incision may be used to apply a Satinsky clamp to the vein after dividing the ureter. This incision allows vascular control and specimen extraction, as well as open vascular repair of the cavotomy.

Hand-Assisted Procedure

The most popular current approach to live donor nephrectomy is the laparoscopic hand-assisted procedure, accounting for nearly 60% of the cases performed in 2005. Hand assist may decrease operative and warm ischemia times relative to purely laparoscopic procedures, but otherwise is equivalent in terms of postoperative complication rates and length of hospitalization. Variations in the time and location of hand-port placement exist, but typically the hand port is placed at the commencement of surgery and is located periumbilically. Colon mobilization and kidney retraction are facilitated by hand assistance, and rapid control of hilar vascular injury is possible by direct manual compression.

When hand assistance is utilized, the abdomen is entered via a mini-laparotomy and the hand port is placed. The abdomen may then be insufflated via a trocar inserted through the hand port and additional trocars can then be placed under direct visualization. The presence of a hand port also eliminates the need for a specimen retrieval bag after the resection is complete, as the kidney can be removed directly by the assisting hand.

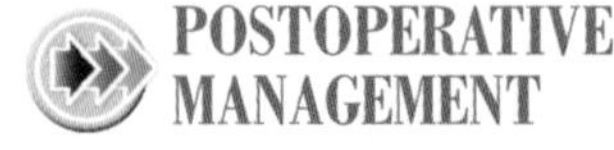

POSTOPERATIVE MANAGEMENT

The patient is recovered in the postanesthesia care unit (PACU) and then admitted to the surgical ward. Sequential compression devices are utilized until the patient is ambulatory, and H_2-blocker therapy is continued until the patient is tolerating a regular diet. Postoperative pain is well controlled with intravenous ketorolac and oral acetaminophen-oxycodone; intravenous narcotics or antiemetics are rarely required after discharge from the PACU. The patient is allowed sips of clear liquids on the day of surgery and continued on maintenance intravenous fluids with 0.45% saline solution. Early ambulation is encouraged, as is incentive spirometry, and typically the patient is out of bed and walking on the day of surgery. If urine output has been acceptable, the Foley catheter is removed at midnight on the day of surgery, and the following morning a liquid diet is instituted and intravenous fluids are discontinued. A complete blood count and basic metabolic profile are obtained on the morning after surgery. When the patient exhibits evidence of return of bowel function, a regular diet is offered. Renal function is again assessed on postoperative day 2; if the creatinine is stable and the patient is tolerating a regular diet, he or she is discharged home on oral analgesics and stool softeners. The patient is seen again 2 weeks postoperatively, at which time a serum creatinine is obtained; if no issues are identified, the patient is allowed to slowly resume normal activity.

Current recommendations are for donor follow-up at 6 and 12 months postoperatively. If no medical or surgical complications or decrement in renal function is detected in that time frame, the donor is returned to the care of his or her primary care physician. Long-term follow-up of living kidney donors in the United States has been less than adequate. Long-term function of the donated kidney has been well documented, but the sequella of kidney donation on the health of the donor has not been as well studied. Extrapolation of data from long-term survivors of unilateral nephrectomy for medical indications or trauma suggests there may be a slight risk for the development of hypertension or renal insufficiency over time. Risk factors for the development of these long-term complications include obesity, tobacco use, and diabetes mellitus; thus these conditions may well be considered relative contraindications to serving as a living donor. As living kidney donation gains popularity, the need for transplant programs to closely follow their donor populations will continue to grow; UNOS is currently considering approaches to improve donor follow-up, including the development of a kidney donor registry.

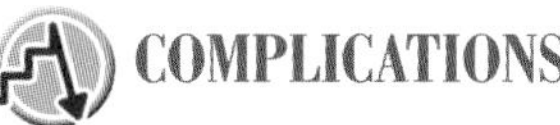

COMPLICATIONS

The complication rate following laparoscopic donor nephrectomy has been remarkably low considering the technical complexity of the operation. This may be due, in part, to the expectation on the part of donors and the insistence on the part of the transplant community that their care and well-being be paramount following their selfless act. After this technique was pioneered, transplant centers from around the country sent their procurement teams to the University of Maryland to learn firsthand the intricacies of the operation. Initial skepticism on the part of experienced transplant surgeons has slowly turned to acceptance as the procedure has been shown to have a complication rate comparable to open surgery. A number of donor deaths early in the LDN experience put the transplant community on notice that this was a difficult procedure to master and that significant training resources would be required to safely institute LDN programs around the country. Despite its eleven-year track record, LDN continues to be a challenging operation that requires thorough preoperative planning to be safely performed. Reported complications from the procedure are listed in Table 60-1 and most commonly include injuries to major vascular structures, which are potentially life-threatening. Each surgeon performing LDN must have the ability to rapidly achieve laparoscopic vascular control or to convert to an open procedure. The best management of intraoperative complications is their prevention. This can best be achieved by having a thorough knowledge of the anatomy preoperatively and performing meticulous dissection, frequently by proceeding one fascial layer at a time. Operating in a bloodless field is critical to recognizing anatomic planes, and even trivial bleeding should be rapidly controlled with the application of an energy source to keep the field dry. Maintaining constant orientation and operating in the correct plane are essential in this operation, as it is easy to wander into vital structures such as the renal vein, adrenal vein, adrenal gland, kidney, pancreas, mesocolon, spleen, or diaphragm without being more than a few millimeters from the Gerota fascia or the kidney.

An intimate understanding of the applications and misapplications of surgical dissectors and staplers is also required. Common mistakes resulting in dramatic complications can result from the inadvertent contact of a hot dissecting blade on a vascular structure, the malpositioning of a surgical stapler prior to firing, or the avulsion of a vessel from torque applied to a stapler while positioning the relatively large device in a tight anatomic location. The development of articulating staplers has alleviated some of the early difficulties in achieving optimal staple line position, but it is important to understand the limitations of the currently available tools in order to be able to use them safely.

When complications do arise, having an established "out" allows the operation to continue without endangering the well-being of the donor. Vascular injuries can often be managed laparoscopically if a clear surgical field can be maintained: ongoing bleeding can be controlled with the application of pressure or the placement of hemostatic adjuncts and suture repair of the bleeding site achieved. Skill with precise suture placement and intracorporeal knot tying are required in these situations. The blind use of surgical clips to control bleeding is often unsuccessful and can result in injury to adjacent structures. Splenic capsular injuries can also be frequently controlled with topical

TABLE 60-1. REPORTED COMPLICATIONS OF PERIOPERATIVE LDN

- **Conversion to open procedure**
- **Vascular injury**
  - Aorta
  - Common iliac artery
  - Renal artery
  - Vena cava
  - Renal vein
  - Mesenteric vein
  - Adrenal vein
  - Lumbar vein
- **Organ injury**
  - Colon
  - Spleen
  - Liver
  - Diaphragm
  - Pneumothorax
  - Bladder
  - Harvested kidney
- **Systemic complications**
  - Bleeding (requiring transfusion)
  - Pancreatitis
  - Pneumonia
  - Urinary tract infection
  - Pulmonary embolism or deep venous thrombosis
  - Rhabdomyolysis
  - Death
- **Wound complications**
  - Infection
  - Incisional hernia

hemostatic agents and gentle pressure application with a blunt instrument against a surgical gauze pad. Rarely will splenectomy be necessary, but if bleeding can not be controlled there is good access to the splenic hilum when the patient is in the lateral decubitus position and the application of a surgical stapler across the splenic vessels should largely control blood loss. Diaphragm injuries can be sutured primarily after debriding any nonviable muscle. A permanent suture such as polypropylene can be employed in a running or interrupted fashion. The use of prosthetic or biologic onlay patches can be considered if the injury is large or can not be brought together easily. The use of an ipsilateral chest tube in these situations is usually unnecessary if all the CO_2 can be expelled from the pleural cavity by forceful ventilation as the repair is completed. Pancreatic injuries may require the performance of a distal pancreatectomy with a surgical stapler followed by the placement of external drains. Bowel injuries prior to specimen extraction typically preclude the harvesting of the organ; after successful repair the case is best aborted, particularly in the face of gross contamination, and rescheduled once the donor has sufficiently recovered. Injuries to the harvested organ should prompt immediate consultation with the transplant surgeon so that the recipient's operation can be cancelled or modified to accommodate any anatomic shortcomings of the donor organ, such as a short vascular pedicle or ureter. Injuries to the kidney parenchyma may be salvageable; consultation with urologist experienced in partial nephrectomy is warranted.

CONCLUSION

In one decade, laparoscopic live donor nephrectomy has gone from a novel concept to the standard of care. The propagation of LDN has been credited with lowering the perceived barriers to live organ donation and increasing the availability of kidneys for transplant. The procedure has been shown to decrease postoperative pain, the length of hospitalization, and the length of convalescence. LDN has also preserved the benefits of live kidney donation for transplant recipients. In 2005 85% of live kidney donor nephrectomies were performed laparoscopically; this number will likely continue to grow as more transplant centers convert to LDN exclusively.

The procedure requires advanced laparoscopic skills and meticulous dissection in an anatomic location that is surrounded by critical structures, including the aorta, vena cava, adrenal gland, colon, spleen, stomach, and iliac vessels. Errant dissection can quickly result in life-threatening hemorrhage, injury to a hollow viscus, solid organ injury, diaphragmatic injury, or damage to the donated organ. Despite these considerable risks, a safe track record has been established due to the diligence of the surgeons performing the procedure. Several case series describing the learning curve for LDN have been published, and a common theme among them is the importance of a multidisciplinary team with advanced laparoscopic skills and an intimate knowledge of the anatomy of the kidney and retroperitoneum.

As the demand for organ transplants continues to grow more rapidly than donor supply, a more aggressive use of living donors is anticipated. Currently donors are being accepted at more advanced ages and with greater medical comorbidities than had previously been acceptable. As the envelope of donors continues to expand, even greater vigilance will be required both preoperatively and in the operating room to ensure that donor safety remains the keystone around which our living donor programs are built.

Acknowledgments

The data on organ transplantation numbers reported here have been supplied by the Organ Procurement and Transplantation Network (OPTN) and are based on OPTN database as of December 29, 2006. The interpretation and reporting of these data are the responsibility of the authors and in no way should be seen as an official policy or interpretation of the OPTN or the U.S. Government.

SUGGESTED READING

Davis, CL. Evaluation of the living kidney donor: current perspectives. *Am J Kidney Dis* 2004;43:508–530.

Derweesh IH, Goldfarb DA, Abreu SC, et al. Laparoscoic live donor nephrectomy has equivalent early and late renal function outcomes compared with open donor nephrectomy. *J Urol* 2005;65:862–866.

Jacobs SC, Cho E, Foster C, et al. Laparoscopic donor nephrectomy: the University of Maryland 6-year experience. *J Urol* 2004;171: 47–51.

Markmann JF, Brayman KL, Naji A, et al. Transplantation of abdominal organs. In: Townsend CM, Beauchamp DR, Evers BM, et al, eds. *Sabiston textbook of surgery: the biological basis of modern surgical practice*, 17th ed. Philadelphia: Saunders, 2004:669–750.

Morrissey PE, Monaco AP. Living kidney donation: evolution and technical aspects of donor nephrectomy. *Surg Clin N Am* 2006; 86:1219–1235.

Su L-M, Ratner LE, Montgomery RA, et al. Laparoscopic live donor nephrectomy: trends in donor and recipient morbidity following 381 consecutive cases. *Ann Surg* 2004;240: 358–363.

Tooher RL, Rao MM, Scott DF, et al. A systematic review of laparoscopic live-donor nephrectomy. *Transplantation* 2004; 78:404–444.

COMMENTARY

Transplantation is one of the fastest growing fields of surgery, the result of breakthroughs in immunosuppression, which, in turn, ever increases the numbers of patients eligible for a new organ. It is also a field in which it would seem that minimally invasive approaches would have little or no application. In fact, as Drs. Catania and Park describe in their review, endoscopy has permeated the transplant field as it has most others. In fact, the only intervention in transplant not directly affected by surgical endoscopy is the actual implantation of the donor organ. Both flexible and laparoscopic endoscopies have a current role in transplant ranging from preoperative screening and evaluation to postoperative surveillance. Many of these uses are indirect, such as screening colonoscopy in pre-transplant evaluation or endoscopic evaluation or treatment for some of the many gastrointestinal complications of chronic immuno-suppression. One must also acknowledge the uses of endoscopy in lung transplant, where both broncoscopy and thoracoscopy have a major role in evaluation and follow-up. More direct uses of laparoscopy include the pretransplant removal of small diseased kidneys, donor organ biopsies to assess for rejection, the postoperative treatment of intraabdominal complications such as seroma drainage, and even, sadly, the removal of failed transplants.

The direct uses of laparoscopy so well described by the authors in this chapter are, of course, exciting developments. Pancreatic islet cell transplant seems to finally be achieving some clinical validation. The ability to obtain pancreatic donor tissue with minimal access approaches may in fact prove critical as it is becoming apparent that successful results require large numbers of islet cells that will need to come from multiple pooled donors, making recruitment of donors more difficult. Partial liver transplants likewise are particularly amenable to laparoscopic approaches; this may eventually make them a viable alternative to cadaveric liver transplant. Of course it has been in kidney transplant that laparoscopy has had the most dramatic and revolutionary impact. The fact that living related donor transplant now outnumbers cadaveric transplants is, to a large extent, a result of being able to offer a "user friendly" surgery to the altruistic donor. It has been well documented that concerns about scarring and the length of hospital stay and subsequent downtime involved with donation has a dramatic impact on the number of volunteer donors. Laparoscopic donation, with its decreased pain and surgical scarring and shorter length of hospital stay, has made it a more palatable choice for family or friends.

So what is the future of surgical endoscopy and transplant? Without a doubt there will be increasing roles for minimal access approaches as they make particular sense in this specialty; providing a marketable advantage to living donors and minimizing morbidity in the immunocompromised recipient population. Eventually we may see a role for transplantation itself, at least for procedures such as islet cell transplant and other cellular-based transplants that may require placement into immunoprotected zones or implanted artificial organ frameworks.

LLS

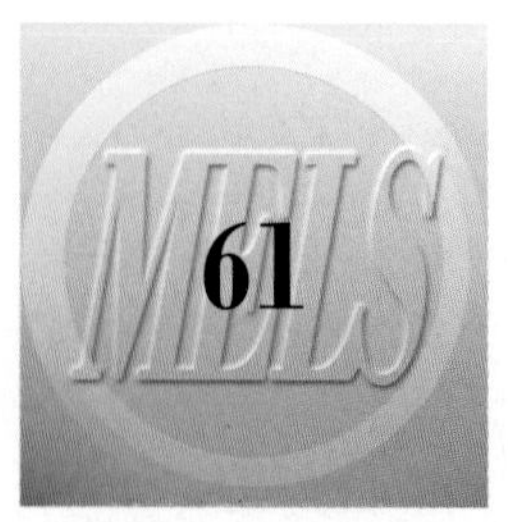

Retroperitoneal Surgery

LEENA KHAITAN

INTRODUCTION

The retroperitoneum refers to that part of the abdominal cavity bordered anteromedially by the peritoneum, posteriorly by the paraspinal and flank muscles, and superiorly by the diaphragm. Inferiorly, this space is continuous with the pelvic extraperitoneal space. This retroperitoneum encompasses organs and conditions that are discussed elsewhere in this book (pancreas, adrenal gland, inguinal and flank hernias, and aortic procedures). Therefore, the discussion in this chapter will be limited to all other retroperitoneal procedures. Many of the procedures that take place in this space are performed by other surgical subspecialties such as urology, gynecology and orthopedics. Some, like the minimal-access spine procedures, require a joint effort by the general and orthopedic surgeon. For other advanced minimally invasive procedures, a general surgeon may be asked to assist or asked to be the primary surgeon, and therefore it is important to be familiar with the pathology within the retroperitoneal space as well as treatment options.

ACCESS TO THE RETROPERITONEUM

The retroperitoneum can be accessed in two ways: either through the peritoneal cavity using a transabdominal approach or directly (also known as retroperitoneoscopy). With the transabdominal approach, the peritoneal cavity is accessed as in any other intraperitoneal procedure using a Hasson technique under direct visualization, a Veress needle, or an optical trocar. To access the retroperitoneal organs on the left (kidney, ureter, testicular vessels, spine) the colon is rotated medially, exposing the Gerota fascia. Below this lie the kidney and adrenal gland. To access the right side, the right colon (duodenum, aorta, psoas muscle, right ureter, right renal vessels) is mobilized in a similar fashion. A Kocher maneuver may facilitate visualization of the right kidney and adrenal gland. To increase working space, the patient position and gravity can be used to the surgeon's advantage. By placing the patient in the flank position, flexing the table, and raising the kidney rest, the working space in the retroperitoneum can be increased almost twofold.

The retroperitoneum can also be accessed directly without ever entering the peritoneal cavity. Using this often virgin plane avoids having to lyse any bowel adhesions and hold the large and small bowel out of the way to get into the retroperitoneal space. The downside is that it is not a natural working space, and is instead created with the assistance of dissecting balloons and insufflation.

To enter the retroperitoneal space, the safest approach is a direct cutdown in the midaxillary line just below the tip of the 12th rib. S-retractors are used to dissect through the muscle layers through the anterior thoracolumbar fascia. After digitally opening up this space with an index finger, a balloon dilator can be passed anterior to the psoas and posterior to the Gerota fascia. After dilation and insufflation of the space, the psoas muscle, Gerota fascia, ureter, peritoneal reflection, and renal artery should be visible on either side, with the aorta seen clearly on the patient's left and the inferior vena cava if accessed on the right. The dissection can be carried caudad for distal ureter procedures. Dissection between the psoas and quadratus lumborum muscles allows better visualization of the spine. With the retroperitoneal approach, even carbon dioxide (CO_2) insufflation can be avoided by using lift devices to provide the needed exposure. Veress needle techniques to enter this space by going through the Petit lumbar triangle have been described. It is difficult, however, to know if the needle has been passed too far or not far enough, and aberrances in either direction can lead to serious morbidity to the patient and compromise of the operative field. Therefore, this technique is not recommended.

Urologic Procedures

The most common procedures in the retroperitoneum involve those performed by the urologists. All of the organs within the urologist's purview, including the kidneys, ureter, and bladder, reside in the retroperitoneum. The field of minimally invasive surgery in urology has advanced rapidly over the last decade. Initially, general minimally invasive surgeons assisted urologists with the advanced laparoscopic procedures. Now, minimally invasive approaches have become the standard of care for many urologists, who are adept at completing most laparoscopic procedures themselves. There still may be situations where the minimally invasive general surgeon is asked to assist, such as with a patient with complex adhesions or with one in need of a concurrent procedure. Therefore, familiarity with the common urologic procedures and port placement is useful. Procedures such as prostatectomy or ureter reconstructive procedures are not discussed, as these procedures are unlikely to involve a general surgeon.

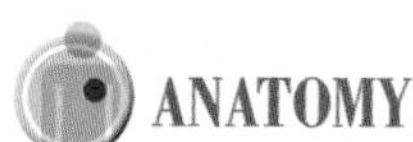

ANATOMY

In order to successfully complete these complex retroperitoneal procedures, a thorough understanding of the urologic anatomy in the retroperitoneum is helpful. The right kidney is situated lower than the left because of the presence of the liver. Within the renal pedicle, the renal vein is the most anterior structure and tends to be longer on the right than on the left. The left renal vein receives direct drainage from the left adrenal, gonadal, and lumbar veins. The renal artery is longer on the left due to the relative position of the aorta. The ureter sits anterior to the psoas muscle bilaterally. On the right, it is to the right of the inferior vena cava and behind the mesentary of the right colon. The left ureter crosses posterior to the left colic vessels behind the sigmoid colon mesentary. The blood supply to the ureters comes from many sources; care must be taken when mobilizing the ureter to avoid any segmental devascularization and resultant stricture.

The bladder is bordered anteriorly by the Retzius space, and the symphysis lies anterior to that. In men, the prostate is contained within this space and the posterior

TABLE 61-1. COMMON LAPAROSCOPIC UROLOGIC PROCEDURES AND THEIR INDICATIONS

Laparoscopic urologic procedure	Indications
Simple nephrectomy	End-stage renal failure, renal artery stenosis, chronic pyelonephritis, xanthogranulomatous pyelonephritis, small tumors
Nephroureterectomy	Urothelial tumors
Radical nephrectomy	Renal cell cancer
Partial nephrectomy	Small tumors
Retroperitoneal lymph node dissection	Testicular cancer (nonseminomatous)
Pelvic lymphadenectomy	Staging for prostate cancer, invasive bladder cancer
Renal cyst decortication	Symptomatic renal cysts
Ligation of varix	Varicocele (usually for bilateral)

aspect of the bladder is separated from the rectum by the Denonvilliers fascia. In women, the bladder and rectum are separated by the uterus.

NEPHRECTOMY

Urologic procedures involve either removal or reconstruction of an organ. Both benign and malignant conditions can be treated with laparoscopic nephrectomy, or kidney removal.

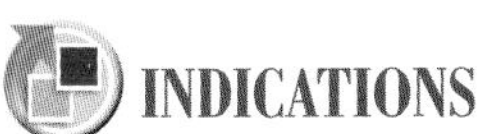

The indication for nephrectomy determines the type of nephrectomy and approach (Table 61-1). Most nephrectomies are approached in a transperitoneal fashion, with a completely laparoscopic or hand-assisted approach. Some benign renal conditions (end-stage renal disease, renal artery stenosis) can be approached retroperitoneally to avoid the increased potential for intraoperative bowel injury and postoperative shoulder pain associated with transperitoneal surgery.

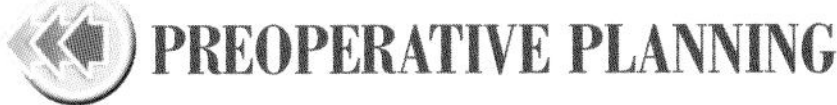

Preoperative workup for laparoscopic nephrectomy includes a thorough history and physical exam, associated serum, urine, and radiologic studies, and an electrocardiogram as indicated. It is important to take a surgical history to know where the patient may have adhesions; extensive prior intraabdominal surgery may sway the surgeon to use a retroperitoneal approach. It is also helpful to define the vascular anatomy clearly with computed tomography (CT) to help with planning of the procedure. A preoperative bowel preparation should be considered in case of an unexpected bowel injury. Preoperative antibiotics are indicated and blood is often made available for transfusion in case of emergency.

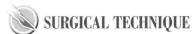

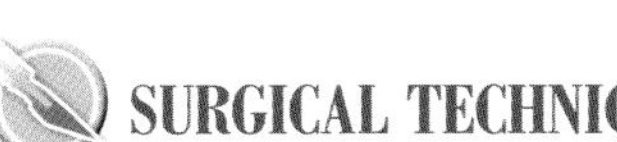

The patient is brought to the operating room and placed in the lateral decubitus position with the side of interest up (Fig. 61-1). The kidney rest is raised to open the space between the costal margin and iliac crest. Care should be taken to pad the arms and legs properly and to secure the patient tightly to the bed with the liberal use of tape and towels. After prepping and draping, pneumoperitoneum is established with a Veress needle, an optical trocar, or with a trocar placed via the Hasson approach. The camera port is placed just lateral to the rectus in the right or left upper quadrant. Two additional 5-mm ports are placed to triangulate the camera with the kidney. The trocar in the subcostal area can be 10 mm in order to facilitate suturing and stapling if needed. An additional trocar or two can be placed for traction in the anterior or midaxillary lines for use by the assistant. This assistant stands at the back of the patient and the other assistant and surgeon stand in front of the patient. Dissection is begun by mobilizing the colon at the white line of Toldt and allowing it to fall medially. Next, to facilitate dissection, the vasculature at the renal hilum should be dissected. The renal artery is shorter on the right and requires very careful dissection. A right-angle dissecting instrument can be helpful for blunt dissection to encircle the artery. Once the artery is dissected, three clips are placed on the patient side and two clips on the other side, and then the artery is divided. Alternatively, the vessel can be tied, but clipping is the easiest laparoscopically. The kidney is allowed to drain into the venous system, after which point the vein can be divided. It may be too large to allow for the placement of a clip, in which case it may be tied and then clipped. As the lower pole of the kidney is dissected with blunt and cautery dissection, the ureter is identified, clipped, and divided. Now the kidney can be dissected circumferentially with the Gerota fascia intact and then removed through a small incision made in the lower abdomen. It is important to remove the kidney in a bag, particularly if it is being removed for malignancy. The adrenal gland is left in place by dissecting in the avascular plane at the superior portion of the kidney.

Alternatively, the whole procedure can be done through a retroperitoneal approach. The retroperitoneum is accessed as previously described just below the costal margin. After the retroperitoneal space is developed, two additional ports are placed. One is placed in the costovertebral angle and the other is placed in the anterior axillary line after the peritoneum is moved far enough forward. An additional trocar can be placed for retraction if needed. The procedure continues similarly to the transperitoneal approach. After the kidney is removed, a muscle-splitting incision is used to remove the specimen.

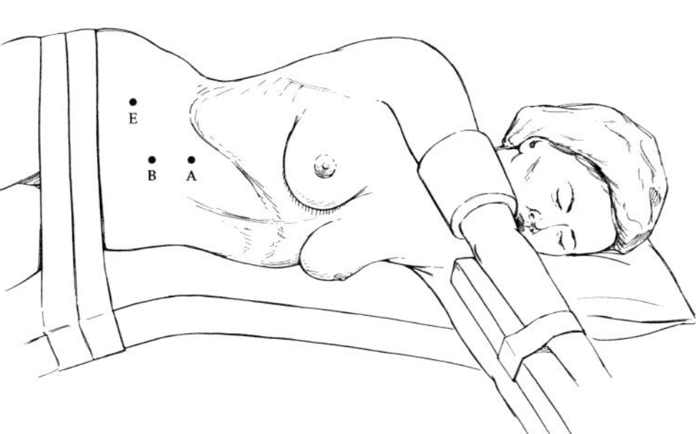

Fig. 61-1. Patient positioning for a laparoscopic nephrectomy. Port B is the camera port and the ports on either side are the working ports for the surgeon. Ports A and B are usually 10 mm, port E is 5 mm.

The major advantage of the retroperitoneal approach is to avoid the peritoneal cavity and any adhesions the patient may have from prior surgery.

The final option is that the procedure can be done using a hand-assisted approach. This is an excellent approach if the kidney must be removed intact. With this approach, the surgeon is able to have one hand in the abdomen throughout the procedure. This decreases operative times and allows many urologists with limited laparoscopic skills to be comfortable with a minimally invasive approach.

The key to maximizing the benefit of the hand-assisted approach is the location of the hand port, whose placement is determined by the surgeon's nondominant hand and the kidney that is being removed. For a right-handed surgeon performing a right nephrectomy, a right lower quadrant incision is used (Fig. 61-2). For a left nephrectomy by a right-handed surgeon, the hand port is best placed in the midline (Fig. 61-3). The hand can help with retraction and blunt dissection. The size of the incision for the hand port depends on the surgeon's glove size. For a surgeon with a size six glove, a 6-cm incision is needed. Typically, with the hand port in place, two additional trocars are required: one for the camera and one for the surgeon's dominant hand. This approach offers the advantages of a laparoscopic procedure while allowing decreased operative times compared to a completely laparoscopic approach. The hand-assist technique may facilitate a more difficult dissection and is easier to learn for those not experienced with laparoscopic techniques.

For the cancer patient needing a ureterectomy in addition to a nephrectomy, the laparoscopic approach offers many advantages. With an open approach this would require a very large incision with the potential for significant morbidity. If a transperitoneal approach is used, the ureter is mobilized as far distal as possible and then the most distal part of the ureterectomy is done open, through a small lower-midline incision. If the hand-assisted approach is used, again the midline incision can be extended to facilitate an open distal ureterectomy. The other approach that has been described is to do this portion minimally invasively as well. With the patient in lithotomy position, cystoscopic assistance is used to dissect the distal ureter. Two small working ports (for 2-mm or 5-mm instruments) are placed directly into the bladder. With cystoscopic guidance, a guidewire is placed into the ureter. A Collins knife is used to incise a cuff of bladder mucosa around the ureteral opening. An endoloop is placed through the trocar around the cuff and the dissection is completed with the Collins knife. Now the ureter is free and the bladder is decompressed with a Foley catheter. The hole in the bladder where the ureter used to be is repaired with sutures. The rest of the nephrectomy is completed.

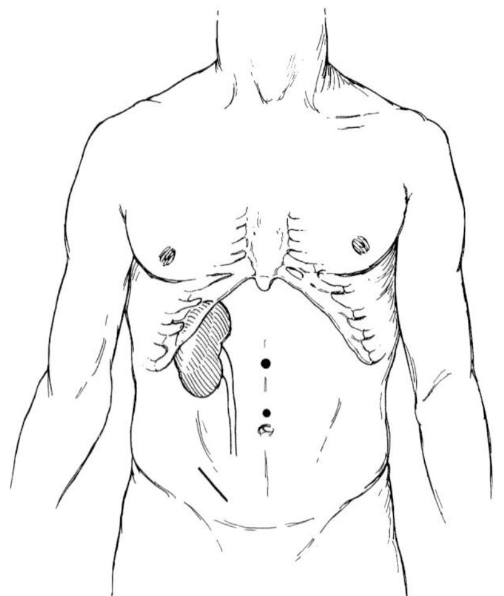

Fig. 61-2. Port placement for a hand-assisted laparoscopic right nephrectomy for a right-handed surgeon.

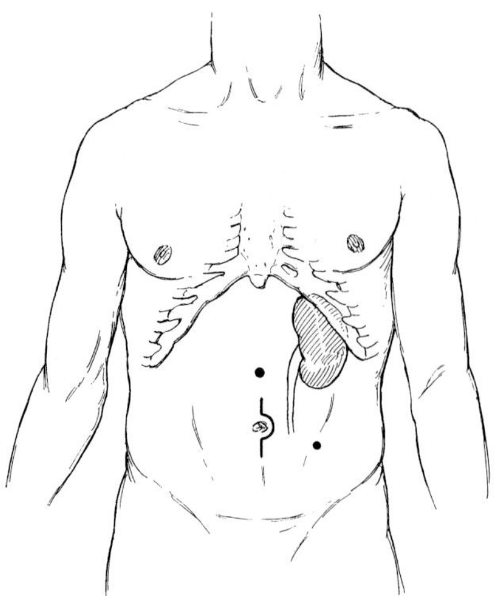

Fig. 61-3. Port placement for a hand-assisted laparoscopic left nephrectomy for a right-handed surgeon.

If a patient requires a partial nephrectomy for a small (<4 cm) tumor, the approach is determined by the location of the tumor on the kidney. Posterior and posterolateral tumors should be approached retroperitoneally, and all others should be approached transperitoneally. Prior to beginning the nephrectomy all patients should have a drainage catheter placed cystoscopically into the ureter. The kidney is approached as previously described. Instead of clipping and dividing the renal pedicle vasculature, a laparoscopic Satinsky clamp is used to control it. Intraoperative use of an ultrasound allows one to confirm the location of the tumor. The goal is to remove the part of the kidney and the overlying fat pad.

The renal capsule is scored. The patient is given mannitol and Lasix for renal protection. The renal pedicle is clamped and the tumor is removed using a J-hook or scissors. No cautery is used on the collecting system. Once the specimen is removed, indigo carmine is injected retrograde through the previously placed ureteral catheter and any leaks in the collecting system are oversewn with absorbable suture. Fibrin glues can be used on the cut surface to assist with hemostasis. Partial nephrectomy allows for the removal of small tumors while maintaining ipsilateral renal function.

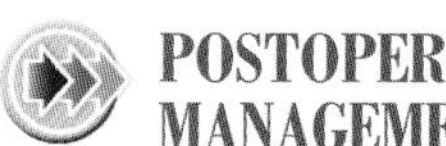

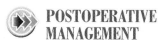

POSTOPERATIVE MANAGEMENT

Most patients have a shortened hospital stay with the minimally invasive nephrectomy. Patients are started on oral intake on postoperative day one. In most series, the majority of patients are home within three postoperative days.

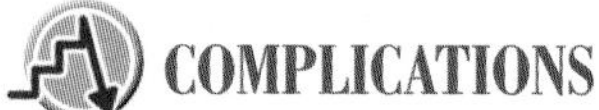

COMPLICATIONS

Laparoscopic nephrectomy is subject to the same complications that can be seen with any minimally invasive procedure. The incidence of bowel injury is low, but it can occur. The potential for injury to major vessels (e.g., aorta or inferior vena cava) is significant and can result in severe injury or death. Prior to completing the procedure, the peritoneal cavity should always be inspected for any signs of bleeding or bowel injury. The retroperitoneal approach allows one to avoid injury to most parts of the bowel, other than the colon. The greatest advantage of the retroperitoneal approach is direct access to the renal hilum. Long-term follow-up of laparoscopic nephrectomy for cancer shows the same oncologic outcomes expected from open techniques.

In a recent prospective, randomized, controlled trial comparing the laparoscopic transabdominal and retroperitoneoscopic approaches, no differences were noted with respect to operative time, blood loss, or patient morbidity. Interestingly, in this study the only difference identified was time to oral intake. Those in the retroperitoneal group resumed oral intake slower than the transperitoneal group. Furthermore, no studies have been able to definitively show any advantage of a completely laparoscopic technique versus an open technique. Therefore, the choice of approach depends on surgeon experience and preference.

DONOR NEPHRECTOMY

The first donor nephrectomy was performed in 1995. It is now the preferred approach in most centers, which has increased the number of people willing to donate exponentially. There is little difference in the donor nephrectomy compared to the procedures previously described. The primary concern in a donor nephrectomy is preserving the vasculature to facilitate transplantation and to minimize ischemia time. For this reason, the kidney is mobilized first and the ureter is then clipped and divided. The vasculature is the last to be taken, with the artery taken first followed by the renal vein. To maximize the length of the remaining vessels, no clips are placed on the kidney side. A thorough preoperative definition of the renal vascular anatomy facilitates this dissection.

One of the most common complications following donor nephrectomy is development of a lymphocele. Several treatments have been tried. Now the most successful treatment is internal drainage of the collection into the peritoneal cavity. This can be done laparoscopically by marsupializing the walls of the lymphocele.

ROBOTICS IN UROLOGY

Urologists have been able to advance the use of robotics in surgery more than any other subspecialty. Laparoscopic techniques have become the standard of care for many urologic procedures. However, the learning curve is steep and not all urologists have the ability to go back and do a fellowship. Robotic technology has facilitated the conversion of many an "open" surgeon to a minimally invasive one. Robotics has most commonly been used for radical prostatectomy, primarily due to the incidence of prostate cancer. Other procedures that have been performed using robotic technology include nephrectomy, partial nephrectomy, and nephroureterectomy; all have been done successfully with reasonable operative times. The port placement with robotic procedures varies slightly from the open techniques. Therefore, one should review the literature carefully prior to attempting this approach. The downside of using this technology is that it is very expensive; for this reason, it is only offered in a few highly specialized centers.

LAPAROSCOPIC TREATMENT OF VARICOCELE

Varicoceles are a result of dilated and tortuous veins of the pampiniform plexus, predominantly on the patient's left side, caused by the retrograde flow of blood through this plexus. Increased retrograde flow develops as a consequence of increased venous pressure, collateral venous anastomosis, and incompetent valves of the internal spermatic vein. The primary concern with varicoceles is testicular dysfunction; the condition should therefore be corrected. It has been observed that the affected testicle generally returns to normal once the varix is ligated.

PREOPERATIVE PLANNING

Most varicoceles are asymptomatic and discovered on routine physical exam in young men. The classic presentation of finding a "bag of worms" is sometimes only evident during a Valsalva maneuver, which should thus be a routine part of any testicular exam. Another important step is to assess testicular volume of the affected side compared to the other. This may have implications toward future fertility. Ultrasound imaging and Doppler flow studies, although commonly ordered, do not provide any additional information that will affect treatment. The primary treatment is varicocele ablation, which is indicated for those patients in whom there appears to be greater than a 2-mm loss of volume in the affected testicle, compared to the other side.

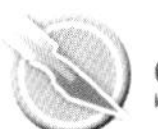

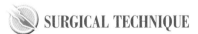

SURGICAL TECHNIQUE

The optimal approach to the treatment of varicocele varies amongst urologists. Multiple approaches have been described, including an open retroperitoneal approach, transperitoneal open approach, laparoscopic approach, and embolization. Since most approaches have equal efficacy, the choice of approach is primarily affected by the experience of the surgeon and the patient age, body habitus, and characteristics of the varicocele. A preperitoneal laparoscopic approach is described.

The primary port is placed at the umbilicus into the preperitoneal space between the rectus and the posterior rectus sheath. A dissecting balloon is used to develop the space as with a preperitoneal hernia repair. After the space is insufflated, two additional trocars are placed. A 5-mm trocar is placed in the suprapubic position under direct visualization and a second trocar is placed halfway between the umbilicus and symphysis. The spermatic veins are identified after the cord is skeletonized. They are then clipped using a 5-mm clip applier. Cautery should be limited to avoid injury to the artery. The patient is sent home on the same day and undergoes routine postoperative follow-up.

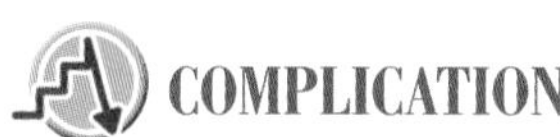

COMPLICATIONS

The primary complications of varicocelectomy are hydrocele formation, varicocele recurrence, and testicular atrophy. Hydrocele and atrophy occur most commonly if mass ligation is used and care is not taken to spare the artery. The laparoscopic approach facilitates preservation of the artery because of the magnified view. These complication rates appear to be the same with the laparoscopic approach as compared to open (5% hydrocele formation, 15% recurrence). The preperitoneal approach offers a short operative time and a quick recovery. The most effective method in terms of avoiding complications is the microscopic approach, with only a 2% recurrence rate, but most are not adept in the microscopic techniques. Therefore, it is important to have the laparoscopic approach in one's armamentarium. Due its increased cost and equivalent morbidity that is noted with other procedures, however, laparoscopy is not usually the primary approach to this disease.

RENAL CYSTS

With the advances in radiologic imaging, many asymptomatic cysts are found on the kidneys. Some patients develop large renal cysts that become symptomatic and require intervention. This may be a solitary cyst or related to polycystic kidney disease. The indications for decortication of the cyst are primarily due to symptoms arising from pressure on surrounding organs. If the patient has a symptomatic cyst, then this is an ideal case for a laparoscopic approach.

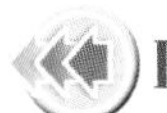

PREOPERATIVE PLANNING

All patients are thoroughly evaluated with a history and physical exam followed by radiologic evaluation. Computed tomography and ultrasound imaging are helpful in defining the location of the cyst and planning the approach. The patient should have a ureteral catheter placed cystoscopically prior to the procedure. This allows for an evaluation of the collecting system during the procedure.

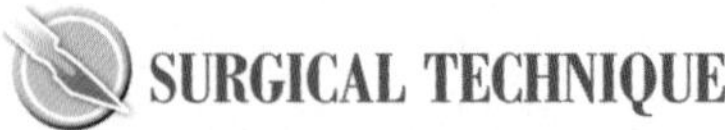

The kidney is approached as one would for a nephrectomy. The cyst wall is identified and opened using cautery. The contents are suctioned and the cavity should be inspected for any suspicious lesions. The bed of the cyst is cauterized to stop continued drainage and connection with the collecting system is evaluated by injecting the ureteral catheter with blue dye. Any connections to the collecting system are oversewn. If this evaluation is not done, the patient may develop a postoperative urinoma. The bed of the cyst can also be covered by perinephric fat or marsupialized to help decrease drainage and recurrence. A drain is placed through one of the trocar sites and removed a few days later if there is no drainage.

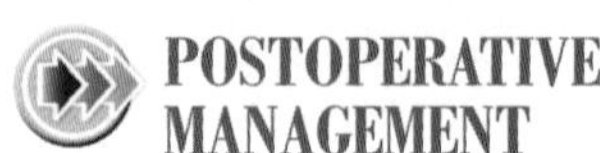

Postoperatively, most patients note improvement in symptoms almost immediately because nearby organs are no longer compressed. Patients can be fed immediately postoperatively. The drain is removed on the second or third postoperative day. Patients should then be followed clinically for any recurrence of disease.

The most common complication is recurrence. With adequate opening of the cyst and removal of a portion of the wall, the incidence of recurrence is decreased.

RETROPERITONEAL LYMPH NODE DISSECTION

Retroperitoneal lymph node dissection is indicated in those patients with nonseminomatous germ cell tumors of the testicle. This procedure is considered both diagnostic and therapeutic. Preoperatively, all patients are evaluated with CT scan of the abdomen and pelvis. The radiologist is asked to pay particular attention to the presence of any retroperitoneal lymphadenopathy. For those with Stage I disease, this is the most sensitive and specific method to detect microscopic metastases. For patients with Stage II disease, this is an acceptable treatment option. It also is a way to stage those patients who would benefit from chemotherapy while also debulking the disease. When performed via an open approach, retroperitoneal lymph node dissection was considered a morbid procedure that did not confer benefit in all patients; for this reason, its use was highly debated. Now, laparoscopic dissections have been done for over a decade and have proved to be as effective as the open approach with significantly less comorbidity.

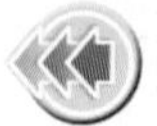

PREOPERATIVE PLANNING

Because this is a transperitoneal procedure, the patient undergoes a preoperative bowel preparation. Appropriately type and crossed blood should be available in the operating room in case of emergency as the dissection is done very close to the aorta and vena cava. The patient is placed supine or in a split-leg position on the operating room table.

SURGICAL TECHNIQUE

The peritoneal cavity is accessed at the umbilicus using a Hasson technique. Three to four additional ports are placed under direct visualization on the side opposite the lymph node dissection. The upper quadrant ports are 10 mm and the other two are 5-mm ports (Fig. 61-4). For patients with disease on the right side, the ports are placed on the left. The nodes to be removed include the paracaval, precaval, retrocaval, and interaortocaval nodes from the renal artery down to the bifurcation. Nodes around the right common iliac and any preaortic nodes are also dissected. For left-sided disease, the corresponding nodes are dissected on the opposite side.

This procedure is tedious; the nodes have to be dissected carefully from the surrounding tissues using blunt, sharp, and ultrasonic scalpel dissection. Advanced skills are required. The laparoscopic approach allows magnification of the tissues to aid in dissection. All of the retroperitoneal organs should be clearly visualized to ensure a complete dissection. The lumbar sympathetic chain should be left intact to avoid complications with ejaculation. The nodes between the aorta and vena cava are the most difficult to dissect and should be addressed early in the procedure so the view is not obscured by bleeding. At the end of the procedure, the lymph node basin should be inspected for hemostasis. The 10-mm ports are closed at the level of the fascia.

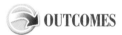

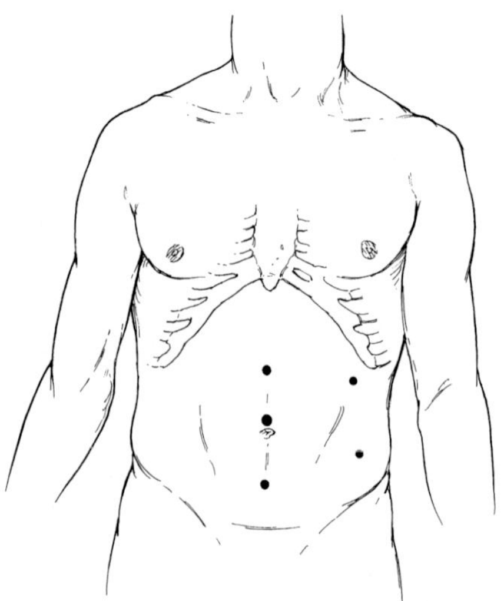

Fig. 61-4. Port placement for retroperitoneal lymph node dissection for nonseminomatous germ cell tumors.

OUTCOMES

This node dissection is essential for those with radiologic Stage I disease, as up to 25% to 30% of these patients will have positive nodes. For those with radiologic Stage II disease, furthermore, as many as 20% will be down-staged to Stage I after the lymph node dissection. This will affect the administration of chemotherapy and is considered a primary treatment for Stage II disease. In a recent study assessing feasibility and outcomes of laparoscopic retroperitoneal lymph node dissection, patients were evaluated at 10-year follow-up. Operative times were 256 minutes for Stage I and 243 minutes for Stage II disease. Blood loss, rate of tumor control, and relapse rates were similar to the open procedure. Complications of ejaculation occurred in only 1.6% of patients. Overall, the laparoscopic approach was found to be equivalent to the open approach for tumor control, while allowing all of the advantages of laparoscopy. The learning curve was noted to be steep, with the authors beginning with left-sided tumors and then progressing to the more difficult right-sided dissection as they gained experience. The authors concluded that the laparoscopic procedure could be done with decreased morbidity and improved quality of life for the patients.

The laparoscopic approach to retroperitoneal lymph node dissection has probably had one of the greatest impacts on patients in terms of urologic procedures. In the past, the open procedure required a large midline incision that resulted in a 5-day hospital stay. Now the procedure can be performed with four to five small trocars, with a resulting hospital stay of only 2 days. The faster recovery also allows for earlier administration of chemotherapy.

PELVIC LYMPHADENECTOMY

Pelvic lymphadenectomy has limited indication in urology. It is used for those patients with prostate cancer in whom the lymphadenectomy might alter treatment. It is also used for patients with invasive bladder cancer. The exception is those with known metastases who are undergoing palliative cystectomy; lymphadenectomy offers no treatment advantage in this subgroup. This procedure is much less tedious than the retroperitoneal lymph node dissection.

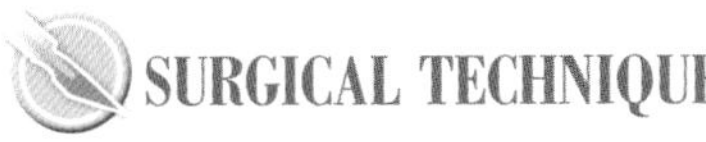

SURGICAL TECHNIQUE

The patient is placed supine and should be secured to the bed well so that the bed can be rotated to facilitate dissection. The umbilical port is placed using a Hasson technique. Two additional trocars are placed laterally on either side above the level of the anterior superior iliac spine under direct visualization. The peritoneum is incised starting at the medial umbilical ligament and extending laterally to expose the obturator and iliac spaces. The peritoneum is peeled back so that the deep insertion of the vas is seen medial to the vessels. The obturator and external iliac nodes are removed on the medial aspect of the vessels. Then this dissection is carried caudad toward the pubic bone. The nodes are removed from this area until the obturator nerve is visualized. The nodes are clipped inferiorly and removed. All of this dissection is done bluntly or with ultrasonic coagulation. The dissection extends from the pubic bone to the level of the bifurcation of the iliac vessels. The patient is then rotated and the dissection is repeated on the opposite side.

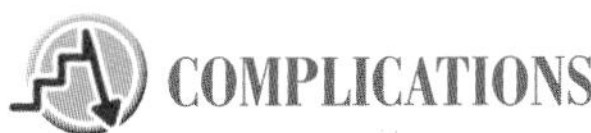

COMPLICATIONS

The most common complication is the development of a lymphocele resulting from the collection of lymph fluid after cutting of the lymphatics during a surgical procedure. This was initially seen more commonly in patients treated laparoscopically as compared to open because oral intake was resumed so quickly. Now we have seen a decrease in this incidence. Lymphoceles are seen in 0.5% to 10% of patients following pelvic lymphadenectomy and 1% to 12% of patients following transplantation. If a lymphocele is noted, it is treated laparoscopically be marsupializing the walls of the collection to allow drainage into the peritoneal cavity. With this technique, recurrence rates are less than 1%.

Gynecologic Procedures

Although most gynecologic organs lay intraperitoneally, several procedures related to the uterus, cervix, vagina, and ovaries involve retroperitoneal dissection. These procedures include retroperitoneal lymph node dissections for cancer staging and those procedures related to a weakened pelvic floor. It is important to know the pelvic floor and the retroperitoneal anatomy to safely perform these procedures. Traditionally these procedures have been performed with a laparotomy. Procedures involving advanced laparoscopic skills including fine dissection next to large vascular structures and laparoscopic suturing have a very steep learning curve. Therefore, gynecologists may ask a minimally invasive general surgeon to assist them with these complex procedures in order to be able to offer their patients the benefits of minimally invasive surgery. In the majority of these procedures, the retroperitoneum is approached transperitoneally with CO_2 insufflation and standard laparoscopic techniques. The procedures are described in detail below.

GYNECOLOGIC MALIGNANCIES

Surgery is a major component of treatment for gynecologic malignancies. The primary affected organ is removed for treatment of the primary malignancy. Gynecologists are well equipped to perform routine gynecologic procedures, even laparoscopically. However, they may not have been trained in more advanced minimally invasive procedures, especially if they did not do a specialized fellowship.

For staging, most gynecologic malignancies warrant a retroperitoneal lymph node dissection. The level of dissection is determined by the type of primary malignancy and its local stage (Table 61-2). Traditionally, these were done open. In 1991, Denis Querleu proposed the transperitoneal laparoscopic approach to these lymph node dissections for staging. Now, many studies have shown that laparoscopic lymph node dissection is feasible and as good as the open dissection. This was key to the acceptance of minimally invasive lymphadenectomy since much of the metastatic disease is microscopic only, and survival is directly related to the extent of dissection. Therefore, the gynecologist may ask for the minimally invasive general surgeon's assistance with this more advanced procedure.

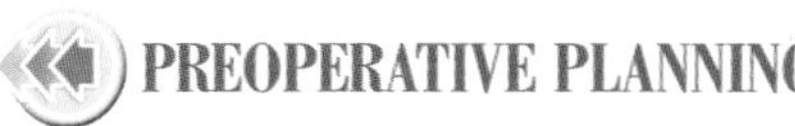

PREOPERATIVE PLANNING

All patients undergo a thorough history and physical examination. Preoperative imaging with CT scan of the abdomen and pelvis is indicated in all patients. The patient should undergo a standard bowel preparation prior to the procedure.

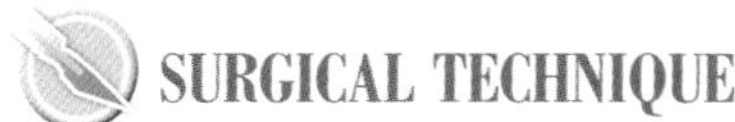

SURGICAL TECHNIQUE

The pelvic lymphadenectomy is the mainstay of lymph node staging for all gynecologic malignancies. This dissection is most commonly performed transperitoneally. The patient is placed in the supine position with lower extremities in the extended split-leg or lithotomy position. The peritoneum is approached at the umbilicus with a Hasson technique and a 10-mm trocar is placed. The abdomen is insufflated to 15 mmHg with CO_2 and the patient is placed in the steep Trendelenburg position in order to allow the bowel to fall out of the pelvis. Two additional trocars are placed at almost the level of the umbilicus just lateral to the epigastric vessels. The surgeon operates from the patient's left and the monitor is placed at the foot of the bed.

First the peritoneal cavity is inspected for any signs of metastatic disease. The dissection is then begun along the pelvic sidewall between the round ligament and the infundibulopelvic ligament (Fig. 61-5, page 622). The external iliac and superior vesicle arteries are then identified. The space between them is the paravesicle space. The Cooper ligament can also be seen and is the

TABLE 61-2. RETROPERITONEAL LYMPH NODE DISSECTIONS FOR GYNECOLOGIC MALIGNANCIES

Gynecologic malignancy	Type of lymph node dissection
Uterine cancer	Bilateral pelvic and periaortic lymphadenectomy
Cervical cancer (early; Stage Ib/IIa)	Bilateral pelvic and periaortic lymphadenectomy
Cervical cancer (advanced)	Bilateral common iliac and periaortic lymphadenectomy
Ovarian cancer	Bilateral pelvic and periaortic lymphadenectomy

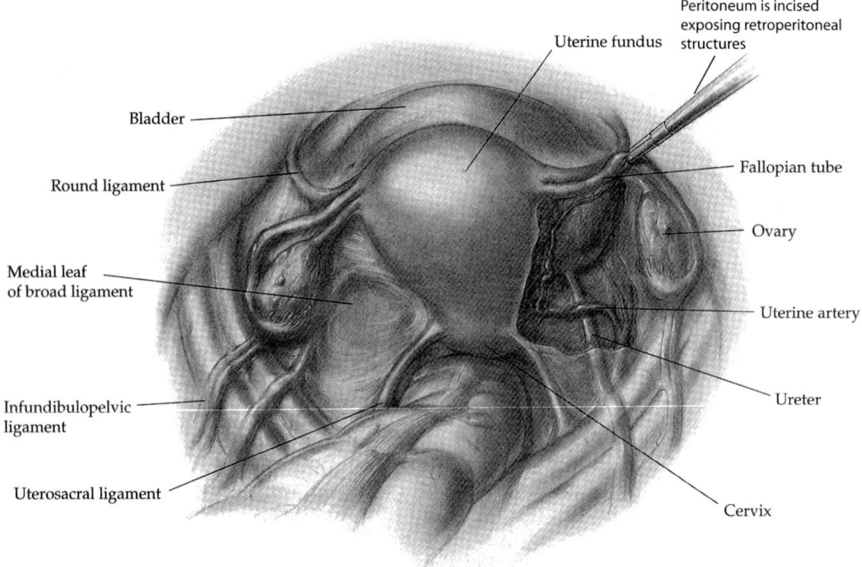

Fig. 61-5. Laparoscopic view of the pelvic anatomy. The anatomy lateral to the uterus is shown with the peritoneum dissected away. This is the location of the nodal dissection.

ventral limit of the interiliac dissection. The interiliac lymphadenectomy involves all nodes along the external iliac extending caudad to the femoral ring. These are the obturator nodes. The nodes are dissected from the pubic bone below the external iliac vein up to the bifurcation. The nodes on the other side of the vein, along the artery and psoas muscle, are easier to dissect. The nodes can be grasped and blunt dissection used to bluntly divide the surrounding tissues. One should avoid violating the capsule of the nodes to minimize bleeding. Avoid the accessory obturator vein as well, as bleeding in this area is difficult to control. It can be seen crossing the Cooper ligament down toward the obturator foramen.

The dissection is then continued up along the common iliac vessels by opening the pararectal space. The peritoneum is divided lateral to the ureter so that all of the tissue lateral to the common iliac can be removed. By the end of this dissection, the obturator nerve and lumbosacral trunk may be visible. The dissection between the common iliac vessels is considered the interiliac lymphadenectomy.

If a para-aortic dissection is warranted, the peritoneum is divided along the root of the mesentery and the dissection is extended to the level of the left renal vein. Both inframesenteric and supramesenteric dissections must be completed to adequately stage the patient. In over a quarter of cases, aortic node metastases are supramesenteric only. At the end of the procedure, the area of dissection is inspected thoroughly for hemostasis. All 10-mm sites are closed at the level of the fascia after the trocars are removed.

POSTOPERATIVE MANAGEMENT

Postoperatively, the patient's diet is advanced as tolerated. Most patients recover much more quickly than they did with the open approach. Many studies have demonstrated the feasibility of this technique. The Gynecologic Oncology Group also did a study that involved open laparotomy after laparoscopic dissection to assess the adequacy of resection. The majority of patients were noted to have a complete resection. The major benefit that has been demonstrated with the laparoscopic approach is a decrease in postoperative pelvic adhesions.

Recently, many surgeons have also experimented with sentinel lymph node biopsy for uterine and cervical cancers to even further decrease morbidity. However, with current techniques, the negative predictive value is too low to replace the systematic lymphadenectomy described.

SURGICAL MANAGEMENT OF INCONTINENCE

Retropubic urethropexy was originally described in 1949 as an open procedure to treat stress incontinence. The urethrovesical junction was sutured to the symphysis pubis to decrease the movement of the urethra. The open approach involved extensive dissection and morbidity to the patient. Since that time the procedure has evolved and now can be done minimally invasively by suturing of the urethra to the Cooper ligament. The most challenging part of the laparoscopic procedure is the suturing. Some have tried to modify the technique by clipping the urethra to the Cooper ligament or by using extracorporeal knots. The effectiveness of these modifications has yet to be determined.

PREOPERATIVE PLANNING

All patients undergo a thorough history and physical exam as well as urodynamic studies to evaluate the etiology of their incontinence. The contrast images usually identify a long, floppy urethra. Therefore the mainstay of the procedure is to fix the urethra in place and restore the proper angle to stop the patient's incontinence.

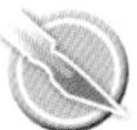

SURGICAL TECHNIQUE

The patient is positioned supine on the table in the lithotomy position. A three-way Foley catheter should be placed to allow better visualization of the bladder intraoperatively. A 10-mm trocar is placed at the umbilicus as the initial port using a Hasson technique under direct visualization. The abdomen is insufflated to 15 mmHg and three additional trocars are placed in the standard positions for most pelvic procedures (Fig. 61-6). The suprapubic 10-mm trocar provides a place to bring the suture into the field and to help facilitate the dissection. The preperitoneal space is entered by incising the peritoneum

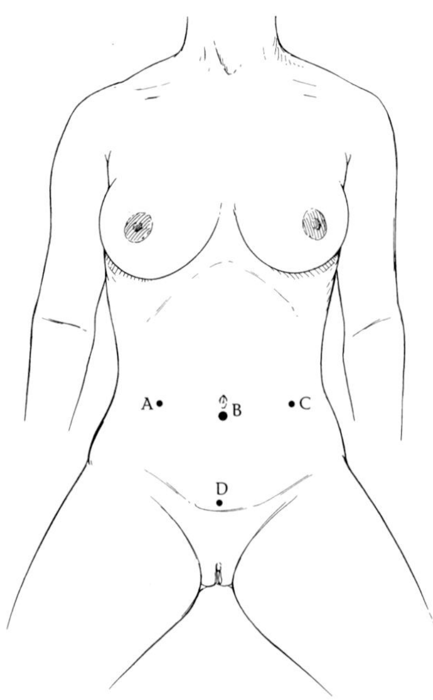

Fig. 61-6. Port placement for retropubic urethropexy; B and D are 10 mm, A and C are 5 mm.

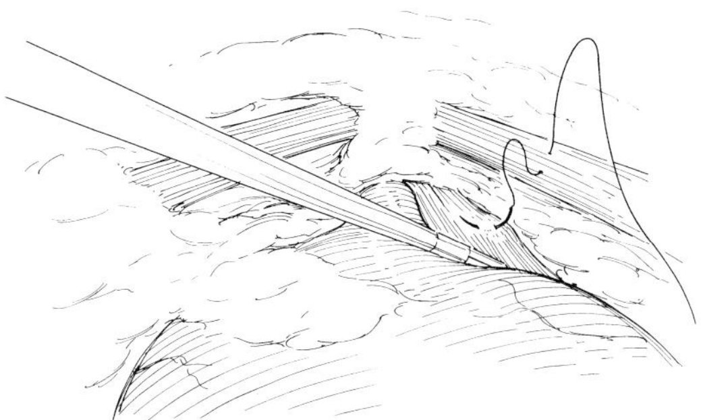

Fig. 61-7. View of the preperitoneal space and the Cooper ligament.

between the umbilicus and pubis and dissecting down to the symphysis. The white, shiny surface of the Cooper ligament should be evident, with the bladder creating the floor of the field. This is the retropubic space (Fig. 61-7). The vaginal fascia is cleared with blunt dissection, after which two fingers can be placed in the vagina to place gentle traction on the Foley catheter to identify the urethral neck. The bladder can be distended (150 to 200 cc of sterile water or saline) to facilitate identification of the anatomy. A permanent suture is placed securing the vaginal fascia at the urethrovesical junction to the Cooper ligament. Two permanent sutures are placed on each side. To be sure these sutures are not too lax, manual pressure is maintained upward from within the vagina. The 10-mm sites are closed at the level of the fascia with absorbable sutures and the procedure is completed.

For patients who do not have midline incisions, a preperitoneal approach can be used. The preperitoneal space is entered anterior to the posterior rectus sheath. The two working ports are placed lateral to the epigastrics on either side at the level of the anterior superior iliac spine.

Cystoscopy should be performed to be sure the sutures did not enter the bladder. Suprapubic tubes can be placed at the end of the procedure. Alternatively, patients can be taught to straight catheterize themselves in the immediate postoperative period. The bladder should be distended at the end of the procedure to identify any evidence of leaking. Prior administration of indigo carmine facilitates this examination.

POSTOPERATIVE MANAGEMENT

Suprapubic tubes can be removed when the residual volume is less than 100 cc. Traditional suturing of the urethra has an 85% to 90% success rate. The most common complication is bladder injury. With concomitant cystoscopy, this complication can be minimized. If it does occur, it can be recognized and repaired immediately. The downside of the minimally invasive approach is that it results in an enterocele in 15% of patients, so a prophylactic culdoplasty is often performed to avoid this complication.

LAPAROSCOPIC PROCEDURES FOR VAGINAL VAULT PROLAPSE

Prolapse of the pelvic organs, which may cause substantial discomfort to the patient, can result from childbirth, chronic increases in abdominal pressure, or estrogen deprivation. It is very important to understand the support axes in the pelvis to exact the best repair. The pelvis has apical, lateral, and distal support regions. It is important to define the defect preoperatively to determine the best treatment via which, simply put, the vagina is secured to another pelvic structure. The most commonly used support structures include the sacrum, the sacrospinous ligament, and the fascia over the iliococcygeus muscle. Suturing of the vagina alone has not proved as effective as using a bridging material to promote scarring in the retroperitoneum and increase the longevity of the repair. Therefore, various mesh materials have been used to facilitate this repair.

PREOPERATIVE PLANNING

The patient undergoes a thorough history and physical exam. The most common cause of the enterocele is a hysterectomy in which the cardinal-uterosacral complex was not reattached to the pubocervical fascia and rectovaginal fascia at the vaginal cuff. It is important to distinguish the enterocele from a cystocele and rectocele, as the treatments are different. The defect in the enterocele is related to a defect in apical support.

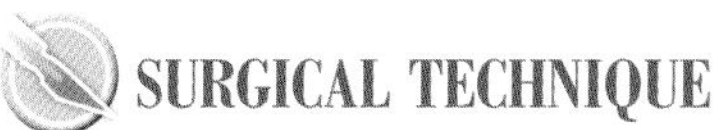

SURGICAL TECHNIQUE

The patient is placed in the lithotomy position with a probe in the vagina. Trocars are placed as described for the retropubic urethropexy. The vagina is elevated using the probe so that the peritoneum can be incised at the vaginal cuff and the rectovaginal fascia exposed. Anterior dissection is then carried out to define the pubocervical fascia. The separation between these fasciae is the enterocele and this can be primarily repaired by imbricating these fasciae or by placing a purse-string around this region. Leaving too much of the enterocele sac behind places the surgeon at risk of only securing the sac to the sacrum and not the fascia, which may result in early surgical failure.

Next, the sacral promontory is exposed by incising the overlying peritoneum. Blunt dissection with the application of clips and some cautery for hemostasis are used to obtain adequate exposure. Next a 12- × 3.5-cm piece of mesh is made into a Y shape. The two top ends of the Y are secured to the rectovaginal and pubocervical fasciae. The sutures should incorporate the entire vaginal wall except the epithelium and three sutures should be placed on each side. The free end of the Y-shaped mesh is then secured to the anterior longitudinal ligament of the sacrum or the periosteum. Any excess mesh is trimmed. The peritoneum is then closed over the mesh to avoid any mesh-related complications. The abdomen is deflated and the trocars removed.

POSTOPERATIVE MANAGEMENT

Intraoperative cystotomies are one of the most common complications with this procedure. Therefore a three-way Foley catheter should be used to help define the margins of the bladder. One of the most devastating complications is a mesh infection. This can be avoided by employing a careful sterile technique, not allowing the mesh to come in contact with the skin, and closing the peritoneum over the mesh at the end of the procedure. There is a potential danger of bleeding from sacral veins, which can be very difficult to control.

The sacral colpopexy has a 95% to 100% success rate and is an excellent enterocele repair. With the laparoscopic approach, patients do have less pain and a shorter recovery time. The limitation is that these procedures have a steep learning curve and should only be performed by surgeons who have a thorough understanding of pelvic floor anatomy.

Spinal Access Procedures

Usually one would not imagine the spine to be in the purview of the general surgeon. However, general surgeons have been assisting spine surgeons since the 1950s. Posterior spinal approaches to the lumbar spine involved a long incision, stripping of the paraspinal muscles from the posterior spinal elements, and prolonged retraction on the deep paraspinal muscles to gain adequate visualization. The posterior approach also led to epidural scarring, nerve traction injuries, and dural lacerations. It was recognized that diseases involving compression of the neural elements with documented anterior compression could more easily be accessed anteriorly. Multiple pathologies lead to this anterior compression, including trauma, neoplasm, inflammation, and degenerative disease. Because the abdomen or chest cavity had to be entered to allow this approach, anterior approaches to the spine were developed as team procedures performed at well-coordinated specialized centers.

As the laparoscopic revolution took place in the 1990s, spine surgeons began to see a need to perform their procedures minimally invasively. Much of the morbidity related to the anterior spinal approach includes injury to the surrounding organs and vasculature as well as the pain from the incision. Minimally invasive transperitoneal approaches and retroperitoneal approaches have greatly decreased the morbidity of these procedures by decreasing blood loss and recovery time. Minimal-access techniques to the spine have been shown to have a high learning curve; however, once they can be done well, the patient greatly benefits.

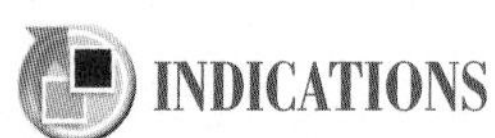

INDICATIONS

Spinal pathologies that the minimally invasive general surgeon can assist with involve the procedures in the distal lumbar and proximal sacral spine (Table 61-3).

Patients with a single level of disease are ideal candidates for a minimally invasive approach. The laparoscopic approach is determined by the level of disease and the pathology involved. Via a retroperitoneal approach, one can expose vertebrae L1 to L5, whereas a transperitoneal approach can be used to approach levels L5 to S1. Disease at the L4 to L5 or L3 to L4 levels may fall under the bifurcation of the aorta and vena cava and thus be difficult to approach anteriorly. Similarly, pathology at L1 to L2 may fall under the renal vessels and may also be difficult to approach.

PREOPERATIVE PLANNING

Preoperative radiologic delineation of the spinal pathology and its relation to the surrounding vascular anatomy is critical. The spine surgeon and abdominal surgeon must both evaluate all of the preoperative workup and have a detailed discussion with the patient. Then, with cooperative effort and communication between both surgeons, the patient can best be cared for. The spine surgeon will determine which spinal procedure would be best for the patient. A joint discussion between the laparoscopic surgeon and the spine surgeon will determine the approach. When considering the approach, the surgeons must consider the level of disease, the pathology, patient anatomy, and the patient's prior procedures. Dense intraabdominal adhesions may be a contraindication to the transperitoneal approach, for example.

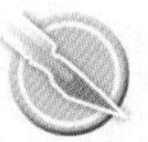

SURGICAL TECHNIQUE

The laparoscopist's primary function is to provide exposure of the spine anteriorly so that the spine surgeon can then use dilators directed toward the intended working space and complete the procedure minimally invasively. In order to provide the needed exposure, the procedure is performed as follows.

The patient is positioned supine on the operating room table. Fluoroscopy should be available in the room (Fig. 61-8). The peritoneal cavity is accessed at the level of the umbilicus using a Veress needle or Hasson technique. The abdomen is insufflated to 15 mmHg and two additional 5-mm working ports are placed in the right and left midclavicular lines under direct visualization. The ports are placed to triangulate the sacral promontory (Fig. 61-9). The patient is placed in steep Trendelenburg position to allow the bowel to fall out of the pelvis and into the upper abdomen. The sigmoid colon is retracted laterally to more clearly expose the posterior peritoneum in the midline. The sigmoid can be held in place by placing a preformed endoloop around an epiploic appendage and pulling the end of the suture through the abdominal wall. The suture can then be secured at the skin with a hemostat to maintain adequate retraction.

Next the peritoneum is incised sharply or with ultrasonic shears to expose the anterior longitudinal spinous ligament. The medial sacral artery and vein can be clipped and divided or divided with the ultrasonic shears if visualized. Next the spine can be visualized with the iliac vessels lying close on either side. These may need to be dissected extensively, particularly if the L4 to L5 disc space is being exposed. To see L5 to S1, the hypogastric nerve plexus may also need to be mobilized.

Now the disc space can be identified radiographically. Fluoroscopy is used to (1) confirm the disc space, (2) identify the midline of the disc space, and (3) determine the exact insertion angle. At this point the spinal surgeon can enter the case and place an additional trocar over the level of pathology at the point predetermined fluoroscopically. This working angle is critical to a successful outcome of the procedure and must be precisely

TABLE 61-3. SPINAL PATHOLOGIES THAT CAN BE TREATED WITH AN ANTERIOR APPROACH

Indications	Procedure	Approach
Herniated intervertebral disc	Discectomy	Transperitoneal or retroperitoneal
Infectious disease	Biopsy or debridement and anterior strut grafting	Transperitoneal or retroperitoneal
Degenerative vertebral disease	Stabilizing procedure with insertion of cage, screws, bone grafts or bone morphogenic protein, spinal fusion	Transperitoneal or retroperitoneal
Neoplasm	Biopsy or excision	Transperitoneal or retroperitoneal
Deformity with scoliosis or kyphosis	Fusion	Transperitoneal or retroperitoneal
Spondylolisthesis	Anterior lumbar fusion	Transperitoneal (L1–L5) or retroperitoneal (L5–S1 or L1–L2)

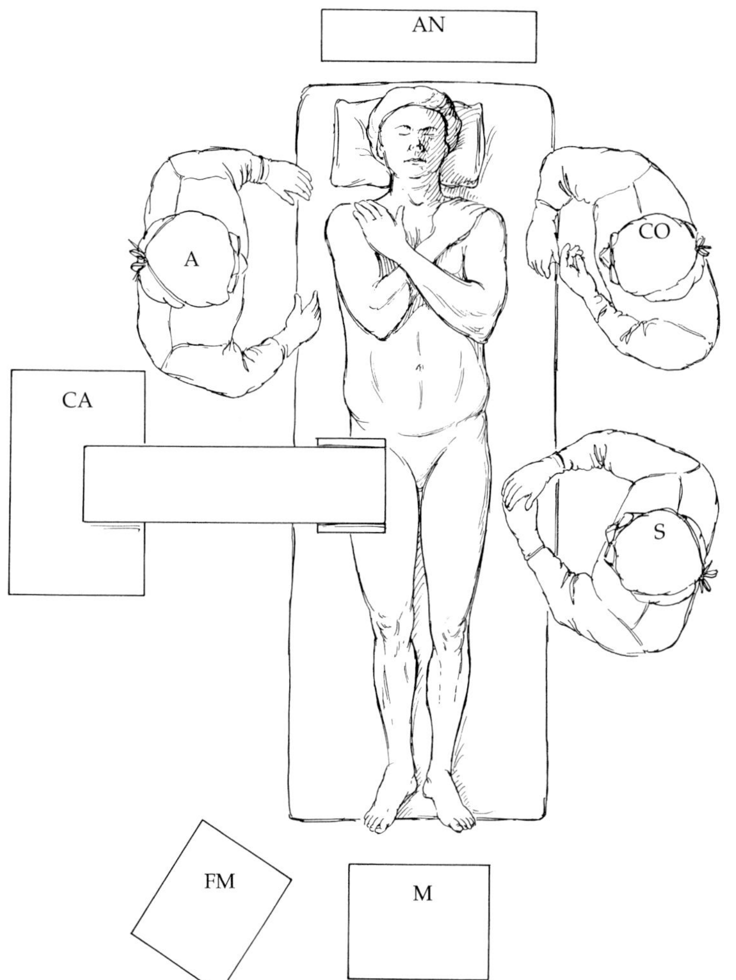

Fig. 61-8. Room setup for spinal access procedures. S, surgeon; CO, co-surgeon; AN, anesthesia; A, assisting surgeon; CA, C-arm; FM, fluoroscopy monitor; M, monitor.

determined by the spine surgeon. Spinal surgeons have developed extensive instrumentation for the insertion of spinal cages and bone graft materials (Fig. 61-10). These instruments are long and narrow so they can fit down traditional trocars.

The spine surgeon preoperatively determines the size of the cage that is to be used. An overtube is placed under direct visualization and the point of cage insertion drilled. Using retraction to their advantage, the cage is placed allowing decompression of the posterior neural foramina. A similar process is completed on the opposite side. All of this is done with the overtube in place.

For those patients who have already had extensive intraperitoneal surgery, a retroperitoneal approach may be preferred. This approach allows access to several different levels for excision, debridement, and grafting. The patient is placed in the lateral decubitus position with the table flexed to open the space between the iliac crest and costal margin. The retroperitoneum is accessed as described in the earlier section. The dissecting balloon is placed in the space between the kidney and the psoas muscle. The psoas can be further separated from the quadratus lumborum muscles to have adequate visualization of the spine. The ureter is allowed to fall anteriorly with the retroperitoneal fat. The psoas muscle is elevated off of the lumbar vertebrae and retracted laterally to the level of the transverse process. The lumbar vessels overlying the vertebrae may need to be clipped and divided. An overtube can again be used for the spine surgeon to do his or her portion of the procedure. The spinal procedure is then completed, the trocars removed, and the skin closed.

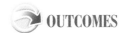

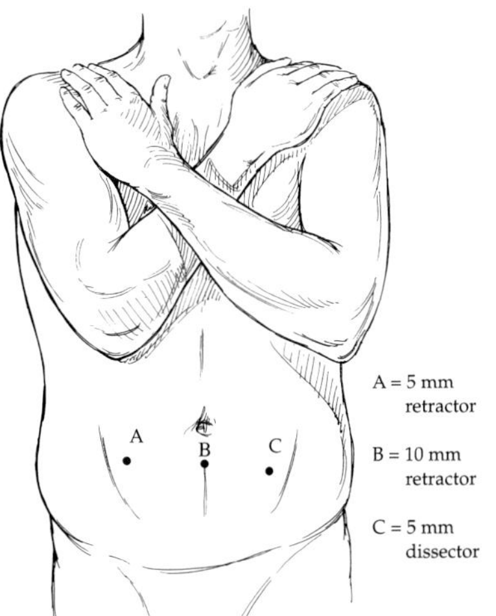

Fig. 61-9. Trocar placement for an anterior approach to the lumbar spine.

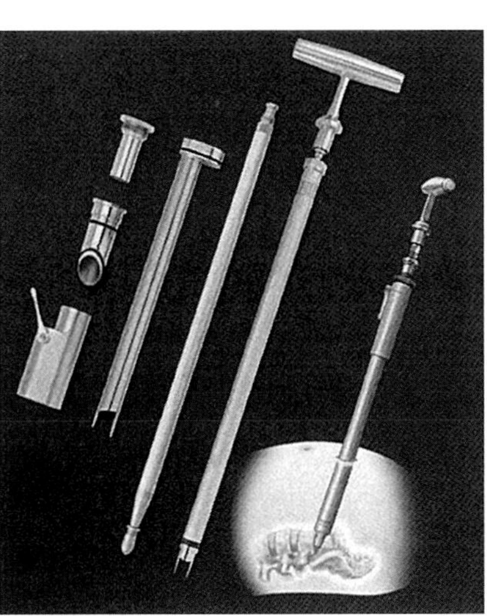

Fig. 61-10. Instrumentation for minimally invasive anterior spinal access procedures.

OUTCOMES

Multiple studies have shown that the minimally invasive techniques can achieve results as good as the traditional open anterior and lateral approaches. Decreased hospital stay and blood loss have been clearly demonstrated at the expense of initially longer operating room times. As experience has increased, however, the operative time is not significantly longer than the open techniques. Additionally, complications of postlaminectomy syndrome, epidural fibrosis, and muscular atrophy are seen less with the minimally invasive techniques. Since the laparoscopic procedure for lumbar fusion was first described in 1995, many new technologies have been developed for lumbar degenerative disc disease. In a recently published review of the literature, results of laparoscopic anterior lumbar fusion were reviewed. For disease at the L5 to S1 level, no significant differences were noted between open, laparoscopic, or mini-open anterior fusions with short-term measures including operating room time, blood loss, and length of stay. The primary long-term complication noted with the laparoscopic approach was retrograde ejaculation. If disease involved the L4 to L5 level or both the L5 to S1 and L4 to L5 levels, then complication rates were noted to be much higher. The complication rate also appears to be related to the experience of the surgeon. As a result of the learning curve and the emergence of new technologies, many surgeons are turning to mini-open techniques. With these techniques, sequential dilators are placed over the desired location. Then, with the assistance of an endoscopic light source, the spinal anatomy is directly visualized and the procedure is performed.

The other technique that has been described as having success is the retroperitoneal approach to the spine. In bypassing the peritoneal cavity, the risk of postoperative adhesions is avoided. Additionally, in early series, patients have no retrograde ejaculation since the hypogastric plexus is avoided. There also appears to be less great vessel injury and implant migration. Again, mini-open retroperitoneal approaches have superseded the initial enthusiasm for the laparoscopic retroperitoneal approach.

Sympathectomy

CELIAC PLEXUS BLOCK

Many patients with pancreatic cancer present with symptoms of pain or develop abdominal pain at some point in the course of their disease. To help improve patient quality of life, multiple approaches, both surgical and nonsurgical, have been used to help control the pain. One of the most effective methods is the neurolytic celiac plexus block. Techniques utilized for this block include percutaneous injection with a long needle under CT guidance, injection at the time of laparotomy, endoscopic injection under the guidance of endoscopic ultrasound, and thoracoscopic neurolysis. Injection under direct laparoscopic visualization has only been described a few times in the literature. Although all of these techniques have proven effective for pain relief in most patients, injection at the time of laparotomy appears to be the most effective.

Laparoscopic neurolytic celiac plexus block offers several advantages. Most patients will undergo abdominal exploration with a staging laparoscopy. For those patients found to have unresectable disease, the block can be done during the same procedure for palliation. Lillemoe et al. have shown in a randomized trial that those patients who are injected at this point in the course of their disease have improved pain relief, mood, and life expectancy compared to those who are not. The conclusion was that many of these improved quality-of-life parameters were observed as a result of these patients not having any substantial abdominal pain during their subsequent course.

SURGICAL TECHNIQUE

The celiac plexus consists of two ganglia that lay on either side of the aorta at the level of the celiac trunk. There is a complex network of neural fibers at this level within the periaortic fat pad. Both sympathetic and parasympathetic fibers to the viscera are within these tissues and it is thought that the neoplastic invasion of these fibers is the etiology of the pain associated with pancreatic cancer. Disruption of the autonomic pain signals from these fibers is the goal of the neurolytic celiac plexus block.

The laparoscopic approach to this block was first described in a swine model in 2000. In the described technique, laparoscopic ultrasound guidance was used to guide the placement of the injection needle in the periaortic tissues. There is only one reported case series in humans.

In the procedure, four 5-mm ports are used, with one port for the camera at the umbilicus and two working ports triangulated toward the lesser sac and celiac trunk. An additional 5-mm port is placed in the right upper quadrant and used for retraction of the caudate lobe of the liver (Fig. 61-11). The patient is placed in the steep reverse-Trendelenburg position. The gastrohepatic omentum is incised with the harmonic scalpel and the stomach is retracted anterolaterally to expose the left gastric artery down to its base. At this point the celiac trunk and the fat surrounding the aorta can be identified. While maintaining exposure, an additional small stab wound is made directly anterior to the celiac trunk and a 23-gauge needle passed through the introducer sheath into the abdominal cavity. Under direct visualization the needle is passed into the periaortic fat pad on both sides and 20 cc of 50% ethanol injected as a sclerosing agent. One must aspirate before injecting to be sure the needle tip is not in a vessel. Laparoscopic ultrasound can also be used to help needle guidance in the periaortic area. Other landmarks that can be used are the bases of the right and left crura. The aorta can be exposed at this level, similar to the technique used for Nissen fundoplication, and the celiac trunk identified. Injections can then be made into the periaortic fat pad under direct visualization or with ultrasound guidance. Once the injection is completed, the abdomen is deflated, the trocars removed, and the skin closed.

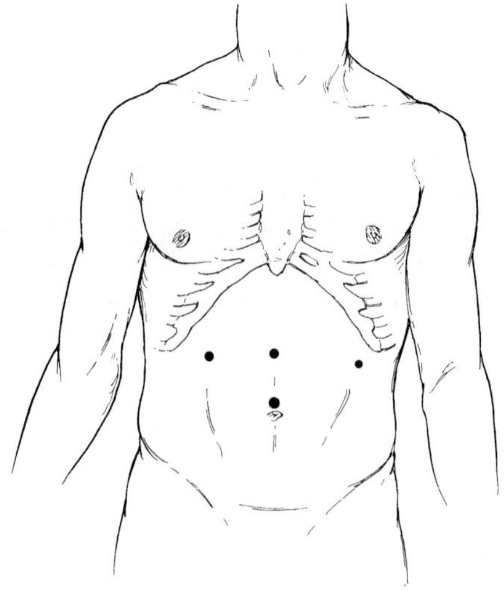

Fig. 61-11. Trocar placement for a laparoscopic celiac plexus block. The camera is placed at the umbilicus and can be a 5- or 10-mm port. The right lateral port is for retraction of the liver and the remaining two 5-mm ports are the working ports.

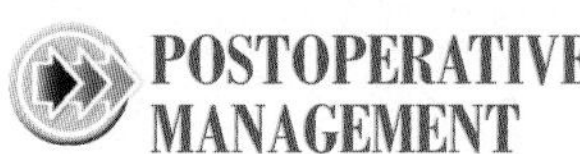

POSTOPERATIVE MANAGEMENT

In the only reported case series in humans, no patients approached with this technique complained of any pain postoperatively. No transient hypotension was noted, as has been seen with some of the nonoperative celiac injections. Some patients will develop a transient diarrhea, which lasts several days and resolves spontaneously. The mechanism is unclear. For patients found to have unresectable disease at the time of laparoscopy, this is an excellent palliative procedure.

LUMBAR SYMPATHECTOMY

Lumbar sympathectomy has been used to treat multiple conditions, including hypertension, arterial occlusive disease, Buerger disease, causalgia, muscular dystrophy, hyperhydrosis of the lower extremities, and Raynaud syndrome of the lower extremities. This procedure has had mixed results in these different disease processes and is now primarily reserved for those patients with arterial occlusive disease, causalgia, and the small group of patients with hyperhydrosis or Raynaud syndrome of the lower extremities. Now symptoms before and after sympathetic blockade can be assessed to better identify those patients who would be benefit from sympathectomy. This has allowed a better success rate overall for this procedure.

Sympathetic denervation as a treatment option for patients with arterial occlusive disease has been known since 1889. Because revascularization techniques below the inguinal ligament have improved for occlusive disease, sympathectomy has fallen out of favor and is considered a palliative option in a limited group of patients. Several case series of patients with Buerger disease have showed positive results. In rare cases, sympathectomy may also benefit those with incipient gangrene if the blood vessel pathology is not too severe.

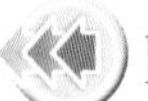

PREOPERATIVE PLANNING

All patients should undergo preoperative lumbar sympathetic block to identify those who would maximally benefit from sympathectomy. All will have some pain relief with sympathectomy; however, those who respond well to the blockade are almost assured pain relief with sympathectomy. Patients should undergo a thorough history and physical exam followed by an electrocardiogram and chest X-ray as indicated based on the their comorbidities to determine their tolerance of general anesthesia.

SURGICAL TECHNIQUE

In the past, lumbar sympathectomy involved muscle cutting and muscle splitting, which lead to high morbidity and a prolonged recovery time. Now, with minimally invasive techniques and an intimate knowledge of the anatomy of the retroperitoneum, the procedures can be done with fewer complications for the patient. A retroperitoneoscopic approach is used. The patient is placed in the lateral decubitus position with the table flexed to open the space between the 12th rib and the iliac crest.

An incision is made halfway between the iliac crest and costal margin in the anterior axillary line. Dissection is carried down through the oblique muscles into the retroperitoneal space. After some finger dissection is used to open the space and the peritoneum is pushed forward, a balloon dissector is placed and insufflated to the equivalent of a 1000-cc, saline-filled balloon. A 30-degree scope can be placed within the balloon so that the dissection can be done under direct visualization. The dissecting balloon is removed and a blunt-tipped trocar placed into the space. The retroperitoneal space is insufflated to 12 mmHg. Two to three additional trocars are placed in the mid and posterior axillary lines and are used for retraction and dissection (Fig. 61-12).

In order to effectively denervate the targeted regions, one must understand the anatomy of the lumbar ganglia. There are technically five lumbar ganglia, but often the ganglia at L1 and L2 are fused. To achieve complete denervation, particularly of either extremity, all of the preganglionic fibers, relay ganglia, and intercommunication fibers must be interrupted or resected. Outflow of the lumbar sympathetic fibers originates from T10 to L3. Sympathetic innervation of the foot and lower leg is primarily though the L2 and L3 ganglia, whereas the proximal leg is primarily innervated from L1 to L4. In most patients, ganglionectomy of L2 and L3 will suffice, but concomitant removal of L4 can avoid collateral reinnervation.

With the surgeon standing on the front side of the patient, the peritoneum is pushed farther away to increase the working space. Any holes made in the peritoneum should be repaired. The psoas muscle can clearly be seen with the genitofemoral nerve running along it, and the gonadal vessels and ureter should all be clearly identified. Intraoperative fluoroscopy or still radiologic studies should be used to identify the location of the lumbar spine and guide the level of sympathectomy. After the location of the spine is confirmed by palpation, dissection is begun on the medial border of the psoas close to the spinal column. The sympathetic chain is located on the front of the vertebral column and lies over the transverse processes of the lumbar spine. On the left these ganglia lie adjacent and lateral to the aorta. On the right they are just behind the edge of the inferior vena cava. To complete the sympathectomy, the communicating rami and vessels should be clipped and divided. Cautery must be used very judiciously as there are several large vessels in the area that would be difficult to control. The level of sympathectomy can be confirmed with radiologic guidance, or the crossing lumbar vessels at the sacral promontory can be used as a landmark. Alternatively, the entire lumbar sympathetic trunk can be excised. Once the procedure is completed, the trocars are removed after the space is deflated, the 10-mm incision is closed at the level of the fascia, and finally the skin is closed.

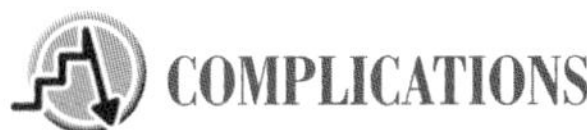

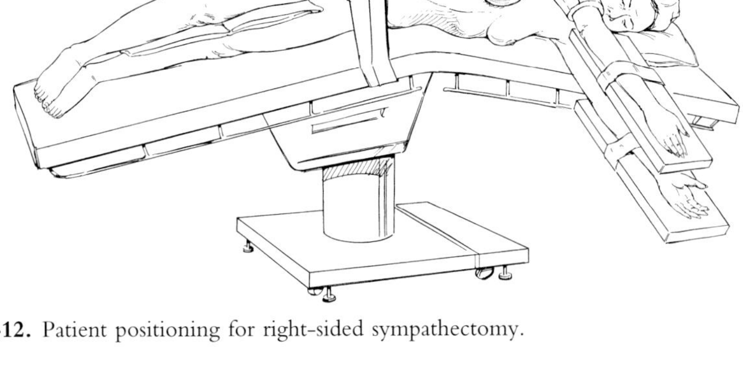

COMPLICATIONS

The most common causes of failure are incomplete denervation and poor patient selection. Incomplete denervation can be avoided by removing at least two ganglia, their accompanying rami, and their lateral connections. Although some have advocated removal of all lumbar ganglia, the removal of L1 can lead to ejaculatory dysfunction or impotence. Another more common complication is neuralgia, which presents as a dull ache in the thigh and usually spontaneously resolves in 8 to 12 weeks in most patients. Preoperatively, this should be discussed with patients so that they are not surprised by this sensation.

Patients who benefit the most from lumbar sympathectomy are those with causalgia, hyperhydrosis of the lower extremities, and vasospastic disorders. Patients with non-bypassable occlusive disease with rest pain and Buerger disease benefit only moderately with this procedure (Table 61-4, page 628). All other conditions have very

Fig. 61-12. Patient positioning for right-sided sympathectomy.

TABLE 61-4. INDICATIONS FOR LUMBAR SYMPATHECTOMY AND OUTCOMES

Indications	Condition	Outcomes
Causalgia (reflex dystrophy)	Positive results to block	Excellent late response in 95% of patients
Raynaud syndrome	10 points distal vasospasm refractory to medical management	Hypothermic toe plethysmography normalized
Ischemic rest pain (inoperable occlusive disease)	ABI >0.3, no neuropathy on physical exam, limited forefoot tissue loss	86% without rest pain after 82 months
Buerger disease	Chronic pain	Pain resolved in 100% of patients

ABI, ankle/brachial index.

poor results and should no longer be considered indications for sympathectomy. Alternative treatments should be explored.

CONCLUSION

Minimally invasive surgery of the retroperitoneal structures traverses many subspecialties. The laparoscopic general surgeon should be familiar with the anatomy and surgical techniques so that he or she can be of assistance if the primary surgeon comes across a difficult case. Furthermore, for those surgeons who practice in lower-volume centers, these described techniques can be used for straightforward retroperitoneal pathologies.

SUGGESTED READING

AbuRahma AF, Robinson PA, Powell M, et al. Sympathectomy for reflex sympathetic dystrophy: Factors affecting outcome. *Ann Vasc Surg* 1994;8:372.

AbuRahma AF, Rutherford RB. Lumbar sympathectomy. In: Rutherford, ed. *Vascular surgery*. 6th ed. Philadelphia: WB Saunders, 2005.

Chander J. Retroperitoneoscopic lumbar sympathectomy for Buerger's disease: a novel technique. *JSLS* 2004;8(3):291–296.

Haznek A, Hubert J, Antiphon P, et al. Robotic renal surgery. *Urol Clin N Amer* 2004;31(4): 731–736.

Inamasu J, Guiot BH. Laparoscopic anterior lumbar interbody fusion: a review of outcome studies. *Minim Invasive Neurosurg* 2005;48(6): 340–347.

Kung RC. Laparoscopic treatment of urinary incontinence. *Obstet Gynecol Clin N Am* 2004; 31(3):539–549.

Lavelle W, Carl A, Lavelle ED. Invasive and minimally invasive surgical techniques for back pain conditions. *Med Clin North Am* 2007; 91(2):287–298.

Lehman RA, Vacarro AR, Bertagnoli R. Standard and minimally invasive approaches to the spine. *Orthop Clin N Am* 2005;36(3): 281–292.

Marchiole P, Dargent D. Laparoscopic lymphadenectomy and sentinel node biopsy in uterine cancer. *Obstet Gynecol Clin N Am* 2004;31(3):505–521.

Miklos JR, Moore RD, Kohli N. Laparoscopic pelvic floor repair. *Obstet Gynecol Clin North Am* 2004;31(3):551–565.

Nambirajan T, Jeschke S, Al-Zahrani H, et al. Prospective randomized controlled study: transperitoneal laparoscopic versus retroperitoneoscopic radical nephrectomy. *Urology* 2004;64(5):919–925.

Querlu D, Lablanc E, Cartron G, et al. Audit of preoperative and early complications following laparoscopic lymph node dissection in 1000 geynecologic cancer patients. *Am J Obstet Gyn* 2006;195(5):1287–1292.

Rieger R. Retroperitoneoscopic lumbar sympathectomy for the treatment of plantar hyperhidrosis: technique and preliminary findings. *Surg Endosc* 2007;21(1):129–135.

Strong VE, Dalal KM, Malhotra VT, et al. Initial report of laparoscopic celiac plexus block for pain relief in patients with unresectable pancreatic cancer. *JACS* 2006; 203(1):129–131.

Taylor GD, Cadeddu JA. Applications of laparoscopic surgery in urology: impact on patient care. *Med Clin North Amer* 2004;88(2):519–538.

Walsh. *Campbell's urology*. 8th ed. Philadelphia: WB Saunders, 2002.

COMMENTARY

The author has covered numerous topics touching on multiple specialties in a chapter that is extremely useful to the surgeon who must occasionally work within the retroperitoneum in conjunction with a surgeon of another specialty. The author covers procedures related to urology, gynecology, neurosurgery, and even vascular procedures. The chapter is extremely helpful in planning a procedure and in highlighting potential pitfalls common to such procedures. In certain areas, one would supplement this chapter with additional materials. However, the breadth of topics under the umbrella of this chapter is significant.

Procedures within the retroperitoneum can run the spectrum from extremely simple and straightforward to some of the most complex laparoscopic procedures devised. The patient's anatomy, prior operations, and disease process and the experience of the surgical team are important factors in the ease or difficulty of such procedures. Developing a clear understanding of the roles that each team will play prior to the initiation of the operation is of utmost importance. Furthermore, a discussion of potential complications and their management between the various teams can avoid conflict or delay should an adverse event occur. Of course, the patient should be fully informed of the potential complications or sequelae of these operations. Finally, a clear understanding of the postoperative management plan is also important. One cannot simply assume that other team members will participate equally in the postoperative care of the patient; these roles should be clearly delineated.

This particular area of surgery continues to evolve and has transitioned significantly over the past 10 to 15 years. The author of this chapter has provided a state-of-the-art update on these procedures, but it is anticipated that within the next 5 years we will continue to see evolution of these operations.

WSE

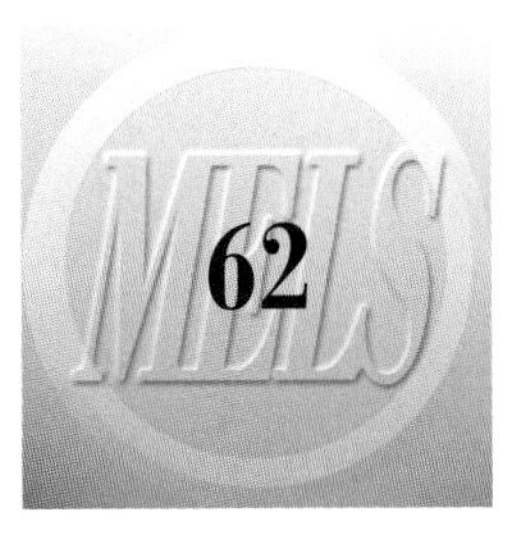

New Developments in Surgical Endoscopy: Natural Orifice Transluminal Endoscopic Surgery (NOTES)

LEE L. SWANSTRÖM AND NATHANIEL J. SOPER

INTRODUCTION

It was perhaps inevitable that minimally invasive surgery would eventually evolve beyond the laparoscope and explore new technologies of visualization. Likewise, one could easily have guessed that flexible endoscopy would become a more therapeutic entity as instrumentation and energy sources evolved. In 2004, Kalloo et al. described a novel approach in a porcine model using a standard flexible endoscope to access the peritoneal cavity (Fig. 62-1). In fact, this concept had already been captured in a U.S. method patent dated 2003 describing transgastric and transcolonic flexible peritoneoscopy (Fig. 62-2). This novel approach quickly caught the attention of surgeons and gastroenterologists and has led to a gold rush phenomenon among clinical innovators and the medical device industry seeking to capitalize on the latest evolution in surgery. In 2005 a small group of surgical endoscopists and gastroenterologists interested in advanced endoscopic procedures met under the sponsorship of both the American Society of Gastrointestinal Endoscopy (ASGE) and the Society of American Gastrointestinal and Endoscopic Surgeons (SAGES) to explore issues related to intraperitoneal endoscopy (Fig. 62-3). This group, which coined the acronym "NOTES" for natural orifice transluminal endoscopic surgery, made recommendations to the medical community on developmental needs and charted a responsible course to guide clinical introduction.

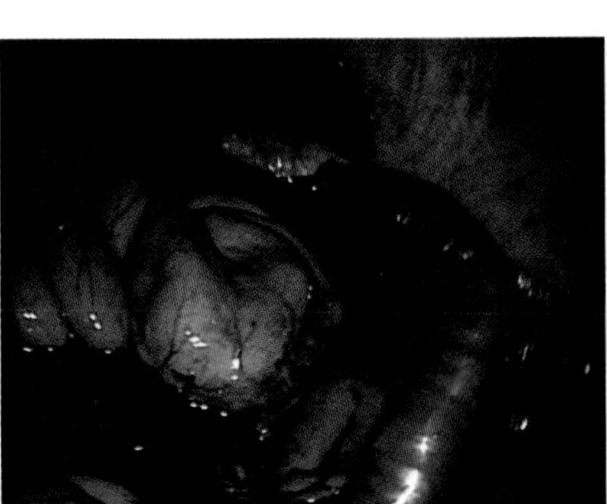
Fig. 62-1. A transgastrically placed flexible endoscope within the peritoneal cavity of a porcine model.

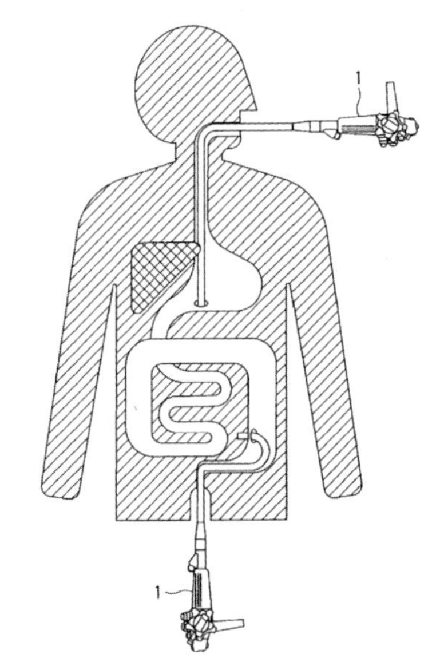

Fig. 62-2. A 2003 patent for the NOTES approach.

THE CONCEPT

The basic concept of NOTES involves the use of flexible endoscopes introduced into the body through a natural orifice (mouth, anus, vagina) and advanced out of the gastrointestinal (GI) tract (transluminal) to perform procedures within the abdominal cavity, the retroperitoneal space, or the chest. This, by necessity, involves several discrete steps to accomplish: safe exit of the GI tract, insufflation of the working space, intracavitary localization and visualization of the target organ, retraction and exposure, dissection and hemostasis, tissue retrieval and/or tissue approximation, endoluminal closure of the enterotomy, and tissue removal. It is hoped that the avoidance of incisions in the skin, subcutaneous tissues, muscle, and peritoneum will provide direct patient benefit: less pain, decreased complications, fewer hernias and adhesions, less immunosuppression, shorter hospital stays, a quicker return to work, and improved cosmesis. These possible advantages are currently only theoretical and are being actively investigated by multiple groups.

TOOLS

As a result of hands-on experience in the laboratory, there is an intense scrutiny of current endoscopic instrumentation, both of the flexible endoscope itself and associated tools, regarding their suitability for NOTES. Opinion is divided regarding

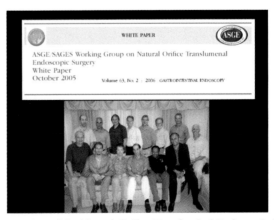

Fig. 62-3. A 2005 meeting of the Natural Orifice Transluminal Endoscopic Surgery (NOTES) group and the subsequent publication of their proceedings.

TABLE 62-1. CURRENTLY AVAILABLE TOOLS FOR NOTES

Endoscopes	Dual-lumen therapeutic scope Standard single-channel colonoscope/upper scope Endoscopic ultrasound (EUS) scope
Endoscopic instruments	Guidewires Balloon dilators Needle-knife cautery knives Sphincterotome Clips Graspers Endoloops Roth retrieval nets Snares

NOTES, natural orifice transluminal endoscopic surgery.

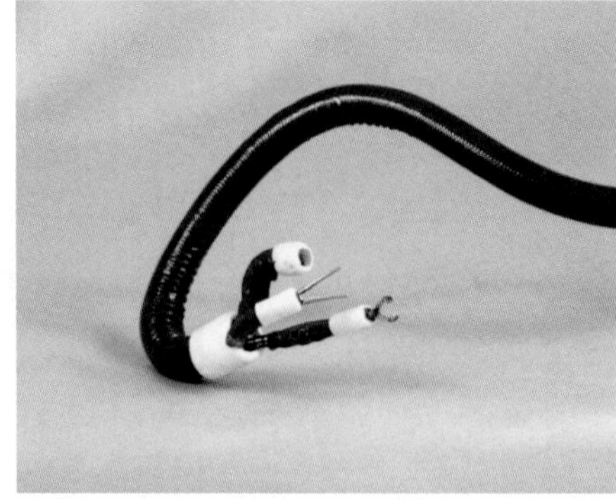

Fig. 62-5. The Cobra scope (USGI Medical; San Clemente, CA).

the need for a totally new generation of endoscopes and instruments. Gastroenterologists often feel that slight variations in current therapeutic scopes and tools are all that is needed, arguing that endoscopists have well honed skill sets developed using current technologies and that pushing the transluminal envelope is demanding enough without relearning the instrumentation. Indeed, at least in animals and very early clinical reports, amazingly complex procedures have been described using commonly available dual-channel endoscopes, cautery devices, clips, endoloops, etc. (Table 62-1). Many investigators, however, and surgeons in particular believe that a new generation of scopes and tools will be needed to safely perform extirpative and reconstructive procedures. Characteristics of a new generation of operating endoscopes that have been proposed include multiple large-instrument channels, horizon-correcting optics, an insufflation port that connects to a laparoscopic CO_2 insufflator, and the ability to firmly fix the scope in position. Many also postulate that in order to replicate laparoscopic techniques with a flexible platform, there should be triangulation capabilities at the tip to permit traction/countertraction and perhaps ultimately the ability to even suture and perform intracorporeal knot-tying. Some prototype devices that have been developed are illustrated in Figures 62-4 to 62-6. In addition to operating endoscopes it will be necessary to develop more "laparoscopic-like" flexible instruments such as graspers, dissectors, needle holders, scissors, energy sources, tissue retrieval bags, endoloops, and other tools to make the procedure both more efficient and safer. These development efforts are taking place in laboratories and engineering centers worldwide and the end results are beginning to be clinically available; a process that will certainly increase in the immediate future.

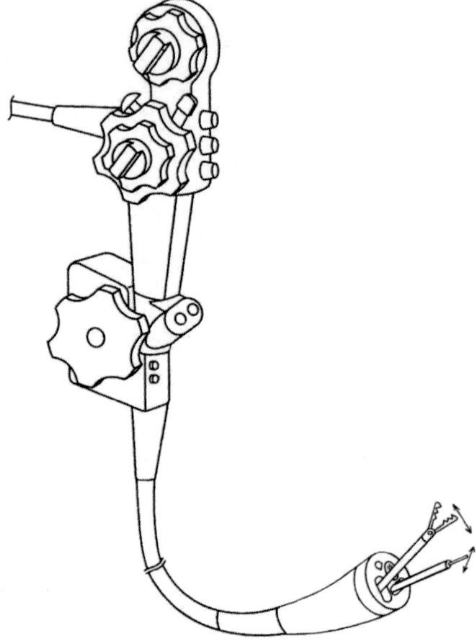

Fig. 62-4. An R-scope (Olympus Optical Co, Ltd; Tokyo, Japan).

CURRENT STATUS

For some time a small progressive segment of the GI community, along with an equally small group of surgeon endoscopists, have been pushing the boundaries of therapeutic endoscopy with procedures that heralded NOTES in many ways (Table 62-2). These experiences made it almost inevitable that NOTES would enter the clinical repertory at some point; in fact, at the annual meeting of the American Society for Gastrointestinal Endoscopy (ASGE) in 2005 Rao and Reddy, stimulated by a 2004 publication on animal experiments by Kalloo, described a small series of transgastric appendectomies performed in humans. This experience stimulated

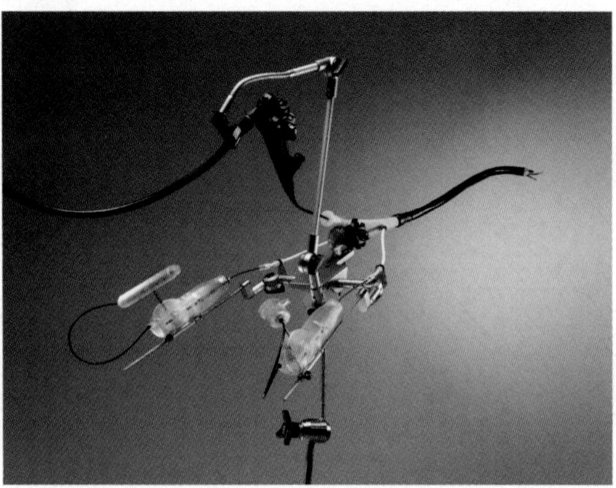

Fig. 62-6. The DDS system (Boston Scientific; Natick, MA).

TABLE 62-2. ENDOSCOPIC PROCEDURES THAT WERE PRECURSORS TO NOTES

- Percutaneous endoscopic gastrostomy (PEG)
- Endoscopic drainage of pancreatic pseudocyst
- Transanal endoscopic microsurgery (TEM)
- Endoscopic mucosal resection (EMR)
- Perforated ulcer repair
- EUS-directed extraluminal biopsy
- Transrectal cholecystectomy

NOTES, natural orifice transluminal endoscopic surgery; EUS, endoscopic ultrasound.

intense laboratory investigation by several individuals, who have performed a number of NOTES procedures that might be possible to approach clinically (Table 62-3); the majority of these procedures have been performed only in acute and survival animal models. Anecdotal reports of human NOTES procedures began to surface in early 2007, including some transgastric and transvaginal cholecystectomies from South America and some interesting Institutional Review Board (IRB)-approved forays into the field such as salvage procedures for percutaneous endoscopic gastrostomy (PEG) tubes and staging peritoneoscopy in patients undergoing pancreatectomy. Finally, in April of 2007 the first widely reported case of an endoscopic cholecystectomy was reported at the annual meeting at SAGES by a joint group of surgeons and endoscopists at Columbia University. This first procedure was done transvaginally with laparoscopic assistance for retraction. Two weeks later a second case from Strasbourg, France that used only a single laparoscopic port for retraction was reported. Within months, other groups reported on transgastric cholecystectomies and there was even a Japanese report of a transrectal gallbladder surgery. One suspects that this was only the first trickle of what will rapidly become a flood of clinical cases. It is hoped that as these approaches are disseminated to clinicians that care will be taken to avoid patient harm. To this end, both SAGES and ASGE have formed a joint committee, called the Natural Orifice Surgery Consortium for Assessment and Research (NOSCAR) to try to prospectively influence some of the critical issues that inevitably will arise, such as credentialing, training, patient selection, documentation of outcomes, and reimbursement. A priority of the NOSCAR group is to mandate that all clinical procedures must be approved by the local IRB, and a registry is being developed to prospectively accrue all NOTES procedures. Other groups have formed in Europe (EuroNOTES and EATS, or European Association for Transluminal Surgery) and Japan (NOTES-Japan) with similar mandates.

TABLE 62-3. NOTES PROCEDURES DESCRIBED TO DATE

Laboratory reports	Cholecystectomy
	Splenectomy
	Tubal ligation
	Gastrojejunostomy
	Pyloroplasty
	Staging peritoneoscopy
	Liver biopsy
	Diaphragm pacing
	Distal pancreatectomy
	Ventral hernia repair
	Gastric sleeve resection
	Colectomy (right and left)
Human cases	Transgastric appendectomy
	Transvaginal cholecystectomy
	Transgastric cholecystectomy
	PEG salvage
	Cancer staging
	Transrectal cholecystectomy

NOTES, natural orifice transluminal endoscopic surgery; PEG, percutaneous endoscopic gastrostomy.

METHODS

Even with fewer than 25 human cases having been performed (as of the middle of 2007), there have been a variety of methods used. The majority of cases have used a dual-channel upper endoscope, although our own experience with transgastric NOTES cholecystectomy utilized the 18-mm TransPort device (USGI Medical; San Clemente, CA). Transvaginal and transrectal NOTES have the advantage of allowing access to, and subsequent closure of, the peritoneal cavity using open techniques or transanal endoscopic microsurgery (TEM). Transgastric procedures require new technology to securely close the required gastrotomy. For transgastric cholecystectomy, the procedure is currently done in the operating room under general anesthesia. The left arm is tucked and the patient's head is turned to the left. Surgeon and endoscopists will stand on the left side of the operating table at the top while an assistant will be positioned on the right at the mid-table level. Finally, an endoscopy nurse will be positioned at the head of the table on the patient's right (Fig. 62-7, page 632). Full-thickness pledgets with sutures are placed in the anterior stomach wall at the midgastric level. A needle-knife cautery is then used to incise between the two sutures. A balloon dilator is used to stretch the gastrotomy and the scope is advanced out of the stomach immediately behind the balloon. After exploration, the scope is turned 90 degrees to the right and the gallbladder located. Under direct vision, a 2.5-mm grasper is directly introduced into the patient's right upper quadrant and is used to grasp the fundus of the gallbladder, allowing the assistant on the patient's right to retract it upwards. Working in concert, the surgeon and endoscopists begin dissection with a toothed endoscopic grasper and a monopolar hook cautery. The dissection, including ligation of the cystic duct and artery, is performed as it would be during a laparoscopic cholecystectomy (Fig. 62-8, page 632). Once free, the gallbladder is withdrawn into the stomach. The gastrotomy is closed endoluminally using the g-Prox system (USGI Medical). The repair is tested by instilling 500 cc of methylene blue saline while watching with a 2.5-mm laparoscope inserted through the

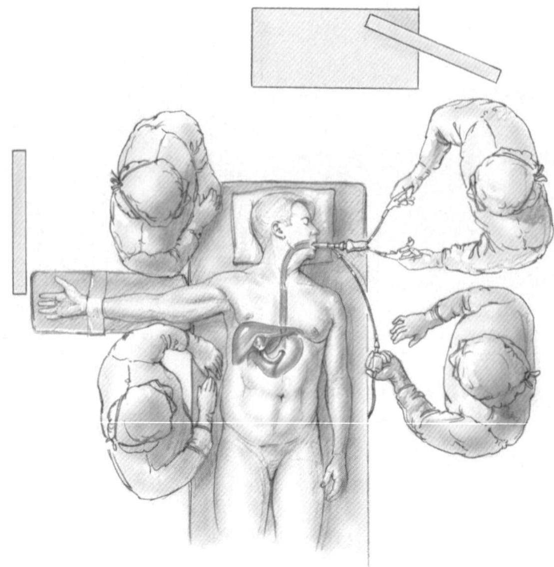

Fig. 62-7. Room setup for a transgastric Natural Orifice Transluminal Endoscopic Surgery (NOTES) cholecystectomy.

site of the retracting grasper. Once a good closure is assured, the gallbladder is once again grasped and withdrawn with the scope out of the patient's mouth. Postoperative care is the same as for a laparoscopic cholecystectomy.

CONCLUSION

Surgery continues to evolve further along the lines of less-invasive access. NOTES represents a fusion between therapeutic endoscopy and laparoscopic surgery in an effort to achieve what is perhaps an archetypal desire of man to be cured of disease without a scar—and without any pain. The hope is that this new approach will in fact represent such an advantage to patients, but we need to be careful to avoid subjecting our patients to harm while we adapt to this new paradigm. If the visceral closures are not secure, patient disasters will occur and the potential of NOTES will go unfulfilled.

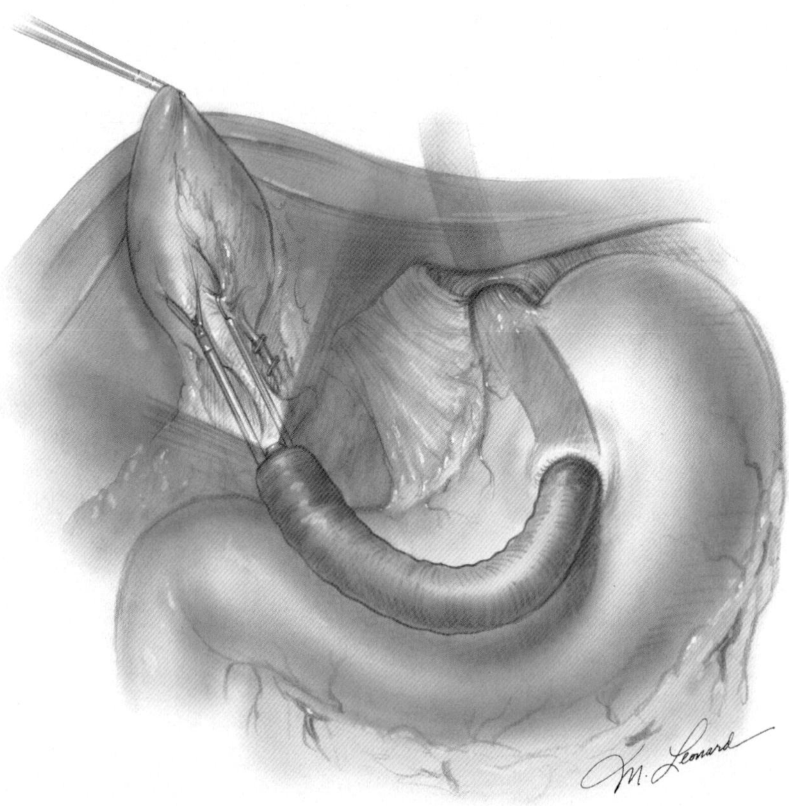

Fig. 62-8. The flexible endoscope and two endoscopic instruments are used to dissect out the gallbladder, as it would be done laparoscopically.

SUGGESTED READING

ASGE/SAGES working group on natural orifice translumenal endoscopic surgery: white paper 2005 *Gastrointest Endosc* 2006; 63(2): 199–203.

Chak A, Mcgee M, Faulx AL, et al. EUS guided natural orifice transvisceral endoscopic surgical (NOTES) approach to the retroperitoneum (abstract). *Gastrointest Endosc* 2006; 63(5):AB 264.

Fong DG, Pai RD, Ryou M, et al. Transcolonic access to the peritoneal cavity using a novel incision and closure device (abstract). *Gastrointest Endosc* 2006;63(5):AB233.

Fong DG, Pai RD, Fishman DS, et al. (2006) Transcolonic hepatic wedge resection in a porcine model (abstract). *Gastrointest Endosc* 2006;63(5):AB102.

Hu B, Chung SC, Sun LC, et al. Endoscopic suturing without extracorporeal knots: a laboratory study. *Gastrointest Endosc* 2005;62(2): 230–233.

Jagannath SB, Kantsevoy SV, Vaughn CA, et al. Peroral transgastric endoscopic ligation of fallopian tubes with long-term survival in a porcine model. *Gastrointest Endosc* 2005;61: 449–453.

Kalloo AN, Singh VK, Jagannath SB, et al. Flexible transgastric peritoneoscopy: a novel approach to diagnostic and therapeutic interventions in the peritoneal cavity. *Gastrointest Endosc* 2004;60:114–117.

Kantsevoy SV, Hu B, Jagannath SB, et al. (2006) Transgastric endoscopic splenectomy: is it possible? *Surg Endosc* 2006;20:522–525.

Kantsevoy SV, Jagannath SB, Niiyama H, et al. Endoscopic gastrojejunostomy with survival in a porcine model. *Gastrointest Endosc* 2005; 62:287–292.

Matthes K, Yusuf TE, Mino-Kenudson M, et al. Feasibility of endoscopic transgastric distal pancreatectomy (ETDP) in the pig (abstract). *Gastrointest Endosc* 2006;63(5):AB229.

Merrifield BF, Wagh MS, Thompson CC. Peroral transgastric organ resection: A feasibility study in pigs. *Gastrointest Endosc* 2006; 63(4):693–697.

Pai RD, Fong DG, Bundga ME, et al. Transcolonic endoscopic cholecystectomy: a NOTES survival study in a porcine model (with video). *Gastrointest Endosc* 2006; 64(3):428–434.

Park PO, Bergström M, Ikeda K, et al. Experimental studies of transgastric gallbladder surgery: cholecystectomy and cholecystogastric anastomosis. *Gastrointest Endosc* 2005; 61:601–606.

Park PO, Bergstrom M, Swain P, et al. Measurements of intraperitoneal pressure during flexible transgastric surgery and the development of a feed-back control valve for regulating pressure (abstract). *Gastrointest Endosc* 2006;63(5):AB101.

Pasricha P, Kozarek R, Swain P, et al. A next generation therapeutic endoscope: Development of a novel endoluminal surgery system with "birds-eye" visualization and triangulating instruments (abstract). *Gastrointest Endosc* 2005;61(5):AB106.

Sclabas G, Swanstrom LL. Secure closure methods in NOTES. *Surg Innovation* 2006; 13(1):23–30.

Swanstrom LL, Kozarek R, Pascriha P, et al. Development of a new access device for transgastric surgery. *J Gastrointest Surg* 2005;9: 1129–1137.

Wagh MS, Merrifield BF, Thompson CC. Endoscopic transgastric abdominal exploration and organ resection: initial experience in a porcine model. *Clin Gastroenterol Hepatol* 2005;3:892–896.

Wagh MS, Merrifield BF, Thompson CC. Survival studies after endoscopic transgastric oophorectomy and tubectomy in a porcine model. *Gastrointest Endosc* 2006;63(3): 473–478.

COMMENTARY

The authors, my fellow editors, have described one of the most exciting and rapidly emerging areas in surgery. Many experts anticipate that the current efforts with NOTES will lead to a major paradigm shift in care that could rival the changes seen with modern laparoscopy. There is little doubt that we will experience advances in endoluminal therapies and it is likely, but less certain, that transluminal procedures will be widely adapted.

Numerous challenges face those who wish to further the field of transluminal surgery. The development of secure closure methods for the enterotomies required in many approaches is of utmost importance. An inability to reliably close the gastrointestinal (GI) tract at the conclusion of these procedures could lead many to abort efforts in this field. Much has been learned and much more will be learned regarding the ability of the body to tolerate contamination from the GI tract. The stomach is capable of remarkable behavior, including transluminal migration of large devices in a seton-like manner without leakage. We will likely advance our understanding of the body in many unanticipated ways through our research in NOTES. The challenges of obtaining appropriate reimbursement from payers for emerging procedures remain a significant obstacle to the advancement of medical care. Adequate documentation of patient safety and benefits is reasonable, but the obstacles needed to overcome the lethargy of bureaucratic agencies can be deleterious to patient care.

The advances in instrumentation, visualization, and understanding of the human body as a result of research in NOTES are currently emerging and promise to multiply in the near future. Cautious application of these techniques in patients is warranted, but aggressive study of the issues raised by this field is advised.

WSE

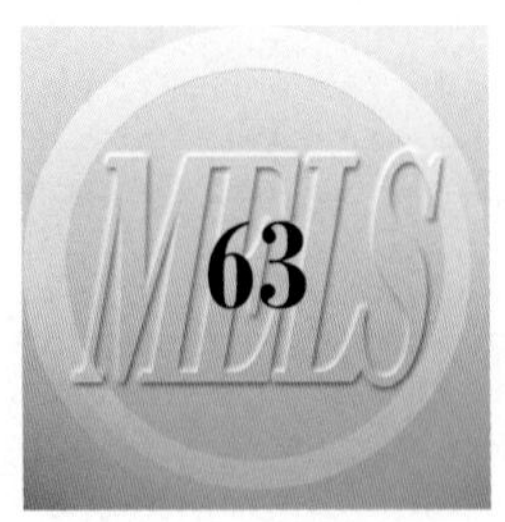

Hybrid Natural Orifice Transluminal Endoscopic Surgery (NOTES) Cholecystectomy

ERIC S. HUNGNESS AND KHASHAYAR VAZIRI

INTRODUCTION

Advances in therapeutic endoscopy and minimally invasive surgery have led to the development of a new and emerging field called natural orifice transluminal endoscopic surgery (NOTES). Therapeutic endoscopy has been extremely useful in the diagnosis and treatment of intraluminal gastrointestinal disorders. Recent advances in equipment and technique have resulted in a broader therapeutic application, allowing physicians to expand the range and complexity of diseases treated through an endoscope. Similar advances in gastrointestinal surgery are evident in the successful completion of complex abdominal operations using a laparoscope and small incisions. Currently, complex general surgical procedures are performed routinely in this minimally invasive fashion, preventing the morbidity of conventional open operations and resulting in shorter hospital stays, earlier return to normal activity, and more benefit to the patient. Continuous refinement of both of these techniques has led to a new and potentially even less-invasive field called NOTES.

NOTES is an emerging field in minimally invasive surgery that is driving the development of new technology and refining operative techniques. The process uses natural orifices such as the mouth, vagina, or anus as an access point to the abdominal cavity, where operations on gastrointestinal or solid organs can be performed through the use of specialized flexible endoscopes, thus avoiding the morbidity of abdominal wall incisions and conventional surgery. A variety of NOTES procedures have been performed in survival and non-survival animal studies. The safety and feasibility of a transgastric endoscopic approach to the peritoneal cavity was shown in a long-term porcine model by Kalloo et al. in 2004. Since that time, many other operations, including liver biopsy, salpingo-oophorectomy, fallopian tube ligation, peritoneoscopy, partial hysterectomy, splenectomy, nephrectomy, cholecystectomy, and gastrojejunostomy have been performed via transgastric, transrectal, and transvaginal approaches. Similar procedures have been performed in cadaveric models. Experience in living humans is much more limited, although some would argue that transluminal surgery has been performed for years. Examples of these procedures include culdoscopy for infertility or tubal ligation, transgastric pancreatic debridement, and transgastric and transduodenal drainage of pancreatic pseudocysts.

Aside from these examples, the current NOTES initiative developed after Kalloo's 2004 publication. The first reported human NOTES procedures were performed in India, and Rao et al. have presented cases of successful transgastric appendectomies and tubal ligations at meetings, though their experience remains unpublished. As others in Europe, South America, and the United States gained experience through animal models, these groups began to venture into human hybrid NOTES cholecystectomy.

Recent hybrid NOTES cholecystectomies have been performed in the U.S. via a transvaginal route by Bessler et al. and Talamini et al. and transgastric routes by Swanstrom et al. and Soper et al. The first hybrid NOTES cholecystectomy was performed by Bessler et al. with an operating endoscope, a 5-mm laparoscopic port, and two 3-mm laparoscopic ports. The laparoscopic instruments were used primarily for retraction and clip placement. Most of the dissection and visualization was completed endoscopically. Similarly, Swanstrom et al. and Soper et al. have performed multiple transgastric hybrid NOTES cholecystectomies with the use of one or two laparoscopic ports, mainly for retraction of the gallbladder and control of the cystic duct and artery. As experience grows, laparoscopic ports are slowly eliminated. Similar hybrid procedures have been reported in Brazil and Peru. The first "pure" NOTES cholecystectomy was recently performed by Marescaux et al. in France using a transvaginal approach and completing the cholecystectomy with the aid of a 2-mm needle port to establish pneumoperitoneum and aid in retraction. As with other emerging technologies, enthusiasm and intellect has led to great advances in NOTES in a relatively short period of time. In order to avoid unchecked and potentially dangerous implementation of the NOTES technique, the Natural Orifice Surgery Consortium for Assessment and Research (NOSCAR) was established.

The NOSCAR body was created in a collaborative effort by the Society of American Gastrointestinal Endoscopic Surgeons (SAGES) and the American Society for Gastrointestinal Endoscopy (ASGE) in order to regulate and ensure the safety of future NOTES applications. All information from human procedures will be reported to a central registry and disseminated by NOSCAR with the purpose of identifying trends, successful techniques, and complications more expeditiously than individual investigators could. This working group serves as a reference for all investigators to gain the most knowledge and avoid unnecessary complications from each and every case. As more NOTES procedures are performed the collaboration and sharing of information through NOSCAR will foster faster advances and establish standardized techniques. The NOSCAR group recommends that all NOTES surgery should be performed under approval of Institutional Review Boards with full disclosure.

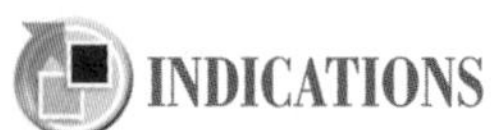

INDICATIONS

In the future, the indications for NOTES cholecystectomy may be similar to laparoscopic cholecystectomy. These indications include symptomatic cholelithiasis, acute cholecystitis, choledocholithiasis, and gallstone pancreatitis. Laparoscopic cholecystectomy remains challenging in situations of active inflammation and carries a higher risk of conversion and complication. Early in the NOTES experience these patients should be excluded. Patients with active inflammation are not good candidates for the NOTES procedure as dissection is more difficult and risk of conversion and complication increases. Similarly, patients with choledocholithiasis and complications of gallstones should be avoided as cholangiography and ductal exploration is not currently possible.

Patients with previous surgery should be approached with caution. The route of NOTES can be tailored based upon the patient's previous procedures. For example, patients with previous gastric or esophageal surgery, dysphagia, large hiatal hernias, severe peptic ulcer disease, and esophageal strictures should not be approached via a transgastric route. Reoperative fields in the lower abdomen and pelvis can be avoided via the transgastric approach. Previous surgery in the right upper quadrant remains a relative contraindication to NOTES, as does cholecystectomy, especially early in a surgeon's experience. As newer equipment is developed and experience grows NOTES can become applicable to a larger patient group.

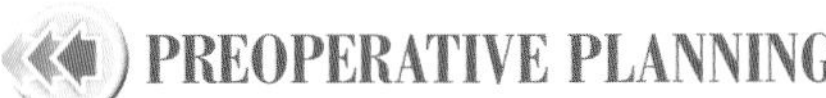

PREOPERATIVE PLANNING

Patient preparation for a NOTES cholecystectomy mirrors the preoperative planning for a laparoscopic cholecystectomy with respect to prophylactic antibiotics and prophylaxis against deep venous thrombosis. Patients should be fully informed of the potential complications and the chance of conversion to a laparoscopic cholecystectomy. In addition to the complications of laparoscopic cholecystectomy, specific risks of NOTES such as access site leak or dyspareunia should be discussed. The operative team should review the history and physical examination carefully in order to prevent any foreseeable complications.

NOTES Access Location

The entry point to the abdominal cavity should be based upon the individual patient and surgical history. The two most common approaches are transvaginal and transgastric. Each of these approaches has distinct advantages.

Transvaginal peritoneal entry though a posterior colpotomy has been established and performed by gynecologists for decades. This eliminates most concerns with closure of the access site. A standardized and safe method of vaginal wall closure has been established and performed for many other procedures. Furthermore, the morbidity of a colpotomy leak is minimal compared to a gastrotomy leak, as studies of vaginal hysterectomies have shown minimal differences between single-layer, double-layer, and open vaginal cuffs. A gastrotomy leak carries a greater morbidity and should be closed. Another advantage of the transvaginal approach includes a direct "straight shot" for the operating endoscope to the gallbladder. Avoiding flexion and retroflexion of the operating endoscope allows for easier passage, manipulation, and articulation of instruments through the working channels and prevents inversion or rotation of the endoscopic image. Challenges of gallbladder retraction may be easier to overcome with a transvaginal approach. A second endoscope or a long laparoscopic instrument can be introduced transvaginally through a colpotomy and used for cephalad retraction of the gallbladder, obviating the need for a needleport. Finally, the vagina may allow for easier removal of larger specimens compared to the esophagus.

The transgastric approach can be used to avoid previous operative fields in the lower abdomen and pelvis. Transgastric operations and upper endoscopy have been performed in the past and many surgeons are more comfortable with this approach based upon these experiences. The transgastric approach is more applicable to the general population as the transvaginal approach is not available to the male gender. Gastrotomy closure and specimen removal remain preeminent concerns of the transgastric approach, but with improvement of technique and equipment these will soon be overcome. NOTES surgeons should be comfortable and facile with both access points in order to be able to tailor the approach to best benefit the individual patient.

Laparoscopic Port Positioning

Early in the NOTES experience three laparoscopic ports are used. One port is dedicated to the laparoscope for aid in visualization and documentation, and the remaining two ports are used for retraction and control of the cystic duct and artery. These ports are slowly eliminated as the surgical team gains experience. Currently, NOTES hybrid cholecystectomy is performed with one or two ports. A dedicated port for the laparoscope remains and is considered essential to ensure the safety and to confirm secure closure of the gastrotomy until a standardized and safe internal technique is established. One other laparoscopic port or needle port can be used if needed to aid in retraction of the gallbladder. Laparoscopic ports can be added throughout the procedure in order to ensure the safety of the patient. Preoperatively, the surgical team needs to plan their access and port sites to ensure a safe and successful operation.

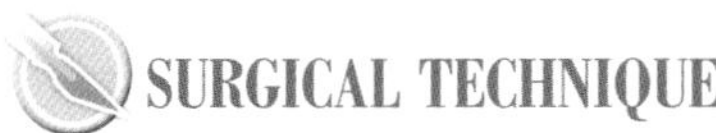

SURGICAL TECHNIQUE

Operating Room Setup and Patient Positioning

Hybrid procedures require both laparoscopic and endoscopic equipment. The equipment requires more room and a larger operative team to ensure proper setup and function. Careful planning and communication with members of the team are needed to ensure proper position and visualization throughout the procedure. In the transgastric hybrid NOTES cholecystectomy the patient is positioned supine on the operating room table. The operating endoscopist stands above the left shoulder of the patient along with the endoscopy nurse. The laparoscopic surgeon stands to the patient's left in order to control the laparoscope along with the scrub technician. An operating assistant stands to the right of the patient. The main laparoscopic and endoscopic monitors are positioned side-by-side at the level of the patient's right shoulder. This allows an unobstructed view for the operating endoscopist and the laparoscopist. Figure 63-1 (page 636) demonstrates the operating room setup for a transgastric hybrid cholecystectomy. Operating room setup for a transvaginal hybrid NOTES cholecystectomy is slightly different and depicted in Figure 63-2 (page 636). The patient is placed in a low lithotomy position with the operating endoscopist between her legs. The endoscopy nurse is positioned to the right of the operating endoscopist. The laparoscopist and operating assistant are to the left and right of the patient respectively. The scrub technician stands at the left shoulder of the patient. The endoscopic and laparoscopic monitors are in the same position as for the transgastric procedure.

Pneumoperitoneum and Endoscopic Access

A Veress needle is inserted through a small infraumbilical incision to establish the pneumoperitoneum prior to placement of the 5-mm trocar. A carbon dioxide pneumoperitoneum is then established with a pressure limit of 15 mmHg.

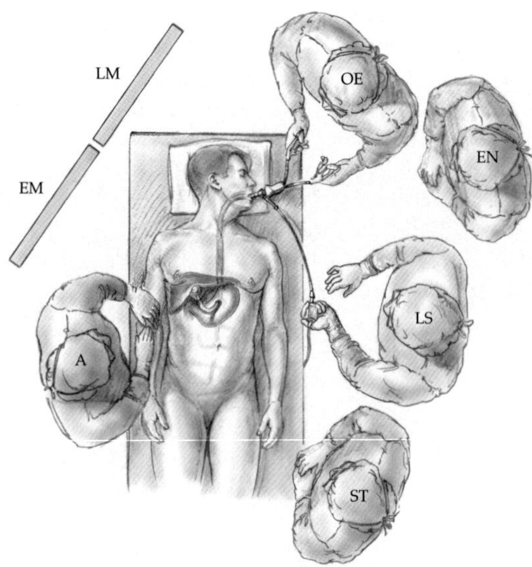

Fig. 63-1. A typical room setup for a laparoscopic-assisted transgastric natural orifice transluminal endoscopic surgery (NOTES) cholecystectomy.

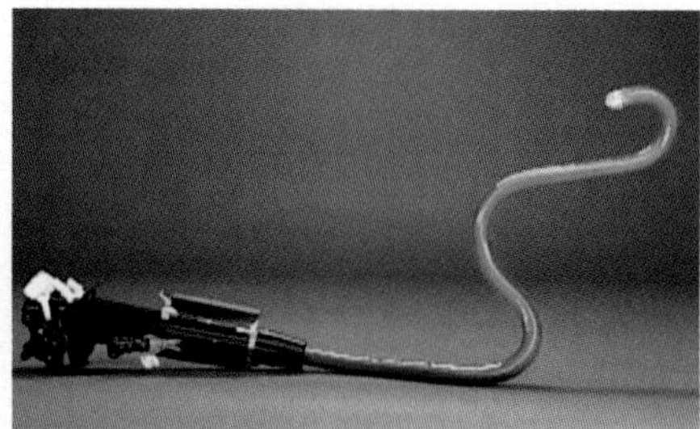

Fig. 63-3. The TransPort is an 18-mm operating endoscope currently available on the market.

A diagnostic endoscopy is then performed to ensure normal anatomy and a disease-free stomach and esophagus. A topical antibiotic is applied to the gastric mucosa with a spray catheter prior to removal of the diagnostic endoscope. Next, the operating endoscope is passed through the mouth, down the esophagus and into the stomach. The operating endoscope or endoscopic operating platform is approximately 18-mm or 54F in diameter, provides a stabilizing or shape-locking feature, and sacrifices one channel to accommodate the visualizing flexible endoscope, leaving the remaining two or three channels for passage of operating instruments (Fig. 63-3). Care is taken during the passage of this large endoscope in order to avoid damage to the oropharynx, posterior pharynx, and esophagus, or the vagina in a transvaginal approach. The stomach is insufflated and a location for the gastrotomy is identified.

The optimal location for the gastrotomy is on the anterior aspect of the stomach at the level of the incisura and midway from the lesser and greater curves. A gastrotomy created too close to either curvature of the stomach may lead to excessive bleeding from the gastric or gastroepiploic vessels. The location of the gastrotomy should be confirmed laparoscopically, should allow the endoscope to reach the gallbladder with a gentle curve, and should be in a location that will allow easy visualization for eventual gastrotomy closure. A needle-knife is passed down one of the two operating channels of the endoscope and a 20-mm dilating balloon is passed down the other. A full-thickness gastrotomy is made with the needle-knife and the dilating balloon is passed through the gastrotomy. The balloon is dilated to a full 20 mm and then retracted to the hub of the endoscope allowing passage of the endoscope and balloon as a single unit through the gastrotomy.

Transvaginal access to the peritoneal cavity can be achieved through an incision in the posterior vaginal cul-de-sac under direct visualization. Eventual closure of the incision is performed in a similar manner. Once access to the peritoneal cavity is achieved, a complete peritneoscopy is performed. Figures 63-4 and 63-5 demonstrate the transgastric and transvaginal approaches, respectively.

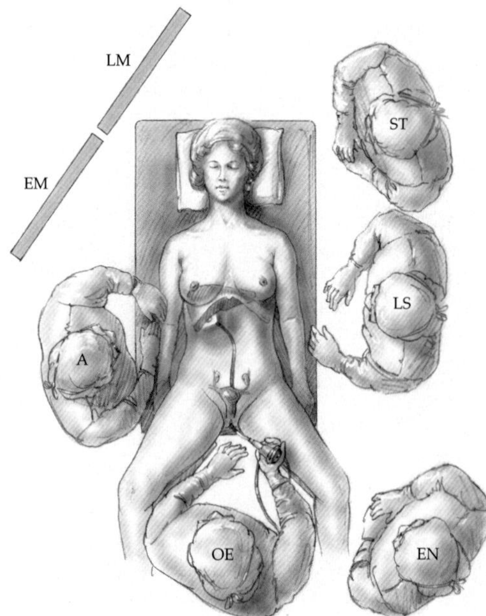

Fig. 63-2. Room setup for a transvaginal natural orifice transluminal endoscopic surgery (NOTES) cholecystectomy.

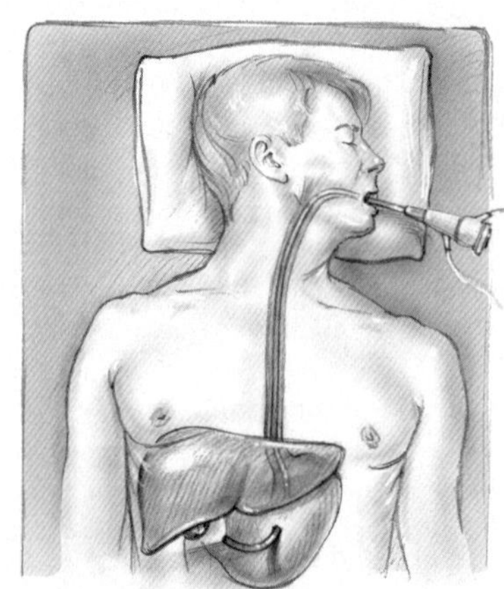

Fig. 63-4. The operating endoscope is inserted by mouth and then exits the mid-stomach and centers on the gallbladder.

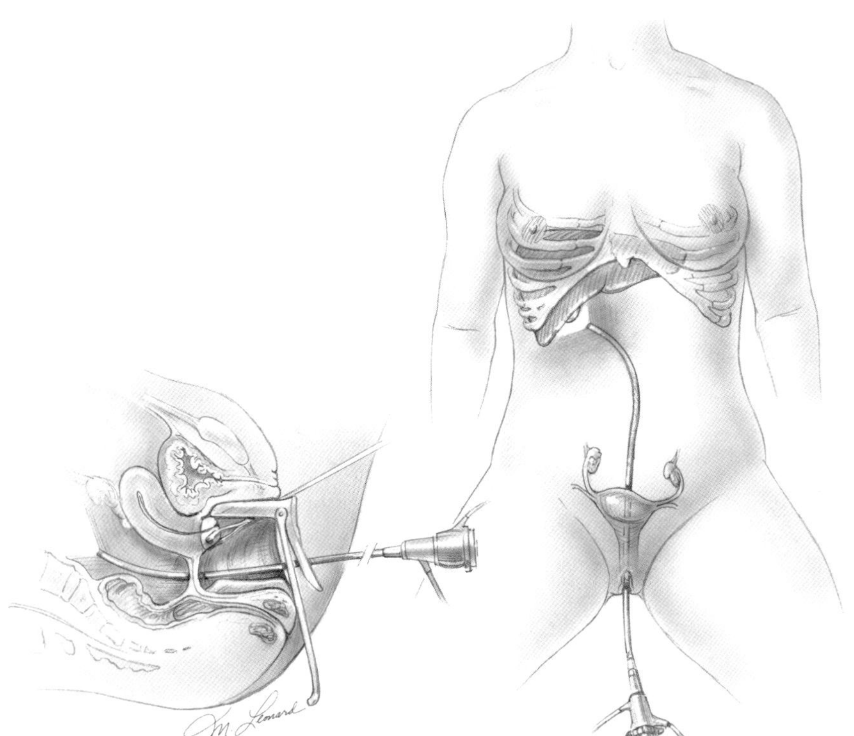

Fig. 63-5. For transvaginal natural orifice transluminal endoscopic surgery (NOTES) cholecystectomy, the scope is inserted through a culpotomy and directly access the right upper quadrant.

Dissection

Endoscopic dissection of the cystic duct and artery is approached adhering to the principles of laparoscopic cholecystectomy. Retraction of the gallbladder and proper exposure remains a challenging obstacle. The laparoscope is removed and the port can be used to aid in retraction. Additionally, a second laparoscopic port can be placed in the right subcostal area to aid in retraction. Use of a needle port or suture passer can obviate the need for this second laparoscopic port. The fundus of the gallbladder is retracted in a cephalad direction exposing the infundibulum and Calot triangle. An endoscopic grasper, endoscopic scissors, and a needle-knife are used to provide countertraction and perform the dissection under endoscopic visualization. The infundibulum is retracted laterally in order to open the angle between the cystic and common bile ducts. Deflection of the endoscopic channels at the end of the operating endoscope allows for more range of motion of the endoscopic scissors and grasper. The peritoneum overlying the neck of the gallbladder, cystic duct, and cystic artery are divided. The cystic duct– gallbladder junction is carefully dissected. This allows for identification and circumferential dissection of the cystic duct. The cystic duct is dissected to an extent only to allow placement of clips. The cystic artery is identified cephalad to the cystic duct and can be dissected circumferentially after the overlying peritoneum is divided. The surrounding connective tissue is dissected, the cystic duct–common duct junction is avoided, and the critical view of safety is established.

With the critical view established, the anatomy can be correctly identified and confirmed laparoscopically. If the ductal anatomy or the dissection can not be safely performed at any time, additional laparoscopic ports should be placed and the dissection should be completed laparoscopically. Control of the cystic duct and artery can be achieved endoscopically or laparoscopically. Endoscopic clips and endoloops are not designed to control the cystic duct and artery, so these structures are controlled via 5-mm laparoscopic clips. Once ligated, the cystic duct and artery are divided with the endoscopic scissors or needle-knife. The gallbladder is dissected free of the liver bed using an endoscopic grasper for countertraction and the endoscopic scissors or needle-knife. A combination of endoscopic scissors, needle knives, or biopsy forceps can be connected to electrocautery and used to dissect the gallbladder off the liver bed. Prior to the completion of this dissection, the liver bed is inspected for hemostasis. Once hemostasis is ensured, the gallbladder is dissected free.

Gastrotomy Closure and Gallbladder Removal

The gallbladder is grasped with an endoscopic grasper and the endoscope is pulled back with the gallbladder into the lumen of the stomach. The gallbladder is then released and remains in the gastric lumen while the gastrotomy is closed. In the case of a transvaginal approach, the gallbladder is removed with the endoscope and the colpotomy is closed primarily under direct vision. Gastrotomy closure is another challenging obstacle in NOTES hybrid cholecystectomy. The gastrotomy is closed using an endoscopic closure device. These devices deploy full-thickness sutures or fasteners and reapproximate the edges of the gastrotomy (Fig. 63-6, page 638). This closure is inspected laparoscopically and the adequacy of the closure can be tested with endoscopic insufflation. Once the gastrotomy is closed, the gallbladder is grasped and removed with the endoscope through the mouth. The laparoscope is removed and the pneumoperitoneum is released.

POSTOPERATIVE MANAGEMENT

The postoperative care of the NOTES hybrid cholecystectomy patient is similar to patients who have undergone laparoscopic cholecystectomy. Patients who have undergone a transgastric procedure should be monitored for signs and symptoms of enteric leak. Routine postoperative tests and extended use of antibiotics is unnecessary. Patients are generally kept overnight as a matter of caution until more experience is gained. Postoperative pain is adequately controlled with oral analgesics, and it has been our experience that NOTES patients experience less pain compared to their laparoscopic counterparts. Patients are started on a liquid diet after the procedure and advanced to a regular diet as tolerated. Antiemetics are given intravenously as needed. Patients are ambulatory shortly after the procedure and are discharged the following morning. They return for a follow-up appointment in approximately 2 weeks.

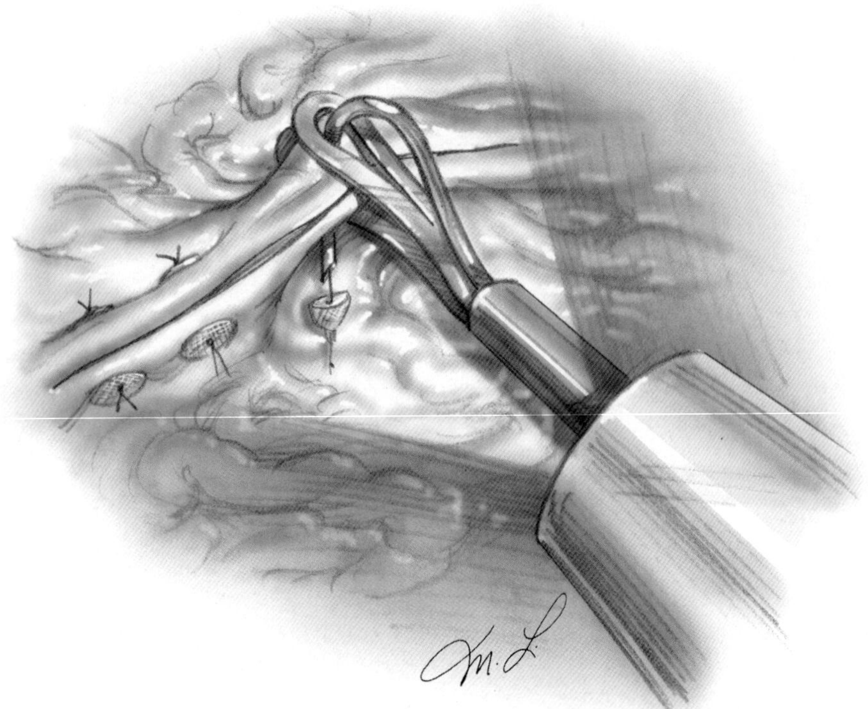

Fig. 63-6. The gastrotomy is closed with an endoscopic full-thickness suturing device with pedgeted sutures.

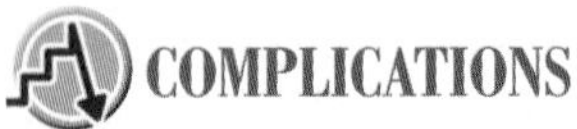

COMPLICATIONS

Similar to other emerging fields or technologies, there are many fundamental challenges to the NOTES approach. Among these are peritoneal access, prevention of infection, spatial orientation, platform development, refinement of operating instrumentation, and visceral closure. Access to the peritoneal cavity is necessary to perform intraabdominal procedures. Whether the access point resides in the stomach, colon, or vagina, a standardized, safe and easily reproducible technique needs to be established. This technique would ensure the proper location and size of the puncture for visualization and completion of the procedure.

Infectious concerns arise from accessing the sterile peritoneal cavity through the lumen of the gastrointestinal or genitourinary tracts. Current research is being conducted to quantify the intraluminal bacterial load of different organs and the subsequent risk of intraabdominal infection. Although the overall risk is low, maneuvers to decrease the total amount of bacteria prior to creation of the enterotomy and techniques for control of spillage into the peritoneal cavity during the procedure are being investigated.

Adequate visualization and creation of a platform from which to operate remains a significant challenge. Improvements to endoscopes for better visualization and development of endoscopic instruments with additional and greater degrees of freedom are needed. Shortcomings of endoscopic retraction can be overcome with the development of this stable platform and triangulation of operating instruments. Finally, an expeditious, safe, and easily reproducible method for enterotomy closure has yet to be established. With modification of surgical technique and advancements in endoscopic instrumentation, these obstacles are likely to be overcome.

CONCLUSION

The NOTES hybrid cholecystectomy requires a unique combination of endoscopic and laparoscopic skill, good communication, and a well-trained surgical team. The NOTES surgeon must have excellent surgical skills, a well-founded understanding of abdominal anatomy, and clinical expertise in perioperative management. Laparoscopic skills will remain necessary as limitations and complications will require periodic laparoscopic intervention. As with any new procedure, a significant learning curve will need to be overcome. With the creation of NOSCAR and collaboration of surgical investigators around the globe, standardized techniques will be established and learning curves will become shorter. Surgical procedures will continue to evolve toward less-invasive approaches and the boundaries between surgery and endoscopy will become less evident. Techniques such as NOTES should be met with enthusiasm but studied cautiously, keeping the safety and best interest of the patient paramount.

SUGGESTED READING

Bessler M, Stevens PD, Milone L, et al. Transvaginal laparoscopically assisted endoscopic cholecystectomy: a hybrid approach to natural orifice surgery. *Gastrointest Endosc* 2007;66(6):1243–1245.

Branco AW FA, Kondo W, Noda RW, et al. Hybrid transvaginal nephrectomy. *European Urology* 2008 Jan 22 (epub ahead of print).

Buyske J. Natural orifice transluminal endoscopic surgery. *JAMA* 2007;298(13):1560–1561.

Marescaux J, Dallemagne B, Perretta S, et al. Surgery without scars: report of transluminal cholecystectomy in a human being. *Arch Surg* 2007;142(9):823–826; discussion 826–827.

Narula VK, Hazey JW, Renton DB, et al. Transgastric instrumentation and bacterial contamination of the peritoneal cavity. *Surg Endosc* 2008;22(3):605–611.

Pearl JP, Ponsky JL. Natural orifice translumenal endoscopic surgery: A critical review. *J Gastrointest Surg* 2007 Dec 5 (epub ahead of print).

Rattner D, Kalloo A. ASGE/SAGES working group on natural orifice translumenal endoscopic surgery. *Surg Endosc* 2006;20(2): 329–333.

Swanstrom LL, Whiteford M, Khajanchee Y. Developing essential tools to enable transgastric surgery. *Surg Endosc* 2008;22(3):600–604.

Shen CC, Hsu TY, Huang FJ, et al. Comparison of one- and two-layer vaginal cuff closure and open vaginal cuff during laparoscopic-assisted vaginal hysterectomy. *J Am Assoc Gynecol Laparosc* 2002;9(4):474–480.

COMMENTARY

Once the concept of transvisceral endoscopic surgery captured the interest of surgical endoscopists and endoscopic surgeons, a major debate began regarding the most probable initial widespread clinical application for this new approach. This debate was watched closely by surgeons—who had a vested interest in knowing what their future might hold—but also by industry, who was weighing the potential impact of NOTES before investing heavily in equipment development. It was largely felt by those who initiated research into NOTES that the "killer app" for the approach was unlikely to be a minor surgery such tubal ligation as the added cost and complexity would make it hard to justify, but equally unlikely was something so complex that it would overwhelm the fledgling technology and "learning curve" process for practitioners. Initial thinking was that cholecystectomy, while a tempting target, probably fell into the latter category. Well, we were certainly wrong. Although appendectomy was the first human case reported, almost all subsequent human cases worldwide have been cholecystectomy, either transvaginal, transgastric, or as a single-port laparoscopic procedure. Why is this, and is it indeed the future of cholecystectomy?

The answer to that question is multifactorial. First, familiarity played a role. The leading NOTES investigators were either advanced laparoscopic surgeons who had cut their teeth on the laparoscopic cholecystectomy in the early 1990s or interventional gastrointestinal surgeons with a large practice base of endoscopic retrograde cholangiopancreatography (ERCP). Institutional memory also is a prominent factor. Cholecystectomy played a prominent role in the development of laparoscopic general surgery and for that reason has an almost mythic stature for surgeons and industry. The fact that cholecystectomy is a very common and mostly an elective procedure also makes it a great candidate to conduct meaningful pilot studies. Surgeons, too, were well aware that if the field of NOTES was to develop that it would require large investments in medical technology research and development. Both established medical device companies and venture-funded start-ups are much more likely to put money into this field if a common procedure is involved as opposed to an esoteric and rare one. Finally, patient preference plays a role. Patients don't typically care about the surgical approach if the case is truly emergent such as acute appendicitis or ruptured diverticulitis, or if it is for cancer. Biliary cholic is a more indolent and less emergent disease overall; patients know, after 20 years, that treating it should involve a minimally invasive procedure.

Regardless of the reasons, it appears that NOTES cholecystectomy will at least receive a thorough and early investigation. Whether it becomes the new gold standard will depend on its scientific validity, its ability to be universally taught, its risk/benefit ratio and, perhaps most importantly, on the public's impression of it. If the public declares that it wants gallbladders done without incisions, I have little doubt that that will be the way they will be done.

LLS

Subject Index

Page numbers followed by "*f*" indicate figures. Page numbers followed by "*t*" indicate tables.

B

C

D

E

F

G

I

J

K

L

M

P

T

U

V

W

X

Y

Z